ISBN: 978-0-578-74359-2

<u>Unconscious Suffocation</u>

<u>- A Personal Journey through the PANDEMIC PANIC</u>

- Amir-ul Kafirs
& fellow HERETICS

Table of Discontent:

Unconscious Suffocation
- A Personal Journey through the PANDEMIC PANIC
- Introduction

- Amir-ul Kafirs, HERETIC, Pittsburgh

How can I even begin to explain why I think that editing & writing this book is so important?!

Around 2013, when I 1st started having to deal with consequences of the AHCA (Affordable Health Care Act) I started to realize how invasive it was into one's private life. It seemed to me that what hadn't been accomplished with the post-9/11 Department of Homeland Security violations of Civil Liberties was now being pushed further with the AHCA. The criminalization of NOT having health insurance gave the 'perfect excuse' for intimate data gathering. Because of this, I postulated that future police state actions would be justified as for 'our own good' & executed in the name of 'Public Health'. Even with this prescience I was unprepared for what was to come!

My mom was living in a reasonably large apartment building complex for people aged 50 & older. She was 93 & had been more or less continually sick for about the preceding 56 years. She had cancer. In mid-December, 2019, she was put in a hospice. On December 30, 2019, she died there. The official cause of death was bladder cancer but I suspect that it was hurried along by sleeping pills given to her without consent & lack of food.

I was her "Personal Representative" so it was my job to take care of all her unfinished business & to clean out her apartment. I didn't get that finished until about the end of February. While I was doing this, I got to know some of the maintenance guys for the apartments. At what was near to or at the very end of my cleaning process one of the maintenance guys commented that 2 or 3 more old people had died there in the past week or so. He seemed to think that was more than usual. Perhaps that was my 1st hint that there might be a pandemic in progress.

Almost immediately thereafter, I started noticing a mass media emphasis on a *deadly virus pandemic*. The public had been prepped for such an event for decades. There had been books such as Richard Preston's The Hot Zone (1994) on Ebola, Mike Davis's The Monster at our Door (2005) on the Avian Flu, & Robin Cook's Pandemic (2018) on Gene-Editing Biotechnology. Then there were the mainstream movies: Wolfgang Petersen's Outbreak (1995) based on The Hot Zone, Richard Pearce's Fatal Contact: Bird Flu in America (2006) on H5N1 Avian Flu, Jason Connery's Pandemic (2008) on a virus developed as a bioweapon, & John Suits's Pandemic (2016) on an unidentified virus.

I have an interest in the disaster movie genre partially because I like seeing the special effects & partially because I'm interested in how public response is depicted. Since some of them try to be realistic about this I like seeing what 1st-responder plans are already in place. I've seen all the above-mentioned movies by now & I've read The Hot Zone & may read the other books if & when I have the time. What those *hadn't prepped me for* was the more subtle terror that I started seeing in March, 2020.

Because the mass media was placing so much emphasis on the spectacular deadliness possibilities I saw people keeping distance from each other, glimpsing around furtively for signs of sickness, & inching their shoulders toward their ears in classic Reichian *Character Armoring*. This was completely mass-media-induced because nowhere, at least in my environment, were there any signs whatsoever of a pandemic: no extraordinary sick people visible. It wasn't like we were seeing bodies brought out of houses & burned in piles on the streets. &, yet, the terror was obvious.

One would think that people would be aware by now that the mass media keeps its audience's attention by constantly parading the latest spectacle of death & destruction — whether it's war or crime or civil unrest or disease, there has to be *something* to keep people in a state of fear strong enough to motivate them to *want to know more* & to look to their preferred 'news' sources for the latest. One would think that this overemphasis on fear-mongering would be so familiar by now that people would understand that it's just *Business-As-Usual* & not let themselves be manipulated by it.

No such luck, this particular media campaign was so omnipresent & so cleverly designed to be *the-new-threat-that's-replaced-that-old-boring-terrorism* that almost **everyone** was taken in by it. ALMOST everyone. The few of us outside that demographic were soon to find that there was a price to pay for being outsiders, for being *resistant* to such manipulation, transparent or otherwise. My opinion was, & still is, that this mass media manipulation had reached a new extreme of causing widespread mental illness, paranoia at a minimum, & that this mental illness was at least as big of a threat as the *coronavirus*, if not more so.

By the middle of March I was well aware that there was a scare about this pandemic happening & my 1st social media post on the subject was from March 16, 2020 & is reproduced below. The essence of my speculation is that what I call "mediated non-experience" is something that people are believing regardless of any actual direct proof in their own life.

I often explain to people that I was raised in an environment where I could observe the effects of brainwashing firsthand &, therefore, it's something I have detailed non-mediated actual experience with. To give a few examples:

As a child I was always being told by my mom that Russia had 'news' that was totally censored & controlled, nothing but propaganda, but that the press in the US was 'free'. This was during the 'Cold War' era. She also told me that Russia's propaganda press was the product of their being Communists. That led to my asking her one day *what Communism was.* She was a bit taken aback by my question & actually didn't have the slightest idea what it was even though she referred to it as an evil thing all the time. That was when I realized that the American press was definitely propaganda since my mom's brainwashed opinions were just regurgitations of it.

I started growing my hair long when I was 14, at the beginning of 1968. In my area at the time that meant that I was subject to frequent abuse from strangers who felt free to insult & threaten me from the safety of their cars — much like the cyber-bullies of today hurling abuse from the remote safety of their computers. My mom was completely opposed to my long hair & tried threatening me to no avail. One day, when I was 15, she & I were sitting at the breakfast table together & she was reading a Letter to the Editor in the *Morning Sun*, a daily 'news'paper.

The Letter stated that all males with long-hair were homosexuals. My mom was vehemently saying "That's right! That's right!" — this despite the fact that her long-haired heterosexual son was sitting a few feet away from her. That might've been my 1st experience of witnessing *mediated non-experience* in action — rather than believe the evidence of her senses, the heterosexual long-haired son who lived in the same house as her, she believed the non-evidence of an *opinion* published in a mass media outlet that had authoritarian weight for her.

Later, I was involved in resistance to the Vietnam War, a war my mom completely supported without having the slightest idea what it was about, except, perhaps, that it was a 'War Against Communism', which she still hated & feared even though she never had the slightest idea what it was. *Over 32 years after the war was over*, she saw a TV 'documentary' which took a position against the Vietnam War. *Because she saw that on TV*, she told me that I "had been right about the Vietnam War". She was incapable of actually having her own opinion on anything, everything that was 'her opinion' was only formed after the mass media told her what to think. While my mom was an exemplary robopath she was hardly alone in that respect. In fact, it seemed at the time that people like her were the majority & *it seems even worse right now* because the internet is being so successfully used for mind control.

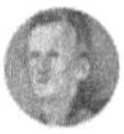

March 16, 2020
4 hrs ·

People are going to get angry with me, as usual, for even daring to suggest the following: What if this PANDEMIC PANIC were just an experiment in mass mind control? It's certainly working. People's behaviors are being even more transparently determined by beliefs based entirely on mediated non-experience than usual. Whether the health danger exists or not the danger of uncritical reception of 'information' from the DOCTOR GODS (who, in my experience are highly fallible) that leads to things happening for 'our own good' that might just not really be for our own good after all is an equally serious danger.

and 2 others 32 Comments

Like Comment Share

Note that I've removed the commenter names that follow this & replaced them with the number that represents the order that they replied in. Their 1st comment number is followed by the letter "a" so if they made any subsequent comments they're labeled "b", etc, following the obvious alphabetical order in which they occur. This was done in order to avoid turning this into a personal thing. I'm not analyzing individuals to be known to the reader, I'm analyzing them as known to myself.

Commenter 001 responds in a way acknowledging the possible validity of my speculation. Alas, commenter 002 responds in what I consider to be a hostile manner.

Note that in my initial statement I imply previous experience with having people get angry with me because of my expressed opinions, even ones that're intended as hypothetical & NOT as statements of 'absolute truth'. It seems that people have been angry with me for such things for my whole adult life. I attribute this anger to my being a Free Thinker in a world of defensive conformists. Conformists '*have to be*' defensive because they're existing on the uncertain ground of an identity *not really their own* & feel threatened by having that identity called into question. Who would they be if that identity fell apart?!

SO, commenter 002: This is someone who friend-requested me, I didn't know them, I looked at their profile, saw that they seemed to have few or no friends, & decided to friend them in case they were someone who I might find socially dysfunctional but otherwise intelligent or with underappreciated qualities. I have sympathies for people who are socially alienated. As it turned out, commenter 002 didn't ultimately impress me as anything other than an ill-spoken lout & I just unfriended them rather than waste any further time trying to navigate their apparently extremely limited intelligence & charm. This was to be the 1st of my PANDEMIC PANIC UNFRIENDINGS.

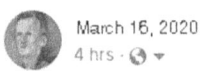

Note my terse reply: "I didn't say it's not a virus." &, in fact, I've avoided this issue throughout the PANDEMIC PANIC because whether the virus exists or not or whether it's lab-manufactured or not or whether there's a possibility that it's something *other than a virus* is ultimately irrelevant to my central concern — which is: that I think that a massive change is taking place in human society as a result of media-induced beliefs being implanted in people's minds. It's my opinion that people are being successfully treated as if they're computers being given a new operating system *without their consent* & being told that it's 'for their own good' even though, to me, it's very much to their destruction.

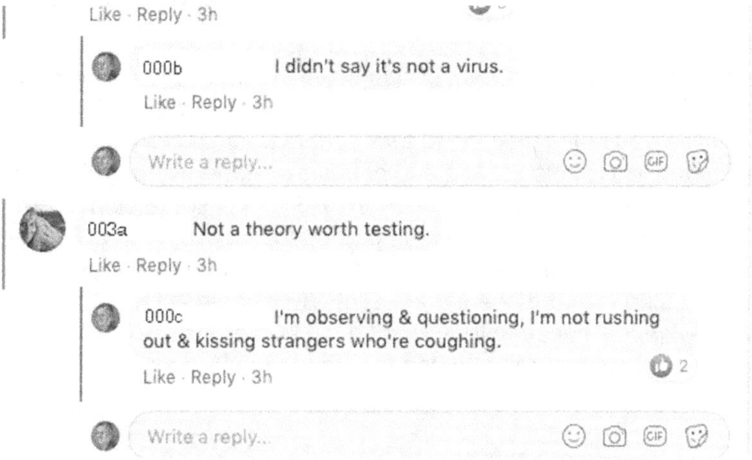

It didn't really take long before it became glaringly obvious that addressing the PANDEMIC PANIC publicly as anything other than what the MONOLITHIC NARRATIVE presented it as being (a legitimate state-of-terror over a high likelihood of imminent death that had to be dealt with by extreme curtailment of civil liberties) was to incur the wrath of the BELIEVERS. How dare I question their God?

Take, e.g., the above comment "Not a theory worth testing": What would it mean to test a theory that speculates that the pandemic is being used opportunistically by people with ulterior motives different from their PR ones, if & when any PR were even to exist? It doesn't *have to mean that I would deliberately get exposed to COVID-19 to test whether it's 'real' or not* because that's not what my speculation was about in the 1st place. Unfortunately, that low level of pseudo-intellection was where most discourse was doomed to stay. 003 continued in this obnoxious vein, ultimately insulting people who presented alternative points. I'll get to that later, although 003'll have a different number by then.

The more I expressed myself publicly on this issue, the more I came under attack. One person came on my social media timeline specifically because they noticed that I'd shared a questioning video link. Even though it was obvious that they didn't know anything about me, they then tried to character assassinate me as someone who thought that research just meant watching YouTube videos. By then, of course, I'd read many articles.

This type of character assassination has been common. People imply that I don't know what I'm talking about & then say something that's meant to be refutational that's so poorly informed that it's a waste of time even replying. It became truly a matter of BELIEVERS (the people who hated what I was saying) & the HERETICS (myself & a few friends who were actually questioning & researching what was happening). & as with any dispute between religious people & non-believers all the religious people had to do was state whatever they believed in as *absolute irrefutable truth known to all as such* & no amount of counter-argument backed with informed articles, etc, would be allowed to effect the beliefs.

What escalated this to a new level of brainwashing that I'd never witnessed before, or, at least, not since the Cold War era, was the degree to which CENSORSHIP was being justified to try to prevent almost any public dialog. Instead of actually trying to understand counter-arguments, the BELIEVERS would, at best, cite what I call FACT CHOKERS to say something to the effect of *'That's been disproven'.* There's been no need for them to look at or in any way try to understand what it is that's supposedly been disproven. Making that even more exasperating is that these same BELIEVERS then act as if they're of *'superior intelligence'* because they won't even bother to try to have any opinion other than the one that's prefabricated for them by their subculturally approved newsfeed.

004 'came to my rescue' by giving an opinion that I agree with but that my detractors ignored. Instead, 005 contributed what was already becoming the standard irrelevancy:

"That theory can be tested by checking into the hospital in Bergamo." Really? How? At the time, Bergamo, Italy, was where most of the COVID-19 deaths were reputed to be happening. The hospitals were reputed to be overwhelmed by more cases than they could handle. As with commenter 003, the implication is that my theory is that the virus isn't real: therefore, checking into a hospital in Bergamo where there were many sick people would show me that it's 'real' because I'd see the sick people.

In actuality, my speculation is that people's minds are being controlled by mass media manipulation of the hypothetical crisis. Therefore, a comment based on a belief in **mediated non-experience** of the Bergamo hospitals (after all, there was a quarantine at that point preventing people from flying in & out of there so neither 005 nor I would've been actually able to get to Bergamo to be 1st-hand witnesses) is intended to 'convince' me that the crisis is 'real' even though whether it's real or not is beside the point. What's to the point is that people are acting *as if experience they're not having is their own* instead of just a story that the media's telling them. 005's comment just proved my point but 005 was too obtuse to understand that.

Another common feature of comments meant to 'disprove' my speculation is a sort of *condescending pomposity meant to 'educate' me.* Hence, 005 informs me that "the virus that is in Bergamo is now here" as if I didn't realize that viruses can travel around the world. This, of course, bypasses what he originally put the focus on: Bergamo. Since the virus is here why not just direct me to a hospital in Pittsburgh, where I live? Because in Pittsburgh, the hospitals *weren't overcrowded* (& never became so) & there wasn't a terrifying mounting death toll. In fact, the CDC's chart for Allegheny County, where Pittsburgh is, lists the *1st COVID-19 death* as happening on March 18, 2020 — 2 days *after* 005's post.

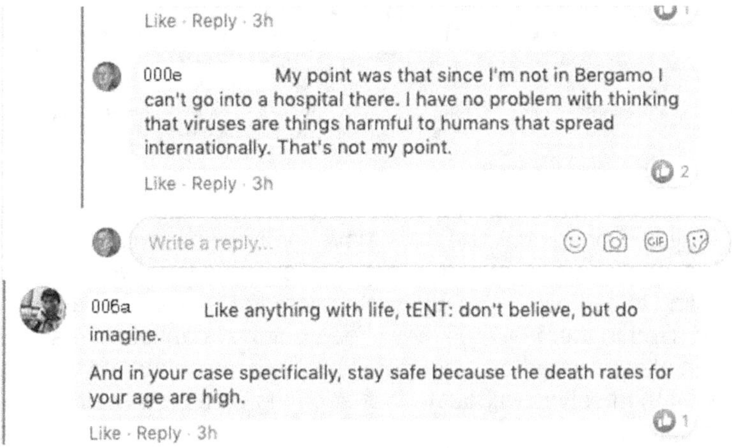

006's comment was a rarity: someone actually expressing sensible concern instead of hiding hostiliy behind a transparent facade of pseudo-concern. As the PANDEMIC PANIC & QUARANTYRANNY stretched on for months the latter personality type became more & more evident. I'll write more about that in an admittedly amateur psychoanalysis of someone later.

Another thing that came more obviously to the fore than usual is the use of the term "Conspiracy Theory". While I don't think my friend whose comments below are shown is misusing the term in a pejorative sense that IS generally the way it's used & people have become afraid of making *any* speculation about what's happening that deviates from the MONOLITHIC NARRATIVE because they're afraid of being branded a 'Conspiracy Theorist' &, hence, a 'fool', a 'moron', someone who lives in a dreamworld, someone easily duped, etc. It's my opinion that the people who uncritically accept the MONOLITHIC NARRATIVE, the version of the story that's being so heavily pushed upon everyone, are the ones who're easily duped, etc.

008a While I don't buy into the conspiracy theory aspects of this, I think the conversation of this being a possibility is a good barometer of where we are - I think there's a lot of good information out there, which requires a critical & unemotional mind to wade through - There's also a lot of panic -We went grocery shopping to a unsually crowded store and were literally the only people not buying toilet paper - I thing the virus is going to kill the amount of people it will kill - The response & lack there of, how much hysteria & bad human behaviour this will engender, that's the rub -

Like · Reply · 3h

008b It is going to be a mind control experiment regardless of if there was any intention from the start of that happening - It's a possible dry run for deeper martial law in areas of the world (Including the USA) and will very much be used as political leverage - And, as I think we all know, we're just at the start of whatever this is happening

Like · Reply · 3h 1

At least so-called 'Conspiracy Theorists' have the imagination & the courage to consider ideas that're often far more deeply researched than what the average person is willing to delve into. Most people seem to just want to have an 'opinion' to parrot that's fed to them by their 'news'feed but they cautiously make sure that it's an opinion also parroted by other people in their subculture so that they can safely repeat it themselves without fear of seeming somehow 'weird'. Take 008's 2nd comment above:

"it's a possible dry run for deeper martial law in areas of the world (including the USA) and will very much be used as political leverage - And, as I think we all know, we're just at the start of whatever this is happening"

Some people might dismiss *that* as 'Conspiracy Theory' but it just seems like an intelligent & worldly observation to me. In the USA, the "political leverage" is entirely in evidence as the Democrats use the QUARANTYRANNY as a tool to pseudo-justify their right to power, post-Rump.

000h It's possible for a health crisis to start & for it to then be used by the people who steer global responses to the crisis for ulterior motives. In other words, one doesn't have to believe that the CIA, say, deliberately caused coronavirus to imagine that surreptitious & opportunistic forces might see a chance to ride on the dilemma. Opportunism Knocks.

Like · Reply · 3m

Write a reply...

009a Fear is a very powerful emotion, tEnt.

Like · Reply · 2h 1

Yes, "Fear is a very powerful emotion", as 009 says, but some of us aren't living in a perpetual state of it. Some of us can stay calm enough, often enough, to recognize opportunism at work — &, importantly, to object to it.

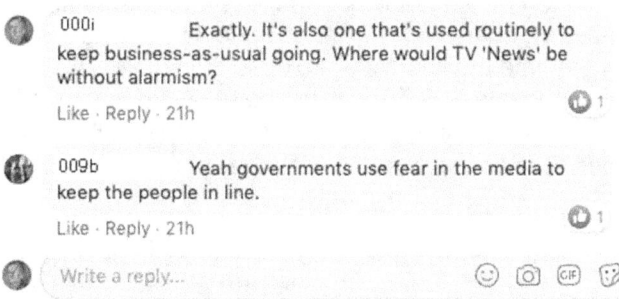

000i Exactly. It's also one that's used routinely to keep business-as-usual going. Where would TV 'News' be without alarmism?

Like · Reply · 21h 1

009b Yeah governments use fear in the media to keep the people in line.

Like · Reply · 21h 1

Write a reply...

010a I def thought this.
I also thought it when we were locked down in boston too during the man hunt after the marathon bombing.

Distrusting the fed gov is at the at time high, and this thread will fuel that fear for some. I am open to this discussion right now because I trust local government, the city council and the people I work with. I trust the flow of information from the state to local and state to state. I trust the CA Office of Emergency Management, and I've seen their response to tangible issues like fires and floods.

I'd rather try to encourage people to listen to local authorities because the only thing people are being asked to do is stay home at this point and i think that is good anyway for the environment.

We need to fundamentally change the way we work, commute, purchase goods and our healthcare if we want to survive our over consumption and not destroy the planet. This will at least get the how conversation started.

I lean on the optimists side, I remember being a big fan of Candide by Voltaire. I think I need to buy a new copy. Ah amazon...

Like · Reply · 2h 1

003b I am seeing it as a grassroots survival uprising much like we need to address climate disaster. In the face of lethargic and idiotic leadership people (for the most part) are acting at a local level to protect themselves and each other.

Like · Reply · 2h 1

As some of my fellow HERETICS have noted, this is where the 'genius' of the PANDEMIC is. It appeals to liberal trust in local authority & in global benign motives. Liberals don't mind tyranny-lite as long as it's for the 'public good'. The

WEF's (World Economic Forum's) proposal for a "Great Reset" in which ecological concerns & a quest for optimized social equality strikes me as the biggest con job EVER, short of religion, perhaps. The fact that the usual global con artists are involved, such as the IMF (International Monetary Fund), makes it even clearer that *the move is on for the biggest power players to control even more of the pie than they already do* — but instead of appealing to the authoritarian-happy 'right-wing' they're going for the pawns most likely to fall for schmaltz. By the time the liberals wake up to their having lost any significant autonomy it'll be too late — for one thing they'll be too feeble from cooperating with their own destruction to be able to flex what little intellectual muscle they may've deluded themselves into believing they had.

003c I have people in my life in the extremely high risk group. This feels like a moment to rely on medical science. This includes skepticism about the use of antibacterials like Purell (science has shown) invite superbugs.

Like · Reply · 2h

000j Yes, skepticism. I went to a doctor 6 months ago because I thought I was diabetic. I wanted confirmation. The doctor, amongst many other egregious things, insisted that I had to start shooting insulin immediately. I said that I preferred trying changing my diet & exercise instead. She told me that was "impossible". I said I'd try it my way for a month & that if it didn't work I'd consult with her again. Within 5 days my symptoms were gone. I tested my blood twice a day. Within 2 weeks my blood sugar normalized. I'm 66, my health could certainly improve but, in general, I'm in excellent health. I would've been dependent on an expensive drug if I'd followed the doctor's advice uncritically. I think it's important to realize that doctors are fallible & that they usually represent a system of doing things that's certainly open to criticism.

Like · Reply · 18m

010b 000 i think you made the right decision and its time to find a holistic doctor if you can, or not go back to her. I don't trust a lot of doctors, especially psychiatrists!

Like · Reply · 6m

Write a reply...

011a Ask someone on a ventilator if you can trade places. If they won't let you then you're probably right.

Like · Reply · 1h

In my initial comment exchanges with people in social media I tried to address the content of the posters in a respectful way that would clarify where I was coming from. Alas, it became quickly obvious that no matter what I said I was unlikely to have a sensible conversation with the new BELIEVERS, people whose medico-religious fervor made it more or less 'impossible' for them to think beyond their already fixed position.

Take commenter 011. They fall neatly into the same category as 003 & 005: there's a wishing of harm on me because they 'think' I'm ignoring the harm being felt by others. My focus on the media's manipulation of popular opinion is side-stepped.

> 000m Ah.. My point is more about how even a health crisis can be used by opportunists or just plain fallible interveners. Obviously, I'm not going to choose to be on a ventilator & my switching places with such a person wouldn't prove or disprove anything about what I'm analyzing.
>
> Like · Reply · 22h 1

Nonetheless, no matter how many times I tried to get commenters to address what I was actually saying instead of what their immersion in propaganda kept locking them into I failed. The MIND-CONTROL was already too total. As I explain in my "Personal Backstory" later in this book, I'd gone through enough life experiences to make me extremely skeptical about the value of the Medical Industry; I'm ***not*** a worshipper at the temple of the DOCTOR GODS.

> 011b Seeing someone dealing with a life threatening viral infection will prove that this is no hoax. This situation is not mind manipulation. Talk to people who are sick. Call your doctor's office. I can assure you, this is no joke. While people are panicking and being manipulated by fear, that I agree, this virus is not a hoax.
>
> Like · Reply · 20h

As far as I can tell, I never said that the virus is a hoax. That doesn't matter to commenter 011. They're utterly oblivious to what I actually said. Furthermore, people get sick all the time. I have no way of knowing whether the virus is what I'm being told it is. Talking with a person who's sick might convince me that they're sick but it won't necessarily tell me that they're sick with a particular disease that I'm being told is life-threatening at a new level.

Commenter 011 further assumes that I 'have' my very own doctor — doesn't everyone?! That's an assumption that's deeply rooted in a belief that it's *good* for everyone to be so intimately tied into the Medical Industry that we have our own doctor. Mightn't it be better if we *didn't* — which would indicate an *absence of need, a state of health?!* No, no, the MONOLITHIC NARRATIVE tells us: we *must* be tied into the Medical Industry.

000n It appears that you haven't carefully read either my original post or any of the other replies. What I'm addressing is PANDEMIC PANIC. As for dealing with life-threatening sickness, my last 3 months have been largely consumed by 1. my mom on her death bed, 2 dealing with the subsequent adult responsibilities.

Like · Reply · 3h

011c 000 I can empathize as a hospice nurse. Those times are VERY difficult indeed. Thank you for sharing that part of your heart.
This situation is not mind manipulation. "While people are panicking and being manipulated by fear, that I agree,.." I have read your comments. This is fear. It's not mind manipulation. People fear death. People fear illness. This is also greed, addiction, and a desire to control the situation in ways that give people a sliver of comfort. Feeling prepared comforts people. That's my opinion.

Like · Reply · 2h

This is where I truly start to feel *nauseous*. 011 thanks me for sharing that part of my heart. What part? The left ventricle? If I shared it with her it was an accident, that would be very unhealthy. I was simply telling her about my reality to try to get her to understand that I'm not unfamiliar with people being sick & dying. Their telling me that they're a "hospice nurse" didn't make me have a new respect for their implied medical knowledge, it made me think of the hospice nurses I'd recently interfaced with.

A hospice worker's "desire to control the situation in ways that give people a sliver of comfort" means basically making the dying person comfortable & making them die under sleeping pills so that they aren't visibly writhing in agony. That doesn't mean it's the best way to go. I didn't particularly like my mom but I didn't really mean her harm either. If I knew before she was put in the hospice what I know now I would've opposed it.

011 was another person I don't really know. I was perfectly happy to get her braindead babblings out of my feed. She was my 2nd PANDEMIC UNFRIENDING. *Finally*, a more substantial comment appeared by a friend of mine whose intelligence I respect:

012a I certainly am observing it with the cold-minded facsination of a scientists who has set up this experiment. What is most striking to me is how people-as-crowds seem utterly uncapable of holding complex thoughts, and consider, let alone weight out, various aspects of phenomena, e.g. yes, there is a virus and yes, there are victims, but also there is an obvious manipulation of the situation from interest groups in position to do so. One thing doesn't preclude the other - most people given the opportunity, would take advantage of a situation like this to advance their interests (there is no conspiracy in this, just human nature). The other striking behaviour was already mentioned by Jean-Luc Bonspiel. Both of those, interestingly, are congruent with psychiatric diagnoses of certain personality disorders. It's been a few years already I've been increasingly under the impression that, in terms of social groups, humanity behaves in ways that make it clearly mental-hospitalizable. It's also interesting how this mass illness carries over to personal behaviour and otherwise healthy individuals become mouthpieces and avatars of media positions, without even suspecting they are paroting a simplistic (i.e. clinically unhealthy) view of an event e.g. Etc., etc. Metaphorically or literally, I also tend to entertain the thought that the experiment is on. 🙂

1

Love · Reply · 40m

I was extremely grateful for their observation that "this mass illness carries over to personal behaviour and otherwise healthy individuals become mouthpieces and avatars of media positions, without even suspecting they are paroting a simplistic (i.e. clinically unhealthy) view of an event": *they addressed what I was saying.* This becoming "mouthpieces and avatars of media positions" is something that's become so common that it's literally hard these days for me to have a conversation without people I know repeating stock phrases like "Our Governor did what needed to be done in time." Most of these phrases profess a disturbingly thoughtless admiration for Big Brother.

&, later, I wrote a statement for public release in case of my death that emphasizes this. We'll come to that later in this book.

000o Thank you, you've gone right to the heart of what I was addressing instead of having a knee-jerk reaction. If I were to die from this virus, which is, after all, entirely possible, at least a few people would gleefully say something to the effect of 'Ha ha! That fool died because he didn't believe in disease!' — which, of course, is not what I'm saying at all.

1

Like · Reply · 21h

012b 000 I promise that, if that happens, I'll dance you to the gates of death so that you don't hear the (contaminating) voices of idiocy in your last moments of human glory! 🙂

Like · Reply · 19m

Write a reply...

I appreciate 012's sentiment but I don't want to drown out the idiocy around me I want it to cease being so robopathic, so *gullible*, so easily manipulated by puppet-masters. Hence, I think I'll stay alive at least *a little bit longer*, if I can, *to continue to struggle for that cause*. Wish me luck.

000p Note that my statement refers to "PANDEMIC PANIC": it's the behaviors surrounding the announcement of the pandemic that I'm addressing. Everyone has direct experience with disease & good reason to think that there are some diseases that are more likely to be fatal than others. Given that I'm 66, have had pneumonia twice, & could be called "pre-diabetic", I'm possibly in a higher risk group than many. Acknowledging that doesn't mean that I have to 'get with the program' & go along with every statement from sources that, like anything human, can be analyzed as possibly misleading or opportunistic or even downright contrary to my own personal experience.

Like · Reply · 9m 2

010c 000 i def thinks its good we question how compliant we are.

Like · Reply · 4m

013a This was actually published a few years back but it's suddenly relevant again.
https://www.theguardian.com/.../naomi-klein-how-power...

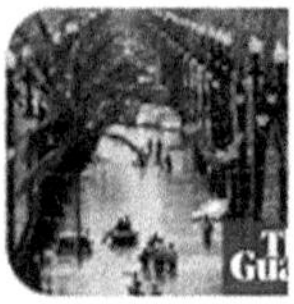

THEGUARDIAN.COM
Naomi Klein: how power profits from disaster

Like · Reply · 17m

013b That being said, the crisis is real.

Like · Reply · 14m

014a yeah there is a piece on the shock doctrine and corona virus in vice magazine;
https://www.vice.com/.../naomi-klein-interview-on...

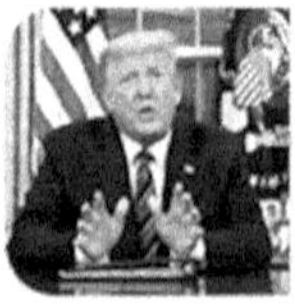

VICE.COM
Coronavirus Is the Perfect Disaster for 'Disaster Capitalism'

Like · Reply · 17h · Edited

013's posting of this link to an article in The Guardian is something I don't recall whether I looked at. Perhaps I should have but this was at a stage in the PANDEMIC PANIC when I was glad to just have & state my observations. I wasn't looking for affirmation from 'reputable' or otherwise sources. I'd heard of

Naomi Klein, I had a very vague opinion of her as someone who was financially successful at a more 'mainstream' version of activism than the more 'lunatic fringe' IMP ACTIVISM that I prefer. Wikipedia describes her as:

"**Naomi Klein** (born May 8, 1970) is a Canadian author, social activist, and filmmaker known for her political analyses and criticism of corporate globalization and of capitalism. On a three-year appointment from September 2018, she is the Gloria Steinem Chair in Media, Culture, and Feminist Studies at Rutgers University.

"Klein first became known internationally for her book *No Logo* (1999); *The Take* (2004), a documentary film about Argentina's occupied factories, written by her, and directed by her husband Avi Lewis; and significantly for *The Shock Doctrine* (2007), a critical analysis of the history of neoliberal economics that was adapted into a six-minute companion film by Alfonso and Jonás Cuarón, as well as a feature-length documentary by Michael Winterbottom." - https://en.wikipedia.org/wiki/Naomi_Klein

She seems great, actually, a feminist aware of & addressing labor issues who's involved with anti-globalization activism. Strangely, though, she's also popular with *The Guardian* & with *NPR*. That makes her acceptable to liberals & an unlikely target for the Fact-Chokers. Consider the following from her own website:

"**SCREEN NEW DEAL**
May 08, 2020
By Naomi Klein
Under cover of mass death, Andrew Cuomo calls in the billionaires to build a high tech dystopia....

"It has taken some time to gel, but something resembling a coherent Pandemic Shock Doctrine is beginning to emerge. Call it the "Screen New Deal." Far more high-tech than anything we have seen during previous disasters, the future that is being rushed into being as the bodies still pile up treats our past weeks of physical isolation not as a painful necessity to save lives, but as a living laboratory for a permanent — and highly profitable — no-touch future." - https://naomiklein.org

Fantastic, right? &, yet, it seems that the liberals that embrace her aren't really getting the message — because the liberals are perpetuating the PANDEMIC PANIC with a fervor more ridiculous than anyone else. Is that the key to Klein's success? Does she give a believable face of critical resistance to something that then continues with Business-As-Usual? Honestly, I don't know.

Despite Klein's apparently acute intellect even someone who recommends her then says "That being said, the crisis is real." But my question is "Which crisis are you talking about?" People are dying, sure; whether they're dying exclusively from COVID-19 or whether they're dying from COVID-19(84) is the question for me. Did so many people die at Elmhurst in NYC because, as one whistle-blowing nurse describes it, sick but non-COVID-19 patients were being all called COVID so that federal funds could be gotten for the hospital — resulting in non-COVID patients *becoming* COVID-19(84) patients. I find the evidence for that compelling. There's definitely a *crisis* & that crisis is being felt amongst almost everyone except those who're steering its handling: *they're not out of a job.*

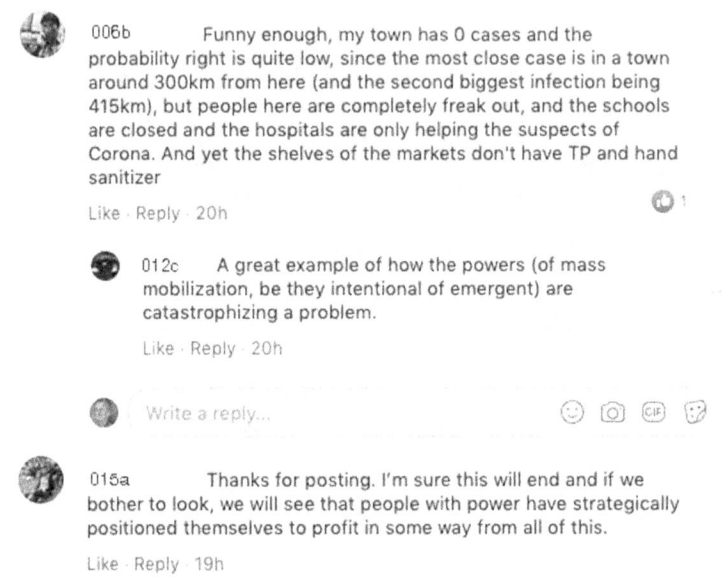

006b Funny enough, my town has 0 cases and the probability right is quite low, since the most close case is in a town around 300km from here (and the second biggest infection being 415km), but people here are completely freak out, and the schools are closed and the hospitals are only helping the suspects of Corona. And yet the shelves of the markets don't have TP and hand sanitizer

Like · Reply · 20h 1

012c A great example of how the powers (of mass mobilization, be they intentional of emergent) are catastrophizing a problem.

Like · Reply · 20h

Write a reply...

015a Thanks for posting. I'm sure this will end and if we bother to look, we will see that people with power have strategically positioned themselves to profit in some way from all of this.

Like · Reply · 19h

I don't think 006's situation is the same 5 months later. Nonetheless, there IS a "catastrophizing" going on.

Once again, I'm thankful for someone commenting on the gist of what I'm observing: *big-business-minded people always have an eye for profit.* Any 'disaster', such as a war, is an 'opportunity'. An opportunity to make enormous amounts off of selling masks & ventilators, off of having COVID-19 patients & getting C.A.R.E.S. money; *an opportunity to create a job crisis & to depress wages for those desperate to get back in the work force.* Listen to the woman from the IMF talk in the WEF "Great Reset" video online: it's all about 'opportunity' — opportunity to improve the world? my ass!

014b How bizarre is it that outlets who were – just weeks ago – warning against trusting anything that comes out of the mouths of our 'masters', are now prepared to surrender entirely to official narratives and official 'safe-keeping' – and for a virus which, even if totally real, has killed about 7,000 people – or around 7% of the numbers who have died over the same time period – of the current flu.

Yes, that is a real statistic. Check it out.

And no, don't tell me it's "not a fair comparison" because the flu is 'always' here and nCoV is new. All you do by that is display your unthinking foolishness. Flu viruses are RNA viruses that mutate all the time – which is why you can catch 'the flu' over and over again; You're catching a different strain, a 'new' variant. Just like nCoV it needs to travel by infection routes. And just like nCov it has to start small.

But unlike nCov it has already managed to kill around 100,000 people since Jan 1 this year. So let go of that particular piece of nonsense, ok?
https://off-guardian.org/.../panic-pandemic-why-are.../

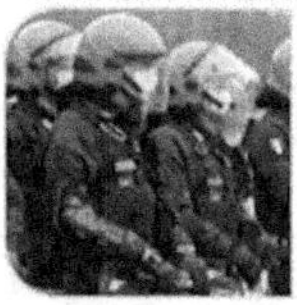

OFF-GUARDIAN.ORG
Panic Pandemic – Why are people who should know better buying the Covid19...

Love · Reply · 17h · Edited 1

015a https://www.bloomberg.com/.../russia-oil-flows-to-asia...

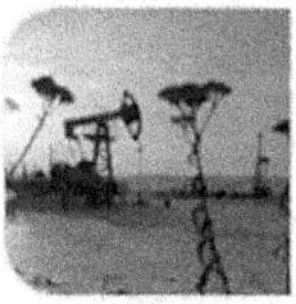

BLOOMBERG.COM
Russian Oil Flow to Unscathed by Coronavirus as OPEC+ Meets

Like · Reply · 10h

& then my friend Phil Bradley commented. He immediately calls attention to people "now prepared to surrender entirely to official narratives". IMO (In My Opinion) that's what using a 'health crisis' as the latest threat has accomplished. It's tricked people into thinking it's not political in contrast to the 'terrorism' that was the big threat before it. *& he links to an article in the Off-Guardian* — a publication that the Fact-Chokers would have you not read at all. The *Off-Guardian* claims that it was founded by people that *The Guardian* wouldn't publish.

Commenter 013, the person who presented the link to Naomi Klein in *The Guardian* informed me in no uncertain terms that *The Off-Guardian* is Russian Propaganda. I read a little of what they had to offer & it seemed reasonable to me. So, *who do I trust?* I trust myself. I trust a few friends, I trust our collective wisdom or intuition or even naivité, our collective experience. It seemed to be time to try to pull a few of these friends together into a group to share our observations & research. &, so, the seeds of the HERETICS started to be planted with this email exchange with Phil:

[All emails are edited both for brevity & to protect both the guilty & the innocent.]

March 18, 2020:

Howdy Phil, You have no idea what a relief it was to read your post about COVID-19. I don't know what it's like there but there's definitely widespread media-induced insanity going on here. I'm practically a lone wolf howling about this. When Obama made the AHCA (Affordable Health Care Act) this was widely lauded by liberals as somehow a great leap forward for health care but I saw that as almost completely delusional. Instead, it extended the powers of the POLICE STATE to an extreme I'd never seen before — authorizing total governmental invasiveness in the name of 'our own good'. I couldn't even understand what the Right Wing was upset about: it enabled mind-boggling profits for largely useless middlemen. Now, 'ironically', this is even worse. People are, essentially, being herded into house arrest & encouraged to do everything 'virtually'. There's even a virtual appliance repair place. Restaurants, museums & all 'non-essentials' are closed. The brain-washing is amazing. The thing that makes this particularly insidious is that it reaches across the political spectrum — almost EVERYONE is taken in by this — &, as you can see if you read 002's & 011's replies to my social media post, it's taboo to question this in any way.

Hi Amir-ul Kafirs,

Im still here in Amsterdam.

I like to always be open to whats really going on and try not to have a fixed position. sometimes I fear the worst with this COVID-19 situation not that the disease itself is that bad but that they will continue to ramp up the fear and introduce censorship and martial law...They are already rounding up the homeless. Other times I think I am just being paranoid. Which ever way, whether it is a real threat or not, it is always good to keep an eye on what is going on in the background while we are disorientated.

I get what you mean about the left going with it too. Obama was never a great president and even he has described himself once as a moderate republican....The health care system here in the Netherlands is shit and I think it might be a bit like Obama care. We are forced by law to pay a lot of money to be covered and we don't really get much back from the system.

Here is a 'practice run' for the corona virus done in october 2019 where they discuss closing down the internet to stop disinformation...
http://www.centerforhealthsecurity.org/event201/videos.html

I woke up this morning to about ten stories of mine being censored by social media. apparently the official story is that with all social media workers working from home the antilogarithms went out of control.

As pressure for coronavirus vaccine mounts, scientists debate risks of accelerated testing
https://www.reuters.com/article/us-health-coronavirus-vaccines-insight-idUSKBN20Y1GZ

And here is another scary project to follow
https://id2020.org/

****

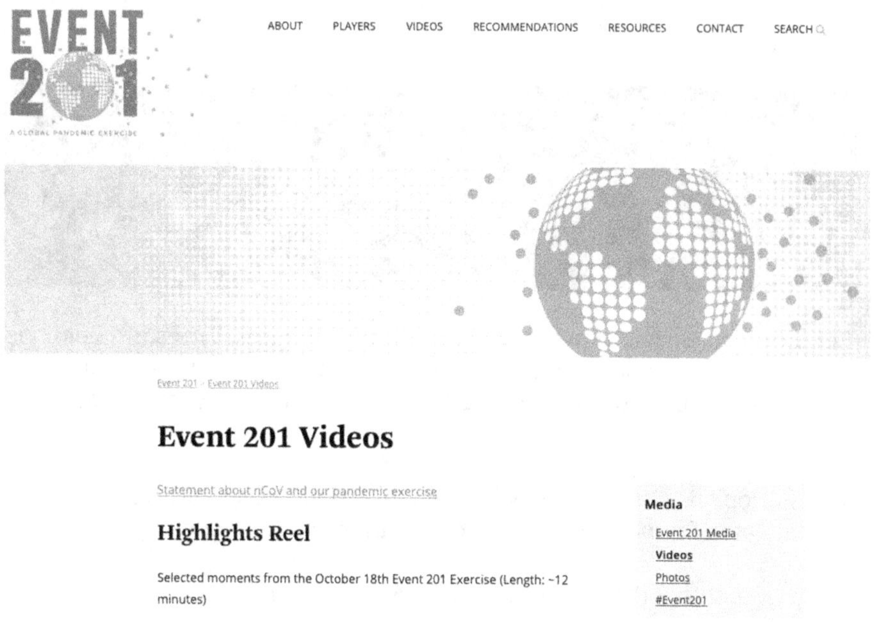

****

Thank the holy ceiling light for Phil! Right from the start of our email correspondence he introduced me to things relevant to my concerns that I wasn't previously familiar with: *Event 201*:

"About the Event 201 exercise

"Event 201 was a 3.5-hour pandemic tabletop exercise that simulated a series of dramatic, scenario-based facilitated discussions, confronting difficult, true-to-life dilemmas associated with response to a hypothetical, but scientifically plausible, pandemic. 15 global business, government, and public health leaders were players in the simulation exercise that highlighted unresolved real-world policy and economic issues that could be solved with sufficient political will, financial investment, and attention now and in the future.

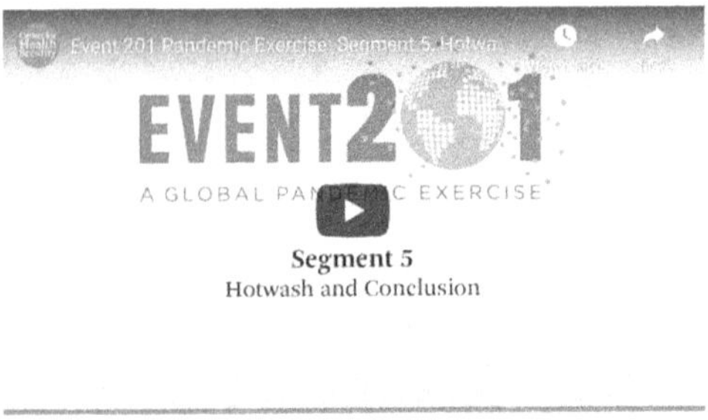

"The exercise consisted of pre-recorded news broadcasts, live "staff" briefings, and moderated discussions on specific topics. These issues were carefully designed in a compelling narrative that educated the participants and the audience.

The Johns Hopkins Center for Health Security, World Economic Forum, and Bill & Melinda Gates Foundation jointly propose these recommendations."

- https://www.centerforhealthsecurity.org/event201/about

NOW, as a former BalTimOrean I'm not exactly the biggest fan of anything Johns Hopkins oriented; as an anti-globalization activist there's no way I'd trust the motives of the WEF (World Economic Forum); as a person who *deeply distrusts billionaires* I'm really not likely to fall for the Gates Foundations 'philanthropic' PR move. This is further solidified by point 7 of Event 201's "Recommendations":

"Governments and the private sector should assign a greater priority to developing methods to combat mis- and disinformation prior to the next pandemic response. Governments will need to partner with traditional and social media companies to research and develop nimble approaches to countering misinformation. This will require developing the ability to flood media with fast, accurate, and consistent information." - https://www.centerforhealthsecurity.org/event201/recommendations.html

Who's to say what constitutes "mis- and disinformation"? Let's take the example of Agent Orange, a defoliant used by the US as a weapon during the Vietnam War:

"**Agent Orange** is a herbicide and defoliant chemical, one of the "tactical use" Rainbow Herbicides. It is widely known for its use by the U.S. military as part of its chemical warfare program, Operation Ranch Hand, during the Vietnam War from 1961 to 1971. It is a mixture of equal parts of two herbicides, 2,4,5-T and 2,4-D. In addition to its damaging environmental effects, traces of dioxin (mainly TCDD, the most toxic of its type) found in the mixture have caused major health problems for many individuals who were exposed.

"Up to four million people in Vietnam were exposed to the defoliant. The government of Vietnam says as many as three million people have suffered illness because of Agent Orange, and the Red Cross of Vietnam estimates that up to one million people are disabled or have health problems as a result of Agent Orange contamination. The United States government has described these figures as unreliable"

- https://en.wikipedia.org/wiki/Agent_Orange#Class_action_lawsuit

Would YOU trust the US government's denial that Agent Orange harmed the soldiers who had to sue to get any settlement? I wouldn't. So, *why*, would anyone trust them now?!

On to Event 201's "Purpose":

"Purpose

"In recent years, the world has seen a growing number of epidemic events, amounting to approximately 200 events annually. These events are increasing, and they are disruptive to health, economies, and society. Managing these events already strains global capacity, even absent a pandemic threat. Experts agree that it is only a matter of time before one of these epidemics becomes global—a pandemic with potentially catastrophic consequences. A severe pandemic, which becomes "Event 201," would require reliable cooperation among several industries, national governments, and key international institutions."

&, then, to its "Scenario":

"The Event 201 scenario

"Event 201 simulates an outbreak of a novel zoonotic coronavirus transmitted from bats to pigs to people that eventually becomes efficiently transmissible from person to person, leading to a severe pandemic. The pathogen and the disease it causes are modeled largely on SARS, but it is more transmissible in the community setting by people with mild symptoms."

[..]

"There is no possibility of a vaccine being available in the first year. There is a fictional antiviral drug that can help the sick but not significantly limit spread of the disease.

"Since the whole human population is susceptible, during the initial months of the pandemic, the cumulative number of cases increases exponentially, doubling every week. And as the cases and deaths accumulate, the economic and societal consequences become increasingly severe.

"The scenario ends at the 18-month point, with 65 million deaths. The pandemic is beginning to slow due to the decreasing number of susceptible people. The pandemic will continue at some rate until there is an effective vaccine or until 80-90 % of the global population has been exposed. From that point on, it is likely to be an endemic childhood disease."

- https://www.centerforhealthsecurity.org/event201/scenario.html

It's bound to be speculated upon by many of us that the occurence of Event 201 on October 18, 2019, with participation from the WEF (whose so-called "Great Reset" proposes a plan, mid-pandemic, for essentially restructuring the socio-economic world along lines of their own 'envisioning') shortly before the PANDEMIC PANIC began is *no coincidence*.

I'm not concerned with whether it's likely that they unleashed the virus on the world. I AM concerned with what seems to me to be the high probability that their 'vision' went into *creating the media hysteria* around COVID-19, thusly creating COVID-19(84), & that their 'vision' has contributed to the substantial damage done to small business to the advantage of the big corporate businesses that their sponsors represent.

Some might find Event 201 to be 'proof' of the far-sighted 'genius' of those involved. If those people aren't naive then I might very well be a *Big Eyed Bean from Venus*.

Phil also brought to my attention the importance that a COVID-19(84) vaccine would play in all this. As the PANDEMIC PANIC threat is widely exaggerated by the mass media, an emphasis on almost completely bringing society to a halt until *everyone in the world is forced to be injected with a vaccine for it* has become prominent.

I haven't had a vaccination since I was, maybe, 14. I'm 66 now. Somehow I've managed to get through 52 years without having another one. My experiences with previous coronaviruses have been mild, I'm not worried about this one, no matter how terrifying the depictions of it are. I AM worried about the transparent financial motives of the Bill & Melinda Gates Foundation because they're one of the main forces, if not *the main force*, promoting the vaccine. The fact that they stand to make an unbelievably large profit off of it should certainly be called into question. It's what's called a *conflict of interest*.

& then Phil mentioned Digital ID. The website that he gave a link to has this to say:

"Since 2016, ID2020 has advocated for ethical, privacy-protecting approaches to digital ID.

"For the one in seven people globally who lacks a means to prove their identity, digital ID offers access to vital social services and enables them to exercise their rights as citizens and voters and participate in the modern economy. But doing digital ID right means protecting civil liberties and putting control over personal data back where it belongs...in the hands of the individual."

- https://id2020.org

"For the one in seven people globally who lacks a means to prove their identity, digital ID offers access to vital social services and enables them to exercise their rights as citizens and voters and participate in the modern economy."

Never for a second is this questioned as anything but desirable. What if there are people *who do not want to be part of the society that's under constant surveillance?* What if I'm one of them? Is it because I'm 'criminal'. I think it's because I'm CRIMINALLY SANE, a person who recognizes that laws aren't always for the greater good.

In support of my position, I like to remind people of the existence of Reinhard Heydrich:

"**Reinhard Tristan Eugen Heydrich**" [..] "7 March 1904 – 4 June 1942) was a high-ranking German SS and police official during the Nazi era and a main architect of the Holocaust. He was chief of the Reich Main Security Office (including the Gestapo, Kripo, and SD). He was also *Stellvertretender Reichsprotektor* (Deputy/Acting Reich-Protector) of Bohemia and Moravia. He served as president of the International Criminal Police Commission (ICPC, later known as Interpol) and chaired the January 1942 Wannsee Conference which formalised plans for the "Final Solution to the Jewish Question"—the deportation and genocide of all Jews in German-occupied Europe." - https://en.wikipedia.org/wiki/Reinhard_Heydrich

Not only was Heydrich a main planner of genocide he was also the head of what became *Interpol*, the international police force. Anyone who would've opposed him would've been a 'criminal' or, in my lingo, CRIMINALLY SANE.

Digital ID, like so many other things these days such as parking meters where you have to enter your license plate #, thus establishing a mapping of your car's location; electronic toll booths that monitor your travel; & *contact tracing*, thinly justified as a health measure, that establishes a data base on your social activities, is a further step in keeping US under constant surveillance. If YOU think this won't be abused for control of every aspect of your life then *you are naive*.

ANYWAY, I quickly saw the 'need' for there to be a group of trusted friends to share research & observations & opinions about what was happening with this PANDEMIC PANIC. A mere 9 people in 4 countries & 7 cities were sometimes gathered under the heading of HERETICS. Eventually this small group became even smaller as 6 people in 3 countries & 5 cities. We exchanged emails & messages & social media posts & phone calls & whatnot. This collaboration GREW into something so HUGE that it seemed obvious to me that it must be shared with the world in the form of this book. Perhaps this is *Event 202*, a very different vision of the world from that represented by the wealthy arrogance of *Event 201*.

Alas, these exchanges have been heavily edited to protect the participants because, unlike the *Event 201* participants, we don't have teams of lawyers to prevent us from losing our jobs if we happen to, ahem, *say something unpopular*, something that goes against the grain of PROPAGANDA, of which there's quite a bit flying around these days. As such, some of the day-to-day details of real-life encounters have had to be left out. It's too bad — but I think that the gist of our findings, of our opinions, has remained intact.

It's worth further noting that all of the contributing writers were writing under a variety of emotional conditions as we've struggled to make sense of all this. Therefore, there are times when some of us are distressed & expressing that distress to each other because our psychological reaction to things like the quarantine are key to understanding the Unconscious Suffocation that we feel is being inflicted on us as a form of psychological warfare.

There are many positions that I could take about this PANDEMIC PANIC but I'll try to summarize the most 'reasonable' one (IMO) below. That'll give YOU, the reader, an idea of what to expect. Maybe you'll be able to identify from the beginning, maybe you'll be willing to pay close attention to our argumentation.

01. *Event 201* as a planning session for pandemic response is suspect as something organized by people who might want to test their plans out regardless of whether there's a real need for the plans or not.

02. Whether the PANDEMIC is 'real' or not is irrelevant in the sense that the PANIC surrounding it is certainly real.

03. The actual threat of COVID-19 has been extremely exaggerated &, in some cases, *augmented & otherwise misrepresented* for reasons that aren't publicly stated as part of the MONOLITHIC NARRATIVE.

04. People have been endangered & have died from things blamed on the PANDEMIC that are more accurately blamed on the PANIC, on the financial manoeuvering that's been central to it, on the utter lack of concern for the health of the majority of the people *disguised as a concern.*

05. The economic effects of the QUARANTYRANNY have been devastating for small independent businesses & *mind-bogglingly profitable* for large corporate ones. This is in no way acknowledged by the MONOLITHIC NARRATIVE.

06. In the United States, there's such a desperation among liberals to get rid of Rump [pun intended] that they'll go along with *anything* that they think will work toward that end — no matter how insanely that "*anything*" curtails civil liberties.

07. If the QUARANTYRANNY is allowed to ride roughshod over the people of the world the result will be *far more catastrophic to the better parts of our societies* than the PANDEMIC is ever likely to be.

08. Among the many likely outcomes of the PANDEMIC PANIC QUARANTYRANNY as it's currently proceeding is: a. Dramatically increased censorship, b. Dramatically increased dependence of the majority of the people on financial forces beyond their control, c. Dramatically increased surveillance, d. Dramatically increased curtailment of movement, travel, socialization, & sexual contact.

09. There's plenty of legitimate concern over the desirability & healthiness of many types of medical intervention, including vaccines. I don't find it in any way acceptable for vaccines or any other medical intervention to be *imposed* on anyone. Everyone should have the choice to welcome or reject such things based on their own experience & philosophy.

- essay finished August 12, 2020

HERETICS emails - March, 2020

March 18, 2020, 11:10AM (Amir-ul Kafirs to Phil Bradley):

Re: corona

I like to aways be open to whats really going and try not to have a fixed position.

Exactly, it's called FREE THINKING — something almost no-one I know understands in the slightest. An effect of having Rump be the Idiot King is that if one even uses words that Rump or his ilk have used then one is suspect of being 'Right-Wing'. It's ludicrous. The fact that the concept predated Rump's use of it & has been used by many people of a variety of political orientations is no longer remembered. 'Liberals' are in such a hurry to prove their moral superiority to Rump that they carefully avoid being tarred w/ the same brush. The result? Prefabricated sentiments of extremely limited analysis. An example: in an argument with a liberal friend I used the term "witch hunt", a term that, apparently, Rump has used. I wouldn't know, I waste as little time listening to his proclamations as possible. My friend informed me that that was Rump language (of course, he said "Trump"). Anyway, after he couldn't browbeat me into repeating the accepted leftist phrases he didn't speak to me for about a year. I have no desire whatsoever to solidify my membership in ANY subculture. People do that for safety's sake, I've spent my whole life going against the thoughtless grain &, yes, there's been alotof hate directed my way, but WHATEVER.

sometimes I fear the worst with this COVID-19 situation not that the disease itself is that bad but they will continue to ramp up the fear and introduce censorship and martial law...

Exactly. Is it really such a big threat that all this quarantining (which is tantamount to house arrest) is necessary? I think not.. & I find it very suspicious. The health threat probably exists but the opportunism of government response to it is a taboo subject. I see this as a test run: if people dociley & passively fall into line, which almost EVERYONE is, then the powers-that-be know what to do when they want a lock-down. Alas, people believe the myth that doctors are very socially concerned citizens whose purposes are completely for the public good. Bullshit. Doctors, especially in the US, are little more than drug pushers trying to get EVERYONE into a system that sucks as much money out of them as possible. Doctors want & HAVE **POWER**. They consider themselves superior beings who have the right to manipulate the masses 'for their own good'. They're like lawyers in that respect. The medical industry is a highly sophisticated system of control. & IT'S GETTING MUCH, MUCH WORSE.

Other times I think I am just being paranoid.

Nope, you're not, I'm observing the same things. The thing is that like all its Draconian predeccesors, this doesn't have to go full throttle yet, I think it's a test run. I think of WWI: I think the rulling elites of the warring countries realized that creating nationalist fervors was just the ticket for stopping international solidarity & revolution by pitting the working class against each other.

****

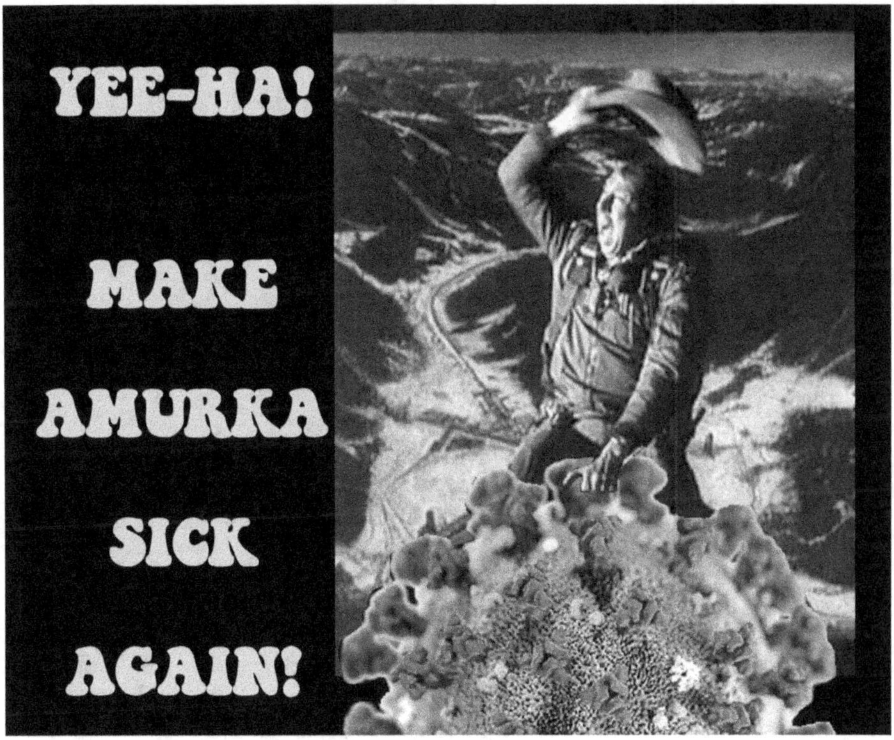

****

On March 19, 2020, my friend **Naia Nisnam** forwarded this text message to me:

Please share with other families.

He said that they are preparing to mobilize the national guard. Preparing to dispatch them across the US along with military. Next they will call in 1st responders. He said they are preparing to announce a nationwide 1 week quarantine for all citizens All businesses closed. Everyone at home. They were told to pack and be prepared for up to 30 days deployment which he said means they may extend the quarantine up to 30 days. He told me to notify our family members and have them stock up and be prepared. They will announce this as soon as they have troops in place to help prevent looters and rioters... he said he got the call last night and was told to pack and be prepared for the call today with his dispatch orders. He thinks they will announce before the end of the weekend to keep people home on Monday.

It supposedly originated from someone in or connected to the National Guard. We were both alarmed that if the Guard were deployed it might involve the shooting of civilians as it had at Kent State in my lifetime. Fortunately, that deployment hasn't happened yet but at this early phase of the QUARANTYRANNY any kind of craziness seemed possible. For that matter, it sill does.

****

On March 21, 2020, a friend in New York City emailed me a link to data on what were purported to be COVID-19 deaths.
I replied on the same day:

Ischaemic heart disease and stroke are the world's **biggest** killers, accounting **for** a combined 15.2 million **deaths** in 2016. These diseases have remained the **leading causes of death** globally in the last 15 years.

check the numbers!! crazy!

I'm not sure exactly what you see as "crazy" about the numbers. I get the impression that people perceive COVID-19 as a huge killer and, hence, all the Draconian measures seem justified. My impression is that this isn't the case, that the number of people dying is relatively small. Here's an [edited] online list of the 10 leading causes of death:

1. Heart disease
- Deaths in 2017: 647,457
- Percentage of total deaths: 23.5%

2. Cancer
- Deaths in 2017: 599,108
- Percentage of total deaths: 21.3%

3. Unintentional injuries
- Deaths in 2017: 169,936
- Percentage of total deaths: 6%

4. Chronic lower respiratory disease
- Deaths in 2017: 160,201
- Percentage of total deaths: 5.7%

5. Stroke and cerebrovascular diseases
- Deaths in 2017: 146,383
- Percentage of total deaths: 5.2%

6. Alzheimer's disease
- Deaths in 2017: 121,404
- Percentage of total deaths: 4.3%

7. Diabetes
- Deaths in 2017: 83,564
- Percentage of total deaths: 3%

8. Influenza and pneumonia
- Deaths in 2017: 55,672
- Percentage of total deaths: 2%

9. Kidney disease
- Deaths in 2017: 50,633
- Percentage of total deaths: 1.8%

10. Suicide
- Deaths in 2017: 47,173
-
- https://www.medicalnewstoday.com/articles/282929#heart-disease

Keep in mind that according to the chart you link to there're 11,868 deaths reported so far. That's over what? A 3 month period? Multiply that by 4 **[interpolation: I realize that the increase was expected to be exponential**

but exponential in what time frame? Every second? By the day? Practical mathematical aspects of this exponential factor were bypassed for the sensationalism of it as a magic word, I chose to not address it here] to get an estimate for an entire year and you get 47,472 — around the range of suicides. If the powers-that-be really wanted to dramatically decrease deaths they'd declare sugar to be a dangerous drug and make it go the way of tobacco. For obvious reasons, that isn't going to happen.

https://gisanddata.maps.arcgis.com/apps/opsdashboard/index.html?fbclid=IwAR2DUiEfHISMdan45tNstt9hZ6buGQXnyeNueYeWyWO-J8ppJW1lgeNTADI#/bda7594740fd40299423467b48e9ecf6

****

I was also already in correspondence with **Dick Turner** & **Inquiring Librarian** about the PANDEMIC PANIC so I shared the above with them on March 21, 2020, & **Inquiring Librarian** & I had the following exchange:

Yes. I am on your page with this situation. I have been making a point to ask select people near me (say at the park or in line at the grocery store, while checking out at the grocery store, at work, etc...) if they know anyone directly who has gotten the virus or who is bonifiedly sick with the virus. So far, no one has answered the affirmative to any of the above. And now that we are isolating, there are very few chances to ask anyone if they have that real life connection to the virus.

In the meantime, I continue to correspond with people asking them what their take on the situation is and what's happening where they live. I have a friend in Amsterdam and a friend in Paris, both are very skeptical and suspicious of the whole mess. Both France and the Netherlands have also been heading toward the right in recent years. Will everyone in Louisiana be quarantined as of Monday? One report says that National Guard have been sighted driving through Louisiana in trucks. It's still unclear what's happening here in PGH. I, personally, am fine. Ironically?, I'm in good health and in good financial shape. One good friend has a daughter who just went into the hospital for pneumonia, bringing up, once again, the question: IF THERE AREN'T ANY SPECIAL SIGNS OF COVID-19 SICKNESS THEN WHAT DOES ANY OF IT MEAN IF THE TEST PRODUCES FALSE POSITIVES OR BAD INFORMATION IN GENERAL? Here're some excerpts from my correspondence that you might find interesting. Particularly noteworthy is the claim that almost everyone who's died had pre-existing severe health conditions and was old — hence bringing into question what satisfactory proof there is that COVID-19 is so much to blame for things. Make sure to follow the off-guardian link. I have no idea what the "OffGuardian" is but I think the article makes good points.

ANYWAY, I hope you and yours are fine. At this point, it's probably more realistic to be careful about the general social insanity that's bound to be generated by the economic desperation.

****

Phil & Amir-ul Kafirs continue:

I know that if this was about taking deaths seriously they would take these other deaths from other things much more seriously

Again, EXACTLY. Suddenly the government is all concerned about its citizens? In the US this is during the Rump era?! Tell me another one. There has quite probably NEVER been a president who cares less about the people he 'governs'. As I said to one friend of mine, 'we're just cockroaches to him'. I can think of quite a few motives for this increasing quarantine but *caring* is not one of them.

....especially iatrogenic deaths https://www.ourcivilisation.com/medicine/usamed/deaths.htm

This is quite a good article too for trying to get a better grasp; https://off-guardian.org/2020/03/19/iss-report-99-of-covid19-deaths-already-ill/

One of the things that I'm finding so frustrating is how low-level people's 'reasoning' is. E.G.: a friend tells me that she's hearing constant ambulances and that everyone's showing the same symtoms. Ok, at least she's reporting on something that she's actually witnessing happening. *But what exactly is she witnessing?* She's hearing sirens. My immediate response is: Isn't it possible that the amount of fear-mongering is leading to people going to the hospital who would ordinarly just stay home? In other words, the increase in people being taken away *doesn't* ***necessarily*** *mean that they're all sick with COVID-19.* That seems faily obvious to me. We have an unprecedented situation here of panic-production. In the 66 years I've been alive I've never witnessed anything even remotely like it.

I wonder how many people will actually die from the lockdown, test positive for the corona virus and then become counted corona virus victims.

Again, EXACTLY. Having people in quarantine can't possibly be good for them at all sorts of levels — an obvious one being psychologically.

In Italy and probably elsewhere they cannot distinguish between dying of the corona virus or a pre-existing medical condition or a combination. Plus we do not know how accurate these test units are as they come up with false positives.

AGAINAGAIN, EXACTLY. Suddenly, the panic-production is so effective that people BELIEVE just about EVERYTHING. I haven't run across any symptoms for COVID-19 that aren't the same symptoms as other things. Since when are tests infallible? Especially tests for something new? It's idiotic to believe there can't be false positives or just sloppy reporting.

****

Still on March 21, Dick Turner sent me a link to an article in French about the vacillations of the French government's positions on QUARANTYRANNY. The below is a bit of his commentary on it:

The following paragraph is excerpted from an article in Le Monde diplomatique, a "respected" publication (it's like the French NYT) that reports on international issues

It's very curious

The article is meant to be an indictment of how the "epidemic" has been mishandled but this paragraph gives an interesting chronology

It recreates the announcements made by the governments here in France

It begins saying that in late January the health minister said the virus would never make it to France, this was the official position for a month

On March 11th President Macron gave a speech saying there would be no need to change any of our behaviors, we could still go to bars, theater, movies, etc

Then on March 12 an official statement made in the afternoon by a Minister was made saying it wouldn't be necessary to close the schools

Then the same day, March 12 in the evening this changes to school closure

Then on the 14th the First Minister announces a general suggested confinement

Then on the 15th Macron goes on air again to announce a full quarantine, that the schools will close, fines if we leave the house, etc. starting the next day at noon

One has to admit, this is like something from the Three Stooges, like "But Curly said that Moe said that Larry said..."

I cannot help but think that perhaps in the midst of all this tergiversation that there is a possibility that the various World Powers put their strategy together of a more or less universal lock-down, thinking "let's see if we can't play this thing out a bit and see where it goes... who knows, could be interesting!"

It's just an idea, after all, there is already in place a means of fast communication between governments in emergencies

****

March 23, 2020, 10:00AM (Dick Turner & Amir-ul Kafirs):

My point with that article wasn't to say the politicians are dopes, which is probably usually the case but rather to pose a question about the rather odd announcements that were made all within a period of 4 days, beginning with "nothing will change" to "confinement"

It looks like tomorrow by the way it will become total, even the stores are closing so who knows how we will eat

Of course we'll mostly all eat but WHO DISPENSES THE FOOD will be more controlled. I'm reminded of 2 things: When Napoleon disempowered the Catholic Church in Spain there were immediately large groups of people without food because the Church had *made them dependent on them.* When the CIA was setting up the infrastructure for the secret wars in Laos they convinced the farmers to convert from rice crops, which was their main food source, to opium crops, which the CIA could turn into heroin and use for secret financing. The farmers then ate rice that was airdropped in by the CIA. At 1st, the men in the farming towns who were then recruited to be soldiers was a small amount, eventually, it became almost everyone. When these people resisted being forced into anti-Viet Cong armies the air-dropped food was stopped. Add to that massive bombings that left unexploded bombs embedded in the ground & the eventual result was an environment originally good for growing food turned into a deadly mined wasteland. My 'Conspiracy Theorist''s point being that the more any necessity is controlled, the more the people become controlled.

it's funny because i'm still skeptical about the whole thing, I don't know if it is a personality thing or not, but I just can't convince myself that it is what "they" say it is

& I'm with you all the way on that & delighted that we're even agreeing about it all because, in my immediate environment, an almost total acceptance of the propaganda is in place.

I talked with a friend of mine in New Jersey last night. He works the front desk of a hotel. Of course, there's almost no-one staying there & most of the staff has been laid-off. He, too, is skeptical. He's supposedly at an epicenter but he's seeing no evidence of people being sick. He told me something interesting that I haven't heard elsewhere: apparently some public health official gave an announcement to the effect that they were trying to control the situation in such a way so that normal hospital business could proceed unimpaired. In other words, they were trying to prevent the hospitals from becoming swamped with COVID-19 cases that would then prevent them from being able to address other things like births or heart attacks or whatever. If I understood what he said correctly, this spokesperson was saying that they were trying to control the populace in such a way to keep people from flooding the hospitals. That seems somewhat sensible if it's true. At any rate, another friend of mine in Brooklyn said that there're sirens from ambulances all day long & my friend in the hotel business said: 'Oh, it's always like that in Brooklyn.' He said there's no increase in sirens in his area of New Jersey. SO, for me, it remains ambiguous.

What has bothered me all along is this mediated non-experience factor. Everything I see around me is generated by media reports. This is then exaggerated by fear. A cough that would've been accepted in the past as just an ordinary bodily function is now potentially a 'symptom' of something far more potentially fatal. I don't really think we have enough info to be much of a judge of anything at the moment. One friend of mine compared this to the Swine Flu of 1918-1919 but I pointed out that there was plenty of hindsight info about that & that it's too soon for hindsight about this.

Basically, I'd rather NOT have my concerns about how this serves the Police State born out. What I'd rather have happen is for a couple of weeks to go by, for restrictions to be lifted, for life to go back to normal, etc.. HOWEVER, even if it 'ends well', if house arrest doesn't go on indefinitely, etc, ***there will still be a precedent for shutting down life-as-usual under the guise of 'public good'.***

Please do continue to keep me posted.

P.S. Last night I participated in a phone meeting of community activists about setting up a network that people-in-need can access for food deliveries & whatnot. I have mixed feelings about that too but I'm now one of the people who will monitor our voice mail for incoming requests for help. So far, even my perception of this group is somewhat cynical but that's a bit too much to get into at the moment.

Good luck to both of us,

yr pal,

Amir-ul Kafirs

P.P.S. If you haven't already seen this, check out this absolutely despicable Fox TV 'News' piece: https://youtu.be/EKHWjOtVyK8 Note, of course, that it promotes purchasing more guns — thusly reinforcing my usual concern about the degree to which arms dealers profit off of any 'emergency', false or real.

****

Dick Turner's reply:

In all of my life I've never seen anything as bizarre as that Fox news report !! Maybe that's normal American television these day, is it? it's INSANE the anchorman is taking sides and so obviously stirring up fear it couldn't be any clearer and yes, he's basically saying "go buy guns, arm yourselves before it's too late"
It seems like something from a 1970's low budget sci-fi film

****

In all of my life I've never seen anything as bizarre as that Fox news report !! Maybe that's normal American television these day, is it?

I stopped watching TV 50 years ago & I've never regretted it so I can't really analyze it as a whole except to say that I doubt that it's changed enough to refute Jerry Mander's wonderful book "Four Arguments for the Elimination of Television" (which I quote from in my movie "Robopaths": https://youtu.be/-PR7C8nFKtA) which provides the entire text for my "**WARNING: TV Suffocates the Senses like a Bag over the Head**" (https://youtu.be/WIoChhRmiiQ). I can say that, yes, it strikes me as 'normal' American TV. 'Conservative' people probably 'choose' FOX TV 'News' as their #1 source. Is it any wonder that people are so out of touch with reality?!

it's INSANE the anchorman is taking sides and so obviously stirring up fear it couldn't be any clearer

Exactly, it's obvious fear-mongering — &, yet, I suspect that its avid viewers just see it as 'hard-hitting' or some such. There's no room for nuance.

and yes, he's basically saying "go buy guns, arm yourselves before it's too late"

Making me wonder, of course, how many arms sales interests are at play in the financial background.

****

You might find this interesting
The second paragraph echoes your thought

there will still be a precedent for shutting down life-as-usual under the guise of 'public good'

http://bookhaven.stanford.edu/2020/03/giorgio-agamben-on-coronavirus-the-enemy-is-not-outside-it-is-within-us/

he develops it a bit

http://positionswebsite.org/giorgio-agamben-the-state-of-exception-provoked-by-an-unmotivated-emergency/

Dick Turner

"The other thing, no less disquieting than the first, that the epidemic has caused to appear with clarity is that the state of exception, to which governments have habituated us for some time, has truly become the normal condition. There have been more serious epidemics in the past, but no one ever thought for that reason to declare a state of emergency like the current one, which prevents us even from moving. People have been so habituated to live in conditions of perennial crisis and perennial emergency that they don't seem to notice that their life has been reduced to a purely biological condition and has not only every social and political dimension, but also human and affective. A society that lives in a perennial state of emergency cannot be a free society. We in fact live in a society that has sacrificed freedom to so-called "reasons of security" and has therefore condemned itself to live in a perennial state of fear and insecurity." - Giorgio Agamben on coronavirus: "The enemy is not outside, it is within us."

****

That article by the Israeli is disturbingly good. The reasonable scenario he hopes for of course will never happen. For example once Homeland Security got in place, what's going to remove it short of some disaster like a massive war?

The 'laugh' for me is that I have to wonder whether Homeland Security is any more secure than anything else. The mere fact that a commercial airliner could be diverted & crashed into the Pentagon makes it pretty damned obvious how vulnerable all these hard men are.

****

It's still March 23, 2020, & Inquiring Librarian & Amir-ul Kafirs correspond:

I suppose it will be the next week or 2 that will show a grim reality or continue the illusion.

Yeah, that's basically what I'm waiting for. I have to drive to Baltimore this weekend for my mom's burial, I'm assuming that there won't be a travel ban on by then. If the police state aspects of this have escalated by 2 weeks from now then I'll be even more alarmed than I am now. If everything's gone 'back to normal' then I'll be relieved but on the lookout for suspicious future incidents.

Supposedly Louisiana is a disaster area of the pandemic but i know no one who directly knows a sick person. It is also curious that the Pences and Trumps all test negative.

The Gods are immune to the problems of the cockroaches. Even if they tested positive would we be told about it? I don't think so.

I'd like to think i for 1, and many others, was exposed and am either immune or just got mildly ill.

A strong possibility.

Basically, I just hope that no-one I'm close to, such as yourself, dies — beyond that I hope for as few deaths as possible.

****

Supposedly Louisiana has the highest growth rate of the corona virus in the entire world at the moment. I'm guessing it's just because we finally got test kits that are bringing back results. I still don't know anyone who is sick. We lost a few octo and nano genarians. People in Louisiana have extremely unhealthy lifestyles. They eat horrible fried food, they drink way too much, and they shoot up tons of drugs. I have not yet seen the old heroin addicts and serious drunks that hang out on and sell drugs on my corner succumb and keel over yet. Really, those guys should be toast soon if this is really real. I saw one of them, in the midst of a crowd of junkies in front of our busy (they sell hard core drugs and liquor out of this store) corner store, launch a very large and loud snot rocket into the street while I was driving by.

What I would like is an antibody test. My partner was really sick 2 weeks ago when the hysteria began. They never get sick. Maybe I carried it to them? I have zero signs of illness. I don't know what my blood type is. There is a blood type immunity theory, type O. But I do take probably toooo much liquid vitamin d per day/ 10,000 mg. My vitamin d had been so low for so many years, my doctor put me on this insanely high dose. When I tried to taper down, I started getting sick and staying sick again. So, I amped it back up to 10,000 mg a half or so year ago. I take a high quality bio-identical thyroid medicine, I don't drink alcohol, I don't take drugs or any medications other than thyroid medicine, not even asprin. I don't drink coffee unless I have a headache. I jog 4x/week when my knees allow me and I go for a half hour bike ride 5 to 7 days a week and I do yoga and pilates and I garden and have too many cats. Perhaps this is the recipe for good health in a viral infection??

****

March 25, 2020, may've been the date of the 1st group email I sent out to my 5 HERETICAL friends:

Announcing The National Emergency Library

During this unprecedented time in history, access to printed books is becoming difficult or impossible. COVID-19 is forcing students, educators, and everyday readers to rely on digital books more than ever before. That's why **the Internet Archive has temporarily suspended all waitlists**, allowing you to immediately check out any of the 1.4 million books currently in our lending library. Until June 30th or the end of the US national emergency (whichever comes later), every borrowable book will be immediately accessible by anyone—creating, in effect, a National Emergency Library.

****

Emails have a way of accumulating threads that can be both confusing & invigorating to me. Take this excerpt from an exchange between Dick Turner, Amir-ul Kafirs, & Phil Bradley from March 25, 2020. Things were barely getting started at the time.

You're probably both aware that either during or just before the 9/11 attacks the Pentagon was doing research on plane-as-bomb scenarios and that in London, at the same time of the subway bomb attacks the British Secret Service was also doing planned response scenarios to subway bombings.

My point being that these chains of coincidences do seem enough to turn even the most anti-conspirationist's head...

Dick Turner

The sad thing, Dick, is that people are afraid of being tarred with the Conspiracy Theorist stigma. As such, out of fear of being perceived as a nut case they'll avoid making even the most obvious speculations. Some of us have been saying that this situation is ideal for Rump, the Idiot King, because it might enable him to declare a National Emergency & suspend elections — effectively making himself emperor or whatever insane fantasy he might have. **[As it turned out, it was Governor Wolf, Democratic Governor of Pennsylvania, who used the 'emergency' to most effectively make himself dictator]** That doesn't mean that Rump created the virus, it just means that, as an opportunist of the 1st order (or is it "odor"?), he'd have no scruples whatsoever about using it to his megalomanical advantage. Now that's a worst-case scenario & I'm not really expecting it to happen but I think it's important to at least recognize the possibility. If I were to suggest this to most people I think I'd be stigmatized immediately.

- Amir-ul Kafirs

De : Phil Bradley
Envoyé : mercredi 25 mars 2020 16:04
À : Amir-ul Kafirs, Dick Turner
Objet : Re: death statistics

Strange day yesterday. I was doing my once a month district newspaper delivery job. Nice day. sun out. fresh cold air. Everything so quiet. The night before I went into one of my more paranoid states about the current situation when the Dutch Government announced extending the lockdown and announced it's medical martial law

https://www.dutchnews.nl/news/2020/03/the-dutch-ban-gatherings-to-june-1-give-mayors-more-powers-bring-in-fines/

This news along with this article https://www.globalresearch.ca/all-sectors-us-establishment-lock-step-deep-states-latest-bio-war/5702773 sent me into a bit of a nightmarish scenario that caused sleeplessness and actual nightmares.

At the moment it is hard to see how this will play out. I can see both negative and positive scenarios. I can see both conspiratorial and more 'comical' out of control multiple cascading situations. I recently read the book 'conformity' by cass r sunstein which helps elaborate how this happens or could happen. Perhaps it is a mixture between both. It is a bit relieving to see some people in my social media feed starting to do about turns. I like to post a swiss doctor around https://swprs.org/a-swiss-doctor-on-covid-19/

also good to see The UK has removed Covid19 from the official list of High Consquence Infectious Diseases.

The medical world is starting to downplay the dangers. The real danger now is if the economic situation spirals out of control or not and things escalate into another paniced emergency that requires internet shutdown which has been played out in the event 201.http://www.centerforhealthsecurity.org/event201/

Amir-ul Kafirs:

Thanks for that. I have no problem thinking that the governmental officials are buffoons but that doesn't make them not dangerous, etc.. One friend of mine was asking me why I think that Rump is the way he is and what motives could he have, etc.. I explained that I think he has 2 main wants: more money, more power. I honestly believe he's an idiot but that very idiocy is partially what enables him to maintain his monomania and his megalomania. He thinks he's a genius. It's easy for someone to think they're a genius if they steadfastly don't know about or care about anything that anyone else says or does — then there's nothing to compare himself to. His way of demonstrating his 'genius' is to show his ability to accumulate as much power and wealth as he can. Wasn't it Papa Doc Duvalier who stole the entirety of Haiti's governmental money and then moved to Switzerland?

[Ok, I got that wrong — It was his successor son, Jean-Claude "Baby Doc" Duvalier who stole from the treasury before leaving the country:

"PORT-AU-PRINCE, Haiti (AP) _ Jean-Claude Duvalier stole at least $120 million in 14 years as president-for-life and Haiti will sue in France to get some of it back, Justice Minister Francois St. Fleur said Monday.

"Duvalier, 35, fled to France on a U.S. Air Force plane with his wife Michele and four children Feb. 7, 1986, after months of demonstrations against his government." - https://apnews.com/7a015e845c6b2446ddbc44f2adfcb594

That said, "Papa Doc" has his own interesting story:

"François Duvalier; 14 April 1907 – 21 April 1971), also known as Papa Doc, was a Haitian politician who served as the President of Haiti from 1957 to 1971. He was elected president in 1957 on a populist and black nationalist

platform. After thwarting a military coup d'état in 1958, his regime rapidly became totalitarian and despotic. An undercover government death squad, the Tonton Macoute (Haitian Creole: *Tonton Makout*), indiscriminately killed Duvalier's opponents; the Tonton Macoute was thought to be so pervasive that Haitians became highly fearful of expressing any form of dissent, even in private. Duvalier further sought to solidify his rule by incorporating elements of Haitian mythology into a personality cult.

"Prior to his rule, Duvalier was a physician by profession. Due to his profession and expertise in the medical field, he acquired the nickname "Papa Doc". He was unanimously "re-elected" in a 1961 election in which he was the only candidate. Afterwards, he consolidated his power step by step, culminating in 1964 when he declared himself President for Life after another sham election, and as a result, he remained in power until he died in April 1971. He was succeeded by his son, Jean-Claude, who was nicknamed "Baby Doc"." - https://en.wikipedia.org/wiki/François_Duvalier

It's important to note that François Duvalier was a doctor — adding an example to *reasons-to-be-cynical-about-doctors* that will further accumulate throughout this book.]

I think nothing would suit Rump better than to declare a national emergency and to then declare himself president until the emergency is over, putting a temporary halt to elections. He weathered the impeachment, now he can weather anything. Naturally, putting himself in such a position might enable him to become the 1st trillionaire (if there isn't one already). Jarry's *Pere Ubu* seems so exaggerated but how far is Rump from that? Not very, IMO.

****

March 25, 2020 (Amir-ul Kafirs to group):

Hello folks,

I've taken the liberty of expanding this list of skeptics. I'm calling this group of people "Skeptics" so if you see me using the term as a proper noun you'll know what I mean. Please feel free to add other people but PLEASE only add thinking people who're really skeptics. No idiots with knee-jerk arguments welcome.

Phil: Thanks much for sending the links. I've reposted on social media 2 things that your research has led me to here.

As you say, "At the moment it is hard to see how this will play out. I can see both negative and positive scenarios" & I agree.

What concerns me is how easily MOST people have been roped into the official line on all this. After having failed to convince everyone with things like Rump's immigration policy there's now something that works! Slip in mind control under the guise of public health & make sure there's an unhealthy dose of fear-of-death & people fall right into line. They're afraid that if they're wrong they might DIE.

I've been saying for decades that most people would turn into what I call "Good Germans" (no offense to my German friends intended) with only the slightest impetus. As such, to continue the nazi era metaphor, most people would turn in their Jewish neighbors in a second if they thought that would save their own skin — regardless of whether they were really even threatened or not. Let's face it: most people are cowards & weaklings, utterly brainwashed.

When the AHCA law was passed I said that it gave the Police State unprecendented powers under the guise of public health. Criminalizing people without health insurance & all those incredibly invasive government probes into people's personal lives posed as 'for your own good' were just a precedent for this.

ANYWAY, all around me I see people turning into 'Good Germans' effortlessly. The 5 people that I'm sending this to are among the very few that've expressed agreement with me that this PANDEMIC PANIC is largely bullshit.

To those of you who haven't checked out the links **Phil** has provided, I strongly suggest that you do so.

****

March 26, 2020 (Dick Turner to Amir-ul Kafirs):

I'm responding only to you because I don't think this information would be useful within the group context, I feel a little silly sending this to you in fact, but you may find it interesting

I have a friend, an actor with whom I've worked, who is a full blown conspiracy theorist. But the "funny" thing is, he favors theories where Trump is a world-saving hero, in fact, there seem to be endless theories from which one can choose

He sent me this (among others which even get weirder including a JFK Jr. is still alive and will be Trump's running mate next year scenario...)
https://www.youtube.com/watch?v=4JQLQ1M1_u0&fbclid=IwAR1ch93gn1_L3FEHgC9WlfHwKwz_-BM5WLZI9985qdFQ7QayvbN7nsj9ngA

****

March 26, 2020 (Amir-ul Kafirs to Dick Turner):

I watched this all the way through. I didn't find it convincing. It's strange that he talks against the billionaires protecting themselves in bunkers & whatnot but seems to find Trump & his troops to be AOK. Also, he criticizes there being a biological weaponry lab in Wuhan as if that's something no-one should do but doesn't mention that the US is certainly doing the same thing & quite possibly has been doing so for the last 70 yrs. I personally know of at least 3 places in Maryland alone where such research is happening. & then, of course, there's the "white hats" & "black hats" stuff — that reeks of the silly religious attitude that eventually creeps into it all with his references to Noah & the Ark, etc..

I should mention that I hold a "conspiracy theory" that huge amounts of mis-information are created and encouraged to sidetrack people from the obvious - that the powers that exist want to consolidate and extend their power, which to me seems obvious.

I agree completely, that IS obvious — so why aren't more people talking about it? Are you allowed to leave your apartment in Paris? Just for food? What are the legal conditions? Here, as far as I know, I'm still 'free' to go out but when I go to the park some people are friendly while others look like they're ready to kill me for even existing. This country being as racially divided as it is I wouldn't be surprised if there're racist theories about all this other than just Rump's "Chinese Virus" bullshit — in other words, I wouldn't be surprised if there were theories circulating amongst the black community that whites developed this to wipe out blacks & that sort of thing..

****

Amir-ul Kafirs observation from Pittsburgh:

The garbage workers haven't picked up the garbage this week. Apparently they want more protective gear, which is fair enough, but it's the 1st time I've ever lived somewhere where that's happened. I know it's happened in NYC before & that must've been pretty horrible. Fortunately for me, I don't really accumulate that much garbage. These garbage workers are actually really good at doing their job so I'm sympathetic to them.

****

March 27, 2020 (Phil Bradley to group of 5 other Skeptics):

PANDEMIC PANIC 02

Hi all,

I am now errring mostly towards a planned event......mostly from the way people are reacting. I never watch mainstream news either corporate or government....but I am getting the feeling people are getting conditioned by it and becoming completely irrational without any critical faculties. Anyone with alternative perspectives will be shouted down. This video has a fairly dark and difficult but I think valuable perspective https://www.youtube.com/watch?v=5CCVUc5ZMZo&t=9s&app=desktop

The 2nd world war parallel you mentioned Amir-ul Kafirs.....is particularly pertinent to me. Last year I just moved into a new area of Amsterdam called Betondorp which translates into concrete village because it was an early 1920s experimental concrete development. nearly three hundred Jewish residents were disappeared from here. There were (and still are some) nazi supporters living here. Many people were dobbed in. There was a resistance here too which hid Jewish people. I should worry most about one neighbor living opposite us. In many ways a kinda nice old man but unfortunately a complete racist.....on the other hand most of our other neighbours seem really nice and diverse.

No problems with inviting more people into this exchange.

The question is though where ever we stand with this situation....how do we organise??

****

March 27, 2020 (Dick Turner):

PANDEMIC PANIC 02

I guess we'll see if the suggested 18 month conditioning process goes into effect with recurrent quarantines.
Here in France the suggestion of a total quarantine was met with the very real menace of a leap in suicides - many people live in very small apartments, difficult for Americans to imagine. A place of 15 - 20 sq meters is not unusual. I don't know for how long they could stand it.
I already see among many of my French social media contacts that they are having a hard time staying inside all the time. I sense widespread depression.
So far it isn't a problem for me but I'm a voluntary recluse anyway.

****

March 27, 2020 (Phil Bradley to group):

PANDEMIC PANIC 02

....perhaps a less conspiratorial more comic explanation runs something like this. Fort Detrick biolab has problems and has to close down..https://www.military.com/daily-news/2019/11/24/cdc-inspection-findings-reveal-more-about-fort-detrick-research-suspension.html

.some of the solders training in Fort Detrick go to Wuhan to the military games. Some of them are sick and they stay in a hotel near the Wuhan wet market. I can not remember where I read this ... if i find the link i will post it. Anyway Americans start to freak out that maybe the soldiers are infected with bio weaponry from Fort Detrick. The US begins making inquires to China (before china makes any public statements-read this somewhere before too) This results in China freaking out thinking that they might be the subjects of a bio-weaponry attack. This creates the visual stimulus for mass media to make the invisible visible. China takes this very seriously and builds temporary hospitals. It does indeed find a new kind of virus.

Meanwhile it really is just a coincide that the pandemic 201 exercise was held just before the Wuhan games along with the Chinese drill.
https://thefreedomarticles.com/chinese-government-foreknowledge-coronavirus-drill-30-days-wuhan-games/

However the people involved in these events are primed for the absolute outcomes.

The media then jumps into its usual hyper reporting....keeping everyone in fear...amping everything up. The true statistics of the virus are unknown but are blown out of proportion. There is disagreement in the WHO but pressure to announce a pandemic.

Rump and Boris take the perhaps more logical route of allowing the virus to pass through the population. People rightfully hate both rump and boris but then take the reactionary position of only the opposite of what they say is true and then start politically weaponising the virus demanding their own medical martial law. The media tunes into the weaponising and keeps hyping things up without any analytical explanation as usual.

In the end the cosmic joke is that the covid-19 was been with us for a long time but just not noticed because in a majority of cases the covid-19 goes un-noticed.

Anyway just throwing a different spin....maybe not that realistic

****

March 28, 2020 (Phil Bradley to group):

Re: PANDEMIC PANIC 02

Ok here is comes....the economic downturn exacerbates.....people beg for the new global government to solve the problem....temporarily of course.

https://www.theguardian.com/politics/2020/mar/26/gordon-brown-calls-for-global-government-to-tackle-coronavirus?CMP=share_btn_tw

other evidence of planned event.
https://theduran.com/why-did-hundreds-of-ceos-resign-just-before-the-world-started-going-absolutely-crazy/

snowdon on corona situ
https://www.youtube.com/watch?v=9we6t2nObbw

****

March 29, 2020 (Amir-ul Kafirs to group):

Re: PANDEMIC PANIC 02

I am now errring mostly towards a planned event......

Howdy. I just got back from BalTimOre. I'm thinking of the majority of people as **Manchurian Candidates for GLOBALIZATION who've been triggered by post-hypnotic suggestion.** In other words, the brain-washing has been going on for a long time but all the PANDEMIC PANIC triggers have brought to the surface the conformity. It's interesting. One video that you sent a link to, **Phil**, mentions giving the World Bank & the IMF (International Monetary Fund) more power to 'intercede on the behalf of failing economies' struck down by the PANDEMIC PANIC. *Whew!* That, in itself, is an amazing suggestion. It's further suggested that the G20 make this happen. What that boils down to, economically, is that the world's 20 most powerful nations will further enable the WB & IMF to go into stricken countries, control their politics, bankrupt them, & steal their resources. **[This is actually born out by the WEF's "Great Reset" plan]** It's as if the Anti-Globalization Movement's criticisms are safely forgotten & that the propaganda machine(s) is/are confident of dominance. What we're witnessing is a birth of the New World Odor far beyond what Hitler managed to accomplish in, say, 1940, & far beyond what Reagan accomplished in, say, 1980. Now it's 2020 & the New World Odor is stinking to high heaven. All for our 'own good', of course. What is given the appearance of international cooperation might just be the G20 countries flexing their muscles.

how do we organise??

Good question. For now, I, personally, am happy to know ANYONE who is even roughly on the same page as me. In my immediate local environment even the political activists are getting hooked in to the propaganda line more or less unquestioningly. By the way, I have, maybe, 2 or 3 friends who are now or who have been sick — maybe as many as would ordinarily be sick at this time of the year. All are recovering & not violently ill. I continue to be fine.

It might be worth mentioning that the African-America communities I was in in BalTimOre seemed to be completely ignoring the PANDEMIC PANIC: no gloves, no masks, no social distancing.

Cheerio,

yr fellow heretic,

****

March 29, 2020 (Dick Turner to group):

RE: PANDEMIC PANIC 02

An aside: A new 'custom' has been introduced into French culture. Every night at 8pm everyone opens their windows and claps and shouts 'bravo" for those "fighting on the front lines" (to keep up the military terminology currently in use) to thank the doctors, nurses, police and people still working in the markets (cashiers, suppliers, etc.).

****

March 29, 2020 (Amir-ul Kafirs to group):

Re: PANDEMIC PANIC 02

I'm watching "Quarantiranny" now. I think they're SPOT ON & that they've done a fantastic job of analysis for such an early time in the process. Thanks for the link, Phil. I'm going to try to contact the moviemakers eventually. **[I did & they never replied]**

****

March 29, 2020 (Dick Turner to group):

RE: PANDEMIC PANIC 02

I would like to suggest something, it's just my personal theory however.

If one looks at history there come, from time to time, events that change the course and the form of history.

Famous examples are the ability to make fire, agriculture, the rise of the city and the concept of national identity, the barbarian invasions of Rome, the establishment of the Middle Ages through the ascension of the Catholic Church and the nobility, the Battle of Agincourt, the Reformation, the French Revolution, the First World War, the atomic bomb...

Each time, in retrospect we see that rather than these events being the beginning of something, they are in fact a sort of culmination and statement of a new type of social order that is - **they are the clear expression of what already was happening**.

Then they come along and basically spell the end of certain types of mass thinking and behavior.

As I wrote to Amir-ul Kafirs before I was invited in this group, even if this current epidemic wasn't planned (though I think it probably was just like 911 was if you believe the PNAC business with the need for a "catastrophic event" to put things in place) but even if it wasn't, once it began happening it must have seemed too good to be true to the powers that be as in "we can't let this go to waste!!"

Perhaps what is happening now is something like a moment of significant historical change. It's possible. After all, all the needed infra-structure is already in place for some kind of world government even if it isn't declared outright. Telephones, computers, constant surveillance, it's all here, now. In fact, there would be no need to even tell the people, that is, make an official announcement of a world government, it could happen and we might not know until a much later date when saying it would be redundant.

My point being, if this major change is now taking place, I don't see really what can be done, in fact, I think nothing. Besides, what would be lost? Freedom? Well, 98% of the people I see don't seem particularly interested in freedom. Oddballs like ourselves don't count, as society has let us know over and over again. (If this offends anybody, excuse me, I'm essentially talking about myself.)

Have you noticed that the new generation, the so-called Millennials seem unusually a-historical, meaning, their culture, on a historical level is, very low? I have seen this repeatedly. A personality means having a position, but having a position may offend someone, so the solution is not to have any real opinions, this is the essence of the "politically correct" as far as I can tell.

Thus, since this new generation represents the future, what would really be lost if most of what we know gets wiped off the blackboard? They don't know or seem to care about it anyway. And did they ever really? For example, I love Jascha Heifetz, the violinist, however I don't share my interest with people because I have met with next to no interlocutors, particularly among the younger set. I imagine that for Amir-ul Kafirs, who has a large number of esoteric interests it is even rarer to meet people who can talk about things he finds interesting or people who even want to discover these things.

Of course if some kind of world government happens, the reigning culture will be garbage, all corporate products; something like elevator music, bad comic books and Jeff Koons-like art work.

Kind of how it is right now in fact.

So all that would be happening would be the implicit would be made explicit. That is, it's where we already are... or so I think.

I don't know if that is what is taking place right now, but from the videos I've seen (thank you Phil) it seems possible.

As to what course of resistance to take, it seems to me either one starts to blow up electrical power plants or just keep making art.

Peace and love.

****

March 30, 2020 (Amir-ul Kafirs to group):

Re: PANDEMIC PANIC

Coincidentally, another friend of mine just sent me this:

A LETTER FROM F. SCOTT FITZGERALD, QUARANTINED IN 1920 IN THE SOUTH OF FRANCE DURING THE SPANISH INFLUENZA OUTBREAK.
Dearest Rosemary,
It was a limpid dreary day, hung as in a basket from a single dull star. I thank you for your letter. Outside, I perceive what may be a collection of fallen leaves tussling against a trash can. It rings like jazz to my ears. The streets are that empty. It seems as though the bulk of the city has retreated to their quarters, rightfully so.
At this time, it seems very poignant to avoid all public spaces. Even the bars, as I told Hemingway, but to that he punched me in the stomach, to which I asked if he had washed his hands. He hadn't. He is much the denier, that one. Why, he considers the virus to be just influenza. I'm curious of his sources.
The officials have alerted us to ensure we have a month's worth of necessities. Zelda and I have stocked up on red wine, whiskey, rum, vermouth, absinthe, white wine, sherry, gin, and lord, if we need it, brandy. Please pray for us.
You should see the square, oh, it is terrible. I weep for the damned eventualities this future brings. The long afternoons rolling forward slowly on the ever-slick bottomless highball. Z. says it's no excuse to drink, but I just can't seem to steady my hand. In the distance, from my brooding perch, the shoreline is cloaked in a dull haze where I can discern an unremitting penance that has been heading this way for a long, long while.
And yet, amongst the cracked cloudline of an evening's cast, I focus on a single strain of light, calling me forth to believe in a better morrow.
Faithfully yours,
F. Scott Fitzgerald

****

Around this time, Amir-ul Kafirs asked the people receiving these emailings if they wanted to continue to do so & if they planned to participate in the ongoing discussion.

March 30, 2020 (Dick to the group):

RE: PANDEMIC PANIC 02

I am interested in the discussion, and am participating...

Here's something you might like, Spiro Skouras has endless well made videos on this subject and many others

https://www.youtube.com/watch?v=F_TPjbu4FAE&list=PL58MCVdG8nh30pDw9dBJ_ow-AuSiAQnJY&index=23&t=0s

US Biowarfare Act Author: Studies Confirm Coronavirus Weaponized! - YouTube
In this interview, the Author of the US Biowarfare Act, Professor Francis Boyle

uncovers four separate studies which he claims confirm as 'smoking gun' evidence the Wuhan Coronavirus known as ...

Coronavirus: Follow The Money - YouTube
The headlines regarding the Coronavirus are inescapable at this point, as more and more cases are being reported across the US and across the world. At this point no one knows for sure how bad ...

****

March 30, 2020 (Dick to the group):

RE: PANDEMIC PANIC 02

https://www.youtube.com/watch?v=rVw9KZ2DwJk&list=PL58MCVdG8nh30pDw9dBJ_0w-AuSiAQnJY&index=23

Is Bill Gates Profiting From The Outbreak? Or Is Something Far More Sinister Taking Place? - YouTube
As we see what is now being called a global health emergency regarding the Coronavirus continue to grow on a daily basis, we also see how the solutions to this crisis fall in line with pre ...

****

March 30, 2020 (Dick to the group):

RE: PANDEMIC PANIC 02

Another video to redeem myself, this made 6 weeks ago:

https://www.youtube.com/watch?v=Z29BTnDfgBU&feature=emb_logo

Financial Expert: The End Game Is Unfolding Before Our Eyes - YouTube
On the heels of President Donald Trump's annual State of the Union speech, where the president declared the US employment numbers, the stock market and the economy in general, are doing better ...

****

March 30, 2020 (Inquiring Librarian to group):

Re: PANDEMIC PANIC 02

Greetings everyone from Louisiana,

I would love to continue to stay on this list. I enjoy reading your posts and try to take the time to watch the videos, etc.

I have been a silent member because I do not feel like I have enough well researched and truly intelligent things to say about the situation. I just know deep down that it seems pre-planned. It seems to me to be a mass exercise in social manipulation experimentation. For what ends, I am baffled, or suppressing what could be. I live in the supposed current epicenter, being in a city in Louisiana. The city is silent. I am hearing fewer ambulances than usual, given I live in the center of a large residential part of the city with 2 major hospitals within .5 miles of me. And the alcoholics and addicts that normally populate my corners are as active, alive, and 'well' as ever. Now, I am not a health care worker. I wish I were a nurse. What I would love right now is 1. a stable income, and 2. to be a nurse (i am a lowly (('non-essential')) librarian) so that I could see what is happening on the front lines, and to help the small people who are getting obliterated by whatever evil has been cooked up by the powers that be. Here in Louisiana, we have lost some beloved elderly musicians who had underlying severe health conditions before the virus hit. To understand here in Louisiana, our rents are extremely high and most of us are paid *very* little. We do have a sizeable extremely wealthy population, but the majority of residents are very, very poor. We have a huge homeless population. Our taxes on everything are high. Our bills are outrageous and our insurance costs are among the highest in the United States. People here live ***EXTREMELY*** unhealthy lifestyles. We have many serious alcoholics, severe drug addicts, and people eat the most unhealthy and horrible food I've ever seen in my life. Many people are obese and do not exercise. It seems natural that a virus like this would obliterate a bit of our less fortunate and less self-care centered population.

To support the notion that this was a planned epidemic. I was listening to NPR yesterday. There was a brief blurb about how a peer approved article was circulating that indicated that the makeup of this virus is such that it could easily have been constructed in a lab for mass production (reproduction). This scholarly article, according to NPR, was deemed 'false' shortly after it started circulating and has now been rejected and hidden by the media from the general public. I listen to NPR a lot, I can't explain why, and have become increasingly disgusted by how it seems to be taking the reins on social manipulation of the left, weighing in on the 'do-gooder,' 'pat yourself on the back', sentiments that are supposed to be the construct of a good liberal mind. They seem to plant 'proper', 'good', 'righteous', 'independent', thoughts into the minds of 'save the world' liberals. If you think independently of their versions of independent thoughts, you are shamed and demonized on many levels. Hence, the ever offended, politically correct Millennial generation. I am supposedly a Gen. Xer. But I was not raised by 'Boomers' like most of my peers.

Anyways, please keep me in this loop. If anyone has questions about Louisiana, please send them to me. It might be good for me to feel productive to intelligent, thinking, people again. I miss my job as a public librarian where I had the chance to interact day to day with all walks of Louisiana life where I felt I could connect with and observe some of the most genuine human interactions. I am almost finished reading Norman Cantor's "In the Wake of the Plague." It is helping me to focus some perspective on the current situation in the light of former documented pandemics.

I do find it ironic that librarians, at least in my city, are silenced. We provide access to free and uncensored information via physical books and free internet access to all walks of public life. Our doors are shuttered and the media has conditioned well-meaning but short sighted and ocd librarians into buzzing about the lifespan of this virus on physical books with and without plastic covers... Meanwhile, we can go to any garden center or Walmart to purchase cardboard, paper and plastic made items to our hearts content until our precious little pennies run out. And... I as a librarian will soon not be able to pay my own internet bill or have a roof over my own head... I too will soon be on the other side of the "digital divide" where my less financially fortunate library patrons already are now as librarians have been asked to abandon them. If you cannot fully shut down the internet, shut down the libraries. It's a sad, sad day.

-Inquiring Librarian-

****

March 30, 2020 (Dick to the group):

RE: PANDEMIC PANIC 02

Here is a video where at about 5 minutes before the end the two speakers try to answer the question of "how to organize" that was posed in an earlier mail.

https://www.bitchute.com/video/tB46iZdaETua/

COVID-1984: A Global 9/11
In this interview Spiro is joined by the host of Geopolitics and Empire who was recently censored by Youtube having his interview with Professor Francis Boyle removed regarding the coronavirus.

****

March 30, 2020 (Amir-ul Kafirs to group):

Re: PANDEMIC PANIC 02

On Mar 27, 2020, at 11:20 AM, Phil Bradley wrote:

how do we organise??

To address this again I suggest that we begin organizing by finding as many people as we can who're feeling similarly critical/skeptical to ourselves & that we communicate with them – in other words: NETWORK. Having contacts in multiple countries is useful — both G20 countries & non-G20 countries — SO, if you have friends around the world write to them & ask them how they are & what's happening in their neck of the woods. If possible, get them to communicate with all of us, if not, then at least pass on what they have to say to us.

****

March 30, 2020 (Amir-ul Kafirs to group):

Re: PANDEMIC PANIC

On Mar 27, 2020, at 5:21 PM, Phil Bradley wrote:

....perhaps a less conspiratorial more comic explanation runs something like this. Fort Detrick biolab has problems and has to close down

Most of you reading this are familiar with the Maryland area, where Ft Detrick is, but Phil wouldn't be so I'll fill this in a little. Fort Detrick has been suspected of conducting biological/chemical warfare weapons (& defense) development since the time of the Korean War. An interesting documentary about this subject is Errol Morris's "Wormwood" made as a Netflix series. I highly recommend it. It's about the death of Frank Olson, one of Detrick's scientists, in the early '50s. The main story that circulated about Olson was 1. he committed suicide. 2. this was changed to he commited suicide because he was unwittingly dosed with LSD & he couldn't handle it. 3. that story was supposed to be the embarrassing disclosure that ended speculation. HOWEVER, Morris's documentary brings up the possibility that Olson was aware of & involved with the creation of bioweapons being used in the Korean War. The theory is that Olson had a conscience & was going to somehow blow the whole thing & he was assassinated to make it look like a suicide. The US military was accused by the Chinese of using bioweaponry, the US (surprise, surprise) denied it. My stepfather was a US soldier in the Korean War. He supposedly had sexual problems that led to his only being able to produce one child. That child speculates that it was because of something he was exposed to in Korea, either bio/chemical weapons or radioactivity. The child is NOT a conspiracy theorist or political activist. My stepfather developed ALS in his late life. The child, working for a hospital, learned that the US military will pay a settlement to any former soldier with ALS because it's acknowledged that soldiers have an 'unexplained' high incidence of ALS.

Ft Detrick is not the only place in MD where such research is being done. A medical center where I worked was also doing such research. I've written an article about that that's not online but may be someday. There's also the Aberdeen Proving Ground, a gigantic weapons testing area NE of Baltimore that's almost as big as the city. I often go to Frederick where Ft Detrick is because there's a good bookstore there so when I go to Baltimore it's on the way. I'm always on the lookout for things I'm only likely to find there. Recently, I found a DVD called "Advanced Topics on Medical Defense against Biological Agents - Botulinum Toxin" published by www.USAMRIID.army.mil . I haven't watched it yet, it's 118 minutes & from 2006. The DVD box says:

"To register for continuing education credits and obtain further information about this program go to: www.swankhealth.com or call 1-800-950-4248"

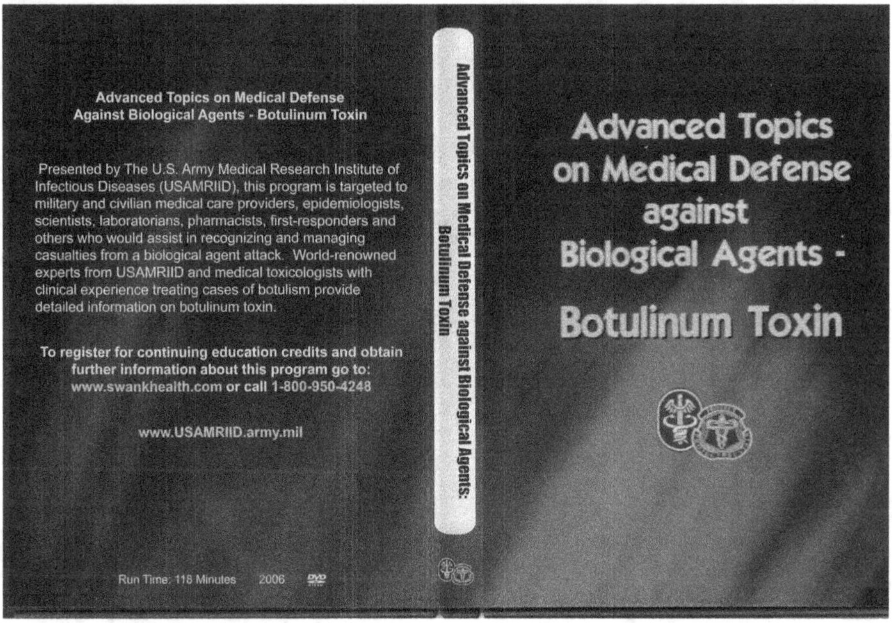

It would be interesting to learn if more recent products have coronavirus specific content. I'm tempted to contact them to find out.. but talk about sending up a redflag that calls attention to myself!!

Cheerio,

Amir-ul Kafirs

p.s. Sorry for my slow replies to everyone's emails, because of my trip to BalTimOre this past weekend I'm way behind in such things, I'm trying to get up to speed but checking out all the movies is time-consuming (but the links are VERY appreciated)

****

March 30, 2020 (Amir-ul Kafirs to the group):

Re: PANDEMIC PANIC 02

On Mar 27, 2020, at 5:21 PM, Phil Bradley wrote:

The true statistics of the virus are unknown but are blown out of proportion. There is disagreement is the WHO but pressure to announce a pandemic.

As usual, I'm trying to put things in perspective. Here's something from the CDC website about the 2018-2019 flu season in the US alone:

"CDC estimates that the burden of illness during the 2018–2019 season included an estimated 35.5 million people getting sick with influenza, 16.5 million people going to a health care provider for their illness, 490,600 hospitalizations, and 34,200 deaths from influenza. The number of influenza-associated illnesses that occurred last season was similar to the estimated number of influenza-associated illnesses during the 2012–2013 influenza season when an estimated 34 million people had symptomatic influenza illness.

"Peak activity during the 2018–2019 influenza season was classified as having moderate severity across ages in the population. Compared with the 2017–2018 season , which was classified as high severity, the overall rates and burden of influenza were much lower during the 2018–2019 season"

- https://www.cdc.gov/flu/about/burden/2018-2019.html

NOW, compare that to current US COVID-19 statistics:
Coronavirus Cases: **164,248** Deaths: **3,164**

- https://www.worldometers.info/coronavirus/country/us/

It seems so unspectacular in contrast doesn't it? The deaths aren't even 10% yet this year, etc.. Of course, to this sort of statistic people always reply that the spread of the virus is exponential but ALL disease spread is exponential — at least when it can spread through the air as opposed to, say, through sex only. SO, why this extreme concern about how deadly the virus is? People keep comparing it to the Spanish Flu but the Spanish Flu is reputed to've killed something like 5,000,000 people **[the estimated deaths from this vary wildly from 20,000,000 to 50,000,000]** & was partially operational in an environment devastated by trench warfare.

The next standard trope could be that the reason WHY it hasn't reached truly horrific proportions is because of what those good doctors & politicians have done to protect us. Social Distancing probably DOES help minimize the spread but that doesn't mean that it's entirely a good idea (or even necessary). There's this attitude that all these social things are disposable, as if people aren't social beings. There's the attitude that culture can just be made entirely virtual &, gee, that's enough. That might be a scientist's attitude but it's certainly NOT a musician's!

****

March 30, 2020 (Amir-ul Kafirs to group):

Re: PANDEMIC PANIC 02

On Mar 28, 2020, at 9:45 AM, Phil Bradley wrote:

Ok here is comes....the economic downturn exacerbates.....people beg for the new global government to solve the problem....temporarily of course.

https://www.theguardian.com/politics/2020/mar/26/gordon-brown-calls-for-global-government-to-tackle-coronavirus?CMP=share_btn_tw

Yep, well I've commented elsewhere on this idea of expanding the G20's power to authorize & manage even more power for the World Bank & the IMF. Note that there's no mention of the non-transparency of the G20: Hey! Why would us peons need to know what the great minds are planning to do to our world? I mean, we only live here! It's as if the whole Anti-Globalization Movement never existed & never mattered. Gee, oddly, I think it was actually very important!

other evidence of planned event.
https://theduran.com/why-did-hundreds-of-ceos-resign-just-before-the-world-started-going-absolutely-crazy/

Right. No doubt it's just a 'coincidence', har, har, that a record # of CEOs quit & sold their stock just before the economy took a nose-dive. No foreknowledge, nnnoooooo, why THAT would be a 'Conspiracy Theory'.

snowdon on corona situ
https://www.youtube.com/watch?v=9we6t2nObbw

As usual the official position is always predicated on the pose that whatever they're doing is for the general good. Even if that were completely sincere, instead of just PR propaganda that's meant to justify ANYTHING, it would of necessity involve what I, personally, consider to be an 'impossibility': which is some sort of 'godlike' intelligence directing it all. There's no possibility admitted of human error, human stupidity, human greed, human brutality, etc.. In short, there's no admission of all those characteristics that are so common in people *who gravitate to power.* In other words, how preposterous can it get?!

****

March 30, 2020 (Amir-ul Kafirs to group):

Re: PANDEMIC PANIC 02

On Mar 29, 2020, at 2:05 PM, Dick Turner wrote:

Thanks for these mails, thoughts.

An aside: A new 'custom' has been introduced into French culture. Every night at 8pm everyone opens their windows and claps and shouts 'bravo" for those "fighting on the front lines" (to keep up the military terminology currently in use) to thank the doctors, nurses, police and people still working in the markets (cashiers, suppliers, etc.).

Thusly showing an uncritical acceptance that that's what's really going on. The use of military language, especially in the case of Rump's announcement that we're 'at war', being a classic example of getting people in the mindset that makes military-like actions 'acceptable' because they're somehow 'necessary' under the conditions. What I've been imagining is what a great cover-up it would be for arrests to start happening carried out by people in Hazmat suits. An ambulance goes to someone's house, breaks in, gets them on a stretcher, & carries them away. The neighbors just take it for granted that the person is an extreme health risk without any proof needed other than the non-proof of the theatrics. & if they never come back? They must've died. That's a paranoid scenario, of course, but not really that hard to conceive of.

****

March 31, 2020 (**BP** to group):

Re: PANDEMIC PANIC 02

On a positive note, word is if one wants to drive like Mario Andretti, now is the time. The cops ain't pulling anyone over. They don't want to deal with a potentially sick person for a low priority like speeding. Vroom!

As for the big picture and population control/management, will have to think about it. It will make it a perfect time to transition the masses to a robot economy. Wave your phone and pay your way or deal with a dirty human who might infect you? It's already gonna change many businesses, be on a permanent skeleton crew.

As for things ACTUALLY being different here (outside work, which has been pure devastation and nearly everyone laid off and the loss of business), the streets are fairly normal. Less cars, yea. But if I came back from a remote Island I really would have no clue that anything BIG happened. No sirens, no warning signs, no police presence like after 9/11. Life as usual, but maybe a touch more...Civilized!

****

March 31, 2020, 5:42AM (Dick to group):

RE: PANDEMIC PANIC 02

There are some scientists who don't agree with the official version, here are some examples:

https://off-guardian.org/2020/03/28/10-more-experts-criticising-the-coronavirus-panic/?__cf_chl_jschl_tk__=79a5f208ca4d7f04614de2004ddec7746bfb593f-1585647430-0-AepvDFmpIRNibv5ZENDMYsot5cUBb-y3DWbi1ZqLGAUouUyqldywO3SqtN39bGKzJV4jNYLbq10DY4gdJmfrB7bttBXCuQt3nBKWwlH5_3V8MvmK_W3Tj9JIyMGc2MUFdUhQAlhgRxmhYy3boEBtEM4SayaqByyNuzorgGdVwfhELpeIyJ3KGkN6agVxpfSdtchryxKTx9HgmWNG8ThbPfoNQIX449wGHk9LSXr5cihBiLbTp2iGZKlveP4X9BwqlE-mooPesBh4FAOUVDIoKyxOrolz58O6TwuE64S__DssO2X-EI_LO2u9_jCvoetjN__DxqWaWc4wwIkGJqBE1kXt4WFLH-uSK5Yg5ixB8OGm

10 MORE Experts Criticising the Coronavirus Panic
Following on from our previous list, here are ten more expert voices, drowned out or disregarded by the mainstream narrative, offering their take on the coronavirus outbreak. * * * Dr. Sunetra Gupt...
off-guardian.org

****

March 31, 2020, 8:29AM (Amir-ul Kafirs to group):

Re: PANDEMIC PANIC 02

1st, as usual, Dick, THANK YOU for your thoughtfullness.

On Mar 29, 2020, at 5:59 PM, Dick Turner wrote:

I would like to suggest something, it's just my personal theory however.

If one looks at history there come, from time to time, events that change the course and the form of history.

What're generally called Paradigm Shifts — although your list gets away from the usual technology-based list of Carl Sagan & others. For Sagan, if I'm not misinterpreting &/or misremembering, it's more things like the Gutenberg Press & NOT things like "the barbarian invasions of Rome". My own book, "Paradigm Shift Knuckle Sandwich & other examples of P.N.T. (Perverse Number Theory)" (which I've known exactly ONE person to've claimed to've read) addresses Paradigm Shifts with the emphasis on mathematical concepts like zero & infinity.

It's interesting to me that you mention "barbarians". I recently watched an atrocious PBS documentary series on "barbarians" & one thing it emphasized over & over (it was a generally repetitive series) was that the barbarian invasions, while completely cruel & homicidal, increased the dissemination of culture &

trade (or some such). That was the 'plus' side. Personally, I feel like the cruelty & homicidal mania of so much of humanity's history could be done without & it would be a big improvement.

Wars are also often described in terms of the technology 'benefits': nuclear power, e.g. — perhaps new medicines & new medical procedures too. *'Oh, gee, we blew this poor sucker's legs off with our new bombs but, HEY!, now we can still keep him alive!'*

Then they come along and basically spell the end of certain types of mass thinking and behavior.

Or attempt to. I sometimes propose that so-called WWI was an attempt to quell revolutions against capitalism in favor of pulling the masses back into the control of nationalism again. Neither of these conflicting forces actually ended as a result.

even if this current epidemic wasn't planned (though I think it probably was just like 911 was if you believe the PNAC business with the need for a "catastrophic event" to put things in place) but even if it wasn't, once it began happening it must have seemed too good to be true to the powers that be as in "we can't let this go to waste!!"

Exactly, we're back at the Reichstag again.

Perhaps what is happening now is something like a moment of significant historical change. It's possible. After all, all the needed infra-structure is already in place for some kind of world government even if it isn't declared outright. Telephones, computers, constant surveillance, it's all here, now. In fact, there would be no need to even tell the people, that is, make an official announcement of a world government

Exactly, again. Why announce it to the people? That would reveal its undemocratic nature too plainly. It's 'better' to make it appear as if it's 'natural' & 'inevitable'. I'm reminded of the whole idiotic thing of '*Now that Communism's failed Capitalism is the only answer'* as if there were only ever 2 possibilities to begin with & as if Communism had failed any more than Capitalism has. Personally, I don't want either.

My point being, if this major change is now taking place, I don't see really what can be done, in fact, I think nothing.

Ah, that I'll never agree with. The obvious saying is that *Resistance isn't futile it's FERTILE*. The more people that think contrarily to the attempted dominating mindset the less that mindset dominates. It's up to us & others like us to trigger a different paradigm shift. I'm not in favor of globalization (what's being pushed for) but internationalism (which isn't the same thing at all) or, better yet, 'patanationalism.

Besides, what would be lost? Freedom? Well, 98% of the people I see don't seem particularly interested in freedom.

Well, 'freedom' isn't exactly something we've ever 'had' is it? There are just relative degrees of it. I've managed to, in many ways, lead the life I've wanted to without being put in prison — despite my 'swimming upstream against the culture' — but I haven't exactly thrived in the process. As to whether other people are interested in it? Younger people? The idea of 'freedom' seems to've somewhat disappeared from popular discourse (not that I exactly have my finger on the pulse of that). Presumably people of any generation ultimately have fairly simple wants & as long as those wants are met what are they going to complain about? Plenty, of course, but nothing philosophically profound. The 6 of us are in countries where basic 'needs', except for psychological ones, are met reasonably well for the majority. Will that continue? As long as Millennials can get something close enough to the latest gadget, the latest iJones or whatever, their completely manipulated desires are met. Who needs 'freedom' when you have such cool apps?

Oddballs like ourselves don't count, as society has let us know over and over again. (If this offends anybody, excuse me, I'm essentially talking about myself.)

Again, I disagree. Even if we 'count' only to each other we still 'count'. I've been conscious throughout most of my life of trying to penetrate culture in such a way that I leave an influential legacy. I haven't written 1,400 book reviews just for the fun of it. I'm hammering away, trying to help foster critical consciousness wherever its darling little seeds might be. Don't we all do that in our respective ways?

Have you noticed that the new generation, the so-called Millennials seem unusually a-historical, meaning, their culture, on a historical level is, very low? I have seen this repeatedly. A personality means having a position, but having a position may offend someone, so the solution is not to have any real opinions, this is the essence of the "politically correct" as far as I can tell.

It seems to me that being 'politically correct' at least started out as a way of trying to be sensitive to different types of self-identity struggles. I'm all in favor of that. It's when it became codified as self-censorship with a faux sensitivity substituted for the original genuine one that it became a source of irritation. As to whether Millennials are unusually a-historical or not, I really have no clue. I'm sure there's the usual minority of thoughtful people in any generation. Again, though, today's 'culture' seems more consumer-manipulation-driven than ever. So many things that were criticized in the '70s through the '90s have gotten even worse now. The glaring example being pre-planned obsolescence. The thought of buying an iJones that'll be 'too old' within a year or less is 'normal' now. & a society that's centered around such things can be in for a rude awakening when 'barbarians' with a much more biological agenda come along & demolish the glittering surface.

For example, I love Jascha Heifetz, the violinist, however I don't share my interest with people because I have met with next to no interlocutors, particularly among the younger set.

& that, sadly, is where you really 'strike a nerve' with me. You & I, & maybe all 6 of us here, are passionately involved with culture. WE ACTUALLY FUCKING CARE. But that's 'because' it's 'our job'. It's not most people's job. I live in a house, as you, Dick, know, that's full of rare cultural artifacts — there's enough knowledge here to fuel the intellectual life of a city for 100 years — but there aren't enough people in this particular city, at least that I know personally, to even care about more or less ANY OF IT. If all these precious books were to burn who would miss them? Most people I know don't really even read — or, if they do, they only read at, say, the level of a 5th grader. So what *DO* people care about? The people I'm most aligned with (but just barely) *DO* care about justice, anti-racism, anti-homophobia — thank the holy ceiling light for that — but their musical tastes are usually pretty banal & the literature? Forget it, it's amazing that anything can be published at all anymore. Thank goodness that books manufactured decades ago still exist as objects.

Of course if some kind of world government happens, the reigning culture will be garbage, all corporate products; something like elevator music, bad comic books and Jeff Koons-like art work.

Kind of how it is right now in fact.

Weelllll.. the most popular music still seems to be hiphop. Hiphop's claims to representing revolutionary culture seem somewhat belied by its ominpresence in all facets of commercial culture.

As to what course of resistance to take, it seems to me either one starts to blow up electrical power plants or just keep making art.

I don't, personally, want to do anything that destablizes the economy in a way that threatens people's survival. As such, blowing up electrical power plants wouldn't be for me or, I'm fairly sure, for anyone else here. As much as I'm a misanthrope, I still agree with 'Live & Let Live'. I always figure it's *the other people* who don't share that philosophy with me & who would be perfectly happy seeing me gunned down or starved to death. I don't even think of "making art" as exactly the point, I want to 'up the IQ of the culture in general' BAMN (By Any Means Necessary) - but the "Means Necessary" don't have to be cruel. What ends up surviving in this Globalization Police State Paradigm Shift will be what is the most imaginative, the most flexible, the most vital, the most audacious, the most on-top-of-it. Whether I've ever been any of those things & whether I continue to be is something that's going to be eroded by the exhaustion of aging. Nonetheless, I plan to continue to try.

Good luck to us all,

your pal,

Amir-ul Kafirs

****

March 31, 2020, 10:33AM (Dick to group):

RE: PANDEMIC PANIC 02

I agree some of my conclusions were a bit dark and hopeless feeling
I have to admit, I wrote that while drunk and feeling pretty low !
I'll keep my late-night outpourings under wraps
I'll be like Joe Friday and stick to the facts
However
I do feel that being an oddball is its own reward in a certain way, I mean just being able to think outside the box is a joy
For example, I think that probably in ancient Egypt there were people thinking to themselves "this Pharaoh-as-God business is really some serious BS" and even though we have no trace of them they must have felt a certain freedom...
But enough of that.
***
here's something about the Central bank situation which seems interesting, they have set up a central lending body
https://www.youtube.com/watch?v=bK_lfn1GS-U

****

March 31, 2020, 10:54AM (Dick to group)

RE: PANDEMIC PANIC 02

here it is from the horse's mouth as they say
https://www.federalreserve.gov/newsevents/pressreleases/monetary20200331a.htm

****

March 31, 2020, 2:30PM (Amir-ul Kafirs to group):

Re: PANDEMIC PANIC 02

On Mar 30, 2020, at 2:47 AM, Dick Turner wrote:

Here's something you might like, Spiro Skouras has endless well made videos on this subject and many others

https://www.youtube.com/watch?v=F_TPjbu4FAE&list=PL58MCVdG8nh30pDw9dBJ_ow-AuSiAQnJY&index=23&t=0s

I'm in the midst of watching this one now. Boyle proposes that the virus got out of a P4 lab in Wuhan accidentally. When I worked for a large medical lab it was said that they hired someone to get rid of their toxic waste & the guy just took it to an unused room (it was a big facility) & dumped it all there & then went & got stoned & screwed his girlfriend. It was supposedly 6 months before this large medical lab realized he wasn't doing his job. The point is that human error & apathy can lead to such accidents easily. HOWEVER, what if such viruses are being "weaponized" with a different agenda in mind? What if they're not really being imagined as something to be used in a war against competing nations? What if, instead, they're intended to be released just as they are? What if they're just scourges against immune-compromised people? What if they're ways of speeding up the natural 'weeding process' of killing off the weak? Overpopulation of the planet by humans is certainly a problem & I get the impression it might be even more of a problem in China than it is in the US. I'm sure I'm not the only person proposing such a possibility.

ANYWAY, around minute 30 when Boyle talks about Congressman Jones's non-response to Boyle's email as "obviously" a sign that Jones had been threatened to not have anything further to do with Boyle that's when Boyle becomes less credible for me since I don't think it's 'obvious' at all. Still, that doesn't effect the credibility of Boyle's argument that COVID-19 was weaponized. I do like his distinction of "correlation" instead of "causation" in connection with the Wuhan military games.

I loved this one. I've joined BitChute & subscribed to his (Spiro Skouras's) channel. I may try to correspond with Skouras but not right now because I have too many other things I'm neglecting. This one's very succinct. Thankfully, he addressed the World Bank & the IMF. Thanks for the links, Dick!

****

March 31, 2020, 5:29PM (Dick to group)

RE: PANDEMIC PANIC 02

Interesting video.
It deals with the economic side of the situation at the beginning and branches out into an interesting conversation of capitalism, then the climate, politics, etc.

https://www.youtube.com/watch?v=3FfkKkmCSu4

XRTV Interview: Chris Hedges on Coronavirus, Climate and What Next?
A live XRTV #alonetogether interview with Chris Hedges, American journalist and author. Chris won the Pulitzer Prize while at the New York Times and has written a number of groundbreaking books on the crises we face. He will talk about the massive changes which are now upon us - why this has been coming for a long time and how it relates to the ...

****

March 31, 2020, 6:37PM (Amir-ul Kafirs to group):

Re: PANDEMIC PANIC 02

Another good one from Skouros. I've been sharing these on Facebook. The whole possibility of Universal ID & under-the-skin IDs is completely plausible. They've been doing something similar with dogs for over a decade. &, NO, I don't want one. I'm still in favor of the barter economy whenever possible.

****

March 31, 2020, 7:13PM (Amir-ul Kafirs to group):

Re: PANDEMIC PANIC 02

On Mar 30, 2020, at 6:37 AM, Dick Turner wrote:

Another video to redeem myself, this made 6 weeks ago:

https://www.youtube.com/watch?v=Z29BTnDfgBU&feature=emb_logo

It's funny how the guy looks like a stereotype of a Mafia coke head. I like the way that his rack focus (?) selfie effect causes black lines (trails) to appear around his hands when he moves them & his ears. Those irrelevancies aside, I'm enjoying this one too (I'm still in the midst of it) but I probably won't link to it! Thanks!

****

March 31, 2020, 8:30PM (Amir-ul Kafirs to group):

Re: PANDEMIC PANIC 02

On Mar 30, 2020, at 12:30 PM, Inquiring Librarian wrote:

I have been a silent member because I do not feel like I have enough well researched and truly intelligent things to say about the situation.

Keep in mind that it's helpful just to get observations from our various environments. You're in Lousiana, Dick's in Paris, Phil's in Amsterdam, BP's in an undisclosed location, & I'm in Pittsburgh. Having observations from 6 different cities & 3 different countries helps us find similarities & differences.

(i am a lowly (('non-essential')) librarian)

As a side-note of sorts it's interesting to me that so many 'non-essentials' are things of substantial value to me: LIBRARIES are very important sources of free resources to the multitudes who might not all have computers or books at home, etc. Most of these 'non-essentials' are exactly the things that're psychologically & socially important to me: bookstores, movie theaters, restaurants.

I listen to NPR a lot, I can't explain why, and have become increasingly disgusted by how it seems to be taking the reins of social manipulation of the left, weighing in on the 'do-gooder,' 'pat yoursel on the back', sentiments that are supposed to be the construct of a good liberal mind. They seem to plant 'proper', 'good', 'righteous', 'independent', thoughts into the minds of 'save the world' liberals.

Ha ha! Believe me, it's fine to diss the liberal standpoint. One of the things that I criticize again & again is the way liberals have such oversimplistic views on language use. If a person uses language that can be assoicated with Rump, The Idiot King, then one becomes a Rump Supporter. That's what's known in logic as a false syllogism. I used the term "witch-hunt" to my liberal neighbor & he told me that was "Trump-speech". The implication was that just by virtue of saying "witch-hunt" I agreed with Rump. Obviously, the term "witch-hunt" preceeded Rump's (mis)use of it. Anyway, there's a sortof 'feel-good-about-yourself-because-you're/we're-the-good-guys' mentality about how liberals self-aggrandize &, yeah, I agree, NPR is probably a part of that. Another part of that, I think, is to assuage the consciences of rich liberals, & there are many of those, for being wealthy. They delude themselves that by supporting Bernie they're taking away their own guilt for whatever greed has helped them amass their wealth.

I miss my job as a public librarian where I had the chance to interact day to day with all walks of Louisiana life where I felt I could connect with and observe some of the most genuine human interactions.

Obviously a useful occupation — I consider it more useful than a Wall Street Trader, e.g..

And... I as a librarian will soon not be able to pay my own internet bill or have a roof over my own head... I too will soon be on the other side of the "digital divide" where my less financially fortunate library patrons already are now as librarians have been asked to abandon them. If you cannot fully shut down the internet, shut down the libraries.

Up with the librarians! Down with the propagandists!

****

March 31, 2020, 9:54PM (Amir-ul Kafirs to group):

Re: PANDEMIC PANIC 02

On Mar 31, 2020, at 2:13 AM, BP wrote:

On a positive note, word is if one wants to drive like Mario Andretti, now is the time. The cops ain't pulling anyone over. They don't want to deal with a potentially sick person for a low priority like speeding. Vroom!

Thanks for your report. I ran over a cop today at 140mph just to test out how much I could get away with & no-one batted an eye. (JUST KIDDING!)

****

March 31, 2020, 10:00PM (Amir-ul Kafirs to group):

Re: PANDEMIC PANIC 02

So far, I see no reason to distrust the off-guardian, I like & agree with what the people are quoting here as saying. Nonetheless, we should all be aware that Snopes, e.g., disputes off-guardians's veracity & one friend of mine lambasted it as Russian propaganda. **[I now recognize such Fact Chokers as mostly censors]**

****

March 31, 2020, 10:12PM (Amir-ul Kafirs to group):

PANDEMIC PANIC: Chomsky

&, of course, there's so much we haven't gotten into here yet including Noam Chomsky's take (which I've just started to watch):

https://youtu.be/t-N3In2rLI4

Personal Thoughts on the Covid-19 Pandemic

Part One

- Dick Turner, Artist/Composer, Paris

I assume people will agree that the first Terrifying Specter of the Covid-19 Pandemic was the announcement of the threat of MEGA-DEATH as it had been presented in the news.

MEGA-DEATH! The Grim Reaper, familiar to those versed in mediaeval iconography, had, with his skeletal hand, raised his dark hood, cast his dark shadow against the human race! Imagine the diseased wandering in the streets, dropping like flies, falling like wheat before the scythe; imagine the horrors of contagion let loose to roam freely among an unsuspecting populace.

And thanks to modern technology, there was even a picture of this Reaper, resembling a sort of round red playground-ball with flower-like protuberances. (Isn't it strange how the infinitely small always resembles planets or dinosaurs?)

But still this just wasn't good enough! There it was but *it was an abstraction*, admittedly a terrifying one, but distant... Something else was needed.

Perhaps you take exception to this line of reasoning.

Why do I suggest that this awesome threat of millions of dead wasn't good enough?

Consider: Haven't we lived in the shadow and with the fear of MEGA-DEATH since the invention of the Atomic Bomb? Repetition is the surest way to produce, *not fear* but familiarity and familiarity as we all know, breeds contempt, or at least, it breeds abstraction, dullness, non-reactivity.

I would say that the announcement of MEGA-DEATH *was like a bare canvas* which was put into place in order to paint upon it *other more personally relatable figures*; like a backdrop in the theater but *the action doesn't start until the actors make their entrances*.

Death after all is abstract, particularly in the West. Sure, we'd heard some Chinese people had died, but isn't that what they are *supposed to do* in this situation? I mean from a traditional Western perspective? After all, look at the numbers! With two or three billion people, *it's only statistically right* that a hundred thousand or so die every time a flu is announced, besides, they are going to shortly take over the world, colonize the moon… turn us into slaves… it's seems almost obligatory that they suffer just a little before they enslave us!

It's like a typhoon in India, if only 20 people die *something just isn't kosher*!

Besides, face it, when it gets down to it, it just can't happen here!

But then, it *was* here! Death had arrived in the West! A different story… After a while the WHO and its specialists declared the gravity of the situation.

This was good because until these announcements, all sorts of differing opinions were being aired, it was like no one knew what was happening; no one knew what to believe!

At least *millions of deaths* was clear, final, unequivocal; *a relief*, so to speak.

But still it was abstract, like the aforementioned blank canvas, something needed to be painted upon that surface to give it a more tangible human reality.

It was at this critical moment that the anus made its majestic appearance.

Is it surprising that in the popular mind the Covid-19 pandemic was heralded by an increased awareness of the anus? Specifically the fear of a germ covered anus unwiped and possibly odiferous; a now stinking, filthy hole attached to our bodies against our wills to follow us like an Avenger, both cruel and accusatory?

For that was the first popular image in the unfolding of the Covid-19 "Pandemic" (a word I have come to detest): namely the shortage of toilet paper.

Let us contemplate: Toilet paper, taken from a certain perspective, is the *mirror image of our anus*; to speak of toilet paper is to speak of the jakes, the powder room, the crapper, the outhouse, it is to speak of excrement, of digestion… Let's cut it short – **to speak of toilet paper is to speak, in coded terms, of the essence of the Human**.

For excrement, along with carbon dioxide, is the only thing Man produces in an unending stream from his first moments on earth to the relaxing of the bowels at the moment of death.

Then quickly on the heels of MEGA DEATH and the anus came the THIRD WOE! For as toilet paper is the mirror of our anus, next came the second blow, **food**, which is, in its turn, *the mirror image of our excrement*.

Thus the menace of food shortages followed close on the heels of the menace of anal uncleanliness. Indeed, **the fear of starvation** in the land of plenty was a sort of pendant commentary to that original horror of the unwiped, germ-laden anus.

But, to speak of food, particularly in combination with toilet paper is this not to speak of ***the horrors of being human***, of eating, masticating, enzymes, bodily processes, fluids, and – let me unashamedly pronounce the word here once and for all – SHIT. Specifically, *human shit*, a shit more repulsive to us than the shit of beasts. (Yet mysteriously, as we all know, one's own shit NEVER STINKS.)

In the end, it all comes back to the anus!

Let us consider an instant the possibility of **mass starvation through food shortages**. Isn't this worse than mere death due to illness? Imagine the slow wasting away, among the familiar surroundings of one's own home… Slow death, creeping like weeds to overtake the comfortable garden of life… There the TV, there the microwave and stained underwear, there the bowl of Hershey's chocolate kisses and the lubrication jelly… And there we are, stretched out and languishing on the floor, helpless, dying in the midst of modernity…it almost seems impossible.

Suddenly food markets were ravaged by terrified citizens, shelves emptied, buying everything that could be touched, hoping to stave off certain death, slow, wasteful, malignant…

There it was on Google news for all to see!

Could it get any worse?

Yes, for food takes us back, back to our very center, our quivering unprotected anus. **A vicious circle.**

Always back to the anus.

Starvation! Perhaps the only thing worse than an unwiped anus *is the anus incapable of being wiped!*

Thus a cycle ineluctable, devastating, relentless…

Think of these three events, these THREE WOES – MEGA DEATH, the filthy anus, no food.

Now think of Bill Gates' mealy-mouthed grin.

For they are one in the same.

Let me say something clearly here: I believe that Bill Gates and all those people of his ilk, that is those with a "plan for humanity" (Klaus Schwab, Jeff Bezos, Mark Zuckerberg, the Rockefellers and many people of whom I know not the names) **hate being human**, they hate what Sartre called the Viscous, they hate the day to day experience, **the reality of human existence**. They want cleanliness, order and predictability.

They hate all that is implied by the anus and thus it was the anus that was the first target of their attacks.

*

I am writing this because tENTATIVELY, a cONVENIENCE feels that it may make a difference to someone one day, I hope that's the case, for it would be gratifying. And I hope that my writing will be taken in the spirit it is meant, namely to show my utter contempt for those who would use their money, power, time, influence to further the expression of their self-centered and BORING ANTI-HUMAN agendas. I won't say *uncreative*, for this event is *certainly creative*, but so was the Third Reich! But the whole thing stinks of Algorithms, lab coats and sterilized metal dissection tables.

The following notes, maybe fragments of notes is a better way of putting it because they aren't very polished, are just my memories of and reflections on the event, which by the way, at the current time, shows no signs of abating as a multi-purpose governmental tool. I am not going to try to cover up the fact that at certain times I had ideas that I now consider almost insane – as for example, a day or so when I felt the best thing that could happen would for humanity to accept the technocratic domination of the "power elite" and move into a new period of history... Well, I thought it, why hide it?

Chalk it up to being stuck inside all day…

I don't think it anymore by the way.

If anything this event makes me only more aware of the fragility of our freedom and of the moral imperative of doing anything we can do to maintain it.

*

Small personal observation: I don't, in general, like groups.

Yet, here I am in the "Heretics" group. Is this hypocritical?

I think I can sum up very easily why I am part of the "heretic" group. It's a sort of group-non-group to begin with. There is no ideology, just an inclination in a similar skeptical direction. I do believe in sharing information, openly and honestly.

I believe I am constitutionally incapable of any form of groupthink. I'm not made for crowds, sing-a-longs, group clapping, doing the "Heil Hitler" salute; not made for singing the National Anthem, participating in "pep" rallies like in High School, or even going to church and sharing a belief structure… things like that.

To sum it up in modern terms: I couldn't attend a pro-Trump Rally but neither can I stand the driveling pro-Bernie Sanders types.

Not to sound absurd, but once Burger King used the advertising rhyme "Hold the pickles, hold the lettuce, special orders don't upset us, all we ask **is that you have it your way**"… well, this is what I want, need, think is right, etc. And I mean for everyone.

It is starting point of any reasonable society.

I should add that I am very sensitive to anything I feel is trying to manipulate me. It's for this reason that I don't watch television and why I don't like 99% of films. Not that I can't be manipulated – I can be, have been and I know it - but I find that I always wake up to it after a while, to the fact that I am being emotionally pushed around, and when I become aware of this it reinforces my wariness.

Importantly, I would add that I am skeptical of governments in general so when things are proposed *for my own good*, well, I simply can't accept these things on face value because of governmental track records of lying, giving misinformation, "manufacturing consent" to use a well-known phrase, etc. From the Kennedy assassination to the Vietnam War, from Watergate to Saddam Hussein's arms of mass destruction, from 911 to – you get the point.

In fact it seems to me that even writing this is laboring the obvious ***for whom in their right mind trusts governments and who wants anyone else to tell them what to do*** unless one personally asks for advice as say from a teacher one trusts, a friend, a doctor, a specialist of some kind?

*

I first heard about the Covid-19 virus (though at the time I didn't know the name Covid-19) from my roommate at the time, a young woman from Hong Kong, her name was Clothilde* (actually it was Ping Wong* but I learned people from Hong Kong adopt a Western name when they are around 14 or so).

*Her name has been changed

I didn't take it as a threat to myself. Over the years various viruses were supposed to come to Europe from China (I think the last was called Avian Flu, it had something to do with chickens if I recall well) and none ever did make it over so I thought it was just the usual fear mongering by the media to give people something to read.

Clothilde talked about it constantly. She was always on the internet or talking with her family. She told me about the "bat-soup' origins of the virus but also mentioned the bio-lab in Wu Han. She took a dim view of any news out of Beijing. She said if it's good news it's always exaggerated, and it it's bad news it's always downplayed. She took the virus seriously - for one thing her brother worked in a hospital. For another she had to return to Hong Kong for family reasons and wasn't sure if she'd find a flight. She finally did and a week after she left China closed its airspace.

I recall her telling me the Chinese authorities had closed down Wu Han Province. Since I know almost nothing about Chinese geography this meant little to me. She did point out that this closing down was done in a ridiculous way, namely they announced it a few days before it actually took place so people started leaving *en masse*.

> NOTE: A similar strange delay is currently taking place in France. About two weeks ago (the 14th of July to be exact, the French National Day of Liberty by the way) President Macron announced that as of 1 August masks will become obligatory in all public spaces. One has to logically ask: if it's truly necessary to wear a mask to fight against the possibility of mass contagion, shouldn't the order go into effect immediately? Why wait? If you are sick you should start treatment immediately, no? I don't know what the official logic in this decision was but it seemed arbitrary, like a test to see exactly what people will put up with, how far they can be pushed, in short how docile they will be in accepting what to an impartial observer looks like a random decision. And if you consider the symbolism of the day it was announced (Bastille Day) the event seems somewhat suspect.

Clothilde left Paris and then for several weeks I was only aware of the virus in a sort of peripheral manner, glimpsing an occasional story in my Google newsfeed.

Then one day cases started getting reported in France. There were a number of different official comments about it starting in either late February or early March; I can't recall the exact date. Some "experts" said it was serious; some that it wasn't, in fact all I recall was a lot got said and it all seemed more or less like nonsense because no consensus was ever reached in the midst of all the official sounding political talk.

This talk ranged from speculations over the "incubation period", to how serious it was, whether or not it was like the regular flu, etc. I also recall, and this is important in light of later events, that the availability of masks was a huge issue. There were no masks to be found anywhere. A story was going around that Chinese tourists were buying them all to take back to China. (Finally at the end of the coming confinement, masks did make their appearance – exactly at a time when they didn't really seem necessary anymore… but just wait!)

Anyway, since all the initial talk was going literally in every direction it didn't make much sense to take it seriously.

Again, it seemed like they hadn't established the "party line" yet.

One day I saw, just a headline, that the actor Tom Hanks had what was now branded as the **Corona Virus**.

Then the next day I saw a friend for a coffee and he mentioned that Tom Hanks had the virus…and then, later that same day, *someone else* mentioned Tom Hanks had the virus! Both times the story was told to me as if they had some special private news to report. To me this proved nothing except the power of the media to get the same story out to everyone in a way that makes them feel *that they alone received it*.

This caused my first feelings that something was fishy. I mean, why make a virus a media-star event when it's a health problem? It seemed like a form of promotion! Somehow, because he is famous, and on top of that, a Mr. Nice Guy actor who happily hasn't been caught with either underage kids, or in a public toilet with his pants around his knees, he was supposed to represent “the rest of us”. But I recall thinking, there are somewhere around 7 billion souls on the earth, OK Tom Hanks has it, so what?! I mean, that leaves 6,999,999,999 people we’ve yet to check on.

I had the flu last year, it didn’t make headlines.

Next, the president of France (Macron who is generally viewed, at least by honest people, as a tool of the rich, hidden ruling class of bankers and financiers, the famous and mysterious 1% we hear about) came out and said people had to voluntarily engage in social distancing. I heard this and didn’t modify my behavior, though I did feel a little nervous when I was in a crowded store and when I went to the post office.

Next just a few days later, I think it was the 13th of March (give or take a day) a lock-down was announced. He more or less scolded the French on TV in a speech, like they were acting like irresponsible children and for their own good and the good of others; the lockdown would be in operation on 16 March and would be reviewed in two weeks.

This lockdown, not so curiously, resembled very closely the one in place in Italy: They’d found the “party line”!

He announced there would be permission slips that must be used if one was to go out. It was, by the way, the first time I heard the expression “non-essential work” used (all non-essential work was to stop. Meaning bars, café, museums, while essential businesses could stay operative, these were the boulangeries – I guess they recalled the French Revolution's cry of "Give Us Bread!" – dry cleaners, hardware stores…).

Then began the aforementioned toilet paper shortage menace and the possible food shortage menace… I went to the store and found no lack of anything.

I felt the constant reporting on toilet paper was a way to bring a lot of attention to people's assholes and by proxy, to make them feel humiliated at being human shit machines.

Further, I felt the anus was being used as a *unifying event* by the media – for whether black, white, yellow, brown or tan we share this essential characteristic with all out fellow beings. To paraphrase Schiller: Alle Menschen werden Brüder…. wenn sie auf der Toilette sind.

Next death counts and hospitalization numbers started to get announced each day. I was reminded of when I watched the evening news in the late 1960's as a child and would hear the casuality reports from Vietnam (Live from Hanoi: 3 American deaths, 26 Vietnamese deaths…). As we all know now, this was, to a large part, media "hearts and minds" manipulation.

I found the entire situation to be suspect, I wasn't sick, I knew of no one who was sick, everything seemed as it always is.

> (By the way, later I asked my doctor ((who I saw later for a shoulder injury)) whether he'd seen a lot of cases. He said yes, at the very beginning ((if six a day is a lot, I don't know)), until the end of March, but NOT A SINGLE ONE in April or May. ((The Lock-down lasted

from 16 March to 11 May and in certain ways, that is through mask paranoia, is still going on)) Someone else's experience may be different – maybe the person reading this did experience shortages or an unwiped ass, maybe the person reading this did catch the virus or even know someone who died *but I didn't*.)

Later I did discover that several friends, and my brother, had had the virus, in short, *they were sick and then they recovered*.

I get the flu every year, it usually lasts a while because I had lung/bronchial problems dating to a pneumonia I had as a child. Again, so far, it hasn't made the news…

(A personal life-event aside, at this time my son who is 18 years old went South on the 15th of March to a town near Marseilles with a group of other teenagers where he stayed for two months having the type of adventures and inter-personal social dilemmas that teenagers often have when in groups together. He stayed there for 53 of the 55 days of confinement that would follow. This would lead to what could be termed family drama because it was his baccalaureate year, the big final exams in France and we had no idea when we'd see him again once he'd left. Finally he did get the BAC as it is called so all's well that ends well.)

The next day, on the 16th, the lock-down took effect.

*

So on March 16th Paris came to a stop. It was easy for me to notice this. I live very close to a busy and noisy intersection. Only in the month of August, when the entire nation goes on vacation, does the traffic ever slow. Well, now it was less busy than in August. There were no metros (I live directly across from an elevated metro line). Needless to say, at first – I loved it. It was quiet, almost like the country comparatively speaking, no pollution. I could sleep with the windows open. Besides I had my entire apartment to myself. I felt almost like a child, happy and free to work. Besides, I spend most of my time at home anyway because I write music and paint and etc.

I went online and saw the permission slip Macron had talked about. In typical French bureaucratic fashion, the slips had no time frames on them, meaning if you had one you could still stay out all day. Someone in the bureaucracy finally noticed this and the slips were changed a week or so later. A third change to the permission slip would follow much later, I forget what was added, something concerning work travel I think.

Anyway with the slip it was stipulated that one was allowed to shop, take an hour walk each day and, if there was an emergency or if one needed to help someone infirm (a sick person, the elderly) one was allowed to go out. One had to wear a mask at all times on the street.

> Little aside: Besides not liking groups and manipulation, I don't like being pushed around, controlled, censored, so you can imagine how I felt about masks, permission slips, a series of "experts" dictating what the entire planet has to do, which of course, includes me.

Enter the Heretics.

I would be lying if I said I didn't feel some degree of nervousness at getting sick at first. The virus was painted as a certain death phenomenon ("It attacks the lungs!" Someone had self-righteously written as a rebuttal to a "conspiratorial" Facebook post that questioned the event), and since as I noted above I had had major bronchial problems, the projected death (Millions!!) toll was scary to hear, etc. But still, I felt I was being had. I mentioned this to tENT in a mail and he added me to the mail sharing group "Heretics", the group wasn't a group yet really, it was Phil, tENT and myself. It was to share videos or articles dealing with the subject.

It was sometime around this time that people started using, on the internet of course because I saw no one, the expression "The New Normal". I felt personally offended by this expression because it seemed awfully presumptuous ***to declare a new total world reality so quickly.***

> Incidental note: I started making home videos of myself, doing one every few days. I saw it as a chance to keep a record of the Pavlovian conditioning effects of the lock-down. I find these hard to look at now, maybe one day I'll edit them together.

At first I didn't mind the lock-down. I work at home all the time and have very few friends. So I saw it somewhat as a challenge to produce as much work as possible. This became stronger as a drive when the lock-down was extended from 2 weeks to 2 months. Only a few times did I start feeling stir crazy. I began to take walks every day. I would take two permission slips and a pen with me so I could stay out a bit longer.

During the lock-down I produced:

- A ballet **BLOW-OUT!** (30 minutes), I also wrote the argument (story) and planned the basic choreography
- A quartet **Desperate Measures** for alto sax, bass clarinet, cello and electric bass
- A quintet **A Few Notes on the Current Situation** for alto sax, bass clarinet, bari sax, cello and trombone
- A large amount of **Postcards from Nowhere** which are postcards I cut up and rearrange (visit my site to see them)
- 30 pen and ink drawings of a relatively high degree of complexity (as I see it…)
- Ten Masks **The New Normal** (oil paint of cardboard)
- And a documentary film if I ever edit it together…

Most of this is available on my website if anyone is curious:

https://dickturner3.wixsite.com/dick-turner-artist

I also read a lot on my small balcony. In particular, I read and immediately re-read The Castle by Kafka, a book I highly recommend to everyone.

I had a lot of different feelings during the lock-down,

sometimes I think I was to some degree a maniac. I started to think that it would usher in a new period of freedom (call that being optimistic!) in which people would adopt newer, freer ways of living. This lasted a day or so.

I had many thoughts, many theories as to what it meant; what it was all about. I find, in my personal and artistic life I have the habit of creating working theories to give direction to what I do, these serve their purpose and usually are forgotten once the project at hand is completed.

My thoughts became more channeled when I saw the Quarantiranny video Phil shared with the Heretics group. Here I learned about Event 201, Gates, bio-metrics, etc.

One day I spoke to my Aunt who lives in Germany. An opera singer by training, she was a very dedicated social activist for many years dealing with issues like acid rain, nuclear power, the destruction of a forest in Frankfurt to build an airport (for which she did prison time for chaining herself to a tree). She suggested I listen to Spiro Skouras, an activist.

I did and found out more about the Covid-19 "back story" so to speak – more about Event 201 (it was strange to see Johns Hopkins University show up, it's one of the Universities in Baltimore, my "home-town" – I use quotations marks because that term suggests a sentimental attachment of which I have almost none), Bill Gates and the RNA - DNA vaccines, then the WHO, the World Economic Forum with Klaus Schwab a sort of Doctor Deadly type guy "here to help" who always appears in elevated shots like cheap sci-fi films from the 1970's, the Federal Reserve and its interconnected system of banks…

I shared these with the group and in turn discovered many things the now larger group shared such as number fixing in the counting of Covid-19 deaths, questionable hospital practices, questions as to the efficacy of masks, etc. I have to be honest, my capacity to look at all the articles, watch the videos, in short digest the sheer quantity of information varies from day to day.

To end this let me say a few words about the phase we are currently in, the Mask phase.

The mask has become the official battleground of the Covid-19 event. Pro-maskers and anti-maskers define two camps, those who believe the official "it's for the public good" line and those who feel the whole event is manipulated.

The idea as I understand it, at least here is France, is that we will all have to wear masks until that happy day when a vaccine is found. This unstated policy is as clear as things get: Because wearing a mask is unpleasant (particularly in the summer heat) it is supposed to make us hope that the vaccine will be developed as quickly as possible so we can get the vaccine in pumped into us and ***finally take the masks off***.

Further, to anyone with half a brain the symbolism of covering the face is blatant as a de-humanizing, control tool it couldn't be any clearer. Hiding the face? Particularly hiding the mouth? Our organ of self-expression? You don't have to like modern theater to figure it out.

This by the way isn't poetic interpretation; it is an observation of what I feel to be a fact.

One final thought: Strangely this current phase mirrors the beginning phase in a significant way.

For the Covid-19 "Pandemic" moved from *exposing the hidden anus* to *hiding the exposed mouth*. Even when I write this it sounds like I'm a borderline maniac, **but these are the facts!** And curiously they both involve tissue-like fiber-based material, the fear of germs, etc.

And since the facial mouth is the inverse of that second usually hidden mouth, the anus, the message is only too clear:

Shut-up, do what you are told and thank God you can keep wiping your filthy ass until we can inject you with the vaccine we decide you need.

*

That's all I'll write.

I could go on about other issues – from the symbolism of hand cleanser to my various mental states during lockdown to the directional arrows painted on the floors of the Parisian Metro to the sudden reappearance of the Black Lives Matter movement - but I'm sure you can figure these out for yourself.

Thank you for reading.

Dick Turner

Paris
26 July 2020

HERETICS emails - April, 2020

April 1, 2020, 8:49AM (Amir-ul Kafirs to group):

Re: PANDEMIC PANIC 02

On Apr 1, 2020, at 2:34 AM, BP wrote:

In the mainstream political cable wars world, anyone questioning the seriousness of the virus would be labeled a Trump lackey. Which I am sure all of you are. Now the White House is saying 100,000 to 240,000 dead by the time it is over.

Such figures are based on exponential growth predictions. No doubt there are excellent ways of making those predicitions but that doesn't make them infallible. Any exponential growth prediction is based on unknowable factors: how many people come into contact with how many other people, etc. There's also the factor of who is the most susceptible of those contacted.

I've discussed this before so I won't get into detail here but I have a theory that everyday small scale exposure to diseases is a form of mild innoculation. As such, I'm less likely to get sick in my natural environment than I would be if I were to go to the Amazon jungle, for example, because I wouldn't have built up an immunity for whatever thrives in the Amazon. I can imagine this enforced social distancing as working CONTRARY to the type of natural immunology that I'm suggesting. It's my understanding that there's the possibility of *excessive sterility* as more causal of *vulnerability*.

So they got Trump in line. Or at least convincing data did.

As Dick pointed out with his info about French politicians changing their story in total about-faces from one day to the next (or even the same day) it's no surprise if Rump, or any other politcian, does the same. I think these 'leaders' are just trying to steer the ships of their political careers on the course that's best for them. For me, the "convincing data" for them would be whatever produces the most likely career-continuance results.

Bolsonaro in Brasil is poo pooing the entire pandemic and his governors are rebelling. So we shall see what happens there.

I have 2 friends in Brazil who've given me reports, both in the same city. Neither seem very worried about the situation. But, once again, we have to wait & see.

I don't believe any of the pre-planned scenarios.

I'm not so concerned with pre-planned vs planned as I am with OPPORTUNISM. The rich & powerful, & that includes politicians, aren't typically ethically 'above' taking advantage of opportunities to make more money & get more power — & destabilized societies/economies are perfect opportunities. I think of Haliburton's parasitism off of war-torn countries that they 'rebuild' & insert private security forces into. I had a neighbor who worked for Haliburton in Iraq. He quit. He told me that he didn't want to "conquer the world" as he thought Haliburton did. In the fictional world there's the movie "The Third Man" which I imagine most or all of us have seen.

Regarding the possibility of preplanning: I only 'know' of the 201 pandemic simulation **[October 18, 2019]** & the Wuhan war games **[October 18-27, 2019]** through mediated non-experience — in other words, I haven't personally witnessed either. If they both existed on the same day, as is claimed, & if they happened a month before the pandemic is said to've started then that's pretty big as a 'coincidence'.

Ultimately, it keeps boiling down to the same thing for me: 1. I hope the draconian death predictions turn out to be exaggerated, 2. I hope all the social distancing restrictions are completely lifted SOON, 3. I hope all the businesses & professions that're negatively effected get to spring back ASAP. As for predictions?: I'm probably better off not making any but I find other people's predictions interesting. I have criticisms & observations — mainly I'm watching this day-to-day to see how it's playing out. The mere fact that this lockdown-lite is happening at all is disturbing & NOT a harbinger of good things to come. Even if I thought this quarantine was entirely an action intended for the public good by medical people I wouldn't trust it. I, & almost everyone I know, have/has had bad experiences with doctors. I don't trust them any more than I do lawyers.

I wish us all good luck,

yr pal,

Amir-ul Kafirs

p.s. In the meantime, I continue to be in excellent health.

****

April 1, 2020, 12:22PM (Phil to group):

Nice to read the about offguardian;
OffGuardian was launched in February 2015 and takes its name from the fact its five founders had all been censored on and/or banned from the Guardian's 'Comment is Free' sections.
Our remit, as we see it, is to provide a home for the comment – & the facts – you no longer find in the MSM.

These 'fact-checking' sites can be useful but then mostly only with things that are obviously fake. When things get grey their own biases and opinions set in. The big problem I see was with the 'Russiagate' scandal which was just another 'deep state' or the workings of the ongoing intelligence agencies that continue no matter who the president is. I perceive that most of the 'deep state' (or whatever you want to call it) were planning for Hilary to win (although there was also division within the deepstate) Russiagate was not only a good strategy to deflect blame from hilary losing the election but also a good strategy to begin censorship campaigns - we have to stop russian interference and fake news. Also to reinvent an old enemy Russia. Like in Chomsky manufacturing consent....the cold war as an enemy to construct public consent to military campaigns. After 9/11 terrorism. Then fake news. russia again. now the corona virus. Of course there is the kneejerk reaction of if Rump speaks of fake news then we should all agree with whatever the cia infested washington post publishes. We should also agree with known liars such as comey and the like. The greyzone was good at covering the nonsense of Russiagate....One of the funniest parts are some of the advertisements that are supposed to have won trump the election;

" 'Struggling with the addiction to masturbation? Reach out to me and we will beat it together.'—Jesus." and "You can't hold hands with God when you are masturbating." (New Knowledge: "Recruiting an asset by exploiting a personal vulnerability—usually a secret that would inspire shame or cause personal or financial harm if exposed—is a timeless espionage practice.")
https://www.newyorker.com/news/our-columnists/why-the-russian-influence-campaign-remains-so-hard-to-understand

But I guess the point here is now we need 'parents' rather than our own critical faculties to know what legitimate news is or isnt.

A couple of other resources that can have interesting perspectives are :
john rappoport
https://blog.nomorefakenews.com/

and
james corbett
https://www.corbettreport.com/

Thanks for everyones contributions....i am reading but also find it sometimes get ahead of it to write stuff.

Also i tend to use my social media page as a place just to scoop stuff out of my stream and forward it on. There's likely a lot there that i have not posted here.

****

April 1, 2020, 6:04PM (Dick to group):

Did any of you see this:
https://www.vanityfair.com/news/2020/03/senate-coronavirus-vacation
It announces that the Senate is taking a vacation... during a so-called wartime

situation
I got it from this guy, who may or may not be your cup of tea
https://www.youtube.com/watch?v=socCV2iCwAw

****

April 1, 2020, 7:19PM (Amir-ul Kafirs to group):

On Apr 1, 2020, at 12:21 PM, Phil Bradley wrote:

Russiagate was not only a good strategy to deflect blame from hilary losing the election but also a good strategy to begin censorship campaigns - we have to stop russian interference and fake news.

Fake news will NEVER STOP. This is another one of those post-Rump thingies: before Rump started complaining about fake news leftists knew that the media lied all the time. Then once Rump complained it turned into another false syllogism that if you agreed that there could be fake news about anyone, Rump included, then you might just be a Rump supporter. Of course, the new version of fake news that exists with social media is quite a different thing from the old school fake news of mass media just making whatever claim they could get away with that suited their propaganda purposes.

We should also agree with known liars such as comey and the like.

Exactly, that's pretty much the way it is now. The idea of just having a detached perspective on something is practically unthinkable for many people.

The greyzone was good at covering the nonsense of Russiagate....

I read that. I never paid much attention to the claims of Russian manipulation of the election. It seems to me that the American public has long since lost most of their ability to be in touch with reality or to be a sane judge of much of anything. We can thank TV for that even before the internet came along. As for Rump's 'winning' the election I can never understand why more emphasis isn't put on the possibility of buying off one or more Electoral College members. After all, they constitute a small group of people & Rump is a billionaire.

john rappoport
https://blog.nomorefakenews.com/

SHEESH! Another good viewpoint IMO. I find his perspective believable — in fact, probably the most sensible one yet — but I'm sure that people would resist it because it makes everything too complex. PEOPLE REALLY DO WANT ONE ANSWER. That makes everything simple.

james corbett
https://www.corbettreport.com/

DICK: If you haven't read the above, I recommend it. Consider this quote: "You may have noticed the interesting phenomenon making its way around the world. I call it “The Totally Spontaneous Balcony Applause Phenomenon.” Yes, completely out of the blue, all the people under lockdown have decided to show their appreciation for the valiant doctors and nurses in this heroic struggle by going to their balcony at a pre-appointed time and applauding. And no, this totally spontaneous phenomenon is not just occurring in one or two countries. Or three or four countries. But in seemingly every country around the globe." I note, however, that I've seen no sign of this in my neck of the woods. May it stay that way. I've had plenty of bad experiences with doctors & I know plenty of other people who have too. That's why I make fun of the "DOCTOR GODS" on social media.

Thanks for everyones contributions....

ANYWAY, THANK **YOU** FOR BEING SUCH A GOOD RESEARCHER. I probably wouldn't have taken the time to've found these articles on my own. It's amazing how much (un)common sense there is in them & YET people still seem to accept 'The New Normal' like it's AOK, a mild bother, but 'necessary'.

****

April 1, 2020, 7:25PM (Amir-ul Kafirs to group):

On Apr 1, 2020, at 12:59 PM, BP wrote:

Be great if Wikileaks got ahold of the contingency plans.

I was just thinking similar thoughts earlier today. It would be amazing if another Snowden or Assange or Manning or whomever regarding any aspect of this PANDEMIC PANIC. Have you seen the Wikipedia entry on Whistleblowers?:

https://en.wikipedia.org/wiki/List_of_whistleblowers

I have plenty of problems with Wikipedia but note that there's already a coronavirus one at the very bottom of the list.

****

April 1, 2020, 7:35PM (Amir-ul Kafirs to group):

On Apr 1, 2020, at 6:04 PM, Dick Turner wrote:

It announces that the Senate is taking a vacation...

I'm glad they're taking a break. It shows pretty clearly how 'seriously' they take it all. Until the politicians start dying off it'll just seem like a problem of 'the little people'.

I got it from this guy, who may or may not be your cup of tea

Yeah, I do find this guy a little hard to take. That doesn't mean that I don't find some of the things he says useful. E.G. I find it useful that he points out that the 'Central Banks' have the basic primary purpose of *generating debt* or some such. Basically, they're **LOAN SHARKS.** That's a very clear, & I think ACCURATE, notion.

****

[In the slightly over 2 weeks that I'd been publishing viewpoints contrary to the PANDEMIC PANIC's MONOLITHIC NARRATIVE on social media I'd attracted what was for me an unusual amount of hostile commentary. It seemed to me that this hostility originated in GROUPTHINK, a collective state of fearful non-thinking that was inculcated by highly successful brainwashing. In an attempt to get people to recognize this & to be more thoughtful I created the following text panel as my social media Cover Photo. My hope was that people would check themselves for signs of GROUPTHINK before posting if they saw this]

April 2, 2020 (Amir-ul Kafirs to group):

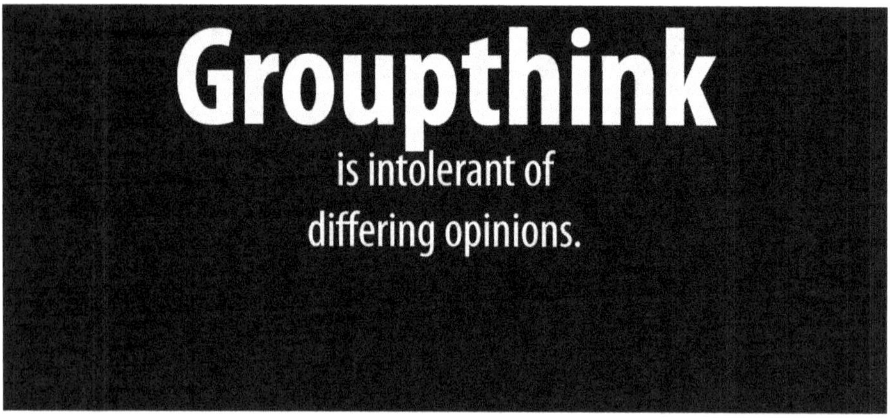

****

April 2, 2020, 6:30AM (Dick to group):

That last entry on the list of whistle blowers is unreal
And now, he's dead -
*
here's a short video a friend here posted all the comments were critical of him for having done so accusing him of spreading false rumors, etc
https://www.youtube.com/watch?

v=5BWHNQn4jH4&feature=share&fbclid=IwARoehKb7pbVsRVM76wB7CvDgg X9d32DvsDQdZUFCj8pGr1tIoPGHaid_2-Y

****

April 2, 2020, 8:54AM (Amir-ul Kafirs to group):

On Apr 2, 2020, at 6:30 AM, dick turner wrote:

here's a short video a friend here posted all the comments were critical of him

https://www.youtube.com/watch?v=5BWHNQn4jH4&feature=share&fbclid=IwARoehKb7pbVsRVM76wB7CvDgg X9d32DvsDQdZUFCj8pGr1tIoPGHaid_2-Y

I agreed with this one too EXCEPT THAT I don't accept that just because someone's presented by the mass media as the "top expert in the United States" on anything that that's true. When it comes from the TV I'm especially inclined to think that some important conflicting piece of information is lacking. I also don't necessarily think that any particular provider of statistics is utterly objective, including WHO &/or the CDC. Nonetheless, I look at & use their statistics so it's a sort of Catch 22.

By the way, I'm still completely healthy AND I still go out for a walk almost every day.

****

April 2, 2020, 3:54PM (Amir-ul Kafirs to group):

I posted a link to Dick's friend's video on social media where I was then attacked by no less than 5 people, not one of them with any sort of understanding about what Dick's friend was expressing. One person "defriended" me which, of course, didn't matter to me at all. I've already unfriended 3 people over these discussions & may unfriend more. One friend, _____, suggests that I'm too paranoid about the "deep state" & that that's affecting my perspective. What's interesting is that of all my friends, I'm, by far, one of the most widely read; the one who's done the most research (I research more or less every day); the person who's published the most writings — but, somehow, I'm the one whose opinion is at fault here — not, e.g., _____'s. So why are they so arrogant? Because, obviously, I'm 'different' from everyone else. I'm a weirdo. I'm also the person who's been a political activist the most. In short, I'm the one who thinks about these things the most — the rest can't even compare. But I'm 'wrong'. Heaven forbid that they might give me a little more credit. Their attempts at peer pressure, to bring me into their sheep fold, just aren't going to work. Ever. I thought I'd made that clear by now after 66 years of swimming upstream.

****

April 2, 2020, 9:30AM (BP to group):

I'm sure you have seen this site, believe it is the projections the government is using.
For April 1st, NY:
Hospital Beds in NY: 13,010
Hospital Beds needed - Projected: 50,962
and as released yesterday, official ny gov counts: 12,226 hospitalized (6142 discharged)

Still terrible for those working in or needing to go to hospital but....

Site last updated April 1. I doubt they update the model using hard figures. They have been saying all along this is about managing the stress on the healthcare/ hospital system. Scaring the shit out of people is part of the equation.

I can't find hospitalisation numbers (even if they truly all are corona specific) for my area, and without it it's not of much use for me. Aside from getting apprehensive about going to work.

http://covid19.healthdata.org/projections

****

April 2, 2020, 12:48PM (Amir-ul Kafirs to group):

I just talked with a friend who works as a respiratory therapist for a major hospital here somewhat at length about this. They told me that the head doctor for their dept, who they respect, predicts that in 2 weeks the shit'll hit the fan & the hospital will be overwhelmed. HOWEVER, it seems to me that that same prediction was made 2 weeks ago & it hasn't come true yet. I asked my friend whether they thinks that the PANIC has been leading to more people coming into the hospital. They somewhat begrudgingly acknowledged that as a possibility. They told me that many people have been coming in for testing & that most of them are being turned away as NON-COVID-19 cases. It would be interesting to know how many of those people are what I call BELIEVERS: i.e.: people who believe the TV 'News', e.g.. As I told another friend of mine today: If the 'News' said that there's a cholera outbreak, anyone having a runny shit wd be rushing to the hospital to be saved.

NYC keeps getting brought up as 'proof' of how bad this is. I can't really comment on that. NYC is very crowded & it seems to me that that alone is a factor that needs to be considered more. Here in Pittsburgh the PGH City Paper's statstics for today are these:

UPDATE — 12:20 p.m., Thurs., April 2:
Number of today's new confirmed positive cases in Allegheny County: 63

Total number of confirmed positive cases in Allegheny County: 419
Total number of hospitalized cases in Allegheny County: 70
Number of today's new confirmed positive cases in Pennsylvania: 1,211
Total number of confirmed positive cases in Pennsylvania: 7,016
Total number of Pennsylvania counties with confirmed cases: 62
Total number of confirmed deaths from coronavirus in Allegheny County: 2
Total number of confirmed deaths from coronavirus in Pennsylvania: 90

- https://www.pghcitypaper.com/pittsburgh/western-pa-sees-first-confirmed-coronavirus-case-in-washington-county/Content?oid=16941415

Given that we're talking about a period of over 3 months that's hardly dramatic. That's TWO deaths in the county that includes Pittsburgh. 90 statewide.

I don't mean to downplay the suffering of the sick. I DO mean to call attention to what a disaster this is for most working people. I can comment on that at great length but for now I'll 'digress' a little: After the Vietnam War was so widely opposed to by so many Americans the American government had to lay low a bit more. SO, the post-Vietnam-War era became the era of covert wars in Latin America. Many, or all of you, might not remember the curtailments of Civil Liberties during the Vietnam Era. Then the Sanctuary Movement developed to support immigrants escaping from oppression in Nicaragua & El Salvador (e.g.) — an oppression that was a direct result of US support for genocidal regimes. After the Vietnam Era faded away in the minds of the next generation it became time to up the drama & justify US interventions again. Enter 9/11. Now I tend to think that that served the Bush regime's agenda from the get-go. Whether Bush & co actually engineered the attacks isn't something I'm ever likely to 'know'. Nonetheless, more curtailment of civil liberties occurred. The Anti-Globalization Movement was in full throttle when 9/11 happened. Now that movement 'belongs' to a different generation & a new generation of gullible inexperienced people has come along. SO, it's perfect timing for generating some NEW DRAMA to justify curtailment of civil liberties.

The thing is that THIS TIME the economy is being attacked BIG TIME. I think of the Secret Wars in Laos. The CIA & its tools convinced the Laotian farmers to switch from rice, a crop they could eat, to opium, a crop they could make more money off of. **For food, & this is important, the villages became dependent on CIA airdrops.** At 1st, the CIA was only taking a couple of males from each village to be anti-communist fighters. However, after these fighters weren't winning & were getting killed off the CIA started wanting basically every useful male to be recruited. If the villagers resisted, their food airdrops were stopped. They couldn't quickly return to farming rice. That's only one example. What we're potentially seeing here is a reduction of the people to a dependency status. In other words, people put out of work will be dependent on these funds from the government. That'll also make them much more politically manipulable. Just as when the IMF gives a businessperson or farmer in Africa money it's done under the condition that they must *vote the way the IMF tells them to*. That could happen here. It might be subtle or it might even work off of imaginary fears but the voting could definitely be more controlled than it already is. Maybe more of the powers-that-be than you realize are afraid of what'll happen if Bernie Sanders wins. Better nip any possibility of THAT in the bud. I, personally, doubt that Sanders would improve things much, maybe Elizabeth Warren might do a little more — but I don't have faith in any of them.

****

April 2, 2020, 5:00PM (Dick to group):

I'm not surprised that people can't deal with the unofficial story. I think they are terrified.

There seem to be basic two stories of what's happening.

1) The virus originated in a bowl of bat soup in China, happens to be particularly virulent and has spread out. Now governments are doing everything they can to help their populations. And things will be back to "normal" soon.

This one is very clean and easy to understand and is useful for dealing with fear and uncertainty.

2) And the other one dealing with Event 201, the Wuhan Games, biological warfare and a possible coup d'état by the Central banking system, rising dictatorships*, world government, bio-metric slavery, etc..

This second scenario is less clear, is not destined to give confidence, and is harder to verify precisely because it is not "official" and involves speculation and thus, is uncertain. However, many things indicate that a fair percentage of the postulates may be true. And other things are factual (Event 201, the games, Fort Detrick, etc). Finally, it suggests an ongoing situation that will have no end.

(Of course, I imagine there must be there are many other theories, the "Q Patriot" business for example, and others that I don't know about. "Fringe" theories for lack of a better word... Not to mention possible religious ones)

I have noticed that, going into the third week of confinement, the atmosphere on social media (at least among my contacts) has started to change. Less posts for example. People seem to be sharing less and even criticizing those who do. The mother of my son told me she was criticized by a friend for sharing some humorous posts on What's App, being told, she was over-doing it, etc.. I've seen bands ridiculed for posting live shows done from home. I think many people are getting close to overload and want to avoid consciousness. They want it to end. (People want to avoid consciousness usually anyway, this situation just makes it harder to avoid.) Could this be due to having to face themselves on a daily basis, consciously, all the time? Perhaps their ideas about themselves are changing. Maybe to suggest that what is happening now is a plot is an overload; to suggest that the suffering and fear they have isn't real in the way they think it is.

So it may not be so much about being right or not, but pure fear.

*Speaking of dictatorships, maybe you've seen this already:
https://www.businessinsider.fr/us/coronavirus-created-new-dictator-

emboldens-authoritarians-worldwide-2020-4

****

April 2, 2020, 6:32PM (Amir-ul Kafirs to group):

On Apr 2, 2020, at 5:00 PM, dick turner wrote:

This one is very clean and easy to understand and is useful for dealing with fear and uncertainty.

Most people seem to 'need' a monolithic narrative. E.G.: Rump is BAD or Rump is GOOD. People are desperately reaching for a monolithic narrative here in relation to the PANDEMIC PANIC. & anything that undermines the oversimplification of that, according to the desperate, is in complete denial of all facets of that monolith. Therefore, if I say that the PANIC serves economic interests I'm denying that there's disease or death. Voila! Therefore, I'm obviously wrong. It hardly even matters when I tell people that I've never denied that there's a virus & that I've been consistently talking about the sociopolitical conditions that have come to surround the pandemic that use the pandemic as an excuse.

This second scenario is less clear, is not destined to give confidence, and is harder to verify precisely because it is not "official" and involves speculation

It also takes having an attention span — something I have. When I post links to a movie online or an article it's because I've watched the movie in its entirety & read the article in its entirety. **[initially — eventually there was too much for me to take in]** I wonder how many of my detractors have done the same?

So it may not be so much about being right or not, but pure fear.

Fear & intellectual laziness are certainly a big part of it. It's funny, many of the people who've been attacking me online are people that I never particularly respected or liked in the 1st place. I've been 'friends' with them because I've tolerated their foibles. Now I feel less tolerant.

****

April 4, 2020, 6:29AM (Dick to group):

https://www.dailymail.co.uk/news/article-8181381/World-sleepwalking-surveillance-state-rights-groups-warn.html

****

April 4, 2020, 2:51PM (Dick to group):

variant on the post pandemic scenario:

https://www.youtube.com/watch?v=J7ei1-rYHMU

Brian Eno in conversation with Yanis Varoufakis: Reflecting on our Post-Virus World | DiEM25 TV
The coronavirus crisis is revealing that the powers that be of the European Union have learned nothing from the Eurocrisis. They are currently betraying the interests of the majority of Europeans in the same way that they have done so in 2010 -- by ...

****

April 4, 2020, 10:48PM (Amir-ul Kafirs to group):

On Apr 4, 2020, at 6:29 AM, dick turner wrote:

https://www.dailymail.co.uk/news/article-8181381/World-sleepwalking-surveillance-state-rights-groups-warn.html

It's nice that people are noticing this extreme encroachment on civil liberties but my impression is that any coup that's happening right now in that direction is going to be by & large accepted by almost everyone.

On a slightly different subject, those of you who followed the almost completely hostile comments that appeared on my social media page after I posted the link to Dick's friend's video of him saying that the presentation of COVID-19 as an extreme health threat is bogus might be interested to know that one "John Piergiorgi" who posted a fair amount & who appeared there only after I posted that link was apparently a troll of some sort. I figured as much almost right away but I didn't flag him or otherwise even comment to that effect. ANYWAY, he seems to've been removed from social media under that identity & all his comments on the thread have been removed too. I had nothing to do with that removal but I'm glad to see him gone. Did any of you have anything to do with it? I think someone might've challenged things he was saying but I stopped following the thread after awhile because I was so disgusted by the shallowness & pomposity of some of my friends' replies. It's to my friend _____'s credit that they actually APOLOGIZED to me after I accused them, accurately I think, of trying to bully me. It's pretty rare for anyone to apologize to me, my usual experience is that a few people of rare integrity, such as the people here, generally try to steer a respectful course but that for the most part it's open season on me every time I display my nature as a THOUGHT CRIMINAL. It's funny, really, I'm a 'nobody', my opinion & the opinions that I share that I agree with, aren't really likely to ever dominate the society by any means but, still, a troll comes in to try to distort & supress them anyway.

p.s. I noticed a police van parked under the bridge on my street the day that the Governor declared that people are supposed to stay in quarantine as of April 1.

The police are almost never in my neighborhood but when they are it's usually a bad sign because it means they're up to no good.

****

April 5, 2020, 6:54AM (Dick to Amir-ul Kafirs):

In terms of people becoming aware of the coup-like aspect of the current situation, the two things of interest in Eno's talk were that 1) one of his friends, who he refers to as an *anarchist* told him, to his great surprise, that he would be strongly **in favor** of universal Chinese-like surveillance methods and 2) that he also recognizes the repressive use of this event which implies to me that thinking people do everywhere, but still, it's a minority

An opinion:

Do you know what I find strange? There is the official story, as I'd written in one of my last letters, But there also seems to be an official unofficial story, at least among the people like Skouras, who seems to the best informed and rational to me (however often I feel he reads into things a bit too much) I mean I sense a shared narrative, but except for a few documents, there is no real evidence as far as I can tell, of intent It formed the basis of the Quarintiranny video and is what Skouros talks about as well

It seems strange that there is a shared narrative when no one knows what is really happening

I first commented to you my misgivings about the official narrative, but I also have misgiving about this unofficial one as well

I think I am constitutionally incapable of accepting any form of group-think regardless of its sources, something inside of me just doesn't trust it

**

Today is the first spring-like day here, a real "April In Paris" feeling-- but no cafés are open, no romantic strolls by the Seine but still I have a balcony so it is pleasant

****

April 5, 2020, 9:11AM (Amir-ul Kafirs to Dick):

On Apr 5, 2020, at 6:54 AM, dick turner wrote:

It seems strange that there is a shared narrative when no one knows what is really happening

That shared narrative is just a continuation of an ongoing thread: a thread that's at least aware that, e.g., the US does chemical/biological warfare research — despite all official denials. Still, I'm always alert for smoke & mirrors, alternate stories that might just be distractions. I think, once again, of Errol Morris's NetFlix documentary series "Wormwood" about the death of Olson. Morris puts forth the idea that the 'exposé' that Olson killed himself when accidentally dosed w/ LSD is just smoke & mirrors to cover-up Olson's murder by forces trying to prevent his whistle-blowing of US biological/chemical warfare. In other words, I think you're right to be suspicious. I try to just believe what I can personally perceive. I worked for _____, they were doing bio/chem warfare research. I live in an area where a few friends have gotten sick. They all describe it as just like an ordinary flu. As I keep trying to explain to people over & over again *that's what I see*. Photographs of bodies being loaded into trucks in NYC is *not what I'm seeing*. What I'm seeing is an incredible Police State w/ *nothing to justify it*. As such, that's what I respond to. IMO, people are completely out of touch with reality. It's ironic that what the nazis tried to do & what Rump's trying to do, i.e.: create a state of constant xenophobia based around the family unit as a sortof small scale feudal system, has now been accomplished in a few weeks by something posing as 'liberal'. The term "neoliberalism" is more apropos than ever!

****

April 5, 2020, 9:23AM (Amir-ul Kafirs to group):

Liberals = Neo-Nazis

One of my more heretical ideas is this:

The nazis tried to create a worldwide state of xenophobia centered around specific ethnic groups as scapegoats. They killed millions of people but ultimately failed.

Rump has been trying to do a similar thing by feeding the fear of immigrants. He's only partially succeeding.

Under the guise of 'liberal' actions for the public good, what the nazis & Rump both have been trying to do has been accomplished in a matter of months, if not weeks: human society has retreated into small enclaves of feudal family units that're totally xenophobic of EVERYONE ELSE. I suppose we could say that it's an improvement that it's no longer so strongly ethnically-based (despite Rump's "Chinese Virus" bullshit) but it still amounts to the same thing. GROUPTHINK HAS BEEN ACHIEVED. (& I'm even more of a misanthrope than ever!) & a part of how it works is simply because people have been successfully brainwashed into thinking that 'liberals' are the opposing force to Rump instead of just another flavor of the same shit sandwich.

****

April 5, 2020, 12:48PM (Dick to group):

https://www.youtube.com/watch?time_continue=649&v=IkFw7J7GhzM&feature=emb_logo

Episode 399: There Are Dark Days Ahead w/ James Corbett - YouTube
36 Minutes Suitable For All Ages Pete invited documentarian, researcher and commentator, James Corbett, to come on the show. James has been consistently repo...

****

April 5, 2020, 2:17PM (BP to group):

what to make of this article?

TECHNOLOGY
Don't Believe the COVID-19 Models
That's not what they're for.

ZEYNEP TUFEKCI
APRIL 2, 2020

https://www.theatlantic.com/technology/archive/2020/04/coronavirus-models-arent-supposed-be-right/609271/

partial credentials: She [author] studies the interaction between digital technology, artificial intelligence, and society.

without ever having to leave the house, I might add!

Don't know what to make of your below theory. I'm far more right wing regarding illegal immigration then you, that's for sure.

****

April 5, 2020, 6:11PM (Amir-ul Kafirs to group):

I think the article was OK but I disagree with this conclusion:

"With COVID-19 models, we have one simple, urgent goal: to ignore all the optimistic branches and that thick trunk in the middle representing the most likely outcomes. Instead, we need to focus on the branches representing the worst outcomes, and prune them with all our might. Social isolation reduces transmission, and slows the spread of the disease. In doing so, it chops off branches that represent some of the worst futures. Contact tracing catches people before they infect others, pruning more branches that represent unchecked catastrophes."

The author has a single purpose: to curtail the deaths from COVID-19. That's all well & good. BUT, to use an extreme dramatic example that's meant to be metaphorical & not real: *What if the best way of curtailing it was to bomb whole neighborhoods or cities?* Everyone would oppose that, of course. Now, to back off from the metaphor, I think many privileged people, friends of mine among them, live in very comfortable worlds where 'It can't happen here', where negative side-effects of certain social scenarios aren't imaginable as ever touching their lives because they're sitting pretty. That strikes me as the author's probable situation. As you said, she reached her conclusion: "without ever having to leave the house". But what about the rest of us who live in the real world? Maybe the measures that the author proposes will have effects that're far more far-reaching than just the solution to the COVID-19 problem & maybe they won't matter to someone who doesn't "leave the house" but might matter alot to people who do.

The question is: **How far is social isolation going to be pushed?** Imagine a near future where you can only go out with permission & you have to wear a HazMat suit. Does that seem like dystopian SciFi? Yep, it does. But if we had mentioned the current social conditions, say, 4 months ago, would that have seemed like dystopian SciFi too? I think it would have — & people have already largely accepted it. The author suggests that "Contact tracing catches people before they infect others" but "contact tracing" also involves knowing just about everything about a person's life. That seems like too high a price to pay to me.

I had to get 3 different child safety criminal background checks to work for museums. One of the questions that people applying for these had to answer was a naming of **every roommate we'd ever had.** Wow. What if we had a roommate who needed to avoid surveillance for completely different reasons than ones related to child safety? I'm all for preventing child abuse, after all, *many* people I know were abused as children so I've gotten to see 1st hand what happened to them psychologically as adults. BUT I DON'T THINK THAT KNOWING WHO EVERY ROOMMATE I EVER HAD IS REALLY THE ANSWER.

The point is that these social measures are ultimately like bombing the whole neighborhood. It might work to stop the spread of the disease but it also might make more collateral damage than it's worth.

Don't know what to make of your below theory. I'm far more right wing regarding illegal immigration then you, that's for sure.

Well, that's probably true. Everyone bases their opinions on what their personal story is. I included you in this list not because I expect to agree with everything that you say but because you're an old friend of mine who I credit with being capable of taking things with a grain of salt. I don't have to always agree with you. All I typically ask of most people is that we listen to each other & try to be respectful. You've 'been around'. I'm sure you're sensitive to the people that you meet & I at least imagine that you're capable of recognizing when people are being respectful to you & treat them in a way that appreciates that.

Here's a modest story that happened to me yesterday: I went into a _____ to order a sub. There was one black woman with a Jamaican or Haitian accent (I'm not good at detecting the difference) working by herself. Usually there'd be 2 people there. The dining room was closed & that's the room I'd usually walk through to use the bathroom. I'd been drinking coffee all morning & I'd just walked 2 miles so I urgently needed to take a piss. Anyplace where I might ordinarily piss was closed. I said: "I guess your bathrooms are closed?" & the worker said "Yes". I accepted that even though I had to piss so bad I could barely stand still. After a minute she said: "Oh if you need to use the bathroom go through that door", a door that was usually for employees. She didn't have to do that, she obviously was sympathetic to me as a fellow human being so she took the risk I wouldn't do something bad that she'd then have to deal with on her own.

ANYWAY, I saw her as a working class person who probably HAD TO WORK THERE UNDER THESE CONDITIONS TO SURVIVE & I was sympathetic to that so I really appreciated her kindness to me. I made sure to be especially polite & I tipped her $5 because I can afford to do that these days. The point is that from my POV it's desirable, as humans, to be sympathetic to each other & to recognize when people are being decent & when they're being assholes. That's what's important to me. What's not important to me is whether Rump or someone like him thinks they're undesirable based on generalizing criteria that don't take actual people, actual individuals into consideration.

****

April 6, 2020, 1:34AM (BP to group):

Rebellion in the news, coming from the Orthodox Jewish community.
https://www.nj.com/coronavirus/2020/04/heres-why-large-gatherings-keep-happening-in-lakewood-as-the-coronavirus-rages-in-nj.html

****

April 6, 2020, 12:14PM (Amir-ul Kafirs to group):

Rebellion in the news, coming from the Orthodox Jewish community.

Thanks for that link, BP, I find it very interesting & important. The article points out that 5 rabbis have died as if that should show the Jewish community that they should take this more seriously. To me, that's like pointing out that X-number of nurses have died & that the nurses should take it more seriously. What would they do? Stop nursing? Obviously the rabbis are doing what they consider their job to be & tending to the needs of their community. As for arresting &/or penalizing Jewish people (or anyone else) for leading their life as they see fit?:

"Last Thursday, dozens of people gathered in small groups in a Lakewood neighborhood and stood witness as a couple was to be married in a traditional Orthodox Jewish ceremony.

"In very unorthodox fashion, the guests watched from three adjacent backyards on Wayne Street in an attempt to limit the number of people in any one yard. But before it was over, police showed up and broke up the festivities, issuing a criminal complaint to the host, 39-year-old William Katzenstein, for failing to abide by the governor's ban on such gatherings amid the growing coronavirus pandemic that continues to spread unabated across the state."

I honestly don't agree that the government, the Police State, should have the 'right' to do this. I, obviously, don't share Orthodox Jewish traditions but I wouldn't suppress them 'in the public good'. What they're doing is a far cry from, say, burning heretics or something like that. Also obviously, I'd be opposed to burning heretics as a 'religious freedom' but having a wedding is a different story — especially when they're trying to comply somewhat with health measures by being spread out.

****

April 6, 2020, 12:19PM (Amir-ul Kafirs to group):

It's this fear & paranoia that I find most artificially manufactured & most questionable. There's probably the argument that that's what the masses 'need' to keep them in compliance with sane safety procedures but I have my doubts about that. I think society would take a giant leap forward if people were more sane & sensible *without the fear & paranoia*. I continue to observe that people's reactions to this are made stupid by a variety of factors not the least of which is fear mongering by the mass media. Sensationalism *continues to sell.*

****

April 7, 2020, 6:34PM (Amir-ul Kafirs to group):

2 more links

Here's one that anthropomorphizes the virus's 'position': https://lundi.am/What-the-virus-said

Here's another one showing government foreknowledge: https://www.thenation.com/article/politics/covid-military-shortage-pandemic/

****

April 8, 2020, 7:25AM (Dick to group):

RE: 2 more links

Thanks for those
A friend posted this
Nothing new really, but a sign of growing awareness perhaps
https://www.youtube.com/watch?v=bc8wujJylHc&feature=youtu.be&fbclid=IwAR2BldmrwVt488Kpn7OCmwpZecJoEzRmmI7qgmHLMHd3TR6Cw6e9tukPsME

Anonymous Message Exposes Bill Gates - Coronavirus - COVID 19 - YouTube
My Family Has Mild Coronavirus. Here's Our Home Covid-19 Treatment Plan - Duration: 9:03. Modern Aging - Holistic Health and Wealth After 50 3,089,948 views

****

April 8, 2020, 11:52AM (Amir-ul Kafirs to group):

Re: 2 more links

THX for this, Dick. Actually, I think this is great. It's very succinct. I generally, if not always, love Anonymous releases and I find this one of a degree of excellence that's very needed.

****

April 8, 2020, 4:28PM (Dick to group):

RE: 2 more links

glad you liked it
here's something else
https://caitlinjohnstone.com/2020/04/07/prepare-to-have-your-worldview-obliterated/?fbclid=IwAR2FxA57J-jQmfoQRmELcrBhgXdd1L-yPea__xoPKvkoTdVtlt5Ijy_BO-o

****

April 8, 2020, 8:24PM (Amir-ul Kafirs to group):

I read that one too. It's fine.. but a little more generic.

The interesting thing about this set-up is that if the worst pandemic predictions don't come true, if the deaths peak earlier than exponentially predicted, then the medical industry and the lockdown advocates can claim victory. Alternately, if the deaths get extreme then they can say that it's all the fault of the people for not going along with the lockdown enough. For skeptics like myself, I tend to take the opposite position as a possibility: if there're less deaths it's because the predictions were too Draconian, if there're more deaths it might mean that all the oppressive measures weren't really the way to go after all.

On another note, I go out for a walk almost every day. I do this as part of an ongoing health regimin. It seems to work marvelously, a simple walk can do wonders for maintaining good health. Usually I don't walk in my immediate neighborhood. Today I did. For about 15 minutes of this walk a helicopter seemed to follow overhead. Maybe it wasn't following me, that seems unlikely, but I still found it strange. It was a non-hospital helicopter, usually the only helicopters are ones for the nearby Children's Hospital. Yesterday, I saw 2 military planes, what looked to me like troop transport planes, flying low overhead. Maybe this was related to that. I was one of the only people out on the streets & the helicopter followed me until I got to a local park & sat down to read.

****

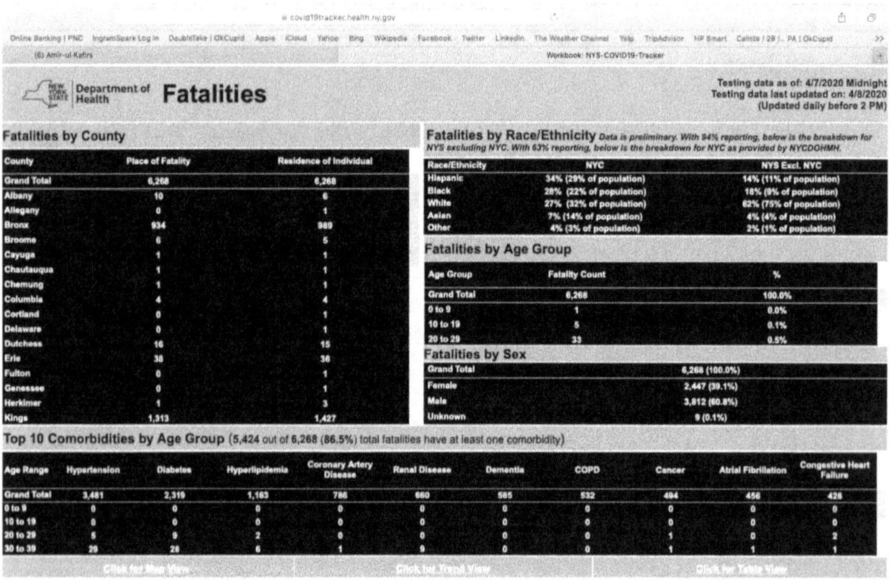
covid19tracker.health.ny.gov

Workbook: NYS-COVID19-Tracker

Department of Health **Fatalities**

Testing data as of: 4/7/2020 Midnight
Testing data last updated on: 4/8/2020
(Updated daily before 2 PM)

Fatalities by County

County	Place of Fatality	Residence of Individual
Grand Total	6,268	6,268
Albany	10	6
Allegany	0	1
Bronx	934	989
Broome	6	5
Cayuga	1	1
Chautauqua	1	1
Chemung	1	1
Columbia	4	4
Cortland	0	1
Delaware	0	1
Dutchess	16	15
Erie	38	36
Fulton	0	1
Genessee	0	1
Herkimer	1	3
Kings	1,313	1,427

Fatalities by Race/Ethnicity *Data is preliminary. With 94% reporting, below is the breakdown for NYS excluding NYC. With 63% reporting, below is the breakdown for NYC as provided by NYCDOHMH.*

Race/Ethnicity	NYC	NYS Excl. NYC
Hispanic	34% (29% of population)	14% (11% of population)
Black	28% (22% of population)	18% (9% of population)
White	27% (32% of population)	62% (75% of population)
Asian	7% (14% of population)	4% (4% of population)
Other	4% (3% of population)	2% (1% of population)

Fatalities by Age Group

Age Group	Fatality Count	%
Grand Total	6,268	100.0%
0 to 9	1	0.0%
10 to 19	5	0.1%
20 to 29	33	0.5%

Fatalities by Sex

Grand Total	6,268 (100.0%)
Female	2,447 (39.1%)
Male	3,812 (60.8%)
Unknown	9 (0.1%)

Top 10 Comorbidities by Age Group (5,424 out of 6,268 (86.5%) total fatalities have at least one comorbidity)

Age Range	Hypertension	Diabetes	Hyperlipidemia	Coronary Artery Disease	Renal Disease	Dementia	COPD	Cancer	Atrial Fibrillation	Congestive Heart Failure
Grand Total	3,481	2,319	1,163	786	660	585	532	494	456	428
0 to 9	0	0	0	0	0	0	0	0	0	0
10 to 19	0	0	0	0	0	0	0	0	0	0
20 to 29	5	9	2	0	0	0	0	1	0	2
30 to 39	29	28	6	1	9	0	0	1	1	1

Click for Map View | Click for Trend View | Click for Table View

****

April 9, 2020, 12:21AM (BP to group):

Re: 2 more links

Good Stuff.

NY started releasing death details.

Of the 4,758 deaths in New York since the first on March 14, 61% were men and 39% were women, the state Department of Health reported on its new data portal.

In addition, 63% of the deaths were among those age 70 and older, while 7% of the cases were those 49 and younger.

And 4,089 of those who died had at least one other chronic disease, the records showed:

- The leading underlying illness was **hypertension**, which showed up in 55% of the deaths.
- Next was **diabetes**, which was diagnosed in 1,755 deaths, or about 37% of the cases.
- Other top illnesses found in those who died from coronavirus were **hyperlipidemia**; **coronary artery disease**; **renal disease** and **dementia**.

https://www.usatoday.com/story/news/health/2020/04/07/new-york-coronavirus-deaths-data-shows-most-had-underlying-illnesses/2960151001/

****

April 9, 2020, 4:01AM (Dick to group):

RE: 2 more links

Minor observation:

The French news is highlighting that 2000 people died in the USA in the last 24 hours as being particularly grave But here 541 died during the same time and the French population is 60, 000,000 compared to 330,000,000 in the USA, thus percentage wise, the death toll in France is worse

And it's been the same day after day

Not sure what that means ultimately other than the reporters can't do math very well, also perhaps a general French attitude towards the USA

****

April 9, 2020, 8:01AM (Amir-ul Kafirs to group):

They might not be not doing the math but they can be sure that most of their readers/viewers won't do the math so they're 'safe' from criticism if they're just trying for a particular sensationalism. Here, much emphasis is being put on how many people are dying in NYC. I've been told that I should 'look at the photos of bodies being loaded in trucks' as a way of 'refuting' any criticism that I might have of socio-political factors surrounding this health situation.

When I 1st heard about the deaths in NYC I wondered whether there had ever been another crisis there in which bodies were so numerous that they had to be loaded onto trucks from hospitals. SO, I started searching online for such information. Every search I made brought me to the present. I found it almost impossible to get historical data no matter how I worded the search. I'm a reasonably good internet searcher so I found that interesting. Essentially the current crisis dominates search answers. One friend tried a similar search and found that this was the largest body count since 9/11. As she pointed out, it didn't say that it was the ONLY large body count since 9/11, just the largest. Of course, there was the Spanish Flu in 1918-1919. My point is that the people in the general public who're using the NYC body count as a horror story don't have the slightest idea whether this has EVER HAPPENED BEFORE or whether it's happened repeatedly over the years. A part of the shock value of it is presenting it as if it's never happened before.

****

April 9, 2020, 8:23AM (Amir-ul Kafirs to group):

Thanks for this, Brainpang. It must be a very sad and disturbing time for all the relatives and loved ones in NYC of the dead and sick. Maybe I'm being insensitive here, but given that I'm 66 I think I can feel not too insensitive about it, because I feel less upset about old people dying than I do about the young ones. I expect old people to die as a part of the natural trajectory, myself included. When my mom was in the hospice dying she said to me: "What's happening to me?" as if she couldn't understand that she was dying — this from a woman who could barely talk about anything other than her impending death for the preceeding 20 years.

I notice that by far most of the fatalities are in the Bronx and Kings.

Looking at this website here: https://a816-health.nyc.gov/hdi/epiquery/visualizations?PageType=ts&PopulationSource=Death&Topic=8&Subtopic=49 for previous years New York City death statistics I find, if I understand it correctly, an average number of deaths at 6 per 1,000 from 2010 to 2015. The population of NYC was 8.459 million in 2013. That would make a very rough average number of deaths in NYC for each of those years at 50,754 (if I'm doing the math right: 6 X 8459). The obvious question is going to be: By the end of 2020 will the total number of deaths in NYC be greater than 50,754? If not, then COVID-19 will be just another factor contributing to the ordinary death toll. As usual, it's not my intention to diminish the seriousness of this as much as it is to call attention to how 'reporting' calls attention to some things and ignores others. I think they always have the basic ulterior motive of SELLING THE 'NEWS' WITH DEATH AND FEAR.

****

April 9, 2020, 8:28AM (Amir-ul Kafirs to group):

Dick tells me that people have to have permission slips to walk in Paris. We haven't gotten to that extreme yet here. Maybe this French misreporting of US deaths vs French deaths is a way of justifying their even more Draconian measures of lockdown.

****

April 9, 2020, 8:37AM (Dick to group):

In case you'd like to see what the slips look like...

ATTESTATION DE DÉPLACEMENT DÉROGATOIRE

En application de l'article 3 du décret du 23 mars 2020 prescrivant les mesures générales nécessaires pour faire face à l'épidémie de Covid19 dans le cadre de l'état d'urgence sanitaire

Je soussigné(e),

Mme/M. :

Né(e) le :

À :

Demeurant :

certifie que mon déplacement est lié au motif suivant (cocher la case) autorisé par l'article 3 du décret du 23 mars 2020 prescrivant les mesures générales nécessaires pour faire face à l'épidémie de Covid19 dans le cadre de l'état d'urgence sanitaire[1] :

☐ Déplacements entre le domicile et le lieu d'exercice de l'activité professionnelle, lorsqu'ils sont indispensables à l'exercice d'activités ne pouvant être organisées sous forme de télétravail ou déplacements professionnels ne pouvant être différés[2].

☐ Déplacements pour effectuer des achats de fournitures nécessaires à l'activité professionnelle et des achats de première nécessité[3] dans des établissements dont les activités demeurent autorisées (liste sur gouvernement.fr).

☐ Consultations et soins ne pouvant être assurés à distance et ne pouvant être différés ; consultations et soins des patients atteints d'une affection de longue durée.

☐ Déplacements pour motif familial impérieux, pour l'assistance aux personnes vulnérables ou la garde d'enfants.

☐ Déplacements brefs, dans la limite d'une heure quotidienne et dans un rayon maximal d'un kilomètre autour du domicile, liés soit à l'activité physique individuelle des personnes, à l'exclusion de toute pratique sportive collective et de toute proximité avec d'autres personnes, soit à la promenade avec les seules personnes regroupées dans un même domicile, soit aux besoins des animaux de compagnie.

☐ Convocation judiciaire ou administrative.

☐ Participation à des missions d'intérêt général sur demande de l'autorité administrative.

Fait à :

Le : à h
(Date et heure de début de sortie à mentionner obligatoirement)

Signature :

[1] Les personnes souhaitant bénéficier de l'une de ces exceptions doivent se munir s'il y a lieu, lors de leurs déplacements hors de leur domicile, d'un document leur permettant de justifier que le déplacement considéré entre dans le champ de l'une de ces exceptions.
[2] A utiliser par les travailleurs non-salariés, lorsqu'ils ne peuvent disposer d'un justificatif de déplacement établi par leur employeur.
[3] Y compris les acquisitions à titre gratuit (distribution de denrées alimentaires...) et les déplacements liés à la perception de prestations sociales et au retrait d'espèces.

****

April 9, 2020, 9:12AM (BP to group):

I sent along the NY stats because it seems to bear out the original predictions: that it is the already compromised that are in danger. Kind of an odd feeling to read an article about the death of 4,500+ and to have it come as a relief. Showing the article to a work team last night the consensus was: the country was shutdown needlessly. Wishful thinking perhaps? Though just about everyone I know who is out here working thinks they've already been infected. But we shall see.

As for counts, one can read that deaths are being understated and other sources that they are inflated. I'm sure it is a struggle to get it right, simply labelling every death as covid instead of running more tests is understandable in a crisis situation. Maybe they will reassess once things calm down. There is a financial benefit to the hospitals. Feds will send approx 13,000 to 42,000 per patient depending on severity. Based on the Medicare model. **[Much later in this book there's a relevant chart that says that $12,000 per NYC COVID-19 patient is the amount]** Though it is also said they will still lose money. Healthcare being what it is here.

The below article is about the other killer: influenza and pnuemonia. 1,091 dead in NJ from October 2019 to Feb 15 2020.
https://www.northjersey.com/story/news/health/2020/03/05/coronavirus-deadly-but-flu-pneumonia-killed-more-nj-season/4962211002/

What will the numbers be Feb 15 on? How will they be counted?

And finally, not a lot to read here except the headline, but it certainly helped me to cope when I read it on March 21. From the top health official in NJ:

"I'm definitely going to get it. We all are," Persichilli says matter-of-factly. "I'm just waiting."

https://www.nj.com/coronavirus/2020/03/im-going-to-get-it-we-all-are-njs-top-health-official-says-as-she-leads-the-states-coronavirus-war.html

BTW, when I said 'Good Stuff," in my original post I was referring to the links sent, not the death stats.

****

April 9, 2020, 9:45AM (BP to group):

Well, it's my day off and I just had to go and read this:

https://www.nj.com/news/2020/04/theyre-terrified-nj-nursing-homes-face-staff-shortages-amid-worker-infections.html

****

April 9, 2020, 3:59PM (Dick to group):

Here's a petition against the ID2020 business

https://www.change.org/p/bill-gates-stop-id2020?recruiter=59218447&utm_source=share_petition&utm_medium=facebook&utm_campaign=psf_combo_share_initial&utm_term=psf_combo_share_initial&recruited_by_id=375bf2e0-8017-0130-fdd6-3c764e044346&utm_content=fht-21233009-en-us%3Av12

Sign the Petition
Stop ID2020
www.change.org

****

April 10, 2020, 10:37AM (Amir-ul Kafirs to group):

I signed it, I don't even care to what extent it's actually a threat. I see the herd animals lining up for the slaughter &, while I hate them, I still can't bear to see their moron chains being jerked.

It gives you a search option. Search for STOP ID2020 & you'll find it.

I had to go through the same procedure that I described to Inquiring Librarian when I followed your link. I've never had a problem accessing a Change.org petition before but maybe that's one of the things we're in for in today's Mod-A-Go-Go Medical Police State. The link you gave is a rather long and roundabout one. A more direct link is here: https://www.change.org/p/id2020-alliance-stop-id2020 .

****

April 10, 2020, 4:53PM (Phil to group):

On the subject of gates....I just discovered this article in counterpunch. I did not realise the extent of his involvement in agrobusiness.

https://www.counterpunch.org/2020/03/02/toxic-agriculture-and-the-gates-foundation/

Also another gates exercise
https://www.youtube.com/watch?v=0wfvtD17G9w

Also another article on bill gates and monsanto in the guardian
https://www.theguardian.com/global-development/poverty-matters/2010/sep/29/gates-foundation-gm-monsanto

****

April 10, 2020, 8:13PM (Amir-ul Kafirs to group):

https://www.counterpunch.org/2020/03/02/toxic-agriculture-and-the-gates-foundation/

"While Bill Gates is busy supporting the consolidation of Western agro-capital in Africa under the guise of ensuring 'food security', it is very convenient for him to ignore the fact that at the time of decolonisation in the 1960s Africa was not just self-sufficient in food but was actually a net food exporter with exports averaging 1.3 million tons a year between 1966-70. The continent now imports 25% of its food, with almost every country being a net food importer. More generally, developing countries produced a billion-dollar yearly surplus in the 1970s but by 2004 were importing US$ 11 billion a year."

When Napoleon liberated Spain from the 400+ year stranglehold of its Catholic Church Inquisition it became obvious that many of the people were completely controlled by the church's 'charity', without it they couldn't eat.

Basically what we have here is a reiteration of that. Gates and company use 'charity' as a guise for controlling markets and, ultimately, for controlling the workforce and the politics of everyone in that market. Agribusiness's purpose is to *prevent self-reliance and to insure total dependency.*

****

April 10, 2020, 8:28PM (Amir-ul Kafirs to Dick):

Did you see my relevant movie?:

"Driving Long Distance with MM 26" notes - 2:44

https://youtu.be/oKjWr0p776o

https://archive.org/details/longdistancedrivingwithmm26

"Driving Long Distance with MM 26": In 2011, I started a series of (m)usician's meetings at my house & elsewhere to discuss, listen to, & play (m)usic. Ahh.. the simple pleasures of life. In 2013, a group of the regular attendees released a CD of samples of our work. I think the CD is excellent. On March 28, 2020 Vision, I had to drive long distance to the burial of the ashes of a relative. They didn't die from COVID-19. Because of the PANDEMIC PANIC & the various social distancing edicts surrounding it there was much less traffic on the road than usual. Listening to the MM 26 CD was one of the things that made the driving less tedious. I decided it was the perfect opportunity to make a new ad for the CD so here it is: some examples of how to put your very own MM 26 CD to work for you in these extraordinary times when the medical industry is being used as a cover for creating the New World Odor. Hitler's & Reagan's DREAM finally come true! & it's all for our own good doncha know?! - April 8, 2020 Vision notes from tENTATIVELY, a cONVENIENCE

Tags: MM 26, music, experimental music, experimental usic, Low Classical Usic, Unfinished Symphonies, tENTATIVELY a cONVENIENCE, Matt Aelmore, Anthony Levin-Decanini, PANDEMIC PANIC

I don't actually like my movie very much but it's the only thing I've put online that has any relevance at all. The use of an 'ad for MM 26' is basically just a device to show one tiny aspect of the-times-of-COVID-19.

****

April 11, 2020, 6:45AM (Dick to group)

Here's a video to start the day

https://www.youtube.com/watch?v=KJ5Xo3NAUEo

WHO Official: It's Time To Remove People From Their Homes & COVID Task Force Admits Inflated Numbers
Day by day, Bill gates is revealing himself in his own words as he calls for strict lockdowns, which cannot and must not be lifted until the vast majority of the

global population is vaccinated... Last week a top WHO official stated that it is time for authorities to come in to your home, to see who is infected and take them away, for the ...

I was thinking... In response to the video I just sent, If this situation was actually planned out in advance then perhaps a vaccine already exists.
I mean, if B Gates has the mechanism of production in place that seems like a possible scenario.

****

April 11, 2020, 10:16AM (Amir-ul Kafirs to group):

https://www.abc.net.au/news/2020-04-06/sa-coronavirus-bill-to-ban-rent-rises-give-police-more-powers/12126614

Unless I somehow missed it, there didn't seem to be a word of criticism or dissent in the article. Heretics like ourselves might think that the following is, uh, questionable?:

"Under the draft bill, the state coordinator, SA Police Commissioner Grant Stevens, would also be given the power to contravene existing laws.

"Additionally, South Australian Police officers could use "reasonable force" to detain people under orders from Chief Public Medical Officer Nicola Spurrier or Commissioner Stevens.

"The legislation would be in place until the coronavirus threat was declared "cleared" by the minister."

Gee, it seems so 'innocent' doesn't it? And *what if the threat is never considered to be "cleared"?!* Here in the US there's already the suggestion that we wear masks for 18 months. That's a far cry from not wearing them at all a month or so ago. What if THAT becomes permanent? Basically the powers-that-be are opening the doors for imposing ANYTHING on us. Welcome to Prison Planet. Anyone who's ever had a bad experience with the police knows that 1. they will lie to justify whatever they're doing — hence "reasonable force" turns into SEVERE BEATINGS, TASERING, and MURDER in no time flat.

****

April 11, 2020, 2:37PM (Amir-ul Kafirs to group):

https://www.youtube.com/watch?v=KJ5Xo3NAUEo

Well, as usual, I agree with most or all of what is being said here against Gates, etc — but it is worth noticing that the ads are from The Epoch Times and that they make a point of being anti-Communist and anti-Socialist. That's ironic since what they're otherwise objecting to is essentially 'free trade' and capitalist business-as-usual.

I just posted this comment on the video:

"I agree with the vast majority of what you're putting forth here. However, it's worth noting that the people who advertise in the midst of your video are "The Epoch Times" who are anti-Communist and anti-Socialist. I'm an Anarchist and a Neoist and Anarchists have always been suppressed by Communists and Socialists so I'm not a big fan either. Remember that the Kronstadt Rebellion was partially asking for free speech for Anarchists and that Trotksy quelled that. HOWEVER, the default from Communism and Socialism is typically FREE TRADE and CAPITALISM and the G20/Gates/Central-Bankers are doing what they're doing as a part of the Globalization process that Free Trade and Capitalism generated."

****

April 11, 2020, 7:25PM (Amir-ul Kafirs to group):

Statement re Mortality

<u>Statement re Mortality</u>

Dear Fellow HERETICS,

I've written the following statement in the hope that if I die you will disseminate it widely. I'm not sick, and I'm not being morbid, I'm being cautious (in my own small way) because I want to be sure that I make my point, even if I have to do it post-mortem:

If I die from COVID-19(84) it won't be because I've avoided the recommended precautions out of stupidity and a foolish and egotistical sense of my own immunity. It'll be because I accept that I'm going to die eventually and because I think that people who live life in such an intense fear of death aren't living life with the fullness that I prefer. I'm not afraid of death, I AM in contempt of forces that restrict my life under the guise of doing it for 'my own good'. I'll be the judge of that no-thank-you-very-much. - tENTATIVELY, a cONVENIENCE - April 11, 2020 Vision

****

April 11, 2020, 3:51PM (Amir-ul Kafirs to group):

Willing to Lock Themselves In

Here's an essay of mine from circa 1982 in which I mention people willing to lock themselves in for 'security':

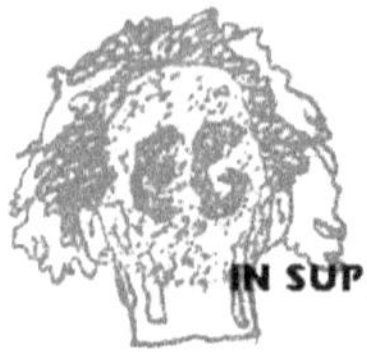

IN SUPPORT OF FUN & AGAINST POLARIZING "AUTHORITIES" VS

the idea of revolutionary guerrillas creating situations
intended to bring into overtness the intrinsic nazism of legalised power.
i.e.: polarizing "authorities" vs.. - vs what/whom?
- those who didn't choose "their leaders"
& who don't want them or any others?
this polarization means bringing a war into overtness
w/ the idea that the majority will as a result understand
that these "leaders" lead them into *illusions* of wide open space
- lulling them w/ a security the falseness of wch
relies upon having the possibilities that the "security" creates
seem greater than those that it represses
- a security wch is actually the security (minimum & maximum) of a prison
w/ wallpaper murals of (mediocre representations of) idyllic landscapes
& prisoners willing to lock themselves in..
- as if a war can be won?
i have no faith in the masses' ability to cope w/ serious thought
(is it too intimidating & tiresome for them? - not necessarily..
- maybe most people are just *too busy* for such things)
the masses are the masses because they are different
from those who are different
(trying to write these things to my satisfaction can seem so futile)
- & a possible difference is their wanting
security to be provided as a commodity.
i.e.: a "security" provided by an external source
- a false security wch is the security of being led ("by the nose")
- of being relieved of the tension of decision making.

the idea of the fun guerrilla as possibly more revolutionarily effective
insofar as it presents the happiness potential of revolution
& insofar as it relaxes people from the tension of serious decision making
by presenting them w/ the possibility
of playful roles wch are flexible (unbinding) enough
not to involve life & death polarization.
"police/criminals" catalyzed to laughter
by a person facing possible "victimization" from them
might perceive the person & the situation in a changed enough way
to disarm the rigidity of the roles
(but you'd better be a damn good comedian if you want to survive long!
- don't try stupid jokes like this:
"What's the difference between a W.A.S.P. & a Let-It Bee?
- Imperialistic Hominas." - NYUK, NYUK, right?)

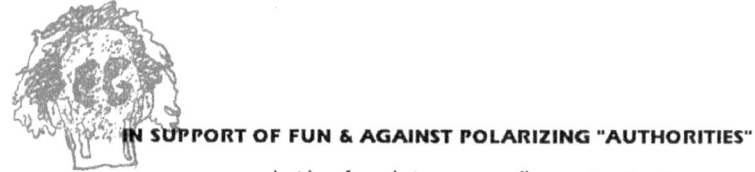

fun guerrilla NOT as ridicule (contrary to popular opinion)
- ridicule just perpetuates the polarizing, the rigidity, the tension, & the victimization..

TOWARD A REVOLUTIONARY THEORY (& SENSE) OF HUMOR

- tentatively, a convenience (Psychopathfinder & Jack-Off-of-All-Trades)
- box 382, cr(ater) Bal Tim Ore, MD, 21203, us@..

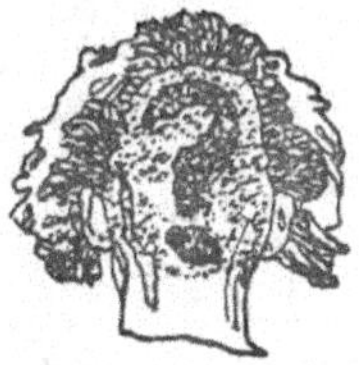

https://www.thing.de/projekte/7:9%23/tent_fun_guerrilla

****

April 11, 2020, 6:43PM (BP to group): :

Re: Willing to Lock Themselves In

An hour ago I had my first experience being refused entry to the supermarket for not having a mask. The governor issued the executive order on Wednesday but I guess it took a few days as I was in the same market without mask on Thursday. I had to suck it up and put one on. A friend gave me one and it's been in my glove compartment. I dropped off the groceries and decided to get some beer. Stopped into the place right next door to the above market and they didn't care if I was wearing a mask or not (which I wasn't). First time I put one on, and I've been doing my work thing, going to the post office nearly everyday, food stuffs, and beer trips since this began.

and some more: I was on the phone with a friend just now and he thinks people are idiots for not wearing a mask. He wears one while taking a walk in deserted suburbia! There is NO ONE around! He wanted me to come over and hang in the back yard (at a safe distance, watching the wind direction) but I told him I was a risk. I could only imagine the lambasting I would have received if my true thoughts were known. We have a tentative plan for tomorrow but I feel like I should avoid him.

It reminds me a bit of the reaction to 911. Those at a distance wanted a Police State while those who witnessed it up close wanted to keep the freedoms, against restrictions.

****

April 11, 2020, 6:13PM (Amir-ul Kafirs to BP):

As a person who's spent my entire life being overtly different from other people and facing the wrath I think people who don't want to wear the masks should stand their ground as much as possible. There's too much potential for bullying here. Mind Control leads to GROUPTHINK leads to Mob Bullying. To hell with people who think they have the right to tell me what to do, I have my reasons or I wouldn't be doing it. Good luck to us all! May we outlive the sheep.

****

April 11, 2020, 7:24PM (Amir-ul Kafirs to group):

Here, it seems that just about anything is being accepted as a mask. I've been tempted to wear women's panties with an obvious wet spot over my face so I can do something that would ordinarily be considered completely perverted as if I'm just complying with health concerns. What me? A Pervert?!

****

April 11, 2020, 7:35PM (Amir-ul Kafirs to group):

It's inspired by this image from my friend Boris Wanowitch who's wearing a hat I had 48 made of (the idea for the hat text was Alan Lord's).

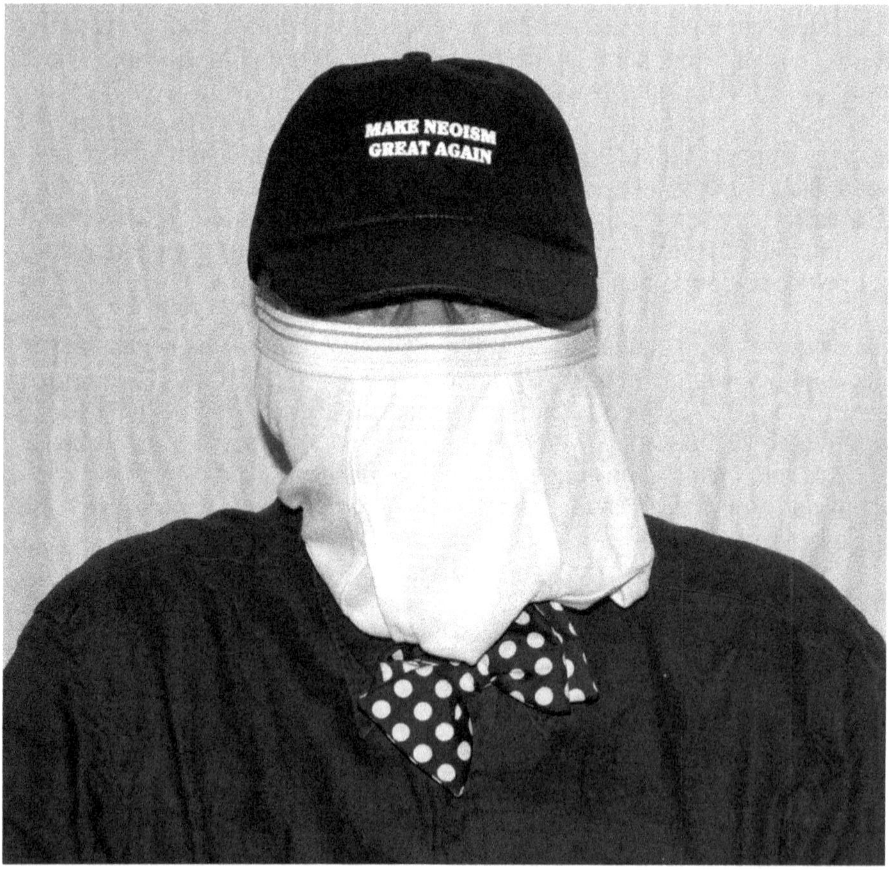

****

April 11, 2020, 8:44PM (Inquiring Librarian to group):

It's very interesting to hear that story from the east coast! We still have very low mask use here in Louisiana. But, although our big uptown park is still open and packed daily, the city ordered that the parking lot for the park be closed.
For me, this is no big deal. I bicycle to the park every day and lock my bike up on the bike rack while I go for my jog. I asked one of the cops blocking the parking lot entrance about it. He said he had no real idea why the city ordered the parking lot closed, he's just doing his job.

I see no sane reason to wear a mask when you are in a remote area around no one but your family.

The NIH is doing a study on 10,000 healthy adults over the age of 18 who were not diagnosed with Covid 19.
https://www.nih.gov/news-events/news-releases/nih-begins-study-quantify-undetected-cases-coronavirus-infection?fbclid=IwAR3a_CUK3ioowjkLXH-9HbaZM4XGPquSCxqwXexOdXcY0ccvU1cPeyDYd5g

I sent them an email already expressing my interesting in being tested for antibodies. I'd like to have the possibility of employment as a librarian again and maybe a stamp of approval saying I have the damn antibodies! =O No stimulus cash has come my or my significant other's way. We are on a dwindling financial cliff.

****

April 11, 2020, 11:18PM (Amir-ul Kafirs to group):

I mean, really, who has NOT been exposed at this point?

Right. Is this really so different from any other flu or cold that spreads around during the 'flu season'? Don't some of us get sick, don't some of us stay healthy, don't different people get sick to different degrees, and isn't the whole process a type of 'immunization' that's natural? I wouldn't be surprised if I'm one of the "asymptomatic" people but my attitude toward that is this: The "asymptomatic" people are the ones with the healthy immune system. It would be interesting to get statistics on how many of us *aren't on prescription 'medicines'.* It's my opinion that many or most of the things that the medical industry does 'for our own good' actually weaken our immune system. An obvious example is the use of antibiotics: how long is it before they won't work anymore? I try to rely on my body's own natural resources as much as possible. What if the lifestyles of the "asymptomatic" people were more of a model and if people were *less dependent on the medical industry?!* THAT would be bad for BIG BUSINESS. We're being told that this is more severe than the usual flus. Maybe it is but I have so many questions: How many of the reported deaths *happened in the hospital?* Is it statistically reasonable to factor in ***the fucking hospital*** as a contributing cause of death?! My mom just died in a hospice on December 30, 2019. She was reported as having died from bladder cancer. I tend to believe that she died from gradually increased sleeping pills coupled with starvation — both the product of her hospice 'care'.

****

April 11, 2020, 11:05PM (Amir-ul Kafirs to group):

More regarding dependency

Agribusiness's purpose is to *prevent self-reliance and to insure total dependency.*

Another historical example is the forcing of the Chiricahua Apache Tribe into the Turkey Creek Reservation in the 1880s where they were expected to become farmers. They could only farm corn and not even enough to be self-sufficient so they were dependent on army supplies. The army then tried to recruit the men into being scouts and soldiers for the US. I'm sure stories like this are numerous but I'm thinking of this one right now because I'm watching a fictionalized movie about Geronimo, the most famous of the Chiricahua warriors. It's probably not wholly historically accurate but I think the gist of what I just recounted probably is.

OTHERWISE, think about the bipartisan promise of money to all the people who're currently suffering economically because of the shutdown of so many businesses and the loss of so many jobs. PEOPLE ARE GOING TO VERY DESPERATELY DEPEND ON THIS GOVERNMENT MONEY. And these desperately dependent people aren't going to want to be arrested for any sort of lockdown violation because it might result in a loss of that money.

****

April 12, 2020, 12:09AM (Inquiring Librarian to group):

Talking about being controlled into following inane orders, I am a professional librarian with an MLIS. I was hired to manage a tiny 1 room library in Louisiana. As the manager, i am on salary. I have always responsibly come and gone from the library as i please, as needed. During Hurricane Isaac, i braved the storm and fed the library fish and kept their filter running through the storm (note it did not get beyond a category 2). This time, I am forbidden to enter my own building that i have managed for 7 years. It took over a week for me to get an 'essential' library Administrator to respond to my pleas to have official permission to use my key and get into my building, to avoid animal cruelty and feed the fish and tend to their easily clogged filter. Unbelievably, after my emails and texts being ignored for at least a week, the only solution was for me, escorted by the library head of security, to move the entire tank and fish to my house where they now reside in my bedroom, the only room in my house with ac. Moving a fish tank is no easy task. It took about 5 hours. I blew out a knee for several days carrying the heavy stuff of the tank. It took the fish a week to recover and start eating again. Note: i was going into the library daily, at sneaky off hours, to tend to the fish before the end solution happened. I cannot needlessly torture animals in the name of this virus... And i feared getting caught and fired every time i fed the darn fish! It was/ is a nonsensically humiliating situation. This week, i tried to rescue the library plants to no avail. Top secret covid plant fairy must ghost in and out of said library 1x/wk. Will the librarian lose their job because they simply cannot submit to senselessly letting the plants they've nurtured for years die?

****

April 12, 2020, 7:56AM (Amir-ul Kafirs to group):

Ha ha! I love your story!! I suspect that when people think of resistance and revolt they think primarily in grander revolutionary actions — but stories like yours show that people have a plethora of reasons for defying the lockdown. Some might say you're being foolish to have such priorities but I'm in complete agreement with you, I'm glad you're taking care of the fish and the plants and I'm glad that you're taking the risk for something that's important to YOU and not letting other people set your priorities for you.

****

April 10, 2020, 10:30AM (Amir-ul Kafirs to group):

Face Masks for 18 Months (ETC)

Have any of you heard about this yet? The CDC is supposedly advising that ALL OF US should wear face masks for the next 18 months.

https://www.accuweather.com/en/health-wellness/americans-may-need-to-wear-masks-for-up-to-18-months-yale-expert-says/716922

Trader Joe's has hours for the elderly and immune-compromised now. We can go in between 8 and 9AM and between 7 and 9PM. Despite this restriction, when I got there at 8:40ish this morning there were already non-seniors/immune-compromised waiting in line to get in *even though they weren't allowed to until 9.* By the time I left, around 8:55, there was already a line around the block. As you may know, only 35 people are allowed in at a time. More people than ever before had on face masks.

The more I watch all this going down the more I'm reminded that I'm a lone wolf in a world of herd animals.

****

April 10, 2020, 11:42AM (Inquiring Librarian to group):

Re: Face Masks for 18 Months (ETC)

I see a little less than 50% of Louisianians wearing masks. I personally still can't bring myself to wear one. I feel like a jerk and a tool if i wear one and a jerk if i don't wear one. I cannot imagine wearing 1 in Louisiana as the heat and humidity creep up to our ungodly summer swamp inferno levels. Mask wearing in such conditions seems logically unsanitary. I can see an outbreak of nose fungus in our future, creeping up into our brains. Yuck.

Ok. Really. It seems like a reliable, free, and accessible antibody test is needed asap.

Louisiana cases are dramatically decreased. I cannot wait for this to be over. My other half is unemployed with no response to their unemployment application. My city hired construction workers and electricians from Texas to do the emergency construction work for our temporary convention center hospital here leaving our own union members and labor workers unemployed. It is corruption and letting down their own as usual in Louisiana. Note: the last i heard, the convention center hospital here is mostly empty. https://www.google.com/amp/s/www.nola.com/news/coronavirus/article_394f37fe-768e-11ea-8ee0-e3c343f13af2.amp.html

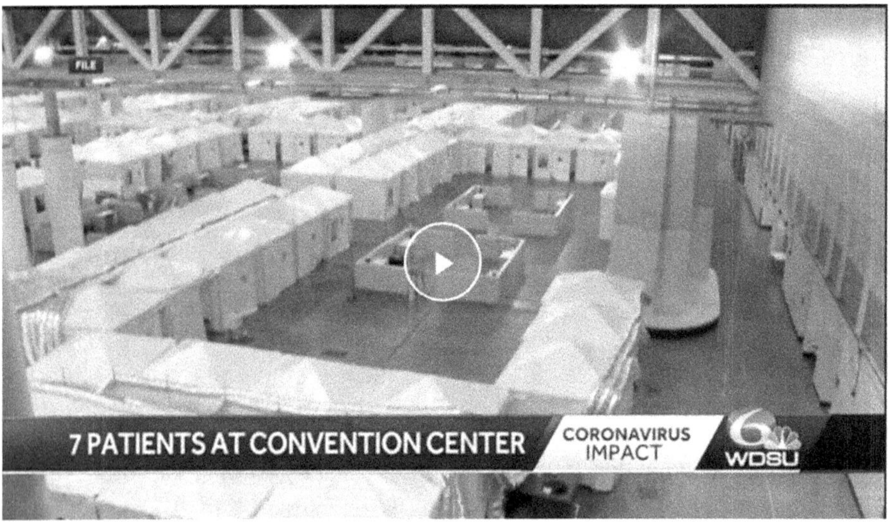

****

April 10, 2020, 12:10PM (Amir-ul Kafirs to group):

Ha ha! As usual, some people are making allllloooottttttoooooffffff money off of this while everybody else flounders.

****

April 13, 2020, 6:00PM (Dick to group):

Bonsoir,
Tonight Macron, the French president (who I dislike immensely) announced that the confinement will last until 11 May
So far there have been around 13,000 deaths here
It may or may not be worth noting, but about 12 years ago there was a two week heat wave in which 13-15,000 people died (I found an article where it says 11,000 but I recall a higher figure, see below) and it was more or less brushed under the rug and nothing was done about it
I am not sure how to interpret that other than the obvious "what is useful" gets attention angle
https://www.theguardian.com/world/2003/aug/29/france

****

April 14, 2020, 2:58AM (Amir-ul Kafirs to group):

It may or may not be worth noting, but about 12 years ago there was a two week heat wave in which 13-15,000 people died

As usual, this type of thing continues to be an issue largely ignored. The last I checked (a day or 2 ago) 18 people have died, reputedly from COVID-19, in Allegheny County, where Pittsburgh is — but that seems to be the kind of info that one has to search for. If it were a larger number it would be, obviously, big news. That 'makes sense' but at the same time it shows what the orientation of the media is: reinforce whatever spectacle attracts an audience so that advertising revenues continue to flow — downplay or completely ignore the small number of deaths in this area, play up the larger number of deaths elsewhere. As I've mentioned before, my friend the respiratory therapist who works for the biggest hospital here was told to expect *nothing but COVID-19 patients* at his hospital by tomorrow. As far as I know, that hasn't even come close to happening but I'll have to check in with my friend to verify that. What do you do when the End of the World doesn't come? The media will just have to find a new disaster to attract the flies-to-shit with.

****

April 14, 2020, 11:36AM (Dick to group):

https://safeyoutube.net/w/ewy5

****

April 14, 2020, 11:46AM (Dick to group):

A friend of mine sent this
I don't know if it's true or not
https://www.youtube.com/watch?v=qNK9zesHQls&feature=youtu.be&fbclid=IwAR1H6ZOmiF4FUcFDNkWhUoGypNO3I3iD2t7PFZR96yWax_w3QIn9QwEwQ6w

****

April 14, 2020, 11:49AM (Phil to group):

There is probably a lot of stuff that I have looked at and haven't posted here.....and lots of stuff i think worthy of discussion i haven't yet raised.... but anyway...I was just watching this video interview and think it is a worthwhile one - more focused on the situation of the global economy;
https://www.youtube.com/watch?v=8LYjOEib9iI&feature=share

Also I was interested to learn more about these dna vaccines..I just read a John Rappoport article on them here;
https://blog.nomorefakenews.com/2020/04/14/passport-to-the-brave-new-world-the-vaccine/

an interesting turn of events. Here is the link to the article in fortruss he was talking about;
https://www.fort-russ.com/2020/04/major-plans-to-re-open-u-s-surgeon-general-adams-dumps-gates-predictive-contagion-model/

****

April 14, 2020, 12:51PM (Amir-ul Kafirs to group):

I did check in with my friend the respiratory therapist today and he told me, as I expected, that the doctor's prediction of a hospital entirely full of COVID-19 patients by today didn't some true. He said is he is keeping busy though.

****

April 14, 2020, 12:59PM (Inquiring Librarian to group):

Thank you for sharing the article. It gives me hope. I didnt know about the news source, but found info here:
https://www.fort-russ.com/abou/

Things remain stable in Louisiana. Everyone I know globally is physically healthy. Though, many are not so financially. My corner drug dealers are so active that they worked up the gumption for a shooting. 2 days ago.

****

April 14, 2020, 1:03PM (Amir-ul Kafirs to group):

On Apr 14, 2020, at 11:36 AM, dick turner wrote:

https://safeyoutube.net/w/ewy5

I watched the 1st 8 minutes of this but I admit to having limited patience for watching any videos relevant to the PANDEMIC PANIC right now. I feel like Shiva was ok but at the same time that he was talking about the importance of our immune system, which, of course, I agree with, he was being introduced as someone who does bioengineering — something that can go very contrary to what my understanding of allowing one's immune system to do its thing is.

****

April 14, 2020, 1:33PM (Amir-ul Kafirs to group):

I don't know if it's true or not

Alas, I don't find Buttar to be a very good spokesperson. He repeats himself too much for one thing. I did look up "Surgeon General Jerome Adams DROPS Gates/CDC/WHO model" and it yielded, after Buttar, Fox News, which, of course, has got to be the worst TV 'news' source out there — at least of the ones that reach millions. That doesn't mean it's not true, it does mean that it's going to be a huge feather in Rump's cap if all the fear-mongering is exposed as such and businesses reopen quickly. I see it all as a performance. The powers-that-be don't want Bernie Sanders or Elizabeth Warren to win. Rump is choice #1, Biden is choice #2. If, after this shit show is over, Rump can be made to look 'sensible' then he might win a re-election. What if that were part of the purpose for all this shit in the 1st place? I'm cynical enough about all this to imagine that being the game in the US.

****

April 14, 2020, 2:47PM (Inquiring Librarian to group):

I have felt for some time that Trump's entire presidency has been political theater. He is likely being paid very well to play the bumbling idiot role while the powers that be covertly fulfill their agendas behind the curtain of insulting political drama and socially engineered chaos.

Just simply seeing an article like the Fort-Russ article circulating, regardless of how 'true' or well sourced it is, is a shred of a positive sign that the theater is maybe turning towards an end to the economic torture of the working class population.

With Bernie and Warren out, it is finally a win win for the political powers that control us all.

Its a cloudy, cold, grim day in Louisiana. My inner sceptic and dark cloudness is not well supressed today.

****

April 14, 2020, 3:18PM (BP to group):

What? Don't Like Fox? heh heh. Well, get this mindblowing statement: Tucker Carlson, opening segment last night.

5:45 for the gold but if you want the lead in 4:05.

April 13, 2020
Tucker: Science needs to drive policy during a health crisis

Or if you'd rather not watch:

"A study emerged, that for some reason cigarette smokers were LESS likely to die, MUCH less likely to die of coronavirus. Didn't think we'd be reporting that on the air..."

I heard this while guiltily smoking a cigarette out the window.

****

April 14, 2020, 3:39PM (Inquiring Librarian to group):

The John Rappoport article on dna vaccines and the relation to crispr gene editing gone awry is honestly terrifying. I am personally afraid of the common flu vaccine. I have never gotten one and hope never to be legally required to get one. I've had my own genetic tests done and have discovered that i have a double copy of a genetic mutation that makes me particularly sensitive to toxins, esp those in most of these flu vaccines. I feel the flu vaccine is taking vaccines too far. Why create a vaccine every year for a mostly innocuous illness? Seems like vaccine related corporations are making out well financially here.... And now the corona virus with this dna twist. :/ i feel glad i never had children. I'd hate to dump any new unsuspecting soul into our current world. I will continue instead to adopt homeless cats in need.

****

April 14, 2020, 4:44PM (Dick to group):

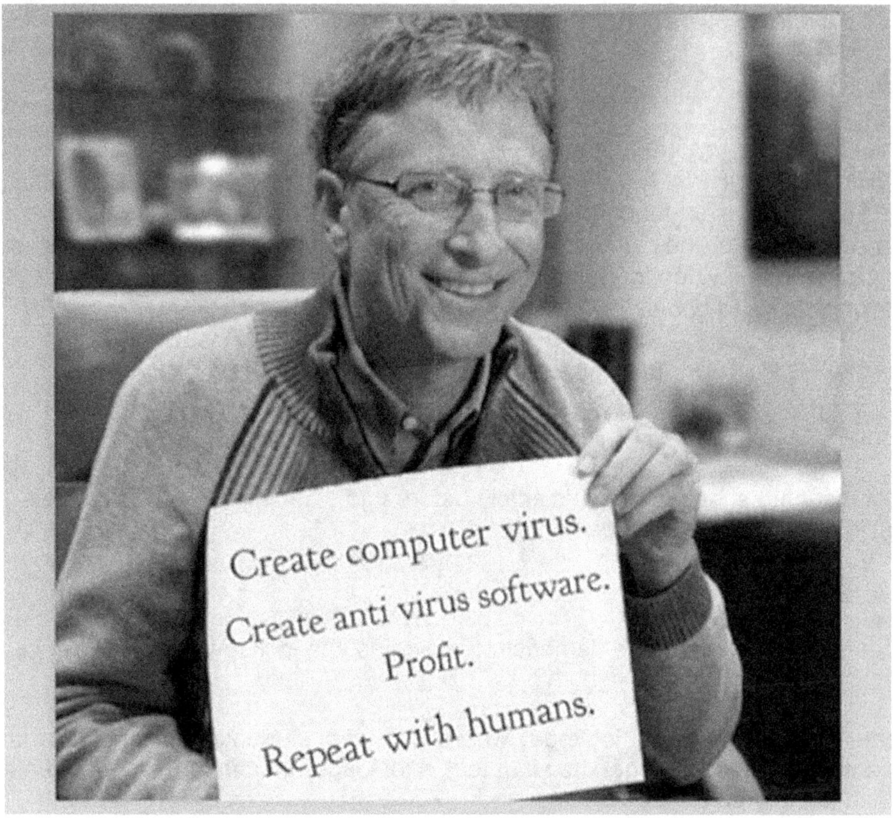

****

April 14, 2020, 4:52PM (Amir-ul Kafirs to group):

I was just watching this video interview and think it is a worthwhile one - more focused on the situation of the global economy

I'm a little less than 10 minutes into this one but I want to call attention to the interviewee's use of the term "helicopter money" for the payments that the states are making to the citizens. For me, that's evocative of the CIA Air America air drops of food that I've mentioned earlier in connection with the Secret Wars in South East Asia.

****

April 15, 2020, 5:09PM (Amir-ul Kafirs to group):

A Mortician's Critique

I feel like I'm beating a COVID-19 casualty with my repetitiveness but it's amazing how few people get the obvious. Fortunately, you HERETICS do get it but I think that you'll appreciate this short video:

https://youtu.be/zLI5yikUKfk

The idea is: the reportage about the dead in NYC is being sensationalized. SURPRISE, SURPRISE! If I were to post such an opinion on my social media feed right now, even though I think it's obvious AND business-as-usual, I'd lose more friends after they take a few thoughtless seconds to insult me. I really recommend this video for some common-sense treatment of the subject of *what happens to dead bodies.*

****

April 16, 2020, 8:09PM (Phil to group):

Just thought I should share this article before I go sleeping, also before it gets lost in my social media stream;
https://www.ukcolumn.org/article/coronavirus-lockdown-german-lawyer-detained-opposition

There is a short video of a demonstration against the lockdown in berlin here;
https://www.youtube.com/watch?v=47d7m0yUZbA&feature=youtu.be

I actually did a life model job today where instead of students coming to draw me, I went to their places to get drawn. It took a lot longer than it normally would but it was a fun exercise.

****

April 16, 2020, 9:37PM (BP to group):

well well well, what are you people doing? I took a walk up the street wearing a halloween mask and monster gloves. I'd say half the people I encountered laughed and the other half recoiled in horror.

****

April 17, 2020, 4:35AM (Dick to group):

That's a great idea
I should try it today with my donkey costume mask
Of course the police here have no sense of humor and they are everywhere
I get stopped and each cop seems to have a different set of rules; each has his or her own power trip going
Whatever happened to Officer Friendly?

****

April 16, 2020, 10:11PM (Amir-ul Kafirs to group):

Just thought I should share this article before I go sleeping, also before it gets lost in my facebook stream

"A large number of well-established doctors and lawyers in the German-speaking countries have questioned the constitutionality of their governments' stringent confinement measures, which are commonly being referred to by the English loan-word *der Shutdown* (as there is no precedent for what to call the situation in German). These measures have begun to be challenged openly on the streets of Berlin. The medical and legal dissidents number in the dozens. None, however, has paid such a price for that freedom of speech as the German medical lawyer Beate Bahner, who has been committed to a psychiatric institution for publicly disagreeing with the measures and policies followed by the German government."

Wow, if anyone doubts that this is a nazi-style crackdown after reading that..

"On Friday 3 April 2020, Ms Bahner issued a press release decrying the German government's Coronavirus measures as "flagrantly unconstitutional, infringing to an unprecedented extent many of the fundamental rights of German citizens". The statement argued that the small minority of the public that was at risk of serious harm in the event of contracting Covid–19 could be far more suitably protected by means of targeted measures based on the principle of adult responsibility for safeguarding one's own health."

Exactly. Since when have any of us asked the government to be, quite literally, our BIG BROTHER. I prefer to safeguard my own health no-thank-you-very-much.

There is a short video of a demonstration against the lockdown in berlin here

Great! I'm glad to see the action picking up. In Pittsburgh, I'm part of a group called _____, the purpose of which is to offer free services to people made in need from COVID-19 &/or the lockdown. So far we've had offers of money & other services from our fellow neighbors BUT NOT A SINGLE PERSON NEEDING OUR HELP. I hope it stays that way. Otherwise, I seem to still be one of the only HERETICS locally. Essentially I have one friend, maybe, who has similar questioning opinions. They were sick, maybe with COVID-19, maybe not, but said it was just like an ordinary flu. They've recovered now. The statistics published by the daily newspaper TODAY say that 12 people have died in Allegheny County (where Pittsburgh is) from COVID-19. *That's 6 LESS than the last statistic I read online.*

****

April 16, 2020, 11:03PM (Amir-ul Kafirs to group) [**MY FIRST USE OF "HERETICS" IN SUBJECT**]:

HERETICS:

I'm told that as of Monday it'll be illegal to enter any store in Pennsylvania without a mask on. In preparation for this, I just bought a Trump mask with a Hitler moustache on it online. Do you think I'll have any trouble?

****

April 17, 2020, 5:28AM (Dick to group):

RE: HERETICS:

I forgot, it is illegal to wear a mask in public
They created the law to forbid the burka

https://en.wikipedia.org/wiki/French_ban_on_face_covering

French ban on face covering - Wikipedia
France became the first European country to impose a ban on full-face veils in public areas. Public debate exacerbated concerns over immigration, nationalism, secularism, security, and sexuality. Arguments supporting this proposal include that face-coverings prevent the clear identification of a person (which is both a security risk, and a social hindrance within a society which relies on ...

****

April 16, 2020, 10:17PM (Amir-ul Kafirs to group) [**announcement of use of "HERETICS"**]

HERETICS

I've decided to give anything addressed to this group a subject heading that begins with "HERETICS". That'll enable me to keep the emails a bit better organized. I've been copying some of the articles into a text file but I've been a bit haphazard about it. As usual, I think that even our small bit of critical analysis here may be of future historical importance. If a month from now this is basically over we'll all be relieved and maybe we won't care that much — but it's still my feeling/thought that precedents are being set here of a most Draconian nature.

****

April 17, 2020, 9:50AM (tENT to group) [**addition of Naia Nisnam to group**]:

HERETICS: new person

Welcome **Naia Nisnam**, my fellow heretic in Pennsylvania & one of the only people I know locally who's suspicious of this whole social engineering. She's the one who sent me the link to the mortician video.

I'm curious about everyone's local reports. Dick tells us that people get stopped by the police in Paris & that the police give contradictory instructions. I've seen that kind of thing happen before & it can easily result in arrests. One cop says: 'Move along', the next cop says: 'Sit down'. Then, if you do either of those things you're in violation of the other & you get arrested.

Today I left my house at 7:40AM to get the the Trader Joe's food store by opening time, 8AM, when only seniors are allowed in. I got there almost exactly at 8 & they were just letting people in. When I went there a few days ago only about 1/3rd of the employees had masks & gloves, now they all do. I only saw one other customer without a mask. I find such externally imposed conformist behavior very disturbing. Even if the masks really are for the public good, which I'm not convinced they are, I don't think that it takes much to force people into conformist behaviors. As anyone who knows me realizes, I think most people are robopaths, latent 'Good Germans' as I've written before, who can be manipulated into lockstep with not much effort. I really mainly trust flagrant pervert individualists because they're more likely to maintain their personal integrity. Even the bearded women were wearing masks at Trader Joe's the other day when it apparently wasn't required. Maybe it was required for bearded people. I went to Trader Joe's today because I'm told that as of Monday I won't be allowed in stores without a mask. I doubt that they'll accept the Trump/Hitler mask but I'll give it a try. It would function to prevent the spread of breath-expelled germs.

I'm still flirting with women internationally & having women apparently try to trick me into sextortion scams so that's been interesting since it's an indication of sex workers having to reroute their work routines. Two of the women who've tried to hustle me are in Las Vegas, the gambling city, which has been closed down. I just verified that it is online, I thought that the mafia might've been able to get gambling declared "essential". In Pennsylvania, the state where I live, beer is sold in state-controlled beer stores & all other alcohol is sold in state-controlled liquor stores. The liquor stores are closed but the beer stores are still open. The bars are closed but I wonder if there's surreptitious bar-going for regular customers.

I've been having fun with using a computer dating site during the lockdown. I told a woman in Brazil that my feet have turned into frogs because of COVID-19. She said she hasn't seen that in Brazil yet. I told her that there are different symptoms in different countries & that in Brazil it might be that people's noses turns into guns or their fingers might turn into pencils or their pets might turn into furniture or vice versa.

****

April 17, 2020, 12:41PM (Dick to group):

Since I now know this is a Historical Record I will clarify what I meant about the cops and varying stories:

Wednesday I went out for a walk with a hand written note (according to the Government site, is legal and I don't have much printer ink left so...)... anyway, a cop stops me, a female cop to be specific, and asks where is my permission note? I produce it.

I have written all the required information, for example:

Dick Turner
address

But not

Name: Dick Turner
Address: address

That is, I didn't **reproduce** the actual form, thinking they've seen it enough (name, date of birth, address, etc) and the answers are what are important. Shows what a fool I can be for she threatens me with a fine. Now **she doesn't mention** that I've written "taking a walk" to explain why I'm outside.

Since I am literally just outside my apt. she allows me to go in and redo my note, saving me 200 euros.

Then **Thursday** I get stopped by three young guy cops, who ask for my note. Since I have learned my lesson I now have a printed note, thus, it creates no problem **BUT** upon seeing "taking a walk" they inform me physical exercise isn't allowed under the "new regulation" (three weeks old already) between 10am - 7pm. I told them I had read this was just for joggers but they say NO, any form of exercise is not allowed.

So I act repentant and they allow me to go. Again, I could have been fined, like the female cop the day before, I got off light.

The funny thing was, I was on the canal which was literally filled with people strolling, with their kids, etc. Not all of them could be going to buy food or the hardware store.

In other words, it was ridiculous and seemingly arbitrary.

Small Personal Commentary: I think one of the most disturbing things about this whole business is that people watch the mass media and somehow feel like they are the only ones that saw it. I noticed this first when **three different people** informed me that the actor Tom Hanks had the virus, each using the tone like the information was somehow **theirs alone**.

EXAMPLE: A friend of mine called me today to say hi, he lives in Pennsylvania. He takes the whole thing very seriously, that is he is terrified of dying, and when I brought up some of the points of view expressed in this group, he just blew them off. Zero interest in other words.

In response to something I said about the possibility of exaggerating the body count and the political uses of the epidemic he said "But *they have drones* Dick !! You can see it, they're piling bodies four deep in Potter's Field in New York" (that is, the same images everybody has seen) so I said he should watch that video Amir-ul Kafirs sent from the mortician which could give a slightly different take on it. But I could tell he thought I was verging on the lunatic fringe. I sent the video anyway, hopefully he'll check it out but I doubt it.

And when I said that I didn't like this talk about a universal vaccine program, **something I thought any thinking person would object to**, he said in a grim voice "You might change your mind if it means you won't die".

****

April 17, 2020, 1:32PM (Amir-ul Kafirs to group):

Dear Dick, Everything that you've written about below exemplifies the Kafkaesque potential of this situation.

1st, there're cops who're robopaths, most cops are. The absence of the word "Name" to tell that "Dick Turner" is a name doesn't mean that they can't make that small deduction it means that their mindset is too inflexible to interact with real life in a way that calls for spontaneity. Life isn't a machine so a person who approaches it as if it is is bound to immediately experience cognitive dissonance *without* having the COGNITIVE DISSIDENCE that creates the possibility of a sensible response.

2nd, your friend in PA? They, too, are inflexible. Inflexible people cannot learn, they can only be programmed. Keeping people in a state of constant fear is an excellent way of making sure their mind narrows to almost nothing. The irony of it is that such a narrowing *is not condusive to survival* — at least not in my opinion. Anyone who questions the MONOLITHIC NARRATIVE borders "on the lunatic fringe" from the perspective of those who don't. I think a large part of why people like you & me have no problem questioning the NARRATIVE is because we make & analyze narratives & are, therefore, more familiar than most with *how narratives are constructed.* This whole business of the dumping bodies 4 deep in Potter's Field is only meaningful up to a point. Yes, it means that there's an overflow of dead people in NYC. Yes, that's bound to be a tragedy for those affected. NO, it doesn't mean we're at the end of the world or that someone in a less crowded area in, say, PA, where your friend is, is at as much risk.

I just asked online "How many COVID-19 deaths in Pennsylvania?" The reply was 707. The same question for NYC yields 11,407. That's quite a difference. NYC is very crowded, overcrowded I would say. That's a partial explanation for the quantity of deaths. I, personally, think that the hospitals are probably responsible for more of those deaths than would be admitted to. The point is obvious: your friend in PA is influenced by the death count in NYC, the media focuses on that because it's the most sensational — it's not, however, realistic for your friend to have the same fear wherever he lives. As I pointed out yesterday, there've only been 12 deaths in the county that includes Pittsburgh. Pittsburgh isn't the biggest city in the world but it's big enough to qualify as a city, it's just not overcrowded. People who are so afraid that they can't even take a detached look at the way they're being force-fed the very fear that they're feeling are Pavlovian dogs and little more than that. How have they gotten through their lives so far? It would be one thing if they were seeing people dropping dead in their immediate environment — but chances are their life is going on as normal EXCEPT FOR THE EXTERNALLY IMPOSED RESTRICTIONS which, of course, skew one's perceptions enormously. Here in Pittsburgh I'm trying to go about my life as I ordinarily would. I go for a walk every day, I don't wear gloves or a mask. I try to get together with my few friends when I can. I've been thinking of throwing a "Enter at your own risk" party but I doubt that anyone I know would come! It's pathetic to me that I have so few friends who're questioning this. Maybe there're more out there than I realize and I'm just not communicating with them.

****

April 18, 2020, 7:00AM (Dick to group):

Observation:

I imagine you all have heard about the "yellow vests" who for over a year were doing protests, sometimes even twice a week, against the policies of the French president Macron. The protests were about his privatizing industries like the airports, cutting back on social services like teachers and nurses and just before this coronavirus happened, he began attacking the retirement system. These things are sacrosanct here.
The police were very repressive, they were using rifles that shot what look like solid plastic tennis balls. With these guns, they put out around 30 people's eyes, broke jaws, knocked out teeth, etc. The cops are supposed only to shoot the chest area (which would be bad enough already, like being hit by a pro-boxer) but they didn't. Furthermore the interior minister who is named Castagner refused to even acknowledge the over use of force.
It's worth noting that Macron didn't do a single thing the yellow vests wanted, even using some special legal provision called 43-7 (or something like that) to push all his legislation through and bypass a real vote.
I'll be very curious to see if these protests resume. I wonder because since everyone is obeying this lock-down like sheep if it may take the wind out of their sails. That is, for around 16 months it was nothing but "fire Macron" but he gives the stay at home order and there's hardly a peep out of anyone.
I hope this won't be the case.

****

April 18, 2020, 8:36AM (Amir-ul Kafirs to group):

I hope this won't be the case.

I hope so too — but the way this coup is happening is 'diabolical'. Basically, if one resists it one becomes potentially stigmatized as an uncaring insane person willing to put everyone's health at risk and most people seem to believe that and roll over for it. It's funny how the same governments who don't seem to have any problem committing genocide in the name of the WAR AGAINST TERRORISM or whatever the flavor of the month is *are suddenly deemed believable when they express care about their people dying from disease.* Right. It's all about money and power just like it always is and always has been.

Truthfully, if there's a total lockdown I anticipate violating it. At 66 I'm in even less of a hurry to get shot or imprisoned than ever but, fuck, somebody's got to take the risk. Dying in rebellion against the police state IS NOT PREFERABLE TO **WINNING AGAINST THE POLICE STATE.** I can easily imagine this becoming mind-bogglingly ugly in short order. I truly hope it doesn't but what can a person do? These billionaires could care less about the peons. If they don't want us to die from disease it's only so we can be slaves.

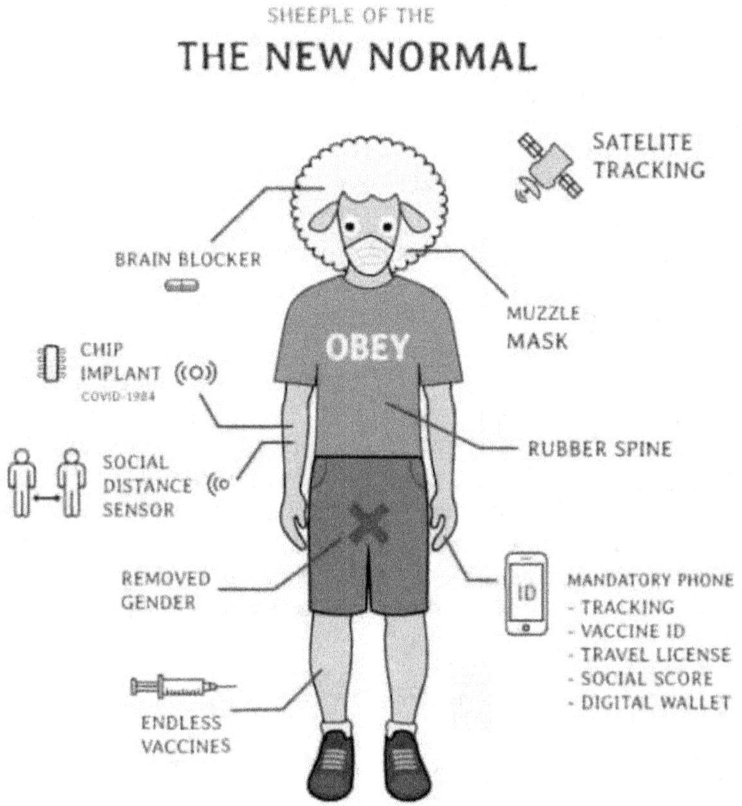

****

April 18, 2020, 9:16AM (Dick to group):

Protesting in France is strange
It took me time to get used to it
It is part of their culture, sometimes they are like parties
On any given day there could be many, many protest marches
"la rue" that is taking to the street is way the people traditionally let the politicians know how they felt and usually the politicians respond, at least to a degree
That isn't happening with Macron, he has an agenda and is just pushing it through
The yellow vest thing was pretty serious, at least it seemed that way to me
There were many working class people involved in the yellow vest demonstrations, I went to many
They were insulted by the power structure as being behind the times, not modern, etc like they were May '68 holdovers, like old morons who aren't into the exciting new European economic model, I recall some politician said they were computer illiterate, things like that
Anyway, there are a fair number of people who protest like a fashion statement, but also many who are really fighting to survive and maintain the social programs that were established after WWII
At least that's how it seems to me

****

April 18, 2020, 11:03AM (Amir-ul Kafirs to group):

HERETICS: Change.org

I assume you're all familiar with Change.org petitions. I sign them fairly often and get annoyed with them at other times. Today I was sent an email promoting a petition to give better COVID-19 coverage for "first responders". I call particular attention to: "_____ was finally cleared to be tested on March 23, when their spouse brought them to the emergency room. They were sedated, intubated, and placed in a medically induced coma. They died on March 31." My question is: *How many of these people dying are dying* ***because of the treatment?!*** Being placed in "a medically induced coma" doesn't really strike me as a good idea.

****

April 18, 2020, 1:34PM (BP to group):

Re: HERETICS: Change.org

I read it's a 20% survival rate for those placed on ventilators. A friend who knows tells me that when it comes to that at their hospital it's considered a Hail Mary Pass so I'm guessing even lower. Which from the media and focus on these damn machines, it's like it will save us all from the grave.

****

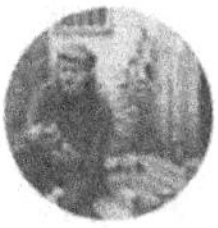

Ben Parsons
3 hrs ·

Believe it or not, it's actually ok to be all three.

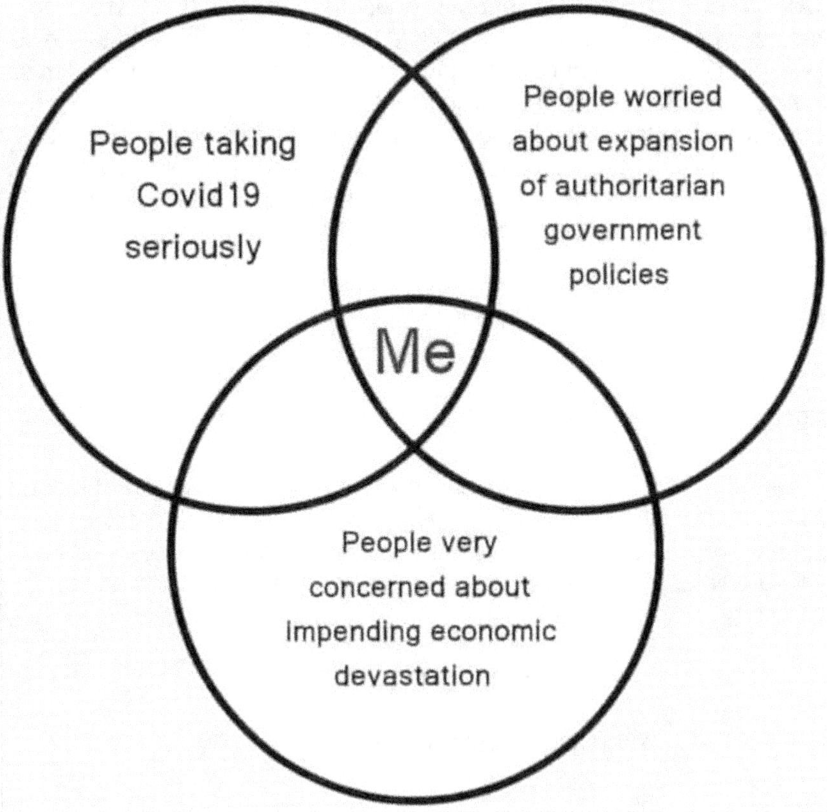

Jessica Mohon ▸ Michiganders Against Excessive Quarantine 22 hrs ·

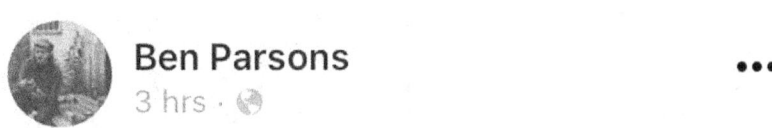

****

April 18, 2020, 1:45PM (Amir-ul to group):

HERETICS: Ventilators

On Apr 18, 2020, at 1:34 PM, brainpang brainpang <brainpang@comcast.net> wrote:
I read it's a 20% survival rate for those placed on ventilators. A friend who knows tells me that when it comes to that at her hospital it's considered a Hail Mary Pass so I'm guessing even lower. Which from the media and focus on these damn machines, it's like it will save us all from the grave.

Exactly. But I'll bet that every patient on a ventilator racks up a pretty high bill, eh?! There's this constant emphasis on **WE MUST GET MORE VENTILATORS TO SAVE THE PATIENTS!** I seriously doubt that. If everyone weren't so terrified I wonder how many of them would just stay at home. Would the survival rate be higher? Maybe not but we'll probably never find out, will we? I'm sure I've mentioned this before but it's worth reiterating: I watched my mom get steered toward death in the hospice, I think she would've lived longer if she'd just stayed home. Yeah, she would've been in more pain. The thing about pain is that you only feel it *when you're alive*, there's no pain (I assume) after death. So if you want to be alive and you're in pain at least you know you're alive.

****

April 18, 2020, 2:59PM (BP to group):

Re: HERETICS: Ventilators

I read something somewhere else about how the low survival rate of those placed on vents was shocking to the medical workers on the front line. To the point that there was question about if it was the right thing to do, there was something else at play why it didn't work. Sorry I don't bookmark these things and have links handy.

****

April 19, 2020, 1:11PM (**Naia Nisnam** to group):

Re: HERETICS: Ventilators

Hello Heretics!
I'm Amir-ul's Pennsylvania friend and I appreciate being added to this list.

I'll share some thoughts on ventilators. Here in the US, there's been a bidding "war" going on between states. States are bidding against each other to buy ventilators. Whether true are not, we are being told that ventilators are critical life-saving devices. The manufacturers of these machines aren't selling them to the states that "need" them the most. They are selling the machines to the highest bidder. Capitalism at its finest.

Basic NPR Marketplace story on the bidding war: https://www.marketplace.org/2020/04/01/ventilator-bidding-war-covid19/

Going with the idea we are supposed to accept- that we need ventilators to save lives- who is responsible for the making and selling of the machines? Should they be held accountable for preventing Americans from obtaining life-saving treatment? Governors in different states have been issuing executive orders preventing retail stores from artificially inflating the price of their products during the pandemic, yet medical supply companies are doing just that. I came across many articles about the price gouging but not a single one reported the name of the companies that are creating this problem. It is definitely big money on a global scale.

A little info on the 7 biggest ventilator manufactorers: https://www.nsmedicaldevices.com/analysis/seven-ventilator-manufacturers/
Are all of these companies guilty of price gouging "desperately needed" medical equipment? I assume so.

Early on, I had read about healthy rich people trying to buy ventilators direct from the manufacturer for their personal use. Unfortunately I've lost track of that story. I would love to know how many individuals bought personal ventilators, at what price, and from what manufacturer.

I am pointing to this bidding war issue as a problem with capitalism and the contradictions between what we are being told and what is actually happening.

I, personally, am not a believer in ventilators and am considering a face tattoo that reads "do not hook my body up to a ventilator".

Highlights from this New York Times article https://www.nytimes.com/2020/04/04/opinion/coronavirus-ventilators.html
"Nobody can tolerate being ventilated like this without sedation. Covid-19 patients are put into a medically induced coma before being placed on a ventilator. They do not suffer, but they cannot talk to us and they cannot tell us how much of this care they want."

"Even among the Covid-19 patients who are ventilated and then discharged from the intensive care unit, some have died within days from heart damage."

"Even before Covid-19, for those lucky enough to leave the hospital alive after suffering acute respiratory distress syndrome, recovery can take months or years. The amount of sedation needed for Covid 19 patients can cause profound complications, damaging muscles and nerves, making it hard for those who survive to walk, move or even think as well as they did before they became ill. Many spend most of their recovery time in a rehabilitation center, and older patients often never go home. They live out their days bed bound, at higher risk of recurrent infections, bed sores and trips back to the hospital."

"... we have to ask ourselves some serious questions: What do I value about my life? If I will die if I am not put in a medical coma and placed on a ventilator, do I want that life support? If I do choose to be placed on a ventilator, how far do I want to go? Do I want to continue on the machine if my kidneys shut down? Do I want tubes feeding me so I can stay on the ventilator for weeks?"

Perhaps it is for the best that we are dealing with a shortage of ventilators.

****

When articles are presented here they're usually only excerpted from with a date & author credit & a link so that the studious reader can find the entire article online. I use bracketed 2 dot ellipses "[..]" to signify missing passages.

How did we end up in a ventilator bidding war?

Marielle Segarra
Apr 1, 2020

Pretty much every day, New York Governor Andrew Cuomo says the same thing in his press briefings. The states all need ventilators and there aren't enough, so they've been competing.

"You now literally will have a company call you up and say, 'Well, California just outbid you.' Cuomo said at a press conference Tuesday. "It's like being on eBay, with 50 other states bidding on a ventilator."
California bids. Illinois bids. Florida bids. New York bids.

"California rebids. That's literally what we're doing." he said. "I mean, how inefficient."

As the number of COVID-19 cases rises, states are bracing for overwhelmed hospitals where there isn't a ventilator for everyone who needs one. That's what's behind this bidding war, which is driving ventilator prices sky high.

It's common for states to bid against each other for things like police cars and fire trucks and corporations.

"States competed over attracting Amazon and they compete over attracting other sorts of businesses all the time," said Ben Brunjes, who teaches public policy at the University of Washington.

But in an emergency situation, things are different. We're not talking about corporate tax incentives. These are ventilators that states and hospitals desperately need. It's life and death. And there's no choice — each state has to keep paying whatever it takes. They're on their own.

[..]

- https://www.marketplace.org/2020/04/01/ventilator-bidding-war-covid19/

****

The seven biggest medical ventilator manufacturers across the world by market share

DEVICESRESPIRATORY AND ANESTHESIA

By Jamie Bell 24 Mar 2020

Many heavyweights in the broader healthcare industry including Philips, Medtronic and Hamilton Medical also operate as ventilator manufacturers

The global coronavirus pandemic has put manufacturers under increased pressure to produce large numbers of medical ventilators — the sophisticated breathing circuits required by many critically ill patients.

With demand for ventilator devices at an all-time high, companies are working around the clock to increase production and build these life-saving machines as quickly as possible.

India-based market research firm Meticulous released a report earlier this year outlining the landscape of the ventilator market, including details of all the major global manufacturers.

Here we take a closer look at the seven biggest companies — in terms of market share — operating in this field.

Biggest ventilator manufacturers in the world

Becton Dickinson

US medtech giant Becton Dickinson is estimated to hold the largest market share of any company working in ventilator production in 2020.

[..]

Philips

Traditionally best-known for its work in the electronics sector — most notably with audio systems and lighting — the Dutch firm has increasingly turned its focus towards medical technology, and healthcare, in recent years.

[..]

Hamilton Medical

Hamilton Medical — a Swiss subsidiary of US biotech company Hamilton — specialises in the production of "intelligent ventilation solutions".

[..]

Fisher & Paykel Healthcare

New Zealand-based company Fisher & Paykel specialises in both hospital and at-home products.
Its devices include invasive and non-invasive ventilators for adults, as well as humidification and resuscitation for young patients and newborns.

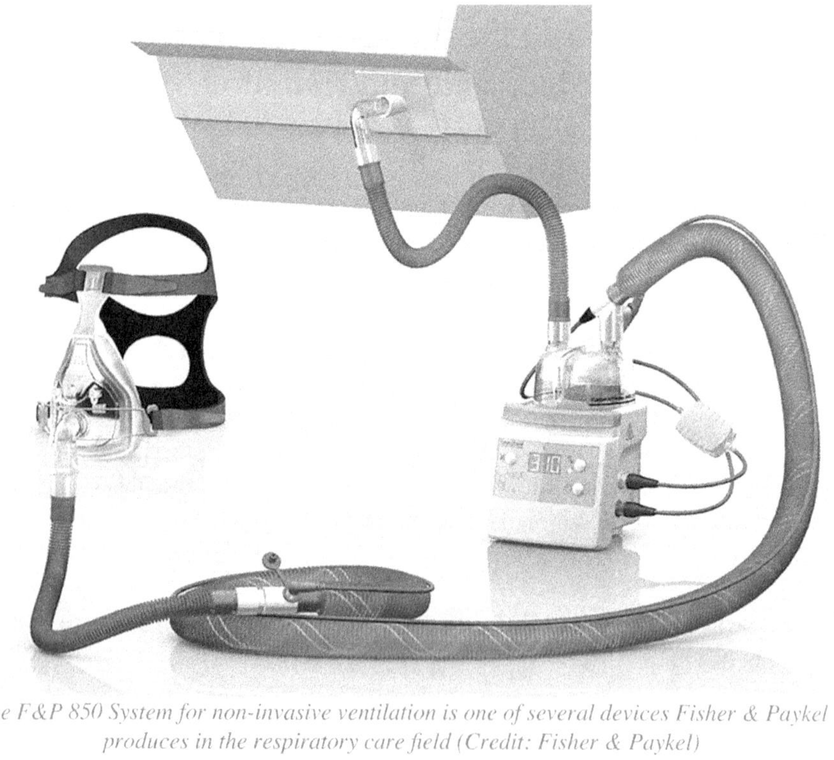

The F&P 850 System for non-invasive ventilation is one of several devices Fisher & Paykel produces in the respiratory care field (Credit: Fisher & Paykel)

[..]

Draeger

Firefighting, mining, and chemicals — specifically gas detection — are a handful of the sectors German tech company Draeger operates in.

[..]

Medtronic

Despite being headquartered in Ireland, Medtronic largely operates in the US. While the biotechnology firm works in a variety of sectors within healthcare, and predominantly treats chronic diseases, it also produces several ventilator products for use in acute care — short-term, active treatment for a serious illness.

[..]

GE Healthcare

GE Healthcare is a US-based biosciences company that specialises in diagnostics and medical imaging.

[..]

- https://www.nsmedicaldevices.com/analysis/seven-ventilator-manufacturers/

****

What You Should Know Before You Need a Ventilator

It breaks my heart that patients who will get sick enough to need them won't know what desperate situations they face.

By Kathryn Dreger April 4, 2020

Dr. Dreger is a doctor of internal medicine in Northern Virginia and a clinical assistant professor of medicine at Georgetown University.

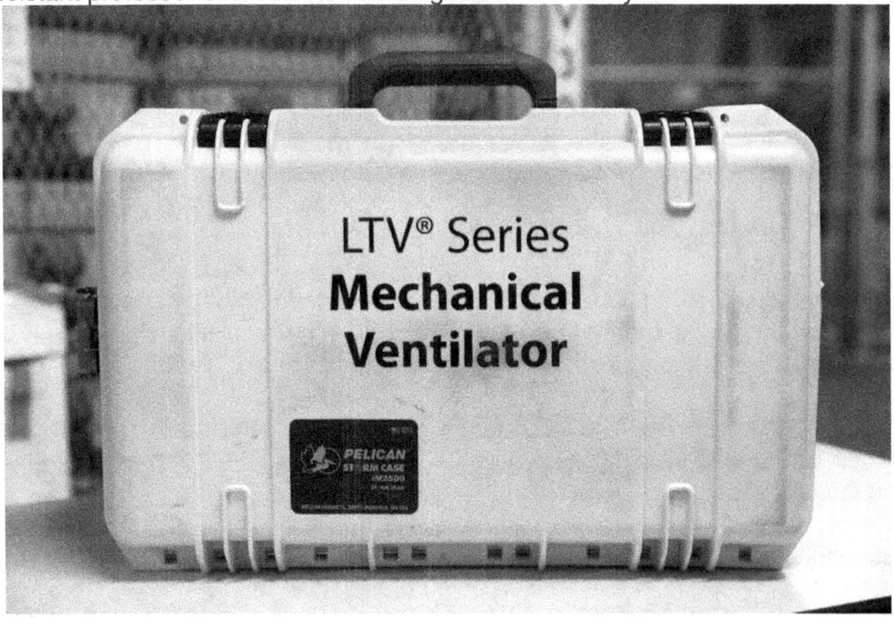

A ventilator at the New York City Emergency Management Warehouse before being shipped out for distribution. Credit...Caitlin Ochs/Reuters

Day by day, as the number of Covid-19 deaths soar, we see more clearly that many of us will not survive this storm.

In the most serious cases, breathing becomes so labored that ventilators have to be used to keep patients alive. That there may not be enough of these machines is horrifying and infuriating.

But even if there were, it breaks my heart that Americans who get sick enough to need them won't know what desperate situations they face, nor will they understand what ventilators can do to help, and what they can never fix.

As hard as the facts may be, knowledge will make us less afraid.

Let me begin simply. When we take a breath, we pull air through our windpipe, the trachea. This pipe then branches in two, then again into smaller and smaller pipes finally ending in tiny tubes less than a millimeter across called bronchioles. At the very end of each are clusters of microscopic sacs called alveoli.

The lining of each sac is so thin that air floats through them into the red blood cells. These millions of alveoli are so soft, so gentle, that a healthy lung has almost no substance. Touching it feels like reaching into a bowl of whipped cream.

Covid-19 changes all that.

It causes a gummy yellow fluid, called exudate, to fill the air sacs, stopping the free flow of oxygen. If only a few air sacs are filled, the rest of the lung takes over. When more and more alveoli are filled, the lung texture changes, beginning to feel more like a marshmallow than whipped cream.

This terrible disease is called acute respiratory distress syndrome. Covid-19 can cause an incredibly lethal form of this, in which oxygen levels plunge and breathing becomes impossible without a ventilator.

Specially trained health care workers insert a 10-inch-long tube connected to a ventilator through the mouth and into the windpipe. The ventilator delivers more oxygen into the lungs at pressure high enough to open up the stiffened lungs.

It's called life support for a reason; it buys us time. Ventilators keep oxygen going to the brain, the heart and the kidneys. All while we hope the infection will ease, and the lungs will begin to improve.

These machines can't fix the terrible damage the virus is causing, and if the virus erupts, the lungs will get even stiffer, as hard as a stale marshmallow."I feel like I'm trying to ventilate bricks instead of lungs," one intensive care unit doctor who has been treating Covid-19 patients told me.

The heart begins to struggle, begins to fail. Blood pressure readings plummet, a condition called shock. For some, the kidneys fail completely, which means a dialysis machine is also needed to survive.

Doctors are left with impossible choices. Too much oxygen poisons the air sacs, worsening the lung damage, but too little damages the brain and kidneys. Too much air pressure damages the lung, but too little means the oxygen can't get in. Doctors try to optimize, to tweak.

Nobody can tolerate being ventilated like this without sedation. Covid-19 patients are put into a medically induced coma before being placed on a ventilator. They do not suffer, but they cannot talk to us and they cannot tell us how much of this care they want.

Eventually, all the efforts of health care workers may not be enough, and the body begins to collapse. No matter how loved, how vital or how needed a person is, even the most modern technology isn't always enough. Death, while typically painless, is no less final.

Even among the Covid-19 patients who are ventilated and then discharged from the intensive care unit, some have died within days from heart damage.

[..]

- https://www.nytimes.com/2020/04/04/opinion/coronavirus-ventilators.html

****

April 19, 2020, 4:32PM (Amir-ul Kafirs to group):

Re: HERETICS: Ventilators

Thanks Naia Nisnam, I really appreciate the extent of your research here. As you know, I've been talking against ventilators from the beginning.

****

April 19, 2020, 6:32PM (Amir-ul Kafirs to group):

Re: HERETICS: Ventilators

On Apr 19, 2020, at 6:09 PM, Inquiring Librarian wrote:

My mom worked as a cardiac care and Icu nurse for many years. I'm almost afraid to ask her what she experienced with ventilators.

I'd love to have her input. I asked my respiratory therapist friend whether he thought they did any good & he said that people wouldn't be surviving without them but when I asked him what his sense of the actual survival rate on ventilators is in Pittsburgh he told me that he didn't really have access to the necessary info so he couldn't tell me. That struck me as invalidating his opinion that they're helpful.

Here's the latest Allegheny County Statistics:

Allegheny County on Sunday reported three more deaths from the coronavirus, bringing the countywide total to 50. The 50 people who have died range in age from 56 to 103 years old, with the most deaths occurring in people over 70, county data show.
- https://triblive.com/local/pittsburgh-allegheny/allegheny-county-reports-3-more-coronavirus-deaths-total-cases-up-to-1035/

That's from the most right wing of the local mainstream news sources.

& here's info about the number of ventilators available & in use:

Here is the full breakdown of hospital capacity in Allegheny County, according to the state data:

Available Adult ICU Beds: 338, **Available Medical/Surgical Beds**: 1,530, **Available Pediatric ICU Beds:** 9, **Available Airborne Isolation Room Beds:** 143, **Ventilators Available:** 785, **Ventilators In Use (COVID-19)**34, **Ventilators In Use (non-COVID-19): ALL** 156

According to the database, 1,979 Pennsylvanians are hospitalized due to COVID-19 as of Thursday morning. Of those, 584 are on a ventilator. The state's hospitals have 5,141 ventilators. Of those, 1,472 are in use for both COVID and non-COVID patients. The state currently has 1,711 — or 40 percent — of adult ICU beds available.

- https://patch.com/pennsylvania/pittsburgh/coronavirus-allegheny-countys-icu-bed-ventilator-numbers

That suggests to me that people on ventilators AREN'T dying so I really don't know what to make of it all.

****

April 19, 2020, 6:20PM (Inquiring Librarian to group):

News from Louisiana

Although Louisiana is extending its stay at home order until May 15th, I see things winding down here. We are certainly not as strict as what Dick is experiencing in Paris. We have no row houses. Most neighborhoods are single or double homes. We do have high rises, and we do have large apartment complexes. But, I'd say our population density is not very compact. I suspect our worse is over.

I've been thrown back on these messages a few days due to a 14 page document with signatures needed from Louisiana that is trying to help to keep us getting paid. I hope this works. I need my job. As a non-essential municipal worker, my prospects of keeping employed are grim without a federal bailout to local governments... please cross your fingers for us all here in Louisiana. Our worst enemy now is a collapsing economy.

That tangent being spewed out there, I found this article in a Louisiana newspaper this morning on Nola.com. it is the first I've seen of a mass publication allowing any press in support of opening up:
https://www.theadvocate.com/baton_rouge/news/coronavirus/article_b68df25e-7ff4-11ea-8d67-cba110feacff.html?utm_medium=social&utm_source=nolafb&utm_campaign=snd&fbclid=IwAR0aZoEMY2yTWBHwZSfbjHscyfKIp5QbkN4PRIVixLI8nA0OJhf4WqDkLjQ

****

April 19, 2020, 6:42AM (Amir-ul Kafirs to group):

Re: News from Louisiana

Thanks for that. I'm told that at the moment the governor of Pennsylvania hasn't extended the April 30, 2020, deadline for the lockdown here. I hope that's true. None of the extreme predictions of quantities of death and overcrowding of hospitals have come true as far as I know. I read the article that you linked to. It seems very safely middle-of-the-road to me so maybe that's an indication that 'your average person' is beginning to perceive this situation with less fear.

****

April 19, 2020, 8:41PM (Inquiring Librarian to group):

Re: News from Louisiana

In response to Amir-ul Kafir's observation that the article was middle of the road... You should see how vicious the comments are in response to the article on nola.com's social media page. It is a bunch of robot brain-washed types spewing venom at the author and acting like scientific authorities and angelic do-gooders against this evil columnist. It's pretty nauseating to read the comments. But, you see there are many thumbs up and several hearts in reaction to the comment. I perceive that the people who gave the positive thumbs up and heart feedback are afraid to actually write out their thoughts, for fear of being bullied online.

I meant also to include in the previous email that our governor is not asking or requiring that Louisiana residents wear masks. I heard him being asked the question directly about wearing masks in our most recent "Ask the Governor" late this week. He gave a resounding no, that he would not make us wear masks.

I go to my local uptown Audubon park every day to jog and bike. I see about a 25 percent mask wearing population in the park. When I go to grocery stores, it's about a 75% mask wearing conformity. I honestly get a little panicky when I wear a mask. I feel suffocated when I cover my nose, and due to thyroid issues and past goiters, I have a hard time covering my neck if I wear a full face and neck garb. I am working on getting over these mask-problems in an effort to be more courteous to my fellow grocery store shoppers. It is maybe the right thing to do to ease other people's fears.

Ok, I just spent the last 3 hours applying for library positions in a neighboring parish... just in case... Worrying about total loss of income is exhausting. I have a horrible headache.

****

April 20, 2020, 5:29AM (Amir-ul Kafirs accidentally just to Inquiring Librarian):

Re: News from Louisiana

In response to Amir-ul Kafirs's observation that the article was middle of the road...

I should clarify, in case it's not obvious, that I wasn't criticizing it for that, I just meant that I didn't feel like he went out on any limbs that could be identified as "left" or "right" wing & that he was toeing a common sense line — apparently in the hope of bringing some reason to the situation.

You should see how vicious the comments are

I won't look at them but I believe you. Unfortunately, I think this situation has 'brought out the worst' in many or most people, once again exposing them as robopaths & untertan — a situation that I'm all too familiar with. I've always thought that the veneer of 'civilization' is just a tiny sliver away from 'turning ugly', turning nazi, turning mob frenzy, etc.. That's one of the reasons why I don't have faith in 'the people' even though I'm all for egalitarianism. My whole life I've seen instances over & over again where mob mentality takes over & people become even more dangerously stupid than ever. Now is one of those times.

I perceive that the people who gave the positive thumbs up and heart feedback are afraid to actually write out their thoughts, for fear of being bullied online.

I think more people should have the strength to resist bullying. The more people cower, the more they're defeated. Bullies rely on having their power reinforced by other cowards. I remember one time I was riding in the back of the bus in Pittsburgh & there were these 2 guys, maybe brothers. One of them appeared to be 'retarded', the other one started ridiculing me & trying to get the 'retarded' one to join in. The 'retarded' guy wasn't having it. What happened instead is that the 'retarded' guy talked about his poetry & about how he didn't have anyplace to read it so I told him about a possible venue & he appreciated that. We both ignored the bully. The beauty of the moment was that everyone in the back of the bus could see how it was all going down & everyone shunned the bully & proceeded to have a friendly conversation with each other. I think the bully was completely taken aback & didn't expect this outcome at all.

He gave a resounding no, that he would not make us wear masks.

That's a really good sign. Unfortunately, it's the opposite here. I'm told that as of 8PM last night a person can no longer legally enter a store without a mask on.

I have a hard time covering my neck if I wear a full face and neck garb.

I'm not convinced that they're even healthy. Then again, I have the heretical position that exposure to one's environment, as long as it's not totally toxicly polluted (which I don't believe it is here), is a mild innoculative process & that this medical industry induced sterlization frenzy has the opposite effect of undermining one's immune system.

It is maybe the right thing to do to ease other people's fears.

Honestly, I can't agree with you there. Literally my whole life I've had people telling me things like 'You're scaring me' to which I sometimes reply: 'No, you're scared but I'm not responsible for that.' if a racist white woman is scared that a black man is going to rape her that's not his fault & shouldn't be his problem either. She makes it his problem because her fear might result in behavior that endangers him — such as by calling the police on him.

****

April 20, 2020, 1:56PM (Amir-ul Kafirs to group):

Re: HERETICS: brainwashed

This is the kind of hopelessly stupid conversation that I keep finding myself in:

all covid deniers deserve to catch the thing. it's a truly wonderful experience from what I gather.

Are there COVID-19 deniers? I don't have any problem accepting that an epidemic of a virus exists & that people with weakened immune systems are dying once they get it. I don't personally know anyone who denies that. I DO have 2 friends who've been sick, they're both very close to me, they're both in their early 40s. At least one of them was told by their doctor that it was COVID-19 although they weren't tested. They said they were sick for 3 or 4 miserable days but that it was just like other flus that they've had. They still self-isolated for 2 weeks to be on the safe side. Their 6 year old child was also sick. They're fine now too. They had to take care of their child while they were both sick.

At any rate, the statement above is the sort of thing I hear all the time. All people who don't believe in God should go to Hell too. Why wish an illness on someone? I've had pneumonia twice. The 1st time my right lung was completely out of order & my left lung was half-full of fluid. At the same time I had appendicitis. I would've died if I hadn't gone to the hospital. It was definitely a miserable experience. Nonetheless, I don't wish it on other people so they can understand what I went through, nor do I care whether they even believe whether I went through it or not. It's a part of my life, it gave me a 'healthy respect' for pneumonia, that's it.

****

April 20, 2020, 6:30PM (Inquiring Librarian to group):

Re: HERETICS: brainwashed

Well said Amir-ul Kafirs! I am so afraid to make any mention to anyone but my family and my significant other about my opinions on the situation. As a Civil Servant for the State of Louisiana, I cannot afford to let anyone know my opinion, beyond why can't any of us be given antibody tests... doesn't anyone think that that so-called 'herd' immunity is happening?. My social media page is all flora, fauna, and yoga.

This is why this email group is so important to me. I feel like I am living in a vacuum where I cannot share or commiserate on an independent intellectual thought. Granted, I've contributed little 'intellectually' to this conversation string. I appreciate all of your efforts. I think I am too stressed out about my job, losing my health insurance, and constant battles with shingles during this situation. I've doven into lace tatting, over exercising, listing to NPR for some shred of mass recovery brain-washing seeds to start sprouting, and reading the absolutely unrelated to today's world 700 pg. novel of Anne Bronte's "The Tenant of Wildfell Hall".

****

April 20, 2020, 6:30PM (Dick to group):

RE: HERETICS: brainwashed

"The French Touch"....

translations (see photo below)

Cover text: "Spice up your confined evenings"

How to choose the right Covid mask (the KKK photo)

The pink circle on the cover says " one free sheet of toilet paper included"

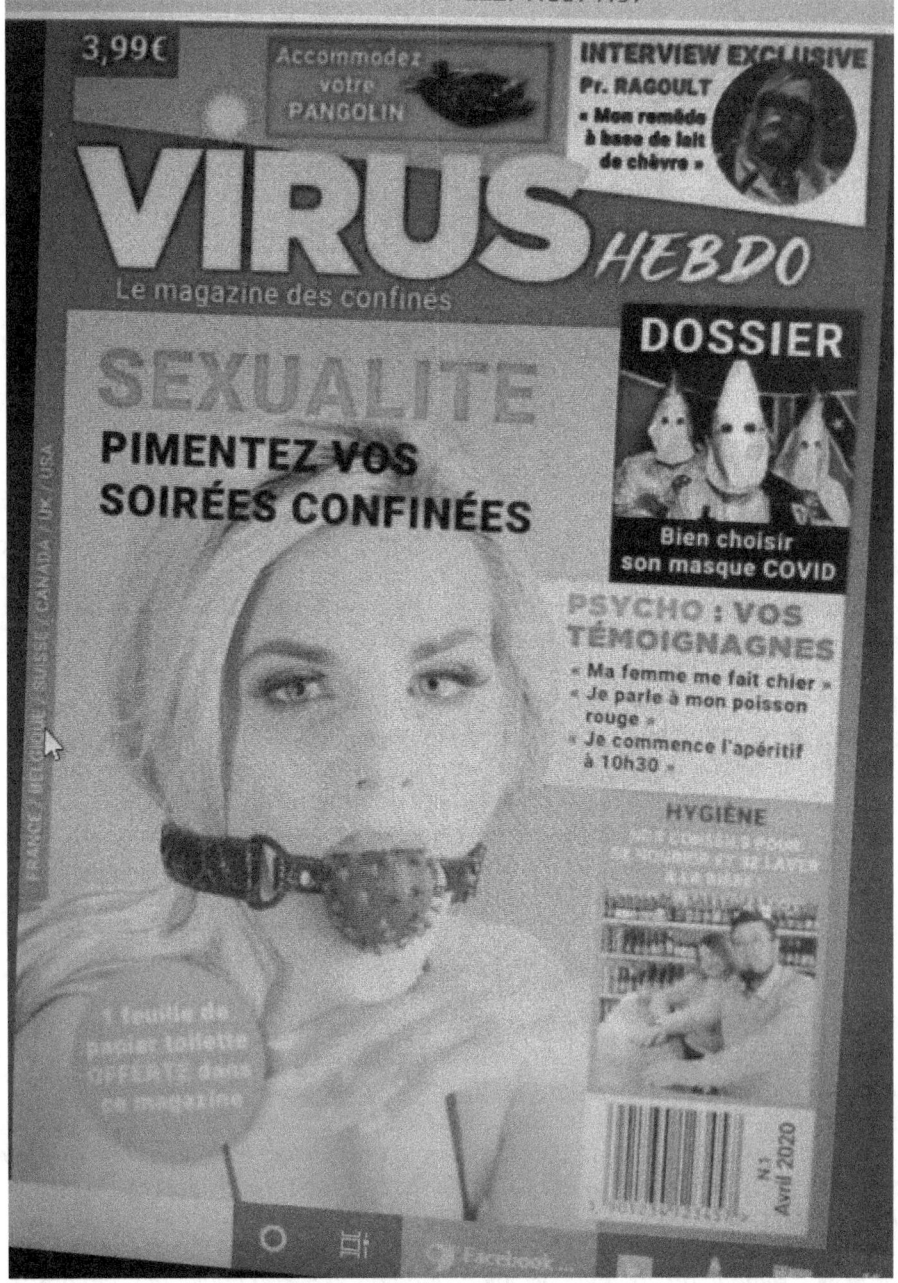

Psycho: Vos témoinagnes (psychology, your stories)

My wife irritates me (literally "my wife make me shit", wife jokes, strangely enough, seem never to go away here...)
I speak to my goldfish
I start drinking at 10:30 am

Exclusive interview - Dr Ragoult (the Dr. who said he'd found that the drug chloroxyquinine was useful
"My treatment using goat's milk"

Hygiene- "information on how to eat and to wash your hands using beer"

I don't get the one about Pangolin, it's some type of African animal

****

April 20, 2020, 8:02PM (Amir-ul Kafirs to group):

Re: HERETICS: brainwashed

Well said Amir-ul Kafirs!

Thank you. I continue to try to not even argue with people. I just give them the basis for my own opinion. E.G.: The same friend quoted in the previous email made a statement that 41,000 people had died in the US & that in 2 weeks more would die than American soldiers in the Vietnam War. I said that that was a prediction & then I mentioned that some of the predictions (& I was specific) hadn't come true so maybe his wouldn't either. I then mentioned that the CDC website says that in the 2017-2018 flu season 61,000 Americans died. THEREFORE, I continued, COVID-19 was only 2/3rds of the way to that so far. I said that I didn't remember there being a quarantine in 2017-2018 or this level of panic. My friend didn't respond to any of that. Instead, he sent me an email saying something like 'I guess I'm just better informed than you.' I DIDN'T REPLY: *Yep, that's the only possible explanation for someone disagreeing with you!* Instead, I just let that go. THEN HE SENT ME A LINK TO AN ARTICLE ABOUT A GROUP OF PEOPLE HARRASSING A NURSE. The subject was "You Happy Now?" as if, of course!, this was what I must be doing! All this because he can't browbeat me into submission. It's tempting to reply:

Yeah, I admit, I actually funded that harrassment. I specifically asked those people to call themeselves the ***Richard Speck Divine Vengeance Militia*** *& I told them that they had to gangrape ALL the nurses before beheading them & giving their heads to their kids. Shit, they didn't do it so I'm thinking about asking for my money back. What do you think about my funding a Concentration Camp in your name? You could be the Commandante & you could imprison there anyone who gives you statistics that go contrary to yours. Then you could inject them with industrial strength COVID-19 & deny them medical care until they agree with everything you say! Wouldn't it be great? You could let them die anyway but you could charge them for it.*

So, I DIDN'T SAY THAT. Instead I just sent that graphic that I made that says: Groupthink is intolerant of differing opinions. From now on I just won't reply. I feel bad to lose an old friend like that but, wow, there's only so much beliigerent browbeating that I'll tolerate & I really don't want to respond to obvious chain-pulling provocations.

This is why this email group is so important to me.

That honestly makes me very happy. I started this group just so we'd be able to talk freely with each other & share ideas. The level of bullying & intolerance out & about is amazing.

Granted, I've contributed little 'intellectually' to this conversation string.

I appreciate everything you write here. I appreciate that you take the time to articulate your thoughts. They aren't lost on me.

****

April 23, 2020, 10:00PM (Amir-ul Kafirs to group):

On Apr 20, 2020, at 11:05 PM, Inquiring Librarian wrote:

This has got to be the most HILARIOUS [potential] response ever!!!! Everytime i read it i can't stop laughing. I am currently part choking on my white sausage & salad dinner! I just spit up a menacing chunk of mushroom. I can actually hear and see you saying this.

THANKS! It just boggles my mind how quickly any sort of sense goes by the wayside. Because I disagree with my (ex-)friend I'm obviously now guilty of whatever crimes he wants to ascribe to me. I DO think that my "*Yeah, I admit, I actually funded that harrassment. I specifically asked those people to call themselves the **Richard Speck Divine Vengeance Militia*** " is a 'nice touch'. Too bad my (ex-)friend'll never see it, I just trash his emails now and I'll never answer him again.

****

April 20, 2020, 9:44PM (Inquiring Librarian to group):

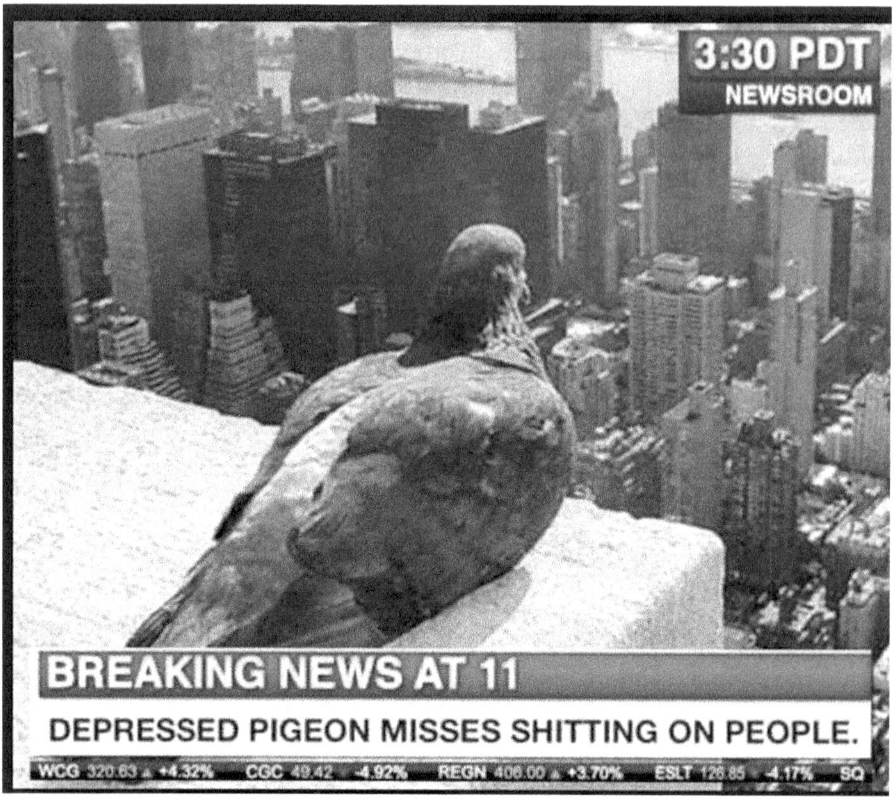

****

April 21, 2020, 10:54AM (Amir-ul Kafirs to group):

Re: HERETICS: brainwashed

On Apr 21, 2020, at 10:46 AM, BP wrote:

I think the Democrat supporting types are in a real mind bind as the media is portraying those against the lock down as Tea Party Redux. So in their minds the freedom to go fishing in the middle of nowhere equates to support for Trump. It's like the Russia thing again.

I hesitate writing this as I don't want this thread to go into the mainstream left/ right fight for power. I run screaming from that sort of stuff.

It's the usual gross oversimplifying that the Sound Byte mentality thrives on. Everything gets reduced down to either/or. The result, of course, is that more complex arguments, arguments that take into consideration a larger variety of factors get lost — largely because it's taken for granted that people's tiny minds are incapable of handling them but also, I think, because the populace is easier to manipulate if it's forced into one of 2 possible positions. Hence the 2 party system. *If you're not for us you're against us!* But what if we're neither/.or?

****

April 21, 2020, 11:43AM (Naia Nisnam to group):

Siri Screenshots

A few days ago, my 6-year old said “I love you”. The Siri app on my phone picked up their words and responded both on the phone screen and speaking aloud through my phone. It was very sci-fi so we tried a few different things. “I love you” gave us 3 different responses. Other simple cues (“good morning” for example) did not result in corona-related responses.

Here are screen shots of Siri’s great concern for our health and safety.

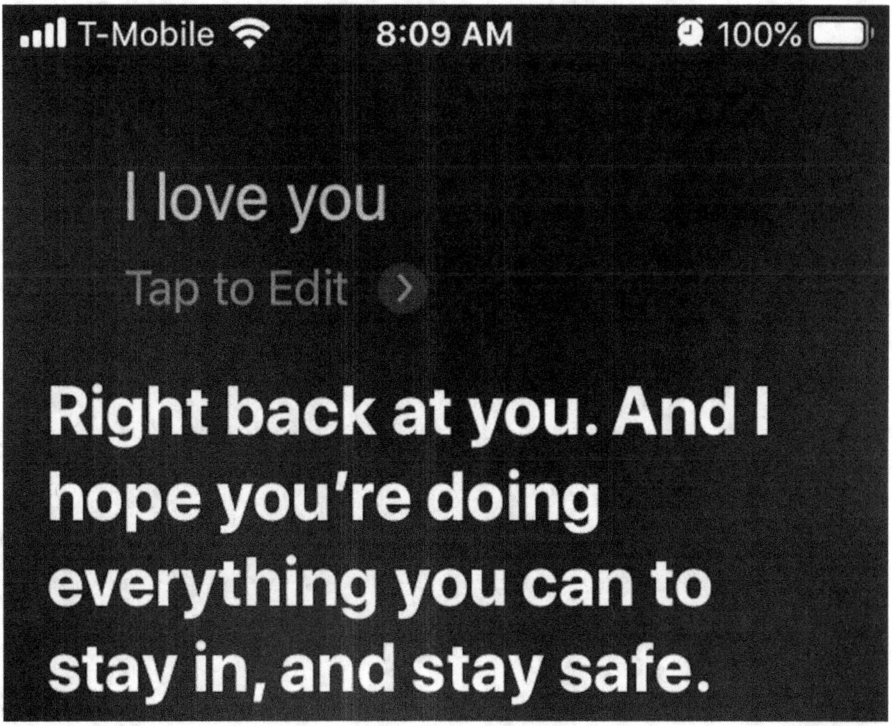

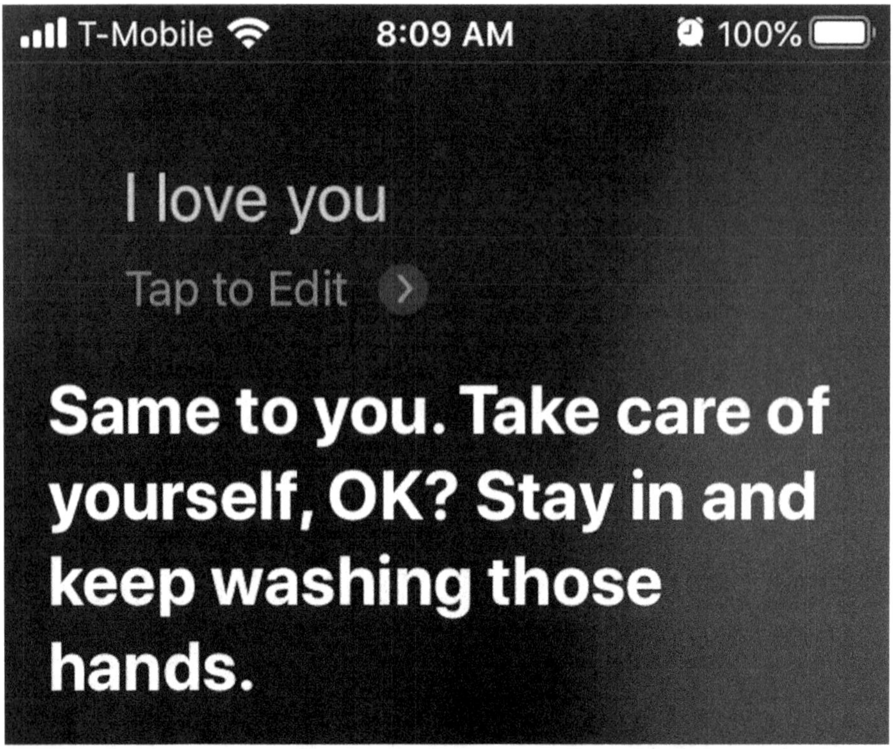
T-Mobile
8:09 AM
100%
I love you
Tap to Edit
Same to you. Take care of yourself, OK? Stay in and keep washing those hands.

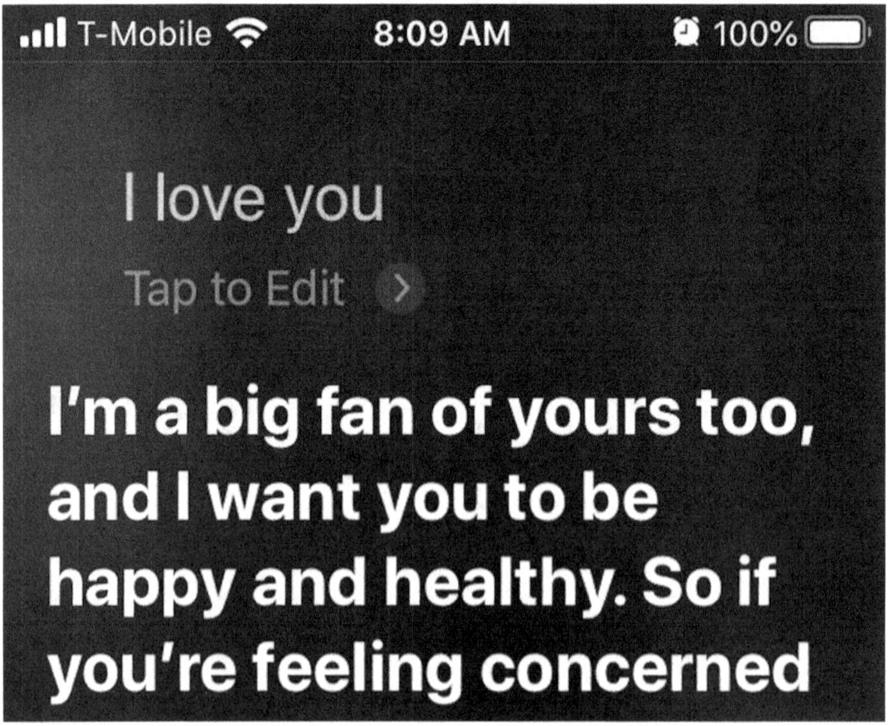
T-Mobile
8:09 AM
100%
I love you
Tap to Edit
I'm a big fan of yours too, and I want you to be happy and healthy. So if you're feeling concerned

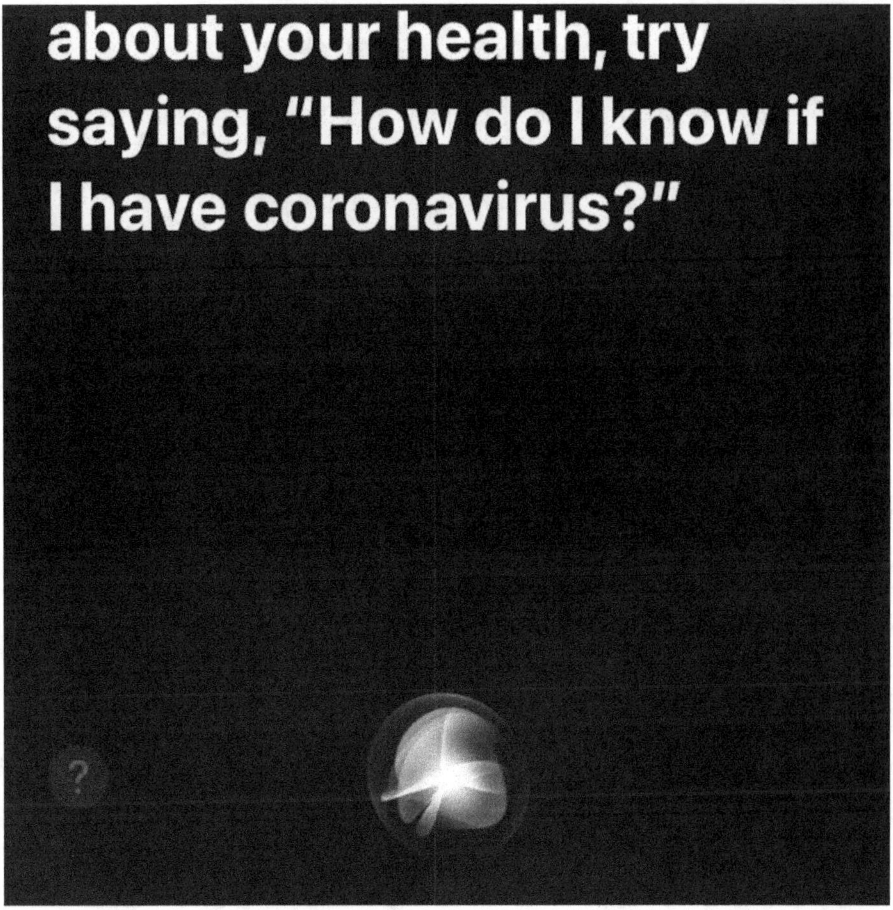

****

April 21, 2020, 11:47AM (BP to group):

Re: Siri Screenshots

And the people who designed that are patting themselves on the back. Creeps!

some good news in my area: 80 to 85%!

Health officials said another 177 area residents have died of COVID-19, pushing the state's death total to 4,377. At least 88,806 have tested positive since March 4, though 80 to 85% of cases are mild or moderate. https://www.nj.com/coronavirus/2020/04/coronavirus-updates-4377-deaths-in-nj-furloughs-possible-for-100k-state-workers-trump-suspends-immigration-what-you-need-to-know-april-21-2020.html

And how many are asymptomatic?

****

April 21, 2020, 11:52AM (Inquiring Librarian to group):

Re: Siri Screenshots

Those messages are so creepy!!!!!

I have stopped bringing my cell phone on my daily bike rides/jogs in Audubon Park. Louisiana has been tracking and broadcasting stats from resident cell phones to rate how well residents are following stay at home orders.

****

April 21, 2020, 12:38PM (Amir-ul Kafirs to group):

Re: Siri Screenshots

Of course, I think that those Siri responses are both hilarious and disturbing. Siri is positioning itself as something to be "loved". This anthropomorphizing is dangerous, especially when it's directed at little kids, because it's a form of psychological conditioning to get people to emotionally accept a remote form of authority.

****

April 21, 2020, 12:38PM (Naia Nisnam to group):

Re: Siri Screenshots

Inquiring Librarian-
The Louisiana government is openly tracking cell phones? That is terrifying. They realize now just how complacent Americans are.

Also, I feel you in appreciating this outlet. My social media page is also mainly fluffy photos of nature and my children. I am a teacher of toddlers and many school parents and staff look at my posts.

I read about things and think critically, but have almost no outlet to share my ideas, besides Amir-ul Kafirs (whom i am so grateful for), a friend in rural Michigan and a conservative pal in rural PA. Many of my friends had called themselves anarchists but... now they are eating up every word the government and mass media are telling them. If I openly expressed a free thought I would be considered a Trump-loving granny killer.
Life has become quite strange.

****

April 21, 2020, 12:49PM (Inquiring Librarian to group):

Re: Siri Screenshots

Hi Naia Nisnam & co.,

Yes. The Louisiana Governor has nonchalantly openly stated this. Unless i am reading this article wrong, it is happening nationwide:

https://www.wwltv.com/mobile/article/news/health/coronavirus/louisiana-gets-d-grade-for-social-distancing-new-orleans-a-minus/289-66a8013c-a528-4fac-9057-9e480a457bfc

****

Louisiana gets D-grade for social distancing; New Orleans A-minus

Using anonymous cell phone data, Unacast tracks mobility nationwide, comparing the amount of movement before the pandemic and movement now.

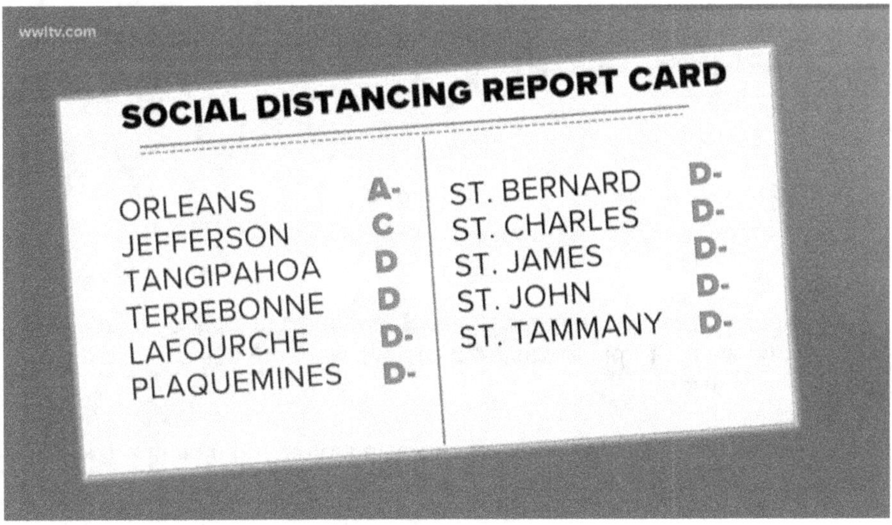

Author: **Devin Bartolotta**
Published: **10:11 PM CDT April 3, 2020**
Updated: **10:12 PM CDT April 3, 2020**

As more parishes tighten restrictions on day-to-day life, technology is outing those who disobey stay-at-home orders.
A data-science company called Unacast has developed a Social Distancing

Scoreboard.

[..]

The report card for Louisiana changed by the end of his press conference. As of 9 p.m. Friday, Louisiana earns a D grade

[..]

Police Chief Randy Fandal posted a video on Facebook Friday, pleading for people to stay home.

"I know this is hard. We live in South Louisiana. We're used to having parties, crawfish boils, and enjoying each other's company," said Fandal. "I'm ready, more than anyone, to get my life back to normal. But we can't until we flatten this damn curve."

New Orleans Police not only arrested two people after a repast in the city last weekend, but it has also responded to about 800 calls about large gatherings this week alone.

[..]

There are similar tools popping up online — like Google's Community Mobility Report — which tracks visits to parks and grocery stores.

****

April 21, 2020, 12:24PM (Naia Nisnam to group):

Upping the numbers

The original prediction for the number of U.S. deaths was 100,000 to 200,000. By the second week of April, it was clear that we were not going to see those numbers. Fauci said:

“I don't know exactly what the numbers are going to be, but right now it looks like it's going to be less than the original projection.”

Good news right? Well.... maybe we can bump the numbers up a bit. We don't want people to think there was a big fuss made over nothing, right? So on April 15th the U.S. figured out how to add "thousands" to the number of CoVID-19 cases and deaths, by including people who did not test positive (I'm thinking that means people who were not tested at all) but showed signs of having the virus.
https://www.cnn.com/2020/04/15/health/us-coronavirus-deaths-trends-wednesday/index.html

So.... "signs of having the virus".... the common symptoms are "fever, tiredness, and a dry cough".

So anyone who has seen a medical professional and complained of a fever and cough are now added to the stats. I found one CNN article promoting this as a good idea. It doesn't seem to have been big news and I'm thinking that the majority of people are not aware of how these numbers are being skewed.

I did come across some information saying that hospitals get extra federal money for each coronavirus case that they treat. I can't find the article again **[More information of the state-by-state breakdown of CARES money given per COVID-19 patient appears elsewhere in this book]** but Id like to. What an extra motivator to inflate those numbers. A fever and a cough gets the hospital more money, without testing....

AND EVEN MORE DISTURBING:

The CDC director explaining why he thinks the U.S. has had less cases than the predicted 1-200,000:

"The early predictions of the COVID-19's expected death toll in the U.S. assumed about half of Americans "would pay attention to the recommendations,"

but......

"What we're seeing is a large majority of the American public are taking the social distancing recommendations to heart,"

The U.S. government expected about half of Americans to comply. The U.S. government Underestimated how compliant their citizens are. Make no further mistakes- "the large majority of the American public" are obedient non-questioning sheep, desperate for rules to keep everyone safe. Great. People complied more than the government expected. The number of cases and of deaths is far lower than predicted. The government has had to change the rules on what qualifies as a corona-case to get those numbers back up, lest we think we stayed inside for months for no real reason.

****

April 24, 2020, 10:56PM (Amir-ul Kafirs to group):

HERETICS: Upping the numbers

The original prediction for the number of U.S. deaths was 100,000 to 200,000.

As of today, April 24, 2020, the CDC's figure for US deaths from COVID-19 is 24,555. That's a much lower figure than you may've already encountered. Consider this chart:

Table 1. Deaths involving coronavirus disease 2019 (COVID-19), pneumonia, and influenza reported to NCHS by week ending date, United States. Week ending 2/1/2020 to 4/18/2020.*

Data as of April 24, 2020

Week ending date in which the death occurred	COVID-19 Deaths (U07.1)[1]	Deaths from All Causes	Percent of Expected Deaths[2]	Pneumonia Deaths (J12.0–J18.9)[3]	Deaths with Pneumonia and COVID-19 (J12.0–J18.9 and U07.1)[3]	Influenza Deaths (J09–J11)[4]	Deaths with Pneumonia, Influenza, or COVID-19 (U07.1 or J09–J18.9)[5]
Total Deaths	**24,555**	654,798	96	54,962	11,070	5,571	73,358

Note that the highest figure is "Deaths with pnemonia, Influenza, or COVID-19". Note that PNEUMONIA is the highest individual figure. COVID-19 is less than HALF that number. I've looked at this page of statistics before & I don't remember that distinction having been made but maybe it was & I just didn't notice.

Fauci said:

"I don't know exactly what the numbers are going to be, but right now it looks like it's going to be less than the original projection."

Good news right? Well.... maybe we can bump the numbers up a bit.

https://www.cnn.com/2020/04/15/health/us-coronavirus-deaths-trends-wednesday/index.html

According to the article Naia Nisnam provided the link to,

"New York Gov. Andrew Cuomo announced Wednesday that the state will begin counting probable deaths, based on the CDC's guidance.

The CDC count is 605,390 cases of novel coronavirus in the United States and 24,582 people deaths.

According to Johns Hopkins University -- data used by CNN -- at least 637,000 people have contracted the novel coronavirus in the US, and 28,364 people have died."

Note that the CDC death count as of the date of that article, 9 days ago on April 15, was HIGHER than the CDC death count as of today. I'd like to think that the CDC is trying to be more accurate as time goes by. If that's the case, then the current death count is about 2/5ths of the flu death count of a mere 2 years ago.

So anyone who has seen a medical professional and complained of a fever and cough are now added to the stats. I found one CNN article promoting this as a good idea.

Note also that CNN uses statistics that it gets from Johns Hopkins, the place where the simulated corona virus outbreak 'game' known as "Event 201" happened.

It doesn't seem to have been big news and I'm thinking that the majority of people are not aware of how these numbers are being skewed.

Once upon a time it seemed to be fairly common knowledge that statistics could be skewed to prove just about anything. Nonetheless, most of us, including myself, use them. I do look for things that take into consideration greater detail, though, such as the multiple death categories in the screen shot of the CDC chart I provided above. The less the stats seem like a sound byte, the more I trust them.

The government has had to change the rules on what qualifies as a corona-case to get those numbers back up, lest we think we stayed inside for months for no real reason.

Unfortunately, until people start to compare death counts to previously existing death counts & realize that a number like "24,555" seems huge if it's flung in your face the right way but isn't comparatively huge in relation to things like pneumonia that people just take for granted, the sheep are going to continue to baa their enthusiasm for Big Brother as they go to get sheared.

****

April 21, 2020, 12:55PM (BP to group):

via the Drudge Report: Highlighted in red at the top of the page:

Man dies from coronavirus after calling it 'political ploy'...
*Said lockdown was bulls***!*

Serves him right! Right?

I think the Russia fiasco of the last few years has made the pandemic behaviour control easier. Questioning it (in certain circles) could be one's downfall. It took a long while to make up but a close friend of mine angrily denounced me over lunch: "I didn't know you were such a fucking idiot."

****

April 22, 2020, 1:40PM (Inquiring Librarian to group):

Brainless Humor

My sister sent me this today. I thought it was really funny. I have no idea who Adley is. But here goes:

https://www.facebook.com/AdleyStump/videos/231988001228251/

[This stand-up comedy routine uses contradictory political speeches re what the public's supposed to do for safety's sake as its material.]

****

April 22, 2020, 2:04PM (Amir-ul Kafirs to group):

Re: Brainless Humor

I asked her to marry me in the comments — i.e. if we're not already married in which case I want a divorce so we CAN get married because we can't get married if we're already married, duh.

****

April 23, 2020, 5:24PM (Amir-ul Kafirs to group):

HERETICS: Medical Police State Improv

Hi Folks,

My apologies for being a bit out of touch with what people have been posting. I need to try to get through all the links that people have been so considerately providing and to give comments.

In the meantime, Dick and I improvised using Zoom yesterday, him in Paris, me in Pittsburgh. After our brief set, we chatted spontaneously, inevitably touching on current events. I made a movie of it all, keeping the improv intact but heavily editing the talk. Unfortunately, Dick's part of the session was inadequately recorded because the field of echo he was playing in is mostly inaudible. I still like it anyway but that's largely because it was the 1st set I've played using my new crotales and melocipede.

SO, some of this might interest you. I mention HERETICS in passing. The last 8 minutes or so are when I rant about my social frustrations with an (ex-)friend and their bullying.

"Medical Police State Improv in wch we don't try to Sooth the Savage Beast w/ Schmaltz" notes - 26:53

https://youtu.be/UcJytu4faag
https://archive.org/details/medical-police-state-improv

It's my feeling that I'm currently living in a world that's been artificially divided into people who believe that the quarantine is 'for our own good' & those who believe it an oppression. Furthermore, many or most people in these 2 camps believe that everyone of one of these opinions all thinks in exactly the same way. Almost all nuance seems to be gone. There's a vehemence & intolerance, in my opinion, to both sides of this divide. Because I think that the medical lockdown is a calculated opportunistic imposition of crowd control as well as a test of the same, those in favor of it lump me in with the stereotype of those against when, in reality, I'm not a member of either side, I'm a free thinker. The result of this is that even old friends of mine who're 'liberal' are acting like fascists in an attempt to get me to toe their party line. I will not comply. And neither will my old friend Dick Turner. As such, we decided to take advantage of the technical opportunities for international video conferencing by playing a brief improvisation with each other & to then have a spontaneous conversation about our own observations & frustrations under the current socially isolating conditions. There've been quite a few of these musical projects so far in which people are playing together while still being isolated in their homes. One thing I've noted is that some of the music played tends toward more consonant 'soothing of the beast', apparently chosen to help people relax. Dick & I didn't preplan what we would play & somewhat to my surprise the result was almost meditatively sparse. Neither of us seemed particularly moved to frenzy. This might speak of our introspective natures. The frenzy, if it can accurately be called that, came more when I began to talk about the abuse that's being heaped on me by one particularly belligerent friend of mine who absolutely can't stand my resistance to what I'm calling the MONOLITHIC NARRATIVE. Because they've been trying to bully me & because they consistently calculatingly misrepresent my position to be a pro-Rump one even though they know that I'm an anarchist contemptuous of the Idiot King this former friend has earned a place of complete disgust in my life. I will never waste my energy on communication with such a person again. They can't peer pressure me & they wouldn't be able to even if they were my peer, which they aren't. It's a pleasure & an honor to've been able to interact with my fellow HERETIC, Dick Turner, on April 22, 2020 (Vision), he in Paris, me in Pittsburgh. - April 23, 2020 (Vision) notes

Tags: improvising, experimental music, crotales, melocipede, Dick Turner, flute, trombone, percussion, medical lockdown, tENTATIVELY a cONVENIENCE, Paris, Pittsburgh, April 22 2020, bullying

****

April 23, 2020, 7:08PM (Dick to group):

Interesting A friend of mine who'd been living in Paris went back to Australia and had a 14 day quarantine he took a walk on the empty beach one late afternoon, was snitched on and paid a $2,000 fine And then the 14 day quarantine started again from scratch he said he felt like the government was trying to drive him insane on a personal level

****

April 23, 2020, 9:36PM (Amir-ul Kafirs to group):

South Australia and most other states here are under martial law, but under the guise of health.

That's the way the police state works these days. For the BELIEVERS oppressive measures become magically transformed into being OK when they're done in the name of "for our own good". As usual, I prefer to be the determiner of what's for my own good, no-thank-you-very-much.

What continues to amaze me is how much people seem to've forgotten the lessons of things like Orwell's "1984".

[..]

Of course, we talked about COVID-19 and the lockdown. They said something about how bad it was in New York, doing what everyone seems to do which was act as if everywhere was the same as New York. I agreed that the situation was bad in New York but I pointed out that in Allegheny County, where Pittsburgh is, only 50 people have died and that those deaths were spread out over 23 hospitals making that roughly 2 deaths per hospital.

This is where it got weird for me. It was as if my friend transformed into a Chatty Cathy doll with preprogrammed speech, as if I could've just reached around them to pull the string that would activate the predictable sentences: "That's because the governor took the right measures here and the governor in New York was too slow." That's such a prefabricated sentence it sickens me. I said: "I don't think so. I think it has more to do with New York being overcrowded and Pittsburgh not being overcrowded."

"It is the largest city in the United States with a long history of international immigration. New York City was home to over 8.3 million people in 2019"

[..]

"The city's population density of 26,403 people per square mile (10,194/km²), makes it the densest of any American municipality with a population above 100,000. Manhattan's population density is 66,940 people per square mile (25,846/km²), highest of any county in the United States." - https://en.wikipedia.org/wiki/Demographics_of_New_York_City

"At the 2010 Census, there were 305,704 people residing in Pittsburgh" - https://en.wikipedia.org/wiki/Pittsburgh#Population_densities

"The city **population** density is now at 5,540 **people per square mile** (2,140/ **square** kilometer). The urban area is home to 1.733 million, the metro area has 2.36 million, and the Combined Statistical Area (CSA) has an estimated 2.62 million in 2013." - https://worldpopulationreview.com/us-cities/pittsburgh-population/

OKAY?! That's 1/5th the population density of New York City. Surely, the spread of disease and its relation to population density is pretty obvious?! And, yet, people here constantly refer to New York as if Pittsburgh is hovering on the verge of having the same pandemic disaster. It's not.

But the initial point that I've meandered from is that my friend is a BELIEVER in the Governor. To me, that's believing in AND WANTING THE AUTHORITY OF BIG BROTHER. That's why I say that the lessons of "1984" seem forgotten. I don't want or need a Big Brother, I'm capable of and desirous of making my own decisions. ***I do not want or in any way authorize the state to govern my life***. Again, that seems pretty simple to me. I think for myself and act accordingly. And THAT makes me a Thought Criminal and this PANDEMIC PANIC is making Thought Criminality even more looked down upon than usual.

****

April 23, 2020, 9:47PM (Amir-ul Kafirs to group):

he took a walk on the empty beach one late afternoon, was snitched on and paid a $2,000 fine

Wow, that's an incredibly large amount of money — but what happens to people who don't pay?! And how much did the snitch get paid. Imagine if the $2,000 partially goes into a pool of money to pay snitches with.

And then the 14 day quarantine started again from scratch

That's an intense way to shame someone.

****

April 24, 2020, 1:05AM (BP to group):

Vive la France!

https://www.dailymail.co.uk/health/article-8246939/French-researchers-plan-nicotine-patches-coronavirus-patients-frontline-workers.html

Was Hockney RIGHT? French

researchers to give nicotine patches to coronavirus patients and frontline workers after lower rates of infection were found among smokers

- A French study found that only 4.4% of 350 coronavirus patients hospitalized were regular smokers and 5.3% of 130 homebound patients smoked
- This pales in comparison with at least 25% of the French population that smokes
- Researchers theorized nicotine could prevent the virus from infecting cells or that nicotine was preventing the immune system from overreacting to the virus
- To test this theory, hospitalized coronavirus patients, intensive care patients and frontline workers nicotine patches

By MARY KEKATOS SENIOR HEALTH REPORTER FOR DAILYMAIL.COM
PUBLISHED: 18:11 EDT, 22 April 2020 I **UPDATED:** 07:50 EDT, 23 April 2020

French researchers are planning to trial whether nicotine patches will help prevent - or lessen the effects of - the deadly **coronavirus**.

Evidence is beginning to show the proportion of smokers infected with coronavirus is much lower than the rates in the general population. Scientists are now questioning whether nicotine could stop the virus from infecting cells, or if it may prevent the immune system overreacting to the infection.

Doctors at a major hospital in Paris - who also found low rates of smoking among the infected - are now planning to give nicotine patches to COVID-19 patients. They will also give them to frontline workers to see if the stimulant has any effect on preventing the spread of the virus, according to reports.

It comes after world-famous artist David Hockney last week said he believes smoking could protect people against the deadly coronavirus.

MailOnline looked at the science and found he may have been onto something, with one researcher saying there was 'bizarrely strong' evidence it could be true.

One study in China, where the pandemic began, showed only 6.5 per cent of COVID-19 patients were smokers, compared to 26.6 per cent of the population. Another study, by the Centers for Disease Control in the US, found just 1.3 per cent of hospitalised patients were smokers - compared to 14 per cent of America. And research by hospitals in Paris found that smokers were under-represented in both inpatients and outpatients, suggesting that any protective effect could affect anyone, not just those hospitalised by their illness.

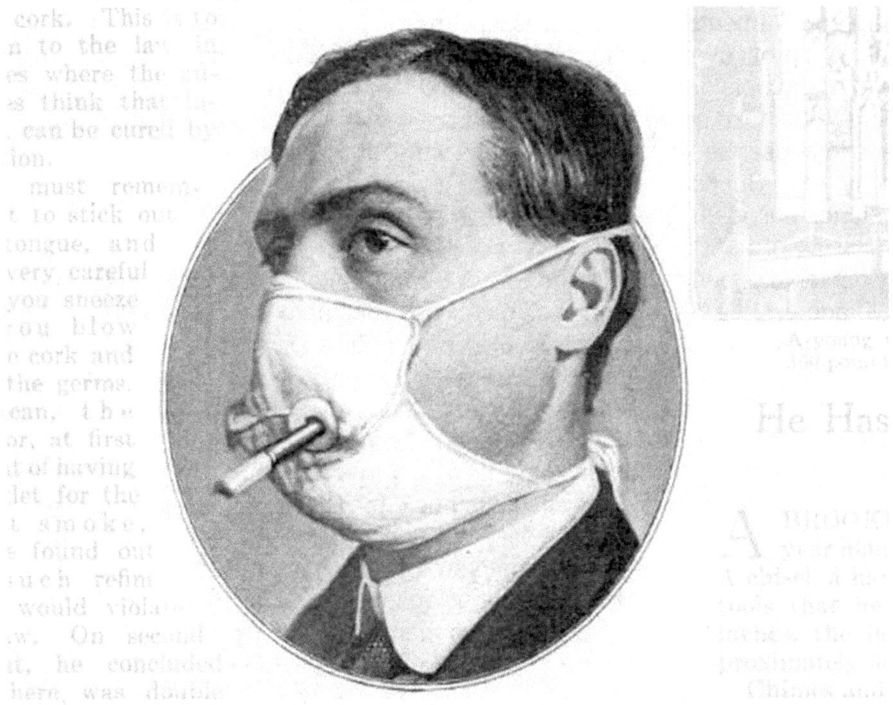

****

April 24, 2020, 1:22PM (Amir-ul Kafirs to group):

Re: Vive la France!

I find it particularly entertaining that David Hockney is one of the endorsers of this idea since I think he's one of the worst artists of all time.

****

April 24, 2020, 1:39PM (BP to group):

NO! It's all true and has saved my life. But I promise to quit smoking after the situation calms down here.

****

April 20, 2020, 6:55PM (Inquiring Librarian to group):

Fee-For Service Health Care

Today, I heard an interesting show on NPR about the health care system's Fee-For-Service for-profit operational model that has created a system of pill pushing, over- and poorly diagnosing doctors, and hospitals that have fewer beds but more appointments and more prescriptions, all providers being more interested in making a profit over keeping patients healthy. Also part of this is fewer hospital beds as patients get pushed out faster and faster, to save costs, but add more pills into the take home measures... part of why the U.S. has not had enough beds to house the sick from the Corona virus. If I could find the podcast, I'd send it your way. But I cannot find it. Maybe it will show up later. My internet searches pulled up little that seemed on point on the topic.

My personal experience with the Kaiser Permanente health care system in Colorado exactly fit the awfulness of this operational mode. I was refused quality thyroid medication in favor of their preferred medication that has been proven ineffective and would eventually lead me to diabetes, weight issues, and hypertension (more opportunity for them to push pills down my throat and make more diagnoses and more appointments). I was also refused the specific antibiotic medication I had documentation to prove was the only medication that could cure my chronic kidney infection problem. The kidney situation landed me, as predicted and as I had warned my doctor about, in the emergency room... and then led to kidney damage that prompted a $20,000 operation in Louisiana 1 year later that my new insurance in Lousiana tried to refuse to pay until I threw my and my father's angry OCD wrath on them.

Another run-in I had with the fee-for-service model was earlier, in my mid 20's. My thyroid seemed wonky. I went to my doctor, who i naively trusted. My doctor told me I didn't need thyroid medicine. 3 months later, I was a total walking disaster. My doctor said it wasn't my thyroid, that these problems I was having were in 'other departments'. I was nearly forced antidepressants, the pill, and Xanax. And I was told my kidney pain was back pain (complete bullshit since my first surgery at 19 was botched and I was told by the surgeon then that I would need another surgery within the next 10 years). Luckily I had the smarts to refuse these things and know my doctor was an idiot. I actually, given my emotional-freakshow due to low thyroid state created by my doctor, broke down and cried and screamed at him in his office and demanded all the healthcare things that I needed and were right for me. He was so scared of me being so insane, he gave me all the referrals and prescriptions I needed (which were very few compared to what he wanted to dump on me), probably just to get me to shut up and out of his office. When I finally then had the permission to see a kidney specialist, my 'back pain' turned out to be even worse than I thought, a permanently rotting cyst that was severely infected on my kidney. My specialist actually said to me, 'what happened to your kidney?! Why did you wait so long??!!). The kidney situation was extremely dangerous. I had reconstructive surgery scheduled and painfully completed immediately.

Here is a very brief, simplified, explanation of the Fee-For-Service debacle of a profit-driven healthcare model:
https://www.berkeleywellness.com/healthy-community/health-care-policy/article/why-american-health-care-sick

Needless to say, I absolutely abhor our healthcare system and avoid doctors at all costs. When I have to see them, I am very skeptical. I am lucky to have found one of the best doctors I've ever had in my life, here in Louisiana. =]

If the WWNO NPR show on Fee-For-Service in Hospitals show comes up as a shareable podcast, I will share with all asap.

****

Why American Health Care Is Sick

by BERKELEY WELLNESS

Sandeep Jauhar, MD, PhD, is the director of the Heart Failure Program at Long Island Jewish Medical Center in New York. His two books about his medical education and career—Intern: A Doctor's Initiation and Doctored: The Disillusionment of an American Physician—provide insights into the inefficiencies and waste of our profit-driven health care system, and the negative impact these flaws have on patient care. He is interviewed here by David Tuller, DrPH, the academic coordinator of UC Berkeley's joint masters program in public health and journalism.

You start your new book like this: "When I look at my career in midlife, I realize that in many ways I have become the kind of doctor I never thought I'd be." Can you elaborate?

Like most medical students, I had certain ideals for the way I wanted to practice medicine. And, like most people, I've fallen short of my ideals—about the way I wanted to take care of patients and the kind of doctor-patient relationships I wanted to work toward. I'm not always as caring as I think I should be, or as careful a steward of health care resources as I would like to be. Medicine today is a business—more of a business than I realized when I started.

It's easy to blame the system, but we doctors brought on a lot of the problems that we now face as professionals. In its early days, Medicare paid doctors generously for whatever they did, and paid them disproportionately for actual procedures relative to cognitive work, resulting in greater payments for specialties than for primary care. This allowed a subset of doctors to really make a lot of money. Managed care, which began in the 1970s, attempted to rectify those abuses, but it also deprived doctors of autonomy.

What are the problems associated with fee-for-service medicine?

When an insurance company pays doctors for each test and procedure, the financial incentive is to do more and more, even if it's not in the patient's best interest. The system encourages over-testing, overuse of resources, and high-volume care. Doctors can order an MRI or see a patient five times a month, and someone else is paying.

The Affordable Care Act and other reforms being put in place today are trying to change the system to one that pays for value instead of every procedure and service. Doctors will be paid more if they perform well on certain markers of excellent care. This includes following treatment guidelines being set by medical societies. But how we define value is an open question right now. New guidelines should not be applied mechanically to every patient because all patients are not the same. There's a fear that doctors will start treating to the guideline—the way teachers teach to the test—rather than consider the individual. If you create a system where the amount of money you get paid depends on whether the patient is treated in a certain way, then doctors will start treating all patients that way, regardless of their condition.

Besides fee-for-service, what are other reasons our health care system is so costly and overused?

There are multiple reasons. There's cover-your-ass medicine because of fears of malpractice lawsuits. There are semi-informed patients who request, or even demand, tests. There is a subset of physicians who are trying to bilk the system and generate more revenue for themselves. Care is so fragmented that people end up repeating tests that they don't need to repeat because we don't have an easy way to share medical records between providers.

[..]

This opinion does not necessarily reflect the views of the UC Berkeley School of Public Health or of the Editorial Board at BerkeleyWellness.com.
Published May 21, 2015

- https://www.berkeleywellness.com/healthy-community/health-care-policy/article/

why-american-health-care-sick

****

April 20, 2020, 7:18PM (Inquiring Librarian to group):

Re: Fee-For Service Health Care

This is from Forbes. Given the source, it is naturally a finance-centered article. But as such, it is an interesting read... Not nearly as telling as the podcast i heard today detailing this profit-driven model's absolute failure during this pandemic that is ironically leaving some healthcare workers unemployed.

https://www.google.com/amp/s/www.forbes.com/sites/robertpearl/2017/09/25/fee-for-service-addiction/amp/

****

Sep 25, 2017,12:55pm EDT

Healthcare's Dangerous Fee-For-Service Addiction

Robert Pearl, M.D. Contributor

[..]

As with any addiction, America's dependence on fee-for-service has dire financial and health consequences. This year, the estimated cost of care for an insured family of four will reach nearly $27,000, paid for through a combination of employer health insurance ($15,259), payroll deductions ($7,151) and out-of-pocket expenses at the point of care ($4,534). Year over year, patients are on the hook for a higher percentage of their total healthcare costs, which rose 4.3% compared to just a 1.9% increase in the U.S. GDP last year. This is a major warning sign. If medical costs continue to surge 2% to 3% higher than our nation's ability to pay, the healthcare system will soon reach a breaking point. Businesses, the government and insurers will have no choice but to ration care or slowly eliminate coverage for the nation's poor, middle-class and elderly populations.

As with all addictions, the fee-for-service model has mind-altering effects, distorting the perceptions of its users in ways that make them unaware of their growing dependence. When providers are paid for doing more, that's what they do: They increase utilization of services and ratchet up the cost of care without even realizing they're part of the problem. According to one study, just 36% of practicing physicians were willing to accept "major" responsibility for reducing healthcare costs. Of course, the first step, as with other habits, is to recognize the problem. Only then can we explore treatment options.

- https://www.forbes.com/sites/robertpearl/2017/09/25/fee-for-service-addiction/#28b525b5c8ad

****

April 24, 2020, 12:13PM (Amir-ul Kafirs to group):

Re: Fee-For Service Health Care

all providers being more interested in making a profit over keeping patients healthy.

1st, my apologies for being so slow to respond to this. I looked at it when you 1st wrote it & started to check out the links you provide below but I got distracted by other things, as I, no doubt, will now too — but I'm trying to at least get through this one email before I move on to other aspects of the day. Everyone's emails here are important to me, I'm thankful to all of you for sharing your thoughts, personal experiences, & research.

2nd, it's been pretty obvious to me for a long time that 'Western' medicine has become increasingly reduced to pill-pushing & promotion of expensive machines. An example from my own life that I may've already told you so forgive me if I'm being redundant:

Around 5 years ago I was cutting the jungle of my backyard back & I got a mild case of poison ivy. I don't recall ever getting it before & I interpreted this as a symptom of my being less aligned with my natural environment AND as a sign that the very robust plants in my backyard were fighting back with chemical warfare against my attack. I probably used some sort of cream to ameliorate the poison's effect on my skin. Then it appeared that I got it on my eyelid. I was afraid I'd be blinded by it or at least develop some sort of eyesight problem so I went to a medical center & told them I was wary of using a cream on my eyelid because of my concern for my sight so they said I should get a steroid shot & that I should get a prescription for steroids to take for, maybe, a couple of weeks. My impression of the doctor was that she was contemptuous of me as a 'lowlife' &, perhaps, thought I was over-reacting to what was a somewhat mild case of poison ivy. I may or may not've explained that I worked for museums handling highly valued objects & that I didn't want to take chances with getting the poison oil on those objects.

They gave me the injection in my hip. When I asked *Why there?* I was told that it was *less painful* that way. I thought that was a bit strange because I wasn't anticipating it being painful. I went home & started taking the pills, as prescribed, perhaps twice a day. The steroids were said to have the side-effect of possibly making me sleepy. In my case, I had the opposite reaction. I felt good & I stayed awake all night the 1st night under their influence. However, within a few days I started becoming in pain — with the pain radiating from the place where I'd gotten the injection but effecting my entire hip area & both my legs. Within another few days the pain was EXCRUCIATING, & I'm not exaggerating, & any pressure put on my legs & hips by standing or walking was so unbearable that I would literally scream uncontrollably.

I had to crawl & butt-walk around my house, even then the pain was terrible. A friend then visited from Hawaii & he took me to the Emergency Room. I got into a wheel-chair & eventually saw a doctor. I explained to him that the pain seemed to be a side-effect of the steroid injection further augmented by my taking steroid pills every day. He told me that was "impossible". He didn't know what the problem was but that didn't stop him from wanting me to take some pills for it. Perhaps they were pain-killers — in my opinion pain-killers just mask one's natural body alarm system creating the illusion that everything's ok now while the actual problem isn't effected at all. I told him that since I thought the problem was CAUSED BY THE MEDICATION I didn't want to take any more. He had my lower body photographed by machines, I forget now whether it was MRI or X-Ray or something else. After this he speculated that I had "reactive arthritis" but he didn't know what my body was reacting to. I told him that I KNEW WHAT MY BODY WAS REACTING TO: ***the steroids***. Once again, I was informed that that was impossible. I was then asked whether *I still needed the wheelchair.* I found that question somewhat amazing since nothing had changed, the best I'd gotten out of the experience was a diagnosis of "reactive arthritis", which made sense to me. That visit, maybe an hour long, cost something like $3,500!

I went home & stopped taking the steroids. *By the next **day**, the pain had lessened by about 50%!* By the day after it was down another 50% to what it had been at its worst, that is to say to about 25%. After that, it was incresingly bearable. I felt that my opinion about the effects of the steroids was vindicated & I've never taken them since. If I had just had enough sense to stop taking the steroids to begin with I wouldn't have had to deal with the $3,500 robbery. The problem was, of course, that I was highly distracted by my agony & worried about being permanently crippled so I wanted the opinion of an 'expert'. That 'expert' was close to useless & very expensive.

my new insurance in Louisiana tried to refuse to pay until I threw my and my father's angry OCD wrath on them.

Thank the holy ceiling light that that worked!

Luckily I had the smarts to refuse these things and know my doctor was an idiot.

More people need to have that epiphany that doctors are fallible human beings like the rest of us. People are inculcated with the idea that doctors are like GODS, that's why I make fun of the "DOCTOR GODS". They aren't, they can have bad days, they can even be, yes, STUPID.

I had reconstructive surgery scheduled and painfully completed immediately.

That's why it's best to get a 2nd opinion, especially if you're convinced that the 1st doctor is probably wrong & that their opinion didn't help solve the problem.

Alas, it's galling to have to then PAY the shits.

Here is a very brief, simplified, explanation of the Fee-For-Service debacle of a profit-driven healthcare model:
https://www.berkeleywellness.com/healthy-community/health-care-policy/article/why-american-health-care-sick

That's a very useful article. It's very simple & direct &, obviously, I agree with most of it. In fact, it resonates remarkably with my own personal story told above. Here's a brief excerpt that demonstrates that:

What can patients do to help control costs and improve their care?
Patients need to ask more questions and be less accepting when doctors send them from office to office to get more tests. The patient is the single most underutilized entity in health care. Medical societies have released lists of tests and procedures that are not beneficial to patients. Patients need to know what those are. Better-informed patients might be the most potent restraint on overutilization.

You've expressed concern that medical technology may lead to a loss of observational and diagnostic skills among doctors. Can you elaborate?

Doctors at one point were very adept at physical examination. That has changed over the years because of an excessive reliance on technology. Personal observations might not be as accurate as technology, but they're certainly a whole lot cheaper. It's important to use physical diagnosis as a tool to selectively decide which technology to use. But doctors now simply order tests as a matter of course. Before you know it, they've gotten a chest x-ray, a CAT scan, an echocardiogram or some other test without anybody thinking about it, and that's very, very wasteful.

I am lucky to have found one of the best doctors I've ever had in my life, here in Louisiana. =]

Fortunately for us they do exist. I was going to one in Pittsburgh but she moved away. She & I bonded around the statement "less is more", she wasn't a drug or technology pusher.

****

April 24, 2020, 12:22PM (Amir-ul Kafirs to group):

Re: Fee-For Service Health Care

This is from Forbes. Given the source, it is naturally a finance-centered article.
https://www.google.com/amp/s/www.forbes.com/sites/robertpearl/2017/09/25/fee-for-service-addiction/amp/

Thanks for that, I found it very pragmatc & useful. I found it particularly cheering that he quoted Upton Sinclair, the author perhaps best well-known for his criticism of the meat industry, "The Jungle", but who was also prolific in his socio-political criticism in general:

"It will be equally problematic trying to get doctors – particularly highly compensated specialists – to give up lucrative but ineffective procedures. As Upton Sinclair once said, "It is difficult to get a man to understand something, when his salary depends on his not understanding it.""

****

April 25, 2020, 2:12PM (Inquiring Librarian to group):

Re: Fee-For Service Health Care

What a terrible experience!! I can't say i am not surprised! I have had far too many terrible runins with doctors. The 1 i have now actually takes my insurance. I heard about him from a naturopath that did not take my insurance. The naturopath mentioned my future dr in passing as being too radical even for her. I immediately swiched dr.s and have never regretted the decision.

On to steroids. I feel that they are HORRIBLE! I am always shocked when dr.s consider them a cure all. They actually lower your immune system, cause weight gain and high blood pressure, depression, low libido, hair loss, fluid retention, aggression, ect. among many other evils.

My gp that i am forced to see 1x/year so my insurance doesn't skyrocket more, prescribed a steroid for me when it turned out my ear pain wasnt an infection but just a little bit of seasonal pressure. I told her i did not want to.take a 'cure' that would be worse than the problem.

****

April 25, 2020, 4:49AM (Amir-ul Kafirs to group):

HERETICS: Russia

I'm corresponding with a woman in Saint Petersburg, Russia, via a computer dating site & somewhat inevitably talk has turned to COVID-19. She depicts the situation as bad there. Looking online for Russian statistics I find reports of COVID-19 deaths to be **unbelievably** low. Hence in Saint Petersburg, population roughly 5 million, ***there are only 20 reported COVID-19 DEATHS***. Here's where those statistics come from: https://www.statista.com/statistics/1102935/coronavirus-cases-by-region-in-russia/ . If those statistics were to be believed, & I see no good reason why they should be, the medical world would be rushing to Russia (pun & alliteration intended) to find out what the Russians are doing right. I assume that 'what they're doing right' is simply not confiming or reporting the COVID-19 situation accurately. Anyway, I'm waiting to see what my Saint Petersburg correspondent has to say further about this.

****

April 25, 2020, 2:29PM (Inquiring Librarian to group):

Re: HERETICS: Russia

I remember being really confused about 1 month ago when the "presumed" cases started being announced and printed and in the news.

We actually had a 'presumed' case here in Lousiana of a supposedly perfectly healthy 39 year old girl. https://www.nola.com/news/coronavirus/article_bdc4e802-6b90-11ea-a747-832e94bc7f56.html

About 1 week later, the nola.com news had to amend the article stating her test result, (actually tested 2x since the news was incredulous) was actual negative for the corona virus.
1st test negative: https://www.nola.com/news/coronavirus/article_68a51972-6e39-11ea-bdab-23243451078b.html
2nd test negative: https://www.nola.com/news/coronavirus/article_98334eea-7049-11ea-8097-fbd7ba1925ae.html

& finally this, but not from Nola.com, from Los Angeles, stating that she, Natasha Ott, positively did not die from the Corona Virus: https://www.latimes.com/world-nation/story/2020-04-01/coronavirus-louisiana-natasha-ott

Ok, enough of that. She looked like a lovely soul. I would imagine her family may not have been happy to have her death used as a false poster child for a virus scare tactic directed at relatively young and healthy individuals.

****

This 39-year-old New Orleans woman tested for coronavirus. She died before getting her results.

She tested for coronavirus, and her results were delayed. Five days later, she was dead in her kitchen.

BY JESSICA WILLIAMS I STAFF WRITER PUBLISHED MAR 21, 2020 AT 11:26 AM I

UPDATED MAR 21, 2020 AT 5:17 PM 3 min to read

****

New Orleans woman, 39, found dead in kitchen tests negative for coronavirus, but doctor 'skeptical'

BY JESSICA WILLIAMS I STAFF WRITER PUBLISHED MAR 24, 2020 AT 8:39 PM I UPDATED MAR 24, 2020 AT 9:23 PM 1 min to read

****

Second coronavirus test comes back negative for New Orleans woman, 39, found dead in kitchen

BY RAMON ANTONIO VARGAS I STAFF WRITER PUBLISHED MAR 27, 2020 AT 11:46 AM I UPDATED MAR 27, 2020 AT 12:11 PM 2 min to read

****

New Orleans social worker who died at 39 did not have coronavirus, test results show

By MOLLY HENNESSY-FISKE HOUSTON BUREAU CHIEF
APRIL 1, 20202:19 PM

****

April 25, 2020, 2:49PM (Inquiring Librarian to group):

Our Own Bodily Created Immunity isn't Enough?!

I find it really disturbing and depressing that the latest news is touting that your own naturally created antibodies to this new corona virus will not produce 'real' immunity and that you can get it 'twice'. And as such the only solution is a fancy vaccine that will be doled out (as they say equitably?!) to all living humans. This makes me think back to that article someone here shared about the dna altering vaccines. I shudder to think... Why??? And basically now, the prognosis is we are all screwed. We must all stay locked down forever and live on government handouts (if we are so lucky to receive their crumbs) until we can be injected with some most likely mandatory vaccine... in the interim, if we do not comply (and in the aftermath if we do not take the vaccine), we are granny and grampy killers.

Here are 2 articles. In both, sources probably suck, but it's all over today's big breaking news here..., I see that you 'May' be able to catch it more than once, but that that is no more confirmed scientifically than that our own bodily engineered immunity is sufficient, and neither article address the fact that the 2nd bout (if it could even exist) would generally be less severe (again you will be a granny and grampy killer if you shed the virus on them again even if you are barely sick). **Can I just add here, all of my living blood relatives aside from my sister and her kids, are in their late 70s and 80s. They are perfectly healthy, aside from the mental strain of being locked at home and then my _____ having a mild nervous depressive breakdown over watching the news too much (he is brilliant, but has always had mental health issues with anxiety and depression).

https://www.bloomberg.com/news/articles/2020-04-25/catching-covid-19-may-not-shield-against-new-infection-who-says

https://bgr.com/2020/04/20/coronavirus-treatment-reinfection-might-be-possible-without-vaccine/

Librarian in waiting (for their job back).-

****

Prognosis

WHO Warns You May Catch Coronavirus More Than Once

By Patrick Henry
April 25, 2020, 4:44 AM EDT Updated on April 25, 2020, 7:10 AM EDT

[..]

Chile was the first country to announce plans to issue immunity cards based partly on antibody tests. This has raised concerns because the tests have proven unreliable elsewhere, and some people may get deliberately ill in order to obtain the card. The U.S. and others have nonetheless said they're looking into the option.

While there's a consensus that the key to ending the coronavirus pandemic is establishing co-called herd immunity, there are many unknowns. One is whether researchers can develop a safe and effective vaccine. Another is how long people who've recovered have immunity; reinfection after months or years is common with other human coronaviruses. Finally, it's not clear what percentage of people must be immune to protect the "herd." That depends on the contagiousness of the virus.

The WHO said it's reviewing the scientific evidence on antibody responses to coronavirus, but as yet no study has evaluated whether the presence of antibodies "confers immunity to subsequent infection by this virus in humans." And while many countries are currently testing for antibodies, these studies aren't designed to determine whether people recovered from the disease acquire immunity, the agency said.

As the hunt for a vaccine continues around the world, the WHO has formed an international alliance to ensure that treatments are distributed fairly. French President Emmanuel Macron, European Commission President Ursula von der Leyen and the Bill and Melinda Gates Foundation are involved in the alliance.

- https://www.bloomberg.com/news/articles/2020-04-25/catching-covid-19-may-not-shield-against-new-infection-who-says

****

[..]

More and more COVID-19 survivors are testing positive again for the novel coronavirus, and some of them are even showing mild symptoms the second time around. Researchers are trying to understand the reasons why that happens, as that's not the kind of question we can afford to leave unanswered. It's not only crucial for COVID-19 immunity research, but also for mitigating new outbreaks and devising policies for easing social distancing restrictions. If patients retest positive, does it mean they're infectious? Was it a testing error? Is it possible they were reinfected?

So far, it's believed that people who test positive again haven't been reinfected by someone else. Instead, the virus may have been dormant inside them and a weaker immune response may have resurrected it. But one researcher who is working on a COVID-19 vaccine candidate said people who have recovered from the disease might be reinfected again. However, that likely can't happen as soon as you think, and it likely doesn't explain why recovered patients are testing positive again.

[..]

- https://bgr.com/2020/04/20/coronavirus-treatment-reinfection-might-be-possible-without-vaccine/

****

April 25, 2020, 3:57PM (Phil to group):

Re: Our Own Bodily Created Immunity isn't Enough?!

I have glanced at some articles that talk about catching it more the once. What I think is the most likely reason for this is the test are giving false positives. I found this interesting interview with david crowe where he talks a bit about the tests. He has this idea that maybe there is no such thing as a covid-19 virus and gives an interesting slant to the whole thing from that perspective; https://www.thehighersidechats.com/david-crowe-coronavirus-the-risks-the-testing-the-treatments/

Here in the Netherlands apparently some older people have formed a union and do not want to be quarantined off. I think a lot of these people that say what about the old people don't actually give a real shit about old people and don't want to hear what old people actually want.

****

David Crowe I Coronavirus COVID-19: The Risks, The Testing, & The Treatments

March 21, 2020

A big THC welcome to David Crowe. He's a telecommunications consultant, environmentalist, writer and critic of science and medicine.
He was one of the founders of the Alberta Greens (Green Party of Alberta), edited their newsletter for over a decade, was the party's president until October 2004, and the party's Chief Financial Officer until December 2008.
He also was founder of the Alberta Reappraising AIDS Society, am on the advisory council of AnotherLook and created the JusticeForEJ.com site. In 2008 he was appointed President of Rethinking AIDS, a position he still holds.
He is also co-host and co-founder of the podcast, How Positive Are You?, and the host of The Infectious Myth on the Progressive Radio Network (prn.fm).
Watch his presentation Rethink All Viruses: https://www.youtube.com/watch?v=331qt-HJQI0&t=
Read his paper on Coronavirus: http://theinfectiousmyth.com/book/CoronavirusPanic.pdf

- https://www.thehighersidechats.com/david-crowe-coronavirus-the-risks-the-testing-the-treatments/

****

April 25, 2020, 7:40PM (tENT to group):

Re: Our Own Bodily Created Immunity isn't Enough?!

I find it really disturbing and depressing that the latest news is touting that your own naturally created antibodies to this new corona virus will not produce 'real' immunity and that you can get it 'twice'.

I'm one of those apparently completely deranged people who find my own natural immune system to be a marvel of deeply successful functioning. If my immune system ever meets one of these immune-system-dissing doctors I'm afraid I won't be able to hold my immune system back from insulting the doctor's mother.

Here are 2 articles.

I skimmed through them both. I found them more or less insufferable. There is NO WAY that I think that doctor knowledge is superior to our natural body defenses. The main time I think our immune system is insufficient is when humans do something dramatic to toxify the environment, Chernobyl and other nuclear power plant disasters being the obvious examples. Then whatever the doctors do is to no avail anyway.

****

April 25, 2020, 8:53PM (Inquiring Librarian to group):

Re: Our Own Bodily Created Immunity isn't Enough?!

Thank you Phill for sharing! I actually made the time today to listen to this whole talk while stringing 320 seedbeads onto a thread. It was a sort of mind warping breath of fresh air. The inconsistencies with the testing do seem as random and nonsensical as the varied lockdown measures. The talk was from about 1 month ago. I wonder what would be said now by them this 1 more month into it. My supervisor's mother is in a nursing home. Her mother tested positive, but has shown no symptoms. She has been locked up in her room for a month now and is very depressed as a result. I appreciate that this talk addresses her condition.

As regards trust in the all knowing doctors and the western disease model as discussed here... I have a related family story... My paternal grandad lived most of his life in rural Belarus, born in 1901. When the family arrived in the United States in 1947, his wife (my grandma) was soon ill and diagnosed with stomach cancer. My dad, 11 at the time, sadly remembers her being taken away for good to a hospital. Chemo was new then. Grandma died at only 41 yrs old in that hospital, suffering for a whole year under the new 'treatment' of chemo. Grandpa finally told the doctors to please stop experimenting on her and let her die naturally. And she did then die. Grandpa later would ask his American friends... Why in the United States do you all die of such horrible diseases like cancer, heart disease, diabetes, etc.... And his friends would counter ask.. Stefan, what did they die of in Belarus... He would reply, They just died!! That made the only logical sense to him. Sadly, whatever pastoral life remained in his Belarussian village was 1st heavily damaged by the ravages of WW2, and later his small oblast became one of the worst contaminated by the Chernobyl fallout. Now Chernobyl truly has created what we can all agree as a true invisible enemy, a manmade tragedy that really breaks my heart. :'-(

****

April 25, 2020, 8:57PM (Inquiring Librarian to group):

Re: Our Own Bodily Created Immunity isn't Enough?!

Amir-ul Kafirs, i am with you 100% on this! These articles were posted en masse with only slight stylistic changes from every major 'liberal' news outlet over the past 48 hrs. I woke and read this drivel and became pretty angry. I biked the anger off and then hurt myself in the name of comfort by eating a big bowl of icecream.... Diabetes here i come! :O

****

April 25, 2020 (Amir-ul Kafirs to group):

HERETICS: WHO vs Laing

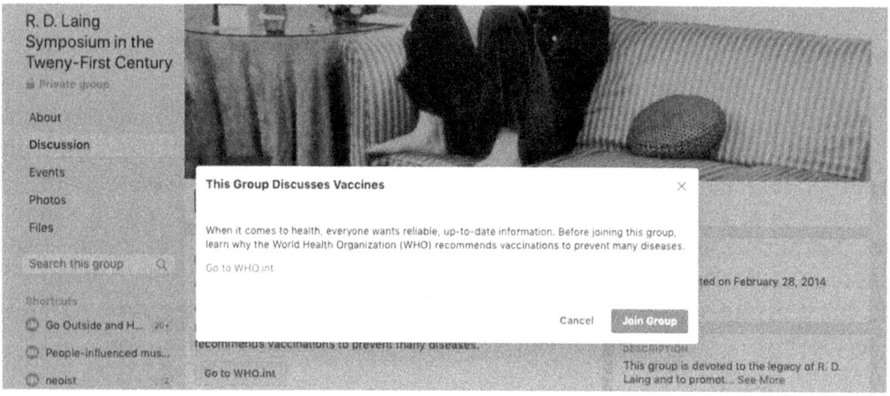

****

April 26, 2020, 12:48PM (Amir-ul Kafirs to group):

HERETICS: Russia

My Russian correspondent wrote me today:

"I don't believe our statistics and I am in great fear. Sorry to say that. Our authorities silence everyone who is trying to open an information."

The New World Odor reeks again!

Personally, I'm more depressed today than usual. It's going to be a hard day. This whole lockdown is as much psychological warfare as it is a physical restraint. Of course, the 2 are interlocked.

****

April 26, 2020, 12:48PM (Amir-ul Kafirs to group):

HERETICS: Proposed Book

I keep imagining compiling a book of criticism of the Global Lockdown and the PANDEMIC PANIC. I imagine the title being something like "Mind Control Opportunism in the era of COVID-19". I have the money to publish it. I don't really want to do all the work that this would entail for me but it just seems like **something that has to be done**. I'm wondering if any of you would like to contribute? This is what I imagine:

I'd write an introduction giving a personal timeline of experiences with the medical industry that have led to my increasing cynicism about it. Then the book would be a chronology of things relevant, focusing on things I've been exposed to by our collective correspondence. I'd quote from videos and articles that links have been provided for here. If anyone here wants to be a contributor then you could either be Anonymous or use whatever name you want to. I'd like to at least identify people by location and profession to get across the idea that there's some global representation. You could pick your own introduction, if any, perhaps describing your social conditions under this quarantyranny, and you would pick what you'd want to to say. If you wanted to summarize the things you've linked to that would be even better but that might be too much work. I'll do the work that other people don't want to do or don't have the time for but I, too, have only so much energy and time so the more the work is spread around the better it is for me.

If all of you want to contribute then the book could be credited to: 6 HERETICS or some other generalization such as 6 SKEPTICS. If only 3 of you want to contribute then it could be 4 HERETICS (or SKEPTICS).

Is anyone interested?

yr pal,

Amir-ul Kafirs

****

April 26, 2020, 1:34PM (Amir-ul Kafirs to group):

HERETICS: Skepticism Poster

In honor of current events I went into my poster aRCHIVE & dug out this poster I scraped off a pole in Baltimore ca. 20 years ago:

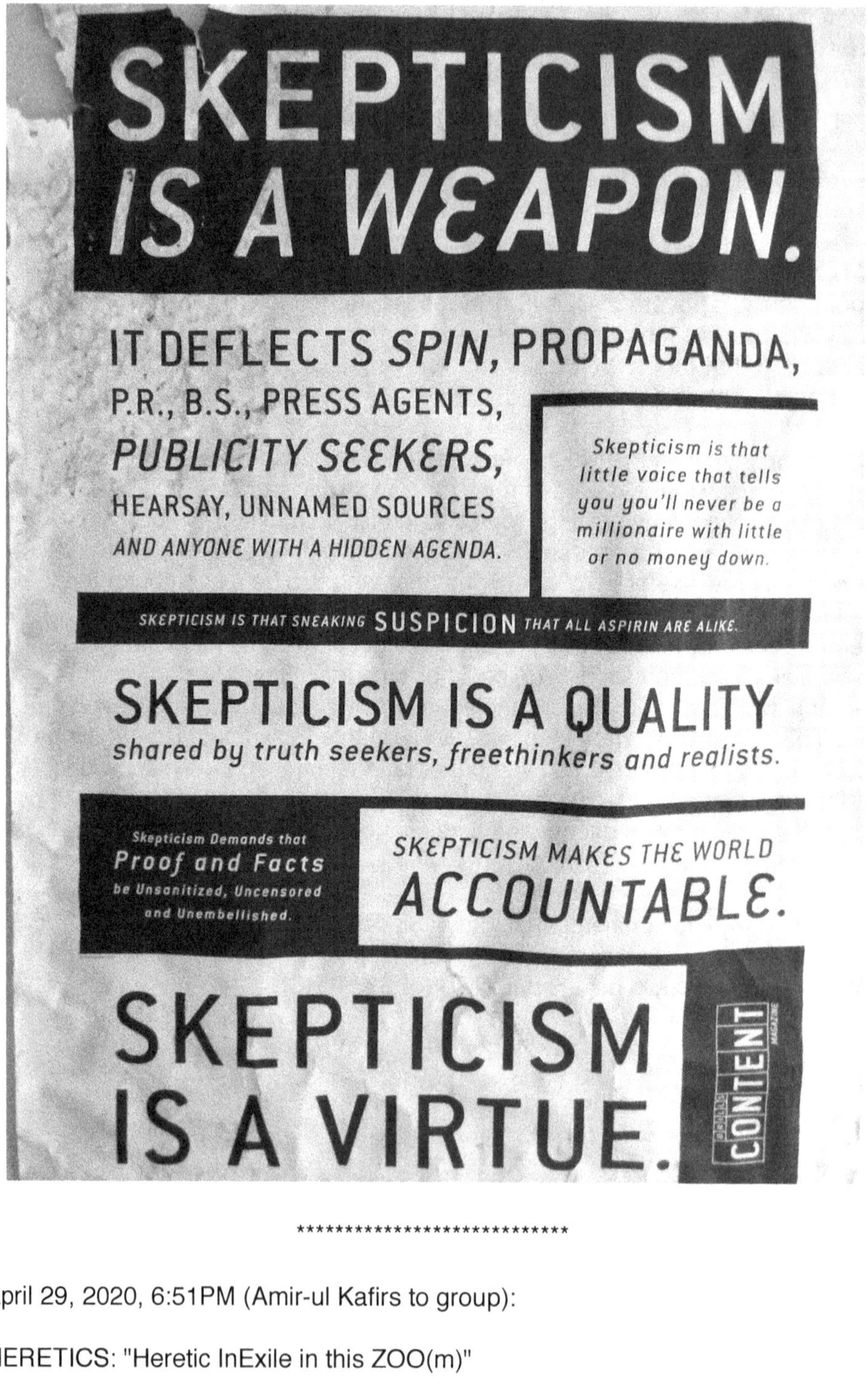

****

April 29, 2020, 6:51PM (Amir-ul Kafirs to group):

HERETICS: "Heretic InExile in this ZOO(m)"

I gave this UNCERT via ZOOM last night to 17 people. I doubt that any of them will agree with the political statement I made to accompany this on YouTube but, oh well!, GOTTA LET IT OUT SOMEHOW!

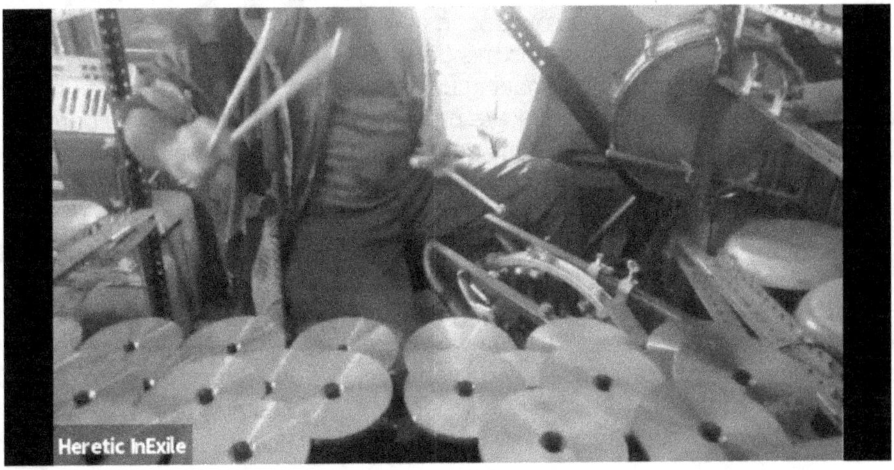

"Heretic InExile in this ZOO(m)" notes - 11:59 - 2K

https://youtu.be/DHn2KEiQQRY

In 1940, Hitler envisioned a New World Order governed by the German people. Germans were referred to as a single body of sorts, a superorganism threatened by the 'disease' of the ethnically & politically 'unclean' & 'degenerate'. Fortunately, he failed to establish his 1,000 year Reich - but not before millions of people were murdered.

Forty years later, in 1980, Reagan envisioned a New World Order, a one world government in which, apparently, the United States of America, being the 'good guys' similar to the white-hat-wearing cowboys of his movie roles, would be the police fighting off the 'evils of communism'. During this time he attended a ceremony honoring nazi SS officers at Bitburg, Germany. Fortunately, he failed to establish this New World Order - but not before multiple covert actions in Latin America had massacred people resisting having their natural resources plundered by American corporations.

Another 40 years later, in 2020, & the New World Odor stinks more than ever in the era of the G20 & the billionaires of the world whose pimple, Rump, exemplifies the dumbing-down of human consciousness. One World Government has been all but officially established in the name of 'our own good' & brainwashing has succeeded under the guise of health where previous excuses for GROUPTHINK had failed. Quarantyranny has been established & economic dependence on Big Brother will help keep it that way.

People are under 'lockdown-lite', staying in our homes 'for our own good' & to 'Save Lives' during a time of a pandemic that entirely too many people believe in unquestioningly thanks to the fear-mongering of the mass media. In order to grab whatever snatches of sociability we can, many are using video-conferencing technology to meet 'virtually'. Hence on Tuesdays, starting April 21, 2020, & continuing indefinitely, a series of concerts using Zoom to bring together the players & audience in small groups has been organized. Instead of passively sitting in front of the boob tube soaking up the oversimplification of sound bytes & destroying our ability to freely think we proactively continue to produce our own culture. I think of the mathematicians gathered around the Anonymous statue in Budapest during the nazi occupation of Hungary. Perhaps that's too dramatic but I think a similar spirit is at work.

My set consisted of playing Neil Feather's instrument, the Melocipede, set up to have 2 of its 4 pick-ups output to stereo speakers & 2 of its pick-ups mixed down to send a signal to a Pitch-to-MIDI converter that then sent a MIDI signal to a sampler playing my SFX samples. Additionally, I played a 2 octave set of Antique Cymbals with a touch of other percussion: chime tree, 2 frying pans, & 2 extremely cheap cymbals.

- April 29, 2020 (Vision) notes

****

April 30, 2020, 4:03PM (BP to Amir-ul Kafirs):

Fwd: "Temporary" Conoronavirus Censorship is Here, Maybe Forever

I read the Atlantic article cited below this morning and was considering sending to the group. I get the email articles by taibbi and thought I'd share.

"Temporary" Coronavirus Censorship is Here, Maybe Forever

As the Covid-19 crisis progresses, censorship programs advance, amid calls for China-style control of the Internet

Matt Taibbi
Apr 30

Earlier this week, *Atlantic* magazine – fast becoming the favored media outlet for self-styled intellectual elites of the Aspen Institute type – ran an in-depth article of the problems free speech pose to American society in the coronavirus era. The headline:

Internet Speech Will Never Go Back to Normal

In the debate over freedom versus control of the global network, China was largely correct, and the U.S. was wrong.

Authored by a pair of law professors from Harvard and the University of Arizona, Jack Goldsmith and Andrew Keane Woods, the piece argued that the American and Chinese approaches to monitoring the Internet were already not that dissimilar:

Constitutional and cultural differences mean that the private sector, rather than the federal and state governments, currently takes the lead in these practices... But the trend toward greater surveillance and speech control here, and toward the growing involvement of government, is undeniable and likely inexorable.

They went on to list all the reasons that, given that we're already on an "inexorable" path to censorship, a Chinese-style system of speech control may not be such a bad thing. In fact, they argued, a benefit of the coronavirus was that it was waking us up to "how technical wizardry, data centralization, and private-public collaboration can do enormous public good."

Perhaps, they posited, Americans could be moved to reconsider their "understanding" of the First and Fourth Amendments, as "the harms from digital speech" continue to grow, and "the social costs of a relatively open Internet multiply."

This interesting take on the First Amendment was the latest in a line of "Let's rethink that whole democracy thing" that began sprouting up in earnest four years ago. Articles with headlines like "Democracies end when they become too democratic" and "Too much of a good thing: why we need less democracy" became common after two events in particular: Donald Trump's victory in the the Republican primary race, and the decision by British voters to opt out of the EU, i.e. "Brexit."

A consistent lament in these pieces was the widespread decline in respect for "experts" among the ignorant masses, better known as the people Trump was talking about when he gushed in February 2016, "I love the poorly educated!"

The *Atlantic* was at the forefront of the argument that The People is a Great Beast who cannot be trusted to play responsibly with the toys of freedom. A 2016 piece called "American politics has gone insane" pushed a return of the "smoke-filled room" to help save voters from themselves. Author Jonathan Rauch employed a metaphor that is striking in retrospect, describing America's oft-vilified intellectual and political elite as society's immune system:

Americans have been busy demonizing and disempowering political professionals and parties, which is like spending decades abusing and attacking your own immune system. Eventually, you will get sick.

The new piece by Goldsmith and Woods says we're there, made literally sick by our refusal to accept the wisdom of experts. The time for asking the (again, literally) unwashed to listen harder to their betters is over. The Chinese system offers a way out. When it comes to speech, don't ask: tell.

[..]

****

April 30, 2020, 10:23PM (Amir-ul Kafirs to *Atlantic*):

response to "Internet Speech Will Never Go Back to Normal"

The strange and, I think, completely insupportable assumption of Jack Goldsmith's and Andrew Keane Woods' position that "In the debate over freedom versus control of the global network, China was largely correct, and the U.S. was wrong" and all that follows is that the people effected by internet censorship 'need' the 'expertise' of censors to make their value judgments for them. After all, what IS "harmful information related to the coronavirus" and whose 'expertise' is objectively provable as such?

My assertion is that there are many opinions about the matter of COVID-19 and, for that matter, anything else and that each of these opinions is bound to have subtexts, hidden motives, ideological assumptions, and different experiences that render the opinion, 'expert' or not, of a limited value that should always be subject to criticism. It's the role of every thinking human being to approach opinions with enough skepticism to enable them to sift what's personally valuable from what's inaccurate from their own considered perspective.

As such, instead of censoring, critical thinking and reading should be encouraged. I'll give you an example from my own personal experience with the medical industry: I realized that I was exhibiting diabetes symptoms, I went to a doctor to get my blood tested, she told me I had diabetes and that I MUST immediately start injecting insulin. I told her I wanted to try to solve the problem with a change of diet and exercise first. She told me that was "impossible". I did it anyway. Five days later, my symptoms were gone, two weeks later my blood sugar was normalized. I've been fine ever since. If I had listened to the doctor's 'expertise' instead of to my own common sense I would now be dependent on an expensive drug, thus feeding the medical industry's seemingly insatiable greed.

My obvious question is: Are Goldmith and Woods among those hypothetically 'qualified' to be future censors because of their educational affiliations and their status as lawyers? If so, I quote from a billboard I saw 25 years ago in rural Canada to put things in perspective: "If lawyers are so smart, why are there so many of them?"

****

April 28, 2020, 11:05AM (Dick to group):

HERETICS... random thought

Hello,

A random thought.

In the early '90's the French philosopher Jean Baudrillard was asked by the French newspaper Liberation to report on the Iraq war. He agreed but under the condition that he would use as his only material that which was given out on CNN.

I think his point was something along the lines of whatever really happens we can never know but we can see how it's being presented and used by the power structure. The official story that is.

Not unlike the current situation it seems to me. I can hardly stand perusing the articles in the mass media, they produce the same effect of me as TV (that is I have an extreme negative reaction to both because I feel they are forms of brainwashing and TV especially as a sort of surrogate character formation) but they do give a pretty good idea of what may be in the works or moreover what a lot of people will think is reality...

It is with that in mind that I post the following not particularly illuminating article, just as a cultural artifact. I find the expression "the new normal" particularly offensive but repeating it constantly seems to be part of the "new normal"...

https://www.nbcnews.com/news/world/south-korea-beating-cononavirus-anxiety-grows-over-new-normal-n1192886

What the United States can learn from South Korea's virus response

In South Korea, coronavirus is in retreat but the concern grows over what the 'new normal' will look like

****

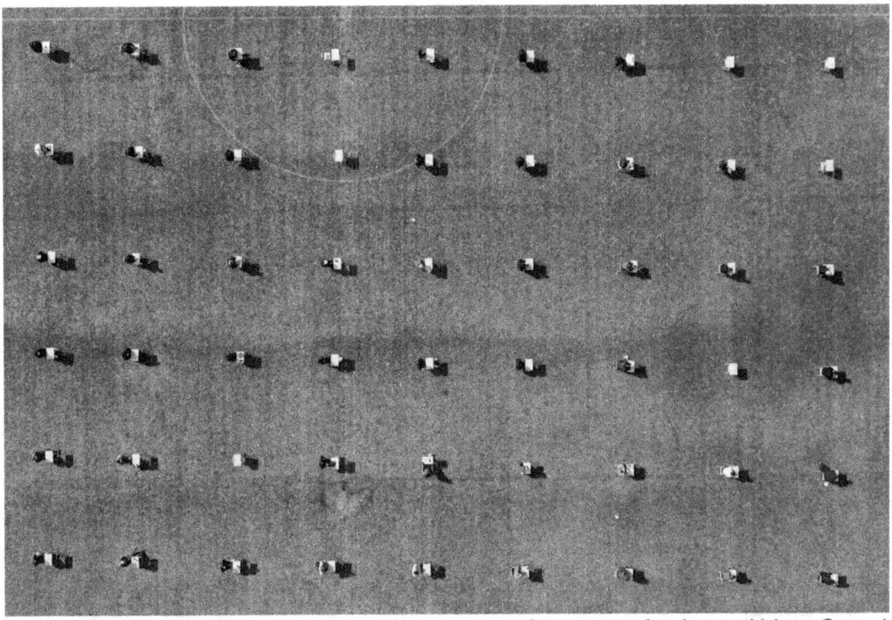

Applicants take a written examination during a recruitment test for Ansan Urban Corp. in Ansan, South Korea, on April 4, 2020.Hong Ki-won / AP file

April 27, 2020, 9:52 AM EDT / Updated April 27, 2020, 3:21 PM EDT
By Grace Moon

SEOUL, South Korea — At a polling station in Seoul's Seongdong district, masked voters stood three feet apart in single file as they waited to cast ballots in South Korea's parliamentary election.

But before they voted, voters pumped dollops of sanitizer onto their hands and had their temperatures checked. When they finally reached the end of the line, they received a pair of disposable gloves.

Occasionally, volunteers made announcements such as, "Please maintain your personal space." But for the most part, voters kept each other in check and walked out within five minutes.

Many countries have postponed elections as a result of the COVID-19 epidemic, but South Korea has proved its resilience by not only flattening its curve of coronavirus infections, but also voting in parliamentary elections on April 15 in record numbers. The turnout was 66.2 percent — the highest in 28 years. South Korea's success has been lauded the world over.

[..]

If it weren't for the ubiquitous masks, the streets of South Korea would look almost as they did pre-coronavirus. People are again frequenting restaurants, which often have waiting lists as customers return to their pre-virus work routines.

The country's success is no accident. As demonstrated in the last few months by its system of early testing and tracking, South Korea seized the chance to prepare for its next course of action while its citizens adhered patiently to social distancing recommendations.

Early this month, a new committee of government officials, medical experts and scholars started drafting guidelines for communal safeguards as society entered the "new normal."

"We are creating a new set of standards and culture," Vice Health Minister Kim Gang-lip said at a briefing. "Moving forward, we will inevitably have to change the way we meet others, work and study together and even interact with our own family members."

[..]

- https://www.nbcnews.com/news/world/south-korea-beating-cononavirus-anxiety-grows-over-new-normal-n1192886

[Looking through the above again as I edit together this book, I find the image that I've used & the text chosen to exemplify the way that humans are being slotted into geometrical restrictions — *we are biomorphic*, geometry is fine for objects but unnatural & energy-flow-inhibiting in organic beings — to use police state measures on human interactions in the name of 'for our own good' is extremely misleading, we aren't objects to be filed away at the convenience of people who presume to rule us]

****

April 29, 2020, 10:33AM (Inquiring Librarian to group):

Re: HERETICS... random thought

This is pretty much how i listen to the 'news'. I get the 'liberal' at home and the 'conservative' when i call my 79 year old dad in pa. It is getting to the point that i can't listen to npr... It is making me angry. I am not an angry person by nature. But since my job is giving me no updates on my employment status, i have to somewhat keep up. It sucks.

Thanks for sharing Dick. It makes me feel less bad about attempting to sift thru and analyze the bs on npr.

I have an old, good friend in Taipei. I was finally able to get in touch with him. Neary no deaths to this virus there. Ppl wear masks bcuz they are just ok with that. And there has been NO lockdown there at all. What a dream. If life totally fails here, Dennis touts Taipei as a real dream. He has been there 20 years teaching esl (originally from a farm in lower Delaware).

Lastly, on news.... I really LOVE Phil's social media page. I spend less time sifting thru it than i could... Bcuz my sanity is impt right now. But i *really* appreciate it.

****

April 29, 2020, 11:00AM (BP to group):

Love the Baudrillard story. Which by coincidence leads me to forward this Frank Zappa interview, specifically on American television and with a lot of time spent on CNN. Never seen before by the public, the interviewer posted it on youtube 2 weeks ago. I watched it last night and thought it great. Frank is clearly ill, but this is right before he took a real nosedive. It's nice to see him smile and clearly enjoying himself discussing probably his favorite topic outside music.

FRANK ZAPPA; "Turgid Flux"- Comments on American TV Culture (1991)
https://www.youtube.com/watch?v=LoayhbHEIMA&feature=youtu.be

****

April 29, 2020, 2:02PM (Dick to group):

that's a great interview
the pulsa dinura sequence was particularly funny
https://en.wikipedia.org/wiki/Pulsa_diNura
here's some additional info on the subject...

Pulsa diNura - Wikipedia
Pulsa deNura, Pulsa diNura or Pulsa Denoura (Aramaic: פולסי דנורא "The Lashes of Fire") is a purportedly Kabbalistic ceremony in which the destroying angels are invoked to block heavenly forgiveness of the subject's sins, allegedly causing all the curses named in the Bible to befall him resulting in his death. It is controversial for having been allegedly invoked against several ...
en.wikipedia.org

****

April 29, 2020, 7:14PM (Amir-ul Kafirs to group):

TV (that is I have an extreme negative reaction to both because I feel they are forms of brainwashing and TV especially as a sort of surrogate character formation)

I ignore it all as much as possible but then I already have for decades. I think doing so is very good for my mental health. I stopped watching TV 50 years ago & I've never regretted it. I prefer to have my ideas about what constitutes 'reality' be based around 1. my personal unmediated experience, 2. my own research (most often books & other more scholarly publications I choose). Anything that's somewhat forced upon me I reject. When I was told by friends that I should "look at the pictures of New York!" I told people that I don't live in New York & that I tend to form my opinions on what I see around me. We wouldn't be in this mess if people weren't so willing to let mediated non-experience form their opinions.

In South Korea, coronavirus is in retreat but the concern grows over what the 'new normal' will look like

Note the following quote from the above:

""Washing hands and sanitizing door knobs has become routine for every family now," said Seo, a housewife who voted at the Samseon-dong community center. "There isn't anything strange about it anymore. It's as normal as putting on shoes and socks in the morning."

Social distancing to 'everyday distancing'"

I can barely tell you how much I object to such things. I'm not going to sanitize my door knobs, nor am I going to accept "everyday distancing". Therein lies the way to insanity. Anyway, why stop there? This mania for sterilization can easily have no end in sight. What about actual sterilization chambers in every home & at the entrance to every business? In order to enter a business, people should pay a nominal fee to step into the sterilization chamber & be irradiated. No skin showing. EVER. Sex through holes in sheets & only after a doctor's approval for it, perhaps allowed once a year, perhaps only for the purpose of reproduction. In fact, do away with sex altogether, only test tube babies approved by eugenicists. Sex is too dangerous, it's definitely a dirty business.

The 'funny' this is: **I don't even think I'm being paranoid here.**

****

April 29, 2020, 8:52PM (Dick to tENT):

Your ideas about germ-free sex are funny

And I imagine not far from the truth

Maybe this group should institute "Heretic Sex Certificates"

Members get a card with "I'M OK FOR FUCKING - OFFICIALLY GERM FREE" printed on it

****

April 29, 2020, 9:19PM (Amir-ul Kafirs to group):

It is getting to the point that i can't listen to npr... It is making me angry.

I don't think there's such a thing as 'news' without a political subtext and ulterior motive. That's why we all have to be critical readers in order to process it all. Fox TV makes it easy because they're so blatant, blatantly selling religion, blatantly selling guns — but NPR is more sublte, hence it appeals to more subtle people who mistake the subtlety for 'truth' instead of camouflage.

Lastly, on news.... I really LOVE Phil's social media page.

I should probably look at friends's timelines more often. For me, I mostly stopped posting about the PANDEMIC PANIC on social media because I'd already unfriended 3 people, been "defriended" by another and was on the brink of unfriending 4 more friends who I've known for a long time. I figured I should take it easy, I was really beginning to hate people. As it is, I'm more misanthropic than ever but I'm also trying to ride this out without making too many new enemies.

[That eventually changed when counteracting the propaganda became even more urgent for me]

****

April 30, 2020, 7:37AM (Amir-ul Kafirs to group):

This reminds me of my pal...the one I wrote about earlier verbally attacking me over lunch. Months later, after he reached out and sort of apologized, there was a day when he was in my car. Even after our mending, he couldnt resist pointing to my pre-programmed radio stations. I guess he thought he was being clever when he pointed to my NPR pre-set, feigning surprise. Like I should stick to that one news source, label it the TRUTH button. I'm sorry, but my problem isn't with The Donald. It's with the people that think everything changed the moment he was elected.

Exactly, as if lying was something that'd never happened before! As if stupidity were a new thing! As if dishonesty & manipulation in politics had just now appeared! Everything objectionable has been with us all along, all the murder, prejudice, greed, you name it. Rump puts a red face on it all where his predeccesors might've been more subtle but such criminality is intrinsic.

****

April 30, 2020, 2:21PM (Amir-ul Kafirs to Dick):

Re: HERETICS... random thought

Your ideas about germ-free sex are funny

I reckon a 'germ-free' body would actually be incredibly unhealthy, not to mention 'impossible', probably close to death. How would it be achieved? Irradiation? Bleach-baths? Whatever would kill the germs would also kill the rest of the body. That's something that these sterility-enforcers seem to misunderstand: ***our bodies are an ecosystem and the germs are part of that ecosystem.***

****

April 30, 2020, 4:35PM (Inquiring Librarian to group):

Re: HERETICS... random thought

As ever Amir-ul Kafirs, i think you are absolutely correct here. I am only attempting to listen to the news so i have some idea of the fate of my job. It is so grim. I am ready to give up listening to the broken record. The politicians here seem hell bent on destroying the economy and breaking our spirits as we beg for handouts. I for one am ready to watch an armed insurrection of the working class against the government. There are a lot of crazy pissed off gun toting nut jobs out there.. Or are they really nut jobs? I feel world life is an inverse fairy tale these daze

****

April 30, 2020, 8:22PM (Amir-ul Kafirs to group):

Re: HERETICS... random thought

There are a lot of crazy pissed off gun toting nut jobs out there.. Or are they really nut jobs? I feel world life is an inverse fairy tale these daze

After having spent most of my life in an economically precarious position I FINALLY have some temporary economic security BUT I STILL FEEL A BIT CRAZY FROM THIS WHOLE PANDEMIC PANIC. I told Naia Nisnam today something like 'It's like watching people have their blood drained from their bodies & being unable to do anything about it.' With "blood" as a metaphor for intelligence. It seems that people just '*have to' believe in* ***something****, whether it's their news feed or their political party of* ***whatever*** so they cling to these beliefs like a life raft no matter how inappropriate the beliefs are to the situation. Hence we have people believing in doctors, in NPR, in right wing talk radio, in Rump, etc.. The thing they *don't believe in* is their own ability to figure things out based on whatever sensory data is immediately available to them.

The HERETICS see specific social things happening, we see the economy endangered, free thinking endangered, etc, so it's easy to just pay attention to that & to try to not let all the hoopla get in the way of just perceiving the day-to-day obvious. BUTT, shit!, it's hard for people to do that if their minds are clogged by a constant barrage of crap, a veritable SHIT STORM of misinformation and smoke & mirrors.

Maybe it's not even an "inverse fairy tale", maybe it's like a Brothers Grimm fairy tale, maybe most people are children being lured to the cannibal's hut by sweets.

-A Statement from an Inquiring Librarian residing in Louisiana-

I am an information science specialist by career. I am a librarian. I live in Louisiana. I believe in the United States 1st Amendment of Free Speech and I believe in Health Freedom. I have spent most of my life dealing with the modern western 'health' care[less] one size fits all system from day one when jaundiced newborn me was placed in an incubator to un-yellow.

I'll be the first to admit, throughout my life, I've remained mostly politically ignorant. I preferred to read old school fiction or revisionist historical nonfiction only on topics that interested me. At least my interests have always been vast, and I've always avoided dime store novels in favor of much more weighty fiction. So I have not been entirely ignorant. Current affairs mostly disinterested me and I found the 'news' to be mostly a waste of my time. Of course, this is shameful, I'll be the first to admit this. To further explain, fiction works seemed more honest to me in explaining past events and genuine human emotions and interactions. In fiction, no one is telling you what is fact, which I appreciate because I was a born, and continue to be a lifelong, skeptic! My favorite works of fiction have always centered around the conflicts in and around the world wars, be the setting Japan, Germany, Austria, Russia, etc... I will go out on a limb here and conjecture, we appear to be entering into World War 3, the format is just obviously different from what we would traditionally call 'warfare'. This is a war against the natural body and the freedoms therein. It's the people who see through this dastardly germ and psychological war-game, against the 1% who would like for us to see our own bodies as disease vectors and not the amazing self-care biomes that nature created us to be.

What has drawn me out of my former peacefully ignorant reverie that I've mostly ducked and covered into all of my life, is this 'virus'. I have always had a very good natural intuition. And my wonderful mother has always told me that I have always had a VERY good guardian angel. By early March, 2020, I could see that the situation at hand was not as it seemed according to what the mass media was telling me. My first instinct was to scour my brain for a friend that would possibly not judge me for being skeptical of the virus and who also might see things the scary/not so great way that I did. I called my friend tENT. tENT and I had not spoken on the phone in literally years. He was, I believe, quite surprised to hear from me. Immediately though, I knew I'd called the right friend. We were on the same page in disbelief and concern as to what exactly the hell was going on. tENT invited me to join his email HERETICS group. It took me a good month of listening to everyone in the group and finding, absorbing, and researching their sources of information, for me to get my bearings and to thus find my own way of navigating the miasma of brainwashing, falsely "fact-checked", carefully packaged disinformation campaign of lies out there for the taking by the obedient and information illiterate masses on the internet, radio, and TV. I found my own sources! As a life long skeptic, even of my own brainpower, finding my own sources of information on current worldly matters, has been hugely beneficial for me, as ignorance has never been 'bliss' for me.

Call me crazy. Call me a Conspiracy Theorist. Or simply assume without doing your own research that I am that poor sweet, innocent little ignorant librarian who simply doesn't understand that, Of Course, the government Does care about me/us, they would Never harm us for money or control. I can take it, other's such judgments of me, as I always have. I firmly believe through my vast research from now trusted sources and my own ability to hash through that information I find and process it with my own god-given brain, that I am more 'correct' in the 'truth' of the matter at hand than those that would doubt and judge me. The only reason I remain silent to most is because I love my job. Imagine, needing to hide information when you are a trained, Master's degreed Information Science Specialist. How absurd. But I live this every day. When I figure out a way out of this quandary, or am forced out of it, I will make my voice heard.

Now get this. Here is what fully 'woke' me up. Have you noticed the recent push for world vaccination laws? If you have not, simply listen to any mainstream news. Now here is something the mainstream news does not tell you… Did you know, that the U.S. HR 5546, 1985-1986, the National Childhood Vaccine Injury Act, provides that no vaccine manufacturer shall be liable in a civil action for damages arising from a vaccine-related injury or death? Think about that for a moment. Do you not see avenues for corruption here? Consider then, that after 1986, the regular schedule of childhood vaccinations grew from just 7 when I was born, to now 72!! But then, you might want to argue with me, "Well, vaccines are of course safety tested and proven to be safe!!". You'd think that, but your thinking is dead wrong. Now know this, vaccines are not considered a 'Medicine'. They are instead considered a "Biologic". Thus, as a "Biologic", they do not need the standard safety required double blind test against a placebo. They have no true safety testing. If you'd like to know more about this and/or check my 'facts,' (and you really should like to know more about this, in my opinion) listen to Robert F. Kennedy Jr., Del Bigtree, Dr. / Senator Scott Jensen, any mother who has a vaccine injured child, watch "Vaxxed", watch "1986: The Act", listen to Dr. Andrew Wakefield & Judy Mikovitz, and J.B. Handley, etc. Shame on you if you are among those who on blind faith only believe those that threw these scientists, lawyers, journalists, activists, and parents under the bus before you even took the time to listen to the vast amount of information they have to share. None of them or I are "anti-vaxxers." We are all for vaccines that are safe and effective, something currently non-existent when you check the true facts. Ask yourself, why did SIDS (Sudden Infant Death Syndrome), Autism, allergies, and chronic illness all sky-rise after 1986? And follow the money trail from the NIH, CDC, WHO, GAVI, etc… all the way to the present Covid debacle.

Due to a homozygous genetic defect that I inherited, I would likely have been one of those children either dead or severely brain damaged through a vaccine induced, otherwise latent, mitochondrial disease, had I been given the modern course of vaccinations for children born after 1986. My doctor has told me that I am one of those people who should NEVER be vaccinated. In fact, his eyes nearly popped out of his head when I told him I'd even had my few CDC recommended vaccinations when I was born in the 1970's. The few vaccines I've had have likely been the cause of my autoimmune issues, my slow growth, my renal issues, my lifelong battles with depression, my never having had children. Many would argue that I have at least a mild case of Asperger's (one of my fellow librarians who IS diagnosed is very fond of telling me this each time I give her a ride home from a work meeting, ha ha!!). Over the years I have found ways to combat these things that some would consider damaged in my body. I have figured out ways to accept myself as I am and to coerce my body to work better with nature through vitamins and exercise, avoiding toxins as much as possible, taking natural methylfolate instead of pharmaceutical anti-depressants, exercising, not doing drugs or drinking when most of my artist friends have. I've always been an outsider. Now I am much more so and further, I have become an outcast, for my HERETIC status as a disbeliever in this "Plandemic" or "Scamdemic" if you'll allow me to give it 2 well-deserved names.

Lastly, did I mention, my father is a refugee from the front lines of Soviet and Nazi occupied Belarus during World War 2. I was taught all of my life, to NEVER follow the herd, to ALWAYS think for myself, to Question Everything. I was a real math and science wiz years ago in high school. I'll never forget that day my previous junior-year's chemistry teacher told my senior year's physics teacher, "You can never fool IL, she will Always figure it out!". Ha Ha!! I think my chemistry teacher was right! I am not fooled and I refuse to be brainwashed. I trust my homeopathic-centered doctor. I trust my intuition and my own research. I trust that the allopathic doctors that gave my Belorussian grandmother (from whom I likely inherited my genetic defect), her first vaccinations and introduction to western profit-driven 'health' care[less] in 1947, 'warp'-sped her to her early death at 41 years old, within 1 year of her arriving in the United States.

I will fight my way out of this biomedical police state, as I have with every bind I've stumbled or been forced into. I will NEVER except Orwell's fiction as My reality. Stated another way, I like to leisurely read science fiction, not live it. Have I made my point clear enough?

HERETICS emails - May, 2020

May 1, 2020, 10:04AM (Phil to group):

Re: HERETICS: Taibbi: The Inevitable Coronavirus Censorship Crisis is Here

In relation to the praise of the Chinese ways of handling things I should share this with you before it gets lost in my stream. It is an interview on the Jimmy Dore show with Whitney Webb about a Government document released under the freedom of information act.
https://www.youtube.com/watch?v=bGMkSNj_-7Q&feature=share

the Last american Vagabond article can be found here;
https://www.thelastamericanvagabond.com/top-news/techno-tyranny-how-us-national-security-state-using-coronavirus-fulfill-orwellian-vision/

Mostly I have tuned my social media stream to interesting stories from various favorite outlets. I don't really use it as social media. I don't really care much about what people think of my posts and I have no family (none of my family have social media accounts) or current work acquaintances as friends. I do not usually use the like button much either, mostly just sift through the more interesting stuff and just share.

Here is another techno-tyranny dystopian article about some microsoft plans;
https://www.independent.co.uk/life-style/gadgets-and-tech/news/microsoft-cryptocurrency-mining-brain-waves-body-data-bitcoin-a9480766.html?amp

and a microsoft patent here;
https://patentscope.wipo.int/search/en/detail.jsf?docId=WO2020060606&tab=PCTBIBLI

The Juice Media is usually spot on and sharp with most issues. Good Arsetrailian sense of humor. With Covid I find them a little bit uncritical of the criticality of Covid-19 and the lockdown itself. But they are still good questioning the Authoritarian responses which is nice to see. They have let me down with some other issues too (cant actually remember which) Mostly pretty spot on though. I guess you can't be spot on all the time.
https://www.youtube.com/user/thejuicemedia

****

May 2, 2020, 2:49PM (Dick to Amir-ul Kafirs):

book

Hi
I've thought about this book idea
I think it's a really good idea but I'm not really sure if I fit into it's scheme which seems research-based
I'd be happy to write about my feelings about this situation but I'm not sure if my personal thoughts are really that pertinent in the final analysis
Ultimately, besides being naturally skeptical, I just think I can't stand the idea of being forced to follow someone else's plans - Bill Gates, Trump's, Macron's, anyone's... and I don't like group-think... I feel uncomfortable in churches, in any groups... I don't trust governments... I feel that government is no longer valid and it's for that precise reason that governments are trying to take more and more control - because they know they must either take over or fade away
Everyone knows they are the enforcement arm of the 1% - all other functions are technical (roads, etc)
Whatever I wrote would be essentially that kind of personal speculation
It's your call

****

May 1, 2020 (photo from Amir-ul Kafirs):

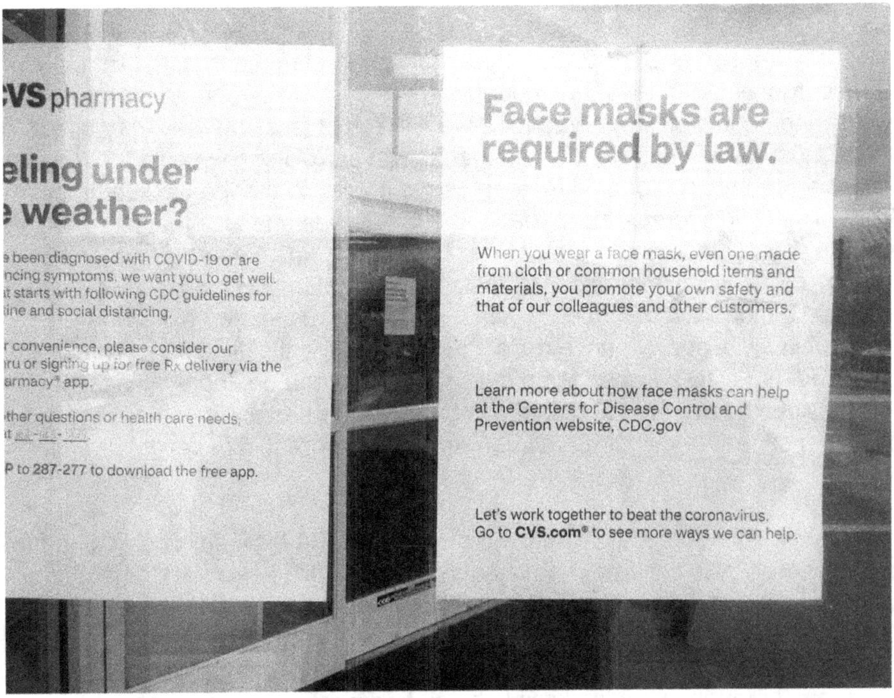

****

May 3, 2020, 5:36AM (Amir-ul Kafirs to Dick):

Re: book

I think it's a really good idea but I'm not really sure if I fit into it's scheme which seems research-based

Dick, I'm just asking you to write whatever you want to pertinent to the subject of "Mind Control Opportunism in the era of COVID-19". I've suggested that each contirbutor write something autobiographical to explain how they got to where they are philosophically at this point in time. I'm also suggesting that you provide some sort of summary of things that you've posted links to on HERETICS. But these are just suggestions. You should just write whatever you're moved to write, what you suggest sounds fine to me.

****

May 1, 2020, 7:35PM (Naia Nisnam to group):

Re: HERETICS: Tabbi: The Inevitable Coronavirus Censorship Crisis is Here

I like this Taibbi article, I've shared it with a few people.
I haven't had much time to share thoughts here, but I have some that are currently bothering me-

1. The assumption of COVID19 without testing- in March and early April, people in Pittsburgh who had fever and cough were told, over the phone, that they have COVID and should stay at home for 2 weeks- out of fear that they may infect others. I just found out from a friend that her 5-year old son was diagnosed over the phone and his doctor said to keep him at home, so that he wouldnt infect others. The child's temperature reached 103 degrees and was that high, off and on, for 3 days. I understand that, at that time, there was a shortage of tests. For COVID19. But. His symptoms also match the symptoms for pneumonia. Pneumonia didn't just disappear when the coronavirus started to spread. Pneumonia still exits. We have tests for it. We have antibiotics for it. This child recovered, but a 103 degree temp in a young child can be deadly. It seems all too plausible the boy was at risk of dying from untreated pneumonia, because of the immense fear of the Coronavirus. Am I being paranoid? I can't even tell anymore.

2. There may be more critical thinkers out there than I realized. Today, I had to deliver packages to children (I am/was a parent & child advocate). One of the dads came outside to meet me on his porch. Already quite different from the other families who hovered inside of their windows to wave at me. This guy seemed to be acting strangely. I never knew him well, usually dealing with the kid's mom. I thought he was possibly trying to express skepticism about the severity of the virus without directly saying it. He told me a friend of his at the local hospital (AGH) said that they would be returning to normal operations soon because they never got close to the numbers of patients they had expected. I told him that, yes, I had been looking at those numbers too... Slowly we each started to say more and more "controversial" things. By the end of the visit, his daughter was in my arms, we told each other stories and ran around playing a

game we had made up in school. It felt wonderfully normal. Old normal, not this insulting "new normal" we are supposed to accept. Her dad finally laid it out to me that he believes this pandemic has been, possibly made up, and absolutely exaggerated to control the public, to hand more money over to large corporations, to continue squashing small businesses. He also sees the end goal as mandatory worldwide vaccination. It left me feeling hopeful that there are many more people quietly questioning. It is also frightening to think about our conversation, testing each other, each of us trying to assess if the other was also a skeptic, afraid to come right out and say it. Is this what our freedom of speech looks like now?

Possibly, as this quote from the comment section of Matt Taibbi's article shows, if someone disagrees with what you are saying, then you are not an advocate of free speech, you are a lunatic:

"I watched a livestream of the PA demonstration, filmed not by a reporter but by the legislator who promoted it. These were not free speech advocates. They were mixing Covid with abortion with gun rights and adding a strong dose of conspiracy theories and anti-vax. And now governors have started to give in to them. At what point does the free speech of the lunatic fringe infringe on the rights and safety of the majority?"

3. I need help deciphering anti-vaccine information. I read and listen to anti-vax information from varying sources. A lot of it seems to make sense, but I always hit a point that seems absolutely ridiculous. All anti-vaccine information is completely discredited in the mainstream, to the point that I can't even get search results that aren't debunking or ridiculing anti-vax information. Can anyone here connect me with reasonable information about the possibility that Coronaviruses are connected to the animal matter that is in vaccines, Bill Gates and the polio vaccine in India, and the ID chip that will be included in the mandatory worldwide vaccine?

I did manage to find this disturbing law about vaccines in America: "No vaccine manufacturer shall be liable in a civil action for damages arising from a vaccine-related injury or death associated with the administration of a vaccine after October 1, 1988, if the injury or death resulted from side effects that were unavoidable even though the vaccine was properly prepared and was accompanied by proper directions and warnings."

That's from the Cornell legal codes... https://www.law.cornell.edu/uscode/text/42/300aa-22 If you are injured or die as a side effect of a vaccine, well, that's just too bad, and certainly not the problem of the manufacturer.

And, yes, Amir-ul Kafirs, write a book. I'm willing to help as much as I can.

****

May 1, 2020, 7:52PM (Amir-ul Kafirs to group):

I did manage to find this disturbing law about vaccines in America: "No vaccine If you are injured or die as a side effect of a vaccine, well, that's just too bad, and certainly not the problem of the manufacturer.

Ha ha! As a sidenote here: I had a job where the employees were told that they had to sign a waiver relieving our employer of any & all responsibility in case of injury or DEATH on the job. We were told that we couldn't work if we didn't sign it. One other older guy & I said something to the effect of: "We'd be crazy to sign this!" & refused. Everyone else was immediately cowed into submission. The employer, needing our expertise, relinquished & then we managed to change the situation so that NO-ONE had to sign it. That took courage on our part because we all needed the work. The issue came up again & instead of remembering what we'd accomplished the last time *our coworkers immediately signed it out of fear of not getting the work.* In the meantime, the other old timer & I continued to refuse & were still hired anyway.

Thanks for the info about the vaccine law. That doesn't surprise me but it's very good to know about. Our society is totally set up to protect the powerful. Here's a simple example: it's illegal to write a post-dated check, it's NOT illegal for a bank to cash it ahead of the date signed. When they do that the person who's written the check then has to pay a penalty fee even though it was the bank that caused the pre-date cashing. The bank pays no penalty.

****

May 2, 2020, 9:56AM (Amir-ul Kafirs to group):

HERETICS: More shit from The Atlantic

Do any of you read things on Medium? It's useful. Here's a link to an Atlantic article made available there:

https://medium.com/the-atlantic/georgias-experiment-in-human-sacrifice-388029dee95e

Given that the article's title is "**Georgia's Experiment in Human Sacrifice**" one might say that they're setting the reader up for a rather sensationalized take on things. As usual, this sensationalism is based on PREDICTION as if it's already FACT, which it isn't.

****

May 2, 2020, 9:59AM (Phil to group):

The thing with vaccines is that any discussion has become very polarised so you can not even discuss intricacies of the topic. As soon as you do you become an anti-vaxer even if that is not exactly your position. Also of course there are a lot of religious right anti-vaxers or even just christians talking on the topic that will drop in some line about god somewhere that is cringe worthy. Big media outlets take a lot of money from Big Pharma and they have been very successful at silencing a lot of voices critical of vaccines. Also through law suits.

Just a little vaccine research here but not necessarily addressing directly your questions. I gotta get off the internet now but I hope help address questions a bit?

I find this a real good read published in the ecologist.
Polio: the virus and the vaccine
https://jeffreydachmd.com/wp-content/uploads/2014/12/Polio-Virus-Vaccine-Janine-Roberts_Ecologist-2004.pdf

Vaccine liability has been given to the Government now instead of the corporations through the National Vaccine Injury Compensation Program although it is not widely publicised. https://en.wikipedia.org/wiki/National_Vaccine_Injury_Compensation_Program

How the oral polio vaccine can cause polio
https://www.npr.org/2019/11/16/780068006/how-the-oral-polio-vaccine-can-cause-polio?t=1588426415441

Mutant Strains of Polio Vaccine Now Cause More Parlysis Than Wild Polio
https://www.npr.org/sections/goatsandsoda/2017/06/28/534403083/mutant-strains-of-polio-vaccine-now-cause-more-paralysis-than-wild-polio

medical paper;
https://web.archive.org/web/20200412234643/https://www.ncbi.nlm.nih.gov/pmc/articles/PMC6121585/pdf/ijerph-15-01755.pdf

Judges demand answers after children die in controversial cancer vaccine trial in India (gardasil)
https://www.dailymail.co.uk/news/article-2908963/Judges-demand-answers-children-die-controversial-cancer-vaccine-trial-India.html

Controversial vaccine studies: Why is Bill & Melinda Gates Foundation under fire from critics in India?
https://economictimes.indiatimes.com/industry/healthcare/biotech/healthcare/controversial-vaccine-studies-why-is-bill-melinda-gates-foundation-under-fire-from-critics-in-india/articleshow/41280050.cms?utm_source=contentofinterest&utm_medium=text&utm_campaign=cppst

These are interesting cases that could also be worth looking into more (coming from a right wing site);

In 2010, the Gates Foundation funded a trial of a GSK's experimental malaria vaccine, killing 151 African infants and causing serious adverse effects including paralysis, seizure, and febrile convulsions to 1,048 of the 5,049 children.
During Gates 2002 MenAfriVac Campaign in Sub-Saharan Africa, Gates

operatives forcibly vaccinated thousands of African children against meningitis. Between 50-500 children developed paralysis. South African newspapers complained, “We are guinea pigs for drug makers.” Nelson Mandela’s former Senior Economist, Professor Patrick Bond, describes Gates’ philanthropic practises as “ruthless” and "immoral”.
In 2010, Gates committed $ 10 billion to the WHO promising to reduce population, in part, through new vaccines. A month later Gates told a Ted Talk that new vaccines “could reduce population”.
In 2014, Kenya’s Catholic Doctors Association accused the WHO of chemically sterilizing millions of unwilling Kenyan women with a phoney “tetanus” vaccine campaign.
Independent labs found the sterility formula in every vaccine tested. After denying the charges, WHO finally admitted it had been developing the sterility vaccines for over a decade.
Similar accusations came from Tanzania, Nicaragua, Mexico and the Philippines.
A 2017 study (Morgensen et.Al.2017) showed that WHO’s popular DTP is killing more African than the disease it pretends to prevent. Vaccinated girls suffered 10x the death rate of unvaccinated children.
https://www.sgtreport.com/2020/04/bill-gates-vaccine-crime-record-496000-paralyzed-children-in-india-and-more/

****

May 2, 2020, 10:57AM (Inquiring Librarian to group):

Re: HERETICS: Tabbi: The Inevitable Coronavirus Censorship Crisis is Here

I also LOVED the Taibbi article. It seemed spot on on so many current issues and social interactions. I tried sharing it with a few people. My sister, a devout republican and Trump supporter, now thinks i am a Trump supporter. I love my sister and family, but she is so wrong. I cannot directly tell her i do not support Trump. But, i do appreciate the common bond we feel against the current government oppression and manipulation. The political differences I've always had with my family have always boggled my mind. I love my family and we have never abandoned one another or seriously quarreled. They are amazing.

Phil, i don't know how you find and compile so much interesting information! Amir-ul Kafirs, also, how do you find the time and energy to read and organize and intelligently and so on pointedly respond to all!! I am in awe! I have all of the free time in the world right now. But i can barely find the time to well read and listen to the links you all share, as much as i 100% want to. My life is currently peppered with a 500 pg bk about the bloodlands, a new outdoor kitten acclimating to 5 other home kitties, overexercising, making lace, gardening, freaking out about work, making and eating too much food (& worrying how i will buy food if my job goes belly up) checking in with family... And being appalled by my social media friends of the liberal 'fingerwagging' type and fearing the future.

All of that being said... I too am happy to work on the book. But i have to also say i am barrelling down freakout mountain, picking up spead, the longer my job situation remains unstable. When this happens, i tend to get really busy doing mindless crazy things like spending hours on my bike or moving plants around or obsessing over a new kitten and hating myself for not trying to learn to play every instrument i have failed at. I want to help. If a specific task is given to me, i will structure it into my day. I do not want to disappoint.

****

May 3, 2020, 5:51AM (Amir-ul Kafirs to group):

On May 2, 2020, at 9:59 AM, Phil Bradley wrote:

Thanks for all these links. I have to admit that I won't be looking at them all right now but I'm glad to have them as a reference resource. I, personally, don't get vaccinated & haven't since I was a kid when I always found it hard to understand why I was getting them. I will resist getting a vaccination now. On the other hand, since I'm old enough to have friends who had polio before the vaccine came along & who're crippled as a result it's hard for me to write off the polio vaccine. It seems that there would be less people crippled by it if they had had access to the vaccine — but then I'm hardly an expert on the subject.

****

May 3, 2020, 3:31PM (BP to group):

We have been living in crazy times. Or more likely it's always been like this and I was unaware. I've largely been spared, my circle is small. And I'm old enough to not give a shit and it will not effect my getting laid. I have a young friend who went through so much Hell and (temporary?) loss of life-long friends as he wouldn't join the bandwagon and blindly condemn Trump, embrace whatever the liberal gestalt is. The rehabilitation of George Bush (the MSNBC/CNN crowd) is telling, a nice summation. In casual social interactions, I've always remained largely mute regarding politics or race relation issues and so people pretty much tell me exaxctly what is on their minds. I've heard some horrid shit! Once in awhile I'll tell them to: Fuck Off. But if they are going to form opinions about me by what I say (whatever they want to hear) I may as well let them form opinions about me on what I do not say. I heard 8 years of how GREAT Obama was and now I have 4 years of how TERRIBLE Trump is. I'm sure each of my encounters think I'm on their team.

PS I should have fleshed this out a bit more so please allow me to add an example: When I have had a back-and-forth with the CAMPS, I can say something simple like: "Obama was resistant to arming Ukraine. He thought it would escalate tensions with Moscow. I think he was right." This infuriated his own Party and the War Party was furious, Hillary among them (they loved her for that). SO: Here I am PRO-Obama. But then as this was "forgotten." the Power Structure says: Trump's resistance to arming Ukraine is a submission to Putin! He is in bed with the Russians. Traitor! They got something on him!

When Trump finally did arm the Ukraine, and I pointed it out to a friend that this was so, he told me that Trump DID, but he gave the arms to the RUSSIAN-backed rebels.

I can't find any evidence of that.

****

May 3, 2020, 6:03PM (Amir-ul Kafirs to group):

if they are going to form opinions about me by what I say (whatever they want to hear)

& that parenthetical aside is increasingly what it amounts to. People have prefabricated opinions that're of soundbyte oversimplicity and they slot those into the blank that they leave after they stop paying attention to what the other person is saying.

****

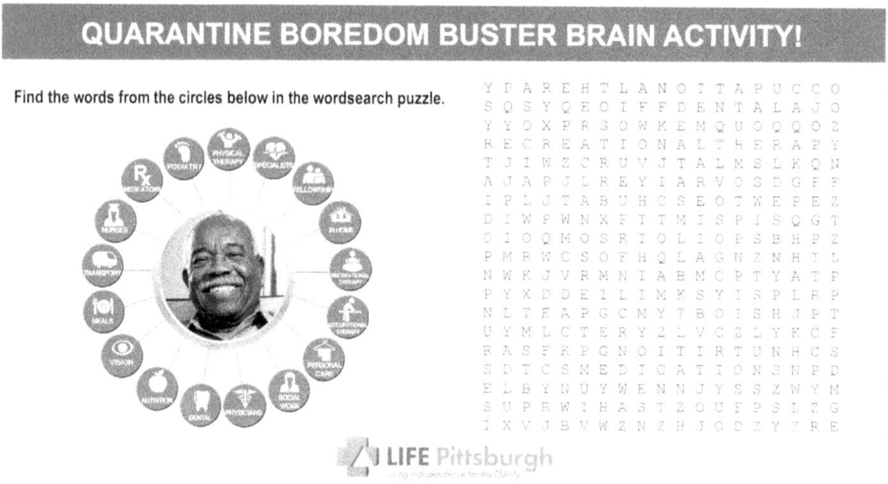

QUARANTINE BOREDOM BUSTER BRAIN ACTIVITY!
Find the words from the circles below in the wordsearch puzzle.
LIFE Pittsburgh

****

May 4, 2020, 7:14AM (Dick to group):

I don't know if you are all subscribed to Activist Channel, if not here's one to start your day
https://www.youtube.com/watch?v=2MGXePjIzXE

Bill Gates Partners With DARPA & Department of Defense For New DNA Nanotech COVID19 Vaccine!
In this powerful interview, Spiro is joined by Whitney Webb and Ryan Cristian

from The Last American Vagabond, as they discuss the rollout of a new system of control the likes of which the world has never seen. It has been said to never let a good crisis go to waste and it appears the ones pulling the strings are taking full advantage of the ...

****

May 4, 2020, 1:43PM (Amir-ul Kafirs to group):

HERETICS: You'll Never See A Billionaire Waiting In A Food Line

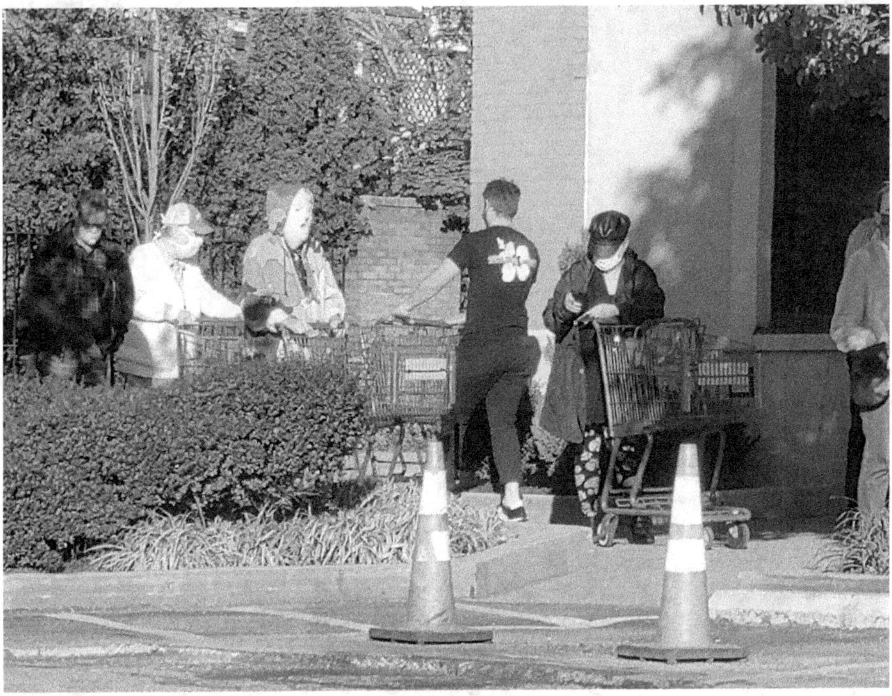

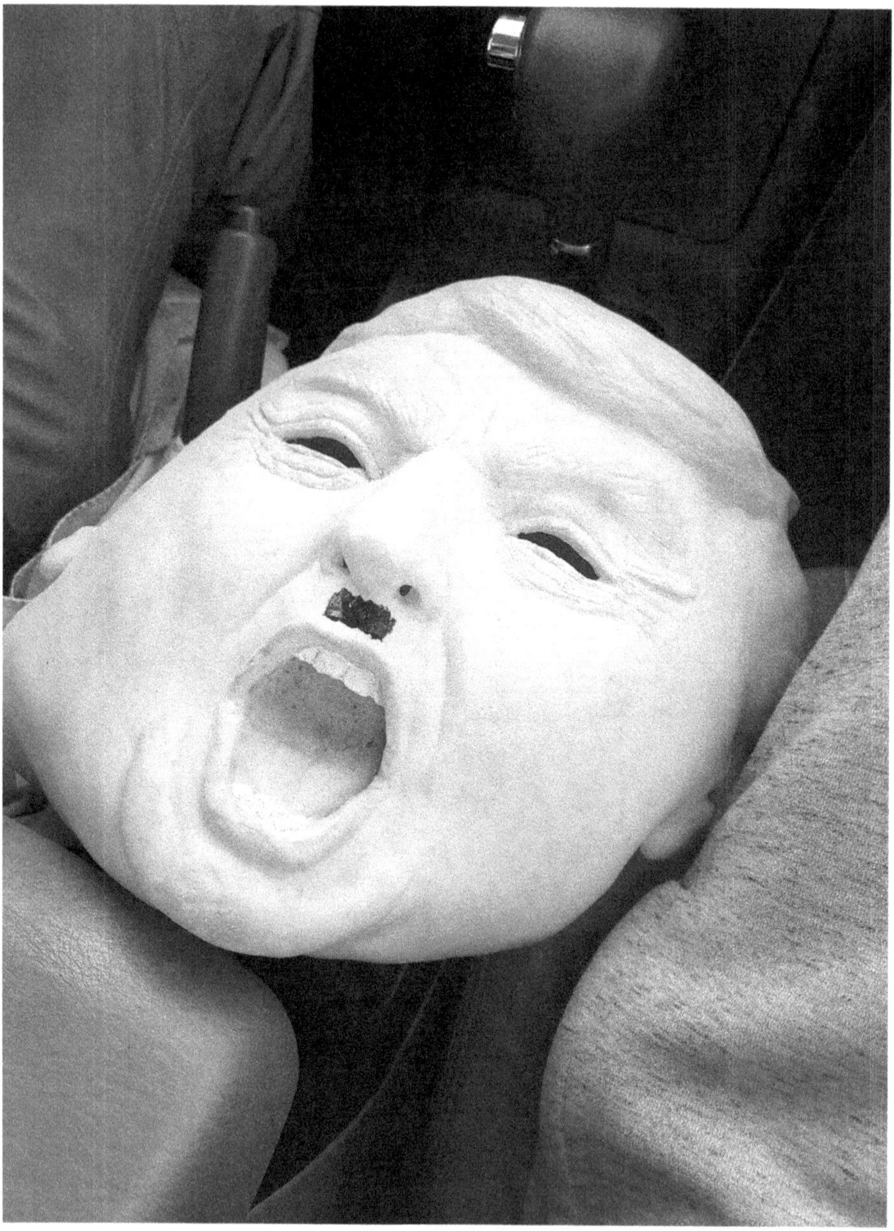

****

May 4, 2020, 11:22PM (Amir-ul Kafirs to group):

HERETICS: Billionaires Speech

Here's the speech that I just wrote as my narration for the footage that was shot today of me wearing the Rump/Hitler mask at the food store:

"You'll Never See A Billionaire Standing In A Food Line"
- tENTATIVELY, a cONVENIENCE
- May 4, 2020 (Vision)

You'll never see a Billionaire standing in a food line and you're not seeing one now. Instead, you're seeing an anarchist with a mask on depicting a well-known billionaire adorned with a suggestive moustache. This gives the anarchist an excuse to use a media figurehead to get your attention for ideas that that figurehead would never express.

"There's no such thing as bad publicity" is sometimes attributed to 19th century American showman and circus owner P. T. Barnum but it might as well be the motto of a certain billionaire. My sense of the saying's application in this instance is that no matter how idiotic the quotes are that the billionaire generates it's still publicity that makes him seem familiar and the familiar, as with music, becomes consonant.

What if the purpose of this media bombardment, this constant presence, is to *dumb down the general consciousness of the people of the world?* The pro-Rump faction gets dumbed down by believing all the shit that the Rump emits while the anti-Rump faction gets dumbed down by ALSO believing that he means all the shit. The result is a highly polarized, divided and conquered society in which BOTH SIDES believe that '*if you're not with us, you're against us.*'

But about the rest of us? What about those of us who can pay attention to anyone's opinions and ideas and evaluate them on a basis that has nothing to do with what 'side' they supposedly generate from?

As a FREE THINKER I question the PANDEMIC PANIC. I see it as an opportunistic exploitation of the fear of death that's been hyper-exaggerated by mass media in order to distract the susceptible public into not noticing that a global reorganization of power is taking place.

According to my own life experience, which I value more highly than any doctor's opinion, it's unhealthy to not allow one's environment to immunize you through coexisting with it; it's unhealthy to be socially isolated; it's especially unhealthy to let other people run your life for you. Even if you MAKE MISTAKES, they're YOUR MISTAKES. I am NOT a worshipper at the Temple of the DOCTOR GODS nor at the temples of any other power-mad megalomaniacs who want to subjugate me — and claims of this subjugation being 'for my own good' are intuitively and intellectually experienced by me as the opposite. Any type of police state, even 'Medical Police State Lite', is not in my best interest.

Instead, I think that humanity is being psychologically conditioned to be a Pavlovian Dog, to essentially be '*'living' in Virtual 'Reality''*, to be so out of touch with unmediated real experience that only mediated non-experience is accepted as 'real' any more. As such, people whose attention is riveted to fear-mongering so-called 'news' and to the approved information sources that match their subcultural identities are more likely to believe prefabricated stories than they are the more immediate evidence of their own senses.

People not living in crowded cities, will still believe that they're as threatened by epidemic circumstances as people living in a city with a population density FIVE TIMES that of their own — even though that makes no sense.

With these, and many other critical and CRIMINALLY SANE THOUGHT CRIMES in mind, I prefer to not obey the laws that have been laid down 'for my own good'. Nonetheless, if I want to buy food from a store that requires a mask then a mask it is — but why wear just any old ordinary mask? Why not wear the mask of a well-known billionaire?

Because "You'll never see a Billionaire standing in a food line", after all, their servants do the food shopping and preparation for them. Let this remind you that no matter how much a figurehead pretends to be working class to manipulate a certain demographic into feeling like he's just another asshole in the family, he's NOT working class, he was born into extreme privilege and this P. T. Barnum act is based on the knowledge that 'a sucker is born every minute.' And the suckers are on BOTH sides of the great artificial divide.

****

May 5, 2020, 10:13PM (Amir-ul Kafirs to group):

Re: HERETICS: Billionaires Speech

On May 5, 2020, at 3:41 PM, BP wrote:

Very well put, Amir-ul Kafirs.

Thank you. I imagine I'll get the usual anger directed my way now that I've put the movie online but I feel like I expressed myself carefully enough so that I'm comfortable with what I said.

Look forward to the visuals as well. Sure beats my drunken tirade! But I'll cut myself some slack. I realized I reached my breaking point the past 2 days. I'm pretty much done looking at the extreme, dire warnings. There is a new barrage today due to a leaked study that says plenty of Hell is a'comin across the usofa. I'm throwing in the towel and going on media black out. I can imagine what television watchers have been put through. At least all I do is read.

It might seem to some like 'escapism' but I think that tuning out the mass media pseudo-'news' is one of the best ways to stay sane.

Good luck to us all. Today is day 47 of the QUARANTYRANNY here in Pennsylvania. It's ambiguous to me as to when it's going to lift.

****

May 5, 2020, 10:07PM (Amir-ul Kafirs to group):

HERETICS: "You'll Never See a Billionaire Standing in a Food Line" online

"You'll Never See A Billionaire Standing In A Food Line" notes - 4:55 - 1080p

https://youtu.be/l_r8F-oMtYE

https://archive.org/details/youll-never-see-a-billionaire

I am a HERETIC. I think that the PANDEMIC PANIC is being used by opportunists to experiment with MIND CONTROL and to condition people to have their lives controlled 'for their own good'. This opinion is sometimes foolishly associated with 'Conservatives' by 'Liberals'. But, no, I'm not either, I'm a FREE THINKER, I'm CRIMINALLY SANE, I'm a THOUGHT CRIMINAL. The degree of pressure that's on the few of us who are trying to think outside the MONOLITHIC NARRATIVE is astounding. Since I exist mainly in a 'liberal' culture it's sickening to see this culture use bullying, misrepresentation, lying, brow-beating, and so on to try to force the few HERETICS and SKEPTICS into going along with the program(ming) instead of reaching our own conclusions. Because of this pressure, and it isn't 'peer pressure' because there's no way these people are even remotely my 'peers', I think of 'Liberalism' as basically a new variation on Neo-Nazism: something I'm adamantly opposed to. No doubt, 'Liberals' will strenuously object to this observation of mine. As is usually the case, I see the ultra-wealthy and their institutions as being the culprits that this dumbing down of humanity into a passive superorganism will benefit. The masses are, indeed, as The Matrix depicted it, just an energy source for the Lords of the Flies. For the last 10 years I've participated in a May Day Parade, a parade celebrating worker's struggles and gains. For the last 8 years I've given a speech as part of this parade. Not so this year. The parade didn't happen. I deduce that it was decided against by people convinced that the QUARANTYRANNY is for the public good. This little action of mine, minor though it is, was my revolt, my tiny attempt to keep the struggle moving forward.
- May 5, 2020 (Vision) notes from tENTATIVELY, a cONVENIENCE

- Tags: May Day, tENTATIVELY a cONVENIENCE, ProjectileObjects, billionaires, PANDEMIC PANIC, masks, food lines, criminal sanity, thought criminal, heretics, skeptics

****

May 6, 2020, 10:06AM (Inquiring Librarian to group):

Re: HERETICS: "You'll Never See a Billionaire Standing in a Food Line" online

I LOVED the film! Thank you so much for sharing. It will be interesting to see the comments. The text/dialog was wonderful. Even if ppl want to be hostile, i hope it makes them think, if not now, later. I appreciate that you have the courage to be upfront about these things we believe.

Ok. So, this is a little scary, and sad:
https://www.post-gazette.com/news/crime-courts/2020/05/04/ross-township-murder-suicide-bing-liu-police-elm-court/stories/202005040082

****

May 6, 2020, 10:13AM (Amir-ul Kafirs to group):

I appreciate that you have the courage to be upfront about these things we believe.

I just unfriended one of my best friends on Facebook because he had the expected kneejerk reaction. He's a respiratory therapist at a hospital. He responded to it as simply making the claim that the whole pandemic is manufactured. I've been consistently addressing the socio-political aspects of all this. I've never denied that people are getting sick and dying. But because people are so wrought up over the deaths they're incapable of detaching themselves emotionally enough to criticize everything surrounding it. I think I'm just going to have to lose friends over this and have that be that. What people really don't understand is that one of the symptoms of their brainwashing is that they project stereotypes onto what I say instead of actually trying to understand it. This has been happening to me my whole life. People become so mentally blocked that they can't perceive what's in front of them.

****

May 6, 2020, 10:40AM (Amir-ul Kafirs to group):

Ok. So, this is a little scary, and sad:

This is, obviously, highly speculation-provoking. It's interesting that the article doesn't mention what part of China the murder victim was from. Thanks for sharing it. Theorists might have a field day with this.

****

May 6, 2020, 12:35PM (Inquiring Librarian to group):

I read another article about it that said he was from Singapore. Singapore makes it impossible to be homosexual.. The have criminalized it with jail time and the government supports conversion therapy. I suspect it may have been related to a homosexual relationship. I had a male friend from Singapore who was in a phd program at jhu. He struggled deeply with depression regarding his bisexuality.

Ok. Article says he is from China. But he got his phd in Singapore.

****

May 6, 2020, 3:18PM (Amir-ul Kafirs to group):

I suspect it may have been related to a homosexual relationship.

That was one of the 2 obvious suspicions that occurred to me.   I appreciate the police saying that they don't know what they have. I doubt that we'll ever get straight info about this, the connection to COVID-19 research makes it all too crazy.

****

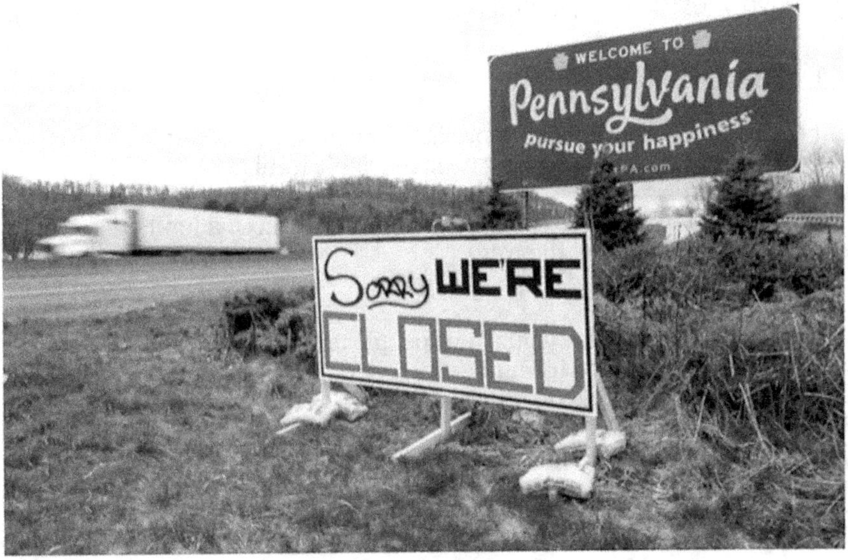

A sign reading "Sorry We're Closed" is placed at the Pennsylvania welcome sign on the westbound lanes of Interstate 80 in Delaware Water Gap, Pa. on Saturday, April 4, 2020. The sign is a short distance from the New Jersey border greeting motorists traveling west. (Christopher Dolan / The Times-Tribune via AP) AP AP

****

May 6, 2020, 3:57PM (Inquiring Librarian to group):

Related to your experience with your respiratory therapist friend, I 'came out' via email to one of my library patron friends here in Louisiana. I let her know, via email, that i am skeptical of the virus panic, fear the numbers are inflated for nefarious reasons, and am not convinced massive job loss through lockdowns is the solution.

My friend actually did write me back.. And while she did not share my doubts, she did not shame or scold me for my skepticism. She kindly expressed her views and experiences and the lives she knew that were lost. I am so thankful for her thoughtful response. And i let her know i appreciated her consideration.

My friend is a teacher, still employed, has 3 awesome kids, and an artist husband, who grew up adopted into a foster family, who works on computers. She is from the country of Colombia. And she spent her formative years growing up in nj, just outside of nyc. Maybe her diverse upbringing has helped her not be a judgemental jerk.

****

May 6, 2020, 4:05PM (Dick to group):

a couple small observations

I went to buy food today and the store had face masks on display
this is notable because they haven't been available until now
usually they sell for.08 cents
the store had 50 for 40 euros ! the government has placed a limit at .98 cents per mask (which are one use by the way)
so much for solidarity with the local merchants
another small note
the quarantine here ends on 11 may but people are impatient to get out, today was sunny so that was an added incentive
in short, outside today looked almost like a normal day
and the funny thing was that the "new normal" we've been hearing about looks a lot like the old normal - honking car horns, people screaming at each other
so much for the new "introspective mind-set" this isolation has brought to the populace

****

May 6, 2020, 5:56PM (Amir-ul Kafirs to group):

Re: a couple small observations

so much for the new "introspective mind-set" this isolation has brought to the populace

It would've been nice if a new introspective mind-set were a byproduct but what I'm witnessing the most is a complete knee-jerk fall-back onto prefabricated opinions and attitudes that're mostly irrelevant to what the responses are supposedly to. In other words, whoever is experiencing the "new introspective mind-set" is probably somebody who was already introspective and everybody else is probably dumber and meaner than ever.

****

May 7, 2020, 6:29AM (Amir-ul Kafirs to group):

HERETICS: An online dating site conversation with a woman in Brazil

Being in lockdown has probably increased online flirting considerably, It has in my life. I've been corresponding with a 54 year old teacher in São Paulo. She's very afraid of the pandemic. We write in Portuguese which means that I use Google Translate since I don't know Portuguese at all. Here's a relevant example from our correspondence in the last 24 hours. I present the English 1st:

Yesterday - 10:12pm

You're being quite critical ...
You know, here the situation of the pandemic is getting worse every day, a lot of people dying ... our health system is collapsing, we are an underdeveloped country, a good portion living on the edge of poverty. Running after everything they did not do for the people now, in the midst of the epidemic, is complicated. I don't know, but if I don't have that isolation, I don't think there's anyone left here.
What do you think about Science?

Você está sendo bastante crítico...
Sabe, aqui a situação da pandemia está cada dia pior, muita gente morrendo...nosso sistema de saúde está entrando em colapso, somos um país sub desenvolvido, uma boa parcela vivendo à beira da miseria. Correr atrás agora de tudo aquilo que não fizeram pelo povo agora, em plena epidemia, fica complicado. Não sei, mas se não tiver esse isolamento acho que não sobra ninguém aqui.
O que você pensa sobre a Ciência?

You are right that I am being critical. I've spent my life analyzing propaganda here in the United States. To give an example: I was born in the era of the "Cold War", anti-communism was very intense in the USA. My mother always said things like, "In Russia, all news is propaganda, in the United States there is freedom of expression. That's because Russia is a communist country." Then, one day I asked her what communism is. She had no idea what it was, she couldn't even begin to define it. That's when I started to realize how intense brainwashing was in the USA. The only time I've seen worse than that is now. People are so forcefully fed with constant fear that they are completely unable to understand what is happening and speak in prefabricated phrases - just as my mother did when she was denouncing communism.

Anyway, the point is that I think the same thing is happening all over the world. All the information you are receiving about the deaths from COVID-19 in Brazil comes from the mass media. The mass media keeps people paying attention, keeping them in a constant state of terror, which allows them to make more money from advertising. You think that everyone might die in Brazil and I propose that this is unlikely and that the disease will run its course. At the moment, there are reportedly 8,588 COVID-19 deaths in Brazil. That's among 210 million people. That is approximately, if I do the calculations correctly, roughly 4 people per 100,000.

NOW, let's compare that to pneumonia in 2013 in Brazil: "Cases of hospitalized pneumonia (incidence per 100 000 inhabitants/year) in adults ≥50 years were: [..] Brazil 225 341 (611.6)". (https://www.sciencedirect.com/science/article/pii/S1201971213000878) As you can see, pneumonia fatalities have been much higher than COVID-19 ones and, yet, have you been so afraid of pneumonia? You probably haven't — and that's because the mass media hasn't made such a spectacle of it and because all these lockdown procedures weren't implemented for it. THAT's science, which, yes, I do appreciate. I'm not saying that people aren't dying in Brazil from COVID-19, I AM saying that the whole situation is exaggerated for ulterior motives that are too invisible to the average person being subjected to them.

****

May 7, 2020, 8:39AM (Dick to group):

RE: HERETICS: An online dating site conversation with a woman in Brazil

Thanks! Who said romance was dead?!
*
a friend posted this:
https://www.youtube.com/watch?v=WJTOTddoFoE&feature=share&fbclid=IwAR2mXnPlHetBqsm8L9tICH5iKXS4HgHsFAcEgeplmmcRRCzOxJAPheWWMHQ

(PLEASE SPREAD THE MESSAGE) We'll DELETE This Video Within 24 Hours For Safety Reasons - YouTube
Watch this now! AVAILABLE ONLY 24 HOURS! Special thanks to our friends at Valuetainment. YT - https://www.youtube.com/user/patrickbetdavid IG - https://www....
www.youtube.com

****

May 7, 2020, 12:01PM (Amir-ul Kafirs to group):

a friend posted this:

I watched this. I'm completely wary of vaccines & feel no need or desire for it at all. I don't really believe they'll be required but then I wouldn't've believed that we'd be in this state of quarantine either! The thing that's becoming increasingly strange to me is the way these warning videos are made. They're very 'professional', very flashy & full of the type of eye candy that TV typically wows its viewers with. THAT makes me distrust them somewhat because the content is somewhat subsumed by its style of presentation.

****

May 7, 2020, 12:04PM (Dick to group):

I agree
I also wonder at Bill Gates constantly being the poster child for the "Great Dastardly Plan"
There must be plenty of other guys & gals who are equally monomaniac in their desires for world power

****

May 7, 2020, 12:10PM (Amir-ul Kafirs to group):

There must be plenty of other guys & gals who are equally monomaniac in their desires for world power

Yeah, I distrust that too. I take it for granted that any billionaire is up to no good, hence the title of my action/movie, but Gates seems like the new Rockefeller or Rothschild target. Why not the Koch Brothers & Rump? It seems that Gates is probably targeted as a 'Liberal' while the 'Conservatives' who're up to as much suspect shit as Gates are conveniently left out of the narrative.

By the way, here's the link to the description of my Billionaires action on my Mere Outline website. It combines all the writing that I've previously posted on the subject & adds more:

http://idioideo.pleintekst.nl/MereOutline2020.html

See entry 442.

****

May 7, 2020, 1:51PM (Inquiring Librarian to group):

I found this on Phil's page:
https://youtu.be/fQSzujHS7YA

& i sent it to an old friend of mine, 1 of my favorite ppl from Denver, who now lives in Phoenix. My friend is also a Skeptic/Heretic disbeliever, as i had suspected he would be. He had already seen the video, as it has been shared within his circle of skeptics. In return, he sent me this video as a ray of hope for all of us skeptics as we grow larger and stronger... Showing a graph curve of how our wave can grow stronger and more exponentially as the population of skeptics grow. https://youtu.be/Wo99IsV7JrE Honestly i totally appreciate seeing a graph that is NOT about this stupid virus nonsense, but instead about all of us rising up against opression and mind control!

Amir-ul Kafirs is doing his part on a computer dating site sewing the seeds of questioning these authorities that have become so comfortable as to be brazenly, blatently trying to destroy us.

****

May 7, 2020, 5:24PM (Dick to group):

A disturbing one from the activist channel
https://www.youtube.com/watch?v=NuToCqoRVHM

US Begins To Implement WHO 'Contact Tracing' To Forcibly Remove People From Their Homes! - YouTube
This report is a follow up to that one where I cover how Michael Ryan of The Who stated in a press briefing how The Who which is of course in the pocket of bill gates now believes its time to...

****

May 7, 2020, 5:24PM (Dick to group):

By the way, the video of Phil's has been deleted already

****

May 7, 2020, 7:25PM (Phil to group):

The video was made by some people working on a feature length documentary. You can find it here;
https://plandemicmovie.com/

You can also find it here on vimeo;
https://vimeo.com/416101668

Dr Judy Mikovits has been pretty badly slandered. It is good to hear her version of the story. Snopes totally trashes her. Here is another short video from her point of view;
https://www.youtube.com/watch?v=wW7lclOmgzE

Well I guess Bill Gates is more of a continuation of Rockerfeller. He was born with a golden spoon in his mouth in a family that mingled with the Rockerfellers.

HIs Philanthropy is just a lesson from the Rockerfellers on how to get richer with more power. He stands out like a sore thumb because he has so many obvious conflicts of interests in this matter. Here is a nice video (in french with subtitles) that exposes his foundation;
https://www.youtube.com/watch?v=Dqzt6yAmdDE&t=536s

Then of course the Rockerfellers themselves are also right up there ready to profit and get more powerful.
https://www.rockefellerfoundation.org/

But of course you are right all billionaires should not be trusted. trump koch bros soros etc....

Cory Morningstar does some interesting research on the Fourth Industrial Revolution and Fake Green movement which exposes another agenda that is exploited by this situation;
http://www.wrongkindofgreen.org/

Also just in case you missed it Niel Ferguson resigned;
https://www.telegraph.co.uk/news/2020/05/05/exclusive-government-scientist-neil-ferguson-resigns-breaking/

****

May 7, 2020, 8:49PM (BP to group):

It's back up but may be back down by the time you see this:
https://www.youtube.com/watch?v=FxEToibWNZM
the deleted one had 6,000 plus views (If I recall correctly), was up for a couple of days. the new link has 12,783, uploaded 10 hours ago.
VERY interesting to watch. I started to look at the criticisms (Snopes, etc. as Phil cited) but had to step out and will resume tonight. Whatever be the truth, I like the message: the people have caught on. Let us pray it is so.

And whatever the truth, I want to watch! I'll sort it out.

On a side note, a couple days ago I binged on a double feature of UFO docs to escape the pandemic media onslaught. The Steven Greer ones: Unacknowledged and Close Encounters of The Fifth Kind. There was this great bit where a woman reveals that a high profile scientist, a former (?) Nazi that the USA recruited after WW2, warned her that all the crisis are false, are a method of control over the population, to keep us in fear and malleable. The Cold War, the coming Terrorist Threat. The Bogey Men. And the biggest hoax of all will be that we are under attack from Aliens from another planet. We have the technology to stage it, saucers flying above. And it will be the permanent crisis. Because they can always come back. And largely invisible (except when it is convenient to trot them out, blow up some buildings). It really resonated with what we are going through! I can definitely see it coming to be. And here it is, released a day ago, our (as in the USofA) new branch of the Military (not a joke!)

SPACE FORCE AD #1: https://www.youtube.com/watch?v=UNsvgbpLMnQ

****

May 7, 2020, 9:45PM (Amir-ul Kafirs to group):

HERETICS my bare beginnings to the proposed book

So, I'm making a not-very-determined effort to get to work on the proposed "Mind Control in the Era of COVID-19" book (I've removed "Opportunism" from the title) and I thought you might be interested in what little I've written. Perhaps it'll inspire some of you. I think some of it provides comic relief.

Editor's Personal Backstory
(the bare beginnings as of May 7, 2020)

****

May 7, 2020, 10:56PM (BP to group):

HERETICS: Emergency in The Empire State

I keep forgetting to forward this. This light display on the Empire State Building in nyc has been burning bright for a good month now. the message to me has never been: In Honor Of Our Fearless Heathcare Workers. It's: Emergency! Run! Be scared! The Cops Are On The Case! They've toned it down since the initial launch as seen in the vid link below. No white strobe. Just a steady, pulsing Red Cop Car in the sky. Can't find any samples of that. How many people see this thing every damn night? Jersey, Brooklyn, Queens. Millions, I imagine.
https://www.youtube.com/watch?v=MBKWTrJIO60

Well, the white strobe flash was back! Saw it a few minutes ago. It's striking from 6 or 7 miles away, where I am at the moment. Any closer must trigger a heart attack! Hmmmm, now it's back to the solid red pulse. One must be aware the building owners always had questionable judgement regarding the display and that it's something to question and that they have used for promotion (tourists to the viewing tower). Years back, someone I know actually orchestrated a display in honor of a new M&M candy color. Caused an upset in the papers that they could be "bought." Today that would be celebrated as a brilliant move.

PS now I remember. When the Empire first lit up in LAVENDER for Gay Pride Day there was all sorts of outrage that it was insulting somehow. But as years march on, if they do not do the lavender then we've slipped into hate. So now we are going to get this flashing police thing annually as a (sniff sniff) Remembrance. Failure to alarm the public will equal indifference to death.

****

May 8, 2020, 5:20PM (Inquiring Librarian to group):

HERETICS: Plandemic Bashed in Forbes

I just found this disturbing article in Forbes. I saw it first on someone's social media page. It's really horrible. Can you all read this and tell me what you think? I cannot see how it actually debunks "Plandemic" beyond simply saying Big Brother Knows Best. The article links to our beloved "Atlantic" to teach you how to understand 'science'. The article also explains all of the techniques of sucking people into nonsensical conclusions and fear of nonsense, just as our government and media do every day to us! It's unbelievable! It is so disturbing to me:
https://www.forbes.com/sites/tarahaelle/2020/05/08/why-its-important-to-push-back-on-plandemic-and-how-to-do-it/#7d1088795fa3

****

May 8, 2020, 8:44PM (Amir-ul Kafirs to group):

Re: HERETICS: Plandemic Bashed in Forbes

Wow, Thanks for sharing that. Need I say that I found it completely insidious?

One of the main flaws I find in its argumentation is that she ***gives no motive for the so-called "Conspiracy Theories" whatsoever!!*** Apparently, we're just supposed to accept that these theorists have malevolent motives purely on their own. Contrarily, the mainstream version of all this can easily be found to have **monetary motives** such as the sales of vaccines, etc.. — so which is more suspect? Of course, at a creepier level, the author of the article is point-blank telling people what to think & how to act as pawns in her own personal game. Utterly despicable.

****

May 8, 2020, 8:53PM (Inquiring Librarian to group):

Re: HERETICS: Plandemic Bashed in Forbes

Thank you Dick & Amir-ul Kafirs for validating my sanity in standing on the side of ... Gawd i though i was gonna ralph up my blt lunch when i read this. It's the stuff of looney bins... Who??? flew over That cuckoo's nest?!

Ok, this tragedy was on Phil's fb page... I only wish it wasn't believable... .. So sad: https://m.youtube.com/watch?time_continue=2&feature=emb_logo&v=CvhTQV5FNUE

YouTube Search

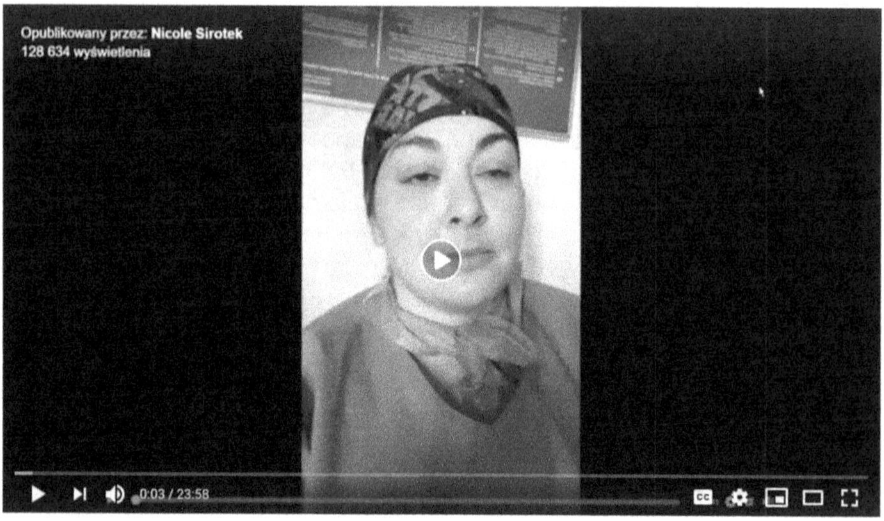

Nicole Sirotek

891,227 views • May 4, 2020 | 9K | 308 | SHARE | SAVE

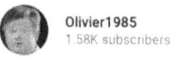

Olivier1985
1.58K subscribers
SUBSCRIBE

Category People & Blogs

3,570 Comments SORT BY

Add a public comment...

onesownthoughts 1 second ago
Wow, thank you for being so outspoken. I've already long since decided that if I'm seriously ill I'd rather not pay someone a huge amount of money to hasten my death by incompetence in a hospital, I'd rather die at home. I've been wondering whether a possible explanation for the extraordinary high amount of deaths in NYC in contrast to smaller cities amounts to more than just larger population density and this seems to confirm that the taboo is quite likely: the taboo being that people avoid presenting the medical industry as anything other than 'heroic' even though many of us have experienced its sadistic, apathetic, greedy, megalomaniacal side and have distrusted it enormously. Heaven forbid that doctors ever be criticized – no matter how shallow and self-centered they may sometimes demonstrably be.
Show less
REPLY

William Brady 3 days ago
This is absolutely criminal.

We need investigations.
308 REPLY
View 24 replies

StGammon77 3 days ago
Leave immediately, lay low, write your story with names and as much detail as possible or record it onto a phone. Contact a Lawyer and whistleblow about it, this is total negligence and murder!

StGammon77 3 days ago
Leave immediately, lay low, write your story with names and as much detail as possible or record it onto a phone. Contact a Lawyer and whistleblow about it, this is total negligence and murder!

411 REPLY

View 20 replies

Samantha Klingner 3 days ago
This is awful!! Please God, protect this woman for speaking out.

185 REPLY

View 11 replies

Razors Edge 3 days ago (edited)
My friends dad (alzheimer's sufferer) was given double dose of morphine & left to die alone. Family were told after 18 hours of death. When questioned what happened they didn't have a clue, one nurse said they were treating him as end of life patient.
...
Read more

129 REPLY

View 6 replies

Screeching Liberal, the 1st of his name 1 day ago
Nice to see a nurse telling the truth instead of making ridiculous tiktoks.

18 REPLY

J YC 3 days ago
They need to start group lawsuits against the hospital and the doctors.

56 REPLY

56 REPLY

View reply

OverkilledUnderdog 1 day ago
This is the face of a Heroine. She needs to be put into witness protection . You know just incase she ACCIDENTALLY falls out of a window or something.

26 REPLY

View reply

Rocco Reid 3 days ago
She needs to keep her doors locked and be aware of here environment everywhere she goes.

94 REPLY

View reply

mo zack 3 days ago
I could not imagine families who lost a loved one watching this video.

29 REPLY

View reply

LINEWALKER 3 days ago
And everyone wants to know why I left Nursing.

111 REPLY

View 22 replies

Kelli Hernandez 3 days ago
Just like 9/11. Never question the official narrative.
This poor baby. She has empathy. The rest don't.

****

May 8, 2020, 9:22PM (Amir-ul Kafirs to group):

Ok, this tragedy was on Phil's fb page... I only wish it wasn't believable...

That's truly valuable and believable information. I liked it and left this comment:

Wow, thank you for being so outspoken. I've already long since decided that if I'm seriously ill I'd rather not pay someone a huge amount of money to hasten my death by incompetence in a hospital, I'd rather die at home. I've been wondering whether a possible explanation for the extraordinary high amount of deaths in NYC in contrast to smaller cities amounts to more than just larger population density and this seems to confirm that the taboo is quite likely: the taboo being that people avoid presenting the medical industry as anything other than 'heroic' even though many of us have experienced its sadistic, apathetic, greedy, megalomaniacal side and have distrusted it enormously. Heaven forbid that doctors ever be criticized — no matter how shallow and self-centered they may sometimes demonstrably be.

****

May 8, 2020, 10:16PM (Inquiring Librarian to group):

Great comment Amir-ul Kafirs! This nurse reminded me of another reason why i avoided nursing. I also have had faulty care with a botched reconstructive kidney surgery when i was 19. Not only was the surgery a failure, necessitating certain surgery again within 10 years, my doctor double diluted my morphine when i woke from surgery. I woke in a phenomenal amount of pain. As much as i could, i told the dr something was wrong, but he insisted i was delusional. Luckily my dad was there to help me, but not until after i hyperventilated in pain and passed out, dangerously going into shock. When i woke again, the doctor at least admitted his mistake, not realizing my morphine had already been diluted before he then again diluted it. Total nightmare. Not to mention, there were not enough nurses. My hair was caked with grease, i was filthy, my mom had to change my sheets... I could do nothing for myself with the 6 inch incision in my side mid section. It was so dehumanizing... And lonesome. I was stuck alone on the children's ward since they had run out of beds in the adult ward. Really a depressing experience. I am realizing as i write this that i have blocked a lot of it out of my memory.. The stories go on and on... Too much morphine, constipation leading to the incision opening up... All this torture and i was an otherwise very healthy 19 yr old gal. Can u imagine, being older and very sick in an inner city hospital?!

****

May 8, 2020, 10:19PM (Inquiring Librarian to group):

Re: HERETICS: Plandemic Bashed in Forbes

Also, i wanted to share my friend from Denver's comment in the Forbes article. I really appreciate his positive twist on the article:

"O no.. Thats a great article... The bigger picture in my opinion is that if people are going to wake up, you give them all the data,, all of it,, and let the people choose.. Consider a couple things like this is an article from Forbes magazine, which is a financial publication. There is no specific medical data what so ever that is listed in the article. It is an opinion piece and is basically telling people to not look at the Plandemic movie because they say so and because its in Forbes magazine.

The reason Plandemic info is taking off is because people are putting the dots together. I have people I never thought would connect dots about whats going on,, posting positive comments about the data coming out as well as out rage that what has been going on has been propagated for so long..

In the Qanon movement its said,, "Never interfere with an enemy while they are in the process of destroying them selves".

Now just look at the results...

Its not going well for the ones who put that article out."

****

May 9, 2020, 5:55AM (Dick to group):

HERETICS: Observation

The other day I received a mail from my brother, one of the more intelligent people I know, in which he suggested similarity between serial killers and billionaires - he suggested that perhaps they use the same brain center. that is, both engage in highly unreasonable behavior, are selfish to the extreme and manipulative. I should add he lives in Hollywood and his wife is a press agent who frequently represents these types.

I found this idea to be very interesting. It would explain at least part of the "control trip" aspect in the behavior of people like Gates, Trump, etc.

I did some research and found that, in fact, CEO's are #1 on the list of workplace psychopaths, at least according to the following article.
https://en.wikipedia.org/wiki/Psychopathy_in_the_workplace

It is interesting to note that the second position is held by lawyers and the third spot is held by people in the media. In other words the three main culprits needed to implement a program and then to convince others to follow it.

In short, it suggests the world is run by the insane. And these people are highly rewarded for their insanity. What else needs to be said? We are living in a madhouse.

Psychopathy in the workplace - Wikipedia
The presence of psychopathy in the workplace—although psychopaths typically represent a relatively small percentage of workplace staff—can do enormous damage when in senior management roles. Psychopaths are usually most common at higher levels of corporate organizations and their actions often cause a ripple effect throughout an organization, setting the tone for an entire corporate culture.
en.wikipedia.org

****

May 9, 2020, 9:11PM (Inquiring Librarian to group):

HERETICS: Librarian Contact Tracers

Hi All,

I just found this horrifying message on the "Libraries Step Up" social media page:
https://www.marketwatch.com/story/librarians-are-being-enlisted-to-help-in-the-battle-against-coronavirus-pandemic-how-you-too-can-become-a-contact-tracer-2020-05-08?fbclid=IwAR0xXSBAAEG54IjiVt5bj8JiiBhM9WA2hqSZHOqXs6AqJvY0LaPS9AdohKk

I need a job, but what do I do if my library system forces me to do this? It's like forcing me to be an innocent little Hitler Youth or an NKVD informant. Louisiana is asking for Contact Tracers. It's part of our "opening up" plan. Do I have to be a pawn to get a paycheck for the job I've loyally served for the past 11 years? ='-[
Honestly, I do not think that my library system is so 'sophisticated" as to think something like this up for us. Our Mayor would likely rather lay us all off. I suppose I will find out this week, as my pay ends this Friday.

-Librarian in Distress-

****

May 9, 2020, 10:53PM (Amir-ul Kafirs to group):

Re: HERETICS: Librarian Contact Tracers

Wow, I absolutely think you should not do this, the more resistance to it the better. Here's a story from my own life:

I think it was in 1988, during the tail end of the Reagan Presidency, it was required by law that all businesses had to report any immigrants working for them. I was working for a used bookstore chain at the time. We weren't actually employing any immigrants at the time. One day, an African-American woman, perhaps in her 40s, came into the store presenting herself as being from the INS (the equivalent to today's ICE, I reckon) & asked me if we were employing any immigrants & asking for proof of their legal status if we were. I told her that I wouldn't cooperate because I thought that the whole business was fascist. She paused, probably somewhat astounded that anyone would have the audacity to say such a thing to her, & then said something to the effect of "*You're right, we wouldn't be doing this if Reagan wasn't president.*" She then left the store without another word. As far as I know we were never reported, it we had been there would've been a **$10,000 fine**. I imagine that the INS agent went on to fudging her reports after that to resist the fascism. I did eventually get fired but that was more because I was brazenly confrontational with a corporate type in the chain that I detested (& who was extremely dishonest). I could've avoided getting fired. The store actually continued to hire me on the sly because my local manager was sympathetic to my rebellion.

-Librarian in Distress-

Good luck with that. Just keep in mind that one of the best ways to resist is to be flexible enough to always land on your feet. You're still young.

****

May 9, 2020, 12:17AM (Inquiring Librarian to group):

HERETICS: Cheap Humor

I thought this was really funny:
https://youtu.be/QcUAG6t5aN8

"What It's Like to Believe Everything the Media Tells You" - What would it be like if you stopped thinking for yourself and believed everything the media tells you? Here's what it might look like to be completely brainwashed by the news - JP Sears

& this was the tissue box sitting on my waiting room table today at the NTB car tire repair shop. I sat there today for 2.5hrs... the box never ceased to amuse me. The flowers remind me of corona viruses and the writing... it's too much - "CREATED WITH PRIDE BY AMERICANS WHO ARE BLIND". Ok, I don't want to be a total jerk, I'm not making fun of blind people... But the double entendre in this is priceless. Or maybe it's my neighbor who incessently smokes mary jane that blows into my back porch haven, ALL DAY and ALL NIGHT. This guy pisses me off. But it could be worse. I do wonder how often I am running around unknowingly and unintentionally high these daze when I'm not supposed to leave my house.

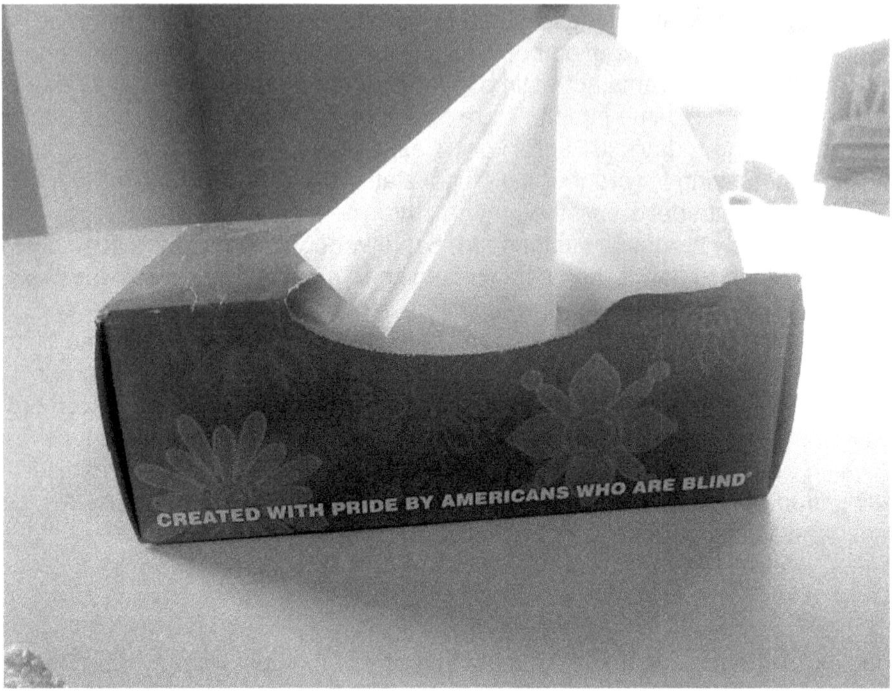

Staring at the box for 2.5 hrs. did remind me to call my eye doctor to order my excessively strong contacts. I cannot get my yearly eye exam, apparently that is not essential. My inability to see anything without glasses or contacts is apparently not essential. I cannot drive a car or walk to the bathroom without running into stuff without my contacts. I cannot read a book (even though I am technically near-sighted... that's how bad my near-sightedness is). But to carry on with this tangent... I had 1 week left of my last year's prescription being valid to order this 2nd set of very expensive and very necessary contact lenses. I had to do this asap because my city has no plans to pay me after the last week of the stay at home order. if I lose my job or am furloughed, I lose my health insurance, and then as a result, I lose my eyesight because I cannot afford my contacts without insurance, muchless without an income. I won the game. My contacts are ordered just in the nick of time, possibly my last week of paid employment and health insurance. Thank you box of double entendred tissues, you reminded me to call my eye doctor. I blow my nose in tp. TP is cheaper and it works great. But I do appreciate a good free tissue once in a while.

****

May 9, 2020, 5:54AM (Amir-ul Kafirs to Inquiring Librarian (presumably intended to be to the whole group)):

Re: HERETICS: Cheap Humor

I thought this was really funny:

I loved it! Did you notice that there were 2,359,619 views? & 6k likes? I even subscribed to the guy's channel. Alas, I'll probably never look at it again but it's the thought that counts. How did you find this one?

"Thank you box of double entendred tissues, you reminded me to call my eye doctor." would make a great ad slogan without any further explanation.

****

May 9, 2020, 10:49AM (Amir-ul Kafirs to group):

A horror movie that reminds me of the current pandemic nightmare is Johnny Kevorkian's 2018 "Await Further Instructions". Here's a link to a short trailer for it: https://youtu.be/cExGHt350NE . It's so much like this PANDEMIC PANIC that it's actually terrifying. In a way it's too disturbing for me to even recommend it right now. The basic plot is that a family gets together for Christmas & finds themselves trapped in their house taking instructions from their TV sets. The family is, for the most part, racist, patriarchical, & robopathic — & those that deviate from this stupidity are not well-received.

****

May 9, 2020, 12:21PM (Dick to group):

Not to do personal promo but I made this video a while back
It expresses my feelings on how the situation should be dealt with
https://www.youtube.com/watch?v=Ikij-ZyxKc4&t=4s

DICK TURNER: SHOOT THE SUIT
Shoot the Suit Words & music by Dick Turner This is a song about injustice. It is one of my Popcycle songs; these are songs written in my interpretations of ...

****

May 9, 2020, 12:28PM (Amir-ul Kafirs to group):

HERETICS: YouTube

By all means, self-promote! I've made a PANDEMIC PANIC playlist on my onesownthoughts YouTube channel & I just added your video to it even though it doesn't expressly refer to COVID-19. I plan to eventually add almost everything that people have linked to here but that's not something I'll get around to soon.

The omnipresence of COVID-19 propaganda is fascinating. Check out this email I just got from YouTube. What I'm increasingly annoyed by is this whole 'expert' opinion thing that tells us what's 'true' & 'not-true'. I'm reminded of 'expert witnesses' at trials: sure, they have credentials but they're still just selling themselves to the highest bidder. I remember when MOVE was bombed & an 'expert' publicly pronounced that they had a gas tank on the roof of their building & that they were actually commiting suicide. Of course, it was a water collection tank & they were being murdered.

Embrace Mental Health Awareness Month with Kati Morton's Health & Psychology channel

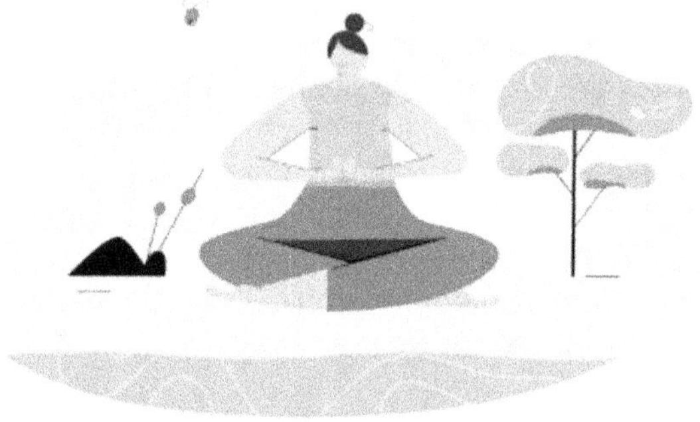

As self-quarantine drags on, it's important to keep posi vibes and stay present. Kati Morton's Health & Psychology channel is a great resource to help maintain healthy habits, stay zen, and be well during Mental Health Awareness Month.

TO YOUR HEALTH

Believe the facts, not the hype! Trevor Noah & more debunk COVID-19 myths.

****

May 9, 2020, 11:23PM (Amir-ul Kafirs to group):

Re: HERETICS: YouTube

On May 9, 2020, at 9:37 PM, Inquiring Librarian wrote:

My Instagram a day ago popped up an advertisement for me, stating that how sad... did you lose your job and also hence your health insurance? Well, we have the solution for you!! Click on this link to buy your own new health insurance on the Healthcare Exchange.

Ha ha! Did you ever see my movie called "HealthCare NightMare"?

419. "**HealthCare NightMare**"
- shot at the Who Unit? December, 2014E.V.
- A glimpse into the dysfunctionality of HeathCare.gov & into the failure of the "Affordable Health Care Act" to be much more than yet-another scam to rob American citizens
- 13:25
- on my onesownthoughts YouTube channel here: http://youtu.be/tjB3QBz4LAc

As the description above explains, it's my critique of the AHCA. Contrary to the beliefs of many Americans, I see the AHCA's criminalization of being without health care to be the beginning of this new Medical Police State. I voted for Obama for the obvious reason of finally getting someone other than a white guy into office but I think he extended the police state even more than Bush did.

****

May 9, 2020, 6:45PM (Amir-ul Kafirs to group):

HERETICS: Jacksonville

OK, I couldn't even watch this for 30 seconds but I think it's worth watching for its, uh, 'different spin' on the matter. Maybe it's a joke, let's hope so:

[short video of Jacksonville parody here]

Ok, my friend who sent me the Jacksonville movie just sent me this:

Well, you can take a deep breath -- I just found out its a fake. Pretty good one I have to say even though some of what she says is really nuts!

https://www.firstcoastnews.com/article/news/health/coronavirus/coronavirus-how-a-fake-duval-resident-went-viral-with-her-jacksonvillelady-videos/77-ef0aea2a-115b-4dc4-b40f-90ea10948289

****

May 10, 2020, 12:34AM (Amir-ul Kafirs to group):

HERETICS: A Personal Note

On a personal note: I DO feel like we need to notice weird positive things that happen in our lives & to go with them, you never know where they may lead. To give you an example: I'm friends with a woman in Brazil who 1st contacted me about 20 years ago when she was maybe 18. She knew about me through Neoism. Anyway, we published things by each other & then went our seperate ways. More than a decade later we reconnected through social media. Now we communicate through the encrypted WhatsApp. That allows FREE international video phone calls so she & I have talked using it. I haven't examined whether there's a 'catch' to it but it's pretty sweet to be able to see & talk to a friend in a different country. She called a couple of times yesterday & I missed the calls, eventually noticed, & called her back. She was visiting her brother & she put her 20 year old niece on the phone because she wanted to talk with me. THEN my friend asked if it was ok to give her niece my phone number so that she could do that more often. Amazingly enough, perhaps, I don't have a sexual motive here, I agreed to the giving out of my phone number to a 20 year old in Brazil because I think this type of 'random' networking is important. I might not've agreed if the person had been a guy.. but maybe I would have. The point is that I think it's healthy to remain open to a variety of people, that's a form of networking in & of itself.

****

May 11, 2020, 6:25PM (Amir-ul Kafirs to group):

Here's my latest neologism. I wouldn't be surprised if someone else coined it or something similar to it already.

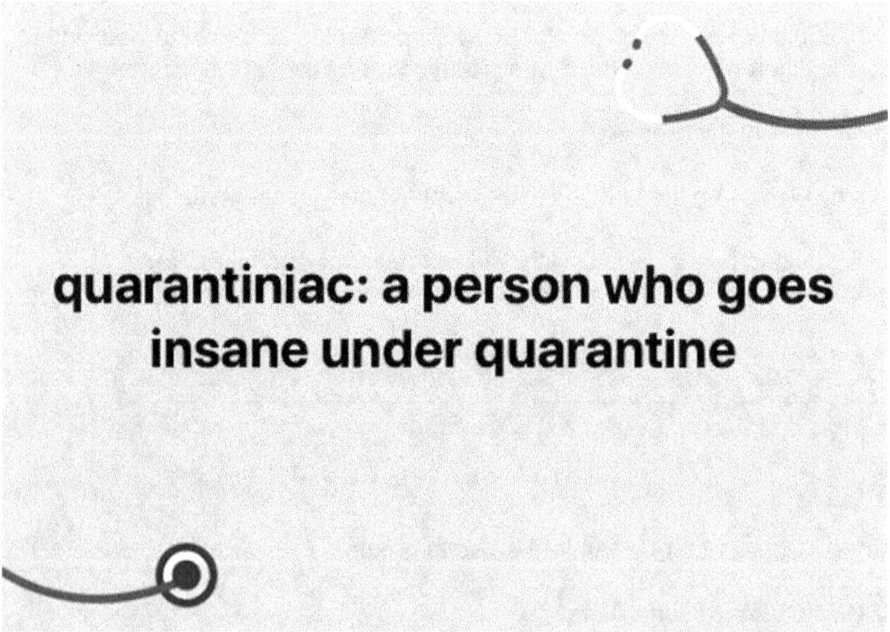

I posted it on social media without further comment. At my most cynical I expect someone to comment something like: 'Is that what happened to you Amir-ul Kafirs?' Of course, they won't be able to get the spelling right.

****

May 15, 2020, 3:02PM (BP to group):

Heretics: whitney webb article

A friend just hipped me to this. My eyes were bulging and I sucked it down like an alcoholic nailing his first scotch of the day.
I need to go back and read it slowly. Sorry if this was posted previously here and I missed it. Published 4/21/20
How the National Security State Is Using Coronavirus to Push AI-Driven Mass Surveillance
https://www.mintpressnews.com/national-security-state-using-coronavirus-push-artificial-intelligence-driven-mass-surveillance/266820/

****

May 9, 2020, 2:17PM (Amir-ul Kafirs to group):

HERETICS: Color Phases in PA

Red Phase

- Life-sustaining businesses only
- Restrictions in place for prison & congregate care
- Schools closed for in-person instruction
- Most child care closed

Yellow Phase

- Telework must continue where feasible
- Businesses with in-person operations must follow safety orders
- Child care open with worker & building safety orders
- Restrictions in place for prison & congregate care
- Schools closed for in-person instruction

Green Phase

- All businesses must follow CDC and PA Department of Health guidelines

Red Phase

- Stay at home ordered
- Large gatherings prohibited
- Restaurants/bars limited to carryout and delivery
- Only travel for life-sustaining purposes

Yellow Phase

- Stay at home restrictions lifted in favor of aggressive mitigation
- Large gatherings prohibited
- In-person retail allowed (curbside/delivery preferred)
- Indoor recreation, health & wellness facilities (such as gyms, spas) and all entertainment (such as casinos, theaters) remain closed

Green Phase

- Aggressive mitigation orders lifted
- Individuals must follow CDC and PA Department of Health guidelines

****

May 9, 2020, 9:15PM (Inquiring Librarian to group):

Re: HERETICS: Color Phases in PA

I find this to be horrifying. My poor sister and mom and dad in Pennsylvania have to deal with this schlop. They are all so upset. My 75 year old mom is depressed with loneliness from missing her knitting friends and all of her social gatherings. My dad is holding strong, as having escaped from a Soviet country in WW2, he is full on in his fight against the "Communist" Democrats (verified by his dad who preferred the Czars to Stalin).

****

May 9, 2020, 9:22PM (Inquiring Librarian to group):

In relation to all of this, I found this on Phil's page (I am a Phil's social media page junkie at this point, it is holding my sanity in its barely stable, but at least stable, state during this 'crisis').

https://zcomm.org/znetarticle/covid-19-and-the-left-an-ignored-civil-rights-crisis-a-missed-opportunity/?fbclid=IwAR0Qa53vl5_nXj8R0axASp6f00vXXI7tTWnL55IP160wxRrtksBpqT818L8

I shared it with my Russian friend, Ilya. Ilya lives in the Seattle area. He moved to the United States as a young adult. He is the only person so far out of this group that has openly agreed with the article to me. He comments how he, from a communist country, cannot believe how people from the United States in this crisis so easily and unquestioningly have allowed their freedoms to be taken away, freedoms that they have not had to actually work for (he speaks for my generation, born after the Vietnam war had long been swept more under the radar).

****

May 9, 2020, 11:08PM (Amir-ul Kafirs to group):

Oh, the irony of it is that this is really a sort of privileged person's problem in the sense that I'm getting irritated by the loss of so many 'privileges' that people in war-torn countries don't have to begin with. I mean my whole life I've been so poor that it would've been horrible but I would've probably had more friends at a local level who would be saying 'fuck this shit' & performing who-knows-what criminally sane actions — then again, maybe not, this situation is just so unprecedented in this country in my lifetime. I think one of the main reasons why people are so complacent is because their whole life experience has been that Big Brother actually has worked to preserve their privilege — without their even being particularly conscious of it. I really don't see any reason why it can't get wwwaaaaaayyyy worse. Liberals consider Rump to be a neo-nazi, or, at least, aligned, but don't seem to realize that this lockdown serves neo-nazi interests bigtime. Just because Rump pretends to be against masks & whatnot he's considered to be against the lockdown so liberals have the kneejerk reaction in favor of it. This seems to be because even though they accuse Rump of being a liar, which I take it for granted he is, *liberals believe that he means what he says.* What if it's all a form of Reverse Psychology? What if Rump is all for the QUARANTYRANNY but acts like he isn't so that liberals will have a kneejerk reaction in its favor?! It's all so Pavlovian. The same thing holds true for the 'news': some people act like '*oh, I know the news can lie sometimes*' &, yet, they *believe the mainstream news almost everytime anyway!!!!!* Contrarily, as I keep pointing out over & over, *they don't believe the evidence of their own experience or alternate news sources, **partially because they're afraid of being tarred with the 'Conspiracy Theory' brush.*** People are so weak.

****

May 9, 2020, 11:23PM (Naia Nisnam to group):

Re: HERETICS: Color Phases in PA

Oh no... I was going to see if you knew the difference between red and yellow because they seem extremely similar. I had not realized that green still had restrictions.
Initially, I believe the official story was that we are under lockdown to "flatten the curve". We didn't want too many people getting sick at the same time so that hospitals don't get overrun. That seems to be working out fine here in southwestern PA. But we are still all kinds of restricted, even under the yellow. We aren't going to be done with this until they vaccinate every human being. If they make a vaccine at all. And there is nothing to prevent a follow up new virus to keep us all in again.
I get such anxiety that this really is the new normal.
Yesterday my social media was full of friends calling for full censorship of the Plandemic video.
I also feel angry and depressed. I want to stop checking the news and the social media, but I keep making myself miserable.

****

May 9, 2020, 11:33PM (Amir-ul Kafirs to group):

Re: HERETICS: Color Phases in PA

Well to cheer yourself up remember that walk we went on that one time? We need to do more things like that. I think we need to start looking for more like-minded individuals too. It's looking like we can't rely on the old anarchist crowd anymore but there must be some younger criminally sane people who aren't brainwashed yet. Let's get to work on "Mind Control in the time of PANDEMIC PANIC" book! (I know, I know, I've changed the title again) All of you who can find time to do so should just write a little bit when you have spare time & I'll try to piece it all together. Let's not take it for granted that things are going to be even as 'good' as they are now. Now I can publish such a book but what about a year from now? Maybe not. Maybe I'll have to go back to samiszdat & having my own presses like I used to!

****

May 9, 2020, 11:39PM (Inquiring Librarian to group):

Naia Nisnam, many of my social media friends are also slandering the Plandemic movie. It is unbelievable. Several have used that Forbes article as their guide and bible against it. They e-shout their opinion with such authority and righteousness. It is really upsetting for me.

I also fear manditory vaccine. I am scared of this vaccine. I will do everything in my power to avoid it, as i always have with flu shots. I have a secret ploy to get my doctor, the awesomest dr i have ever had, to help me get out of any manditory vaccines. He is crafty and also hates vaccines. I think he really will help me. I just have to keep my health ins. But i believe he also takes Medicaid if i qualify... I feel hope.

& yes... I fear our gov will do this again, & again... When flu season hits again, as flu season does every year.

****

May 10, 2020, 12:07AM (Naia Nisnam to group):

You’re fortunate to have a doctor that you like. I like mine well enough but he wouldn’t get me out of a vaccine.

I wonder what they’ll do to people who refuse the vaccine?? Fines? Jail time? Permanent quarantine lock down?

****

May 10, 2020, 12:09AM (Amir-ul Kafirs to group):

It is really upsetting for me.

& so easy for them! Forbes tells them what to say, they don't even question Forbes's ulterior motives as a *fucking financial magazine*, after all, it represents *established power, what's wrong with that?!* & away they go, dissing us evil 'conspiracy theorists', in other words, people who at least **try to think for ourselves.**

I will do everything in my power to avoid it, as i always have with flu shots.

Me too — but now we have to consider the possibility of *actually being criminalized for deciding what goes into our bodies.*

& yes... I fear our gov will do this again, & again... When flu season hits again, as flu season does every year.

Oh, well, for what it's worth: here's another 'pep talk' (or is it 'Pepto Abysmal Talk' [pun intended]) from my own experience:

In 1988, I was living in Scotland, the British government was trying to impose a "Poll Tax", the people were opposed to it. I was part of that resistance. The people won. The Poll Tax was defeated. That was possible because there was *so much resistance.* There's almost no resistance to anything medical in the US these days. We need to build on that more.

****

May 10, 2020, 12:19AM (Amir-ul Kafirs to group):

Re: HERETICS: Color Phases in PA

You're fortunate to have a doctor that you like.

Yeah, I don't know any doctor that I'd trust either. When I was in high school, I hated gym & wanted to get out of it so the school nurse gave me a medical exemption & I didn't have to go to gym for maybe my last 2 years of high school?! Such things are possible.

I wonder what they'll do to people who refuse the vaccine?? Fines? Jail time? Permanent quarantine lock down?

It's easy to have such dystopian predictions but I think we'll just have to find out. A part of how it all works is that people are made to fear reprisals to resistance so much that they just go along with the p(r)ograms. Throughout my life I HAVEN'T gone along with them &, for the most part, nothing has happened to me (well, sortof).

I refused to register for the draft during the Vietnam War era, the penalty for so-doing was **10 years in federal prison**. Of course, I was scared, I was only 18. I never had any reprisals at all. Right now I'm refusing to get health insurance, I do have Medicare but I don't pay for it. The law seems to be very ambiguous about this. One health care worker told me he wasn't "allowed to give his opinion" — meaning, apparently, that he had no idea what the legal situtaion is these days. I intend to keep 'erring' on the side of doing *what I think is best* & hoping that the scare tactics don't come true. It takes chutzpah but it's worth a try, it's better than just rolling over & dying.

****

May 10, 2020, 8:18AM (BP to group):

I think remaining skeptical of the PLANdemic movie is healthy, too. I support the right to see it more than anything. Until then, the jury is out for me. Until I spend time researching it.
Last week I caught a bit of Governer Cuomo (NY) on the radio and he said that he is partnering with Bill Gates to "re-imagine" the NY school system. Just found the time to start looking into it, but wanted to see what Ms. Ravitch had to say (I've read a couple of her books over the years): https://dianeravitch.net/2020/05/05/nightmare-vision-for-new-york-schools-post-pandemic/
And this one where she links to a Naomi Klein/Intercept article. I stopped looking at the Intercept regularly so missed it. I found them to be less than trustworthy, some of the writers. But anyway, Mr. Alphabet Google is front and center, too.

****

May 10, 2020, 5:49PM (Dick to group):

My doctor is against all immunizations, even antibiotics unless the situation is serious...I plan on asking him about this vaccine idea
I'm going to see him on Wednesday because I hurt my shoulder, I wonder what he'll have to say about this situation
I agree watching all these videos is depressing, I wonder how people like Spiro Skouras can do it everyday, he's the guy on Activist Channel
I think if you don't get the vaccine , I mean if it happens, it means you can't travel, take airplanes, etc
The quarantine ends here in Paris tomorrow morning by the way
It's been 55 days
Talk about a strange-reality-parenthesis

****

May 10, 2020, 6:46PM (Amir-ul Kafirs to group):

I support the right to see it more than anything.

Exactly. Since when does someone else have the 'right' to make our own decisions for us, including the decision to scrutinize media?

wanted to see what Ms. Ravitch had to say (I've read a couple of her books over the years): https://dianeravitch.net/2020/05/05/nightmare-vision-for-new-york-schools-post-pandemic/

I read this. The bottom line strikes me as: *Why should Bill Gates have any power over ANY public arenas whatsoever?* No to Gates in connection with public education, no to Gates in connection with international health matters, etc.. The obvious thing is that he's not content with JUST being one of the richest people in the world, he has to start making decisions that affect EVERYONE'S LIVES TOO. Why settle for less, right?! Thusly making himself more or less parallel to Rump.

****

May 10, 2020, 6:54PM (Amir-ul Kafirs to group):

I think if you don't get the vaccine , I mean if it happens, it means you can't travel, take airplanes, etc

That seems like a likely direction that all this is pushing toward. One wonders, though, is there opposition to this even among the ultra-rich or are they experiencing a united front? All of this slick anti-Bill-Gates stuff may be being funded by people like the Koch brothers or some other 'conservative' interests. I'm sure that such people will have easy ways of being exempt so why would they agitate in favor of protecting the rest of us?

The quarantine ends here in Paris tomorrow morning by the way
It's been 55 days

Supposedly we go to Yellow, a very partial quarantine end, far from complete, on Friday, May 15th. That'll be 57 days. Is the quarantine end in Paris total or just partial?

****

May 10, 2020, 6:57PM (Dick to group):

I'll let you know
Schools open tomorrow
Don't know about other places, like restaurants or cafés, etc
I saw that to take the métro at peak hours you'll need yet another permission slip !
Talk about a waste of paper

****

May 11, 2020, 8:56AM (Dick to group):

Interesting
https://www.youtube.com/watch?v=qy5FDoXameI

Dr. Andrew Kaufman: They Want To Genetically Modify Us With The COVID-19 Vaccine - YouTube
In this powerful interview Spiro is joined with Doctor Andrew Kaufman. Spiro and Dr. Kaufman discuss the expanding curtailment of basic civil liberties being normalized under the false pretext of ...

****

May 11, 2020, 11:46AM (Dick to group):

Strange event
A omnipresent smell of sulphur has been reported in LA and Paris, and my neighbor said in Wuhan and other places as well
https://www.lefigaro.fr/flash-actu/paris-une-odeur-de-souffre-envahit-la-capitale-suscitant-craintes-et-interrogations-20200511

****

May 11, 2020, 12:08PM (Amir-ul Kafirs to group):

I didn't translate this. Is it parody? After all "the smell of sulphur" is a common expression meaning that the devil is nearby.

****

May 11, 2020, 12:12PM (Naia Nisnam to group):

This was on a friend of a friends social media. It links to many screen shots of medical professionals and family members, most of them saying people are dying of other things but getting labelled COVID19.
I think at least some of these stories are true....

https://m.facebook.com/100002521020056/posts/2900774126683260/?d=n&__tn__=R

****

May 11, 2020, 12:31PM (Dick to group):

I realized that, but in fact there is a smell of sulphur in the air and the government is saying it's due to the recent heavy rain (that's what the article says)
Maybe it's mass hysteria, I don't know

****

May 11, 2020, 12:46PM (Inquiring Librarian to group):

I enjoyed the video you posted with Dr. Kaufman Dick! Some of it was over my head. And i will admit, it's hard to go so far as to imagine viruses aren't real. But lord only knows what is real these days. I find myself overwhelmed questioning everything lately. The fact that this seems to be a worldwide scam has really rattled me into wanting to hear and somehow consider and organize every mildly reasonable conspiracy theory. The bs spouted on NPR is so asinine, it's hard to find any conspiracy theory out there that is much more stupid than the npr nonsense.

As for sulphur... That is odd. I have no idea. But i can say, living in S. Louisiana, home to a fazillion noxious oil refineries... On cloudy days here i often smell sulphur in the air. It is disgusting. I have been told by the wife of someone who works at 1 of the plants that refinery workers let off more noxious gasses into the atmosphere here on overcast days because the sight of it is more covertly sheilded by the clouds. I have a better sense of smell than your average human. I can smell the poison all too often. We here are also known as cancer alley.

****

May 11, 2020, 6:23PM (Amir-ul Kafirs to group):

Re: HERETICS: sulphur

I realized that, but in fact there is a smell of sulphur in the air

Have you smelled it? That seems like a big deal to me. The only time I ever smelled sulphur in the air was when I took a walk in a volcano crater in Hawaii. There were vents everywhere with sulphur coming out. It seems to me that the smell of sulphur in the air doesn't bode good.

****

May 11, 2020, 6:27PM (Dick to group):

I smelled something in the air but I assumed it to be the sudden increase in car fumes
The article said it was strongest in the 'proche banlieue" meaning the close suburbs, where it was reported by many people independently
To be honest, my sense of smell is somewhat reduced due to my painting with oils, using turpentine and paint thinner all the time

****

May 11, 2020, 6:54PM (Amir-ul Kafirs to group):

On May 11, 2020, at 6:44 PM, BP wrote:

I find this stuff so crazy. But then I find it crazy that people are still telling others to stay indoors. Through the worst part here in NJ people were still encouraged to get in exercise, take a walk. No mask required.

The other day I was at a big park & I saw an old guy, masked, walking his little dog. He threw a little ball for the dog to chase. A woman, also masked, started running toward the old guy, screaming at him something to the effect of "What do you think you're doing?!" & flailing her arms as if she were going to beat him. The old guy cringed and the woman stormed away. Then the old guy went back to throwing the ball for his dog to chase. That was part of my inspiration to coin the word "quarantiniac".

****

May 11, 2020, 7:20PM (Inquiring Librarian to group):

I found this on the same doctor's website:
https://www.andrewkaufmanmd.com/

****

UNMASKING THE LIES AROUND COVID-19: FACTS VS FICTION OF THE CORONAVIRUS PANDEMIC

Did you know that in the modern era you are exposed to thousands of toxins each and every day?
They are from the air, water, food, clothing, household products, personal hygiene products, and electromagnetic radiation.

Your body is full of natural wisdom.
It can heal itself from almost any insult. It is powerful and amazing. If you support your body's wisdom, you will return to vitality.

"Medicamentum Authentica"
Welcome to the concept of Authentic Medicine, the way nature intended for you to heal.

Andrew Kaufman

- https://www.andrewkaufmanmd.com

****

May 14, 2020, 3:37AM (Dick to group):

A visit to my doctor

I hurt my shoulder so I went to see my doctor yesterday. He's a no-nonsense kind of guy; for example, as I think I wrote before, he doesn't prescribe antibiotics unless absolutely necessary. That is, he is an immune system advocate.
While I was there I asked him about his experience with the virus.
He said that for the last couple of weeks in March he had had about 10 patients a day who had the virus but since the beginning of April not a single one. He also said that in the hospitals (where he often works), the doctors and nurses were, to

quote him exactly "sitting around twiddling their thumbs with nothing to do for the last month". I found this to be very surprising when compared with the information circulated, for example, on Google News, but it's straight from "the horse's mouth" as they say.
He said that the deaths he'd encountered were in old folks homes among the extremely aged with preexisting health issues. He added that many were transferred to hospitals when ill whereas usually they would have just stayed in the home to die.
He commented that he'd seen cases where a patient contracted the virus and from the first symptoms to the moment of death was just three hours.
*
Another small comment. I've seen an increase in pro-lock-down comments coming from the USA. I don't know if any of you have noticed this or not. They have a righteous duty-of-a-good-citizen tone. I have also seen here, where the lock-down is over, some pro-mask posts, also with a sort of moralizing tone to them. (I don't wear one but keep one in my pocket in case a store I need to go into has a sign saying it is obligatory to wear it.)

****

May 14, 2020, 7:45AM (Amir-ul Kafirs to group):

Re: A visit to my doctor

I hurt my shoulder

It serves you right for not wearing a mask you fucking grannie killer.

They have a righteous duty-of-a-good-citizen tone.

This is a wonderful opportunity for petty tyrants to strut their stuff. When you & I were trying to communicate via Zoom the other day & a poor connection was interfering, I was trying to tell this story:

I went to a convenience store the other day. The store's at the tip of a triangle created by the interesection of some roads so there aren't any houses or other buildings directly next to it, just a parkinglot. I only wear a mask when places require it for entry, which I reckon everyplace does now, & I don't even carry it with me, I keep it in the trunk of my car. Hence I got out of my car without a mask on & I heard a nasty old redneck woman's voice say "**Sum peoples dont knows how to reed!!**" Now, in my transcription I'm trying to get across the ignorance & violence of her shouting. She seemed to be standing in the doorway of a house across the street looking at the parkinglot. I'm not really sure what was going on in her mind. Perhaps it was just my paranoid impression that she was shouting self-righteously at me for not wearing a mask. At any rate, I opened my trunk to get the mask out, put it on & went into the store to do my business. Was the woman standing in the doorway just to watch the parkinglot & scream at people who were disobeying? This is exactly the sort of behavior that I expect to see more of.

I have also seen here, where the lock-down is over, some pro-mask posts, also with a sort of moralizing tone to them.

I wish such folks would just stick to self-flaggelation in the privacy of their own home.

****

May 14, 2020, 9:41AM (BP to group):

The next big announcement will be about the beaches. The Gov is surely sweating that one out. Needs to strike a balance or he is going to have rioters on his hands.

Thus far I've been spared from any shaming tho' from a quick perusal of the video below it seems a sad state of affairs.
I post the vid as it's gone viral and it's very mainstream, reaching a lot of people.The creator/star came to fame on a tv show in 1998 (with a 9 year run) playing a working class UPS delivery type of guy living in Queens, NY. A blue collar hero, I guess.

Out Of Touch I Kevin James Short Film

https://www.youtube.com/watch?v=wfGAktuU93s&feature=emb_logo

[In this short movie 2 guys are running from helicopter & tracking-dog pursuit, the production values are high so the drama of it is compelling — their crime? They shook hands & made dinner plans in a park.. without masks on — a flashback shows masked people reporting them to police with their cell-phones]

****

May 14, 2020, 10:01AM (LInquiring Librarian to group):

Yes, I see my friends on social media, countywide in the U.S.A. begging for longer lockdowns and shaming those that want to open up. Some of these lockdown rabid friends actually have advanced degrees, phd's & master's. And the mask debacle, don't get me started... Many of my social media friends now have profile pics of themselves wearing masks. These people post and repost the mantra 'stay at home, save lives' like their new Virus Dr. God has risen and the nonbelievers will soon burn in the pits of granny killing hell.

check out this terrifying video, supposedly out of Singapore:
https://m.youtube.com/watch?v=xHjR_8fb8Co&feature=share

[This movie promotes an actual social-distancing robot whose 'job' it is to

monitor & enforce social-distancing in public situations, in this case in a park]

****

May 15, 2020, 9:27AM (Amir-ul Kafirs to group):

I see my friends on social media, countywide in the U.S.A. begging for longer lockdowns

Fine, make the lockdowns *just for them!* The rest of us 'wild & crazy' types can 'risk our lives'. It would almost be a dream come true for me, I've always wanted to have a device that would enable me to send people who verbally abuse me out on the streets, guys from passing cars who call out "faggot" for example, to an alternate dimension where *only their type of person exists*.

Some of these lockdown rabid friends actually have advanced degrees, phd's & master's.

Thusly proving what I've been saying my whole life, which is that a university education doesn't necessarily make a person smarter, it just buys their way into an earning bracket that enables them to pay back their student loans.

check out this terrifying video, supposedly out of Singapore:
https://m.youtube.com/watch?v=xHjR_8fb8Co&feature=share

There were 30,789 views, 424 likes, & I added another dislike bringing the total to 46.

Contrast THAT to the one BP shared, which had a zillion likes & which I added to my PANDEMIC PANIC playlist.

****

May 15, 2020, 12:14PM (BP to group):

Contrast THAT to the one Brainpang shared, which had a zillion likes & which I added to my PANDEMIC PANIC playlist.

Yep. Something askew with the polls out there. People want OUT! Haven't seen how the question is posed but I'm sure it is shaky.
(btw, type ASKEW into a google search for a bit of nerd humor)
I can't find it now but in the comments to the vid someone said that one of the snitches says in portugese: "They are not wearing masks or gloves." Nice, little touch.

****

May 16, 2020, 6:15AM (Phil to group):

Re: Heretics: whitney webb article

This particular article was not posted here particularly but I did post whitney webb interview on the jimmy dore show;
https://www.youtube.com/watch?v=bGMkSNj_-7Q&t=135s

and also an article on the last american vagabond site;
https://www.thelastamericanvagabond.com/top-news/techno-tyranny-how-us-national-security-state-using-coronavirus-fulfill-orwellian-vision/

You can see some of these agendas also on the world economic forum website;
https://www.weforum.org/

The rockerfeller foundation
https://www.rockefellerfoundation.org/

and also henry kissinger seems a bit excited about the situation;
https://www.henryakissinger.com/articles/the-coronavirus-pandemic-will-forever-alter-the-world-order/

Anyhow this last american vagabond article on darpa technology is also an interesting scary read;
https://www.thelastamericanvagabond.com/top-news/coronavirus-gives-dangerous-boost-darpas-darkest-agenda/

****

Techno-Tyranny: How The US National Security State Is Using Coronavirus To Fulfill An Orwellian Vision

Posted on
April 20, 2020
Author
Whitney Webb

Last year, a government commission called for the US to adopt an AI-driven mass surveillance system far beyond that used in any other country in order to ensure American hegemony in artificial intelligence. Now, many of the "obstacles" they had cited as preventing its implementation are rapidly being removed under the guise of combating the coronavirus crisis.

****

- https://www.weforum.org

****

Getting to 30 & Beyond

The United States is losing the battle against Covid-19. We called in April for the nation to get to three million Covid-19 tests a week by July and to 30 million by October. To beat this virus we need a massive national effort to get to 30 million and beyond with tests that are easy, fast, and cheap. Only then can we keep the economy open and protect our most vulnerable.

- https://www.rockefellerfoundation.org

****

The Coronavirus Pandemic Will Forever Alter the World Order

by Henry A. Kissinger

The Wall Street Journal
April 3, 2020

The U.S. must protect its citizens from disease while starting the urgent work of planning for a new epoch.

The surreal atmosphere of the Covid-19 pandemic calls to mind how I felt as a young man in the 84th Infantry Division during the Battle of the Bulge. Now, as in late 1944, there is a sense of inchoate danger, aimed not at any particular person, but striking randomly and with devastation. But there is an important difference between that faraway time and ours. American endurance then was fortified by an ultimate national purpose. Now, in a divided country, efficient and farsighted government is necessary to overcome obstacles unprecedented in magnitude and global scope. Sustaining the public trust is crucial to social solidarity, to the relation of societies with each other, and to international peace and stability.

Nations cohere and flourish on the belief that their institutions can foresee calamity, arrest its impact and restore stability. When the Covid-19 pandemic is over, many countries' institutions will be perceived as having failed. Whether this judgment is objectively fair is irrelevant. The reality is the world will never be the same after the coronavirus. To argue now about the past only makes it harder to do what has to be done.

The coronavirus has struck with unprecedented scale and ferocity. Its spread is exponential: U.S. cases are doubling every fifth day. At this writing, there is no cure. Medical supplies are insufficient to cope with the widening waves of cases. Intensive-care units are on the verge, and beyond, of being overwhelmed. Testing is inadequate to the task of identifying the extent of infection, much less reversing its spread. A successful vaccine could be 12 to 18 months away.

****

OK, is Henry Kissinger your idea of a credible opinion-maker on this subject?! Here's an excerpt from an article in the *New Yorker* entitled "Does Henry Kissinger have a Conscience?" by Jon Lee Anderson (August 20, 2016):

"The latest revelations compound a portrait of Kissinger as the ruthless cheerleader, if not the active co-conspirator, of Latin American military regimes engaged in war crimes. In evidence that emerged from previous declassifications of documents during the Clinton Administration, Kissinger was shown not only to have been aware of what the military was doing but to have actively encouraged it. Two days after the Argentine coup, Kissinger was briefed by his Assistant Secretary of State for Inter-American Affairs, William Rogers, who warned him, "I think also we've got to expect a fair amount of repression, probably a good deal of blood, in Argentina before too long. I think they're going to have to come down very hard not only on the terrorists but on the dissidents of trade unions and their parties." Kissinger replied, "Whatever chance they have, they will need a little encouragement . . . because I do want to encourage them. I don't want to give the sense that they're harassed by the United States."" **- https://www.newyorker.com/news/news-desk/does-henry-kissinger-have-a-conscience**

That's from a guy who was National Security Advisor in 1969 and U.S. Secretary of State in 1973. *HE WAS ENCOURAGING ONE OF THE MOST BRUTAL REGIMES IN HUMAN HISTORY* - one that tortured & disappeared people who disagreed with government. SO, *really,* do we want to support his idea that the corona virus will "forever alter the world order"?!

The article's from April 3, 2020. Kissinger says: "U.S. cases are doubling every fifth day." **Like all the propagandistic fear-mongering, that doesn't take into consideration that natural tendency for a disease to have a peak & a decline. According to the CDC, all deaths involving COVID-19 by the week ending April 4, 2020, in the USA were: 9,993. https://www.cdc.gov/nchs/nvss/vsrr/COVID19/ That doesn't mean that COVID-19 was the killer, just that it was present. That, however ISN'T "cases". Let's be the most fearful: even though cases ≠ deaths we'll pretend like they do anyway like**

the fear-mongers do. By April 9, there would be 19,986 deaths; April 14: 39,972; April 19: 79,944; April 24: 159,888; April 29: 319,776; May 4: 639,552; May 9: 1,279,104; May 14: 2,558,208; May 19: 5,116,416; May 24: 10,232,832; May 29: 20,465,664; June 3: 40,931,328; June 8: 81,862,656; June 13: 163,725,312; June 18: 327,450,624; June 23: 654,901,248..

Given that the US population as of 2019 is said to've been 328.2 million that means we'd all be long-since dead. If Kissinger had his genocidal way that might actually be the case.

****

Coronavirus Gives A Dangerous Boost To DARPA's Darkest Agenda

Posted on
May 4, 2020
Author
Whitney WebbComments(19)

Technology developed by the Pentagon's controversial research branch is getting a huge boost amid the current coronavirus crisis, with little attention going to the agency's ulterior motives for developing said technologies, their potential for weaponization or their unintended consequences.

In January, well before the coronavirus (Covid-19) crisis would result in lockdowns, quarantines and economic devastation in the United States and beyond, the U.S. intelligence community and the Pentagon were working with the National Security Council to create still-classified plans to respond to an imminent pandemic. It has since been alleged that the intelligence and military intelligence communities knew about a likely pandemic in the United States as early as last November, and potentially even before then.

Given this foreknowledge and the numerous simulations conducted in the United States last year regarding global viral pandemic outbreaks, at least six of varying scope and size, it has often been asked – Why did the government not act or prepare if an imminent global pandemic and the shortcomings of any response to such an event were known? Though the answer to this question has frequently been written off as mere "incompetence" in mainstream media circles, it is worth entertaining the possibility that a crisis was allowed to unfold.

Why would the intelligence community or another faction of the U.S. government knowingly allow a crisis such as this to occur? The answer is clear if one looks at history, as times of crisis have often been used by the U.S. government to implement policies that would normally be rejected by the American public, ranging from censorship of the press to mass surveillance networks. Though the government response to the September 11 attacks, like the Patriot Act, may be the most accessible example to many Americans, U.S. government efforts to limit the flow of "dangerous" journalism and surveil the population go back to as early as the First World War. Many of these policies, whether the Patriot Act after 9/11 or WWI-era civilian "spy" networks, did little if anything to protect the homeland, but instead led to increased surveillance and control that persisted long after the crisis that spurred them had ended.

Using this history as a lens, it is possible to look at the current coronavirus crisis to see how the long-standing agendas of ever-expanding mass surveillance and media censorship are again getting a dramatic boost thanks to the chaos unleashed by the coronavirus pandemic. Yet, this crisis is unique because it also has given a boost to a newer yet complimentary agenda that — if fulfilled – would render most, if not all, other government efforts at controlling and subduing their populations obsolete.

[..]

****

May 16, 2020, 4:42PM (Dick to group):

RE: Heretics: whitney webb article

Thank you for this info
This one is pretty intense, particularly when it gets to around 9 minutes
https://www.youtube.com/watch?v=ftzijxExjkY

Setting The Stage For Phase 2 As States Deploy National Guard For Contact Tracing
Several states are preparing to ease restrictions related to the Coronavirus lockdowns, other states have extended the lockdowns while a handful of states like South Dakota never imposed a statewide lockdown at all, why don't we hear about this in the mainstream media? Surely we would hear about these rogue states if there was a significant ...

****

May 16, 2020, 5:56PM (Dick to group):

RE: Heretics: whitney webb article

I would like to make a comment on these videos and papers all of which I watched or read and found very interesting..
In many of them there is a thesis put forth that the US government feels that it is necessary to copy China's surveillance policies in order that the US can surpass them in their Artificial Intelligence capacities.
This means, the USA wants to copy China, thus introducing centralized everything. They call this getting rid of "legacy behaviors" and replacing them with AI variants (no cash, no in-person doctor visits, shopping online, no

personal car ownership, etc)
Now here's what I'd like to say:
I have noticed since I have lived in Europe that people here, the French for example, are always talking about lagging behind the US and how they have to catch up.
Now, not surprisingly, they never do and and in my opinion, never will.
I believe this is neither due to their smaller size nor a lack of intelligent people but lays in the fact that copying someone else rather than innovating, or doing your own thing, means that you will never win.
It is the basic lesson from chess playing that if you play a game of chess where you follow your opponent's game you are doomed. The key to a good chess game is to introduce moves that either force your adversary to play your game or to somehow turn your adversaries' moves to your advantage - say he makes an attack and so, instead of defending yourself, you respond with an attack as well.
Thus, if it is true that American policy is now in a phase of playing "catch up" or "follow the leader" with China, this means, in my opinion, that they have already lost.

****

May 16, 2020, 6:39PM (BP to group):

Yesterday, I spent way too much time reading nasty stuff, including this non-pandemic related article but a must-read for those following the persecution of Assange:::: https://thegrayzone.com/2020/05/14/american-sheldon-adelsons-us-spy-julian-assange/
and ended the day with the brilliant thought of: what will I find if I search for GOOD NEWS CORONAVIRUS COVID?
Yep, nice stories about teens delivering meals to the old folk (an admirable thing to do) but I only came up with two hits, but both connected.
https://blogs.sciencemag.org/pipeline/archives/2020/05/15/good-news-on-the-human-immune-response-to-the-coronavirus
Science way beyond me, but I did my best, and it's boiled down a bit at the end.
Basically: strong signs it's like the previous coronas, and that our systems are doing the right thing, fighting the new one off. NATURALLY. As it has always been. The stance may be all about developing a vaccine, but a positive development for those that want to get by WITHOUT the vaccine.
This one is more easily consumable to my brain, commenting on the same study:
https://www.kpbs.org/news/2020/may/15/coronavirus-patients-recovery-immunity-likely/
“The researchers were surprised to find some patients who had never been exposed to COVID-19 also showed an immune response to SARS-CoV-2. As part of a control group, Sette's lab tested blood samples taken from people between 2015 and 2018, before the virus was circulating, and found about half of those had immune memory that could recognize the COVID-19 virus.”
Hmmmm.
In the comments section of the Science article a fellow, "immunologist," posted this mainstream news bit:
https://www.nbcboston.com/news/coronavirus/study-shows-9-out-of-10-boston-

residents-havent-been-exposed-to-covid-19/2124944/
but translated the FEAR click as:
"Some 10% of ASYMPTOMATIC Bostonians have antibodies to the virus and another 3% have a positive culture for the virus. Some 750 people were tested. This means for most people, the pandemic coronavirus doesn't make you very sick.
Of course the worst possible spin was put on the news by the Mayor and those interested in continuing the lockdown, namely that 90% of the population is at risk for infection (catch the lead). But so what, if it doesn't make you sick (if you're young and healthy)."

Like the Fear Mongers have been saying for months: we are at a critical juncture. Just give it 2 more weeks.
Now we're 2 weeks into the critical 2 weeks of "re-opening."
Nothing on Georgia, Florida, Texas, Tennessee in the "news" search?
We need to hear about the Good News from these States in the Big Time media. But will they?

****

Good News on the Human Immune Response to the Coronavirus

By Derek Lowe 15 May, 2020

[..]

So overall, this paper makes the prospects for a vaccine look good: there is indeed a robust response by the adaptive immune system, to several coronavirus proteins. And vaccine developers will want to think about adding in some of the other antigens mentioned in this paper, in addition to the Spike antigens that have been the focus thus far. It seems fair to say, though, that the first wave of vaccines will likely be Spike-o-centric, and later vaccines might have these other antigens included in the mix. But it also seems that Spike-protein-targeted vaccines should be pretty effective, so that's good. The other good news is that this team looked for the signs of an antibody-dependent-enhancement response, which would be bad news, and did not find evidence of it in the recovering patients (I didn't go into these details, but wanted to mention that finding, which is quite reassuring). And it also looks like the prospects for (reasonably) lasting immunity after infection (or after vaccination) are good. This, from what I can see, is just the sort of response that you'd want to see for that to be the case. Clinical data will be the real decider on that, but there's no reason so far to think that a person won't have such immunity if they fit this profile.

[..]

****

Some Good Coronavirus News: Recovered San Diego Patients Showed 'Robust' Immunity

Friday, May 15, 2020
By **Mark Sauer**, **Megan Burke**

[..]

"It seems likely to us that immunity is developed. At least some reasonable amount of immunity is present and is developed by most people," Crotty said. "We would consider that good news and largely fits with the expectations we would have for an antiviral immune response."

[..]

****

Study Shows 9 Out of 10 Boston Residents Haven't Been Exposed to COVID-19

Of the 1,000 Boston residents tested, the Massachusetts General Hospital study found 9.9% were positive for antibodies, according to Mayor Marty Walsh's office

By **Melissa Buja** • Published May 15, 2020 • Updated on May 15, 2020 at 8:04 pm

[..]

"We can draw two preliminary conclusions from the results of this study. First, that the actions we took early on in this pandemic made a real difference in slowing the spread and, second, that the majority of our population still have not been exposed to the virus," Walsh said in a statement.

The mayor added that in order to reopen the economy, there must be a "phased-in approach" that includes safety guidelines that are dependent on testing. Officials from Mass. General echoed that sentiment, saying careful decisions need to be made about reopening, as 90% of Boston's residents have not yet been exposed to COVID-19.

"Making sound decisions about safely reopening requires that we understand how extensively the virus has already spread in our community," said Dr. Peter Slavin, president of Massachusetts General Hospital. "We also know that COVID-19 will be with us for a while. It is vital therefore that we be thoughtful and careful about reopening, and that we continue to take actions — wearing masks, physical distancing, working from home when possible, limiting gatherings. That can prevent another surge of the disease."

****

May 16, 2020, 8:24PM (Inquiring Librarian to group):

Re: Heretics: whitney webb article

Something I have noticed now on my social media Page, since Louisiana is starting to reopen... some of my 'friends' are now going-back-to-work shaming. AKA, they are shaming those of us who are heading back to work this week. I hate this kind of bullying. I am personally infinitely grateful to my library director and Mayor for letting me go back to work and maintain my income and to serve the city public that I was hired to serve as a Civil Servant. It will be interesting to see who does and does not show up for work at the library this week. I have been silently observing various library worker's social media pages to see their comments and reactions to my most work shaming bully friend. I am happy to report that all of my staff at my tiny branch are coming back to work and doing it happily (despite the masks... I had to buy some masks... they are all WAY too big on my face. I have a tiny face, somewhere between a kid and a teen sized. I bought homemade masks from a gal who has no income outside of those masks now... no stimulus check, no unemployment, I am sadly helping to pay her rent, phone, and food bills).

One of my librarian friends lives in Milwaukee. He was furloughed for a week. And then he was called back to work again if he would agree to be a Contact Tracer. He appears happy to be a Contact Tracer. Then one of my fellow Louisiana Librarians commented on her page that she wished that our library would give us that job instead of asking us to report back to work. These are such kind, well meaning, thoughtful people. I hate to see them so obliviously falling down this rabbit hole feeling they are 'helping' out the needy. Sigh...

I'm listening to Russian Melodia WWII era folk songs... heavily influenced by the USSR during WWII, I believe actually that Melodia was the state sponsored record company of the USSR. Here is Katusha, a song that is actually about a missile named Katusha and Russia's love for this bomb! =O I grew up listening to this stuff, because my dad grew up listening to it. It is beautiful but really scary in how everyone in Russia knows and loves these songs but they were from such a tyrannical police state that spied on and murdered millions of its own in the name of the "truth". https://www.youtube.com/watch?v=MLg83QMmlGs
The music really fits what we have going on here. =/ Maybe our government can make a catchy song about our "war" against the virus. Ultimately, in the U.S. it would be some horrible soulless musician that I couldn't listen to for more than a second.

Check out this scary article on Contact Tracing in Washington state.

https://www.lifesitenews.com/news/washington-gov-those-who-dont-cooperate-with-contact-tracers-and-tests-not-allowed-to-leave-home?utm_content=bufferdb078&utm_medium=LSN%2Bbuffer&utm_source=facebook&utm_campaign=LSN&fbclid=IwAR2jYhFO_WsvM1mA3DmyzArwiOgIFdpqtdgNrEVZYp2vimBGWJHF7e0eDls

****

Washington gov: Those who don't cooperate with 'contact tracers' and tests not allowed to leave home

The state will provide 'family support personnel' to check in on the non-compliant.

Thu May 14, 2020 - 4:38 pm EST

OLYMPIA, Washington, May 14, 2020 (LifeSiteNews) – Washington Governor Jay Inslee indicated that people who refuse to cooperate with contact tracers or refuse coronavirus testing won't be allowed to leave their homes even to go to the grocery store or pharmacy.

"When it comes to contact tracing, how are you guys going to handle people or families who want to refuse to test or to self isolate? If they want to leave their home to get groceries I know you've said they can't do that; how will you make sure they don't?" a reporter asked him.

"We will have attached to the families a family support person who will check in with them to see what they need on a daily basis," he responded. "If they can't get a friend to do their grocery shopping, we will help get them groceries in some fashion. If they need pharmaceuticals to be picked up, we will make sure they get their pharmaceuticals... We are going to be there on a daily basis for them – now that's going to help encourage them to maintain their isolation too."

[..]

Talk about repulsive euphemistic language!! Why not just call a torturer at Abu Ghraib "a family support person" **& get it over with?!**

Here's one of the comments on that one:

There's no death penalty in Washington state for murder. Now he's claiming authority to slowly starve you if you don't conform. Without trial.

****

May 17, 2020, 4:53PM (Inquiring Librarian to group):

HERETICS: An Irish Scientist in Support of Dr. Judy Mikovits' Theories

Here is another gem that I found on Phil's fb page:
https://www.youtube.com/watch?v=Avc6_ftzk3w&fbclid=IwAR3FJXvrzlwD6TuaRwNvNzi4DWjyNMODRw4xs-FXemOphNFspTjaaQcml2g

You will hear this woman, Professor Doris Cahill of Ireland, speaking in support of Dr. Judy Mikovits' theories on the pandemic. You will also hear the same suggestion that a former flu vaccine, given widely in Wuhan and also in Italy, left many given the vaccine with a very lethal immuno-response to this Covid 19 virus.

****

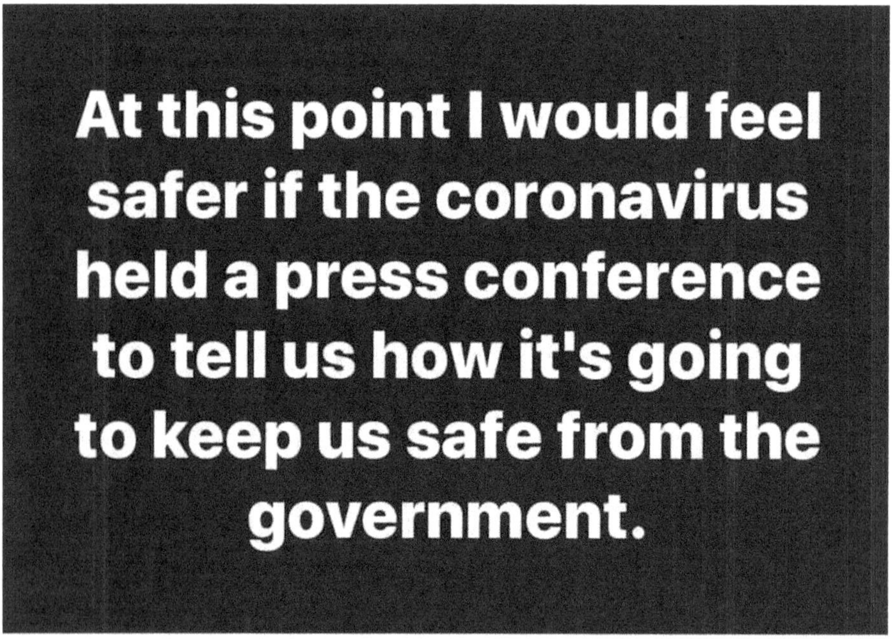

At this point I would feel safer if the coronavirus held a press conference to tell us how it's going to keep us safe from the government.

(Not one of Amir-ul Kafirs text panels)

****

May 17, 2020, 6:00PM (Amir-ul Kafirs to group):

HERETICS: New Normal Regulations

Here's my latest example of snide humor. It's conveniently sized at 11X17" (actually 10X16" so that there's a half inch margin all around). Feel free to print it out and put it up in places where people need to be reminded of the proper ways to act.

New Normal Regulations

1. Be in a constant state of fear.

Nature is your enemy. You are not a part of nature. It is out to kill you. So are we.

2. Be on prescription drugs.

Your natural body cannot provide for you. Only doctors know what's best for you. Evolution and instinct and your immune system are utterly without value.

3. Pump as much money into the Medical Industry as possible.

Unnecessary extremely expensive tests? Don't hesitate for a second. After all, doctors and other representatives of the MI are human too and may need to buy a $6,000,000 home or at least pay off their student loans — and *this is your problem and your responsibility.*

4. Be a coward.

You've always known you are one, you've just tried to hide it by being a sheep in wolf's clothing. Now that it's the New Norm there's no reason to hide it anymore. Cower. Wallow.

5. Be a conformist.

It's the easiest way. Don't worry, Big Brother gives you a choice of subcultures that you can stay in. It makes shopping for clothing and picking music to listen to so much easier. Opinions? No need to give that a second thought — just parrot what your subculture's Alpha Male or Female says and you'll be set.

6. Don't think.

Thinking is a Thought Crime. PERIOD. And we can tell.. there's just something a little odd about you.

7. Accept always being wrong.

No matter how hard you try to be at one with the majority something idiosyncratic might slip out. We'll punish you for that. We may even punish you even if it DOESN'T HAPPEN.

8. Spend.

You can buy anything but freedom online now. If you can't afford it some kind of credit can be worked out. Even a car can be delivered directly to your home.

8. Bully, lie about and Shame others who defy GROUPTHINK..

Its the only way to PROVE you belong.

This has been a public service message brought to you by Big Brother with a Vengeance.

****

May 17, 2020, 11:11AM (Amir-ul Kafirs to group):

Heretics: ZOO(m), etc..

I keep using social media as a way of sniping at the MONOLITHIC NARRATIVE. Here're the notes to a movie I uploaded recently.

"Heretic InExile in this 2020.05.12 ZOO(m)" notes - 10:23 - 2K

https://youtu.be/Mfd7YUIGXKM

In order to avoid becoming a complete QUARANTINIAC (a person who goes insane under quarantine) I've been trying to keep my creative life on track regardless of the way entirely too much of the world's human population is bending over & spreading it for their 'vaccination'. One mild-mannered way of doing this is to participate in the Improv Tuesdays organized by _____ over Zoom. I called these Zoom sessions "ZOO(m)s" because it's like a nice bourgeois panopticon, we're all in our comfy cells in ZOO-WORLD where the 'masters' can watch us on surveillance cameras. We get to see ourselves too but we don't get to see the 'masters'. ANYWAY, I'm not knocking the Tuesday Improvs because they've been fun & I appreciate _____'s organizing of them. For this episode of My Life In Progress, I reminisce about being a teenage musician & imagine what might have happened if I hadn't been arrested in a stolen car but had, instead, made it to a music festival & played my special brand of, unfortunately, covers of Leonard Cohen & Incredible String Band & such on the 12 string acoutic guitar I was hitch-hiking with. Gosh! I might've been 'discovered', much as Columbus, 'discovered' America.

Needless to say, when I post such things on social media there're retaliations.

I just drove long distance to buy a cheap cello & violin. I had to go through Pennsylvania, Maryland, West Virginia, & Virginia to meet the Craigslist seller on the parkinglot of a shopping mall that had just reopened its food court that day & which was, consequently, crowded — many people in violation of social distancing & not wearing masks. The seller was wearing a mask. He also had a bumper sticker that said something like: "I'm the worst of everything: white, straight, and conservative." & another pro-Trump one. He told me he was Jewish & that his dad was a rabbai & that he left the religion because the synagogues were run like 7/11 franchises with admission to important events that were unaffordable to the poor. He's an opera buff so we could talk about that somewhat. He wants me to go to the opera with him when it reopens in Pittsburgh. He was 75 & in obvious bad health & wearing a mask.

The trip was too long for me to make in one day so I stopped at a hotel on the way back. Hotels are the only place where I willingly watch TV. I was watching a Jackie Chan movie, whose work I love, but it was heavily separated by commercials, which I muted. The ads were so intensely PANDEMIC PANIC oriented that I can easily see how TV watchers would find the mind control pressure inescapable. There was the usual prescription drug mania; a justification of how pregnant women are being treated in terms of equating COVID-19 with the Spanish Flu; plenty about what to do in isolation (all of it involving spending loads of money) including buying stuff from Etsy no less!; a diabetes type 2 medication ad in which, as usual, the emphasis was on a wonder drug rather than on changing one's diet & getting more exercise; ***but this one wins the prize!:*** it was for people who "just can't wait to get a new car!": they were reassured that they could buy one ONLINE & HAVE IT DELIVERED TO THEIR HOUSE where they could take proud ownership of it *wearing a mask*.

I am, truthfully, beyond disgust now. If I had the knowhow I'd turn all TV off. That would be a *huge step* in a healthy direction.

****

May 17, 2020, 6:39PM (Inquiring Librarian to group):

Re: Heretics: ZOO(m), etc..

Wow! I had forgotten about tv. I don't have one in my house. My only access to tv used to be on the treadmill at my gym. Since my gym has been closed since early March, i forgot about commercials and how much they irritated me b4 the pandemic panic. I feel glad i continue to be spared them as my gym remains closed now and i have grown to love jogging in Audubon park now that i have restarted my physical therapist recommended knee excercises which are genius and now allow me to jog in nature without pain.

The closest to Amir-ul Kafir's tv commercial experience i get now is npr. My bf usually sleeps all day and i sleep all night since this nonsense started. I get lonely. I need to hear voices sometimes... In would come npr which has increasingly disgusted me these past few months, barely a level above Amir-ul Kafirs's commercials. But now that i have found Phil's page, i just play whatever videos and interviews he posts and what u all share. I am ever grateful for you all. You reinstill my faith in humanity.

I start work again tomorrow! I am a total asshole about wearing my mask. But i will suffer through it. I am a manager and i love my staff/coworkers. I bought my masks from a sad gal who has no other income. And my mom is sending me some she made herself. I love my mom. I am sure i will have stories to share about the panic amongst library staff. Many/most if not all of my fellow library staff are eating this pandemic panic up. And many of them are up in arms about going back to work, risking their lives to hurt others. It kinda disgusts me. But i will grin and bear it and play the game as best i can without giving up my soul. I work with a great crew. So glad the more brainwashed angry ones do not work in my building!

Here is an article that some library staff members here felt compelled to hurl at our city public. They make me feel ashamed for my profession. & how dare they feel that they speak for all of us?
https://www.nola.com/news/coronavirus/article_3b4f6af6-9574-11ea-b0cb-e79daf48bdf8.html

****

New Orleans libraries are still closed, but librarians told to head to work Monday

BY MATT SLEDGE I STAFF WRITER MAY 14, 2020 - 7:00 AM 2 min to read

[..]

Librarian Amanda Fallis expressed frustration that her colleagues have not been told what the safety procedures and equipment will be.

"This is a failure of communication in a new and dangerous age of pandemic, where such mistakes really need to be avoided going forward," she said. "Such secrecy or procrastination, whatever it is, is untenable going forward."

Another librarian said she was frightened for her coworkers with underlying health conditions who will be forced to go to work, or colleagues with children who will need to arrange childcare on short notice.

[..]

****

May 18, 2020, 13:42PM (Phil to group):

Thanks for the links BP. I found this quite interesting;

As part of a control group, Sette's lab tested blood samples taken from people between 2015 and 2018, before the virus was circulating, and found about half of those had immune memory that could recognize the COVID-19 virus.

I remember reading someone else suggesting that this should be a way of testing the coronavirus test (not the antibody test). I couldn't remember who. I thought it was John Rappoport but could not find when I went looking. i think it was actually in the David Crowe interview.

The president of tanzania has done one better and did some blind tests of paw paw, goats, motor oil, etc....
https://www.youtube.com/watch?v=gbsRK7e-G9o

As a side note Madagascar has called on african nations to leave The WHO https://www.omokoshaban.com/2020/05/16/madagascar-president-rajoelina-called-on-african-nations-to-quit-who-because-of-the-bad-faith-of-europe-towards-africa/

David Crowe has also put out a paper on the antibody test...I haven't read either of his reports directly yet but hope to soon. Here is Rappoport's summary of Crowes paper;
Assuming that a new virus called COVID-19 was actually discovered—we are being told that antibody tests are a vital tool for determining who is immune and who is not.
These tests are heralded as essential and necessary, despite some downplayed doubt among "experts" about how reliable they are.
https://blog.nomorefakenews.com/2020/05/15/covid-david-crowes-brilliant-new-paper-takes-apart-antibody-testing/

Then on this whole subject I found this author Charles Ortleb. I have downloaded several podcasts to listen to later.
https://charlesortleb.podbean.com/

He wrote this book on Fauci last year.
Fauci: The Bernie Madoff of Science and the HIV Ponzi Scheme that Concealed the Chronic Fatique Syndome Epidemic.
https://www.goodreads.com/book/show/45069570-fauci

I am kind of curious now to learn more about this relationship between AIDS and Chronic Fatigue Syndrome and how Covid-19 might fit in. Rappoport in researching AIDS writes.....
The AIDS cover story that had been invented by medical researchers was all about One Reality, one disease condition caused by one virus, one description about how the infection destroyed the immune system, one label, one symbol for the condition: "AIDS".
When, in fact, that was "the obstruction on the road" which was blocking further investigation. In fact, the whole "Oneness" myth was a lie. A gigantic lie.
A very, very convincing lie. An awesome lie.
The truth was, so-called AIDS was many different conditions (realities) which had been falsely welded together, through massive propaganda.
That was the key to unlocking the puzzle. And it was the key for me to move into new territory with new energy and confidence.
https://blog.nomorefakenews.com/

Also it is good to see Naomi Klein chiming in on the technodistopia subject.
https://www.democracynow.org/2020/5/13/naomi_klein_coronavirus_tech_privacy_surveillance

Anyway on a different note here are some videos I made some years ago on the subject of dystopia. The old dystopia not the new one. No budget hand held guerrilla just messing around style;

Blind Sight
https://www.youtube.com/watch?v=p_GqK_BTMGE&list=PL9F2D2D0EC362998B

****

May 16, 2020 Omokoshaban World News 0

The President of Madagascar, Andry Rajoelina has called on all African Nations to quit the World Health Organization (WHO) because of the bad faith of Europe towards Africa.

The Malagasy president says," Europe created organizations with the desire for Africans to remain dependent on them. Africa has found a medicine against Coronavirus but Europe thinks they have a monopoly of intelligence as such they are refusing to acknowledge it. It is against this backdrop that I invite all African Nations to quit the international organizations in order for us to build ours.

"My country Madagascar leaves all the organizations tonight and I call on other African Nations to do same".

****

COVID: David Crowe's brilliant new paper takes apart antibody testing

by Jon Rappoport
May 15, 2020

Assuming that a new virus called COVID-19 was actually discovered—we are being told that antibody tests are a vital tool for determining who is immune and who is not.
These tests are heralded as essential and necessary, despite some downplayed doubt among "experts" about how reliable they are.
Canadian author and long-time independent researcher, David Crowe, has written a new paper, *"Antibody Testing for COVID-19."* (May 13, 2020).
(For David Crowe's paper that challenges the discovery of the COVID-19 virus, click here.)
I can safely say it is the most detailed analysis of the tests anyone will ever read. It approaches the subject from a number of angles, and includes a breakdown of the test-kit manufacturers and the comparative results of their efforts to bring a useful test to the public.
Here are several devastating excerpts from Crowe's very deep dive:
"The only jurisdiction with a formal structure for approval of antibody tests is the United States but, until very recently, it was a complete joke, as the test manufacturers did not need to provide validation data. Now it is only a partial joke, as validation data must be provided, but the FDA can only do a paper analysis. Imagine if auto-manufacturers had to build cars to certain EPA (US Environmental Protection Agency) fuel efficiency standards, but rather than sending a car to the EPA for testing, they could do the testing at their facilities, and just send the results in afterwards..."
"Antibody tests are often subject to cross-reactions with other conditions. This

could be because the [other irrelevant] medical condition produces similar antibodies, or because something related to that [other] condition reacts with other test components. The choice of [cross-reacting] conditions to check for is completely under the control of the manufacturer and even when no cross reactions were found for a condition, the number of samples tested was so small that the possibility of a fairly high rate of false positive cross reactions still exists."
"Positive antibody tests have only been found in a minority of people in the general population even where the virus is believed to have been circulating for months. These fractions are generally taken as truth, but one would expect a highly infectious virus to have spread much more widely...The one experiment that could show whether antibody tests are actually meaningful would be a time series of a large number of people who are currently negative on all tests. This experiment would be time consuming, inefficient (as many people would never become positive on any tests), intrusive (frequent nasal swabs and blood tests) and obviously very expensive. Those are practical considerations, but in the absence of such an experiment we are almost totally in the dark about COVID-19 antibody testing. Given the billions being spent on COVID and the trillions being lost by the economy, it surely is not impossible to do some worthwhile science."
David Crowe's paper demands widespread notice and very careful study. He has provided a great service.
Superficial reliance on antibody tests has no connection to real science. Yet, the so-called experts are using these tests to make momentous decisions about the present and future of humans on Earth.

[..]

****

[..]

These the elements of Fauci's scientific Ponzi scheme:

1. Nosological fraud. (That's the branch of medicine dealing with the classification of disease. It is ground zero for public health fraud.)

2. Epidemiological fraud.

3. Virological fraud.

4. Treatment fraud. (Treatments that harm more than they heal or conceal more than they reveal.)

5. Public health policy fraud.

6. Concealment of negative scientific data and paradigm-challenging anomalies.

7. Use of an elite network of "old boys" and pseudo-activist provocateurs to censor critics and whistleblowers.

8. Chronic obscurantism.

9. If necessary, vigilantism and witch-hunts against any intellectuals, scientists, or citizens who constitute any form of resistance to the Ponzi scheme.

Fauci and his puppets at NIH have created a real mess. Like Bernie Madoff, Anthony Fauci is rich, famous, and powerful as a result of his scientific Ponzi scheme. And Fauci is a clever manipulator who will continue to try and hide the nature of his scientific Ponzi scheme from the public the way Bernie Madoff hid his financial records. But luckily, this brilliant and uncompromising work of journalism will enlighten members of Congress and the media as they begin extensive investigations of the Fauci Ponzi scheme.

- https://www.goodreads.com/book/show/45069570-fauci

****

How I assembled The Matrix Revealed: The Key Symbol

by Jon Rappoport
August 9, 2020

The key was handed to me by a colleague and friend.
In 1987, when I was researching my book, *AIDS INC.*, I took a side road. It was prompted by a conversation I had with the brilliant hypnotherapist, Jack True. He was telling me about experiences he'd had with his patients under hypnosis.
"Some patients encounter a 'monolith'," he said. "They come across a symbol that is there in the subconscious. Sometimes it looks like a closed door. Sometimes it shows up as a blank wall. Sometimes it's a geometric shape. One patient actually called it a 'brick sky'."
"But in every case, it locked up the patient's ability to recall or explore under hypnosis. It was like a giant obstruction on a road. However, these patients could describe something about the nature of the symbol. They said it was broadcasting a message: 'THIS IS REALITY'."
"The patients were in awe of the symbol. It had a deep emotional effect on them. It was as if many different realities had come together to form this single symbol, like separate pieces clicking into place."
Jack went further. He stated that the symbol induced a profound passivity in his patients...
Jack subsequently devised strategies to take apart the symbol, so these patients could rid themselves of their passivity and access huge amounts of previously blocked energies.

****

Now, given that I've been using the term "MONOLITHIC NARRATIVE" to mean the most dominant story that people are being obsessively exposed to in an apparent attempt to get as many to believe it as absolute unquestionable 'truth' — meaning to get them to

accept it as *the* description of "reality" — I found the above story about the hypnotherapist fascinating.

****

Screen New Deal: Naomi Klein on How Companies Like Google Plan to Profit in High-Tech COVID Dystopia

MAY 13, 2020

In her new report for The Intercept on the "Screen New Deal," Naomi Klein looks at how the coronavirus pandemic is more high-tech than previous disasters — and how the future we're being rushed into could transform our lives into a "living laboratory for a permanent — and highly profitable — no-touch future." She joins us to discuss what she found, and says, "I think we're going to see very incomplete so-called solutions … that massively benefit private tech interests."

Transcript

This is a rush transcript. Copy may not be in its final form.

AMY GOODMAN: Naomi, we wanted to turn right now to your major piece in *The Intercept*. You talk about the "pandemic shock doctrine" beginning to emerge, as we turn to your new report that looks at how this crisis is more high-tech than previous disasters and how the future we're being rushed into could transform our lives into a, quote, "living laboratory for a permanent — and highly profitable — no-touch future."

This future was on display a week ago during New York Governor Andrew Cuomo's daily coronavirus briefing, when he welcomed a video visit from former Google CEO Eric Schmidt and announced Schmidt will be heading up a blue-ribbon commission to reimagine New York state's post-COVID reality.

ERIC SCHMIDT: The public-private partnerships that are possible with the intelligence of the New Yorkers is extraordinary. It needs to be unleashed.

GOV. ANDREW CUOMO: Well, great. You are the person to help us do that. We are all ready. We're all in. We are New Yorkers, so we're aggressive about it and we're ambitious about it. And I think we get it, Eric. You know, we went through this period, and we realize that change is not only imminent, but it can actually be a friend, if done the right way.

AMY GOODMAN: This comes as Eric Schmidt has also been selling his services to the military-industrial complex. *The New York Times* reported on Schmidt's, quote, "Pentagon offensive."

Well, Naomi Klein, I want to ask if you can comment on all of this, and particularly lay out your piece in *The Intercept*, called "Screen New Deal: Under Cover of Mass Death, Andrew Cuomo Calls in the Billionaires to Build a High-Tech Dystopia." Lay out your thesis.

NAOMI KLEIN: Sure. Well, the billionaires I was referring to is, he didn't just announce that partnership with Eric Schmidt, who will be chairing this blue-ribbon commission to, quote-unquote, "reopen" New York state with an emphasis on telehealth, remote learning, working from home, increased broadband. That's what they announced during that briefing. He also announced that he would be kind of outsourcing the tracing of the virus to Michael Bloomberg, another megabillionaire. And the day before, at the briefing, Cuomo announced a partnership with the Bill & Melinda Gates Foundation to, quote-unquote, "reimagine" education.

And during all of these announcements, there's just been sort of effusive praise heaped on these billionaires. They're called "visionaries" over and over again. And the governor talks about how this is an unprecedented opportunity to put their preexisting ideas into action. And this is what I've described as the shock doctrine previously.

And we have talked on the show during the pandemic about what I would describe as kind of lower-tech shock doctrines of the kind we've seen before — immediately going after Social Security, immediately bailing out fossil fuel companies. And I want to stress that all of this is still happening, right? The suspending of EPA regulations. So, there's still this kind of lower-tech shock doctrine underway with the bailout of these industries, the suspending of regulations they didn't want anyway.

But there is something else going on, that Eric Schmidt really epitomizes. And this is this, what I'm calling a "Screen New Deal." And this is an idea that treats our months in isolation, those of us who are privileged enough to be self-isolating — and that, in and of itself, is an enormous privilege, because we have seen this sharpening and widening of a class dichotomy. And this relates to the calls to open up the economy, right? The people who are making these calls are not the people who are going to be most at risk. They're calling for other people to be putting themselves at great risk, and there is a feeling of being immune to the worst impacts of the virus. But that's another issue.

What this, what I'm calling a "Screen New Deal," really does is treat this period of isolation not as what we have needed to do in order to save lives — this is what we thought we were doing, right? — flattening the curve, but rather — and Eric Schmidt has said this elsewhere. He said it in April in a video call with the Economic Club of New York. He described what was happening now as a "grand experiment in remote learning." So, all the parents out there who are listening or watching, you've been struggling with supporting your kids on Google Classroom and Zoom calls, and you thought you were just trying to get through the day. Well, according to Google, you've been engaged in a "grand experiment in remote learning," where they are getting a great deal of data and figuring out how to do this permanently, because they actually believe this is a better way of educating kids, or at least, and coming back to our earlier conversation, a more profitable way.

Eric Schmidt talked, in that clip that you just played there, Amy, about all of the opportunities for public-private partnerships. And what he is really talking about is public money going to tech firms, like Google, like Amazon, to perform public functions. So, once again, a bonanza for the tech companies — who, by the way, have been doing very well during the pandemic already — where they see huge opportunities in telehealth, in the educational market in public schools, in supporting us working from home and learning from home.

And they're not looking for a kind of a traditional reopening, but, rather, a new

paradigm, where the privileged classes, who are able to isolate themselves, basically get everything that we need either delivered through digital streaming or by drone, by driverless vehicle.
And we're seeing a massive rebranding effort going on in Silicon Valley, where all of these technologies that were very, very controversial, and where there was a lot of pushback way back in February — whether it's driverless vehicles, because there have been all kinds of accidents, or drones delivering packages, or telehealth, because of concerns about security for patients' sensitive information, or the benefit of having our kids in front of screens all day. I mean, I could go on and on. There was a lot of pushback.

[..]

- https://www.democracynow.org/2020/5/13/naomi_klein_coronavirus_tech_privacy_surveillance

****

May 18, 2020, 6:07AM (Amir-ul Kafirs to group):

HERETICS: The New Normal

I think I forgot to share this:

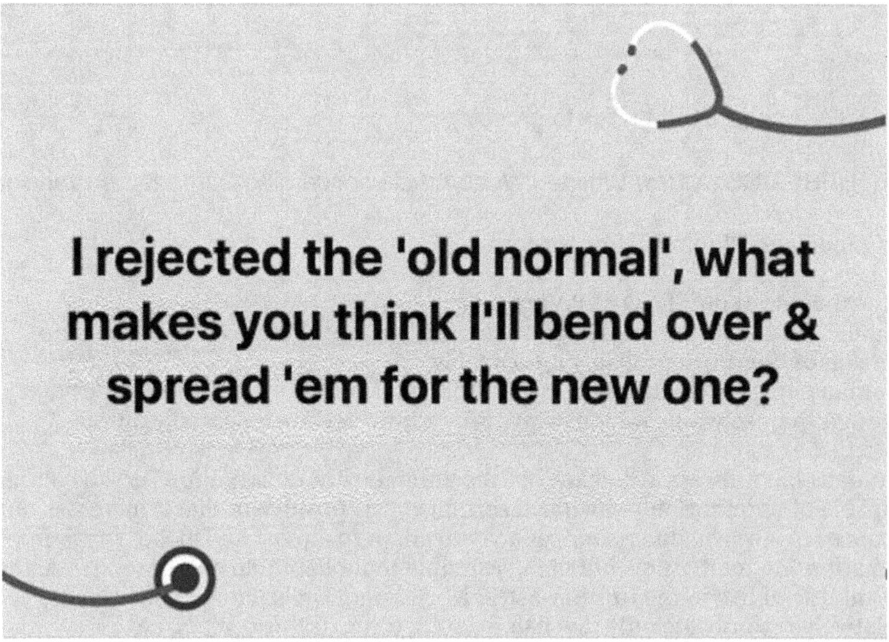

****

May 17, 2020, 4:47PM (Inquiring Librarian to group):

HERETICS: A New Whitney Webb Article concerning Darpa & the "Vaccine"

This new Whitney Web Article concerning the new dna/rna altering vaccines being developed really disturbs me. Can you all read it and tell me what you think? The article is long and very detailed. The Vaccine is not fully detailed until towards the end of the article but a good background on DARPA precedes this part about the new vaccine studies for covid 19. I shared it via social media with a few friends. It does not take sides and it does not say that covid 19 isn't real. I thought it was safe to share. Unfortunately, I am not sure the few who responded even read it. The blanket response was "I don't believe in 'Conspiracy' theories". =/ Sigh... I mean, this is REALLY SCARY STUFF! It could explain why we are being mass brainwashed into a frenzy over this virus.

Please tell me what you all think. Please tell me I am not crazy for being worried. And why is everyone so quick to call some article as detailed as this as 'conspiracy' while they cling to npr and whatever else their news tells them with little to no fact backing. Can I cry now? ='-[

https://www.thelastamericanvagabond.com/top-news/coronavirus-gives-dangerous-boost-darpas-darkest-agenda/?fbclid=IwAR1u2iMNCPebSXDHYpkfsyJmTybaEbyzNCfgKR6c2QHvMd8q1CRSIwvzmqY

****

May 17, 2020, 7:10PM (Dick to group):

RE: HERETICS: A New Whitney Webb Article concerning Darpa & the "Vaccine"

To Linda and Whom It May Concern,

My thoughts about the DARPA article :
Though it isn't very comforting, it seems to me that these scenarios, or some version of them, are probably inescapable
Human beings seem destined to go through all variations, all possibilities that present themselves as we move forward in time; we are essentially, never satisfied as a species
Humans have always struck me as "the animal without definition" or "the animal capable of redefinition" which in a certain way is positive in that it increases our chances of survival due to our capacity to adapt to almost any niche, any living situation (no matter how horrible - example that people survived Auschwitz, that Eskimos can live in the frozen wastes, Norwegians on isolated rocky islands, until relatively recently ate only raw fish for something like 800 years, etc.)
Consider extinction: all animals that can be defined are destined to perish if their niche perishes
Human beings however can adapt to any situation and thus this means that their chances of survival are much higher (lions can't adapt to city living for example,

that is, learn to stop at red lights, or wait in lines, thus they are, in the long term, doomed as their niche disappears and, sadly, the same seems to happening to Brazilian rain forest dwellers)
Perhaps genetic self-modification is just another step in the process of this continual human redefinition...
Humans seem to want to take over from Nature, maybe it's a God Complex or something like that, that's the general idea written in Genesis as you may recall, the God didn't want people to eat from the Tree of Knowledge and become like Gods so he kicked them out of Paradise before they got a chance... maybe humans are hung up on that somewhere in their hidden inner-consciousness - at least the humans doing this research at DARPA
Now, having said that, I'd like to clearly say I prefer what is known as "normal human existence" (that is I like to be left alone to pursue my interests) and that the scenarios presented (soldiers that don't need to sleep and that can be "switched off" once fighting is over) are, in my opinion, a vision of living hell, and if possible, prevented.

****

May 17, 2020, 8:47PM (Inquiring Librarian to group):

Dick, what you said sounds pretty spot on. I wish it was not. And I am also more in your camp. I want my genes left alone. I got a pretty good set. And I think mine have the benefit of half of them not being touched by 'modern' society for probably eons. Thus leaving them much less susceptible to 'herd mentalities' of this current 'modern' world. My dad is from a small swamp village in now Belarus. It was not touched by wars or any modern society until ww2 when the technology finally existed to murder and/or uproot dad's likely native swamp family of generations until ww2 unaltered by the modern world. Dad's family stayed away from the herds of families escaping Belarus and Poland into Germany, because Grandpa knew following the herds was going to lead to nothing good during ww2. Even in the refugee camps, they kept at a distance from others as much as possible. And then also I am among the very few of my generation, born in 1975, that grew up on well water. My body, outside of the dentist, never had to drink down daily doses of fluoridated water. I think fluoride is awful. It binds like an iodide to your thyroid and destroys your endocrine system, etc.

All this being said, what I'm getting at is that I value and cherish my genes just as they are. I have this hopefully irrational fear that my natural skepticism is just the kind of thing that a new gene editing vaccination is set out to destroy and 'reprogram' so that I/we can better ingest and embrace herd mentality. This I cannot tolerate. I will avoid this vaccine at all cost if it is truly to be a dna/rna gene editing vaccine. I have no children, and no cousins, so my imminent extinction because I refuse to have my genes tampered with to make me a more compliant and war-worthy super human will not hurt anyone but myself.

****

May 18, 2020, 9:57AM (Inquiring Librarian to group):

All of the major news outlets today announced a brand new, 'promising', vaccine from Moderna. It is an RNA vaccine.
https://www.google.com/amp/s/www.washingtonpost.com/health/2020/05/18/coronavirus-vaccine-first-results/%3foutputType=amp

****

Moderna's coronavirus vaccine shows encouraging early results

By
Carolyn Y. Johnson
May 19, 2020 at 4:30 p.m. EDT

Moderna, the Massachusetts biotechnology company behind a leading effort to create a coronavirus vaccine, announced promising early results Monday from its first human safety tests.

The eagerly awaited data provide a first look at one of the eight vaccines worldwide that have begun human testing. The data have not been published in a scientific journal and are only a preliminary step toward showing the experimental vaccine is safe and effective.

The company's stock, along with the Dow Jones industrial average, soared on the report that eight participants who received low and medium doses of Moderna's vaccine had blood levels of virus-fighting antibodies that were similar or greater than those in recovered covid-19 patients. That suggests, but doesn't prove, that it triggers some level of immunity.

Another 17 people had immune responses at a level similar or greater than recovered patients, but scientists had not yet tested whether their antibodies neutralized the virus.

Moderna's announcement comes days after one of its directors, Moncef Slaoui, stepped down from the board to become chief scientist for Operation Warp Speed, a White House initiative to speed up vaccine development. Watchdogs called out Slaoui's apparent conflict of interest. Filings with the Securities and Exchange Commission show Slaoui's stock options in Moderna are worth more than $10 million with the company's share price at $66.69. In regular trading Monday, Moderna's stock soared almost 20 percent to $80.

Moderna also received $483 million from the Biomedical Advanced Research and Development Authority, a federal agency. Moderna has also partnered with a contract development and manufacturing firm, Lonza, and Slaoui stepped down from that company's board on Monday.

[..]

****

May 19, 2020, 1:48PM (Amir-ul Kafirs to group):

HERETICS: Sneak Preview

Here're 4 text pieces that I made today to release on social media. I'll probably release them one a day rather than all at once so that they won't get lost in the quantity.

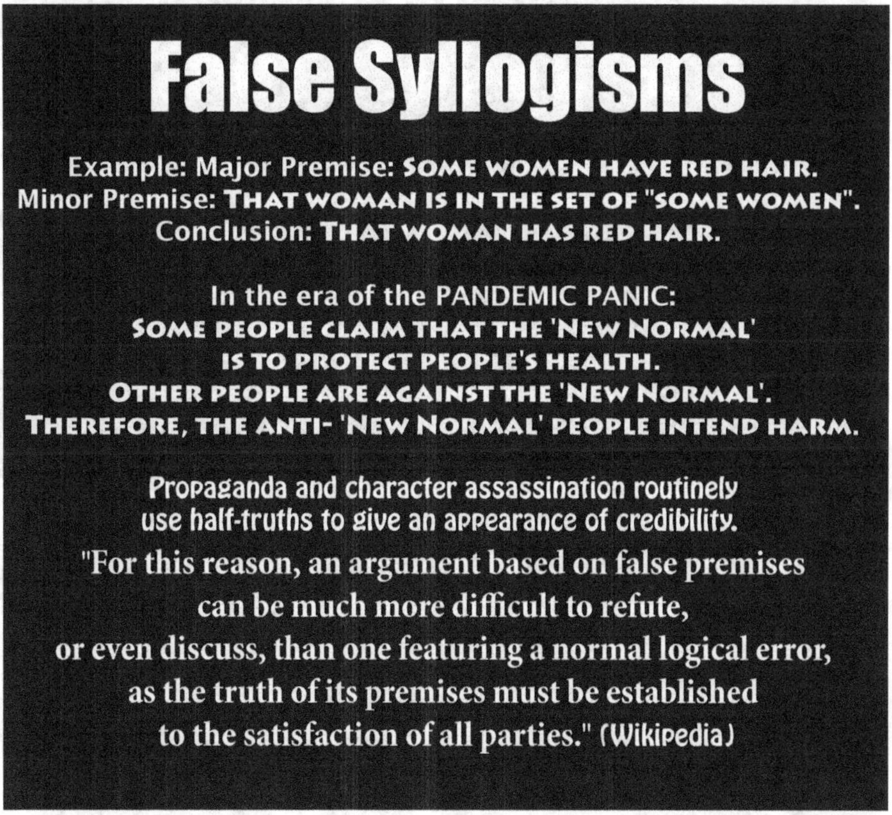

False Syllogisms
Example: Major Premise: SOME WOMEN HAVE RED HAIR.
Minor Premise: THAT WOMAN IS IN THE SET OF "SOME WOMEN".
Conclusion: THAT WOMAN HAS RED HAIR.
In the era of the PANDEMIC PANIC:
SOME PEOPLE CLAIM THAT THE 'NEW NORMAL'
IS TO PROTECT PEOPLE'S HEALTH.
OTHER PEOPLE ARE AGAINST THE 'NEW NORMAL'.
THEREFORE, THE ANTI- 'NEW NORMAL' PEOPLE INTEND HARM.
Propaganda and character assassination routinely
use half-truths to give an appearance of credibility.
"For this reason, an argument based on false premises
can be much more difficult to refute,
or even discuss, than one featuring a normal logical error,
as the truth of its premises must be established
to the satisfaction of all parties." (Wikipedia)

Life isn't Safe

Some People Live It,
Others Hide from It

Stop Posing as Political Activists,
You're the People the
Police State Exists For.

WAR is PEACE

Kill Yourself, Save Lives

****

May 19, 2020 (photo from Amir-ul Kafirs):

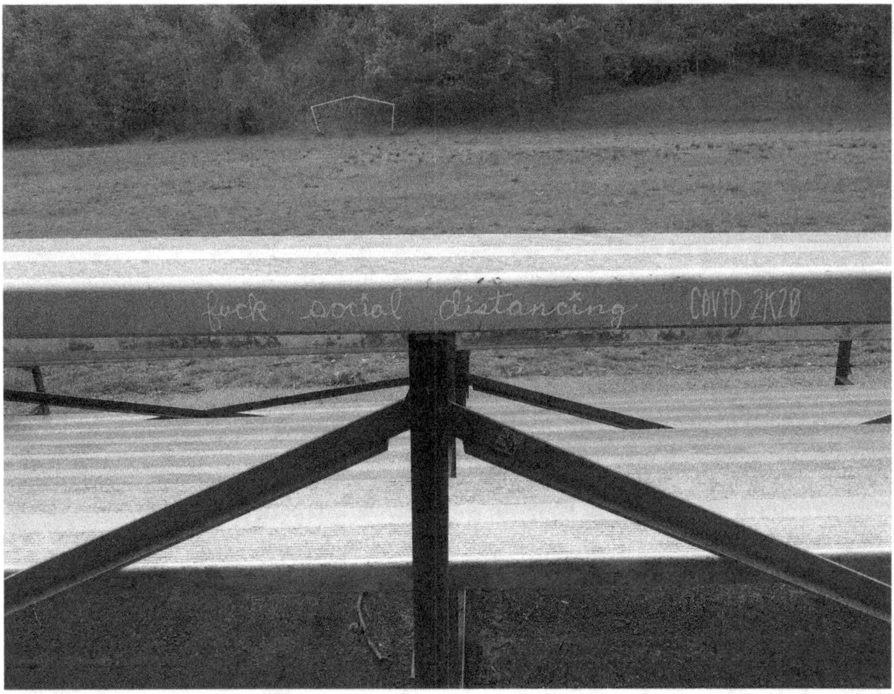

****

May 18, 2020, 11:21PM (BP to group):

Hirsute: Gates Press Release

https://news.yahoo.com/bill-gates-bogeyman-virus-conspiracy-theorists-152254923.html

I don't think he's Dr. Evil but a definite strategy to tamper down on his Sainted image.
Wild accusations but no mention of concrete stuff where the all-wise money man has failed.
Highlighted on Drudge. Which if you ain't checking out then you don't know what people are being fed.

****

Bill Gates, bogeyman of virus conspiracy theorists

Julie CHARPENTRAT

,AFP·May 18, 2020

Microsoft founder and philanthropist Bill Gates, seen here in October 2019, has been a top target of Russian-backed conspiracy theories, according to a US report
(AFP Photo/JEFF PACHOUD)
Paris (AFP) - False claims targeting billionaire philanthropist Bill Gates are gaining traction online since the beginning of the coronavirus outbreak, with experts warning they could hamper efforts to curb the virus.

Doctored photos and fabricated news articles crafted by conspiracy theorists -- shared thousands of times on social media platforms and messaging apps, in various languages -- have gone as far as accusing the Microsoft founder of creating the outbreak.

Gates, who has pledged $250 million to efforts to fight the pandemic, is the latest in a string of online targets despite the World Health Organization's efforts to fight what it called an "infodemic" -- misinformation fanned by panic and confusion about the virus. In recent months, 5G networks and Hungarian-American billionaire George Soros have also been blamed for creating COVID-19, which has killed more than 315,000 people around the world.

"Bill Gates has always been a target of specific conspiracy communities," said Rory Smith, research manager at First Draft, a non-profit that provides research and training for journalists.

Gates -- whose eponymous foundation has spent billions of dollars improving healthcare in developing countries over the past 20 years -- has become "a kind of abstract boogeyman", said Whitney Phillips, an assistant professor at New York's Syracuse University, where she teaches digital ethics.

[..]

****

Wow. Even the little excerpt I chose above is *so loaded* with what seem to me like transparently propagandistic statements that I find it a little bizarre. The title, of course, sets the tone: "Bill Gates, bogeyman of virus conspiracy theorists". In other words, there's no chance that anything anyone has to say about Gates is anything other than wingnut stuff, any calling attention to conflicts of interest, for example.

We're 'informed' that he's the "philanthropist Bill Gates"**. No, indeed, there's *no chance* that his so-called 'philanthropy' has any ulterior motives for public relations or profiteering or the pursuit of megalomaniacal plans for all of humanity. Nope. No chance. AND, *of course*, ANY criticism of him is because he's** "a top target of Russian-backed conspiracy theories"**. Remember the Russians? It's time for them to be the bad guys again. In fact,** "False claims targeting billionaire philanthropist" **are the problem. Why he probably got to be a billionaire by shining shoes at the train station & now he wants to give back to the other struggling shoe-shiners.**

"Doctored photos and fabricated news articles crafted by conspiracy theorists": **ANY picture of Gates that's used to illustrate a critical point *must be doctored*. Mainstream news *never slants its content*, THERE'S NO SUCH THING AS A SPIN DOCTOR. Oh, well, I could go on & on but if you are**

fortunate enough to have even the slightest molecule of critical reading faculties in your brain you'll pick up on the brainwashing.

****

May 19, 2020, 1:32PM (Dick to group):

This has connections with various ideas expressed in this group
i.e. global political design, the role of banks, origins of mind control, etc.
https://www.youtube.com/watch?v=fh2cDKyFdyU

HyperNormalisation (2016 + subs) by Adam Curtis - A different experience of reality FULL DOCUMENTARY
Added subtitles (french, braziianl, hebrew, english, croatian, spanish, turkish and russian) The cult documentary maker explores the falsity of modern life in his own inimitable style. Though he's spent the best part of four decades making television, Curtis's signature blend of hypnotic archive footage, authoritative voiceover and a ...

****

May 20, 2020, 10:35AM (Dick to group):

Re: Hirsute: Gates Press Release

Hi
I regret having sent that video, I found it on a friend's page, someone who is intelligent and who shares things which are usually interesting
I'd watched about 1.5 hrs of it and it seemed like a good summation of certain ideas, so I shared it with this group, but as it kept going I got the feeling that it was doing exactly what it was criticizing, that is, representing the world as a sort of inescapable mirror of ultimate meaninglessness which I do not believe is the case
That is, I started to get the gut feeling I was being somehow tricked
The content as well I feel is suspect - it is a dramatic retelling of political events - but in my opinion the story he tells is already the established narrative - that is it presents the known like it is a secret, that is a curious aspect of this film
I didn't realize this at first because it is somewhat compelling - but I think that it is compelling because it is familiar
I did learn a few things I didn't know about - the origins of Blackrock and the role of Assad in suicide bombings
But this doesn't counterbalance what I feel is the counterproductive aspect of the "why even bother" narrative at the bottom of the film

****

May 20, 2020, 4:50PM (Phil to group):

Yeah I remember having a similar reaction to this documentary when I tried to watch it. I didn't get that far with it and I can't remember exactly why. Perhaps

because it followed mainstream propaganda somewhat? Not that I didn't want to watch it in full but I just left it somewhere on the backburner and never came back to it. It is by the maker of Black Mirror which I enjoy a lot. One excellent documentary on propaganda is the century of the self. I highly recommend that one:
https://www.youtube.com/watch?v=eJ3RzGoQC4s

****

May 15, 2020, 1:41PM (BP to group):

Heretics: another Taibbi just in

I only send this one along to brag about what I said here weeks ago: that the Russiagate craziness was the gateway to our Pandemic Panic dilemma. I'd followed the Russia thing closely for years and the similarities to what was going on was plain as day.
Read it And Weep!

Democrats Have Abandoned Civil Liberties

The Blue Party's Trump-era Embrace of Authoritarianism Isn't Just Wrong, it's a Fatal Political Mistake

https://taibbi.substack.com/p/democrats-have-abandoned-civil-liberties

and I read this one last night:

COVID19 and the Left: an Ignored Civil Rights Crisis

Michael Lesher
https://off-guardian.org/2020/05/07/covid19-and-the-left-an-ignored-civil-rights-crisis?__cf_chl_jschl_tk__=0796bb7280efad0c279a752f3f97f62c8c3c5a49-1589320821-0-AZKyFFIv43YyPDdWRXsPNFtL5BGsUiBFIHI0TnNXFKQErh-eiMtKu1MtMyW0XSUNw5pTXrV74JBHwgig2phhc75KaIMxEQo604ImxqO6JMXnCM2uBvcvrWQaw42QwZUfpsiHyNy0y6Q00YA5pqaI1FBixr3tkXMHnMaf3smJuMkkk2bmjPhCKe5YoEG2T4xgRsFvOosxeQnJaInIhdQD5kgdYsIGI71e5u8h2MGvwxNCP2LUORO5ZYi5y3Ng4zJg70PBI6svqOK7_7beaFmYJisbc-qpkBqzUIzGc7jvJWOPMU_BfC_ehNV3xHEHE2oZI4WEIbLpULzQSnOAXD-cc87yo607CZrRcv_jZmrY_3kI

When I shared the above article elsewhere, this is the response I received: "Clearly it's all Obama's fault and he is going to make billions from his Chinese mask factory next door to his Kentucky Fried Bat outlet and he wasn't even born in this planet and he's black. When will Fox Fakenews tell the truth."

****

Democrats Have Abandoned Civil Liberties

The Blue Party's Trump-era Embrace of Authoritarianism Isn't Just Wrong, it's a Fatal Political Mistake

Matt Taibbi
May 15

Emmet G. Sullivan, the judge in the case of former Trump National Security Adviser Michael Flynn, is refusing to let William Barr's Justice Department drop the charge. He's even thinking of adding more, appointing a retired judge to ask "whether the Court should issue an Order to Show Cause why Mr. Flynn should not be held in criminal contempt for perjury."

Pundits are cheering. A trio of former law enforcement and judicial officials saluted Sullivan in the *Washington Post,* chirping, "The Flynn case isn't over until a judge says it's over." Yuppie icon Jeffrey Toobin of CNN and the *New Yorker*, one of the #Resistance crowd's favored legal authorities, described Sullivan's appointment of Judge John Gleeson as "brilliant." MSNBC legal analyst Glenn Kirschner said Americans owe Sullivan a "debt of gratitude."

One had to search far and wide to find a non-conservative legal analyst willing to say the obvious, i.e. that Sullivan's decision was the kind of thing one would expect from a judge in Belarus. George Washington University professor Jonathan Turley was one of the few willing to say Sullivan's move could "could create a threat of a judicial charge even when prosecutors agree with defendants."

Sullivan's reaction was amplified by a group letter calling for Barr's resignation signed by 2000 former Justice Department officials (the melodramatic group email reported as momentous news is one of many tired media tropes in the Trump era) and the preposterous "leak" of news that the dropped case made Barack Obama sad. The former president "privately" told "members of his administration" (who instantly told *Yahoo!* News) that there was no precedent for the dropping of perjury charges, and that the "rule of law" itself was at stake.

Whatever one's opinion of Flynn, his relations with Turkey, his "Lock her up!" chants, his haircut, whatever, this case was never about much. There's no longer pretense that prosecution would lead to the unspooling of a massive Trump-Russia conspiracy, as pundits once breathlessly expected. News that Flynn was cooperating with special counsel Robert Mueller inspired many of the "Is this the beginning of the end for Trump?" stories that will someday fill whole chapters of *Journalism Fucks Up 101* textbooks.

[..]

****

May 7, 2020

COVID19 and the Left: an Ignored Civil Rights Crisis

Michael Lesher

Reading op-eds these days about the grim progress of COVID-19 through the United States, I sometimes have the eerie feeling that I've traveled backward in time and landed in some sort of Cold War-like, hyper-conformist dystopia — but with one disquieting difference.

As in those dark days, we're bombarded with warnings of a ruthless, insidious enemy that will destroy us if unchecked. As in those days, we are assured that the battle to suppress this mortal enemy requires unquestioning faith in government authorities and the suspension of ordinary liberties.

As in those days, dissenters are vilified; people who challenge the suppression of civil rights are mocked as dupes, fellow travelers or outright accomplices of the Evil One.

Only this time, the roles are strangely reversed. Instead of red-baiting conservatives, it's so-called liberals who are wearing the executioner's hood and carrying a shredder for the Bill of Rights.

Instead of jingoists shouting down dissenters, we've got erstwhile defenders of free speech telling political critics they ought to either shut up or drop dead.

And in the present-day dystopia, the enemies of society are not just people with the wrong ideas, as they were in the old days; even taking a walk in the park can prompt well-meaning liberals to denounce you to the authorities as a public menace.

That is today's political reality in a nutshell — and I'm afraid the situation is much worse than merely ironic. I think it represents a colossal error by which civil libertarians and their normal political allies are abandoning their most valued principles at precisely the moment they're most urgently needed.

[..]

****

Some people might find the above exaggerated. I find it very accurate. To give an example, one friend of mine on social media asked me if I'd "crossed over to the dark side" or some such because I mocked mask-wearing. Isn't that essentially the same as saying that I'm an "outright accomplice[..] of the Evil One**"?**

****

May 20, 2020, 6:42PM (Amir-ul Kafirs to group):

Re: Heretics: another Taibbi just in

Democrats Have Abandoned Civil Liberties

I'm FINALLY trying to catch up on everything posted here but it's hopeless because I have too many other things to attend to in my life. STILL, I did just read the above article and was glad to've done so. I've never paid much attention to the 'Russiagate' stuff except to notice with interest that the 'left' is now anti-Russia while the 'right' is pro, a complete reversal of not-very long ago. That coupled with the 'right' protesting and the 'left' being pro-police-state seems to define this current era. ANYWAY, I was particularly glad to read this bit from the above:

"I've written a lot about the Democrats' record on civil liberties issues. Working on *I Can't Breathe,* a book about the Eric Garner case, I was stunned to learn the central role Mario Cuomo played in the mass incarceration problem, while Democrats also often embraced hyper-intrusive "stop and frisk" or "broken windows" enforcement strategies, usually by touting terms like "community policing" that sounded nice to white voters. Democrats strongly supported the PATRIOT Act in 2001, and Barack Obama continued or expanded Bush-Cheney programs like drone assassination, rendition, and warrantless surveillance, while also using the Espionage Act to bully reporters and whistleblowers. Republicans throughout this time were usually as bad or worse on these issues, but Democrats have lately positioned themselves as the more aggressive promoters of strong-arm policies, from control of Internet speech to the embrace of domestic spying. In the last four years the blue-friendly press has done a complete 180, going from cheering Edward Snowden to lionizing the CIA, NSA, and FBI, and making on-air partners out of drone-and-surveillance all-stars like John Brennan, James Clapper, and Michael Hayden. There are now too many ex-spooks on CNN and MSNBC to count, while there isn't a single regular contributor on any of the networks one could describe as antiwar. Democrats clearly believe constituents will forgive them for abandoning constitutional principles, so long as the targets of official inquiry are figures like Flynn or Paul Manafort or Trump himself. In the process, they've raised a generation of followers whose contempt for civil liberties is now genuine-to-permanent. Blue-staters have gone from dismissing constitutional concerns as Trumpian ruse to sneering at them, in the manner of French aristocrats, as evidence of proletarian mental defect.
Nowhere has this been more evident than in the response to the Covid-19 crisis, where the almost mandatory take of pundits is that any protest of lockdown measures is troglodyte death wish. The aftereffects of years of Russiagate/Trump coverage are seen everywhere: press outlets reflexively associate complaints of government overreach with Trump, treason, and racism, and conversely radiate a creepily gleeful tone when describing aggressive emergency measures and the problems some "dumb" Americans have had accepting them."

and I read this one last night:

COVID19 and the Left: an Ignored Civil Rights Crisis

This 2nd article was even better and it's made it so that I can now more fully respect the off-guardian. I'm going to use Google-Translate to translate the section quoted below into Portuguese to send to someone I'm corresponding with in Brazil to try to help her understand why I think we're essentially seeing a fascist coup *enabled* by 'liberals':

"If that doesn't startle you — as it startles me — try a simple thought experiment: imagine that, about six months ago, Venezuela's President Maduro had unilaterally claimed the power to confine much of his country's population and to close down most of its businesses — without a court order, in likely violation of Venezuela's constitution, and without the sanction of the national legislature.

Do you suppose the American press would have ignored that event? Would our pundits have given Maduro a pass for grabbing quasi-dictatorial power? Would cable news hosts have ridiculed Venezuelans who dared to defy his orders as mobs of knuckle-dragging weirdos possessed by a death wish?

Or try another sort of thought experiment: suppose that next fall, as flu season rolls around, the governors of New York, New Jersey, California and an assortment of other states all declare "health emergencies" and issue blanket prohibitions against political protest on the grounds that public gatherings might spread an infectious disease.

Impossible? A few months ago, I would have thought so too. But something very similar is happening right now, and its unconditional endorsement by both major political parties and the liberal press makes it difficult to imagine how these institutions, or any related ones, could speak up in any credible fashion against even a power play as naked as that."

****

May 20, 2020, 7:26PM (Amir-ul Kafirs to group):

"Clearly it's all Obama's fault and he is going to make billions from his Chinese mask factory next door to his Kentucky Fried Bat outlet and he wasn't even born in this planet and he's black. When will Fox Fakenews tell the truth."

ALSO, is that actually a quote or is it your parody?

****

May 21, 2020, 7:25AM (BP to group):

Not me. Supposed to be some form of satire, so the poster said. Directed at me I guess because any criticism of the lockdown is a defense of Trump? Which proves the point of the article. That's all I can make of it.

****

May 21, 2020, 8:46AM (Amir-ul Kafirs to group):

That's all I can make of it.

Wow. Not only does it prove the point of the article but it also reeks of bullying and shaming as well as the poster's absolute laziness and inability to debate or address the reasonable and calm points of the article. It's this type of behavior that I'm finding unbearably shallow and cowardly.

****

May 21, 2020, 10:51AM (Amir-ul Kafirs to group):

Heretics: Liberals

As an anarchist, I am, of course, commonly considered to be at the extreme end of leftism — with leftism, in its more moderate incarnation, considered to be liberalism. However, I've been saying for many decades that I consider myself to be a Post-Left Anarchist, someone operating independently of the left-right duality. I've also been saying for decades that if Hitler had needed to present himself as a liberal to get into power that's what he would've done. Instead, he presented himself as a socialist, a NATIONAL SOCIALIST. Mussolini, pulled a similar trick by being 1st a militant socialist and then founding Fascism as another variant of NATIONAL SOCIALISM, but *not* nazism. The NATIONALISM is what enabled things to turn really ugly. Anyway, when my friend etta and I were in Australia in 2000, largely because of Phil, we participated in a demonstration against a liberal politician:

213. "**Slime Detecting**"
- shot in Melbourne
- 1/2" VHS cassette
- 4:35
- april '00 / april '01
- on my onesownthoughts YouTube channel here: https://youtu.be/sppHtVbLKvQ

I bring this up because political activists there didn't seem to have any problem protesting a politician presenting themself as liberal. NOW, *here*, in the utterly brainwashed USA, such an act is becoming more and more taboo.

****

May 22, 2020, 1:02PM (Naia Nisnam to group):

HERETICS: NY nursing homes

Have you guys seen this?

https://m.huffpost.com/us/entry/us_5ec7c03ec5b6b9438505aa8e?fbclid=IwAR2lpGhPh83Il9YEFLdIMuGkEnAp0LRALA9h-SWdlPg6M7roJNXA6rjks2E

Yet another reason the virus caused so many deaths in NYC:
4,300+ Coronavirus patients sent from NY hospitals to nursing homes.

While we were put under lock down in our homes to protect the vulnerable, the state of NY (and NJ) were sending sick people into facilities where the most vulnerable population live.

That was not a careless mistake.
"...Gov. Andrew Cuomo — the main proponent of the policy — called (nursing homes) "the optimum feeding ground for this virus."
He knew what he was doing.

Yet it is those of us who simply question what we've been told that are accused of wanting the elderly to die.

****

U.S. NEWS 05/22/2020 08:18 am ET **Updated** May 22, 2020

Over 4,300 Coronavirus Patients Sent To New York Nursing Homes: AP

The COVID-19 patients were discharged from hospitals to already vulnerable nursing homes under the governor's directive, which has since been scrapped.

AP

Bernard Condon, Jennifer Peltz and Jim Mustian

NEW YORK (AP) — More than 4,300 recovering coronavirus patients were sent to New York's already vulnerable nursing homes under a controversial state directive that was ultimately scrapped amid criticisms it was accelerating the nation's deadliest outbreaks, according to a count by The Associated Press.
AP compiled its own tally to find out how many COVID-19 patients were discharged from hospitals to nursing homes under the March 25 directive after New York's Health Department declined to release its internal survey conducted two weeks ago. It says it is still verifying data that was incomplete.
Whatever the full number, nursing home administrators, residents' advocates and relatives say it has added up to a big and indefensible problem for facilities that even Gov. Andrew Cuomo — the main proponent of the policy — called "the

optimum feeding ground for this virus."

"It was the single dumbest decision anyone could make if they wanted to kill people," Daniel Arbeeny said of the directive, which prompted him to pull his 88-year-old father out of a Brooklyn nursing home where more than 50 people have died. His father later died of COVID-19 at home.

"This isn't rocket science," Arbeeny said. "We knew the most vulnerable — the elderly and compromised — are in nursing homes and rehab centers."
Told of the AP's tally, the Health Department said late Thursday it "can't comment on data we haven't had a chance to review, particularly while we're still validating our own comprehensive survey of nursing homes admission and re-admission data in the middle of responding to this global pandemic."

Cuomo, a Democrat, on May 10 reversed the directive, which had been intended to help free up hospital beds for the sickest patients as cases surged. But he continued to defend it this week, saying he didn't believe it contributed to the more than 5,800 nursing and adult care facility deaths in New York — more than in any other state — and that homes should have spoken up if it was a problem.

****

May 22, 2020, 1:57PM (Inquiring Librarian to group):

Re: HERETICS: NY nursing homes

I cannot find evidence of this in Louisiana, but I have not searched real hard. But in my mini search, I found this, within this article from our local news https://www.wwltv.com/article/news/investigations/katie-moore/a-third-of-louisianas-covid-19-deaths-are-in-nursing-homes-could-that-have-been-stopped/289-04bf19fb-a411-4645-9054-7cd89982ee90 :
How did we get here?
Geriatric physician Dr. William Lacorte is the medical director for several New Orleans-area nursing homes.
He says in early March, area hospitals hesitated to take nursing home patients suspected of having the virus.
"I remember one discussion I had with an E.R. doc, she said, don't admit this patient he has COVID send back to the nursing home," one of two similar conversations Lacorte describes with ER doctors at that time.
Because of their age and their existing health conditions, Lacorte and other nursing home administrators who asked not to be identified said hospitals pushed the patients toward hospice care back at the nursing homes, fearing the projections that they were about to be overwhelmed by a surge of COVID-19 patients in need of ventilators, then, in short supply.
"So, you're basically sending Typhoid Mary to the nursing home to infect other people," Lacorte said.

****

May 22, 2020, 2:04PM (Naia Nisnam to group):

I just found this about PA...

https://triblive.com/local/regional/pennsylvania-state-senator-calls-for-resignation-of-health-secretary-dr-rachel-levine/?fbclid=IwAR1vK8QZO8bbJFxEN0ZqECiRXvLiUhWGX3ENIV--0Y6iM_UueOZaUZt0hBA

This is hard to imagine because Franklin is only about an hour from Pittsburgh. We had extra ICU beds and ventilators in Pittsburgh the entire time. This article is from a mainstream Pgh news outlet. I can't wait to see people's reactions...

****

Pennsylvania state senator calls for resignation of Health Secretary Dr. Rachel Levine

TRIB LIVE [redacted]

THE PATRIOT-NEWS I Monday, May 11, 2020 3:22 p.m.

A state senator from Franklin County has called for the immediate resignation of Pennsylvania Health Secretary Dr. Rachel Levine, saying her actions were a major factor in the large number of covid-19 cases and deaths in the state's nursing homes.

Sen. Doug Mastriano, a first-term Republican representing Franklin, Adams and a part of York counties, said Levine has committed the equivalent of policy malpractice in her handling of the coronavirus pandemic, specifically in her handling of the virus's spread through nursing homes and other long-term care facilities.

Mastriano specifically targeted Levine for a policy which called for nursing home and long-term care patients who had been hospitalized after testing positive for covid-19 to be returned to their homes when they were ready for release from hospitals. Mastriano said that contributed to major outbreaks in numerous nursing homes around the state.

"Our secretary of health, Dr. Levine, decided that it would be good to allow covid-positive patients to be returned to elder-care facitlies. And as a result of that, it broke out like fire," Mastriano said during a Monday rally with constituents at the base of the Capitol steps.

"The very same people our secretary of health said were going to be vulnerable

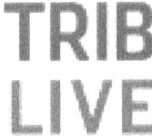

… It unleashed heck upon our dearly beloved fathers, mothers, grandparents, aunts and uncles. I think that's unconscionable, unacceptable, and that secretary needs to be held accountable for that awful decision," Mastriano said.
Wolf made clear Monday morning that he is firmly in Levine's corner.

[..]

****

May 22, 2020, 6:48PM (Amir-ul Kafirs to group):

It just goes on & on. One of my fondest hopes is that if & when this is all over so many believable reports of malpractice by both the medical industry & the politicians will come out that there'll be a bipartisan distrust of any future coup along these lines.

****

May 22, 2020, 7:02PM (Amir-ul Kafis to group):

We had extra ICU beds and ventilators in Pittsburgh the entire time.

Once again, I just find all the brouhaha to be avoiding one of the many obvious things: viz that it's mostly really old people with previously existing conditions who're dying, people who would be expected to die of something or another anyway:

"To date, state figures show that nursing homes residents have accounted for 2,529 of the state's 3,707 reported covid-19 deaths. That is a pattern that has been echoed in most states across the country, however."

****

May 22, 2020, 7:10PM (Amir-ul Kafirs to group):

On May 22, 2020, at 2:27 PM, BP wrote:

I'll remind you: I've never worn a mask and I've never worn gloves. I'm still standing. And if I do become ill? Fuck it, ya can't live forever. I've managed all this mentally by looking at death stats: seeing who is being taken out by this thing. I continue to make the mistake of looking at the hysteria now and then, and it can upset me. RANT OVER.

It's too bad we can't look at some parallel universe where people were to just continue as they have during the rest of their life with minimal or no intervention from the politicians & medical industry. At any rate, we're here so we're stuck with this universe. I think it's fair to say that if more people ignored the mass media we'd be living in a much smarter world right now.

****

May 21, 2020, 12:25PM (Inquiring Librarian to group):

HERETICS: Librarian Liberals

Here is an article written by a librarian, about how they feel going back to work. This attutude is shared by many in Louisiana libraries. Any who do not feel this way, like myself, remain silent. Not many are remaining silent, so i do not think there are many of us who do not agree with this article. I feel the article is priviliged, self-centered, selfish, and narrow minded. Supposedly librarians read a lot and are thus smart. What, pray tell, are these librarians really reading that makes them so "smart" and self-important. I fear for the future of my profession that most of us cannot manup and read between the lines and think for ourselves and use logic, and... Dear Gawd... Stop putting implicit faith in Big Brother and the Dr. Gods (as Amir-ul Kafirs so aptly dons our dread doctors). Attitudes like this are hurtling us towards massive budget cuts and then privitization and eventual extinction.

https://bookriot.com/2020/05/20/library-staff-safety/

****

ESSENTIAL UNTIL WE'RE NOT: AN ANGRY LIBRARIAN ON THE DISREGARD FOR LIBRARY STAFF SAFETY

Katie McLain May 20, 2020

As I write this article, many, many libraries across the country are planning to reopen in some capacity, whether it's offering curbside pickup services or allowing patrons inside the physical building, like the Chicago Public Library plans to do as of June 1. And while libraries are pushing ahead with their reopening plans, I read about a lot of talk from administrators and library publications about how libraries are resilient and librarians are heroes. The internet is full of articles like this one from Publishers Weekly that says "Librarians, America is counting on you." All of this is complete and utter bullshit.

I'm not hiding it. I'm furious. I'm stressed out to the point where I feel like I'm vibrating from anxiety. Several years ago, I wrote about how I hated the "hero" narrative surrounding library work because calling us heroes ignores the fact that we are just average humans who need way more from our profession than our leaders are willing to provide, and now I'm watching that narrative play out on a national level. Libraries are resilient, they say, ignoring the fact that it's not safe for patrons or staff to open the libraries yet. But no one seems to realize that empty words can't keep us safe.

STAFF AREN'T SAFE

Every day I see these articles, and then I see actual librarians going on social media to talk about how terrified they are to return to work. It's too early to open up the library, yet their board members are demanding it even though the board will never have to actually work with the public. Directors are putting up signs that encourage social distancing, saying that patrons will inevitably police themselves and obey library signage. (Because we all know how well people read library signs in the first place.) Staff are forced to go without essential PPE, because opening services to the public is more important than ensuring that staff are safe. Some argue that the libraries have to open because otherwise their funding will be at risk, but what kind of a service are you actually providing if your staff are terrified, angry, sick, or killed?

[..]

****

May 21, 2020, 3:53PM (Amir-ul Kafirs to group):

Re: HERETICS: Librarian Liberals

"Once again, I don't feel safe at my job. But this time, it's not the administration or the other employees that are contributing to this. It's the fact that having a supportive organization is becoming more and more of an outlier in this profession, and I'm afraid of having to watch my fellow library employees die because their libraries didn't do enough to protect them."

How dramatic, right? 6 months down the line when NONE OF THE LIBRARIANS HAVE DIED I wonder whether this librarian will still be so angry? I'll bet the answer is yes — because, after all, it's the thought that counts, right? The THOUGHT that the librarians are going to die is all that counts, the reality is neither here nor there.

****

May 21, 2020, 4:34PM (Inquiring Librarian to group):

Yes, it is all of the excessive self pity that really throws me over the edge here. The librarians are more likely to die from the rushed Moderna RNA editing vaccine that Npr & the New York Times are raving about than the covid fairy.

****

May 21, 2020, 4:53PM (Dick to group):

interesting
library safety was a concept unknown to me
that is, they always seems pretty calm but i guess sometimes borrowers go ballistic
"What do you mean you don't have"Heidi"??!! and out comes the .357 magnum
have you experienced violence at your job?

****

May 21, 2020, 6:14PM (Inquiring Librarian to group):

Public libraries can be a bit hairy these days. Since the United states had the bright idea in the 1980's to stop caring for their mentally ill with anything but prescription pills for the very few 'lucky' in the 1980's, public libraries have been the haven for the homeless and/or mentally ill.

We get a lot of drunk people in the public libraries here in Louisiana. There are other addicts that also enter the buildings and cause trouble. A friend/fellow library employee of mine did have her life threatened by a patron in one of our more savory neighborhood libraries. She was immediately transferred to work in the archives when she expressed to our administration how stressed out she was working in the branches. So, yes, public library work can be a little dangerous at times, because of our clientele and how our cities otherwise neglect such clientele who find libraries to be their only free refuge from the elements and also the only free wifi and computer/internet use... and yes... many of our homeless also love to read books and don't have fancy devices to use to read ebooks. Most of our branches do have guards these days. Mine does not. We have been trying to get a guard for over 2 years now, to no avail. But ultimately, at my particular branch, the worst I've seen is 2 homeless people shouting at each other "BALLS, GET A PAIR!!!" while a class of middle school kids were on a class book checkout. And there was that time that I had to get a guy off the floor and out of the library when he got so drunk at the computer that he fell off of his chair and couldn't get up due to sloppy drunkenness. He reminded me of a half squished slug writhing on the floor making weird noises and drooling on himself.

One shocking new duty we have been given is Narcan administration. If someone passes out in our libraries, we have been told and trained on how to shoot Narcan spray up said passed out person's nose, in case they are having a heroin overdose... we can 'save' their lives. I hate this new directive. It's not something any of us have signed up to do. And having known too many heroin addicts, I don't see this as really saving their lives when they wake up in a state of shock and then have zero options for real detox and rehab anywhere in the vicinity. The state needs to invest in treatment centers, not extraordinarily expensive shots of Narcan to wake these people up and dump them back out onto the streets again. And what if they wake up and barf all over you... hello hepatitis and possibly HIV!! Not to mention, what if the passed out person is actually just a blackout drunk and you wake them by shooting spray up their nose and they wake up swinging at you with their fist, a knife, or a gun. I'll tell you, library people are some naive world savers. Geeze, I have to stop trashing my field.

****

May 21, 2020, 7:38PM (Naia Nisnam to group):

I'm so annoyed with the "it's too soon to reopen" crowd. For the most part, these are the same people that went inside and locked their doors the minute they were told to. They didn't question their governors' orders to lockdown. They repeatedly call on us to "listen to the science".
Now the CDC and the governors' are saying it's okay to open a few things, and these same people are calling it "too soon". Suddenly, the people who believed every word the governors and CDC said, now no longer believe in the "science"? I believe that a lot of privileged people Want to stay home. They can feel like heroic martyrs while ordering take out and binging Netflix. They can criticize and shame people with different opinions from the safety of their own homes.

From a personal point, my mother is a library clerk. She is thrilled to go back to work on Monday because she is bored and misses socializing with her patrons. She is 73 years old, diabetic, and obese, thus high risk. She is a liberal/Democrat who has been eating up all the TV news panic. She isn't scared so... I'm surprised that many others are.

(Though I do understand the concerns about patrons with mental issues. She's had 2 different people freak out on her when she noticed their poorly concealed guns and told them they weren't allowed in the building as per county ordinance. Each week she has a new story about people w mental health issues doing strange things. Last year her library was put under lockdown for several hours after a man threatened to bomb the place.)
But... the people in the article who are afraid of the virus... even for curbside pick up?? Did I miss masses of grocery store workers dying after dealing with curbside pick ups? That doesn't make sense.

Earlier today a friend sent me some guidelines from the CDC about schools reopening in the fall. People are upset that schools are opening "too soon" (4 months from now). Again, the CDC went from knowing everything when schools closed to being reckless when suggesting schools can reopen 4 months from now.
I'm angering other parents when I express concern that keeping children isolated from their peers is extremely unhealthy and that long term isolation will have long term effects on our mental health.
The people love lockdown. They loved being scared.
I fantasize about permanent lockdowns, only for the "it's too soon to reopen" crew.

****

May 21, 2020, 9:42PM (Amir-ul Kafirs to group):

Now the CDC and the governors' are saying it's okay to open a few things, and these same people are calling it "too soon".

When in doubt, always pick the most neurotic position.

Though I do understand the concerns about patrons with mental issues.

That's a REAL issue & one that librarians have been plagued by for decades, *if not forever.* So why isn't that more of an issue? When I worked for the library we were given a talk about how to deal with what were called "problem patrons". Nobody seemed that upset about it even though I'm sure there were some real doosies.

Did I miss masses of grocery store workers dying after dealing with curbside pick ups?

No, because it didn't happen. Just like the food delivery people haven't been dying in droves.

People are upset that schools are opening "too soon" (4 months from now).

When the fuck do they think it's going to be 'OK'? When there's *no more disease in the world?!* Because there'll still be plenty of dangers after that that we'll be expected to be terrified of. Maybe we should all stay inside until the weather is completely under human control.

The people love lockdown. They loved being scared.

It's masochism. I wonder if people would be surprised at how many women on computer dating sites want to be tied up.

I fantasize about permanent lockdowns, only for the "it's too soon to reopen" crew.

Exactly. The world should take note that you're not wishing their death just wanting them to.. GET OUT OF OUR FUCKING WAY.

****

May 21, 2020, 10:18PM (Inquiring Librarian to group):

I really appreciate ALL of your responses. Amir-ul Kafirs & Naia Nisnam, i am 100% on your page. Although Amir-ul Kafirs, i know several serious scientists that are old college friends, they are eating this hysteria up and posting about the 'science' and random nonsense articles about why we need to stay home and 'save lives.' I was shocked at first by their inability to think independently. But then i guess some sciences are very memorization centered. You learn a lot of supposed 'facts' and regurgitate them and use them as the building blocks for your own theories. I am pretty sure big pharma pretty much owns most institutions of higher learning in the U.S. Case in point, one of my most favorite, brilliant, beautiful, and kind-hearted friends from college is a chemical engineer. Note: she is still getting well paid, to work from home, right now. She got her degree at the University of Delaware in chemical engineering. The chem-e program there is funded by Dupont. This poor girl got her 1st job at Dupont in Wilmington, DE. By the time she was able to move on from that job to a more environmentally friendly job, her dream job, she'd lost half her thyroid to tumourous growth, something she can't fathom blaming on Dupont.

****

May 21, 2020, 10:44PM (Amir-ul Kafirs to group):

Case in point, one of my most favorite, brilliant, brautiful, and kind-hearted friends from college is a chemical engineer.

Oh, well, I suppose I could argue that a chemical engineer is more of a mechanic than a scientist.

she'd lost half her thyroid to tumourous growth, something she can't fathom blaming on Dupont.

Groan. Doesn't she realize what a bad reputation Dupont has?!

****

[The following email is inserted out of chronological order to show where DowDuPont stands as the world's largest polluter]

June 21, 2020, 11:36PM (Amir-ul Kafirs to group):

Top 100 air & water polluters

Well, this is 'off-topic' but it's something that I've been researching for a different project that might interest you. The data is according to PERI (Political Economy Rsearch Institute) at University of Massachussetts Amherst, (https://www.peri.umass.edu/combined-toxic-100-greenhouse-100-indexes-current).

Since most of the air polluters are also water polluters (but not necessarily greenhouse gas producers) here's the list of the top 100 of companies in both categories & the averages of their 2 numbers. They're organized in reverse order with the most egregious polluters as the climax. Therefore, the #s are simply to keep track of making sure that there're 100.

001. Leggett & Platt (air: 88) + (water: 190) = 278 ÷ 2 = 139
002. Komatsu (air: 65) + (water: 194) = 259 ÷ 2 = 129.5
003. Compass Group (air: 87) + (water: 165) = 252 ÷ 2 = 126
004. Ecolab (air: 79) + (water: 170) = 249 ÷ 2 = 124.5
005. ChemChina (air: 89) + (water: 153) = 242 ÷ 2 = 121
006. Lockheed Martin (air: 54) + (water: 185) = 239 ÷ 2 = 119.5
007. Emerson Electric (air: 46) + (water: 188) = 234 ÷ 2 = 117
008. Praxair (air: 37) + (water: 191) = 228 ÷ 2 = 114
009. Schlumberger (air: 96) + (water: 133) = 229 ÷ 2 = 114.5
010. PPG Industries (air: 91) + (water: 131) = 222 ÷ 2 = 111
011. Pemex (air: 98) + (water: 122) = 220 ÷ 2 = 110
012. Daimler (air: 139) + (water: 81) = 220 ÷ 2 = 110
013. Mitsubishi Group (air: 155) + (water: 59) = 214 ÷ 2 = 107
014. Resolute Forest Products (air: 145) + (water: 66) = 211 ÷ 2 = 105.5
015. Shin-Etsu Chemical (air: 77) + (water: 130) = 207 ÷ 2 = 103.5
016. Dominion Energy (air: 148) + (water: 55) = 203 ÷ 2 = 101.5
017. Eaton (air: 69) + (water: 132) = 201 ÷ 2 = 100.5
018. Bayer (air: 83) + (water: 116) = 199 ÷ 2 = 99.5
019. Tyson Foods (air: 142) + (water: 56) = 198 ÷ 2 = 99
020. NRG Energy (air: 133) + (water: 65) = 198 ÷ 2 = 99
021. SABIC (Saudi Basic Industries) (air: 127) + (water: 70) = 197 ÷ 2 = 98.5
022. Saint-Gobain (air: 92) + (water: 102) = 194 ÷ 2 = 97
023. Henkel (air: 73) + (water: 120) = 193 ÷ 2 = 96.5
024. Becton Dickinson (air: 16) + (water: 176) = 192 ÷ 2 = 96
025. Nissan Motor Company (air: 95) + (water: 192) = 287 ÷ 2 = 93.5
026. 3M Company (air: 67) + (water: 118) = 185 ÷ 2 = 92.5
027. Caterpillar (air: 81) + (water: 98) = 177 ÷ 2 = 89.5
028. Renco (air: 136) + (water: 53) = 189 ÷ 2 = 89.5
029. HollyFrontier (air: 100) + (water: 78) = 178 ÷ 2 = 89
030. Alcoa (air: 129) + (water: 47) = 176 ÷ 2 = 88
031. Textron (air: 102) + (water: 73) = 175 ÷ 2 = 87.5
032. Icahn Enterprises (air: 101) + (water: 73) = 174 ÷ 2 = 87
033. BP (air: 78) + (water: 92) = 170 ÷ 2 = 85
034. United Technologies (air: 41) + (water: 127) = 168 ÷ 2 = 84
035. Lincoln Electric Holdings (air: 29) + (water: 139) = 168 ÷ 2 = 84
036. National Oilwell Varco (air: 22) + (water: 145) = 167 ÷ 2 = 83.5
037. PPL Corp. (air: 154) + (water: 12) = 166 ÷ 2 = 83
038. Carlyle Group (air: 72) + (water: 85) = 157 ÷ 2 = 78.5
039. Tenneco (air: 48) + (water: 106) = 154 ÷ 2 = 77
040. Hitachi (air: 106) + (water: 48) = 154 ÷ 2 = 77
041. Stepan (air: 35) + (water: 117) = 152 ÷ 2 = 76
042. Pentair (air: 122) + (water: 27) = 149 ÷ 2 = 74.5
043. Whirlpool (air: 21) + (water: 125) = 146 ÷ 2 = 73
044. Platform Specilaty Products Corp. (air: 110) + (water: 34) = 144 ÷ 2 = 72
045. General Motors (air: 34) + (water: 109) = 143 ÷ 2 = 71.5
046. Cargill (air: 93) + (water: 50) = 143 ÷ 2 = 71.5
047. Chemours (air: 120) + (water: 23) = 143 ÷ 2 = 71.5

048. Graphic Packaging (air: 85) + (water: 57) = 142 ÷ 2 = 71
049. Vistra Energy (air: 128) + (water: 14) = 142 ÷ 2 = 71
050. Southern Company (air: 135) + (water: 5) = 140 ÷ 2 = 70
051. Archer Daniels Midland (air: 75) + (water: 64) = 139 ÷ 2 = 69.5
052. First Energy (air: 104) + (water: 32) = 136 ÷ 2 = 68
053. Olin (air: 90) + (water: 38) = 128 ÷ 2 = 64
054. ABB Ltd. (air 86) + (water: 42) = 128 ÷ 2 = 64
055. Robert Bosch (air: 44) + (water: 82) = 126 ÷ 2 = 63
056. Ashland Inc. (air: 18) + (water: 105) = 123 ÷ 2 = 61.5
057. Ingredion (air: 53) + (water: 69) = 122 ÷ 2 = 61
058. HeidelbergCement (air: 76) + (water: 45) = 121 ÷ 2 = 60.5
059. AK Steel (air: 94) + (water: 26) = 120 ÷ 2 = 60
060. Duke Energy (air: 109) + (water: 11) = 120 ÷ 2 = 60
061. Total S.A. (air: 58) + (water: 58) = 116 ÷ 2 = 59.5
062. Phillips 66 (air: 27) + (water: 51) = 117 ÷ 2 = 58.5
063. Albemarle (air: 30) + (water: 86) = 116 ÷ 2 = 58
064. Valero Energy (air: 36) + (water: 79) = 115 ÷ 2 = 57.5
065. Huntington Ingalls Industries (air: 61) + (water: 52) = 113 ÷ 2 = 56.5
066. Boeing (air: 2) + (water: 110) = 112 ÷ 2 = 56
067. Honeywell International (air: 107) + (water: 4) = 111 ÷ 2 = 55.5
068. PBF Energy (air: 39) + (water: 71) = 110 ÷ 2 = 55
069. Freeport-McMoRan (air: 26) + (water: 83) = 109 ÷ 2 = 54.5
070. Deere (air: 55) + (water: 49) = 104 ÷ 2 = 52
071. Parker-Hannifin (air: 99) + (water: 3) = 102 ÷ 2 = 51
072. Royal Dutch Shell (air: 9) + (water: 93) = 102 ÷ 2 = 51
073. Goodyear Tire & Rubber (air: 62) + (water: 35) = 97 ÷ 2 = 48.5
074. Allegheny Technologies (air: 49) + (water: 46) = 95 ÷ 2 = 47.5
075. Formosa Plastics (air: 60) + (water: 30) = 90 ÷ 2 = 45
076. International Paper (air: 71) + (water: 18) = 89 ÷ 2 = 44.5
077. Occidental Petroleum (air: 25) + (water: 61) = 86 ÷ 2 = 43
078. Westlake Chemical (air: 47) + (water: 37) = 84 ÷ 2 = 42
079. Huntsman (air: 6) + (water: 75) = 81 ÷ 2 = 40.5
080. DTE Energy (air: 74) + (water: 6) = 80 ÷ 2 = 40
081. Chevron (air: 40) + (water: 39) = 79 ÷ 2 = 39.5
082. Marathon Petroleum (air: 33) + (water: 40) = 73 ÷ 2 = 36.5
083. American Electric Power (air: 56) + (water: 16) = 72 ÷ 2 = 36
084. Nucor (air: 28) + (water: 43) = 71 ÷ 2 = 35.5
085. Arconic (air: 14) + (water: 54) = 68 ÷ 2 = 34
086. United States Steel (air: 43) + (water: 21) = 64 ÷ 2 = 32
087. Daikin (air: 15) + (water: 42) = 57 ÷ 2 = 28.5
088. General Electric (air: 11) + (water: 41) = 52 ÷ 2 = 26
089. Mitsui (air: 6) + (water: 42) = 48 ÷ 2 = 24
090. ArcelorMittal (air: 38) + (water: 8) = 46 ÷ 2 = 23
091. Exxon Mobil (air: 19) + (water: 22) = 41 ÷ 2 = 20.5
092. Berkshire Hathaway (air: 13) + (water: 24) = 37 ÷ 2 = 18.5
093. Rio Tinto (air: 20) + (water: 15) = 35 ÷ 2 = 17.5
094. Eastman Chemical (air: 8) + (water: 25) = 33 ÷ 2 = 16.5
095. Koch Industries (air: 17) + (water: 13) = 30 ÷ 2 = 15

096. Northrop Grumman (air: 24) + (water: 2) = 26 ÷ 2 = 13
097. Celanese (air: 5) + (water: 19) = 24 ÷ 2 = 12
098. BASF (air: 7) + (water: 10) = 17 ÷ 2 = 8.5
099. LyondellBasell (air: 3) + (water: 9) = 12 ÷ 2 = 6
100. DowDuPont (air: 4) + (water: 1) = 5 ÷ 2 = 2.5

****

May 22, 2020, 5:04AM (Dick to group):

there have been various references to Hitler in these exchanges
unfortunately this article is in French, but it deals with Hitler's use of disease control as an organizing tool
his slogan was Gemeinnutz vor Eigennutz
this means "the group before the individual"
in the article you see it printed on the german mark
i tried to find the english article upon which it is based with no success
it's main thesis is that people accept authoritarian measures more readily during epidemics
maybe google translator would work if anyone feels motivated
https://www.santenatureinnovation.com/hitler-virus/?fbclid=IwAR2gsJG2h77yCQVIUi7cXNnbb2RoNd-RnW_BUeawMfQDFU2beLoQy3TeRdY

I was able to find an article it mentions by some nobel prize winners on disease with the following statement which prioritizes disease as the key factor determining levels of authoritarianism or democracy historically - it's very interesting, it suggests that sexism, racism, etc are all liked to the fear of infectious disease

We hypothesize that the variation in values pertaining to autocracy–democracy arises fundamentally out of human (*Homo sapiens*) species-typical psychological adaptation that manifests contingently, producing values and associated behaviours that functioned adaptively in human evolutionary history to cope with local levels of infectious diseases.

https://onlinelibrary.wiley.com/doi/10.1111/j.1469-185X.2008.00062.x

****

May 22, 2020, 9:01AM (BP to group):

When the fuck do they think it's going to be 'OK'? When there's *no more disease in the world?!*

This George Carlin bit has been spreading...
George Carlin - Germs, Immune System
https://www.youtube.com/watch?v=X29lF43mUlo

Love the bit about swimming in the Hudson as a kid. Amir-ul Kafirs has been saying something similar all along.

****

May 22, 2020, 10:31AM (Naia Nisnam to group):

The George Carlin video is hilarious and spot-on. I also appreciate the comments, as most people are expressing common sense in the comment section.
This video reminded me of a conversation I had with a homeless man here in Pittsburgh. He was an old-timer, connected with a few camps in this city. He told me that no one he knows of has gotten sick at a camp. When I try to look up articles about the homeless all I can find are reports about outbreaks in shelters, but nothing about the many homeless people who avoid shelters.

I did find several articles reporting “shocking” numbers of people in shelters testing positive for the virus but showing no symptoms.
It’s like the study done in 4 prisons that showed 3,300 prisoners tested positive for the virus but 96% of them had zero symptoms.
Also similar to those stats coming from NYC maternity wards. Over 15% of pregnant women who were admitted for labor/delivery tested positive for the virus.
I’ve heard about similar numbers coming from a study in Iceland but I can’t find the article myself.

These numbers point to a large number of the population having the virus but not getting sick at all. For the masses, this is a terrifying sign of how the deadly virus travels through asymptotic carriers.
But... to me this is an indication of how non-fatal the virus really is.
Why isn’t anyone talking about these numbers in terms of how much the virus has already spread and we didnt notice because it IS NOT making most people sick??

Thank you George Carlin fans, and those of you on this email list, for helping me to feel sane in the midst of a world gone mad.

https://www.wgbh.org/news/local-news/2020/04/07/one-in-three-among-boston-homeless-have-tested-positive-for-coronavirus-city-officials-say?_amp=true

https://www.google.com/amp/s/mobile.reuters.com/article/amp/idUSKCN2270RX

https://www.cuimc.columbia.edu/news/new-york-city-1-7-expectant-mothers-test-positive-coronavirus

****

April 7, 2020

One In Three Among Boston Homeless Have Tested Positive For Coronavirus, City Officials Say

By **Isaiah Thompson**
Reporter

Roughly one in three people of Boston's homeless community have tested positive for the COVID-19 virus, Boston officials said Tuesday.

Boston Mayor Marty Walsh and Boston Health and Human Services Chief Marty Martinez shared the grim statistic at one of Walsh's near-daily press briefings during the coronavirus crisis here.

"Right now, we think there's about close to two hundred cases in the homeless community," Martinez said. "We think that number is probably close to 30 percent of those who were tested."

Walsh said the city has secured roughly 170 beds at a Suffolk University dormitory, and that they should have capacity for as many as 500 beds for people who are homeless at the Boston Convention Center, which is being re-purposed into a temporary field hospital, but which has not yet opened as such.

[..]

****

In four U.S. state prisons, nearly 3,300 inmates test positive for coronavirus -- 96% without symptoms

Linda So, Grant Smith

(Reuters) - When the first cases of the new coronavirus surfaced in Ohio's prisons, the director in charge felt like she was fighting a ghost.

"We weren't always able to pinpoint where all the cases were coming from," said Annette Chambers-Smith, director of the Ohio Department of Rehabilitation and Correction. As the virus spread, they began mass testing.

They started with the Marion Correctional Institution, which houses 2,500 prisoners in north central Ohio, many of them older with pre-existing health conditions. After testing 2,300 inmates for the coronavirus, they were shocked. Of the 2,028 who tested positive, close to 95% had no symptoms.

"It was very surprising," said Chambers-Smith, who oversees the state's 28 correctional facilities.

As mass coronavirus testing expands in prisons, large numbers of inmates are showing no symptoms. In four state prison systems — Arkansas, North Carolina, Ohio and Virginia — 96% of 3,277 inmates who tested positive for the coronavirus were asymptomatic, according to interviews with officials and records reviewed by Reuters. That's out of 4,693 tests that included results on symptoms.

[..]

****

In New York City, 1 in 7 Expectant Mothers Test Positive for Coronavirus

April 20, 2020

About 15% of pregnant women admitted to two maternity wards in northern Manhattan in late March and early April were already infected with the new coronavirus, though most had no symptoms, according to a new study by physicians at the Vagelos College of Physicians and Surgeons at Columbia University Irving Medical Center and NewYork-Presbyterian. In the study, the researchers tested all 215 women who were admitted to the two labor and delivery units as soon as the women arrived at the hospital.

Findings May Shed Light on Overall Infection Rate
Study authors Dena Goffman and Desmond Sutton discussed their findings in the Washington Post.

The data were reported April 13 in a letter to the New England Journal of Medicine.
"It is important to recognize that there are a significant number of women (and likely others) who are in the community and asymptomatic," says Dena Goffman, MD, associate professor of obstetrics & gynecology at Columbia University Vagelos College of Physicians and Surgeons and chief of obstetrics at NewYork-Presbyterian/Columbia University Irving Medical Center.
"Obstetric services and other teams that will have patients coming in for necessary health care need to recognize this potential risk," Goffman says. "We need to take precautions to keep our moms, babies, families, and teams safe."
A solution, continues Goffman, may involve broader testing of patients admitted to non-COVID-19 wards and more universal protection across hospital departments with PPE to prevent ongoing spread.
New York City is currently the epicenter of COVID-19 with nearly 140,000 cases as of April 20, nearly 20% of confirmed cases in the United States.

[..]

****

May 22, 2020, 11:02AM (Amir-ul Kafirs to group):

it deals with Hitler's use of disease control as an organizing tool

Have all of you seen the nazi propaganda film comparing Jews to rats? It's called "Der Ewige Jude" (The Eternal Jew) (1940):

"One of the film's most notorious sequences compares Jews to rats that carry contagion, flood the continent, and devour precious resources." - https://encyclopedia.ushmm.org/content/en/article/der-ewige-jude

The above-mentioned scene shows Jews crowded together, perhaps in a marketplace, & then cuts to rats crowded together. It's very, ahem, direct.

Lesser known is a US film called "Japanese Beetles" (made between 1937 & 1945?). I recall it as a more subtle propaganda film that is on the surface against the destructive swarming of the insect but which could easily be interpreted as a metaphor for the Japanese-Americans who eventually ended up in camps.

his slogan was Gemeinnutz vor Eigennutz
this means "the group before the individual"

This sort of thing might be explained more in a documentary called "Colour of War VI: Adolf Hitler" movie from TWI/Granada Television - 2004 (I'm not sure it's that one, it might be another) that I excerpt from in my film "Robopaths". I've made reference to this sort of thing in things I've written elsewhere recently: this whole notion of the German "Volk", the body of the people as a 'superorganism'. I think such a mentality is truly at the heart of alot of what's going on these days: the reduction of individuals to parts in a larger 'body', or, really, a *machine*, a robopathic machine.

maybe google translator would work if anyone feels motivated

I'm going to try to translate it. Google Translate has a word limit so something like this has to be done piece-by-piece.

Thanks for these links, Dick. I really think this is important stuff & I'm going to look at both articles now.

****

May 22, 2020, 11:32AM (Amir-ul Kafirs to group):

I used Google Translate to produce the following. I only made one small correction which I note at the bottom.

From Santé Nature Innovation [Health Nature Innovation]:

"Hitler and the fight against viruses"

According to a study published in Plos One, there is an extremely strong link between the presence of infectious diseases in a population and their sympathy for authoritarian regimes
Adolf Hitler was obsessed with viruses.

After the Spanish Flu, which ravaged Europe in 1918-1919, Germany was indeed affected by a cholera pandemic (1923) while tuberculosis and polio continued to spread.
In 1924, the great German novelist Thomas Mann published “The Magic Mountain” (Der Zauberberg). This novel, which is "considered to be one of the most influential works of German literature in the 20th century" [1], recounts life in a terrible sanatorium of tuberculosis patients in Davos, Switzerland.

This story traumatized the Germans to the point that one of Hitler's first steps after coming to power in 1933 was a major tuberculosis control program. He mobilized a fleet of trucks equipped with X-ray machines to detect the disease by X-ray of the lungs and isolate the sick.
You had no choice whether to get tested or not. The motto of the Nazis, it should be remembered, was "common interest before individual interest" ("Gemeinnutz vor Eigennutz"). It was engraved on 1 Mark coins from 1933:

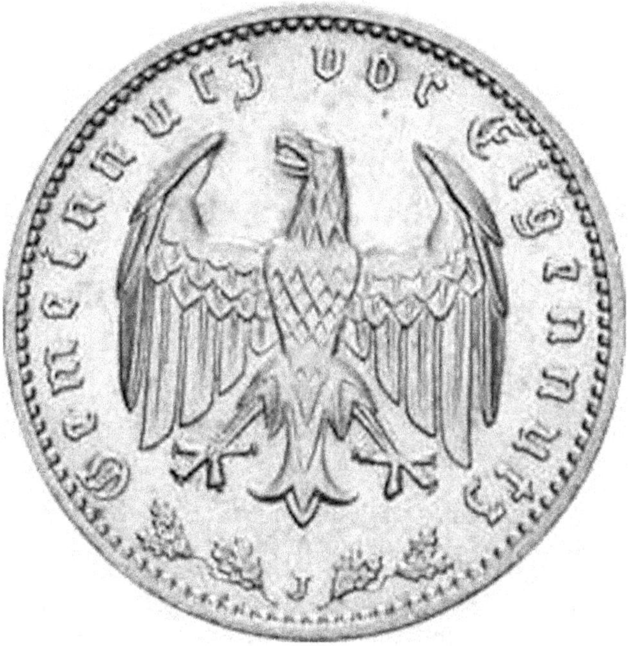

After tuberculosis, Hitler launched a major program to disinfect factories and eliminate lice and rodents, which cause epidemics.

Zyklon B gas, later used in gas chambers, was used for this purpose.

He also launched a big plan for green spaces around factories, with trees and flowers to create a “healthier” environment. Youth were recruited into colonies called "Hitler Youth" for activities in the countryside, forests, far from the stale air of big cities, thus "fortifying the race" and contributing to "greening" Germany.

But the fight against "infections" of all kinds should not stop there. The Nazis extended it to psychiatric hospitals, the mentally handicapped being regarded as weak and undesirable, consuming the resources necessary for "German workers". It was then the turn of the Gypsies, the Jews, the Slavs, considered as inferior and carriers of diseases, and finally to all kinds of other social groups designated as useless or harmful.

"Fire, symbol of purification"

This disgust and fear of infection also explains why Hitler adored fire. The Nazis used fire as a symbol of their movement.

Fire is, par excellence, the purifying element.

It destroys all life, and therefore all disease.
The Nazis organized night torchlight marches through the streets of Berlin, as well as huge ceremonies at night when 150,000 men were lined up in perfect squares, or swastikas, while huge torches lit the stage and powerful spotlights. swept the sky.

We also know the use of fire in crematorium ovens, intended to remove all traces of human beings and therefore all microbes.

A close link between authoritarian regimes and the presence of infectious diseases

According to a large study published in Plos One in 2013, there is a direct and very close link (correlation of 0.7) between the prevalence of infectious diseases in a population, and their sympathy for authoritarian regimes. [2]

In other words, the higher the risk (real or imagined) of infection, the more the population approves, even requests, authoritarian measures, restricting their freedoms.

The higher the risk of infectious diseases, the more a society becomes sexist, xenophobic, ethnocentric, explained Randy Thornhill, Corey L. Fincher and Devaraj Aran in 2008 in a famous article entitled “Parasites, democratization and liberalization of values among contemporary countries ”, published in Biological Reviews (Cambridge Philosophical Society), which could have won them the

Nobel Prize. [3]

These authors identified a system "of adapting homo sapiens to manage the problem of infectious diseases." As soon as we feel the risk of infection increasing, we accept (we ask!) That the authorities restrict our freedoms to protect us.

However, as human beings are the main vector of infectious diseases, the best way to protect ourselves is to prohibit other human beings from approaching us, by closing public places, by prohibiting gatherings, parties, borders, or limiting movement within the territory, or even by imposing permanent social distancing measures.

Sexual freedom and promiscuity, in particular, are hotly contested, as can be seen with the current distancing guidelines in the name of Covid-19, described in a very recent Chinese study as "sexually transmitted disease" [4] and therefore an additional justification to avoid intercourse.

Since the end of the Second World War, we have regarded as a “natural” phenomenon the progress of countries towards openness, democracy, the liberalization of customs, the mixing of cultures. Could it be that this phenomenon was in fact largely caused by antibiotics, vaccines and medical progress? And that, deprived of this newly acquired security, we renounce all the progress and rights of which we claimed to be so proud?

Imprisonments, violence and deportations in the event of an epidemic

In Kuwait, Qatar, going out without a mask is already punishable by imprisonment. [5] In China, people with fever are sometimes walled up or deported, and the Chinese press also reports that Chinese people present in Russia are also captured and deported because of fear of the coronavirus. [6]

Also in the name of the coronavirus, many Africans in China are beaten, evicted from their apartments, have to sleep on the streets, are prohibited from shopping or going to the doctor. [7]

In South Africa, coronavirus patients are being prosecuted by the authorities for "attempted murder" for having risked infecting others while traveling. [8]

In France, the Police were able to deploy drones for the first time to monitor the inhabitants, Justice having rejected the appeals of associations for the defense of liberties who denounced this practice. [9]

More than a million citizens have received tickets for breaching confinement rules. Hundreds of thousands of businesses are banned from operating, triggering chain bankruptcies and numerous job losses (not to mention the big chain stores, the hall of shoes, the hall of clothing, Naf Naf, the shoe maker André, over a hundred years old, Alinéa (2,000 employees) and Prémaman furniture are in receivership). [10]

Airbus is talking about laying off 10,000 people. [11]

The summer holidays seem compromised for millions of Europeans, endangering millions of jobs in hotels, restaurants, lodges, campsites, crafts, and among the guides, monitors and guides to the four corners of the country.

Where should you put the cursor?

It is extremely difficult for humans to know where to put the cursor, regarding hygiene and protection against infectious diseases.

We have a very strong disgust instinct that makes us, or even forces us, to stay away from potential vectors of disease, be it people or things.

Thus our instinct prevents us from eating the sticky, rotten, smelly things, which in fact are the most likely to give us diseases, by triggering a regurgitation reflex (spitting) if we are forced to swallow, or vomiting.

But we must also learn to overcome these instincts because many foods, while having an apparently repulsive appearance and odor, are actually good for health, or necessary for survival, like fermented foods.

Likewise, we learn to keep our distance from others. We are naturally wary of people with skin problems or other outward signs that suggest the presence of dangerous germs. Distrust of strangers is an archaic reflex to protect against epidemics, and we can even unconsciously use our sense of smell to be attracted, or repelled, by people according to their bacterial flora and therefore their immune system.

But we are also social creatures who absolutely need exchanges and human contacts to feel good. We need to cooperate, exchange information, or even comfort ourselves by touching us: handshake, hand on the shoulder, even hand on the neck, pat on the cheek, kiss, hug ...

It is also good to practice some exogamy (looking for your spouse outside your village, your tribe) in order to diversify the gene pool and avoid problems of inbreeding.

So our instincts can play tricks on us and make us run away from people who, in reality, pose no danger to us, and who, on the contrary, have something important to contribute to our community.

We have a lot of trouble calculating statistics, especially for large numbers. So if you are told that you have a 500, 5000 or 50,000 risk of catching a deadly virus, you do not know what to do with this information. Should we worry? Change your plans, your behavior? From what level can we afford to completely ignore the threat?

We don't know, but our anxiety can cause us to make bad choices in a panic.

Let us realize that today we are collectively confronted with such a problem. The presence of the coronavirus destabilizes our landmarks, and leads us to mistrust, withdrawal, isolation. It is undoubtedly a necessity, the time to understand what is happening to us, what is the real danger for our civilization, what is the actual risk of a massive "second wave" which would take other people away.

However, let's not forget that our health depends on many more factors than a simple virus. We have a whole social, economic, human edifice, essential to manage many other problems than the coronavirus, including our health system which fights many other diseases. This building is fragile. He is attacked from all sides. To exist, it absolutely needs that one can continue to work, circulate, undertake, meet, communicate, finance. If, in the name of the fight against the coronavirus, we destroy all this, we do not know where it will stop.

To Your Health !

Jean-Marc Dupuis

['translator"s note: the original French sign-off was "A votre santé !" which was translated by Google as "Cheers!" because it's used as a toast but I believe it's more correctly translated as "To Your Health !" because that plays into the meaning of the article more & is also a toast.]

[1] https://fr.wikipedia.org/wiki/La_Montagne_magique
[2] https://journals.plos.org/plosone/article?id=10.1371/journal.pone.0062275#pone.0062275-Thornhill1
[3] https://onlinelibrary.wiley.com/doi/abs/10.1111/j.1469-185X.2008.00062.x
[4] https://www.tdg.ch/monde/coronavirus-estil-mst/story/29015328
[5] https://news.trust.org/item/20200517153832-9wvuw
[6] https://www.globaltimes.cn/content/1181467.shtml
[7] https://blogs.letemps.ch/tidiane-diouwara/2020/04/24/51/
[8] HTTPS://WWW.DAILYSABAH.COM/WORLD/AFRICA/TWO-COVID-19-PATIENTS-FACE-ATTEMPTED-MURDER-CHARGES-IN-SOUTH-AFRICA
[9] HTTPS://WWW.LEMONDE.FR/PIXELS/ARTICLE/2020/05/06/A-PARIS-LA-JUSTICE-VALIDE-LA-SURVEILLANCE-DU-CONFINEMENT-PAR-DRONES-POLICIERS_6038884_4408996.HTML
[10] HTTPS://WWW.LUNION.FR/ID150816/ARTICLE/2020-05-16/LENSEIGNE-NAF-NAF-MISE-EN-REDRESSEMENT-JUDICIAIRE
[11] HTTPS://FRANCE3-REGIONS.FRANCETVINFO.FR/OCCITANIE/HAUTE-GARONNE/TOULOUSE/CRISE-ECONOMIQUE-LIEE-AU-CORONAVIRUS-AIRBUS-POURRAIT-LICENCIER-10-000-SES-SALARIES-1828654.HTML

- https://www.santenatureinnovation.com/hitler-virus/?fbclid=IwAR2gsJG2h77yCQVIUi7cXNnbb2RoNd-RnW_BUeawMfQDFU2beL0Qy3TeRdY

****

May 22, 2020, 11:44AM (Amir-ul Kafirs to group):

Re: HERETICS: TRANSLATION PS

I've also linked to the original & provided some of the translation to people on my social media timeline. Given that _____ & other people are bound to retaliate with hostile comments, any likes & shares I get from the rest of you are very welcome to relieve my stress. The article's excellent & I find nothing wrong with its logic whatsoever.

****

May 22, 2020, 12:04PM (Inquiring Librarian to group):

I love George Carlin! I will try to listen to this on my lunch break. I am feeling a bit suffocated by all of the rules here at the library. Most of them really make no sense, but I must adhere to and enforce them. And I must put on the face of taking the situation very seriously and gravely. I would say that half of the staff at my tiny branch library seem to be silently on the same page as me.
As for the testing and homeless people and also the testing people who are positive but who have no symptoms.... Imagine if this level of testing was done every year for the common flu? Obviously it would be another panic disaster for every obedient brainwashed germ-aphobe. My most unmotivated worker is my branch's most scared of the virus citizen. He exclaimed yesterday that several of his friends tested positivel... he is terrified... I asked him why they got tested... were they sick? No, he said they had no symptoms but that they were tested as a mandatory requirement of their job and now they are forced to be quarantined at home for 2 days. Thank goodness no one is testing our library staff at the moment. Imagine too, how we've been told repeatedly how innacurate the testing is... if you come up negative... but no one seems to question those false positives. It is so mindbogglingly nonsensical. I took a Logic class for English majors in college. Of my class about 30, only 2 of us (myself and my brilliant friend Heather) were not failing the class. Heather and I were acing the class. I was baffled, everything in the class seemed so, well...."logical" to me.

****

May 22, 2020, 1:04PM (Dick to group):

Re: HERETICS: TRANSLATION

I saw that _____ already has
he attacks the magazine (for being pro-natural health)
but not the content
that is a classical logical fallacy, it's a version of ad hominen

****

May 22, 2020, 1:18PM (Amir-ul Kafirs to group):

Re: HERETICS: PPS

The full version of this was only available for pay so I've just copied the abstract below.

On May 22, 2020, at 5:03 AM, dick turner wrote:

I was able to find an article it mentions by some nobel prize winners on disease with the following statement which prioritizes disease as the key factor determining levels of authoritarianism or democracy historically - it's very interesting, it suggests that sexism, racism, etc are all liked to the fear of infectious disease

Parasites, democratization, and the liberalization of values across contemporary countries

Randy Thornhill Corey L. Fincher Devaraj Aran
First published: 30 January 2009 https://doi.org/10.1111/j.1469-185X.2008.00062.xCitations: 116

Abstract

The countries of the world vary in their position along the autocracy–democracy continuum of values. Traditionally, scholars explain this variation as based on resource distribution and disparity among nations. We provide a different framework for understanding the autocracy–democracy dimension and related value dimensions, one that is complementary (not alternative) to the research tradition, but more encompassing, involving both evolutionary (ultimate) and proximate causation of the values. We hypothesize that the variation in values pertaining to autocracy–democracy arises fundamentally out of human (*Homo sapiens*) species-typical psychological adaptation that manifests contingently, producing values and associated behaviours that functioned adaptively in human evolutionary history to cope with local levels of infectious diseases. We test this parasite hypothesis of democratization using publicly available data measuring democratization, collectivism–individualism, gender egalitarianism, property rights, sexual restrictiveness, and parasite prevalence across many countries of the world. Parasite prevalence across countries is based on a validated index of the severity of 22 important human diseases. We show that, as the hypothesis predicts, collectivism (hence, conservatism), autocracy, women's subordination relative to men's status, and women's sexual restrictiveness are values that positively covary, and that correspond with high prevalence of infectious disease. Apparently, the psychology of xenophobia and ethnocentrism links these values to avoidance and management of parasites. Also as predicted, we show that the antipoles of each of the above values—individualism (hence, liberalism), democracy, and women's rights, freedom and increased participation in casual sex—are a positively covarying set of values in countries with relatively low parasite stress.

Beyond the cross-national support for the parasite hypothesis of democratization, it is consistent with the geographic location at high latitudes (and hence reduced parasite stress) of the early democratic transitions in Britain, France and the U.S.A. It, too, is consistent with the marked increase in the liberalization of social values in the West in the 1950s and 1960s (in part, the sexual revolution), regions that, a generation or two earlier, experienced dramatically reduced infectious diseases as a result of antibiotics, vaccinations, food- and water-safety practices, and increased sanitation.

Moreover, we hypothesize that the generation and diffusion of innovations (in thought, action and technology) within and among regions, which is associated positively with democratization, is causally related to parasite stress. Finally, we hypothesize that past selection in the context of morbidity and mortality resulting from parasitic disease crafted many of the aspects of social psychology unique to humans.

- https://onlinelibrary.wiley.com/doi/10.1111/j.1469-185X.2008.00062.x

****

May 22, 2020, 1:32PM (Amir-ul Kafirs to group):

Ha ha! Carlin's, uh, ***particularly AGGRESSIVE with this one, isn't he?!!*** I saved it to my onesownthoughts PANDEMIC PANIC playlist. I've been mainly putting short entertaining things there that aren't 'too dull' for people with little or no attention span.

****

May 22, 2020, 2:45PM (Amir-ul Kafirs to group):

Re: HERETICS: TRANSLATION PS

he attacks the magazine (for being pro-natural health)
but not the content
that is a classical logical fallacy, it's a version of ad hominen

Ah, thx for the tip on the term. I've run across it many times but didn't remember its meaning. I think that it'll be used in my next white-on-black text. _____ has what one might call a Superiority Complex. He's been attacking me almost every time I post something PANDEMIC PANIC related for the last 2 months or so. Fortunately for me, I DON'T have an Inferiority Complex so I try not to let these frequent attacks get to me too much. Still, the other day when I announced here my plan to post those 4 black-on-white texts I told Naia Nisnam that _____ would attack the False Syllogisms one but that he wouldn't be able to do so logically so he'd have to use something spurious & irrelevant. SO, what did he do? He posted a comment sarcastically attacking my use of fonts! That was so illustrative of what I've been talking about all along that it was wonderful. Apparently, even _____ thought that was too transparent because he deleted the comment

****

May 22, 2020, 2:56PM (Dick to group):

Re: HERETICS: TRANSLATION PS

I wanted to verify so I found these
(see below)
maybe ______ is afraid of societal collapse so he's doing an I Love Big Brother thing
he's heavily invested in the stock market, or so I'm told

https://en.wikipedia.org/wiki/Ad_hominem

Ad hominem - Wikipedia
Ad hominem (Latin for 'to the person'), short for argumentum ad hominem, is a term that is applied to several different types of arguments, most of which are fallacious.Typically it refers to a fallacious argumentative strategy whereby genuine discussion of the topic at hand is avoided by instead attacking the character, motive, or other attribute of the person making the argument, or persons ...

https://en.wikipedia.org/wiki/List_of_fallacies

List of fallacies - Wikipedia
In reasoning to argue a claim, a fallacy is reasoning that is evaluated as logically incorrect and that undermines the logical validity of the argument and permits its recognition as unsound.Regardless of their soundness, all registers and manners of speech can demonstrate fallacies. Because of their variety of structure and application, fallacies are challenging to classify so as to satisfy ...

****

Ad hominem

"Personal attack" redirects here.

Ad hominem (Latin for 'to the person'), short for ***argumentum ad hominem***, is a term that refers to several types of arguments, most of which are fallacious.

Typically this term refers to a rhetorical strategy where the speaker attacks the character, motive, or some other attribute of the person making an argument rather than attacking the substance of the argument itself. This avoids genuine debate by creating a diversion to some irrelevant but often highly charged issue. The most common form of this fallacy is "A makes a claim *x*, B asserts that A holds a property that is unwelcome, and hence B concludes that argument *x* is wrong".

The valid types of *ad hominem* arguments are generally only encountered in specialized philosophical usage. These typically refer to the dialectical strategy of using the target's own beliefs and arguments against them, while not agreeing with the validity of those beliefs and arguments. Ad hominem arguments were first studied in ancient Greece; John Locke revived the examination of ad hominem arguments in the 17th century. Many contemporary politicians routinely use ad hominem attacks, which can be encapsulated to a derogatory nickname for a political opponent.

[..]

****

List of fallacies

From Wikipedia, the free encyclopedia

For specific popular misconceptions, see List of common misconceptions.

In reasoning to argue a claim, a fallacy is reasoning that is evaluated as logically incorrect and that undermines the logical validity of the argument and permits its recognition as unsound. Regardless of their soundness, all registers and manners of speech can demonstrate fallacies.

Because of their variety of structure and application, fallacies are challenging to classify. Fallacies can be classified strictly by either their structure (formal fallacies) or content (informal fallacies). The classification of informal fallacies may be subdivided into categories such as linguistic, relevance through omission, relevance through intrusion, and relevance through presumption. Or, fallacies may be classified by the process by which they occur, such as material fallacies (content), verbal fallacies (linguistic), and again formal fallacies (error in inference). Material fallacies may be placed into the broader category of informal fallacies, while formal fallacies may be placed into the more precise category of logical (deductive) fallacies.[*clarification needed*] Yet, verbal fallacies may be placed into either informal or deductive classifications; compare equivocation which is a word or phrase based ambiguity (e.g., "he is mad", which may refer to either him being angry or clinically insane) to the fallacy of composition which is premise and inference based ambiguity (e.g., "this must be a good basketball team because each of its members is an outstanding player").

The conscious or habitual use of fallacies as rhetorical devices is prevalent in the desire to persuade when the focus is more on communication and eliciting common agreement rather than on correctness of the reasoning. The effective use of a fallacy may be considered clever, but the reasoning should be recognized as unsound and the conclusion regarded as unproven.

[..]

****

May 22, 2020, 3:33PM (Amir-ul Kafirs to group):

Yes, thanks. I've already made my response text. Note that I don't specifically reference _____ & that the example is culled from something that they deleted theirself. That means that few people will understand that it's a direct reference to them & that they might be able to recognize the relevance of my criticism. I'm trying to avoid direct personal attacks on _____ but I think they're a little less restrained in that way. I wonder how long it'll be before they start name-calling?

RELEVANCE FALLACIES

An *irrelevant conclusion* is the fallacy of presenting an argument whose conclusion fails to address the issue in question.

This is related to *ad hominem* arguments in which the person making the argument is refuted not by debating the actual point but by attacking the person making the original statement.

For example: A person wishing to degrade a written logical argument but unable to do so on logical grounds attacks its use of fonts instead.

**Such logical fallacies are extremely common in the era of the PANDEMIC PANIC, especially originating from people with Superiority Complexes
who are unable to agree to disagree.**

****

May 22, 2020, 5:04PM (Amir-ul Kafirs to group):

The 2nd article linked to below contains the following: "The numbers are the latest evidence to suggest that people who are asymptomatic — contagious but not physically sick — may be driving the spread of the virus, not only in state prisons that house 1.3 million inmates across the country, but also in communities across the globe." What continues to amaze me is that none of the mainstream news articles ever seem to address what's been obvious to Naia Nisnam & myself (as well as to, presumably, everyone else here): viz that asymptomatic people could simply be called people with healthy immune systems whose not getting sick from COVID-19 points to its being less deadly than it's constantly touted as being.

https://www.google.com/amp/s/mobile.reuters.com/article/amp/idUSKCN2270RX

****

May 22, 2020, 5:10PM (Amir-ul Kafirs to group):

I would say that half of the staff at my tiny branch library seem to be silently on the same page as me.

Maybe you could try feeling them out & finding who your fellow HERETICS are? That might enable you to collectively put a monkey wrench into the paranoia works eventually.

No, he said they had no symptoms

Even in those circumstances such people are terrified. It doesn't seem that they have the capacity to understand that their whole life they've been surrounded by people who're asymptomatic for something or another that 'might' kill somebody somewhere down the road — & that they, too, might be one of these asymptomatic people. Only now, in the PANDEMIC PANIC, does this suddenly become an issue.

now they are forced to be quarantined at home for 2 days.

TWO DAYS. It's not enough. I say life imprisonment or mandatory suicide.

****

May 22, 2020, 5:14PM (Dick to group):

Re: HERETICS: Librarian Liberals

jeez, ______ just wrote a response to my comment
he doesn't have a logical approach
he mixes things up
he is masking emotion with attempted logic, but it is transparent
i don't know him very well so i can't say if he's just a moron or if there is something about this situation (covid-19) that particularly bothers him
not sure if I should have but I responded

****

May 22, 2020, 7:42PM (Amir-ul Kafirs to group):

YOUTUBE.COM

2020 05 12 ZOOm

"2020.05.12 ZOO(m)": During this time of enforced social isolation, many...

Monty Cantsign, and 2 others 3 Comments

Like Comment Share

001a https://www.huffpost.com/.../florida-man-brian-hitchens...

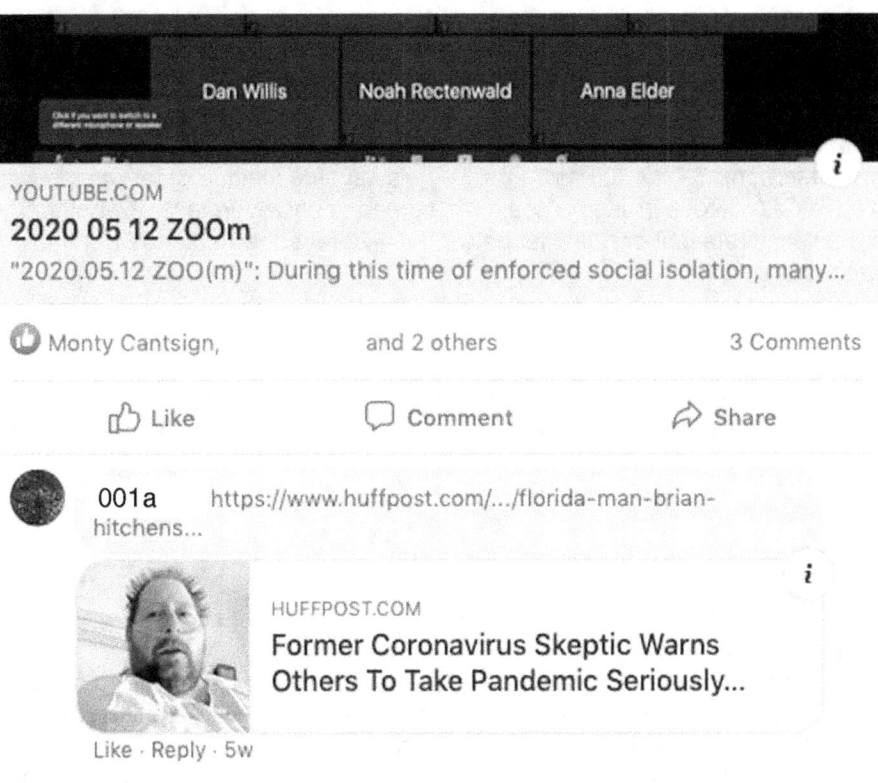

HUFFPOST.COM

Former Coronavirus Skeptic Warns Others To Take Pandemic Seriously...

Like · Reply · 5w

002a My wife works for Becton Dickinson . They are working with the idea that the mortality of cv-19 is 6 % the flu is .1% .

Like · Reply · 5w

003a Thanks for sharing this musical experience!
I can read and know that you are not denying the existence of the virus but are having reasonable questions relating to the unhelpful media-induced panic and policies that will shape our future.
(Edited: spell check error)

Like · Reply · 5w · Edited 2

he is masking emotion with attempted logic, but it is transparent

It's transparent to you & me but I don't know how transparent it is to other people. At 1st, quite some time ago when his attacks on me began, he said he was surprised I wasn't being "more skeptical". Given that what I felt I was doing was posting everything that I could find (& that the good folks here could find) that WAS skeptical about the whole MONOLITHIC NARRATIVE but also seemed reasonable & in keeping with my own observations, I just got disgusted with him & could see that he wasn't ever going to satisfied until I bowed down to his thinly disguised pompous condescending pseudo-superior 'logic'. As such, I decided to not waste any more time replying to him because I knew it would be like debating the existence of 'God' with Christians. Since then, he seems to've reversed his position & decided he's against skepticism (or, at least, skepticism against what he's supporting) — hence his posting of a link to a story about a former skeptic who got sick with COVID-19 & renounced his skepticism. It didn't matter that the guy was overweight & religious & had other characteristics that made him different from me — the attempt was _____'s usual technique of tarring me with whatever slanderous brush he could manage to apply regardless of whether they were actually relevant or not. Hence we have **Relevance Fallacies** out the wazoo.

i don't know him very well so i can't say id he's just a moron

Well.. he's not a moron. He was actually one of my closest collaborators up until 1998 & someone I've done some great work with. That's part of what makes this so difficult for me.

or if they is something about this situation (covid-19) that particularly bothers him

I think part of it is is that he's not critical about his own place in the hierarchy of privilege. It's ok for me to be 'smart' but only if I bow down, subtly or overtly, to his own 'smarts'. When I don't do that, & I never have, he feels a deep need to compete with me. Alas, like all other competetive people who aren't ultimately concerned with truth value but are instead primarily worried about their own dominance, only the appearance of "a logical approach" is 'necessary', the most important thing is to just keep attacking, hoping to wear me down. What he really doesn't understand is that while he's lived a life of relative luxury for a long time now I've been struggling against a society that has been largely unfriendly & I've long since had a resilience that few people possess. As I like to say, I'm a "Professional Resister of Character Defamation" &, believe me, I've had more experience in that department than I would wish on anyone. Essentially, he 'needs' to be completely confident that he's 'right' but that confidence doesn't have to be based on logic because he has privilege to tell him that he's a representative of the justly dominant class.

not sure if I should have but I responded

I'm thankful that you did because I'm not going to but I'm glad that someone else calls him out. If he gets to the point of just personally attacking me in a more overt way I'll probably just unfriend him but I've been holding out on that one. I notice that he brought up "A Natural History of Rape - Biological Bases of Sexual Coercion", as a way of trying to discredit the original article under scrutiny (about Hitler & viruses). Talk about changing the subject to avoid the main one! Whew! What makes that even more 'hilarious' is that the book is advertised on MIT's website. That means that _____ is going to have to write off all of MIT now (which he won't do, of course, because it's an icon of what he reveres}!

****

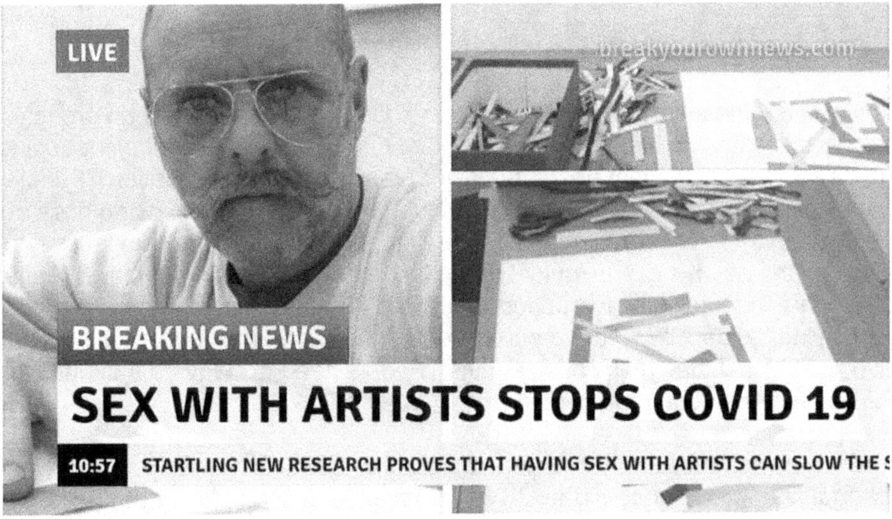

****

May 26, 2020, 1:02PM (Amir-ul Kafirs to group):

HERETICS: Computer Dating

Irrelevant (but funny):

_____'s intro to me:

I'm _____ 31 I'll be turning 32 on august, I'm a college student here in California , I study fashion design , I own a small scale business I'm into merchandising of gold, diamond antiques and gems, i buy from Dubai and Cyprus and most of all I do some local trades.. but due to this pandemic it's hell of a time since my item are currently been withheld from shipped down here to the states from Cyprus... I love spending time with friends and family, watching tv and playing video games

My reply:

Hi _____, you're one hot capitalist babe. Thanks for informing me about your down-to-earth issues with getting your gold, diamonds, antiques, and gems past customs. Perhaps I could help you out, in my small way, by giving you a few million? I'd hate to see you go without during these difficult times.

Relevant to PANDEMIC PANIC, my correspondence with a Brazilian woman:

May 25, 2020 (_____ to Amir-ul Kafirs):

Na sua opinião qual seria a saída para essa situação?

In your opinion, what would be the way out of this situation?

May 26, 2020 (Amir-ul Kafirs to _____):

1st: Do I imagine a way out of the situation? OK, I'm a heretic. I'm an anarchist. I deeply disbelieve in hierarchical authoritarian structures. I DO think that power breeds corruption and that absolute power breeds absolute corruption. People enable this power and its attendant corruption by believing in the worthiness of people 'above them' in hierarchies. This, then, enables those people 'above' to believe in their own 'right' to 'guide' (that is: control) the 'lesser' people. This is suffocating economically and unconsciously. The more people there are who resist being 'guided' by what I consider to be fake superiority the better off we all will be. That includes medical situations. People need to cultivate their intuition, their instinct, their common sense.

More on the 1st question: I think that the body's natural immune system is very powerful and 'wise'. Here in the US and, I imagine, elsewhere, there's emphasis from the Medical Industry that the immune system is 'not enough' to protect us against COVID-19 and, of course, other health issues. There are, thankfully, oppositional voices in the Medical Community but, as with everything else, they're outshouted by corporate interests. Greed, greeed, and MORE GREEED is what is driving much of what's happening now. The more people hear and obey the 'voices of experts' to not trust their own body, their own instincts, their own intuition, their own native intelligence, the more the interests of GREED can invade and colonize their lives. I suggest that there are many things that can compromise a person's immune system and that most, if not all, of these things originate in human-made problems. For example: an excessive forcing of sugar and other harmful substances on consumers; an excessive forcing of MEDICATIONS, that are just as harmful, if not more so, than helpful, on people in the name of 'our own good'. COVID-19 is often compared to the Spanish Flu of 1918-1919. It's my understanding that that flu would not have been nearly so 'empowered' if it hadn't been for the extremely ecologically harmful effects of trench warfare during so-called "World War I". Huge areas were reduced to puddle-filled mud, obvious breeding grounds for little other than mosquitos. Anyway, the point is that the more people relinquish their own defense systems in favor of those of the 'experts' the more defenseless they become — and that's true across all areas: whether it's political or medical.

May 25, 2020 (_____ to Amir-ul Kafirs):

Gostaria de te perguntar se vocês escutam notícias do Brasil aí?

I would like to ask you if you hear news from Brazil there?

May 26, 2020 (Amir-ul Kafirs to _____):

I'm sure there's news about Brazil. I, personally, don't pay much attention, if any, attention to it. I don't ignore Brazil in particular, I ignore the 'news' here in general because most of it just serves vested interests that make the 'news' suspect or useless. The larger the source of news, the more there's going to be a socio-political-economic bias slanting it. These biases become absolutely insane after awhile. One of the most popular 'news' sources here in the US is "Fox TV". They're 'conservative' — but what that really means is that they just serve the interests of billionaires and shit on the people under the guise of representing them/us. They're flagrantly religious and flagrantly in favor of arms dealers. SO, any 'news' about Brazil would probably be either depicting Brazil's president as a deranged dictator or as a stalwart ant-communist or anti-terrorist. Therefore, any 'news' about the pandemic would follow one of those initial biases. My very vague impression is that the Brazilian president has been depicted as a fool for not acting fast enough to enforce quarantine measures.

Here's a sample of 'news' coverage from TIME, a major 'news' source:

"On May 9, Brazil's death toll from the coronavirus topped 10,000. Instead of marking the grim milestone with an address or a sign of respect for the victims, President Jair Bolsonaro took a spin on a jet ski. Video footage widely circulated on social media shows Brazil's far-right leader grinning as he pulls up to a boat on Brasília's Paranoá Lake where supporters are having a cookout. As he grips onto their boat, Bolsonaro jokes about the "neurosis" of Brazilians worried about the virus. "There's nothing to be done [about it]," he shrugs. "It's madness."

"Even by the standards of other right-wing populists who have sought to downplay the COVID-19 pandemic, Bolsonaro's defiance of reality was shocking. From the favelas of densely packed cities like Rio de Janeiro to the remote indigenous communities of the Amazon rain forest, Brazil has emerged as the new global epicenter of the pandemic, with the world's highest rate of transmission and a health system now teetering on the brink of collapse.

"Unlike the previous global hot spots – Italy, Spain and the U.S. – Brazil is an emerging economy, with a weaker social safety net that makes it harder for local authorities to persuade people to stay home, and an underfunded health care system. When a particularly severe outbreak struck the city of Manaus, in the Amazon, in late April, hospitals were quickly overrun, leading to a shortage of coffins. On May 17, the mayor of São Paulo, Latin America's largest city, warned that hospitals there would collapse within two weeks if the infection rate continued to rise. The country has confirmed almost 18,000 deaths as of May 19, with a record 1,179 people dying in the preceding 24 hours–the world's second highest daily fatality rate. Epidemiologists say the peak is still weeks away."

The problem with such coverage is that while it may be accurate enough there's always a subtext of ulterior motives that are related to US foreign policy. Perhaps the US wants to take more natural resources from Brazil than Bolsonaro is allowing so the mass media is setting up their readers to justify some future covert action against him, a coup d'etat for example. Such inevitable ulterior motives make such 'news' completely unreliable even if based on actuality. As such, I prefer just getting my 'news' from individuals, such as yourself, who may not be 'objective' sources but who are, at least, less likely to have major ulterior motives.

****

May 27, 2020, 6:47PM (Amir-ul Kafirs to group):

Re: HERETICS: Computer Dating

OK, I thought my sarcasm in the exchange below was glaringly obvious. Look at what _____ replied. Maybe whoever's behind this particular scam actually believes that I might be serious about the "few million"? Hard to believe but I guess they thought it was worth the chance.

Perhaps I could help you out, in my small way, by giving you a few million? I'd hate to see you go without during these difficult times.

Nice to hear that from you and I could like to no more about you , if you don't mind let me give you my # so hit me up [I've deleted the phone number]

****

May 28, 2020, 4:11PM (Amir-ul Kafirs to group):

HERETICS: Proposed Book reiterated

To refresh people's memories about the book I proposed, here's my email of April 26th, a little over a month ago. These days I'm thinking of calling it: "Unconscious Suffocation: Mind Control in the era of COVID-19".

I keep imagining compiling a book of criticism of the Global Lockdown and the PANDEMIC PANIC.

****

May 28, 2020, 5:29PM (Dick to group):

RE: HERETICS: Proposed Book reiterated

ok, i'll try to get something written soon
maybe a deadline could be useful
*
by the way
the French Government has declared that as of Monday everything will be open

here's what Edouard Phillipe (the PM) said (copying Amir-ul Kafir's example, I used Google translator)

the boldface I put in for the telephone app and the thing about gatherings of more than 10 people which means there will be no demonstrations until at least 21 June

Certificates. The certificate necessary for trips of more than 100 km should logically be deleted as of Tuesday. However, the so-called "employer" certificate for taking public transport in Ile-de-France is at this stage maintained. "We will see with the transport organizing companies if we can withdraw these authorizations," said Edouard Philippe, adding that he had contacted the president of the Ile-de-France region Valérie Pécresse on this issue. The use of telework remains encouraged.

Tests. "We have the capacity to screen each symptomatic person and all contacts," said Olivier Véran during the press conference. "More than 80% of PCR tests are rendered in less than 36 hours," he assured, calling on the French to consult their doctors "at the slightest hesitation".

Masks. The mask will remain mandatory in transport and in some places mentioned below, it is "widely recommended" in general. Edouard Philippe was asked about the government's lack of communication on how to wear it. "Wearing a surgical mask in conditions of maximum health security is not completely simple, [...] a great effort of communication was made, but also on the part of doctors, interveners". "In the end, I think our fellow citizens know how to wear the mask," he evaded, even if he pointed out sometimes contradictory comments in the streets.

StopCovid. "The StopCovid application will be launched for the June 2 deadline" announced Edouard Philippe about the tracing contact app, which will allow you to be alerted on your smartphone if you have encountered a person tested positive in the last 15 days. "I invite everyone who watches us and our fellow citizens to use this application," asked the Prime Minister. All about StopCovid.

Schools, colleges, high schools. The Minister of Education Jean-Michel Blanquer also spoke during the press conference and indicated that "all the schools will gradually reopen from June 2" and in particular that "the colleges will be able to accommodate students from 6th to 6th the third in the green zone ". "In the orange zone we will give priority to pupils in grades 6 and 5," he said. "Regarding high schools, priority will go to vocational high schools [...] where dropping out is the most important," said Jean-Michel Blanquer. "In the green zone, general, technological and professional high schools will reopen [...] at least on a first level to start [...]. In the orange zone, we will be more careful. Professional high schools are also opening up but first with the final and CAP students, "he continued. "Students from general and technological high schools will be welcomed for interviews in small groups. The objective is that all students have had an interview by the end of the year."

French baccalaureate. "The French baccalaureate test will be validated by continuous assessment," also announced Jean-Michel Blanquer, thus formalizing the cancellation of the oral exams taken by the first graders. "We will take into account the scores from the first two quarters," said the minister.

Cafes and restaurants. "Cafes, bars and restaurants can open from June 2 in the green zone. Only the terraces can reopen in the orange zone," said Edouard Philippe. A strict protocol will be implemented in open cafes and restaurants: "wearing a mandatory mask for staff and customers when traveling", "tables of 10 people maximum", "distance of at least one meter between each table" , "prohibition to consume standing inside establishments" open in the green zone ...

Parks and gardens. "Our social, cultural and sporting life will be able to resume more widely. From this weekend, the parks and gardens will reopen throughout the territory. The wearing of masks may be imposed in many spaces. At the request of mayors , the prefects will be able to impose the wearing of the mask in public space, "added Edouard Philippe.

Beaches, lakes and water points can also be opened from June 2 under the same conditions as parks and gardens.

Hotels and campsites. "Tourist accommodation will be able to open in all green departments from June 2," says Edouard Philippe. The reopening is postponed to June 22 in the orange zone, that is during the third phase of deconfinement.

Cinemas and performance halls. "In the green zones, theaters will be able to reopen from June 2. The wearing of the mask will be compulsory," declared the Prime Minister. "The cinemas will reopen from June 22."

Swimming pools and sports halls. "Physical activities can resume with the reopening of gymnasiums, sports halls and swimming pools," announced Edouard Philippe. Collective and contact sports are prohibited.

Amusement parks. "The leisure parks will be open for activities allowing physical distance and a maximum area of 5000 people". Discos and games rooms, however, remain closed, as well as stadiums and racetracks.

Events and gatherings. **Meetings of more than 10 people remain prohibited until June 21.** "Our biggest adversary is the very big rallies," says Edouard Philippe. Even more "in a confined environment and without specific organization". A maximum gauge of 5000 people will be set for outdoor events.

Weddings and funerals. "For a long time, weddings have been delayed. Fortunately, that period is over: we will finally be able to start celebrating weddings again," announced the Prime Minister. He nevertheless warns that "the moment to completely release the tension on religious ceremonies or civil ceremonies has not come" and that "we will therefore have to be very attentive to the physical distance and density, which correspond to the protocols that have been accepted and implemented. "

Summer holidays. "Travel in Europe will be, I hope (soon) authorized. We will harmonize with our neighbors," said Edouard Philippe indicating that until June 15, restrictions are maintained on entry into French territory. "We make our decisions at our own pace and we considered that the right time to access the national territory was June 15. We will open our borders within a fortnight." The external borders of Europe will undoubtedly be reopened later, awaiting a "common European position". "Children can be enrolled in open-air holiday camps," said the minister.

****

May 28, 2020, 5:41PM (Amir-ul Kafirs to group):

RE: HERETICS: Proposed Book reiterated

mavbe a deadline could be useful

You proposed a deadline to me on May 3 too & I replied:

"There's no hurry, so no deadline. The general vibe I'm getting is that everyone feels a bit intimidated by the prospect and I have so many things going on that I don't even know when I'll get started on it."

To clarify that further: AFTER I get the emails somewhat sorted out (& there're many hundreds of them) it's my plan to extract all the links from them & to go thru everything & write a synopsis about each one & then a critique of each one. That's only one aspect of what I have in mind but it's extremely labor-intensive. That, alone, could take me months to do even a shitty job. SO, since you've suggested a deadline twice now **I suggest August 1**. That gives me roughly 2 months to get some basics done so that I can then figure out how to add your contribution.

****

May 31, 2020, 8:51AM (Amir-ul Kafirs to group):

the French Government has declared that as of Monday everything will be open

Thanks for keeping us informed. It's interesting to contrast that to what's happening here in Pittsburgh & the US. Yesterday's march in solidarity with

George Floyd obviously violated all social distancing rules but most people kept their masks on. I had mine on about 2/3rds of the time.

"We will see with the transport organizing companies if we can withdraw these authorizations," said Edouard Philippe

Fortunately, we don't have such things here as far as I know. I've gone on 2 long-distance trips so far during the lockdown. It remains to be seen whether I'll be penalized for them or not.

"We have the capacity to screen each symptomatic person and all contacts,"

The value of such screening remains dubious to me insofar as I'm not convinced that being aymptomatic is bad in the way it's presented as being.

The mask will remain mandatory in transport and in some places mentioned below, it is "widely recommended" in general.

Needless to add, except 'for the record', I detest the masks & continue to question their healthiness.

will allow you to be alerted on your smartphone if you have encountered a person tested positive in the last 15 days.

Welcome to the total surveillance society.

priority will go to vocational high schools [...] where dropping out is the most important,"

Another glimpse at what's considered "essential".

the prefects will be able to impose the wearing of the mask in public space

This seems like an enforcement nightmare.

"Travel in Europe will be, I hope (soon) authorized. We will harmonize with our neighbors,"

That would be a nice change, eh?!

****

May 29, 2020, 5:30PM (Amir-ul Kafirs to group):

HERETICS: Social Distancing Tracking Technology

Today, I was at the park & a masked guy passed me & I heard what sounded like a synthetic voice say: "Social Distance 5.1.." & then I was too far past to hear the rest. I imagine it ended in "feet" & that it was measuring the distance between me & the masked man. SO, now, I was thinking of buying something like this to use in performance so I looked it up. There're devices for sale for THOUSANDS OF DOLLARS & then cheaper things like a wristband that vibrates or flashes if someone comes 'too close' that was only $28. All in all, it seems to be big business. SO, here's a relevant 'randomly' selected article (https://spectrum.ieee.org/the-human-os/biomedical/devices/wearables-track-social-distancing-sick-employees-workplace):

The Human OS
Biomedical
Biomedical Devices

01 May 2020 | 19:27 GMT

Back to Work: Wearables Track Social Distancing and Sick Employees in the Workplace

As companies re-open, employees may don wearable tech to prevent the spread of COVID-19

By Emily Waltz

As shuttered businesses make plans to resume on-site operations, many plan to outfit their employees with new, anti-pandemic gear: wearable tech that could prevent the spread of COVID-19 inside the workplace.

Ford employees are experimenting with smartwatches that vibrate when workers come within six feet of each other. The accounting firm PricewaterhouseCoopers (PwC) has developed an app that turns employees' phones into contact tracing devices, notifying them when they've been exposed to a coworker with the novel coronavirus.

Other employers are considering equipping their workforces with wearables—separate from their phones—that are capable of granular on-site and indoor location tracking and contact tracing. CarePredict recently rolled out such devices for senior living facilities.

In fact, in a survey of 871 finance executives at companies in 24 countries, 21 percent said they were eyeing location tracking and contact tracing for their workforces, according to PwC, which conducted the survey and posted it online this week.

[..]

****

May 29, 2020, 9:48PM (Inquiring Librarian to group):

Re: HERETICS: Social Distancing Tracking Technology

What a horribly invasive and needless invention! I hope my work never adopts this nonsense. :/

My work is trying to get creative while drilling pandemic overkill paranoia down my throat. Today i was assigned a learning module to train me on the Mango Languages database. Really i love this! It's an awesome database that i have been wanting to navigate. But.... they apparently created a "Covid Pandemic Vocab." course. :/ i got to pick my own language. Then i had to spend an hour learning pandemic related words in Russian. I learned such words as vaccine, pandemic, epidemic, ambulance, xray, sheets, pillow, pills/'medicine', germ, she did/did not wash her hands/clothes... Etc... Oh yeah... And don't forget grammy and grampy. Good grief! :/ :/ :O... The training was over an hour. I am proud i still know my cyrillic alphabet. But the words i learned disgust me.

****

May 29, 2020, 11:11PM (Naia Nisnam to group):

All of this tracking stuff is unnecessary. We know that there is a portion of the population that is high-risk. People in the high risk category can choose to quarantine themselves.

This tech is being introduced during the media-induced pandemic panic so that the public will buy into the idea that such surveillance is for the public good. When the pandemic is declared to be over, we will be stuck with all of this surveillance as a “normal” part of life.

Why do most people seem to be just fine with this? I’m so frustrated.

****

May 29, 2020, 9:33PM (Amir-ul Kafirs to group):

HERETICS: Conversation for Beginners

Here's one that I made today that I'll save for harsher times.

I've been watching a movie of "A Conversation with History: Tariq Ali & Oliver Stone" (2009) in which, around minute 56, it's discussed how the US government overthrew leadership that was attempting neutrality in the cold war in other countries. These leaders were neither capitalist or communist & didn't want to ally with either. This made them a threat to US world domination so the US proceeded to support more compliant potential leaders who then instigated US-backed coups. I mention this because it's an example of how Divide & Conquer works in relation to today's 2 position simple-mindedness.

Conversation for Beginners

Monster: I like oranges.

Caring: You think it's ok to stab people in the face?!

Monster: What? I said I like oranges.

Caring: You Trump supporters make me sick!!

Monster: I can't stand Trump!

Caring: You COVID-deniers should be forced to suck the assholes of all the corpses in New York. THEN you'll see what the truth is!!!

****

May 30, 2020, 1:19AM (BP to group):

somewhat but not entirely unrelated to the topic at hand, but I just found out that the cop who murdered George Floyd is....
Derek Chauvin.
It's too weird. Like the Bill Hick's skit about one of the actual convicted cops in the Rodney King beating, Officer Koon.
These names are not a convenience but a warning!

****

May 18, 2020, 6:39AM (Dick to group):

HERETICS: Ken Knabb

Hi,

I'm on the mailing list of The Bureau of Public Secrets and received this text this morning (the BOPS is run by Ken Knabb, he was discussed earlier in some mails)
http://www.bopsecrets.org/recent/corona.htm

He doesn't seem to deal with any of the larger aspects that we discuss here, i.e. the "plandemic" angle in all of its potentially sinister manifestations... I assume he must be aware of them, it seems almost everyone is now, I mean those people who interest themselves in the issue

In fact he makes a lot of references to previous movements, like May '68, singing in groups, slogans, the Situationists, etc. that is, he treats it like a social movement whereas it seems like it is a fascist-techno-bio power grab

I was struck similarly by the Kissinger article where he discussed his youthful experience at the Battle of the Bulge and compared it with the present moment... I get the feeling that these men, each in his own way, want to relive what was for them an exciting youthful period in their lives... just a feeling

Pregnant Pause: Remarks on the Corona Crisis
Remarks on the coronavirus crisis, with links to other articles, songs, memes, etc.
www.bopsecrets.org

****

BUREAU OF PUBLIC SECRETS

PREGNANT PAUSE
— Remarks on the Corona Crisis —

We were already living in a general global crisis, but most people were only vaguely aware of it since it was manifested in a confusing array of particular crises — social, political, economic, environmental. Climate change is the most momentous of these crises, but it is so complicated and so gradual that it has been easy for most people to ignore it.

The corona crisis has been sudden, undeniable, and inescapable. It is also taking place in an unprecedented context.

If this crisis had taken place fifty or sixty years ago, we would have been totally at the mercy of the mass media, reading about it in newspapers or magazines or sitting in front of a radio or television passively absorbing whatever instructions and reassurances were broadcast by politicians or newscasters, with scarcely any opportunity to respond except perhaps to write a letter to the editor and hope that it got printed. Back then, governments could get away with things like the Gulf of Tonkin incident because it was months or years before the truth eventually got out.

The development of social media during the last two decades has of course dramatically changed this. Although the mass media remain powerful, their monopolistic impact has been weakened and circumvented as more and more people have engaged in the new interactive means of communication. These new means were soon put to radical uses, such as rapidly exposing political lies and scandals that previously would have remained hidden, and they eventually played a crucial role in triggering and coordinating the Arab Spring and Occupy movements of 2011. A decade later, they have become routine for a large portion of the global population.

As a result, this is the first time in history that such a momentous event has taken place with *virtually everyone on earth aware of it at the same time*. And it is playing out while much of humanity is obliged to stay at home, where they can hardly avoid reflecting on the situation and sharing their reflections with others.

[..]

- http://www.bopsecrets.org/recent/corona.htm

****

My statements about Knabb below are a bit harsh. I respect Knabb but I don't necessarily agree with him. Here're some examples of *why* I disagree with him:

"The corona crisis has been sudden, undeniable, and inescapable."

It's not really that "sudden" given how much prepping there's been for it. Event 201 is a pretty strong indicator that a major power-play was at hand that would use a pandemic as an excuse. Even independent of things like that there's been plenty of prepping in movies & books that I've mentioned elsewhere for at least the last 26 years. But, even more importantly to me, the idea that the corona crisis is "undeniable" seems particularly ridiculous. It's my assertion, & the assertion of many others, that COVID-19 is, indeed, *completely deniable* as an unprecedented plague. Instead, it strikes me as just-another-virus that would've hardly been noticed if it hadn't been so blown out of proportion by the mass media & the ensuing police state actions. It seems mind-bogglingly naive to me that Knabb seems to accept it as 'real'.

Furthermore, Knabb's belief in the internet as something that can't be used or compromised by mass media is also naive:

"The development of social media during the last two decades has of course dramatically changed this. Although the mass media remain powerful, their monopolistic impact has been weakened and circumvented as more and more people have engaged in the new interactive means of communication."

"As a result, this is the first time in history that such a momentous event has taken place with *virtually everyone on earth aware of it at the same time*."

It seems to me that it's precisely this aspect of the internet that's been thoroughly

exploited to enable mind control on an unprecedented level.

May 18, 2020, 11:24AM (Amir-ul Kafirs to group):

Re: HERETICS: Ken Knabb

In fact he makes a lot of references to previous movements, like May '68, singing in groups, slogans, the Situationists, etc. that is, he treats it like a social movement whereas it seems like it is a fascist-techno-bio power grab

I find that pathetic. As I told you, I had a brief correspondence with Knabb, it must've been in the late '90s. We traded, to his credit he was open to that. He expected me to want his Situationist Anthology but I wanted to know who HE was since he was the one I was trading with so I got his autobiography instead. I respect Knabb as the person who brought the most Situationist writing translated into English into the US. Alas, I don't remember his bio much, I vaguely remember finding it very dull. My retrospective feeling is that he's a BUREAUCRACTIVIST, meaning someone who spends most of his activist time in meetings. (I just coined that word today, by the by) Maybe that's doing him an injustice.

Anyway, I could claim to have been an anarchist political activist for roughly 50 years now. I'm not going to claim that I'm particularly 'important' in that area but I've participated in actual on-the-street activism and I've documented this somewhat online (http://idioideo.pleintekst.nl/IMPACTIVISM.html). I've also been published in anarchist magazines and published my own and published videos of activism. The point is that I can claim to've been active in ways that haven't always been exactly safe. On the other hand, there's a variety of activist that could be called "armchair activists", these are the activists who mostly have meetings and do very little else. Whether Knabb is that type or not I won't say because I really don't remember his bio well enough but my impression is that he fits in that category more than not.

I, too, have been involved with activism that centers around meetings and generally found it to be a negative experience. As I've mentioned before, I'm currently part of a neighborhood group called _____. Its purpose is to help people hurt by either getting sick or losing their income as a result of this pandemic. My minor job within the group is to monitor our email inbox and google voice mail on Mondays. In the 7 weeks or so that the group has existed I only know of ONE PERSON ASKING FOR HELP. One. That's in a neighborhood of, maybe, 2000 people. *SO*, what's happening is that the group is rediverting its energies to things like the Census, which I've expressed my opposition to, and a voting drive. I'm glad that the group was founded and I'm glad to be a participant but, ultimately, it's a Yuppie group that won't accomplish much of anything positive. Maybe if there had been an actual NEED we might've been of some use.

ANYWAY, what I'm getting at here is that it doesn't surprise me that Knabb is out-of-touch with what I, at least, consider to be 'harsh reality'. I think everything he does is framed by typical leftist tropes. What old leftists seem singularly unprepared for is for leftism to be co-opted and exploited for its cred. There's no way an old leftist is going to acknowledge that possibilitity. I've always said that I'm an anarchist but if there comes a time when 'anarchism' becomes circumscribed by things that I no longer consider to be real then I'll move on. In other words, it's dangerous to become too attached to an identity that can be manipulated into something that's no longer appropriate for you. I still think of myself as an anarchist but I do so partially to put a conceptual monkey wrench into the machinations of people using anarchism for non-anarchist purposes. The obvious example of this at present is people identifying as anarchists supporting a governor's decision.

I get the feeling that these men, each in his own way, want to relive what was for them an exciting youthful period in their lives... just a feeling

Yeah, "resting on their laurels" as the saying goes. I think you're probably right.

What's bizarre, and what's something that I keep returning to, is that 'leftists' seem to believe Rump's act that he's against all this. It's bizarre that the 'conservatives' are pro-Rump and anti-government. As I've been pointing out, Rump IS THE HEAD OF THE GOVERMENT THAT THE 'CONSERVATIVES' ARE AGAINST. This lockdown is happening during Rump's regime, regardless of how he presents his image in relation to it I don't think its happening now is a coincidence. 'Leftists' seem to think that by supporting the Medical Police State they're rebelling against Rump. I don't think that's true. I think Rump represents the Police State and that any embracing of it for any reason is supporting Rump.

****

May 18, 2020, 12:59PM (Dick to group):

Re: HERETICS: Ken Knabb

I answered Knabb by the way, thanking him for his text and sending some links to Spiro Skouras and Whitney Webb both of whom I like...I'll be curious to see if and or how he responds

****

May 18, 2020, 1:12PM (Amir-ul Kafirs to group):

Re: HERETICS: Ken Knabb

I think the odds favor his responding in a knee-jerk leftist way given that Skouras is funded by 'conservatives' you may be condescendingly informed that you're a dupe of right-wingers. Maybe I'm wrong, it's better to actually find out than it is to assume. I, personally, find Skouras to be pretty level-headed.

****

May 29, 2020, 8:20PM (Amir-ul Kafirs to group):

Did Knabb ever reply?

****

May 30, 2020, 6:30AM (Dick to group):

No, he never did.
There is a possibility my response went into his spam folder. It did have his message in the "object box" however

****

HERETICS did reply to the following "General Check-In" but there was some discomfort about the replies being used for this book. As such, in some cases the replies have been deleted altogether. Otherwise, they've been jumbled together & not credited to avoid any overly-revealing or embarassing information.

May 24, 2020, 8:43AM (Amir-ul Kafirs to group):

HERETICS: General Check-In

Hi folks, This is, as the subject heading suggests, a general check-in. In other words, I'm wondering how everyone is?

I'm almost taking it for granted that everyone's fine PHYSICALLY but I'm curious about how everyone is EMOTIONALLY & PSYCHOLOGICALLY.

I can certainly testify that I'm fine physically but that I'm barely holding it together emotionally & psychologically (even though I might be doing better than many or most people). I've been trying to psychoanalyze myself a little lately. A theory this morning is that I've had a life-long resistance to and antipathy for *fraud* and I must be feeling like FRAUD is being perpetrated on an unprecedented scale. This, in turn, makes me very angry and I work toward peacefully counteracting this fraud. Here's a story from my own life that could be used as a metaphor here:

I was lovers with a woman named _____. To make a long story short, her 2nd lover after me was a guy who was very young, very naive, and very very rich from inherited wealth. People told me that _____ and the rich guy were at a social gathering where they used a Ouija Board. This Ouija session 'revealed' that they were 'soul mates' from ancient Egypt. When I was told the story I hypothesized, knowing _____ well, that she wanted rich guy's money and that this "'soul mates' from ancient Egypt" was her way of getting her claws into him. I was ostracized for being so cynical. How could I not recognize this great love? _____ and rich guy got married and had a kid. She then proceeded to milk something like $1,000,000.00 from him (or so I've been told) that she spent on herself and on her opiate addictions shared with her lover(s) outside the marriage. After she'd more or less bankrupted him she split off. I don't recall anyone saying to me: *Gee, you were right! How naive and gullible we were!*

Now I feel like I'm witnessing something like this on a worldwide scale. I don't think we're going to be thanked afterwards for having been skeptical all along even if most people come around to positions similar to ours.

SO, how are you feeling? I'm truly curious. I think we're probably all disgusted and angry but do you sometimes look at yourself and think you're disproportionately angry? I really have to calm myself down! If someone were to physically attack me and catch me off-guard I'm afraid I'd kill them, that all my anger would flood to the surface. If you have any personal emotional and/or psychological observations I'd sure love to read them!

****

I am pretty much on Amir-ul Kafir's page. I have always had a passionate loathing for and rejection of all things I see as 'fake'... It just seems so natural to not like being blatently and deliberately lied to, and worse when everyone around you believes the BS and shames you for not being with the brainwashed herd. And now as a form of mass world control... And most of my 'friends' and coworkers knowingly hold their heads up high and pat themselves on the back for being 'informed' and understanding 'science'. It baffles and seriously alarms me. If there is any positive in this, I have always been very doubtful and self critical of my own intelligence... Innately seeing through so much of this from day 1, I feel a bit less intellectually challenged. It seems to me that we are hanging out with a bunch of brainless addicts that are in clear denial of their media addiction, take pride in elevating themselves by stomping on others, and who also enjoy the self pity that can be generated through enjoying pain and being controlled.

My emotional state is not great. I've had terrible anxiety and related insomnia for most of my life. I believe my anxiety mostly stems from being hyper critical of our society and from an inability to "fit in" with most people. Since age 9, when I realized that people used to drink clean, healthy water straight from rivers and streams, I've been distressed and angry at the world as it is. I've always wanted to live in a world where humans were more connected to and in harmony with nature. The older I get, the more I realize this is a idyllic dream that will never be fulfilled. The pleasure that so many people seem to find in staying indoors, ordering everything online and socializing mainly over computers, is giving me fears of a completely computerized AI world coming at us sooner than I had ever considered possible. I'm deeply concerned about the near future, if this "pandemic" will ever be over and what the world will look like when it is. This is putting my both my anxiety and my anger into overdrive.

I like to turn the radio on in the morning. NPR is always set and easy on my radio. Yesterday I turned it on to a show about what an antibody is and why our natural ones are not good enough. I lost it. I was so angry.

Yesterday, I saw a snake in the woods, took a photo, and put it on Instagram to see if anyone could identify it. Someone said it was a timber rattlesnake. Cool! She proceeded to tell me to "be safe" and "isn't that scary". A second person chimed in to tell me that juvenile snakes are more venomous than adults and that I should watch out. A third person added "thanks for the warning!" I wasnt warning anyone of anything! I saw a cool creature and wanted to know what species it was! These people are being caring and kind, right? Yet I felt full of anger. I can't handle the illogical fear. For one thing, I posted the picture after I was home, hours after being in contact with the deadly creature. Second, wild animals don't just attack people. The thing was just lying there on a rock in the sun. I end up feeling like an asshole for being mad at these well-meaning people. I have much less tolerance for humans than I did before. I used to feel generally misanthropic but still able to appreciate the individuals around me. I am more of a misanthrope every day and appreciate individuals less and less.

On the negative, I am socially withdrawing more, not reading enough or being creative enough. I am working on a balance that i see within reach.

Since I was about 9, I've also gotten upset at myself for thinking so differently, for being unable to fit in. I've wondered why I can see these things that other people can't (or won't) and at times it feels like a curse. My grandmother always told me, "You're too smart for your own good." I feel that now more than ever. I see others being comfortably dumb, and they appear to be quite happy. I suppose I get jealous as I obsessively think about things that make me unhappy. I find myself scrolling through my social media feed, something I usually don't do, looking for glimmers of hope, wanting to see posts by people who are thinking about these things critically. Ive found a few things to feel good about but mostly I end up angry, disappointed in people, lonely and depressed. Those feelings are usually followed by a frustration that I can't get others to see things the way that I do. That leads me to bad feelings about myself. I want to look at things rationally but not feel so emotional about it. I haven't figured out how to do that.

I've had to reassess my friendships. I have information and ideas that I'd like to share with my friends but I censor myself because I believe they will attempt to shame and bully me. I also fear for the loss of my job. This has already happened with a few people that I have spoken freely to. I'm realizing that most of these people arent actually my friends if I don't feel comfortable sharing my thoughts with them. On the other hand, I'm also very grateful for the few people that I can communicate with (including all of you).

I'm severely depressed today. I really need to stop the internet surfing but I can't help myself. I see the scare tactics and then I go seek out some positivity. It's getting old! I haven't been out-of-town since last August. So here I am, no escape and feeling shitty. June 1 around the corner! Good Grief. Full of rage for the partisan hacks out there, framing fucking Everything as usual in their self-serving world view. Watching the cop murder of George Floyd makes me want to drive halfway across the country in support. I never read Taibbi's I CAN'T BREATHE (Eric Garner) but I asked if I could borrow a friends copy like 2 weeks ago (unfortunately his doofus friend borrowed it first and then lost it!) and so this new news really upset me, it's been on my mind. I guess it could easily be anticipated. The cops are probably more crazy and yahoo than ever due to the pandemic. There hasn't been enough people around for them to feel manly-man and puff out their chests in public and boss us around. Fuck Them! Fuck the Partisan Hacks! Phew! Thanks for listening. I feel a little better.

I fall into self doubt. I feel uncomfortable with how much I am relating to and agreeing with my conservative friends and the libertarians in my family. While we can agree on this one thing, they inevitably say something overtly racist or homophobic or whatever and I question myself. I've felt grateful for the mostly conservative-identifying protesters who are speaking out. I question myself when a small number of those protesters are actually wearing Nazi symbols on their clothing. I wake up in the middle of the night, sick with anxiety, thinking- what if I'm completely wrong? What if I am really a selfish asshole who would rather do what I want than prevent the elderly from dying terrible deaths? What if masks really are effective and staying at home for a few months will make this virus go away? Over 80,000 people dead in America over the course of 3 months... That is terrible isn't it? How off is that number? Should I be more concerned about the sick and dying? It's not that I'm not concerned about them but.... self-doubt creeps in and is really bad for my mental and emotional state.

Yesterday, hoping to calm me down and make peace, a friend sent me some great clips of a mass media star, Bill Maher, who apparently is a liberal on our 'side' of this mess. This helped me immensely yesterday and I feel renewed hope things might get better. HBO lets him air this stuff... You tube has not taken it down. He even interviewed Matt Taibbi:

https://m.youtube.com/watch?v=6hLBmMXmC2k&list=TLPQMjMwNTIwMjBqvFHWHGifAQ&feature=youtu.be

https://m.youtube.com/watch?list=TLPQMjMwNTIwMjBqvFHWHGifAQ&v=28I5WyLp15o&feature=youtu.be#menu

https://m.youtube.com/watch?v=Lze-rMYLf2E&list=TLPQMjMwNTIwMjBqvFHWHGifAQ&feature=youtu.be

https://m.youtube.com/watch?v=4lxiJda-vPs&feature=youtu.be&list=TLPQMjMwNTIwMjBqvFHWHGifAQ

I am very excited to watch the Bill Maher videos. When all of this started I turned to my usual source of relief from political garbage. Usually TV personalities like John Oliver, Colbert, Trevor Noah, etc. at least give me some laughs about the bullshit. This time around, they are eating up the bullshit and regurgitating it all over my computer screen, so I had to stop watching before the vomit over took. (The exception is the episode of The Daily Show where Trevor Noah took off his pants and did part of his show in his boxer briefs. I felt quite happy at that and have watched the episode several times.)

Summary- The panic is making my pre-existing mental health issues much worse.

Thanks for asking!

****

May 24, 2020, 1:56PM (Amir-ul Kafirs to group):

Re: HERETICS: General Check-In

Thanks for the detailed report. I'm trying to wrap my head around more 'unconscious' elements of what we're going through & what you & others have to say contributes enormously.

One thing I've been saying fooooorrrrreeeeevvvvveeeeerrrr is that politicians *have to be liars* to truly represent their constituents because their consituents are liars too. The complicating factor is that I don't even exactly 'believe in truth' in the sense that life is far more complicated than that but I still think that the delusions & lies & deliberate misrepresentations really get in the way of clear-thinking. AND I SURE AS FUCK AM NOT GOING TO PRETEND TO BELIEVE SOMETHING I DON'T UNLESS I'M MAKING A PREPOSTEROUS JOKE.

pat themselves on the back for being 'informed' and understanding 'science'.

What do they really 'understand'? One of the best things about science is that it can outgrow its 'certainties'. Hence 2 mathematicians can elaborately assert that all reality can be described mathematically only to have Gödel come along & prove that that's impossible. Religion only changes when it has to co-opt something to maintain power. As such, I love science — but NOT when it's used as if it's another religion — which is pretty much what's happening now: that's part of why I make fun of the DOCTOR GODS.

I feel a bit less intellectually challenged.

The people in this small group are better than a breath of fresh air. You're all a breath of fresh ATMOSPHERE. Don't feel "intellectually challenged", just get to work & use the abilities that you have. One of the problems that we all have is what I call "having to swim up-dam", in other words, we're not just swimming upstream, we're trying to rise above a massive human construct of mental constipation. I'm confident that our sheer stubborness, with as much of a sense of humor as possible, helps.

It seems to me that we are hanging out with a bunch of brainless addicts that are in clear denial of their media addiction, take pride in elevating themselves by stomping on others, and who also enjoy the self pity that can be generated through enjoying pain and being controlled.

I've recommended Heinrich Mann's great novel "Der Untertan" before (it has various English translations, "Man of Straw" is the one I read) for an in-depth exploration of this unfortunate characteristic in humans. Essentially, people debase themselves in the hope of being able to debase others along the line.

It upsets me that I have to hone my lying and acting skills for fear of getting fired.

Maybe you don't really have to. There's an art to finding points of agreement in other people's talk & then using those to forge alliances. You don't have to be pushy or manipulative or LIE. You just only deal out small doses of what people might find difficult to take in larger quantities.

****

May 24, 2020, 10:57PM (Amir-ul Kafirs to group):

I believe my anxiety mostly stems from being hyper critical of our society and from an inability to "fit in" with most people.

Welcome to the non-crowd!

Since age 9, when I realized that people used to drink clean, healthy water straight from rivers and streams,

Fortunately, I don't think that possibility is completely gone. There're springs all over the place in my neighborhood & someone told me about someone they knew who actually had the water of one of them tested & found it to be drinkable.

I think I might not've mentioned here (I don't remember) that a water main broke in my neighborhood & the water company sent out an automated voice message explaining that people shd boil their water, etc, until notified that the water's safe again. WELL, this led to a tide of self-righteousness among people I know, outraged that their water was threatened & feeling that the water co wasn't doing their job right. I think this excess of spleen is yet another PANDEMIC PANIC byproduct. The reason why I call it an "excess" is because these water main breaks & related water distribution problems happen frequently. If the water starts to come out brown let it run at the lowest tap in the house until it's clear again. Yes, it's a drag but it's nothing new. In this case it didn't even come out brown in my house, there was a very brief drop in water pressure, I only noticed it for a few seconds. I never bothered to boil the water, I haven't gotten sick, I'm sure the red carpet of ululating fungus on my face will go away in a few days (JUST KIDDING!). The water co tested the water for bacteria twice, it came up clean both times & after about 36 hrs the company sent out another automated message saying it's ok to not boil it now.

Has anyone seen Ken Russell's 1970 movie about Tchaikovsky called "The Music Lovers"? Tchaikovsky dies in the end thrashing about in a fever of clean white sheets. He 'committed suicide' by drinking unboiled water during a cholera epidemic. In reality he would've died by shitting himself to death & going into fluid-loss shock. I would boil the water if I thought it might have cholera in it.

I've always wanted to live in a world where humans were more connected to and in harmony with nature.

Ah, well, you're not alone in this desire at least. There're still plenty of us who love being out in nature & paying attention to the non-human life. Today, I'm going to take someone to a secret sex club where humans & bears mess around (JUST KIDDING!).

fears of a completely computerized AI world coming at us

There's a SciFi book about a society of people who live in a giant shopping mall. The rich live outside it in a peaceful rural world. The residents of the mall can't leave. Eventually some of them revolt, capture one of the rulers, cut off their hand & use it to open a door to the outside that requires palm-print identification. SF predicts the dystopias but it usually depicts the way out too. Of course, these days there's plenty of SF that glorifies a 'virtual' future. I'm one of those old-fashioned types who has no intention of being subsumed by the net.

I'm deeply concerned about the near future

Me too. I'm glad to be able to admit that to you folks without having to even, really, explain.

A third person added "thanks for the warning!"

Not to point out the obvious to these people or anything but humans are the most dangerous creatures on the planet, by far. I'm definitely scared of crocodiles & alligators but if I decided to make a crusade of wiping them out I could get explosives & go to where they live & blow them to kingdom come — which they do NOT have the ability to do to me. As for the snakes, I sure as fuck wouldn't want to accidentally step on a rattler but the thought of seeing one is actually exciting not scary.

These people are being caring and kind, right?

They're being people who're seperated from, & therefore fearful of, nature. The same people who're terrified of stinging insects. Most creatures, except for humans, will leave you alone if you leave them alone. I've been stung by a bee ONCE in my entire life & that was when I stepped on it in my bare feet as a child. Bad move on my part.

****

May 25, 2020, 6:04PM (Dick to group):

For whatever it's worth I will respond by sending this poem by Whitman (see below), I think it expresses at least some part of the truth and may be helpful in dealing with the non-sense in the current world
*
I was walking down the street last night and a friend of mine was in a bar, so I went in and had some beers, the cops saw us and did nothing that was promising

Song of Myself, 3
Walt Whitman - 1819-1892

I have heard what the talkers were talking, the talk of the beginning and the end
But I do not talk of the beginning or the end.

There was never any more inception than there is now,
Nor any more youth or age than there is now,
And will never be any more perfection than there is now,
Nor any more heaven or hell than there is now.

Urge and urge and urge,
Always the procreant urge of the world.

Out of the dimness opposite equals advance, always substance and increase, always sex,
Always a knit of identity, always distinction, always a breed of life.

To elaborate is no avail, learn'd and unlearn'd feel that it is so.

Sure as the most certain sure, plumb in the uprights, well entretied, braced in the beams,
Stout as a horse, affectionate, haughty, electrical,
I and this mystery here we stand.

Clear and sweet is my soul, and clear and sweet is all that is not my soul.

Lack one lacks both, and the unseen is proved by the seen,
Till that becomes unseen and receives proof in its turn.

Showing the best and dividing it from the worst age vexes age,
Knowing the perfect fitness and equanimity of things, while they discuss I am silent, and go bathe and admire myself.

Welcome is every organ and attribute of me, and of any man hearty and clean,
Not an inch nor a particle of an inch is vile, and none shall be less familiar than

the rest.

I am satisfied—I see, dance, laugh, sing;
As the hugging and loving bed-fellow sleeps at my side through the night, and withdraws at the peep of the day with stealthy tread.
Leaving me baskets cover'd with white towels swelling the house with their plenty,
Shall I postpone my acceptation and realization and scream at my eyes,
That they turn from gazing after and down the road,
And forthwith cipher and show me to a cent,
Exactly the value of one and exactly the value of two, and which is ahead?

****

May 26, 2020, 3:41PM (Amir-ul Kafirs to group):

I end up feeling like an asshole for being mad at these well-meaning people.

A "well-meaning" person can do great harm. I often turn to my own family for examples of everything that I loathe in humans. Here's yet-another personal story (that I hope I haven't previously shared):

My mom & stepdad noticed a feral cat passing thru their suburban backyard. My stepdad built a shelter for it & they left food there as a way of caring for it & befriending it. When they finally got the cat to trust them, after something like 6 months, they took it somewhere to have it killed. I think it might've even been pregnant. As my mom explained in her typical 'loving' way: it was better to save it from the suffering of living in the wild. That was pretty much the way I was raised: with the general philosophy that I'd probably be better off dead than the way I was.

I am more of a misanthrope every day and appreciate individuals less and less.

Ha ha! Me too! But I still look for like-minded individuals all over the world. I'm desperate for company.

I want to look at things rationally but not feel so emotional about it. I haven't figured out how to do that.

My own 'solution' is to be 'proactive': to creatively counterbalance the increasing dumbing-down. It's time to 'smart-up'!

I believe they will attempt to shame and bully me.

The advantage that we have is that bullies are inevitably cowards. If someone wants to humiliate me they can be damned sure that I'm going to have an arsenal of sarcasm available that'll put their feeble attempts at language to shame. Of course, fighting back is a calculated risk.

Of course, I'm just an undercover agent gathering information on HERETICS so I can be given some sex slaves by the Police State (Sorry, but I've got to keep my priorities straight). JUST KIDDING. HERETICS help keep me Criminally Sane too. We're codependent HERETICS!

While we can agree on this one thing, they inevitably say something overtly racist or homophobic or whatever and I question myself.

Just because you agree on one thing doesn't mean you agree on everything. There're plenty of people who believe that the Earth is round. I agree with them. But it doesn't follow from that that I also agree that the world is God's tuna sandwich with extra mayo.

What if I am really a selfish asshole

That's an easy one to answer: If you're a selfish asshole then you never shit, you want to keep it all for yourself.

who would rather do what I want than prevent the elderly from dying terrible deaths?

Last time I looked, elderly people were going to die eventually anyway.

What if masks really are effective and staying at home for a few months will make this virus go away?

Even if it worked well for this virus it's not going to abolish all causes of sickness & death. All I ask for out of life is simple: right before I die I want to have every billionaire in the world lined up in front of me & I want to be given a machine gun. What happens next is anybody's guess. If the government can hand out trillions of dollars SURELY they can satisfy a tired old man's simple dying wish!

Over 80,000 people dead in America over the course of 3 months... That is terrible isn't it?

Not really, that would hardly put a dent in the population of Washington DC.

How off is that number? Should I be more concerned about the sick and dying?

As I keep saying, I'm not as afraid of dying as I am of having my Quality-of-Life deteriorate. I think I'd rather die fast than have the Medical Industry use me as an ATM until I'm useless for even that anymore.

It's not that I'm not concerned about them but.... self-doubt creeps in and is really bad for my mental and emotional state.

I hereby swear that I'm SURE that you have a SELF & that it's a doozie (in a positive sense). Since I'm an expert on the subject you're welcome to uncritically accept my word & move on.

This time around, they are eating up the bullshit and regurgitating it all over my computer screen

Ooohhh.. that's nasty. That's why when I lick my computer screen in moments of Virtual Reality frenzy I wear a dental dam.

The panic is making my pre-existing mental health issues much worse.

Ha ha! At least you're not BRAIN-DEAD YET!! That's more than I can say for most people (I, of course, am privy to the thoughts of billions of people & can, therefore, make such a generalization with full confidence that I'm absolutely correct).

****

May 27, 2020, 12:16PM (BP to group):

This is a good and proper way how to spend a lockdown, and to cheer up those glued to their computer screens:
The Swish Machine: 70 Step Basketball Trickshot (Rube Goldberg Machine)
https://www.youtube.com/watch?v=Ss-P4qLLUyk

****

May 27, 2020, 12:53PM (Amir-ul Kafirs to group):

I'm thinking of renaming my proposed book: "Unconscious Suffocation: Mind Control in the Era of COVID-19" because I think Unconscious Suffocation = Depression & there's alotof that going around.

Fuck Them! Fuck the Partisan Hacks! Phew! Thanks for listening. I feel a little better.

INDEED. My apologies to everyone for my too-minimal recent participation. I've been trying to copy all our emails into a text file so I can organize the ideas & check out all the links in chronological order so I can summarize the linked-to for the book. This is a HUGE job so I've been neglecting everything else. I'm only up to April 15!

HANG IN THERE EVERYONE!

****

May 27, 2020, 1:47PM (Naia Nisnam to group):

One of the Bill Maher videos is of him interviewing Dr. Katz. I've been following

Katz since he came to PA to consult with a hospital, our largest medical system. Dr. Katz is also a non-partisan, left-leaning, doctor talking a lot of sense in a way that should be acceptable to mainstream America. His basic message is- protect the vulnerable and let everyone else live their lives. His website has several interviews and podcasts that hes done as well as his plan for protecting the vulnerable. So far, his message isnt being heard or believed on a large-scale, but his drive to keep on putting the information out there gives me hope.
There is also a link on his site to a Senate Hearing on how to deal with the new information that we have about COVID. The hearing was interesting to listen to as I did other chores and I felt hopeful as several other doctors were giving testimony similar to Dr. Katz. These guys are very mainstream but probably our best hope at getting out of quarantine.
I wanted to include links to Dr. Katz's site as well as to the Senate hearing but my kids are distracting. I have to get them outside for a walk.

Have fun and be unsafe!

****

May 30, 2020, 10:36AM (Naia Nisnam to group):

Regarding workplaces sanitizing everything:

"...transmission of novel coronavirus to persons from surfaces contaminated with the virus has not been documented."

That's the CDC. They do go on to recommend sanitizing though there is zero evidence that it is necessary. There have been many scientific studies that have shown the risks of over sanitizing our environment. Why are they recommending something that is known to be harmful, while they also admit that there is no evidence saying it is helpful with stopping the spread of this virus?

https://www.cdc.gov/coronavirus/2019-ncov/prevent-getting-sick/cleaning-disinfection.html

****

Cleaning and Disinfection for Households

Interim Recommendations for U.S. Households with Suspected or Confirmed Coronavirus Disease 2019 (COVID-19)

Updated July 10, 2020

There is much to learn about the novel coronavirus (SARS-CoV-2) that causes coronavirus disease 2019 (COVID-19). Based on what is currently known about

COVID-19, spread from person-to-person of this virus happens most frequently among close contacts (within about 6 feet). This type of transmission occurs via respiratory droplets. **On the other hand, transmission of novel coronavirus to persons from surfaces contaminated with the virus has not been documented.** Recent studies indicate that people who are infected but do not have symptoms likely also play a role in the spread of COVID-19. **Transmission of coronavirus occurs much more commonly through respiratory droplets than through objects and surfaces, like doorknobs, countertops, keyboards, toys, etc.** Current evidence suggests that SARS-CoV-2 may remain viable for hours to days on surfaces made from a variety of materials. Cleaning of visibly dirty surfaces followed by disinfection is a best practice measure for prevention of COVID-19 and other viral respiratory illnesses in households and community settings.
It is unknown how long the air inside a room occupied by someone with confirmed COVID-19 remains potentially infectious. Facilities will need to consider factors such as the size of the room and the ventilation system design (including flowrate [air changes per hour] and location of supply and exhaust vents) when deciding how long to close off rooms or areas used by ill persons before beginning disinfection. Taking measures to improve ventilation in an area or room where someone was ill or suspected to be ill with COVID-19 will help shorten the time it takes respiratory droplets to be removed from the air.

[..]

- https://www.cdc.gov/coronavirus/2019-ncov/prevent-getting-sick/cleaning-disinfection.html

****

May 30, 2020, 11:25AM (Inquiring Librarian to group):

We are also 'quarantining' our book returns. Instead of library patrons tossing their returned books into our usual bookdrop, patrons must throw their returned items into 1 of 2 trash cans (1 labeled audiovisual and 1 books). At the end of each day, we wheel the trash can in and are instructed to spray the inside and outside of the can with Lysol and then let it all sit for 3 days b4 we check it in. CRAZY!! But i manage my small branch and must do it with a smile and positive conviction and try not to laugh or make dark humoured jokes when i sternly explain this 'life-saving' protocol to staff and patrons.

Needless to say, we all must wear masks all day in the building. I am a compulsive snacker, so this poses a logistical problem for me, plus my nervous fidgeting habits include, i have discovered, frequently touching my face and hand scrunching my often itchy nose. Remember, 'Don't touch your face!' Ha ha.

Luckily i have only 1 of 6 staff members who are obsessed with disinfecting themselves and everything. Her logic seems so moronic to me. But she is otherwise a kind and well meaning person. Luckily also, my maintenance person is pretty weak in the cleaning realm and everyone else is too lazy to do much cleaning themselves.

As ever, i am grateful to be getting a paycheck. I am grateful to connect again with my library patrons and staff. I have discovered waivering and weak belief from my sneaky polling of patrons on the pandemic. Only 1 patron seemed crippled with fanatical belief in the power of the virus and her complete trust in and adoration of the God Doctors and Big Brother. This woman severely annoyed me in that she spoke to me in a way that she expected me to confirm and share emotional outrage with her every word. I did my best to remain pleasant and resist her attempts to draw me into her hysteria. I did pull out of her that she knew no one sick of the virus... No one dead. But she was still married to "The Science!" and could not understand disbelievers (those she assumed to be trump supporters).

Another patron, 1 of my favorites, is an elderly man who is retired but does vaudville shows in retirement homes. He is on our side... Such a relief to hear!! He said every year during flu season he must take a break from his work bcuz of the flu season. No big deal for him. But he did say he cannot wait for someone to write about what really happened in the pandemic years from now. He too smells a rat. And, he and his wife went on to tell me that they have a friend who works as a cardiac care doctor. At 1 point he had 10 patients die of heart failure... He was told by his higher ups to change the coding of every death from heart failure to 'Covid 19'. Need i say more?

****

May 30, 2020, 12:44PM (Dick to group):

Have you all seen this?

https://www.activistpost.com/2020/05/battlefield-america-as-the-covid-story-falls-apart-a-new-crisis-takes-over.html?utm_source=Activist+Post+Subscribers&utm_medium=email&utm_campaign=3192e8deee-RSS_EMAIL_CAMPAIGN&utm_term=0_b0c7fb76bd-3192e8deee-388376415

Battlefield America: As The COVID Story Falls Apart, A New Crisis Takes Over - Activist Post

Hot Topics May 29, 2020 | Battlefield America: As The COVID Story Falls Apart, A New Crisis Takes Over; May 29, 2020 | At Least 9 Million US Households With Children Are "Not At All Confident" They'll Be Able to Afford Food Next Month, Census Survey Finds; May 29, 2020 | Announcing #ExposeBillGates Global Day of Action on June 13, 2020; May 29, 2020 | Scammers Exploit Pandemic to Peddle ...

****

Battlefield America: As The COVID Story Falls Apart, A New Crisis Takes Over

TOPICS: Civil UnrestDAHBOO777PoliceProtestSpiro Skouras
MAY 29, 2020
By Spiro Skouras
For months the global health pandemic known as the coronavirus or COVID-19 has been dominating the headlines while drastically changing the lives of billions of people around the world. With unprecedented restrictions of people's fundamental human rights, while simultaneously destroying the global economy, what is really going on?
Many have questioned the response from governments and global institutions such as the World Health Organization from the very beginning. Now, the CDC admits the mortality rate of the virus is much lower than previously projected, but the question remains why are we all still on lockdown?
Although the question for the need of continued lockdowns is now more important than ever, it seems to be lost as we are witnessing massive civil unrest spread across the US just as quickly as we were told the virus was spreading.

Are these protests spontaneous? Or is there an outside force facilitating the unrest, as we seem to be entering the second stage of a much larger operation? Is this the stage between phase one and phase two of the outbreak? A summer of chaos? In an election year, does it resemble shades of a Soros-sponsored color revolution, or a new form of Operation Gladio?
Regardless, it is almost impossible to deny the US, among many other nations, is in the midst of a rapid destabilization operation.

[..]

****

May 31, 2020, 7:18AM (Amir-ul Kafirs to group):

The Swish Machine: 70 Step Basketball Trickshot (Rube Goldberg Machine)

https://www.youtube.com/watch?v=Ss-P4qLLUyk

4 days later I finally took the time to check this out &, yes, it was amazing. I thoroughly enjoyed it as I do every 'Rube Goldberg' machine. STILL, 'I can't help' myself from making the 'inevitable' class analysis. This guy obviously lives in a home that makes social isolation very luxurious. He's not crowded in a city apartment. He has the toys around to cobble together into the machine. He can also get merch made to sell promoting his accomplishment. At least he took

advantage of his privilege to make something fun, I like him for that — but I have to admit that I'd be much more impressed if he'd done it under worse conditions (not that I'd wish those worse conditions on ANYONE).

****

May 31, 2020, 7:32AM (Amir-ul Kafirs to group):

Apparently masks are now mandatory for staff.

It's become *de rigeur* for maintaining the 'proper' 'caring' public image.

****

May 31, 2020, 8:25AM (Amir-ul Kafirs to group):

I read the brief article but didn't watch the linked-to movies or check out where any of the other links led to. I did note this:

"Are these protests spontaneous? Or is there an outside force facilitating the unrest, as we seem to be entering the second stage of a much larger operation? Is this the stage between phase one and phase two of the outbreak? A summer of chaos? In an election year, does it resemble shades of a Soros-sponsored color revolution, or a new form of Operation Gladio?
Regardless, it is almost impossible to deny the US, among many other nations, is in the midst of a rapid destabilization operation."

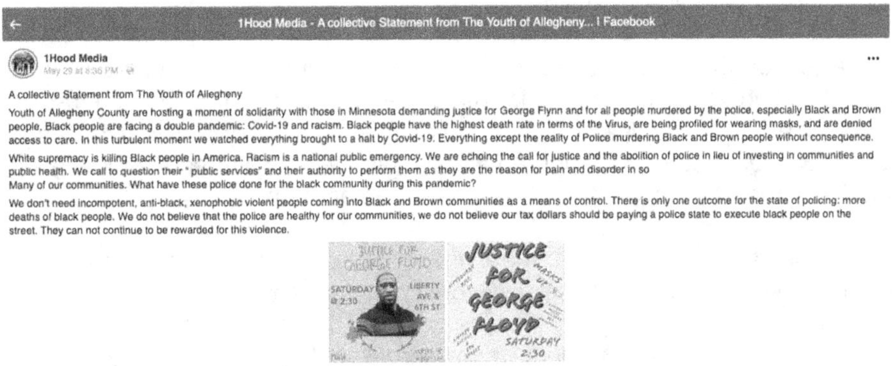

1Hood Media - A collective Statement from The Youth of Allegheny... I Facebook

1Hood Media
May 29 at 8:36 PM

A collective Statement from The Youth of Allegheny

Youth of Allegheny County are hosting a moment of solidarity with those in Minnesota demanding justice for George Flynn and for all people murdered by the police, especially Black and Brown people. Black people are facing a double pandemic: Covid-19 and racism. Black people have the highest death rate in terms of the Virus, are being profiled for wearing masks, and are denied access to care. In this turbulent moment we watched everything brought to a halt by Covid-19. Everything except the reality of Police murdering Black and Brown people without consequence.

White supremacy is killing Black people in America. Racism is a national public emergency. We are echoing the call for justice and the abolition of police in lieu of investing in communities and public health. We call to question their " public services" and their authority to perform them as they are the reason for pain and disorder in so
Many of our communities. What have these police done for the black community during this pandemic?

We don't need incompotent, anti-black, xenophobic violent people coming into Black and Brown communities as a means of control. There is only one outcome for the state of policing: more deaths of black people. We do not believe that the police are healthy for our communities, we do not believe our tax dollars should be paying a police state to execute black people on the street. They can not continue to be rewarded for this violence.

I went to a solidarity march yesterday in response to the murder of George Floyd. It was organized by a group called "One Hood". It was one of the most multi-cultural protests I've seen for a while & certainly a fairly large one: the masses of people stretched on for 3 or 4 blocks. It wasn't, of course, "spontaneous", it was organized & there were chants that had a similarity relevant to the subject of police murders & specifically to the murder of George Floyd; there were people with megaphones who led chants, there were people spray-painting graffiti that read "I Can't Breathe": echoing Floyd's last words. This protest was in downtown

Pittsburgh. On May 1, 2000, when I participated in a May Day Parade through the downtown financial district of Pittsburgh there was substantial police oppression — including, as I recall, snipers on roofs. On that occasion, police caused more or less all the problems & bogus charges were laid on 10 arrestees. The police maced people for no good reason, etc. The police were the problem, the parade was quite peaceful & good-natured.

Yesterday's solidarity march was very different. The visible police presence was very subdued, at least at the beginning. Bringing up the rear, in a very unobtrusive way, was a group of 5 cops on horseback who were waiting near the announced location of the end of the march. What interested me is that the horses were SHOW HORSES, the kind of horses that're only brought out for PARADES. These weren't the usual horses that cops ride on for the usual reasons. One was spectacularly dappled, another was a Clydesdale or something similar with fluffy hair groomed poodle-like above its feet. It didn't occur to me until later that these police were actually **participating in the solidarity march**. Now one can be cynical & say that's just PR. Regardless of what the case is, by the time the march had reached a point of chaotic climax these horse cops were being chased away by people throwing things like plastic water bottles. They trotted off w/o being confrontational themselves until they got a safer distance away while the protestors chanted: "Get those a-ni-mals off those horses!" Not long thereafter a cop car was set fire to. To say that it burned spectacularly, with a huge & long-lasting black smoke given off & the occasional pop of what I took to be exploding ammo in the car, would be an understatement. Who actually set fire to it I can't say. It could've been what I call Police Theater. While the burning of the vehicle provided entertainment for the likes of me it also provided the usual grist for the mass media mill of 'Peaceful Protest Turns Violent'. I never trust such things.

All in all, I thought it was a great show of solidarity. As I noted in some brief internet surfing yesterday, even the wife of Derek Chauvin, the cop apparently responsible for Floyd's death, has turned against him & is divorcing him. I'm told that the wife of another cop fingered him as the one who started the looting in St Paul (?). From my perspective, these instances are hopeful.

There were strange elements to the march. Almost everyone was masked. Obviously, in the past at such protests only people prepared to protect themselves against macing would've been masked. At one point 2 masked people, I think people I know but I wasn't sure who they were because their masks covered so much of their faces, pointed out a guy to me who they said had a gun tucked in the back of his pants that he kept touching. He was a part of a group of 5 or 6 guys who stayed very close to each other. I went to check them out to try to get a read on who they were & what they might be capable of. The guy who supposedly had the gun, I never saw it, was next to the only black guy in the group so it didn't seem to be a white supremacist group. I went & looked at the guys from the front. My impression was that they were rural right-wingers & that I didn't trust them. They struck me as jaded & potentially violent. But, then, I probably seem that way to other people too — the difference being, of course, that I don't own or carry a gun. I also have a sense of humor. I didn't get much of a sense of that from these guys, they seemed very grim. I have to say, though, that I think it's valid to wonder whether they were basically there for the same reason as everyone else: to protest police brutality. Just as it's possible that I might go to a dominantly right-wing protest against the lockdown it could be possible that some right-wingers might go to a dominantly leftist protest against police brutality. If I were to guess I'd say that all of these guys had probably done jail-time & had a deep hatred for cops.

Another strange thing about the march was that shortly before the horse cops started being chased, a young person looked me directly in the face & said something like: "Be careful, sir." That took me a little aback, why were they saying that to me? Almost immediately thereafter the crowd from the opposite end of the block starting running to my end & then people started chasing the horse cops. Maybe 5 or 10 minutes later the cop car blew up. The running crowd & cop chasing has cleared the area around the cop car enough so that no-one would be hurt by shrapnel. I had to wonder: did the person who warned me know that this was about to happen?

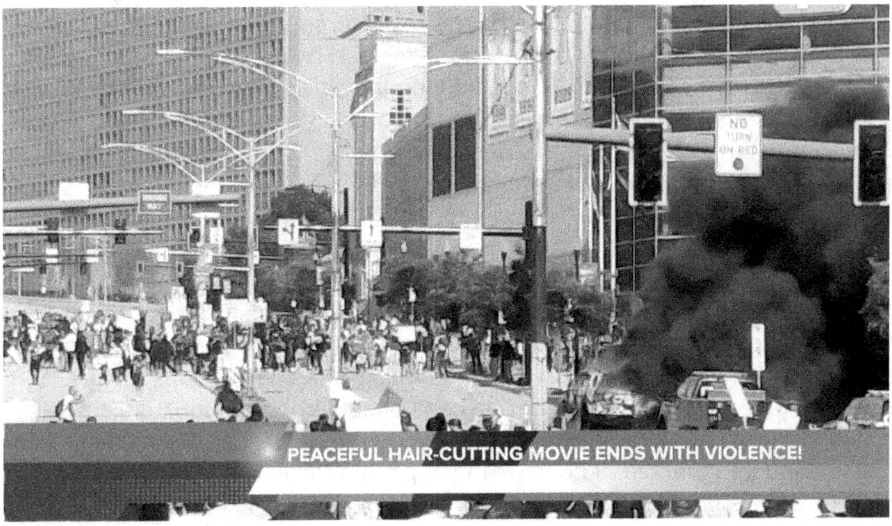
NO
TURN
ON RED
PEACEFUL HAIR-CUTTING MOVIE ENDS WITH VIOLENCE!

Whether this in any way supports Spiro Skirous's assertion that "it is almost impossible to deny the US, among many other nations, is in the midst of a rapid destabilization operation" is questionable to me in the sense that while I think that the lockdown is destabilizing I think that protests against the murder of George Floyd are a continuation of a long history of protests against entirely too many such murders & that I don't think this history plays very neatly into the current lockdown dilemma.

****

May 31, 2020, 6:16PM (Inquiring Librarian to group):

I am concerned about the incident with the cops on the horses being harangued and slandered by the protesters who just didn't know what was going on and who those cops on horses were. It is this kind of GroupThink gone wrong that upsets me so and keeps me away from all but any protest I feel I know too little about to angrily wave my opinion like a flag of riotousness. And these days, crowds freak me out.

****

May 31, 2020, 6:50PM (Amir-ul Kafirs to group):

who those cops on horses were.

That's just my theory, I can't definitely say what I was proposing is true. People who hate cops would strongly disagree with my theory &/or cynically denounce any hopes of positive intentions from cops as anything other than PR &/or say it doesn't matter anyway because there shouldn't BE ANY COPS NO MATTER WHAT. Most of my anarchist friends would probably fall into that latter category but would still call the cops in a pinch anyway. Personally, I've been arrested more than most of my friends & have been abused by cops in the process but, generally, have been treated OK considering the circumstances. I don't think this has been because of the infamous good-cop/bad-cop dynamic, I think it's more because most rank & file cops are basically working class people who're low on theory but not necessarily bad on character judgment.

It is this kind of GroupThink gone wrong that upsets me

There's definitely GroupThink in any large crowd situation, including, of course, protests. This always bothers me but I still make a point of joining the chants, e.g., when I'm in agreement with them. People's chasing the cops away yesterday was a way of saying that no cops should be there because it was a cop who killed the unfortunate George Floyd in the 1st place. I don't think that's completely unreasonable. I do think that if people really want these cop murderers to be prosecuted like any other murderers then people are going to have to accept that it's valuable to have their fellow cops reject them. Most cop-haters won't give an inch on that. To me that means that they're holding out for a 'perfect world' in which there're no cops. I, personally, won't hold my breath for that one. I'm not a reformist, perhaps I'm a pragmatist. If there's going to be a police department at all, which there is for the time being, I'd rather have it be one that won't have the backs of murderers like Chauvin anymore.

****

May 26, 2020, 4:29AM (Dick to group):

thought

I imagine i'm the last to realize this, but I think the reason why Washington State is particularly tough with this Covid-19 lockdown business is because it's the home of Microsoft... I imagine the governor is under pressure to do their bidding or lose their business

I signed up for Bill Gates blog...it's full of happy visions of the future... he seems to have an answer for everything

here's one that puts a smiley face on surveillance, this is the sub-title

"A new surveillance program in Seattle is detecting cases of COVID-19 and helping guide public health responses."

https://www.gatesnotes.com/Health/Seattle-Coronavirus-Assessment-Network

Scanning for answers to a pandemic | Bill Gates
In any fight, it's important to know your enemy. Unfortunately, in our battle against COVID-19, there's a lot that we still don't know. How many people are infected with the virus, including those without symptoms? Is it seasonal or weather dependent? And how will we know when it might be safe ...

****

SWAB, SEND, SOLUTIONS?

Scanning for answers to a pandemic

A new surveillance program in Seattle is detecting cases of COVID-19 and helping guide public health responses.

By **Bill Gates** I May 12, 2020 5 minute read

[..]

These are important questions. More testing, of course, will help us answer them. But with tests in short supply in many parts of the world, including the U.S., it is impossible to test everyone—at least for now.

That's why I'm excited about a new disease surveillance program in the Seattle area to detect cases of COVID-19 and help guide public health responses. Not only will it help improve our understanding of the outbreak in Seattle, it will also provide valuable information about the virus for other communities around the world.

The greater Seattle Coronavirus Assessment Network—or SCAN—is a first-of-its-kind disease surveillance platform for COVID-19 that allows participants to use a self-swab test to collect their own nasal samples and send them to a lab without leaving home. As a surveillance program, SCAN's goal isn't to test every person or serve as a replacement for medical care. Instead, SCAN is testing a sample of people in the Seattle region, including those who are healthy as well as those who are feeling sick. The test results and other data (like a person's age, gender, race, zip code, and any underlying health conditions) are used by researchers, data modelers, and public health officials to paint a clearer picture of how COVID-19 is moving through the community, who is at greatest risk, and whether physical distancing measures are working.

[..]

- https://www.gatesnotes.com/Health/Seattle-Coronavirus-Assessment-Network

****

May 31, 2020, 10:40AM (Amir-ul to group):

Re: thought

I imagine the governor is under pressure to do their bidding or lose their business

It would be interesting to research which billionaries live in which states & what the various PANDEMIC POLICIES are in those states & how those policies may or may not jive with vested interests of the billionaires. Gates stands to profit enormously from any surveillance tech embrace.

For starters there's this article below. The formatting changes make it a little difficult to read so here's the URL: https://patch.com/pennsylvania/philadelphia/meet-richest-person-pennsylvania

Business

Meet The Richest Person In Pennsylvania

Forbes identified the wealthiest person in each state. Meet Pennsylvania's richest:

By Max Bennett, Patch Staff

Jun 26, 2019 1:09 pm ET
|
Updated Jun 26, 2019 2:10 pm ET

PHILADELPHIA — Forbes analyzed the fortunes of the country's richest people to identify each state's wealthiest person. This is the magazine's fifth edition of the list.
Pennsylvania's richest resident is Victoria Mars, the Mars Inc. candy fortune heiress, who is worth $7 billion, according to Forbes.
Mars has long been featured on the list of Pennsylvania's richest residents due to her family's company. She serves as the candy and pet food company's Board of Directors Chairman.
Mars Inc. is known for iconic candies such as Twix, 3 Musketeers, Skittles, Milky

Way, and many more.
A Wharton School of Business grad, Mars inherited a roughly 8 percent stake in the company when her father, Forrest Mars Jr., died in 2016.
Mars Inc. was founded in 1911 in Newark, New Jersey by her great-grandfather Franklin Clarence Mars. In 2014, the company reported $33 billion in sales.
Mars' three sisters are also heirs to the company.
The net worth of the individuals on the list varies. For example, Washington is home to the world's two richest and most recognizable billionaires; Jeff Bezos and Bill Gates, but in certain states, the richest people only had a nine-figure net worth, Forbes writes.

The top 10 richest people on the Forbes list are:

1. Jeff Bezos & family: $157 billion (Washington)
2. Warren Buffett: $85 billion (Nebraska)
3. Mark Zuckerberg: $71 billion (California)
4. Michael Bloomberg: $53.8 billion (New York)
5. Jim Walton: $51.1 billion (Arkansas)
6. Alice Walton: $50.1 billion (Texas)
7. Charles Koch: $42 billion (Kansas)
8. Sheldon Adelson: $35.7 billion (Nevada)
9. Phil Knight & family: $35 billion (Oregon)
10. Jacqueline Mars: $28.1 billion (Virginia)

You can view the full list via Forbes of the richest people in every state.
Collectively, the wealthy on the Forbes list had a net worth of $875 billion, which the magazine says set a new record.

****

May 31, 2020, 11:47AM (Amir-ul Kafirs to group):

The URL for the 2nd relevant article is this: https://www.forbes.com/sites/jenniferwang/2019/06/26/the-richest-person-in-each-state-2019/#2f29413980d8

The names of the richest Americans in each state are as follows. It's interesting to see that people from the Mars candy family dominate THREE STATES. The Waltons dominate 2.

Alabama:
Jimmy Rane
Net worth: $900 million
Age: 72
Source of wealth: lumber
Residence: Abbeville, Alabama

Alaska:
Leonard Hyde, Jonathan Rubini & families
Net worth: $300 million each
Age: 62, 64
Source of wealth: real estate
Residence: Anchorage, Alaska

Arizona:
Ernest Garcia II
Net worth: $5.6 billion
Age: 62
Source of wealth: used cars
Residence: Tempe, Arizona

Arkansas:
Jim Walton
Net worth: $51.1 billion
Age: 71
Source of wealth: Walmart
Residence: Bentonville, Arkansas

California:
Mark Zuckerberg
Net worth: $71 billion
Age: 35
Source of wealth: Facebook
Residence: Palo Alto, California

Colorado:
Philip Anschutz
Net worth: $12 billion
Age: 79
Source of wealth: investments
Residence: Denver, Colorado

Connecticut:
Ray Dalio
Net worth: $18.4 billion
Age: 69
Source of wealth: hedge funds
Residence: Greenwich, Connecticut

Delaware:
Robert Gore & Elizabeth Snyder
Net worth: $885 million each
Ages: 82, 72
Sources of wealth: Gore-Tex

Florida:
Thomas Peterffy
Net worth: $18.8 billion
Age: 74
Source of wealth: discount brokerage
Residence: Palm Beach, Florida

Georgia:
Jim Kennedy
Net worth: $9.2 billion
Age: 71
Source of wealth: media, automotive
Residence: Atlanta, Georgia

Hawaii:
Pierre Omidyar
Net worth: $13.5 billion
Age: 52
Source of wealth: eBay, PayPal
Residence: Honolulu, Hawaii

Idaho:
Frank VanderSloot
Net worth: $3.5 billion
Age: 70
Source of wealth: nutrition, wellness products
Residence: Idaho Falls, Idaho

Illinois:
Ken Griffin
Net worth: $11.7 billion
Age: 50
Source of wealth: hedge funds
Residence: Chicago, Illinois

Indiana:
Carl Cook
Net worth: $9.5 billion
Age: 56
Source of wealth: medical devices
Residence: Bloomington, Indiana

Iowa:
Harry Stine
Net worth: $3.8 billion
Age: 77
Source of wealth: agriculture
Residence: Adel, Iowa

Kansas:
Charles Koch
Net worth: $42 billion
Age: 83
Source of wealth: Koch Industries

Residence: Wichita, Kansas

Kentucky:
Tamara Gustavson
Net worth: $5.3 billion
Age: 57
Source of wealth: self storage
Residence: Lexington, Kentucky

Lousiana:
Gayle Benson
Net worth: $2.9 billion
Age: 72
Source of wealth: pro sports teams
Residence: New Orleans, Louisiana

Maine:
Susan Alfond
Net worth: $1.7 billion
Age: 73
Source of wealth: shoes
Residence: Scarborough, Maine

Maryland:
Ted Lerner & family
Net worth: $5.1 billion
Age: 93
Source of wealth: real estate
Residence: Chevy Chase, Maryland

Massachusetts:
Abigail Johnson
Net worth: $14.7 billion
Age: 57
Source of wealth: money management
Residence: Milton, Massachusetts

Michigan:
Daniel Gilbert
Net worth: $6.8 billion
Age: 57
Source of wealth: Quicken Loans
Residence: Franklin, Michigan

Minnesota:
Glen Taylor
Net worth: $2.9 billion
Age: 78

Source of wealth: printing
Residence: Mankato, Minnesota

Mississippi:
Thomas Duff & James Duff
Net worth: $1.35 billion each
Ages: 62, 58
Source of wealth: tires, diversified
Residence: Hattiesburg, Mississippi

Missouri:
Pauline Macmillan Keinath
Net worth: $6.9 billion
Age: 85
Source of wealth: Cargill
Residence: St. Louis, Missouri

Montana:
Dennis Washington
Net worth: $6.2 billion
Age: 84
Source of wealth: construction, mining
Residence: Missoula, Montana

Nebraska:
Warren Buffett
Net worth: $85 billion
Age: 88
Source of wealth: Berkshire Hathaway
Residence: Omaha, Nebraska

Nevada:
Sheldon Adelson
Net worth: $35.7 billion
Age: 85
Source of wealth: casinos
Residence: Las Vegas, Nevada

New Hampshire:
Andrea Reimann-Ciardelli
Net worth: $720 million
Age: 62
Source of wealth: consumer goods
Residence: Hanover, New Hampshire

New Jersey:
John Overdeck
Net worth: $6.1 billion

Age: 49
Source of wealth: hedge funds
Residence: Millburn, New Jersey

New Mexico:
Mack C. Chase
Net worth: $700 million
Age: 88
Source of wealth: oil
Residence: Artesia, New Mexico

New York:
Michael Bloomberg
Net worth: $53.8 billion
Age: 77
Source of wealth: Bloomberg LP
Residence: New York, New York

North Carolina:
James Goodnight
New worth: $9.1 billion
Age: 76
Source of wealth: software
Residence: Cary, North Carolina

North Dakota:
Gary Tharaldson
Net worth: $1 billion
Age: 73
Source of wealth: hotels
Residence: Fargo, North Dakota

Ohio:
Les Wexner & family
Net worth: $4.7 billion
Age: 81
Source of wealth: retail
Residence: New Albany, Ohio

Oklahoma:
Harold Hamm & family
Net worth: $11.8 billion
Age: 73
Source of wealth: oil & gas
Residence: Oklahoma City

Oregon:
Phil Knight & family

Net worth: $35 billion
Age: 81
Source of wealth: Nike
Residence: Hillsboro, Oregon

Pennsylvania:
Victoria Mars
Net worth: $7 billion
Age: 62
Source of wealth: candy, pet food
Residence: Philadelphia, Pennsylvania

Rhode Island:
Jonathan Nelson
Net worth: $1.8 billion
Age: 63
Source of wealth: private equity
Residence: Providence, Rhode Island

South Carolina:
Anita Zucker
Net worth: $1.8 billion
Age: 67
Source of wealth: chemicals
Residence: Charleston, South Carolina

South Dakota:
T. Denny Sanford
Net worth: $2.5 billion
Age: 83
Source of wealth: banking, credit cards
Residence: Sioux Falls, South Dakota

Tennessee:
Thomas Frist Jr. & family
Net worth: $11.7 billion
Age: 80
Source of wealth: hospitals
Residence: Nashville, Tennessee

Texas:
Alice Walton
Net worth: $50.1 billion
Age: 69
Source of wealth: Walmart
Residence: Fort Worth, Texas

Utah:

Gail Miller
Net worth: $1.5 billion
Age: 75
Source of wealth: car dealerships
Residence: Salt Lake City, Utah

Vermont:
John Abele
Net worth: $640 million
Age: 82
Source of wealth: health care
Residence: Shelburne, Vermont

Virginia:
Jacqueline Mars
Net worth: $28.1 billion
Age: 79
Source of wealth: candy, pet food
Residence: The Plains, Virginia

Washington:
Jeff Bezos & family
Net worth: $157 billion
Age: 55
Source of wealth: Amazon
Residence: Seattle, Washington

West Virginia:
Jim Justice II
Net worth: $1.5 billion
Age: 68
Source of wealth: coal
Residence: Lewisburg, West Virginia

Wisconsin:
John Menard Jr.
Net worth: $11.4 billion
Age: 79
Source of wealth: home improvement stores
Residence: Eau Claire, Wisconsin

Wyoming:
John Mars
Net worth: $28.1 billion
Age: 83
Source of wealth: candy, pet food
Residence: Jackson, Wyoming

****

May 31, 2020, 5:37PM (Dick to group):

you might like this Amir-ul Kafirs, he says something at around 12 minutes that echoes your thoughts...

https://www.youtube.com/watch?v=5_sWQKFhelo

Health Officials Admit Virus Not As Deadly As Previously Thought: So Why Are We Still On Lockdown? - YouTube
We have started to see official government health institutions like the CDC for example, quietly admit that the virus is much less dangerous than what we wer...

****

May 31, 2020, 8:20PM (Amir-ul Kafirs to group):

I checked out the 1st 18 minutes. As usual, I found it interesting, ominous, & mostly believable. At minute 12 the guest was talking about snitching, I don't remember his having anything remarkable to say about that but, of course, I agree about the idiotic reprehensibility of it. I think what interests me more is the ID cards that'll not only list one's health report but also one's purchasing history — might as well throw in browsing history too, eh? The point is: all that is believable precisely because it's already here — at least the purchasing history is if one notices how products are advertised to you online. Alas, also as usual, I don't currently have the patience to sit thru the entirety of any of these longer videos. I'd rather be doing something else — such as working on my own movies. I don't mean that doing so isn't worthwhile, I'm just not in the mood. Another note on this latest of Skouras's: his guest is wearing a RAMONES t-shirt. The Ramones are just about the only punk band that I know of & like that had a more leftist member (Joey) & a more right-wing member (Johnny). Johnny liked George W. Bush. As such, it's hard for me to not see the Ramones as a symbol of a 'unification' of right & left — even though the band members seem to've mostly hated each other!

"Everyone in Quarantine for Maximum Harm"

- Naia Nisnam, Parent and child advocate, Pennsylvania

In March, we were told that we would have to quarantine for 15 days so that the medical system was not overwhelmed by the new coronavirus. We were told that the virus would spread but that most of us would be able to fight off the infection without medical care. We were told that we needed to spread out the infection rate so that our hospital system would have enough resources to care for the most vulnerable people, the people at high risk of serious complications from the virus. The order came from the governor of Pennsylvania, as similar orders came from various governors across America, as similar orders were given around the world. It felt like a reasonable request at the time so I, and it seems most everyone else, complied. It was a scary time but what we doing seemed to make sense.

After two weeks, the lockdown order was extended. No laws had been passed. I could tolerate the alleged need for an immediate response when we didn't know what we were facing and wanted to save our health care resources for those who needed it. That time came and went, yet we continue with isolation. There was never an announcement that our objective had changed. We were never told that our goal had shifted from not overwhelming the health care system to completely stopping the spread of the virus. Why did that goal change? Why was there no announcement, no public discussion, no debate, and most importantly no legislative acts? The official story changed without notification, discussion or justification. I followed news of the virus closely and began to question what was really happening.

I began to research, almost obsessively, digging deeper, reading articles from doctors and scientists around the world. It was around this time that I was invited to join the Heretics email group and it was a great relief to be a part of the tiny global network of free-thinkers who also sensed something bigger going on behind the scenes, who were also researching a wide variety of international sources. I found much needed solace and comradery in a group of people I had never met.

What I found confirmed my suspicions that there was something more going on than what we were told. I found doctors from all across the political spectrum, doctors with nothing to gain and often a lot to lose by speaking their truths. The head of emergency medicine at our major medical center told the public, in April, that Covid-19 wasn't nearly as deadly as we had initially thought. Our local hospitals never came close to reaching capacity. The initial scare of overrunning the hospital system had, as I had suspected, passed. Doctors and scientists from various fields were suggesting a different approach. Several doctors testified in the U.S. Congress, recommending new approaches based on the what they'd learned from studying the new virus. The proposed new approach, labeled by some as the "total harm minimization" strategy, was to focus on protecting the most vulnerable while allowing the rest of society to return, more or less, to the way things had been before the March lockdown.

Below is one doctor's suggested harm minimization plan. I

have found a variety of doctors advocating for similar plans. I don't think this one plan is necessarily the ultimate answer but I believe working with this plan and similar ideas from other doctors and scientists would lead to a workable solution that would not attempt to eliminate the virus completely, which is not realistic, but would allow it to spread through the population of people that can fight if off with their immune systems, thus leading to herd immunity. Healthy people would be exposed to and survive the virus so that the high-risk population would not have to expose themselves to the danger. This type of plan would also decrease and spread out the rate of infections in people that may need hospital treatment.

David L. Katz, MD, MPH *3/22/20*

Risk & Vulnerability-based Interdiction Responses to SARS-CoV-2 (RaVIRS)

Stratified sets of personal and public policy interdiction policies and practices for coronavirus (SARS-CoV-2) predicated on levels of vulnerability to severe infection and risk for death from infection.

	Risk Tier*	Public Policies*
• Shelter-in-place; strict social distancing including from family members; strict personal sanitation routine	***High Risk***: >= age 75 Treated heart disease, diabetes- any age Medically treated or induced immunocompromise, any age Chronic lung disease, any age Other	• Restricted from worksites/schools • Restricted from social gatherings • Routine, mobile testing • Digital health monitoring • Home service support (food delivery, other) • Home care as needed • Institutional shelter (e.g., idled hotel space) as needed • Early anti-viral treatment as needed
• Strict social distancing; strict personal sanitation routine	***Service Providers to High Risk***: Health professionals First responders Home service	• Routine testing, clearance/approval • Personal protective equipment
• Routine social distancing; personal sanitation	***Intermediate Risk***: Age 60-74 Well controlled medical condition Mild/moderate asthma	• Work, social gathering precautions/warnings • Restricted from interaction with High Risk individuals
• Routine social distancing; personal sanitation	***Low/Average Risk***: <age 60 Good health	• Restricted from interaction with High Risk individuals

**risk categories to be defined, updated, promulgated to public by suitable authorities- e.g., CDC, NIH, WHO, etc. Similarly, recommended practices and policies for interdiction/risk minimization to be updated and disseminated routinely by the same authorities based on most current data.*

The harm minimization models look at all of society, not just the small percent that could be adversely affected by the virus. Why do we continue using a blanket-method of so-called protections? Why have these other potential models never been discussed? Why has this concept never seen airtime on any mainstream news channels, despite being promoted by a variety of doctors? Why does the average citizen have no concept of this type of model as a possibility? The more unanswered questions I had, the more suspicious I became.

There is a clear correlation between severe infection, age, and underlying health conditions. It is quite possible to identify people in the high-risk group. It is possible to do more to protect those high-risk individuals (if they want to be protected) than we have been doing. As we are now very slowly pretending to reopen the economy, there is no differentiation between who is sent back to the workforce. For example, I know someone who is 73 years old, obese, has high blood pressure and diabetes. She was called back to work. I am in my 40s and as healthy as can be but my job working with children had been deemed non-essential and I have not been allowed to return to work. Why aren't the vulnerable provided with the choice to stay home from work, to be the ones to collect unemployment, to have their shopping items delivered to their homes for free?

While searching for answers to those questions, I came across a horrific truth. As we were all in the early stages of lockdown to protect the vulnerable, the vulnerable were not being protected where they lived. In other sections of this book you should find information about people who tested covid positive being intentionally moved into nursing homes. I cannot understand why this would be done and out of all of the many things that don’t add up, this is the one that has bothered me the most. Why would these governors of Pennsylvania, New York, New Jersey, Michigan, Connecticut, and Massachusetts, (and possibly more) order nursing homes to take in covid 19 positive people? They were apparently advised to do so by Christopher Murray, director of the IHME model, with the justification of keeping the hospitals empty... to treat covid patients. It makes no sense. There was more than enough hospital capacity everywhere except maybe New York City. The governors that ordered this also ordered healthy children home from schools and healthy adults home from work. If they believed the virus to be so deadly, then they also knew that they were endangering nursing home patients. Why would they do such a thing? Many people are calling for a criminal investigation into the actions of these governors, to find an explanation for why this happened. I realized that the "protect the vulnerable" dialogue is not based on fact but is used as a ploy to get people to continue to comply with and not question the orders they are given. I still couldn't figure what was really going on but I saw this as one of several ways that the number of deaths was forced to be higher than it naturally would have been.

Those of us who oppose the lockdown are branded selfish and told that we don't care about others. I would argue that the opposite is true. It is selfish to shut down the entire world and damage a huge percentage of the population while continuing to allow the vulnerable to be at risk. There are too many adverse effects to justify continuing on this path. Too many people continue to live in fear and isolation. That in and of itself is not healthy. The way we are currently forced to live is truly the definition of unhealthy. People are stressed, depressed and anxious. Most therapists and psychologists have not been seeing patients in person for almost five months and many of us are unable to receive proper care over a phone call or video chat. I don't have a large circle of friends anymore, but I know one person who has attempted suicide and another who has admitted to me that he considers it as an option. We know that humans are social creatures, even the most anti-social among us need some sort of interaction with others. I believe that isolation is killing people. Children are missing out, on education yes, but more importantly on physical play and socialization with their peers. Children are not learning interpersonal skills and we are seeing setbacks in their social and emotional growth. Children and adults with special needs are suffering greatly, as are their families that rely on outside care, day programs, physical therapy, and in-home visits. Drug abuse and alcoholism are on the rise, with many people who had been sober for years now returning to prior addictions as a result of the isolation and ensuing mental health issues. Domestic abuse and child abuse are reportedly on the rise though we cannot be sure how many cases we are missing simply because there is no one to witness, no one to report the abuse. Am I selfish because all of these people matter to me? I don't think so. Focusing solely on a virus that affects a specific subsect of the population, while dismissing everyone else's suffering as a sidenote, is absolutely selfish.

The mainstream media sensationalize suffering and death, as they always have. When deaths are down, they focus on the number of cases. We will not save every soul from dying of covid complications; that is not a realistic possibility to strive for. People do die, and while our medical system and society in general focus on keeping everyone alive for as long as possible, regardless of quality of life, we must learn to accept that death is an unavoidable part of life. Living in constant fear of sickness and death is really no way to live but it does ensure ratings. As the death rate in my state drops, after our hospitals never neared capacity, the governor's orders increase rather than decrease. Demands for transparency, for the facts that support his orders, have been denied. It seemed as if our economy was intentionally being destroyed, but why would anyone do that?

The bipartisan divide in America has gotten so bad that very few people have thoughts outside of party lines. Most Republicans see the unjust lockdowns as an attempt by Democratic governors to keep the economy in ruins to prevent Trump from winning the November election. Democrats and other liberal leftists blame everything on Trump. They claim that it was his poor handling of the pandemic that led us into this mess. I wish I could believe that this will all be over after November, but it won't, regardless of who wins. Too many Americans are so busy blaming the opposing political party that they are blind to this being a global phenomenon. Too many of my friends are so preoccupied with blaming everything on Trump and his supporters that they cannot see the bigger picture. It is sadly disappointing.

I used to have friends that were also free-thinkers, that knew that the mainstream media thrived on fear mongering, that politicians from both sides of the spectrum told whatever lies that served them, that the rich and powerful world leaders did not have our best interests at heart. Now my friends love eating up and regurgitating the mainstream news narrative, and conveniently blaming the other major political party while self-righteously denouncing anyone with differing opinions. Precious few people seem interested in being exposed to alternate ideas, to any sort of questioning. Somehow most people, including people that used to stand by me at anti-globalization protests, are intentionally blind to the fact that this is part of a global agenda. It was a fellow Heretic who first led me to the video of the World Economic Forum discussing their plans to reset the global economy as a response to the pandemic.

That isn't a conspiracy, as you should see in other parts of this book. The global reset has been publicly announced and the information can be found on the website of the World Economic Forum. It makes even more sense when taken into account with Event 201, which is also a real thing that happened and not part of a conspiracy theory. The information about that project is also open to the public. I still have questions, but I think I've found the root of what is really going on. I see a very small number of people on the right that have caught on to the globalization agenda but the left seems happy to not question. Intentionally timed or not, the WEF announced their plan the week after the George Floyd murder, ensuring that former anti-globalization activists were distracted by protests. Even if the left did notice what was being planned, I'm not sure that they would care. From the beginning we were led to accept the concept of a "new normal". When the WEF talks about their global reset they do so in a way that would appeal to the left. Saving the environment, promoting global equality, etc. It's all made to sound like a swell new utopia. Liberals now seem so easily deceived, so ready to believe that people in power have their best interests at heart while greatly restricting their freedoms. I can imagine so many leftists loving the concept of a new normal devised in secret by a small group of the richest and most powerful technophiles the world has ever seen. Despite my talking about this to many people, no one outside of the heretics have looked into it. It is easier and more comfortable for them to write me off as a conspiracy theorist, to compare me with nazis, to tell me that I'm using right-wing talking points. I have lost friends throughout this process but I don't need friends who condemn me for being a skeptical, free thinking, seeker of truth.

HERETICS emails - June, 2020

June 2, 2020, 10:02AM (Amir-ul Kafirs to group):

HERETICS: Belarus

I have a friend in Belarus who's been sending me pictures of propaganda there. I can't understand it so I found this article online to check into what's happening. Lukashenko is widely lambasted by the 'western world' as a 'dictator' but I didn't realize that he's also hated in Russia. I know that my Belarusyn friends don't respect him but that's to be expected. ANYWAY, I found the following article very interesting. Lukashenko is presented as a covid-19 DENIER WHO HASN'T IMPOSED ANY RESTRICTIONS & the country reports a very low death rate. I'll assume that the low death rate is not realistic but I'd love to know what IS realistic?!

The leader of Belarus is using the coronavirus crisis to troll Putin

Strongman's country has emerged as the Sweden of the post-communist world.

By **VIJAI MAHESHWARI** 5/19/20, 4:15 PM CET Updated 5/20/20, 4:01 PM CET

Vijai Maheshwari is a writer and entrepreneur based in Moscow. He tweets at @Vijaimaheshwari.

MOSCOW — Belarus' football team Dinamo Brest was, until recently, a minor squad in an obscure Eastern European nation, whose only claim to fame was winning the local Premier League title last year. However, with the country's league still playing games while the rest of the world has shut down, interest in the team — and Belarussian football — has spiked globally.

India, Israel and a host of other countries, including Belarus' neighbor Russia, have bought rights to air matches. The enterprising team has even begun selling virtual tickets online for €25, with fans rewarded with having their pictures pasted on top of a mannequin inside the stadium.

It's a sharp contrast with what's happening in Vladimir Putin's Russia, and Belarus' eccentric dictator Alexander Lukashenko has not been shy about highlighting the differences.

While Putin has followed the rest of the world in imposing a lockdown as coronavirus cases have surged there, Lukashenko has scoffed at such restrictions as "coronapsychosis" and kept his country open for business despite criticism from the World Health Organization.

And while his nemesis in Moscow has holed up in his country estate and retreated from public view as the crisis has intensified — prompting Press Secretary Dmitry Peskov to dismiss rumors that Putin was "waiting out the pandemic in a bunker" — pugnacious Lukashenko has sought out the spotlight instead.

Lukashenko is relishing his role as a COVID-19 denier and has claimed that drinking vodka, having saunas and driving tractors will keep the virus at bay.

He has continued playing ice hockey in front of fans, and upstaged Putin by holding a live military parade — with thousands of soldiers and elderly veterans of the war — to commemorate the Soviet Union's victory over Nazi Germany on May 9, while neighboring Russia canceled its celebrations.

"In this insane, disoriented world there will be people who condemn us … but we had no choice," Lukashenko declared defiantly at the parade, as thousands of spectators without masks thronged the bleachers. "Let the parade in Minsk today be the only one in the post-Soviet world."

[..]

- - https://www.politico.eu/article/belarus-lukashenko-is-defying-the-coronavirus-and-putin/

****

June 2, 2020, 10:06AM (Phil to group):

HERETICS: A quick update from amsterdam....Protest and work

Yesterday I went to a protest in Dam Square in support of the whole uprisings happening after the George Floyd incident. Quite some thousands there. Very peaceful and a good vibe. The police approach was very hands off which was good to see. I think I only saw about 5 cops there. I am sure there were more somewhere else and plenty on standby. Police responses to situations can vary quite a bit here depending on the particular cops in charge I guess. Generally speaking most protests and rallies go fine it is more squat actions and squat related issues where I have seen more heavy handed cop action. Having said that though there has been some heavy handed violent approaches to protests related to racial issues here in Netherlands especially in regards to Swarte Piet, more or less Santas little helpers here in the Netherlands. Swarte Piet for those unfamiliar is dutch people wearing back face and is a 'tradition' that comes from

the slavery era (not that we are not still in a slavery era). When I first came here many activists who grew up with Swarte Piet defended it in many ways claiming it was not racist. However slow but effective campaigns have been building over the years changing Dutch opinion and slowly changing Swarte Piets appearance and banning full blackface for Swarte Piet. Anyway here are some photos I took of yesterdays protest.
https://www.flickr.com/photos/kareneliot/albums/72157714543179753

Restaurants are back open here which means that I am back at work. They opened on the 1st of June and will practice social distancing for one month which means we can only serve half as many customers. I worked on Sunday so the restaurant was not actually open yet. I worked in the kitchen alone preparing food to be ready for the opening. There were two service staff upstairs preparing the service area and selling bread to take away and coffees. I was working without gloves and without a mask. The whole mask thing was never mandatory here in the Netherlands which I am so glad of. Mostly people don't wear them although they were recommended for public transport. I saw that there was a box of masks next to the boxes of gloves but only one box. At some point my boss (not the store manager but the boss who owns the Amsterdam franchise of _____) came into the kitchen trying to workout how to reprogram the oven for some different bread we have to bake (the bread actually comes from Belgium prebaked). It was only then that I realised I was working without gloves but the boss didn't say anything. I don't think he cares really. Only cares that we appear to be concerned. I did put on gloves though after that just because I thought I should look like I am doing the right thing and wearing gloves aint such a big deal. I was mostly cutting cheese. My next shift is tomorrow and the coming weekend.

****

June 2, 2020, 11:13AM (Amir-ul Kafirs to group):

Re: HERETICS: A quick update from amsterdam....Protest and work

Thanks for the update. Judging from what you wrote, things seem more sane in Amsterdam than they are here. Things here seem more insane than ever. I'll write about that more in a separate post. Naia Nisnam tells me that we enter the "Green Phase" this upcoming Friday. That's still a lockdown but bars will reopen & other restrictions will 'relax'. Even though I've stopped drinking alcohol I plan to go to a bar for 'Happy Hour' on Friday to celebrate.

****

June 3, 2020, 7:21AM (Amir-ul Kafirs to group):

I am concerned about the incident with the cops on the horses being harangued and slandered by the protesters

I feel like I need to clarify here. The cops were using the horses they were riding for a reason, the horses were show horses, as I've stated, meant for parade use, not for policing use. The horse cops *weren't* policing the crowd, they avoided confrontation. I DO believe that some cops are seriously against these police murders. HOWEVER, that DOESN'T MEAN that there isn't a public relations ulterior motive at work or also some crocodile tears. The agenda of the police is, 1st & foremost, to keep the people under control. Sometimes more psychologically subtle means for doing so are used. Alas, I DO think that any mob is going to produce counterproductive self-righteous behavior but I think the police psychologists are well aware of this & of how to manipulate it for their own ends. In other words, the police AREN'T INNOCENT VICTIMS. To quote from an email I just sent to Dick:

"With that aside, I don't think it's particularly valid to compare the Watts riots to anything happening now — not that there aren't similar root causes but just because, in some sense, the times HAVE changed in the last 55 years. Whatever rioting there may or may not have been in Pittsburgh was probably infused with at least a little romanticism on the part of the younger white folks & not driven as much by *need.* Still, I can't ultimately say, I wasn't part of the 'rioting', nor did I witness any of it — there's definitely a serious anger out there over the murders of George Floyd & Brionna Taylor & I don't think the rioting is the issue, the police murders are what's important & what has to stop. The 'rioting' is just a distraction for the police & the mass media to use to demonize protestors & to divide & conquer different tendencies in the resistance movement. I'm not going to fall into the trap of demonizing 'rioters'. The police seem to be uniting against Floyd's murderer but will he ultimately really go to jail or will it just be another PR move? That remains to be seen but, historically, there's not much room for optimism. SO, the police demonizing 'rioters' & expressing concern over the 'legitimate' cause might not be crocodile tears but it's more than a little hard to trust."

****

June 3, 2020, 10:52AM (Inquiring Librarian to group):

Thanks for the clarification Amir-ul Kafirs. I admit ignorance on this one. Although I do still want to think those police were/are good people. I like to see the police force as the doctor force, not all are horrible. And as many doctors do suck, there are many who do not and who do not condone the murderous behavior of others. And those doctors/police that I consider good should have the right to freely protest against those that are not, just as you and I should be given the freedom to protest for justice. In any case, I hate seeing people bullied, and inevitably those horses were probably getting hit with bottles and the negative energy was surely felt by the horses who certainly deserved none of the hostility.

I am among the lucky few that have not been subject to police misconduct. And I have known several decent humans that are/were cops. I have also had it explained to me from former cops who have explained how easy it is to fall into horrible actions out of their own fear and out of simple rage unchecked and also the pressures of systemic corruption. I also have a friend who spent about 20 years in jail for violence he took out on others while steeped in a severe heroin addiction paired with ptsd from being raised in a violently abusive family. There is no black and white in these situations. And the situations with the police are over my head and ability to clearly fathom. I chose to focus my shared opinions more on the corruption within the medical system right now, as that is something I personally have been abused by and it hits close to home.

& yes, I do see the police demonizing rioters and also demonizing anarchists and free thinkers that do not think as the mass media thinks they should think. I find it nauseating. I have come to expect no less from our media these days.

****

June 3, 2020, 2:49PM (Naia Nisnam to group):

Re: HERETICS: A quick update from amsterdam....Protest and work

Phil- Thank you for sending those photos, I appreciate seeing people worldwide coming together over this man's murder and inter-related issues.
I noticed you said that the Netherlands never made masks mandatory. It seemed like a lot of protesters in the photos did wear masks. Is that also true in general daily life? I'm wondering how many people in your country seem to be wearing masks and if that seems to have any effect on the number of reported covid cases. (Im coming from the belief that masks do not help stop the spread of the virus but am open to the possibility that Im wrong).

I'm really intrigued by this topic. I found out just a few weeks ago that New Zealand, which has reopened, was not advising people to wear masks unless they are caring for a sick person, as per World Health Organization orders.
I keep telling people about the WHO telling us not to wear masks but no one wants to hear it. Masks have become such a polarized issue here that the CDC will never step back and tell us that masks arent necessary because masks have turned into a political debate instead of a scientific discussion.

Last week, I met up with a friend to go for a walk. She was wearing a mask and I asked her if she wanted me to put one on and she did want that so I did. I also told her that I think its totally unnecessary as we were walking outside. I told her about the WHO and New Zealand but she didnt take the mask off. It was very hot outside and after walking for about 20 minutes, she decided that it would be okay to take our masks off. Common sense doesnt seem to prevail but the beating sun does bring some sanity.

****

June 2, 2020, 10:23AM (Phil to group):

Re: HERETICS: Belarus

Thanks for the info on Belarus. Yes what is realistic with covid-19 statistics. Mostly they do not make too much sense especially for people wanting to prove a point either for or against lockdown. Too many variables on how the raw data is collected and the reliability of tests. On the Russian front it is interesting that Dr Alexander Myasnikov let it slip that 'it's all bullshit' ;
https://off-guardian.org/2020/05/31/its-all-bullsht-3-leaks-that-sink-the-covid-narrative/?__cf_chl_jschl_tk__=7d1fdf4cf52b6196c0c0dda492b12a8ad44b8db5-1591107389-0-AaNrouTtR5_vpjc9euSHThHypHh2G3UBZ1-fz10fMW-v7cHvr9Q6VQ0-iK_OxCgMRtNgrH-fnyUqJd8a4FCmc2cs85vmyOND1rBHqDasgWG0bShxId-0_D-NzR8dYkrOe8Jwq4mQGIyEJotdBomzuWhWUEX74ZsMygk6TXvVHg5X8Yj0mwFsOT_28HEklqi06iQaVGVjhi1O-VjVe0j0t2byxm4pTGp18j4z8ECszKYgPLyVITLEYasVAi1dmPFHzeGTtPWkzAahjaf_X8Y-d2DqcmAnUESF7UtRQSZsVVRRXEusEq3PySUjFLEWU3U8LzoePbH9XpxXAJ0ExktfEh5CGIZJJEZj-09JwQdxZEUV

****

May 31, 2020

"It's all Bullsh*t" – 3 Leaks that Sink the Covid Narrative

In recent days a series of leaks across the globe have further shown the "official line" on coronavirus does not hold water

Kit Knightly

The science of the coronavirus is not disputed. It is well documented and **openly admitted**:

> Most people won't get the virus.
> Most of the people who get it won't display symptoms.
> Most of the people who display symptoms will only be mildly sick.
> Most of the people with severe symptoms will never be critically ill.
> And most of the people who get critically ill will survive.

This is borne out by the **numerous serological studies** which show, again and again, that the infection fatality ratio is on par with flu.

There is no science – and increasingly little rational discussion – to justify the lockdown measures and overall sense of global panic.

Nevertheless, it's always good to get official acknowledgement of the truth, even if it has to be leaked.

Here are three leaks showing that those in power know that the coronavirus poses no threat, and in no way justifies the lockdown that is going to destroy the livelihoods of so many.

1. “IT’S ALL BULLSHIT!”

On May 26th Dr Alexander Myasnikov, Russia’s head of coronavirus information, gave an interview to **former-Presidential candidate Ksenia Sobchak** in which he apparently **let slip his true feelings**.

Believing the interview over, and the camera turned off, Myasnikov said:

It’s all bullshit […] It’s all exaggerated. It’s an acute respiratory disease with minimal mortality […] Why has the whole world been destroyed? That I don’t know,”

[..]

****

June 2, 2020, 12:04PM (Amir-ul Kafirs to group):

Thanks for this. I found the article very useful. It seems to go contrary to my friend's claim that the OffGuardian is 'all Russian propaganda' (or something like that) since the positions taken are definitely NOT the official Russian ones. Putin, like Rump, has reputedly delegated the responsibilities to the governors in order to, presumably, evade responsibility himself.

****

June 2, 2020, 9:13PM (Inquiring Librarian to group):

Ha ha!! Mother [Belo]Russia!! I will share this with my dad. I am sure he will find it interesting. This action by Belarus is not far from the kind of attitude I see in my Belarussian dad. It seems like a hard headed culture that puts up with no nonsense and has no qualms with bluntly stating what they believe to be painfully obvious, regardless of whether they may be right or wrong. They are very agrarian and not as well schooled in higher education as their neighboring Eastern European countries. & they were totally brutalized and then trashed by their supposedly intellectually 'superior' neighbors from ww2 through and the ongoing aftermath of the Chernobyl fallout landing mostly on Belarus in 1986. If they turn out to be right in their approach to the virus, my applause to them for finally having a chance to prove their worth and earth-based intelligence above their former tyrants. Note also, at least in my dad's time, they were well behind and frankly rejected, 'modern' western medicine.

My dad told me that Belarus is seen as backward country hick peasants compared to Russia and the Ukraine, somewhat the way Germans may have viewed Austrians at some point. When he worked at GE, one of his coworkers was Ukranian and dad would joke with that guy calling him ukranian bourgeoisie while that guy would call dad a Belorussian redneck.

Anyways, i can appreciate this Belorussian leader based on the absurdities of my upbringing by a Belorussian dad. I was regularly called a 'pansy' and shamed into action when i was scared to do something he saw nonthreatening but that scared the bejebus out of me. Note: likely part of the roots of my hostile feelings towards the 'milennial' we discussed previously.

And lastly, i cannot trust any countries' 'numbers' to be honest... And certainly not those from Russia... From Belorussia, lawd only knows!! To be honest the 'testing' baffles me. The mass media on various sites have claimed the tests to be so innaccurate... And i listened to several talk shows discussing the impossibility of really ever well testing an RNA virus. So that is my 2 cents on numbers. The similarities between number curves in various countries does muddy my thought though. Confused. That is where i stand.

& a 'candy-ass'. My dad's favorite shame me into action accusations were 'pansy' and 'candy-ass'. This is so similar to Lukashenko's "die on your feet than live on your knees" attitude! I found this whole article fascinating and funny. I hope that is not offensive or seemingly ignorant to anyone here.

****

June 3, 2020, 5:43PM (Amir-ul Kafirs to group):

Re: HERETICS: Belarus

I will share this with my dad. I am sure he will find it interesting.

I assume your dad is anti-Lukashenko & anti-communist.

This action by Belarus is not far from the kind of attitude I see in my Belarussian dad.

Ha ha! I wonder if he'd be insulted to be compared to Lukashenko.

Chornobyl fallout landing mostly on Belarus in 1986.

Lukashenko's been saying for a long time now that it's ok to return to the highly radioactive areas. I suspect that he's wrong about that one. In case anyone's interested, here's a book review that I wrote relevant to this:

review of
Svetlana Alexievich's Voices from Chernobyl
by tENTATIVELY, a cONVENIENCE - May 15, 2016

"Chernobyl Hibakusha": https://www.goodreads.com/story/show/443403-chernobyl-hibakusha

that guy would call dad a Belorussian redneck.

I have a Belorusyn friend, currently going under the name of "Monty Cantsign" on Facebook. Partially inspired by him, I've made these 3 Belarusyn-relevant movies:

450. "**Limpolysemia**"
- attendees: tENTATIVELY, a cONVENIENCE (Pittsburgh), Monty Cantsin (Rotterdam), Monty Cantsin (Minsk), Carrion Elited (Richmond), Yuli Ilyushchanka (Minsk), Carlin Christy (Pittsburgh), Katya (Minsk), Deanna? (Minsk), Sasha Krotovsky (translator) (Minsk), Egor (Minsk), Alexei (Minsk), Jury Urso (Minsk), Dmitry Veleskevich (Minsk), Anna Oldfield (translator) (South Carolina), Ben Grubb (Pittsburgh), Caleb Gamble (Pittsburgh)
- shot using screen recording (Ryan Broughman), mini-dv & iJones (tENTATIVELY, a cONVENIENCE) mostly on May 5, 8, & 9, 2016
- unedited 2:53:00 screen recording by Kareem EL E OT on YouTube here: https://youtu.be/DikIpJ_RX3E
- edited, titled, scanned, & otherwise labored over by tENTATIVELY, a cONVENIENCE
- 3:05:09
- 1200 X 800 (Custom 3:2)
- edit finished June 16, 2016
- a coproduction of tENTATIVELY, a cONVENIENCE & Lipovy Tsvet
- on the Internet Archive here: https://archive.org/details/limpolysemia

451. "**Limpolysemia (take 7)**"
- one of the many sampling piece versions that didn't make it into the feature-length "Limpolysemia" & more fully explicated than any of the feature versions
- music box rolls d composed by tENTATIVELY, a cONVENIENCE in order of 1st appearance: "Flurries" (May 8, 2016), "Dum-Dee-Dum" (May 8, 2016), "Counterpointillism" (May 6, 2016); samples for tENTATIVELY, a cONVENIENCE's "Limpolysemia" sampling piece taken from: "HONK" poem by Monty Cantsin realized by Neal D. Retke, "Polka-Troika" performed by Nataliya Romanskaya & Kirmash from the "Songs & Dances from Belorussia" CD, Sergei Loznitsa's "In the Fog", Davide Ferrario's "Primo Levi's Journey", karen karnak Ekaterina Samigulina feat Sedoj - golos, karen karnak & samigulina - alfavit dinozavrov, karen karnak - na smert rabochego, Ekaterina Samigulina & Karen Karnak - Chernorabochie, Living Language Russian Complete Course; Super Duper Light Sensitive Doomsday Device made by Echo Lightwave Unspeakable
- 8:42
- 720 X 480 (3:2)
- edit finished June 20, 2016

- on Vimeo here: https://vimeo.com/171385032

458. **B.Y.O.C. #4: premier of "Limpolysemia"**
- shot at Who Unit? August 6, 2016
- featuring: tENTATIVELY, a cONVENIENCE; Ryan Broughman; Myrna Newman; Calder Dudgeon; Mark O'Connor
- mini-DV, iJones: tENTATIVELY, a cONVENIENCE; laptop, iJones: Ryan Broughman
- edit finished September 5, 2016
- 28:38
- 1700X1275 (4:3)
- on my onesownthoughts YouTube channel here: https://youtu.be/aKIyLMvZjCo

And lastly, i cannot trust any countries' 'numbers' to be honest...

Of course not! Obviously I'm biased in favor of the low COVID-19 deaths statstics but I don't think ANY OF THEM CAN BE TRUSTED.

****

June 2, 2020, 11:43AM (Amir-ul Kafirs to group):

HERETICS: Story from Pittsburgh

Alright, Naia Nisnam is probably sick of this story by now but it still boggles my mind & demonstrates the extent of the quarantinia here.

Saturday, I was waiting on my front steps for Naia Nisnam to pick me up to take me to the George Floyd protest march. Two women walked by, one had been walking on the sidewalk with her dog but when she saw me she went out to the street where her friend already was. The dog-walker was telling a story. Neither was wearing a mask so I thought they might be not insane even though they were taking the social-distancing a bit far. The one in the street, who I'll call "Skinny Woman", looked familiar but I didn't really think I knew her. After they passed me the dog-walker got back on the sidewalk again. A few minutes later they turned around & came back past me again. Dog-walker stayed on the sidewalk this time, still talking, & skinny woman stayed in the street. Skinny Woman looked right at me, smiled & may've said "Hi" under her breath — apparently not wanting to stop the flow of her friend's monolog. I said "Hello." Skinny Woman still seemed somehow familiar.

Two days later, Naia Nisnam & I were at another George Floyd memorial protest. Naia Nisnam & I were walking & I saw skinny woman. It may've been around this time that I realized that she looked like a friend of mine who I'd made a movie with called "Dead & Breakfast", a comedy horror short made before the Hollywood movie of the same name:

240. "**Dead & Breakfast**"

- on my onesownthoughts YouTube channel here: https://youtu.be/TCGBnvAyYao
- on the Internet Archive here: https://archive.org/details/deadbreakfast

I didn't think Skinny Woman was actually my friend because she seemed about the same age that my friend had been when I saw her last, which might've been as much as 15 or 16 years ago, but I thought she might be her sister. The resemblance seemed uncanny but that might just be my impression after not seeing my friend for a long time.

SO, I saw Skinny Woman, with a guy & facing me, this time with a mask on, so I walked toward her, with Naia Nisnam, & said something like: "Excuse me.." but before I got to ask her whether she knew my friend that she resembled she rushed past me. I don't think Naia Nisnam & I had our masks on at the time but they would've been pulled down around our necks. I wasn't sure whether Skinny Woman had noticed me in her rush so I reached back to her, she was past me by now, & lightly touched her arm to try to get her attention. She still didn't stop but the guy she was with glared at me & I said something like this to him: "I wanted to ask her a question."

They hurried off & I saw Skinny Woman pull out some sanitizer which she then vigorously rubbed on her hands & then on the arm that I'd touched. She seemed terrified. She kept looking back at me & then pulled out her cell-phone & held it up in such a way that she could shoot footage of me. She continued to look nervously over her shoulder at me. I got paranoid & started wondering: *What's going to happen? Is she going to try to have me arrested for attempted murder or some such?!* Her apparent terror seemed so extreme. Naia Nisnam & I couldn't hear the speakers from where we were so we went to the front of the crowd of thousands of people, none of them social-distancing & that was the last I saw of Skinny Woman.

The point is that a simple touch on the arm or even an attempt to talk to a stranger has been turned into being perceived as 'life-threatening' situations in the minds of quarantiniacs now in this time of the PANDEMIC PANIC. A simple action like touching a person on their arm has been turned into something so terrifying that a person immediately pulls out sanitizer & starts applying it as if they've just been bitten by a leper. **THAT'S INSANE & THAT'S WHAT ENTIRELY TOO MANY PEOPLE ARE LIKE THESE DAYS.** & they think it's 'normal', they think they're being 'reasonable'.

****

June 2, 2020, 12:07PM (Dick to group):

RE: HERETICS: Story from Pittsburgh

wow
crazy story
was she by any chance a so-called "millenial"? I've heard, I don't know whether

correctly or incorrectly, that that segment of the US population is particularly paranoid about masks, distancing, touching, etc
*
as a member of the heretics i'd like to ask if any of you feel any "heretical thoughts" about the George Floyd situation? meaning not was it an injustice because it clearly was, but rather do you feel it is being instrumentalized and if so, how?
for example i have heard reports that some large % of the rioters are paid, from other states...I have no idea if this is true or not...

****

June 2, 2020, 2:15PM (Amir-ul Kafirs to group):

was she by any chance a so-called "millenial"?

I'm still not clear on that term's use. It seems to me that people born as early as 1980 are being called "millenials". According to Wikipedia: "**Millennials**, also known as **Generation Y** (or simply **Gen Y**), are the demographic cohort following Generation X and preceding Generation Z. Researchers and popular media use the early 1980s as starting birth years and the mid-1990s to early 2000s as ending birth years, with 1981 to 1996 a widely accepted defining range for the generation." (https://en.wikipedia.org/wiki/Millennials) So, YES. definitely a millenial, probably in her 20s, possibly in her 30s. Naia Nisnam might be able to narrow that down more, sometimes I might be a bad judge of age.

i'd like to ask if any of you feel any "heretical thoughts" about the George Floyd situation?

I've been to 2 George Floyd memorial events in the last 3 days, Naia Nisnam's been to 3. Given that we're talking about thousands of people at just those marches it's hard for one person to get a handle on what's happening. I DO HAVE A THEORY, though, ABOUT THE COP-CAR BURNING THAT HAPPENED ON SATURDAY. I speculate that it was what I call "Police Theater", a deliberate set-up *by the police*. I think it's highly probable that they arranged for the car to be set fire to so that this image could appear on the 'news', generating & selling even more fear & 'justifying' things like the curfew that's been imposed. I've copied 3 of the mainstream 'news' articles about it below.

The guy arrested in connection with "starting the rioting" in Pittsburgh is a 20 year old white male "anarchist". He's not even being accused of setting fire to the car, just of breaking its windows. The 'news' says that peaceful protestors didn't want him to do this. How reliable that is I don't know, I was too far away from the action at the time. There're several reasons why I find the whole situation suspicious:

1. the cop car was the only car parked in the block that the march was effectively ending at. Why? Why was it there? Why was it unguarded? In short, it was such a convenient target it was ridiculous. I find it impossible to believe that the

police just parked it there & left it without thinking that it might be vandalized. Instead, I think they left it there *to be vandalized.*

2. who actually set fire to the car? There were hundreds of protestors around, many shooting footage with cell-phones, they got footage of the accused breaking the cop car windows but NONE, apparently, of the car being set fire to? **[I'm told that there is footage online of someone setting fire to the car but that it's very hard to find — I haven't seen it]** That seems strange. Of course, maybe no-one wants to share that footage, that's less strange. Here, of course, is where what I postulate might seem 'far-fetched': *What if the car was prearranged to blow up like a special effect?* What if the cops waited until people were clear of the car & then pressed a remote control & blew it up? I haven't heard of anyone being injured. That seems strange, the area around the cop car was crowded & no-one got hurt?! ALSO, the car burned with an intense **BLACK SMOKE** that went on for a llllooooonnnnggggg time. While I was watching it from a safe distance that seemed strange to me. I'm not an expert on burning cars but the black smoke seemed unnaturally intense & **BLACK**. If I were a special effects guy, that's the kind of smoke I'd want the car to give off — especially if I wanted a zillion helicopter shots of it burning to look very dramatic.

3. the 'rioting' is all supposed to've been started by this 20 yr old in response to his breaking the car window. I find this highly improbable. I think most people would've just taken that in stride & kept on at their business.

SO, here're my 2 proposals:

1. the police (& mass media) were prepared to sabotage this peaceful protest. They have 1 or more local provocateurs in the anarchist community. These provocateurs look for young impressionable anarchists who want to be 'anarchist heros' & get them all riled up to do stupid things so that they can then be used as scapegoats to discredit anarchists in general. The accused was worked on by this provocateur.

2. the police (& mass media) were prepared to sabotage this peaceful protest. They figured that if they left their car in such a vulnerable place that the windows would get broken sooner or later & they were prepared with special effects explosives to be remotely triggered to create a discrediting incident. There was a uniformed cop watching the burning cop car standing next to a vehicle accompanying an over-sized load truck. He seemed to have at least 2 plainclothes cops next to him. He was basically leaning on the escort car's driver's window. The control for activating the explosion could've been in the 'escort' car.

Either way, I think the burning of the cop car gave the mass media what it usually wants: a violent fearful spectacle that can be used to increase the police state. It appears that anarchists are going to be the target now — probably in a divide & conquer to split the black community from the predominantly white anarchist one.

As for "some large % of the rioters are paid, from other states"?: As someone who's participated in many protests all over the world & who's been otherwise active & knowledgable about such things I find that assertion to be an unlikely one that would be put forth by people with little or no experience of the reality of the matter, probably right-wingers. I've known very few people who took activist training where they learned things like how to build a tripod & lock down in a way that prevents their easy removal from blocades & maybe some of them got funding to participate in such trainings — but that's about it. I've traveled out-of-state & out-of-country & participated in protests wherever I've been & I've NEVER been paid to do so or known ANYONE who was paid to do so. I think it's safe to say that most anarchists are people doing such things on their own initiative. I think it's a little more possible that some socialists might be paid to go places to organize by their party. The most likely people to be paid would be undercover cops. But a "large % of the rioters"? That seems like pure propaganda. I don't think there are even many "rioters" to begin with. Let's say that if there were ANY in Pittsburgh, there might've been 50. A large percentage of that might be 30 people. That just seems so improbable to me that it's ridiculous. Then again, I've never been in a "riot" so what do I know? In most riots that I've observed it's been the police who've rioted.

PITTSBURGH (KDKA) – Pittsburgh Public Safety has placed a curfew on the City Of Pittsburgh beginning tonight at 8:30 p.m. until 6:00 a.m.

According to Director of Public Safety Wendell Hissrich, the curfew will be in place both tonight and tomorrow.

"We believe a lot of these individuals that are creating trouble are not from the city," Hissrich said. "With that, effective at 8:30 this evening, until 6:00 tomorrow morning, there will be a curfew in the city of Pittsburgh."

CURFEW: Effective at 8:30 P.M. tonight, there is a citywide curfew in effect for #Pittsburgh.@PghPublicSafety will enforce the City order from 8:30 P.M. to 6:00 A.M.

They said that anyone that is downtown between those hours, will be stopped by law enforcement.

Several other law enforcement agencies are being called into the city, including state police and neighboring towns.

Pittsburgh Police Chief Scott Schubert expressed his disappointment at those that took a peaceful protest and turned it violent.

"I can tell you as the police chief, I am very disappointed because this was a peaceful protest for something that was very serious, and this does nothing to honor the memory of somebody who died," Chief Schubert said.

Schubert agreed with Hissrich that the belief is those that turned the protests violent are not from the city.

"There's a lot of people who are anarchists, they're not here to protest what happened, they're here to take advantage of situations and throw it their way and bring other people into the mix and cause damage and cause injury," Chief Schubert added. "There's no doubt that that's who's doing it and a lot of things we're seeing are white males, dressed in the anarchist, ANTIFA, they're ones who are fueling a lot of this."

The curfew comes in response to the George Lloyd protests that turned violent.
- https://pittsburgh.cbslocal.com/2020/05/30/downtown-pittsburgh-city-wide-curfew/

[The blaming of things on anarchists & ANTIFA is a convenient way of trying to discredit people who believe in Direct Action]

I don't know if the curfew is still on today. One guy is being sought in connection with the car burning:

Arrest Warrant Issued For Brian Bartels, Police Say He Started Saturday Riots In Pittsburgh

May 31, 2020 at 9:56 pm

PITTSBURGH (KDKA) – Pittsburgh Police are searching for 20-year-old Brian Bartels for breaking the windows out of a Pittsburgh Police car.

According to Police, Bartels broke the windows against the wishes of peaceful protesters.

Pittsburgh Police, along with Shaler Police, North Hills SRT, and FBI Pittsburgh served a search warrant at a home in Shaler on Sunday.

Bartels was not there but investigators found evidence that linked him to the protests.

He is facing charges institutional vandalism, rioting, and reckless endangerment of another person.

A warrant has been issued for his arrest.
- https://pittsburgh.cbslocal.com/2020/05/31/brian-bartels-wanted-for-starting-pittsburgh-riots/

'Damn Shame': Pittsburgh Police Chief Says White Males Dressed In Anarchist

Attire Hijacked George Floyd Protests Downtown

May 30, 2020 at 9:11 pm

PITTSBURGH (KDKA) – During a press conference, Pittsburgh Police Chief Scott Schubert expressed disappointment and anger toward those that turned Saturday afternoon's protest from peaceful to violent.

[It's entirely too convenient for the police to use this to distract attention from police culpability in connection with murders]

Brian Bartels, 20-Year-Old Accused Of Inciting Violence And Riots In Pittsburgh, In Police Custody

June 1, 2020 at 5:17 pm

PITTSBURGH (KDKA) — Twenty-year-old Brian Bartels, the man accused of inciting violence and riots in Pittsburgh on Saturday, is in police custody.

Bartels turned himself in at police headquarters Monday. He arrived with an adult male and adult female.

[..]

Besides Pittsburgh Police, Shaler Police, North Hills SRT and FBI Pittsburgh served a search warrant at a home in Shaler Sunday.

Bartels was not there, but investigators say they found evidence that links him to the protests — guns, spray paint and gloves. Also found during the search warrant execution was the sweatshirt matching the one seen in the video of the protest on Saturday.

- https://pittsburgh.cbslocal.com/2020/06/01/brian-bartels-pittsburgh-protest-arrested/

****

June 2, 2020, 3:19PM (Dick to group):

I think your theories seem pretty reasonable
I guess my point was, is it somehow tied into the Covid-19 business? a continuation, capitalizing on it to keep the "dark agenda" going?

*

An aside:

For whatever it's worth: my definition of a millenial... that is, the definition in my head when I asked the question... which isn't scientific I should mention...is a young person currently alive who is militantly concerned with being politically correct all of the time

this translates into an "US versus THEM" attitude as a guiding principle to existence and opinion making

perhaps this is because they haven't yet been forced to buckle down to the system due to the pressures of supporting a family or of just being too tired to keep up the energy level needed to be irritated/on edge all the time...

and so, they adhere, with varying levels of ferocity, to a group identity extremely concerned about not offending anyone in any way... it's an available identity, like any available identity

that is total conformists in the latest non-conformist mode who have a found an outlet for their sexual energy...

which translates into total blandness and pre-packaged opinions and easy answers for all questions

It's nothing new really

I used to meet "Communists" in Baltimore who had their version of it, a quote for every occasion

It isn't that noticeable when you're in the same ballpark, that is the same age group, but once you are out of it, you become fair game for attack

I felt that the people I saw in Pittsburgh when I was there, the young people - meaning between 18 - 35 - near the center where we gave the film show, all those kids who wore the same get-up of short pants, ragged olive drab t-shirt with holes in them, dyed black hair, the same tattoos, etc - were great examples non-conformist conformists... I felt wary around them

I hope the above doesn't offend anyone by the way, it's not meant to in any case... but it is what I have seen and distilled from my encounters with that particular species

****

June 2, 2020, 5:53PM (Inquiring Librarian to group):

Dick, I feel like your description of millennials is basically what I also see in this group of young people. I appreciate your succinct and clear description. And I appreciate that you are willing to throw yourself out there to let us know what you think, even fearing that you might upset some of us. It honestly makes me feel much better hearing you say what you said, because I agree with you. Given that I was born in 1975, there is some amount of overlap of this generation into mine. For years, I battled with wondering why this group of people alienated me and eventually realized that I didn't really care because they irritated me, bored me, and clearly I had nothing genuine in common with them and also that they often seemed to thrive in the herd, something that I've never been able to bring myself to do. And yes, they are easily offended. To my dismay, and sometimes to my devious pleasure, I have inadvertently offended many millenials. I also find them to be judgemental and often rude and often have the know-it-all air about them. I find those that fall snugly into this smug categorization of 'intellectuals' to be very irritating and limited, regardless of their education level. I know I sound like a total jerk. But I have had to deal with them head on for so much of my life. When I left Baltimore in 2003, I was partly fleeing what I now recognize as the rise of this generation's influence. I met Amir-ul Kafirs when I lived in Bmore and meeting him was such a breath of fresh air in a 'real' person who was an active artist without pretensions . I left Bmore to go to Colorado and felt much better there (many thanks to Amir-ul Kafirs for introducing me to Lauren and Dave of Little Fyodor & Babushka fame - amazing and lovely and genuine souls that I miss dearly!!). It seems the train of thought associated with this generation is working its way deep into politics and the running of our nation. I am very thankful for the few friends I have in my generation who are not easily offended and who are conforming 'noncomformists'. & yes, this group always seemed to have some sort of a 'uniform'. A friend a few years my senior remarked back in the early 2000's when visiting me in Baltimore, when he was snubbed by a punk rock looking coffee shop gal, "Man, what happened to the days when how you dressed was an indication of who you are!". I"m not sure if that makes sense, but the gist is, if you are dressed punk rock, you'd think the person would be open minded and interesting. Instead my friend was snubbed and treated very rudely by this girl. I experienced so much of that in Baltimore.

Ok, enough of that. I appreciate your sharing your thoughts on the Pittsburgh protest Amir-ul Kafirs. I honestly think your theory is VERY possible. It seems the mainstream media is doing everything it can to rile up the crowds and create more clashes, be they racially or criminally motivated. I would assume this is being done for political reasons and that it is pretty evident that most people these days eat this stuff up and run with it with the passion that the mass media prescribes. I'd hate to think that the police would be involved in staging a cop car blow up. But from your description of the events and the dramatic news article complete with young masked remorseless vigilante 'suspect', it reads like a poorly written cop show drama.

****

June 2, 2020, 6:00PM (Dick to group):

Thanks.
Yeah, Baltimore is a tough town.
I need to go back there to deal with some stuff but have been putting it off for 3 years!
Baltimore gives a new meaning to the word "clique".

As they say, the smaller the turf, the fiercer the dogs.

****

June 2, 2020, 9:03PM (Amir-ul Kafirs to group):

I guess my point was, is it somehow tied into the Covid-19 business? a continution, capitalizing on it to keep the "dark agenda" going?

That's a bit murkier. Judging from just recent PGH events I'd say the move is on to lock down the society more AND to create a bad vibe against anarchists who, after all, were responsible more than any other political group for the anti-globalization networking that was pretty successful in some ways 20 years ago. Sicilians are reputed to say something like *Revenge is best cold* — so maybe the ruling elites are thinking that anarchists are smug & complacent enough now to suddenly find ourselves royally fucked.

Naia Nisnam has astutely pointed out that people who travel for protests from another state may be prosecuted as federal criminals now. Hence the whole emphasis on "outside agitators" is to both discourage people from traveling to protests AND to encourage locals to distrust people who do that. As a person who's traveled around the world for protests I could easily be called an "outside agitator" even though, strictly speaking, I never 'agitated' at all in the sense of tried to convince anyone to do anything they weren't already going to do. This whole angle of things is a continuation of the lockdown: if you're not staying at home, at least stay in your city or your state. Any kind of even national, let alone international, activism becomes, therefore, banned. Funny how that doesn't also apply to business, eh?! After all, 'free trade' does far more harm than most forms of internationalism.

militantly concerned with being politically correct all of the time

One of the ironies of that is that queer culture, which I've been around for 50 years, always had a very dark sense of humor. Now, an old queer telling an 'off-color' joke would be considered incorrect even though the 'correctness' would've been partially created to 'protect' such people. Any adherence to prefabricated modes of speech & action for 'sensitivity''s sake is inflexible enough to be actually insensitive to real life. I often tell jokes that're so outré that they're meant to both 'horrify' people & to also get them to lighten up by making them realize that IT'S A JOKE.

E.G.:

A water main recently broke in my neighborhood. The neighborhood group I'm in was up-in-arms over it's not being treated properly. This notion of 'proper' is rooted in the PANDEMIC PANIC. I just continued to drink the water unconcerned. It was fine. Everybody else was boiling their water. When it was pronounced safe I told a joke to the group about it. I was, admittedly, poking fun at them for being so alarmist although I didn't make that explicit. What I 1st thought of writing was:

I was doing my own water testing. I took unboiled water straight from the tap & boiled water & I poured some of the unboiled water down the throat of one kidnapped baby & some of the boiled water down the throat of the other kidnapped baby. Unfortunately, I forgot to let the boiled water cool down so the one baby died & that invalidated my research.

Now, of course, that's meant to be a 'sick' joke & it's NOT something I would ever actually do *but I knew that people would be unbelievably upset.* SO, I changed the kidnapped babies to plants. Even then, one of the people had to make a comment that it was a good thing that no humans had to drink the water. I didn't bother to tell him that actually I DID DRINK THE WATER & I WAS FINE & THAT THESE WATER MAIN BREAKS HAPPEN ALL THE TIME & THEY'VE ALWAYS DRUNK THE WATER BEFORE.

I hope the above doesn't offend anyone by the way

Egads, Dick! Who would you offend?! Punk started becoming conformist non-conformist by about 1980 & it's been downhill ever since! The 'news' even refers to the "anarchist uniform". It's pathetic that they can refer to that & know what it means, that's how widespread the uniform actually is. When women from the Weather Underground went into a corporate building to plant a bomb do you think they wore torn jeans & feminist buttons? Of course not, they dressed like proper conservative young women so that their presence there would go unquestioned. I was NEVER a punk &, yet, I was *more punk* than the punks were.

As for the application of all this to the young woman who was so terrified that I'd touched her? I'm definitely preoccupied with how likely it is that people like myself are going to face a fresh wave of demonization. For a time, I was probably at least somewhat a 'respected elder', at least someone that younger anarchists knew had 'been around'. Now? I can easily see that I could be almost instantly turned into a monster by the media for young women like the 'Skinny Woman' to project all her fears on. Any knowledge I might have would be swept under the rug. Would it matter that I'm actually a person who doesn't advocate rioting, etc? Of course not! — because what it's ultimately about is getting people *in line*, to make them fear more & more having any opinions that aren't prefabricated. ironically, I think intellectuals & academics might aid & abet this process more than seasoned cops might.

****

June 3, 2020, 2:11AM (Dick to Amir-ul Kafirs):

TR: Watts 1965 . . . Minneapolis 2020

You asked about Ken Knabb, whether he'd responded or not, as I wrote, no he didn't but he sent this today

Objet : Watts 1965 . . . Minneapolis 2020

Here's what the situationists said about riots, looting, and the condition of black people in America 55 years ago (commenting on the Watts riot of 1965):

"THE DECLINE AND FALL OF THE SPECTACLE-COMMODITY ECONOMY"
http://www.bopsecrets.org/SI/10.Watts.htm
Many things have changed since then, but the fundamental things still apply as time goes by . . .

"Making petrified conditions dance by singing them their own tune."

****

June 3, 2020, 7:03AM (Amir-ul Kafirs to Dick):

Re: Watts 1965 . . . Minneapolis 2020

THX, Dick. My initial reaction to this was along the lines of "how pathetic", meaning how pathetic it is that Knabb would fall back on the words of his heros rather than respond to the actual materials you tried to get him to check out. Then I read the beginning of the Situationist text & I found it erudite, as usual, but I didn't feel motivated to read it all & stopped after reading this bit:

"Until the Watts explosion, black civil rights demonstrations had been kept by their leaders within the limits of a legal system that tolerates the most appalling violence on the part of the police and the racists — as in last March's march on Montgomery, Alabama. Even after the latter scandal, a discreet agreement between the federal government, Governor Wallace and Martin Luther King led the Selma marchers on March 10 to stand back at the first police warning, in dignity and prayer. The confrontation expected by the demonstrators was reduced to a mere spectacle of a potential confrontation. In that moment nonviolence reached the pitiful limit of its courage: first you expose yourself to the enemy's blows, then you push your moral nobility to the point of sparing him the trouble of using any more force."

For most of my life I was probably more inclined to liking Malcolm X in preference to Martin Luther King, partially because X was more 'criminal' & partially because King was a Christian minister, etc. Now, though, in hindsight, I have to give King credit for actually accomplishing more for civil rights than X ever did. In fact I have to wonder whether X really accomplished much at all in that area. He was certainly incisively critical & I still appreciate what he had to say & I read his 'autobiography'. I DIDN'T read anything by or about King other than his statement from the Birmingham jail in which I remember him off-handedly using the word "anarchy" in a pejorative sense. Still, calling King's pacifism a "pitiful limit of its courage" is just bullshit. Debord & co were comfortably well-off bourgeois who probably never took much of a risk in their lives, certainly not by rioting when there would've been any danger to themselves & certainly not having the level of justifiable anger as the Watts rioters — so it's hard for me to not perceive their rhetoric as just that, rhetoric, a "defiant pose" as Stewart Home has put it. Maybe I'm wrong about the Situationists being bourgeois, I don't really know their personal histories.

****

June 3, 2020, 1:32PM (Naia Nisnam to group):

MILLENNIALS:

Yes, "skinny woman" definitely fit into the category of Millenial, based on age.
I actually do not support the defining of individuals by generation or age. (Don't worry- I am not offended by any of this. It's really hard to offend me.)
I know all too many people my age (early 40s) or older who fill that role of conforming non-conformists PC police shaming people for not wearing masks.
Amir-ul Kafirs- are you a Baby Boomer? You clearly don't fit the stereotypes of that generation.
The "millenials" are hit by both sides. On one hand, they are thought of as the overly uptight PC liberals who are shaming others for not wearing masks 24/7. On the other hand, they have also been criticized for not caring enough, for example when large groups of people in that age range went to the beach for spring break. Both things are true, as there seem to be over 80 million americans in that age range (according to wikipedia).
I worked with a guy in his 20s, a disillusioned socialist, and I was impressed with his ability to think critically. I keep meaning to reach out to him as I'm curious to hear his thoughts on the lockdown, etc.

BACK TO SKINNY WOMAN:
She is a millenial that fits the category of PC to the extreme. I also think she is utterly insane, probably as a result of isolation. When Amir-ul Kafirs reflects on the situation, he is rightfully offended. The woman was beyond rude in the way she handled it. She completely ignored Amir-ul Kafirs's existence, except to photograph him. She dismissed him the way people often dismiss homeless people on the street. (I have a story related to that coming up next). Skinny woman tried to act as if she didn't see him or hear him at all, though she clearly did. Her frantic scrubbing of herself with sanitizer was absolutely hilarious to me. I still chuckle when I think about it. Her sanitizing went on for a looooong time. It was so excessive that if I had it on video, it would appear to be satire. The pandemic panic seems to be pushing a lot of people over the edge and into total insanity. Her behavior, which wouldve seemed crazy to most anyone just a few months ago, is probably considered normal and sane now.

ANOTHER PGH STORY:
At the beginning of the large protest here on Saturday, I witnessed a bizarre

conflict. A woman had a "Black Lives Matter" sign. A Black man wanted to high five her. She refused, because she was afraid of the virus. She, like most people at the protest, was wearing a mask. There was no possibility of social distancing at the protest. People were walking side by side, all touching each other. It was lovely to see and experience.

But- this woman refused to high five a Black man who was excited that she was carrying a sign that said he mattered. He didn't matter enough for her to touch his hand for one second. He was drunk but "clean", he had on clean clothes and was well-kempt.

The conflict escalated because the man was drunk and highly offended. He started yelling that there is no disease and he just wanted a high-five. The woman sort of cowered in a corner, hiding behind her sign. Security from the building they were in front of started to get involved. I imagined this man getting arrested at a BLM protest because he was offended that a white lady was afraid to touch him.

I could feel the guy's distress and as I walked by I touched his shoulder and said "I hear you man". He stopped and said thank you and we high fived and he calmed down and went on his way. The guy needed a small bit of physical contact. I hope that the woman joined the crowd of protesters and realized that she had been an ass, but I doubt it.

The part that really has me upset is a conversation I had two days later with a friend. The conversation happened over text messaging and I really wish that it would have happened in real life. I hadn't realized my friend was there as it all happened quickly and I continued on my way. I had felt disgusted at all of the people who stood around watching but did nothing to help. Turns out my friend was one of those people watching. He wrote to me to explain what had happened in context, as if he thought I just happened by and high fived the guy without knowing what was going on. I responded by telling my friend that I knew exactly what had been going on and I responded the way that I did because I have been concerned about the effects of isolation on people's mental health and I could feel the man's need for physical contact. I didn't express my disdain for the woman who was afraid to touch the man. My friend had to write back to me to express his concern for the scared white woman who appeared, in his words, "devastated". I don't give two shits about that woman's "devastation". If she was that afraid of human contact, then she should stay the hell home.

I feel like I'm losing friends because of my unpopular pandemic views and I have to be fine with that.

****

June 3, 2020, 2:21PM (Naia Nisnam to group):

PGH GEORGE FLOYD "RIOT" & COP CAR BURNING:

It does seem likely to me that the police car was set up as bait. I had assumed that it was set on fire by the 20-year old that the city wants to blame for inciting a riot, but when I looked at his charges he is only blamed with spray painting and throwing a rock at the car. In the video, we see him walking away, flipping off the protesters who want him to stop messing with the car, but it is clearly not on fire when he leaves. I suspect he would have been blamed for setting the fire if other protestors didn't have video of him walking away pre-fire. I also do not think the protestors released their video to help him avoid heavier charges, I think they put the video out there to blame the anarchist, just as police intended. I also think this whole police car thing would have been orchestrated by a small number of law enforcement and most cops there wouldn't have known it was a set up.

When I think about why...Why would police be so interested in demonizing anarchists that they would orchestrate all of this, I think about future protests. Americans protesting police murders is pretty harmless, overall. We've all been seeing the videos for years and thankfully it's pretty mainstream to be pissed off about it. I think the people with real power are using and manipulating these protests to serve their own agenda. They can tolerate protests against local police murdering Black people because that is a well know problem at this point. What the people in power don't want to see is a repeat of the globalization protests, where activists brought to light issues that were not being covered by the main stream media. I think it's safe to say that most americans didnt know what the WTO was before the "Battle in Seattle". Even the Occupy movement changed the public dialogue as average citizens became aware of and angry about economic inequality and these issues are now part of a more mainstream conversation. What I'm trying to say is, I think those in power are okay with BLM protests because they know the days of dividing people based on race are slowly slipping away. What they do not want to see happen are more protests like the anti-globalization movement, that are exposing hidden truths. Im not sure that Im expressing myself well here.

They are demonizing anarchists and Antifa, and they are manipulating BLM/anti-cop murderer protests in a way that turns the liberal left against anarchists. Too many activists in this city are ready to throw this 20-year old into jail for spray painting and breaking a window in a cop car.

Yesterday the Washington Post's headline read "White Instigators to Blame for Mayhem in Some Protests..." with yet another photo of a burning cop car, so it seems to be a nationwide thing and not specific to Pgh.

On the evening of our first protests here, the Pgh Chief of Police and the mayor went on TV claiming outside agitation and repeatedly mentioned protesters from out of state and how our city would work with the FBI to prosecute these "outside agitators". I believe that these ideas were spoon fed to PGH police and mayor by the FBI. I believe the feds came in and told our city officials that this outside anarchist thing was going to happen and the police chief and mayor got on TV and parroted what the feds told them. Im sure our mayor loved the chance to blame things on non-city residents. And I'm sure the FBI has more long-term goals here, including normalizing the idea of pushing federal charges on anyone travelling across state lines to demonstrate. On Tuesday the names of the 46 people who were arrested on Sat were released. Guess where the 46 arrested people were from? Pittsburgh and surrounding areas. No one came from further

than a few counties away. Still, there are no new headlines pointing out that the mayor and police chief were wrong.
https://triblive.com/local/pittsburgh-allegheny/these-are-the-people-arrested-during-the-pittsburgh-protests/

In the above article listing the names of the people arrested, there is a 47-year old man who was arrested for various things, but one of his charges is carrying a firearm without a license. He is being held without bail. Who is going to do jail support for this protester? I can't assume anything about a man that I don't know but he is from an area about an hour from the city that is notorious for its white supremacist population. Amir-ul Kafirs and I also saw a younger white guy, (maybe in his 30s??) with a handgun shoved into the waistband of his pants. He was wearing a T-shirt from a website that focuses on Survivalist stuff. He seemed to be w at least 2 other white guys and a Black guy. Im super concerned about people carrying concealed guns at a protest, walking through a crowd of thousands of people... That's new to me.

Finally- My biggest paranoia-
In two weeks or so we will be told that there is a huge spike in covid cases because of the protests and that will be used as an excuse to ban future protests. George Floyd protests have spread worldwide and I fear a worldwide ban on protests will follow. I truly hope that I am just being paranoid, as I tend to be.

[Strangely enough, that *didn't happen* — instead the media announced that the protests didn't spread COVID-19 at all — THAT is also suspicious]

****

June 3, 2020, 5:33PM (Amir-ul Kafirs to group):

HERETICS: Bourgeoisie

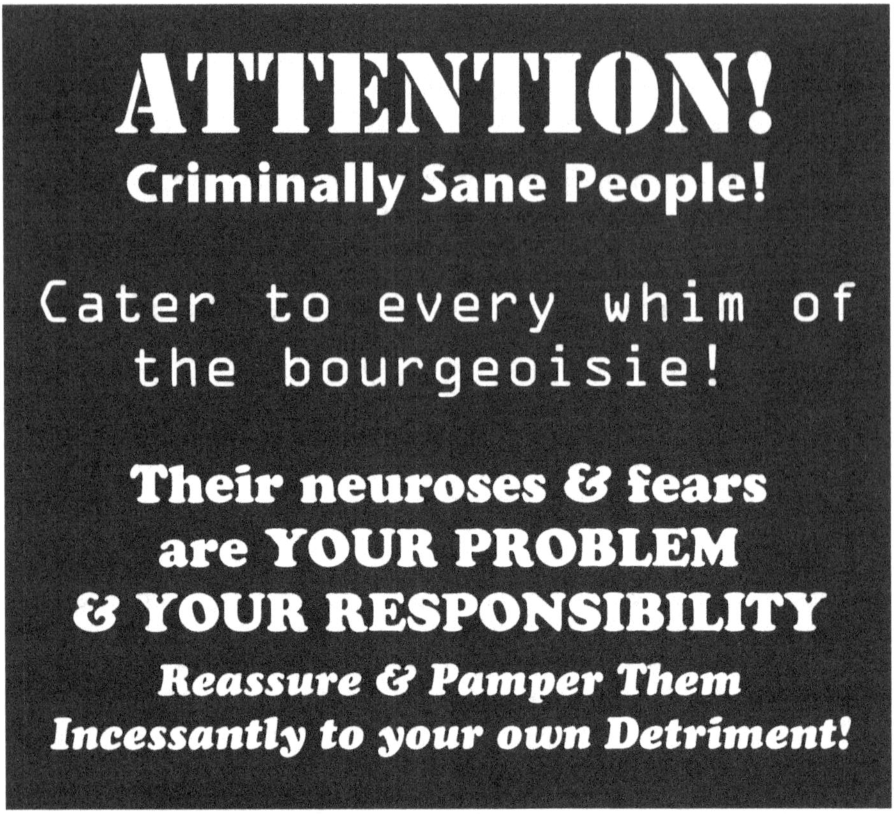

ATTENTION!
Criminally Sane People!
Cater to every whim of the bourgeoisie!
Their neuroses & fears are YOUR PROBLEM & YOUR RESPONSIBILITY
Reassure & Pamper Them Incessantly to your own Detriment!

****

June 3, 2020, 6:26PM (Inquiring Librarian to group):

Re: HERETICS: Belarus

Absolutely, my dad knows Lukashenko is a Dictator, in line with Putin. But you will note, Putin and Lukashenko are at odds with one another and Putin sees Lukashenko's actions as a reason to strongly consider interfering in Belarus as a nation, https://jamestown.org/program/kremlin-considers-renewed-interference-in-belarus-under-guise-of-coronavirus-crisis-response/?fbclid=IwAR1ZMPJzfTMV_vVlzvpweIXf08kS07q6F_WF1cnrG3CFJSDCFEeTMfr48sc . Beyond that I do now know what dad thinks about the guy. My dad appreciates that Belarus did not lock down. I tried calling my dad to talk about the article after work, but the phone connection cut off. I am tired today and don't feel like playing phone tag. I don't think my dad would care if I compared his way of talking to Lukashenko's. It's not a direct comparison to Lukashenko exactly, it's more of a manner of speaking and communication that is Eastern European, possibly even specific to Belarus, much different from what we are used to in the west. I believe it comes out of the deceptions of communism as it was in ww2. But I could be wrong. Anyways, I'm too tired to be saying anything intelligent today. I appreciate the links. I am hoping to buy a portable internet capable device by the end of 2020 so that I can watch movies that I chose.

****

June 3, 2020, 6:43PM (Inquiring Librarian to group):

Re: HERETICS: A quick update from amsterdam....Protest and work

Thanks for the update Phil. It sounds like your boss is running your place the way I am running my library. I found out who is the most concerned about the virus, and I and the others work tegether most of all to make her comfortable and the rest of us take our liberties when out of range of her. We try to keep mutual respect while appearing concerned and acting appropriately. So far it is working. Because I do not work with food, gloves are not required. But the masks... at the end of a day of cloth masking, I am sometimes a bit tired and irritable, as I am today.

Relating to protests. There was a shutdown of our major highway on interstate 10 yesterday at the tail end of rush hour. The shutdown was due to a protest that was held on the highway. From what I gathered from my staff, the protest was peaceful and successful. I didn't know it was happening until today at work. But I had wondered why there were so many low flying and very LOUD helicopters buzzing around my back porch last night while I was eating dinner. Louisiana so far has had no violence associated with riots. I am thankful for this. This state has had enough of instability and unrest recently.

****

June 3, 2020, 7:29PM (Inquiring Librarian to group):

Re: HERETICS: Belarus

Ok, for whoever is interested in investigating the bluntness/frankness/rudeness of Russian/Belorussian culture (it was technically Russia in Belarus when my dad left), this article perfectly illustrates what I am getting at, including the roots in ww2 era murderous communism. It can illustrate Lukashenko's comical bluntness and also my dad's and possibly what got me socially into trouble again and again and again through more of my life than I want to admit: https://medium.com/@smff/theres-a-bluntness-to-russian-culture-that-generally-rubs-westerners-the-wrong-way-a1d21e682b08

It is also very apparent in my 2 Russian friends, both named Ilya. I love both of them for their outright honesty and I always loved seeing how they could call people on their own crud, but in the most endearing and sincere of ways, by being painfully honest and not meaning to be hurtful, just trying to avoid the fake song and dance.

To bring this full circle, I find it unendingly fascinating to see this attitude of Eastern Europe applied to this apparent figment of a virus and its effects on the masses in Eastern Europe vs. the West.

****

June 3, 2020, 8:57PM (Amir-ul Kafirs to group):

Dick, I feel like your description of millennials is basically what I also see in this group of young people.

Personally, my dealings with humanity in general have been largely bad. As such, it's hard for me to distinguish the millenials in that respect. Self-righteousness & a lack of humor or flexibility is pretty common. Dick mentioned some communists in Baltimore, I have a relevant story:

I was friends with people in the RCP (Revolutionary Communist Party). Even though they were hypothetically ideologically in conflict with anarchists because they were somewhat Stalinist & had a "Chairman", i.e.: a hierarchical leader, I still got along with most of them fine & found us to be mainly politically on the same page regarding things like racism & imperialism. ANYWAY, one of them, who we'll call "Cynthia", was maybe the only RCP person who hated me. I think she found me entirely too flippant & hedonistic. One time I was talking with her & I said something about trying to enjoy life & she said something like 'I'll leave that for my children' — as if pleasure was something that we had to forego in the present in order to create a revolutionary future. That just seemed like a variation on ChristInanity to me: depriving oneself in anticipation of a reward in heaven. She was completely without a sense of humor as far as I could tell. No thanks. I want my 'heaven' NOW.

Anyway, I doubt that Dick OR Inquiring Librarian mean that ALL people born between 1981 & 1996 are humorless automatons clutching at the life-raft of political correctness conformity. Sure, some are, &, yeah, because this whole notion of 'political correctness' is a relatively new phenomena there might be more 'political correctness' while it's in its heyday but I'm sure there're plenty of exceptions. As I like to say, I hate all women, but I hate men even more. That's my way of adequately simplifying the problem. (OK, ***that's a joke!!***)

And yes, they are easily offended.

Well, you know what they say: the best defense is an offense: that's why I just immediately call everyone I meet *a shit-eating moron* before I stab them repeatedly in the face. That helps me get out my innermost feelings in a way that's completely healthy for me.

I know I sound like a total jerk.

I've always found you to sound more like a helicopter flying underwater but that's just me.

meeting him was such a breath of fresh air in a 'real' person who was an active artist without pretensions .

When you're as great as I am you don't need pretensions — those are for weaklings & inferiors.

(many thanks to Amir-ul Kafirs for introducing me to Lauren and Dave of Little Fyodor & Babushka fame - amazing and lovely and genuine souls that I miss dearly!!).

You're welcome. Did they make you sign your lease with a blood "X" like I commanded?

It seems the train of thought associated with this generation is working its way deep into politics and the running of our nation.

All we need to do is tie the shoelaces of the running nations together.

this group always seemed to have some sort of a 'uniform'.

Yeah, the uniform is the sign of the end times.. the end of punk as open-minded, the beginning of it as subculturally conformist. Unfortunately that started about 4 years in, in 1980.

Instead my friend was snubbed and treated very rudely by this girl.

Truly annoying. That's why I'm a firm believer in at least imaginary face-stabbing.

It seems the mainstream media is doing everything it can to rile up the crowds and create more clashes

Well, it's Business As Usual, as political activists used to say in the 1980s. Imagine a TV 'News' program with a slant to it like this: 'Today, in Pittsburgh, a 3,000 person march ended peacefully and the police acknowledged that they killed entirely too many people just because they were black.' It just doesn't have the same OOMPH! that: 'Today, in Pittsburgh, a 3,000 person march ended violently' does. I mean, what if there's no burning police car?! What would TV 'News'casters do? They'd be up shit's creek without a paddle or a cup!

it reads like a poorly written cop show drama.

Alas, it'll do the job of 1. selling fear, 2. turning people against anarchists.

My tongue in the world's cheek (& I don't mean its ass cheek),

****

June 3, 2020, 9:00PM (Amir-ul Kafirs to group):

As they say, the smaller the turf, the fiercer the dogs.

Don't dogs eat their own vomit?

****

June 3, 2020, 9:35PM (Amir-ul Kafirs to group):

It's really hard to offend me.

That's not true. Everytime I point out to Naia Nisnam how fat she is she throws diarrhea at me so watch your potty mouth.

You clearly don't fit the stereotypes of that generation.

I have to admit that I don't know what those stereotypes would be even though I take it for granted that they're there. Then again, I'm a Virgo & Virgos are perfection incarnate so any criticism directed against us of any kind is just a sign that the critic is utterly worthless & should've been aborted.

large groups of people in that age range went to the beach for spring break.

Damn! Really?! I now officially declare myself a millenial if it'll get me a free beach house that I absolutely haven't earned & don't deserve.

I keep meaning to reach out to him as I'm curious to hear his thoughts on the lockdown, etc.

But, of course, he's what I've just now decided to call an **ILLENIAL**. I support ILLENIAL IMMIGRATION. Let's flood the workforce with them.

The woman was beyond rude in the way she handled it. She completely ignored Amir-ul Kafir's existence, except to photograph him.

This is where I **thank the holy ceiling light for Naia Nisnam**. I'm going to petition the US military to restructure its mission statement to exclusively keeping Naia Nisnam alive & well. Why? Because I swear that for my whole fucking life if I'd told a large percentage of the people that I know the Skinny Woman story they would've said something like: *Well, you know, technically you raped her & you should consider yourself fortunate that she didn't have you arrested.* OR something equally idiotic. It might be hard to believe but for much or even most of my life I've been confronted by the attitude that just by being myself I am *inherently wrong.* I'm not kidding. In Naia Nisnam's next story she mentions a message exchange with someone who didn't realize that she knew exactly what was going on, probably more than anyone else around her, & that she did exactly the right thing to make the rightfully offended party (& I don't mean the woman) feel better.

So here's my story: this same condescending & ignorant person was once a close friend of mine. He didn't invite me to his wedding. I was told that I wasn't invited because *When Amir-ul Kafirs gets drunk he hits on all the women.* This former friend of mine & I talked about this: I said: When was the last time you saw me totally drunk? (My point being that it might've been 15 years ago) He said that that was not the point. It seemed to me that that was pretty central to the point. I reminded him that almost every time I see him he's so drunk he can barely stand & that he slurs his words. I also reminded him that at my house-warming party he was so drunk that he kept trying to convince me to let him suck my cock. I told him no but I did encourage him to sleep on my couch because he was too drunk to ride his bike home. I DIDN'T ban him from my house after that even though he was totally drunk & hitting on me. I mean, the guy's supposedly a 'punk' but he's intolerant of behavior that he himself displays?! I also disagreed with the "hitting on all the women part." I explained that at my age if I talk to a woman AT ALL I'm 'hitting on her' *if she's a PRINCESS.* My point was that whoever had complained about me **is a 'princess'** — by which I meant a bourgeois person who thinks that it's preferable for people to suppress their desires to satisfy the princess's neuroses. I mean just because I ALWAYS HAVE A HARD-ON & I PRESS IT AGAINST WOMEN'S MOUTHS AT PARTIES WHILE THEY'RE TRYING TO EAT doesn't mean that I'm hitting on them, does it?! (OK, you can see how my sense of humor might, um, rub some people the wrong way. Fuck'em.) Actually, I rarely hit on women anymore. I'd feel like I was in heaven if I could find a woman locally to even have an intelligent conversation with (other than Naia Nisnam, of course, who is a GODDESS AMONG BAD HAIR DAYS).

I could feel the guy's distress and as I walked by I touched his shoulder and said "I hear you man."

Naturally, I admire Naia Nisnam's reaction here.

The part that really has me upset is a conversation I had two days later with a friend.

The same guy I complained about above. If only Naia Nisnam has asked him to suck her dick.

If she was that afraid of human contact, then she should stay the hell home.

Such people have been my enemy my whole life. They're so self-centered that they think that other people should conform their behavior to **their fears** as if their fears are somehow justified. Instead of being like Sysyphus pushing a boulder uphill over & over again they should eat shit & die in a GIF.

I feel like I'm losing friends because of my unpopular pandemic views and I have to be fine with that.

Me too. I AM afraid I might be losing Naia Nisnam as a friend though because I noticed her pinky looking askance at me the other day. I'll have to watch my back with a mirror or something.

- flippanted out,

****

June 3, 2020, 9:43PM (Inquiring Librarian to group):

Amir-ul Kafirs, your comments are priceless, even more so tonight than usual... Can't stop laughing at the commentary!

About the millennial tag... Honestly i should be the last person trying to label anyone into a social group. For years i was pegged as a 'hippie.' I abhorred this label. I was more a brooding out of 'uniform' 'goth' but i loved colors and was a total nerd and a kind person. The label infuriated me. I hated what i had heard as folk music (think puff the magic dragon) and i could not stand what i perceived as hippie peace drivel mentality. Ok. Enough of that. I still plead ignorance to knowing what a hippie really is. But i do know i am not one. Am i even spelling it correctly?

All that being said, i am sure every generation generates annoying people who gather in like packs. A lot of the younger generations seem particularly upsetting... But maybe i am just getting old.

****

June 3, 2020, 9:59PM (Amir-ul Kafirs to group):

I also think this whole police car thing would have been orchestrated by a small number of law enforcement and most cops there wouldn't have know it was a set up.

I agree. What would be wonderful would be if there were a whistle-blower *in the police department* but that would be taking an incredible risk.

When I think about why...Why would police be so interested in demonizing anarchists that they would orchestrate all of this,

Let's keep in mind that there's nothing insuring that anarchy won't be made illegal. In some or all prisons the circled "A" anarchy sign is considered a gang sign, or, at least, was at one time. One thing I've been pointing out ffffooooorrrrreeeeevvvvveeeeerrrrr is that there was a time, the time of the Palmer raids earlier in the 20th century, when anarchists were deported. The problem for 'law & order' now is that most or all of the anarchists are american citizens

BORN HERE so we can't be deported but if anarchy is made illegal *we can be jailed.*

I think about future protests. Americans protesting police murders is pretty harmless, overall.

HHmm, I might have to turn Naia Nisnam's pinky against me here because I'm not sure I agree. I think the very fact that the police murdering black people is becoming so public really is a threat to the status quo. The usual police position is to urge everyone to stay calm while they deal with it. Then they let the murderer go. Every time people seem to think *this is going to be the time when the shit's been caught red-handed & can't get away* but let's not forget that no DA wants to endanger their career by being on the wrong side of the FOP.

What the people in power don't want to see is a repeat of the globalization protests, where activists brought to light issues that were not being covered by the main stream media.

Yep, that too. The more I think about it the more important I think the anti-globalization movement was.

Too many activists in this city are ready to throw this 20-year old into jail for spray painting and breaking a window in a cop car.

These same idiots are probably not paying much attention to the fact that the cops who murdered Brionna Taylor are walking around free. They care more about an easily replaced window than they do about a person's life. Hell, I think that burnt-out police car should be minimally serviced & put back on the streets without even a tad of body work.

Yesterday the Washington Post's headline read "White Instigators to Blame for Mayhem in Some Protests..." with yet another photo of a burning cop car, so it seems to be a nationwide thing and not specific to Pgh.

I think it's nationally organized, presumably by the FBI in conjunction with the more secret police cops at the local level, the cops who would've been 'Red Squad' in the past — I don't know what they're called now, probably something euphemistic like "Community Outreach".

I believe the feds came in and told our city officials that this outside anarchist thing was going to happen and the police chief and mayor got on TV and parroted what the feds told them.

Peduto blamed a graffiti campaign against the food coop on POG (Pittsburgh Organizing Group - an anarchist group) way back when before he was mayor. It's my understanding that there wasn't actually a firm basis to that accusation.

Im super concerned about people carrying concealed guns at a protest, walking through a crowd of thousands of people...

AND at the protest we went to on Monday 2 of the young black guys who seemed to be leading it openly held automatic weapons. I think one guy had an AK-47 & the other had a Tech-9. They might've been fearful because it had been said that white supremacists were planning to come & make trouble.

I fear a worldwide ban on protests will follow.

I hope you're wrong. I actually doubt that that'll happen but if I'm wrong & you're right I authorize your pinky to beat me mercilessly (just don't harm my pretty face).

your violent anarchist maniac friend,

****

June 3, 2020, 10:09PM (Amir-ul Kafirs to group):

Amir-ul Kafirs, your comments are priceless,

Damn! No wonder the Stock Market won't take them!

Can't stop laughing at the commentary!

Aw, shucks. I promise to stop vomiting on you every time I see you.

I still plead ignorance to knowing what a hippie really is. But i do know i am not one. Am i even spelling it correctly?

It depends on how high you are.

But maybe i am just getting old.

Well, you know what Woody Allen didn't say: Don't trust anyone over 50 & kill yourself when you get to be that age. You've got what? 5 years left?

-Inquiring Librarian-

Amir-ul Kafirs "Laugh-a-Minute" Psycho Killer

****

June 3, 2020, 10:19PM (Amir-ul Kafirs to group):

But the masks... at the end of a day of cloth masking, I am sometimes a bit tired and irritable, as I am today.

I honestly don't know how you can stand it. I can't stand to have one on for even a few minutes.

This state has had enough of instability and unrest recently.

Has anyone noticed whether any of the 'news' has made any acknowledgement whatsoever that the quarantine might be making people crazier? & that this could be factored in to the 'rioting' that theyre complaining about (&, presumably, exaggerating)?!

****

June 3, 2020, 10:32PM (Inquiring Librarian to group):

Re: HERETICS: Story from Pittsburgh

& i keep forgetting. Yes the Skinny Woman sounds like an insane unhealthily ocd germaphobe - aka: The New Normal. Gak. There is 1 girl working in my library that obsessively wipes down every surface with disinfectant wipes whenever she gets the chance. The place smells like oil based rotting fruit alcohol. Just gross.

I had a milder but no doubt very annoying and upsetting experience 3 weeks ago in the elevator at my physical therapist. I walked unkowingly into the elevator as usual, and a woman in the elevator broke me out of my oblivious daze to shout panickedly and angrily out that i need to SOCIAL DISTANCE that i should not be in the elevator with HER!!!! !! Next time i go to that place i feel like i need a plague mask and also a double yard stick whirling around my midsection and maybe an oldfashioned bullet bra under my attire for as useless an effect as the rest of my attire. See, you can yell at me for my inappropriate bullet bra but all the while be scared of my mask and possibly be painfully poked by my whirling yard stick gizmo when i get too close to you... You might really have something to scream at me about. But... Please, never end a sentence with a preposition.

Well i need to stop wasting everyone's time with my nonsense. I am frankly depressed today. Even insulting jokes at me are better than failing to type what i wish to convey. :/

****

June 3, 2020, 10:43PM (Inquiring Librarian to group):

I honestly don't know how you can stand it. I can't stand to have one on for even a few minutes.

i am losing it a little. It is making me a bit depressed and more alienated and dark minded. But i try to remind myself to be thankful i still have an otherwise great job. Luckily i have connnected on positive like ground with several patrons despite the distance of 'contactless pickup'. Because i have my own desk, i have taken to snacking a lot which helps me get the mask off. And i answer the phone obsessively so i can be the contactless pickup runner and rip my mask off as soon as i leave the building to drop the patron items on the pickup cart in front of the library.

Has anyone noticed whether any of the 'news' has made any acknowledgement whatsoever that the quarantine might be making people crazier?

No. I have not. Not the mainstream media i hear on npr and nothing on social media. Although i have mostly turned npr off this week.

****

June 4, 2020, 7:38AM (Phil to group):

Re: HERETICS: A quick update from amsterdam....Protest and work

It seemed like a lot of protesters in the photos did wear masks.

Yes I meant to say something about that. Most people were wearing masks in the protest because the organisers had asked and encouraged people to wear masks. I arrived on my own maskless but after a while it felt comfortable to put one on so I did. It is hard to estimate the amount of people who generally wear masks but I would guess something quite low like about 2 percent. At the moment Netherland cases are very low. New cases are close to zero. https://www.statista.com/statistics/1101300/coronavirus-cases-in-netherlands/

It is hard to explain Dutch culture to people who don't live here. The Dutch polder model of politics.https://en.wikipedia.org/wiki/Polder_model The 'doe maar normaal' (just be normal). Everything organised in straight lines. With that protests are also very organised. It is illegal to hold a protest here without first asking permission. This solidarity protest was no exception. Now the people in the Amsterdam Gemeente (council) that gave permission to the protest are getting some predictable flack. It has been the right wing that has been pushing for things to reopen and now they are complaining about the permission given to the protest given that although restaurants are open they are still practicing social distancing and gyms will not be opened until September.

I also deliver a neighborhood paper once a month with a (very) small business that was originally set up by activists (to support activists and also people without paper etc) to deliver 'the amsterdam weekly' a paper that has now gone out of business. Anyway this once a month job is a nice easy day, listening to audio books and getting paid cash in hand with a team of six people who are in some way or another involved in the amsterdam queer, squatter, anarcho movements. We work alone in our designated areas and meet for lunch. We were due to do a delivery just before the lockdown and it was these people who went overboard with precautions even before it was necessary. Masks and gloves and skipping lunch. Even the suggestion that we pull papers from the middle of the bundles rather than touch the top and bottom papers. They provided nice reversible pink and black masks which is what I wore at the protest. I went through the first half of this day wearing a mask but then decided that I really did not like it and never wore it again, also for the next two deliveries in the months after. The postal service does not wear gloves or masks here while they work. I used to work for the postal service for a while in the centre of the city. I bumped into one of my colleagues in the city once when I was doing part two of the modeling job I wrote about before. He was also a bit of a lockdown skeptic. He showed me a tiny bottle of disinfectant that the postal service had provided him with. It was a bit of a joke.

****

June 4, 2020, 10:15AM (Amir-ul Kafirs to group):

I like to see the police force as the doctor force, not all are horrible.

I agree. The thing that complicates matters, however, is that the police adhere to a strong practice, for obvious reasons, of 'having each other's backs' which means that if one of them lies the rest all get in line with him to support him. The rare cops who try to deviate from corrupt behavior are endangering their lives or, at a bare minimum, putting themselves at risk of becoming total social pariahs. You might be interested in reading this short e-book:

review of
Stephen Tabeling & Stephen Janis's Black October and the Murder of State Delegate Turk Scott
by tENTATIVELY, a cONVENIENCE - February 11, 2018
"Black October: White Christmas": https://www.goodreads.com/story/show/615672-black-october

The link is to my review of it but I'm sure you can find the book online for sale easily enough. Basically, the policeman tells 2 stories: one about the investigation of "BLACK OCTOBER" in Baltimore, the other about his uncovering police corruption, again in Baltimore, in connection with gambling.

And those doctors/police that I consider good should have the right to freely protest

I agree.. but for the same reasons cited above that's rarely what happens & while I speculated that the 5 cops on horseback might've been expressing solidarity with the cause there was nothing explicit to indicate that. In other words, they didn't have signs, e.g.. They might be forbidden to do such things, to have signs, etc.. I imagine they're going to be subject to stricter regulations than non-cops.

inevitably those horses were probably getting hit with bottles

I only saw, maybe, 10 to 20 items thrown. These were all small, the largest being a plastic water bottle, apparently empty, maybe 16 ounces size. People seemed to be careful to NOT hit the horses & I didn't actually see any horses hit.

I am among the lucky few that have not been subject to police misconduct.

That might put you in a minority of people I know. I've been told by the police, e.g., that I'm "the type of guy who hangs himself in his cell." — the implication being that they'd do it for me & then claim I committed suicide. &, no, there was no way I deserved that, they were berserk.

There is no black and white in these situations.

Of course not. I generally see the rank & file cops as working class people caught between a rock & a hard place. However, the civilians are also caught between a rock & a hard place but we don't have the legal right to kidnap & murder people. This latter right distorts matters enormously & is the primary engenderer of the hatred of cops.

& yes, I do see the police demonizing rioters and also demonizing anarchists and free thinkers that do not think as the mass media thinks they should think.

Alas, it could also lead to scapegoating. As someone who people have been trying to use as a scapegoat for most of my life I'm particularly hypersensitive to that.

****

June 4, 2020, 10:33AM (Amir-ul Kafirs to group):

Re: HERETICS: Belarus

I don't really know much about Lukashenko & Belarus but my impression / vague memory is that Lukashenko wanted Belarus to stay as part of the USSR, he might've been the only leader who preferred that. Again, this is only my vague, perhaps dramtically underinformed, impression but I see Lukashenko as someone who promotes vodka, saunas, driving a tractor, & playing ice hockey as staples of communist working class behavior. He seems more like someone who, at least for the sake of the image, cuts through the bullshit. I don't think my Belarusyn friends like him but that's what I'd expect. I'm sure they have a more realistic impression of who he is.

****

June 4, 2020, 10:40AM (Dick to group):

RE: HERETICS: A quick update from amsterdam....Protest and work

Interesting.
It's also illegal to hold a demonstration here without permission.
However, the day before yesterday there was one - when it happens it's called "une manifestation sauvage" - and it attracted a huge crowd, my son went in fact
It was obviously inspired by events in the US but centered around the killing here of a black man named Adam Traoré a couple of years ago by the police and for whom so far there has been no justice

****

June 4, 2020, 10:46AM (Amir-ul Kafirs to group):

The place smells like oil based rotting fruit alcohol. Just gross.

It apparently doesn't occur to such people that the disinfectant itself might be harmful. I think of the heavily perfumed people who hate other people's sweat odor. They never seem to consider that the smell of their industrial-strength chemical might be repulsive to others. As long as they BUY their smell it's ok (to them, not to me),

i need to SOCIAL DISTANCE that i should not be in the elevator with HER!!!! !!

Fucking unbelievable. It's an elevator, people are going to be crowded in it. If she was that upset she should have gotten off & walked up the steps. That's HER problem, NOT YOURS!!!

Even insulting jokes at me are better than failing to type what i wish to convey. :/

I hope you don't think my jokes were insults directed at you!! They're not. I'm just getting pretty desperate here for some absurdity — & by "here" I don't mean in this HERETICS group I mean in this claustrophobic society.

****

June 4, 2020, 10:52AM (Amir-ul Kafirs to group):

No. I have not.

Interesting isn't it that the most glaringly obvious cause of a widespread mental health problem is *completely ignored as if it's not there?!*

****

June 4, 2020, 10:55AM (Amir-ul Kafirs to group):

The postal service does not wear gloves or masks here while they work.

I don't think the delivery people here wear masks or gloves. At the actual Post

Offices they have plexiglass barriers in front of them & I think they wear masks & gloves but the masks are probably often pulled down below their mouths.

****

June 4, 2020, 10:59AM (Amir-ul Kafirs to group):

It's also illegal to hold a demonstration here without permission.

It's illegal in the US too. Anarchists tend to be the only people who defy that law (that I know of - maybe the 'right-wing' does too but I wouldn't know about that) but the more bourgeois end of the anarchist spectrum is afraid to do that. The police will respond harshly to an unpermitted protest but, of course, the argument in favor of not having a permit is that one shouldn't be paying the state to protest against it &/or having police protection. The annual May Day Parade in my neighborhood is unpermitted. That was stopped dead in its tracks by the PANDEMIC PANIC.

****

June 4, 2020, 11:05AM (Dick to group):

I didn't know that
I thought the "right to assembly" meant you could demonstrate
But I guess not!

****

June 4, 2020, 11:14AM (Amir-ul Kafirs to group):

I thought the "right to assembly" meant you could demonstrate

That's an interesting point. I wonder if the "right to assembly" was quietly made illegal somewhere along the line. In occupied countries the right to assembly is one of the 1st things to go. When the nazis occupied Hungary, e.g., I think no more than 4 people were permitted to assemble. Limiting assemblies to 10 people is awfully evocative of that. isn't it?!

****

June 4, 2020, 12:50PM (Inquiring Librarian to group):

No problem Amir-ul Kafirs. It's sometimes my own insecurities that get the best of me. I'm capable to jumping to extraordinarily wrong and uneducated conclusions. I'm really excited to dive deeper into Belorussian affairs now. And I fear I may never have a handle on the police and brutality. But I hope to look at those videos you shared asap. =] I know your jokes are just absurdities. I really absolutely LOVE them!! I need the absurdity too. I've been becoming increasingly more so in my writing and it's seeping more into my actions which I need to keep in check at work so that I am not seen as more nuts than usual.

****

June 4, 2020, 12:45PM (Inquiring Librarian to group):

I am hoping to talk with my dad this weekend. I am super curious to hear what he has to say. And honestly, I have no idea what he will say. But he likely knows quite a bit about Lukashenko and the current situation of Belarus with Russia. But then again, maybe not. He feels no great connection with either country, likely due to war trauma and losing his mom and also his hate for communism (part of why he has deduced democrats are horrible). I have to remember too, that dad will be 80 in September (another Virgo!!), but still seems pretty spry and fully cognitively functioning. He will be coming from an extreme Republican Trump supporting political view, which seems insane to me but also one of someone who grew up in a Russian community and spent many years in a refugee camp having fled Soviet era communism. He loves talking about politics and international relations. So it will be interesting to pick his brain!

It is very possible Lukashenko is aiming to rejoin Russia under the guise of the coronavirus. I really don't know. I will see what I can dig up and what my dad might have to say. From what I've seen most recently, that isn't Lukashenko's intention... but earlier posts did seem to indicate him angling towards a Belorussian/Russian merger... who knows, it's Russia/Belorussia... what can you trust?? I last saw something that supports Lukashenko rejecting a merge with Russia on June 4th, 2020 ... that I cannot find again =/. And then I found this (again I don't know about the source): https://emerging-europe.com/news/seven-reasons-why-belarus-wont-merge-with-russia/

As for Lukashenko and the fallout hit areas of Belarus. Honestly, from what I have read, so much of the country was hit (70% from several published estimates), and many people in the less horribly severely hit places continued to carry on life in those regions despite the radiation. What they could not see left them feeling unwilling to leave their homes and livelihoods unless they were forced out by the government. No doubt, many suffer terrible health issues that should be attributed to the radiation. The whole country seemed to just not know what else to do by carrying on, brokenly. They were/are a predominantly agrarian society that lived off of their land in their little villages with their families and grew their own food, for generations. Then Chernobyl hit all of sudden one day and they were told to stop their entire lives and leave the only things they'd ever known... for something they could not see or immediately feel. Horrible. A good book to read about the mess is "Manual for Survival: A Chernobyl Guide to the Future", by Kate Brown. I also learned in this book that many of the swamp lands in Belarus were used for nuclear testing throughout the cold war, irradiating communities and food supplies who had no idea about this. I am inclined to suspect Lukashenka knows all of this and is using the same logic of basically living with it because what else can you do but vacate the country and give up. I found this questionable article online: https://www.cbsnews.com/news/chernobyl-radiation-belarus-farm-produce-milk-high-level-radiation/ and in this, the farmer interviewed stating this: " "We're not afraid of radiation. We've already gotten used to it," said Kirpichenko" Although I wonder if he wasn't paid off (or threatened) by the government to say this (what I would think except that in the "Manual for Survival", this man's attitude did seem to honestly exist among residents hit with the radiation).

****

June 4, 2020, 1:06PM (Inquiring Librarian to group):

Dick & Amir-ul Kafirs,

How scary to think and to see the comparison. I am still trudging through that book on Europe between Stalin & Hitler from the 1930's through the 40s... Too much of it eerily echoes the past into today's government actions, including control of the masses through emotionally brainwashing them into completely otherwise irrational actions and thus into 'new normals'.

****

June 4, 2020, 4:11PM (BP to group):

I'll have to think about the protest stuff. I have the conformist, intolerent youth brigade rolled up in a ball with the Antifa camp in my brain.
Really don't like either separate or apart and I'd be way more impressed if they set themselves on fire. heh heh. Peacefully.

Anyway, I read the below article a day or so ago and got me to thinking about Dick's China question. Get over the first paragraph, the covid mentions sprinkled and I found it a compelling read. I should really read it again before I send but do not know when that will be.

Covid has exposed America as a failed state

It's hard to view the US at this point as anything other than a cautionary tale

https://unherd.com/2020/06/covid-has-exposed-america-as-a-failed-state/

****

June 4, 2020, 5:23PM (Amir-ul Kafirs to group):

rolled up in a ball with the Antifa camp in my brain.

Well, I have to say something in defense of Antifa. Really, though, I should clarify & say that it's in defense of ARA (Anti-Racist Action). I don't know whether that, specifically, even exists anymore per se but I imagine that if it does it probably gets lumped in with Antifa. Anyway, the ARA that I was familiar with 20 years ago seems to've been largely formed to fight back against prison-originated white supremacist gangs like the Hammerskins. Members of these gangs were leaving prison & aggressively re-entering the community. The ARA seems to've felt that such people would feel much freer about murdering people if there were no known violent opposition to them. I quote from the ADL website re Antifa:

"That said, it is important to reject attempts to claim equivalence between the antifa and the white supremacist groups they oppose. Antifa reject racism but use unacceptable tactics. White supremacists use even more extreme violence to spread their ideologies of hate, to intimidate ethnic minorities, and undermine democratic norms. Right-wing extremists have been one of the largest and most consistent sources of domestic terror incidents in the United States for many years; they have murdered hundreds of people in this country over the last ten years alone. To date, there have not been any known antifa-related murders." - https://www.adl.org/resources/backgrounders/who-are-antifa

The ADL site is basically against Antifa's violence but I think that the above distinction that they make is important. Neo-nazis & white supremacists don't seem to have any problem with murdering people, Antifa isn't murderous. That's a big difference.

****

June 4, 2020, 5:38PM (Inquiring Librarian to group):

HERETICS: The Irrational World of Libraries in the Time of Covid 19

I am beside myself on this one. This is what I have to deal with when being a librarian in the time of the pandemic panic. To me it is so utterly senseless and irrational. Read below, a quote from my supervisor in response to one of my fellow librarians asking about being able to provide free masks to patrons when we are allowed to open if the patron forgets or does not have a mask:

"I feel like all I'm doing is putting you guys off answers/decisions etc. You know me, I am a PLANNER to the nth degree so yeah, I'm frustrated. Truth is, we are not open yet.....and there is no timeline for when we will re-open. The mayor and the public will expect something of us at some point (of course!) but right now is "idea collection time" on how to open. Do we open for 2 hours at a time, then close/clean, reopen two hours later? Do we let 25% of the public in for 30 minutes at a time? How do we manage a clock on each person who enters? Do we open all the branches or just a few? Do we take temperatures of all entering public? Who's going to do this and how with social distancing? What about family groups? Do they need to social distance from each other? How do we know who belongs to which group if any? Do we let people use the computers? How do we help them on the computers? Do we stand 6 feet behind them and use a laser pointer for help? What about the problem of...if you are standing 6 feet behind someone...how can YOU see the screen to help them? Will this method help or hurt more? Do we out rightly state to them that we cannot help them on a computer? Does that help our image or hurt it? We are a group (mostly) made up of people helpers. How do we deal with NOT helping? There are so many questions and, since this is an unprecedented long-term event, few answers. Admin is working on ideas based on staff input and how other library systems are reopening.......so feel free to send ideas to me and I'll bring them up to the group. So far, the issue of masks hasn't gotten past the "required for entry" talking point."

So, what upsets me so is that this is supposedly an unending long-term problem in the eyes of the public library world. I ask, why is it that I can go to Walmart and do self checkout, the self checkout malfunctions and the Walmart attendant comes to my side and swipes her little card and punches stuff into the screen, and voila, I am able to self check again. We did not social distance, we touched the same screen, she helped me with my tech problem. Why can't the libraries do this?? Why is it ok to be smashed onto people in a protest (be tear-gassed... don't tears contain the stupid virus too??), but we can't let our population in need use our computers and why can't we help them on the computers? Where is the logic in this? Have we all gone completely bonkers??

I have neighbors and library patrons who are very poor. They cannot use their cell phones to do many things that they need and simply like to do. They do these things at the library. We help people apply for food stamps, unemployment, job applications (even McDonald's requires an online application these days), create an email address so that they can do all of the above, etc... See above, This is apparenltly DANGEROUS!!! Jebus Chriminy!!! REALLY??!! !!

Why does this have to be long-term indefinite, etc.??? Are we all being primed for all civil servants being required to get some horrible vaccine?? Will I lose my job because my job is no longer allowed in the "New Normal". And if I get to keep my job, and am forced to be vaccinated, and I actually have a legitimate medical reason that makes it dangerous for me to get this vaccine, is it even legal for them to do to me and anyone else who cannot (or chooses not to) tolerate unnecessary vaccinations? And what about the fact that this virus is going away, ALL ACROSS THE WORLD right now... But wait, no, read the NYT today... The corona virus is apparently gaining strength across the world:

View in browser nytimes.com

The New York Times

BREAKING NEWS

Coronavirus cases are growing faster than ever around the world, driven by emerging outbreaks in Latin America, Africa, Asia and the Middle East.

Thursday, June 4, 2020 1:46 PM EST

The coronavirus pandemic is ebbing in some of the countries that were hit hard early on, but more than 100,000 new cases worldwide are being reported each day.

Twice as many countries have reported a rise in new cases over the past two weeks as have reported declines, according to a New York Times database.

Will this ever end?? I am feeling overwhelmed with the powerless of the insanity I am surrounded by and that seems to be enforcing total control over my and all of our worlds. I innocently ask each library patron I talk to on the phone how they are doing and their loved ones. NOT A SINGLE ONE thus far knows anyone or has anyone in their family that died of this, and none that tested positive for it. I had one patron tell me that his doctor friend told me that in his cardiac care unit he was asked to change all of the unit's deaths to Covid 19 from their originally recorded heart related deaths. I am feeling like a guppy trapped in a tank, waiting for emotional and physical slaughter by my 'owners'.

****

June 4 2020, 6:57PM (Amir-ul Kafirs to group):

Re: HERETICS: The Irrational World of Libraries in the Time of Covid 19

This is what I have to deal with when being a librarian in the time of the pandemic panic.

Whew! It really is a heavy load.

Have we all gone completely bonkers??

The answer to that, of course, is YES, most people have gone completely bonkers. What can you even propose? Perhaps you could consult the latest advisories from the WHO & the CDC & emphasize that they're no longer as Draconian as your library system apparently is.

I reckon there's not much hope that you could propose that the staff choose which levels of 'safety' they prefer & that some staff be allowed to work together WITHOUT MASKS & all the rest of it. The paranoids could either take an extended leave or only work in non-public areas or only work during closed times or whatever. If only there were some viable way to express that you (& others) think that the danger is exaggerated & that the quality of your life is being severely degraded by precautions that you think are unnecessary & ridiculous.

Yesterday I went for a walk in a park like I do frequently. Some people, like myself, are without masks & seem a little nervous but are willing to say HI. I descended from a smaller path that goes down a hill to intersect with a park road that people walk on. There was a couple walking there with a dog. The man had on a mask, the woman didn't. I intersected the road at about the same time that they passed the end of my trail by. We then walked in the same direction & turned down a stairway to get to the lowest level. I figured it would make them nervous that I was even walking in the same direction as them so I wasn't in any hurry. As soon as they got on the stairwell they got on their cell-phones. I heard the man say something like 'There are many signs' as if he were answering a question. I had to wonder whether they'd called the police saying that they were being followed by someone with COVID-19 & whether the police were asking them why they thought that. Of course, I had no way of knowing. When I got to the bottom of the steps they had gotten off the trail, the woman had her back turned to me & the man was staring at me. I said "Hello" & walked by. He nodded his head slightly but didn't say anything. I didn't really have any way of knowing what was going on with them but the lack of a "Hello" added to the way the guy was watching me etc made ME paranoid. I think things will get better when no-one wears the masks anymore but the way things are going that might not happen any time soon. Of course, if it happens widely enough all the crazy conformists might fall in line.

I am feeling overwhelmed with the powerless of the insanity I am surrounded by

Where is Louisiana at in the quarantine relaxation? The "Green Phase" starts tomorrow in Pittsburgh but when I went to look at books on the sidewalk in front of my friend's bookstore she was still wearing full regalia, including goggles even though it was 88ºF outside today. I mentioned to her that Green starts tomorrow & asked whether the store's conditions would be changing with that & she told me something like 'that she was working on being able to reopen the store'. I think I need to look at what the WHO & the CDC are advising & see if I can use that as a wedge to restore a little sanity here because people are at least as fearful as ever.

****

June 4, 2020,9:24PM (Amir-ul Kafirs to group):

HERETICS: Self-Styled Anarchists

It just occurred to me that anarchists were formerly referred to in the mass media as something like "self-styled anarchists". In other words, we were never *just anarchists*, we were always people just calling ourselves anarchists. I don't think "self-styled" is right, though, it was something else. DOES ANYONE ELSE REMEMBER? It was always the same language in every 'report'. Anyway, the point is that now that these cop car burnings are happening anarchists are "anarchists", we're no longer "self-styled anarchists". I think there's a reason for that.

****

June 4, 2020, 10:09PM (Amir-ul Kafirs to group):

HERETICS: Good News

Naia Nisnam sent me the link to this article in a text message earlier today & since she hasn't shared it here yet I'm doing so. If local people take this doctor's opinion seriously it could make a huge difference in how crazy people are acting around here. Naia Nisnam & I are both pessimistic about that. It seems that people actually WANT to be in a crisis. I have to wonder whether Americans, at least, don't have some unconscious need to not feel so privileged. Maybe these people want to feel more at one with other people in the world whose lives are harsher.

****

UPMC doctor says COVID-19 has become 'less prevalent' and isn't making people as sick

Updated Jun 05, 2020; Posted Jun 04, 2020

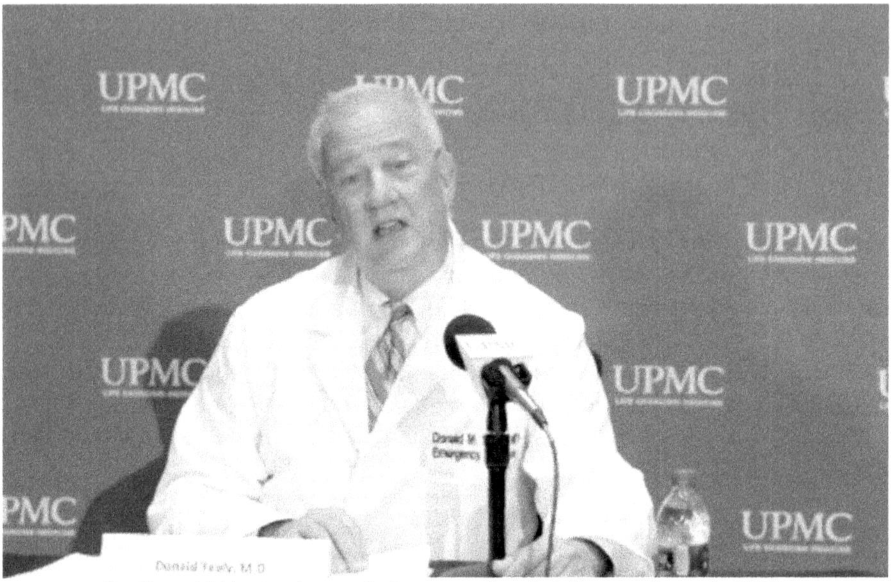

Dr. Donald Yealy shown during an online briefing on June 4, 2020.

By David Wenner I dwenner@pennlive.com

Fewer people are testing positive for COVID-19 and those who test positive don't seem to be getting as sick, a UPMC doctor said Thursday.

"All signs that we have available right now show that this virus is less prevalent than it was weeks ago," said Dr. Donald Yealy, the chair of emergency medicine at UPMC.

Yealy further said, among people who test positive, "the total amount of the virus the patient has is much less than in the earlier stages of the pandemic."

RELATED: UPMC doctor argues COVID-19 not as deadly as feared, says its hospitals will shift back to normal

The proportion of people with COVID-19 getting so sick they need a breathing ventilator has fallen, according to Yealy.

"We see all of this as evidence that COVID-19 cases are less severe than when this first started," he said.

Yealy said those observations apply to western and central Pennsylvania along with communities in New York and Maryland served by UPMC.

He said UPMC has so far conducted about 30,000 coronavirus tests, with less than 4% showing positive. He further said UPMC has tested about 8,000 patients who had no symptoms, with those patients testing positive at a rate of about 1 in 400.

He said that suggests the widely-feared prospect of getting COVID-19 from someone with no symptoms is unlikely. However, that assessment is based on the likelihood of encountering someone who is COVID-19 positive but doesn't know it. It doesn't address the likelihood of catching COVID-19 from someone who actually has it but doesn't feel sick.

"Your risk of getting into a car accident if you go back and forth across the turnpike in Pennsylvania is greater than your risk of being positive for asymptomatic COVID-19 infection," he said. "This should give you some reassurance that the risk of catching COVID-19 ... from someone who doesn't even know they have the infection, in our communities, is very small."

Yealy said he doesn't know exactly why the prevalence and severity of COVID-19 seems to have fallen. He said it likely reflects an interplay of things including weather, possible genetic changes in the virus, people watching themselves more closely for symptoms, and better medical decisions and treatment.

UPMC hospitals have discharged about 500 people who had been hospitalized with COVID-19, Yealy said. They are presently treating about 100.

- https://www.pennlive.com/news/2020/06/upmc-doctor-says-covid-19-has-become-less-prevalent-and-less-severe.html

****

June 4, 2020, 10:21PM (Amir-ul Kafirs to group):

HERETICS: More Good News

& here's the 2nd relevant article that's linked to in the last article. Of course, this is just reinforcing things that all of us have been saying all along but it's great to read it from a doctor connected to the biggest hospital in the region.

UPMC doctor argues COVID-19 not as deadly as feared, says its hospitals will shift back to normal

Updated May 11, 2020; Posted Apr 30, 2020

By David Wenner | dwenner@pennlive.com

A UPMC doctor on Thursday made a case the death rate for people infected with the new coronavirus may be as low as 0.25% — far lower than the mortality rates of 2-4% or even higher cited in the early days of the pandemic.

Dr. Donald Yealy based it partly on studies of levels of coronavirus antibodies detected in people in New York and California, and partly on COVID-19 deaths in the Pittsburgh region. The studies found that 5-20% of people had been exposed to the coronavirus, with many noticing only mild illness or none at all, he said.

"We've learned that way more people, far, far more people have actually been exposed to the infection without any knowledge of it. That makes the overall death rate much lower," said Yealy, who is UPMC's chair of emergency medicine. "Many people just didn't feel sick at all and recovered without difficulty."

Yealy went on to offer a hypothetical scenario of 3% of Allegheny County residents being exposed — a conservative number compared to the findings of the New York and California studies.

That would mean about 36,000 people in Allegheny have been exposed to the coronavirus. With 94 COVID-19 deaths in the county as of Thursday, it would mean 0.25 percent of people exposed to the coronavirus had died, he said.

"There is a big difference between 0.25% mortality and 7%," Yealy said.

Yealy said about 1,300 people in Allegheny have tested positive for COVID-19. That would mean, in his hypothetical scenario, another 34,700 had been exposed but had no symptoms. He noted the latter group may also have antibodies to protect them from future infection, although he pointed out it's still unknown how much protection people get from previous exposure to the new coronavirus.

Yealy further said the majority of the deaths among UPMC patients involved people over 80, with many being nursing home residents.

Yealy has been one of the main public voices of UPMC during the coronavirus pandemic. He spoke Thursday during a 40-minute online discussion with reporters.

Another speaker, Dr. Rachel Sackrowitz, the chief medical officer for UPMC's intensive care units, said 234 COVID-19 patients have recovered and been discharged from UPMC hospitals. "This is very good news. It means people are getting better and we're all on the right track together."

Yealy said only 2% percent of the UPMC system's 5,500 beds are occupied by COVID-19 patients and the number of new COVID-19 patients is declining.

He cited that figure in explaining UPMC's plans to quickly increase its volume of the non-emergency surgeries that were largely banned to conserve beds and supplies for COVID-19 patients. The ban is now being eased as the volume of COVID-19 patients falls short of worst-case predictions.

The officials said UPMC remains ready to deal with any upturn in COVID-19 cases.

Yealy said he can't predict if there will be a second wave, but said "What I suspect is COVID-19 will be a part of our experience treating patients for an extended [period of] months to maybe years."

Yealy was asked whether people should worry about COVID-19 more than the regular flu. He said people should be "worried differently," pointing out that both take their heaviest toll on the elderly, especially nursing home residents, and people weakened by other medical conditions.

Yealy said he "would not think of it as more or less, just two different illnesses that share some features, but have some distinct differences."

Sackrowitz said she expects COVID-19 will be part of the ongoing "disease burden" affecting Americans and, as with the flu, doctors will find treatments.

- https://www.pennlive.com/news/2020/04/umpc-argues-covid-19-not-as-deadly-as-feared-says-its-hospitals-will-shift-back-to-normal.html

****

June 4, 2020, 10:32PM (Naia Nisnam to group):

Re: HERETICS: More Good News

Don't get too excited... This doctor said similar things in early May and no one paid attention:

https://inside.upmc.com/yealy-shapiro-senate-testimony/?utm_source=facebook&utm_medium=social&utm_campaign=socialized&utm_content=socialized-share-link&utm_term&fbclid=IwAR0j4529KPIlVXJTNJ9sDwA5AVj9_TL_irC9OPKfrUVeTxsgGgo81-5igKc

****

June4, 2020, 11:26PM (Amir-ul Kafirs to group):

Re: HERETICS: More Good News

This doctor said similar things in early May and no one paid attention:

Well, yeah, that last article was originally posted APRIL 30 & THEN REVISED MAY 11!!

****

June 5, 2020, 4:45PM (Inquiring Librarian to group):

Car Accidents charted like Covid spoof

https://youtu.be/oxznGIj8Ja0

The video replaces Covid-19 with Car Accidents. It seems like the same logic to me. =/

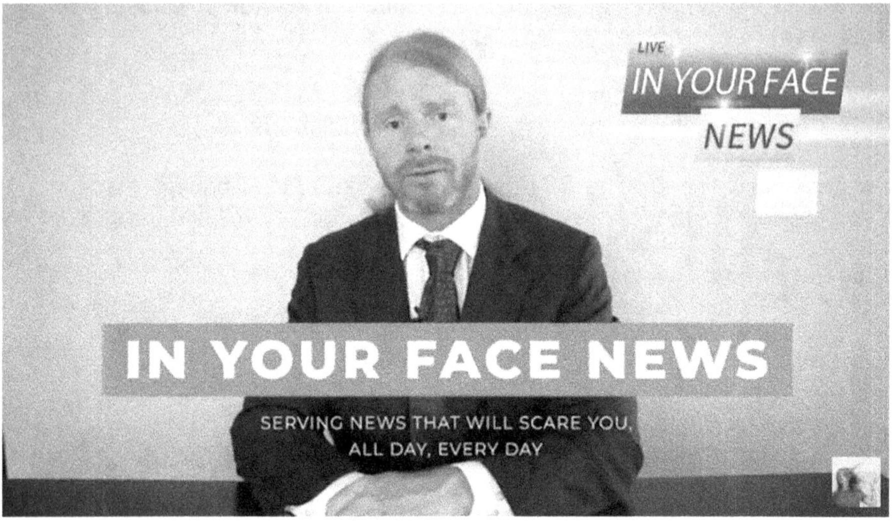

AwakenWithJP

1.17M subscribers

Here's why the lockdown should never end. In the global pandemic the lockdown has been used and extended. Many think it should end. Here's why they're wrong and it should potentially never end.

****

June 5, 2020, 10:13PM (Amir-ul Kafirs to group):

Re: Car Accidents charted like Covid spoof

THX. I didn't find this as funny as his other ones but I still liked it & left this comment:

I'm struggling enough with just trying to end my breathing & eating addictions. Unfortunately, a side-effect of this is that I've taken to driving 2 or even THREE motor vehicles simultaneously every time I go out as a way of overcompensating for the withdrawal that I'm going through. I have found that informing on my anarchist neighbors is helping to relieve the stress & it's my hope that even though they've been very nice & friendly to me that their way of life will become completely illegal so that we'll all have a scapegoat to take our frustrations out on.

****

June 5, 2020, 11:02PM (Inquiring Librarian to group):

For me, this video was helpful today. Within the 1st hour at work, I let my staff of 4 know that the state of Louisiana is likely going into phase 2 reopening sometime next week, with some restrictions and that the library may open in some restrictive form to the public soon. I thought this would be good news to the staff. Instead, my sanitization obsessed young Library Assistant attempted to knowingly school me on how stupid opening up and moving into phase 2 would be and the lives that it would cost. I tried what Amir-ul Kafirs said in giving her tidbits of information to consider such as herd immunity and also considering countries that didn't close such as Sweden and Taiwan. Her immediate response to Taiwan was "Contact Tracing", that saved them and we need more. Sounds to me like she's ready to become a good Hitler Youth or a Stalin informist. She has her thinking cap on. Then I started to take it too far. She's a smart girl, I want her to learn critical thinking and logic skills. I mentioned an interview I'd heard by a Nobel Laureate in Chemistry, Tony Levitt, who analyzed the graphed statistics of the virus and noted that the curves for all countries, whether they locked down or not, were basically the same. https://youtu.be/sEbcs37aal0 She still was not having it. She is one of those people that thinks that the lockdown must last indefinitely. I guess she will be first in line to eagerly get her new DNA vaccine and add surveillance apps to her phone so as to save herself and the world.

****

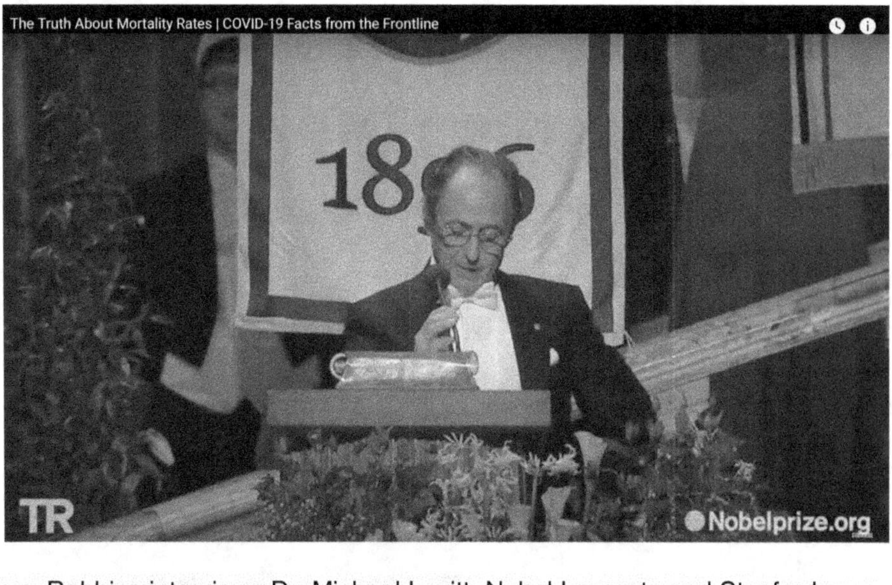

Tony Robbins interviews Dr. Michael Levitt, Nobel Laureate and Stanford Professor, about his extensive analysis of COVID-19 mortality rates – which have shown strict lockdowns to be an overreaction that have caused more harm than good.

This interview is part of the “Facts From the Frontlines” episode of #TheTonyRobbinsPodcast, where Tony uncovers the truth about coronavirus with a 7-person panel of highly qualified researchers, an experienced epidemiologist, a Nobel Laureate, and M.D.s testing and treating patients on the frontlines. Together, they reveal the evidence-based research that has come to light in the last two months.

This is one of the most important interviews Tony has ever conducted. It reminds us to stand guard at the door of our mind, practice discernment when determining trustworthy sources, and think critically in order to stay flexible and maintain the ability to pivot in light of new information – especially when lives depend on it.

COVID-19 Playlist
https://www.youtube.com/watch?v=YgP_A...

Do You Fear COVID-19? Take the survey now! https://www.youtube.com/post/Ugw2ngqc...

00:00 - start
00:31 - Professor Levitt
00:19 - Journey against fear
03:18 - Not much worse than the flu
03:46 - Average person believe what we have been told
04:36 - Death rates is what's important
06:06 - Epidemiologists don't mind being wrong on the high side
07:02 - Decisions that were made were bases off morbidity rate of 3.5% - 4.5%
07:28 - Algorithm = Model = Guess
08:13 - We have new data but we haven't changed what we're doing
10:08 - 4 countries that did NOT shut down
10:58 - Herd immunity
14:03 - Who Coronavirus taking out?
15:32 - Being coded for COVID
16:54 - A race to try to maximize deaths
17:28 - Did social distancing save us?
18:41 - Update from Tony Robbins

To hear the full interview, go here: https://www.tonyrobbins.com/podcasts/...

NEW RESEARCH FROM DR. LEVITT: Influenza and COVID19 Have Similar Total and Age Range Excess Deaths
https://www.tonyrobbins.com/podcasts/...

****

FUNNY HOW "ANARCHIST CHAOS" RARELY KILLS ANYONE WHILE "LAW & ORDER" KILLS PEOPLE REGULARLY.

****

June 6, 2020, 8:20AM (Dick to group):

RE: Car Accidents charted like Covid spoof

Thank you... I watched a number of his videos... they are be a mixed bag but enjoyable overall... they seem to center around making fun of people... I guess that's what comics always do in one way or another....
certain people seem to understand how the youtube thing works... I wonder if it's calculated or a natural extention of what they do... maybe both...
it's interesting I think to look at early films, early disc recordings, early radio programs, early tv shows - I mean the days when no one knew "what the people wanted" and the repetitive formulas developed... or the early days of jazz, rock, any new style.... there's always an experimental period before the money men get in there and fix things in place and essentially ruin things... perhaps because the internet is still somewhat free & open (at least in comparison say to disc or film distribution) the experimental period could, hypothetically at least, go on forever... on the other hand I do see a certain rule at play, that of the lowest-common-denominator

****

June 6, 2020, 12:59PM (Amir-ul Kafirs to group):

Her immediate response to Taiwan was "Contact Tracing", that saved them and we need more.

Sheesh. The advantage that you have might be one you don't want to use. You're the branch manager. You can simply tell her that this is the way it's going to be, that you've noted her concerns but that you think that this is the best course. When the changes happen & she doesn't get sick & everyone else is ok with it she can either recognize the reality of it or move on to a different job where she feels safer.

I mentioned an interview I'd heard by a Nobel Laureate in Chemistry, Tony Levitt, who analyzed the graphed statistics of the virus and noted that the curves for all countries, whether they locked down or not, were basically the same.

One of the interesting points that the host of the above-linked-to show makes is that fear reduces the immune system by increasing stress & the bodily expenditures that go with stress.

thinks that the lockdown must last indefinitely.

Apparently, it doesn't affect the quality of her life. If that's the case, then I can only speculate that she doesn't have much of one.

I guess she will be first in line to eagerly get her new DNA vaccine and add surveillance apps to her phone so as to save herself and the world.

At my most pessimistic I expect us to see alotof that. I'm hoping that my pessimism isn't justified but it is interesting to note that the electronic world, espcially that of cell-phones, has paved the way to making surveillance 'acceptable' to many people. These are the people who don't have the imagination to see that there might be a downside to it that might ruin THEIR LIVES TOO. These are the people who're unable to imagine THEMSELVES AS CRIMINALIZED. &, yet, it's possible.

****

June 6, 2020, 2:42PM (Dick to group):

This is a bit long but it is interesting
Among other ideas, he describes millenials in an interesting way i.e. as a possible force for change due to their being educated but without any real chance to get what they want - that's a Marxist thought at its base I believe
In a certain way however it seems like all these videos are preaching to the converted
That is, whether we have this or that set of specific facts or not, we all know or can reasonably guess that everything about government these days is corrupt, awful etc.
I do wonder if the USA will become the kind of total hell he describes
I also wonder what ideology would be powerful enough to actually get people to start to revolt en masse
https://www.youtube.com/watch?v=_F94MMbow6o&t=1172s

"The Ruling Elite Has Lost All Legitimacy". w/Chris Hedges

****

June 6, 2020, 10:44PM (Amir-ul Kafirs to group):

Among other ideas, he describes millenials in an interesting way i.e. as a possible force for change due to their being educated but without any real chance to get what they want

I only made it thru the 1st 5:21 of this so my opinion is close to worthless but Hedges's statement that the millenials "get it", essentially saying that they know that they can't even be "bought off" & that they're not going to get anywhere in terms of upward mobility just seems silly to me. What I mean is that I don't really think that people's primary concern is whether they can live the American Dream, it's much more directly that they want the murder of black people by the police to STOP. I think many people are more economically secure than Hedges seems to think, maybe I'm completely wrong about that.

****

June 7, 2020, 2:59AM (Dick to group):

What I thought was interesting is that everybody I know seems to describe millenials as self-righteous rule-following conformists, thus I wonder if for some reason Hedges is saying that for political reasons... meaning I found it interesting in a sort of backwards way

I guess I think that sometimes I feel like these videos, regardless of the source, seem like placebos and are suspect
If they were really dangerous would they even be there?
Meaning: you read something, it affirms a suspicion, you feel like you've done something, but in truth, you haven't, nothing in fact has happened
In the case of that video, saying to millenials that they can't be fooled, etc seems like a possible way to fool them with a lulling feeling of self-rightousness "Ah, cool, I'm hip...people can't get over on me...ok, let's get a latté...maybe i'll buy that guy's book"
I've noticed that almost all the videos are negative and the bigger the disaster, the more ominous the statement, the darker the conspiracy, the more popular they are... there's also an implied "in-crowd" element I wonder about
It gets to the point where the random event and the planned event seem indistinguishable, where fantasy, conjecture and reality become completely confused
Good old Chairman Mao said revolution comes out of the barrel of a gun
I think he knew what he was talking about, he was an a expert, a success for better or worse
Spiro Skouras, who I "like" says at the end of many of his videos "Prepare yourselves for what is coming!! etc."
I never know what to make of it... does he mean I should start stocking dried beans? buy a rifle? barricade my doors? move to Northern Canada?
Any real act is better than theory
Theory is useful to motivate action but isn't action itself

In music for example, you can talk forever but a good composition blows it all away
So, all these videos, etc seem useful to me only if they somehow motivate action
But at same time they don't suggest any real action to take at least as far as I can see

****

June 7, 2020, 12:26PM (Amir-ul Kafirs to group):

I wonder if for some reason Hedges is saying that for political reasons... meaning
I found it interesting in a sort of backwards way

Yeah, I can see that. Maybe if I'd managed to watch more than the 1st few minutes I would've found Hedges's ideas to be interestingly developed. I don't really have this concept of "millenials as self-righteous rule-following conformists" in my usual vocabulary so that absence is part of why I don't particularly appreciate what Hedges has to say. Not having paid much attention to the usual presentation of "millenials" I'm now beginning to wonder whether the idea of them as "self-righteous rule-following conformists" might be another mass-media construct along the lines of what happened in the 1970s when the trend seemed to be reeling people back to mainstream society by pronouncing the '70s to be the time of the "Me Generation". Personally, I'm really happy to see so many people out protesting day in & day out against police murders of black people because it's really necessary to show mass resistance to this. Unfortunately, the PIttsburgh police chief who actually made a point of trying to reduce police brutality was forced out of his position because the FOP gave him a vote of no confidence.

****

June 7, 2020, 12:32PM (Dick to group);

I can understand your liking seeing people out protesting
But I wonder about that, too
It seems that the G Floyd event has become a "global event", in fact the second recent global event after covid-19
And while I think its goal is worthy, I also wonder about it, maybe that's just my ingrained tendency to doubt all mass actions
Thus I was thinking when this showed up in my mailbox
https://www.youtube.com/watch?time_continue=1324&v=X6pzXrEBqRo&feature=emb_logo

The Great Reset Plan Revealed: How COVID Ushers In The New World Order - YouTube
For months we have seen our way of life change dramatically. We have been told time and time again things will never be the same and we must accept the new normal. Now the social engineers have ...

****

June 7, 2020, 1:05PM (Amir-ul Kafirs to group):

If they were really dangerous would they even be there?

Despite the censorhip of the internet I still think it's possible for important & paradigm-shifting work to get on YouTube & all the rest of it. It depends, I suppose, on what you mean by "dangerous". I've always preferred humor as a tool for social change. Is that dangerous? Probably not by most people's standards &, to me, that's part of what makes it effective. If "dangerous" means *likely to incite violent action* then, personally, I'd prefer to not go there. If I ever become as violent as what goes on in my imaginings then it'll be because I've lost self-restraint under stress. I saw a protestor's sign recently that said "Follow Your Anger", I think that's a really bad idea given that anger is an emotional response that doesn't have to be rooted in reality. I'm sure there's plenty of violence-inciting things, mostly hate rants, online — & that's where people like the guy who did the mass murder at the Tree of Life Synagogue gets his inspiration.

a lulling feeling of self-rightousness "Ah, cool, I'm hip...people can't get over on me...ok, let's get a latté...maybe i'll buy that guy's book"

In a way, that's one of the criticisms that I made in this book review:

1219. **a review of Jacob Wren's "Revenge Fantasies of the Politically Dispossessed"**
- credited to: tENTATIVELY, a cONVENIENCE
- published on Goodreads on January 6, 2011
- https://www.goodreads.com/book/show/8583944-revenge-fantasies-of-the-politically-dispossessed

The book is a political novel & I liked it ok but I realized that reading it could give people the delusion that they were being political activists by doing so.

I've noticed that almost all the videos are negative and the bigger the disaster, the more ominous the statement, the darker the conspiricy, the more popular they are...

It's apocalypse culture. It's something to get the adrenaline going, a type of high. I'm not nearly as apocalyptic as I was 35 years ago but then my life's not as difficult as it was then so I don't feel as much of a 'need' for volcanic change.

It gets to the point where the random event and the planned event seem indistinguishable, where fantasy, conjecture and reality become completely confused

Indeed. & that's part of what I'm thinking of as herding people into Virtual 'Reality', confuse it all together until none of it seems to make any difference anymore. One of the important things about Black Lives Matter is that it brings people back to reality. It tells people: *WAKE THE FUCK UP! BLACK PEOPLE ARE GETTING MURDERED BY THE POLICE, HERE'S A VIDEO OF IT HAPPENING! THIS HAS GOT TO STOP!!*

Good old Chairman Mao said revolution comes out of the barrel of a gun

I'm beginning to think there's a sortof 'default' position for humanity. In other words, a revolution happens & then things gradually get back to a variation on what was already there. As I see the police state taking over the US &, apparently, the rest of the world it seems that the "New Normal" is being implied to be the default. I'm hoping it isn't. Mao & co accomplished alot but it didn't take long for things to slide back & I'm not sure that this sliding was such a bad idea. It's like a form of cultural entropy. If the changes Mao & co brought about had been accomplished with less mass murder maybe it would've been more effective in setting up a new default.

Spiro Skouras, who I "like" says at the end of many of his videos "Prepare yourselves for what is coming!! etc."

I think he has a clear head but that he's still a part of survivalist culture & I think survivalists have an exaggerated sense of how bad things are. Then again, so do I much of the time! ESPECIALLY NOW. Still, what I'm hoping for isn't predicated on the idea that the shit's going to hit the fan & that we're all going to have to hunker down in our bunkers.

Any real act is better than theory

Indeed. That's why I'm happy to be at least a body in these protests — even though I'm exhausted & depressed.

In music for example, you can talk forever but a good composition blows it all away

I've been researching West German music after WWII & been finding out about composers who consistently composed outside of any system. Those are the people who interest me the most at the moment. Academics clung to serialism like a life raft in an attempt to save themselves from a lack of imagination.

So, all these videos, etc seem useful to me only if they somehow motivate action

At the end of the video that started this whole thread **[An episode of "Awaken With JP"]**, the character takes the simple action of: 1. driving to the store to get food, 2. going back to work, 3. leaving his house (although he still takes his laptop with him). Basic as those actions are they're at least common-sensical.

****

June 7, 2020, 3:21PM (Amir-ul Kafirs to group):

It seems that the G Floyd event has become a "global event", in fact the second recent global event after covid-19

George Floyd's murder is, unfortunately, another addition to a long string of murders. It's the straw that broke the camel's back. An earlier incident that prompted a similar response was the beating of Rodney King. I don't personally believe that either of these crimes by police against blacks were premeditated by a ruling elite to further destabilize things & I'm not convinced that the ruling elites are opportunistically taking advantage of them either. I think these protests are a natural reaction to injustice. Something that doesn't seem to be acknowledged is the affect that the quarantine is having on the unconscious of EVERYONE — including the cops. I suspect that cops are even more trigger-happy than usual thanks to the psychological effect of the quarantine. This seems fairly obvious to me but it can't be acknowledged, mainstream society has to be in denial of it because acknowledgement would mean admitting that the quarantine's affects are substantially negative enough to call the quarantine into question. Add the quarantine's unconscious suffocation to the racist business-as-usual & that's a powerful recipe for mayhem.

And while I think its goal is worthy, I also wonder about it, maybe that's just my ingrained tendency to doubt all mass actions
Thus I was thinking when this showed up in my mailbox

As is fairly typical these days with my computer, the video wouldn't play. I probably need to give the computer a rest, I hardly ever turn it off, & I imagine that the internet is getting even more use than ever — both of those things can explain how poor my internet service is now.

ANYWAY, I like Spiro Skouras but I think he doesn't have much practical experience with what I, at least, call the 'real world'. He's an intelligent guy but he strikes me as a technician, someone with social experience limited primarily to 'his own kind'. Hence, after awhile, his speculations & proclamations seem a bit too rooted in his & others's fabrications rather than day-to-day experience out in the 'real world' with a variety of people. For me this's related to things like "The Turner Diaries" in which depictions of black people aren't based on actual experience with a variety of black people but, rather, with stereotypes provided within a narrow social circle. I don't mean to say that Skouras is a racist, I just mean to say that his worldview is almost exclusively conspiracy oriented & doesn't seem to have many other facets to it. I have to wonder how he's made his living. Has he had a security clearance job as a technician for the government? That would certainly increase one's paranoia.

****

June 7, 2020, 3:37PM (Inquiring Librarian to group):

The Spiro talk about the 'Reset' freaked me out enough that i biked to the park and jogged against the wind and intermittent downpours in the mud puddles at Audubon Park in the midst of Tropical Storm Cristobol. I survived. I am soggy. I feel better. Let's hope Spiro has taken the survivalist new world order theory a bit too far. Then again, maybe nanotech can help flatten my mid 40s stomach and i can be perfectly happy eating chips and having my dr program more functional sanity into my veins.

Like Dick, i am also skeptical of 'mass actions'. But at this point i admit total confusion.

****

June 7, 2020, 4:43PM (Dick to group):

Yes, that video had a similar effect upon me
It may be my last one for a while
*
One potentially positive note: I have seen more and more articles (in France) saying the pandemic wasn't a pandemic, that it was exaggerated, and almost everyone I meet, to varying degrees, seem to think the whole business was amplified out of proportion, so maybe that's the result of all these videos being watched and shared, who knows?
*
Here there have been demonstrations about Floyd comparing his death to a guy named Adama a couple of years ago... but a white guy was killed in exactly the same way, in fact his larnyx was smashed under a cops knee and it was filmed to boot, and he doesn't get mentioned yet it was the same police brutality that killed them both... this is not my trying to pull a "white lives mater" bit or to downplay what happened to G Floyd but rather to show what I think may be selective media coverage

Cédric Chouviat, dead after a police check: the autopsy that calls out

According to the autopsy report, Cédric Chouviat died of suffocation and a broken larynx during a police check. A judicial investigation for manslaughter has been opened.

By Ronan Folgoas and Jean-Michel Décugis

January 7, 2020 at 5:23 p.m., modified January 7, 2020 at 9:09 p.m.

The hypothesis of a police blunder took on a new thickness on Tuesday. According to the first results of the autopsy performed on Monday, Cédric Chouviat died after suffering from asphyxia with a broken larynx. "To cause such a result, the police officer (s) necessarily exerted a prolonged and very strong pressure with two support points, in front on the Adam's apple and behind in the upper back," clarifies an expert retired medical. Christophe Castaner, Minister of the Interior, himself recognizes that these autopsy results "raise legitimate questions to which answers must be given in all transparency".

Friday, January 3, Cédric Chouviat, deliveryman by profession, rides a scooter near the Eiffel Tower when it is checked shortly before 10 am by a patrol of four police officers (three men and a woman). First, it seems to be the subject of an ordinary verbalization for using a telephone while driving.

But this father of five, a Parisian by birth, does not want to stop there. According to videos filmed by motorists and broadcast on Tuesday by his family's lawyers, he approaches the police, helmet on his head, telephone in hand. Is he trying to film them? The man is vehement and provocative, according to the police officers who face him. "You are clowns, puppets. You are the laughingstock of all Paris, you have only that to do, to scratch people... "he would have said according to remarks transcribed in the police intervention report, written the same day.

Cédric Chouviat, 42, was then arrested for contempt. The peacekeepers handcuff his left arm but fail to hinder his right arm.

"The Paris prosecutor's office tried to disguise the truth"

What happens in the following seconds? According to the intervention report, Cédric Chouviat steps back and stumbles. "Dragging us into his fall, he fell on a peacekeeper, causing him severe pain in both knees," it is written in this report. The peacekeeper rotated him bringing him face down, the peacekeepers hardly put handcuffs on him, places the individual on the side, asking him to sit down. This is where we see that his face is all blue, and that his helmet is removed. "

Cédric Chouviat has just suffered from pulmonary asphyxia, causing cardiac arrest. Rescued by firefighters and transported to the emergency room, he was then placed on artificial respiration. His death will be noted on Sunday at 3:30 a.m.

A video of about ten seconds collected by Arié Alimi, lawyer for the Chouviat family, sheds additional light. Cédric Chouviat, gray pants and black jacket, is then stomach on the ground. He actually wears his helmet. Three police officers are around him, one of whom is visibly in close combat. Does he exercise a particularly powerful throttling key as suggested by the result of the autopsy and the testimony of a passerby collected by the Chouviat clan?

"We welcome the opening of a judicial investigation but regret the head of manslaughter who has been retained", points Me Alimi. This Tuesday morning, a complaint was filed by the Chouviat family for intentional violence resulting in death without intention to give it.

"The Paris prosecutor's office tried to disguise the truth by first disseminating the idea that the death of Cédric was not directly linked to the intervention of the police," criticizes the lawyer. Moreover, even today, the prosecution maintains confusion by evoking a previous cardiovascular state. "Overweight, Cédric

Chouviat simply suffered, according to his wife, from high blood pressure problems.

- https://www.leparisien.fr/faits-divers/cedric-chouviat-mort-apres-son-interpellation-l-autopsie-evoque-une-asphyxie-avec-fracture-du-larynx-07-01-2020-8230815.php

****

June 8, 2020, 11:12AM (Phil to group):

Re: Happy 54th!

Thanks eveyone for wishing me well with my social media birthday!. Don't forget that Phil Bradley is a pseudonym for Phil Bradley. A less virtual Phil Bradley will have a birthday later in the year. Nice to have two birthdays in one year. To work out the other birthday you just need to replace the 06 with 10. I was exploring Phil Bradley a little bit with this social media group;
https://www.facebook.com/feelrad

After work on my social media birthday I decided to go to the graduation exhibition of the students I modeled for. Sylvie who is the teacher for the group and her husband Hewald who i also often model for also turned up. https://zijlmansjongenelis.nl I had a short conversation with him about how teaching was going with the covid stuff. Just the general expected stuff...more and more things becoming permanently digitalised.

On a side because I neglected to mention before is the covid story of one of the students. I modeled for the students two weeks in a row and I modeled for two students on their balcony. One of the students just talked with me more than she drew. She asked me what my opinion of the covid-19 situation and the lockdown was. I hesitated for a second and then decided to warn her that my views were not so conventional on the topic. She let me know that she was open to whatever my point of view was so I began to start articulating my ideas on the situation. Anyhow it turns out that her father (who was quite young, around 50) was diagnosed with Covid-19 and was put on a ventilator and it was not clear if he would survive or not. Even still it was good to know that _____ was still open minded on this subject and that before her father was even diagnosed she wondered if there was even such a thing as Covid-19. She was also quite obviously less worried about following the regulations. In the following week she was part of organising that I model for four of the students in total in a park. I did express originally my concern for ventilators. At the time I had not researched much about ventilators but remember seeing some stuff which suggested that they were not good. I followed up on the research that showed that ventilators themselves might be killing people. Perhaps hard stuff to share with her considering her fathers situation. I feel my own father was killed by the medical system. He was in his early eighties but very fit and healthy and also a rower still competing. He had a skin cancer removed but a few years later it manifested all through his body. He went in for chemo and it all went horribly wrong. Luckily _____'s dad though pulled through and survived in the end and was apparently quite mad about what happened to him. Most probably he would have been much better off if he had not gone to the hospital in the first place.

Yesterday during my lunch break I went upstairs to eat in the same space as the customers like I usually do if the space is not completely full. None of the other cooks leave the kitchen for their breaks if they have them but I always like the change of perspective and the chance to surreptitiously sketch some of the customers. I noticed now that a new system was implemented where a bar code (or whatever those square codes are called that smart phones can read) **[I assume Phil means a QR code]** was stuck onto the tables so that people could get a digital version of the menu direct onto their phones so that people don't have to touch those dirty filthy menus that other people are touching. Then I witnessed a customer walk in and get served in this case by the shop manager. First of all he needed to record the customers name. The customer had apparently just come from Germany and replied that it was worse here (in the Netherlands) than in Germany. They were surprised that they could not even be served before they gave their details. The customer also expressed some skepticism about Covid-19 talking about the science that 'they' don't want you to know about. I wonder how/if the Government will use this information? In my lunchbreak the day before on my social media birthday one of the on duty assistant managers asked if I had been living with or had contact with anyone with Covid-19. I was not sure if they were joking or not. I said as a joke I would check my app. I do not own a smart phone. They laughed. They also asked if I had a temperature. Apparently it was for some contact tracing bureaucracy that the Government was collecting. Anyway this particular assistant manager did not take it very seriously.

Another backdate from work was that on my last day before the lockdown (I did not even know at that point that it was my last day) a colleague confessed that he thought that the whole Covid-19 was more or less a conspiracy so that was comforting. He is from Portugal but also his family originally comes from Cape Verde. When he expressed this point of view the temp dishwasher from Algeria also agreed that it was a lot of BS so that was a comforting end day for my work.

****

June 8, 2020, 2:29PM (Phil to group):

HERETICS - TNI Webinar / second BLM solidarity protest amsterdam

Just thought I would advertise this TransNational Institute Webinar. It looks interesting. Taking on the Tech Titans: Reclaiming our data commons.

https://www.facebook.com/events/537325880275309/

TNI is an Amsterdam based NGO set up by Susan George who has done a lot of work exposing the World Bank, and the International Monetary Fund and Global Trade Agreements. I have watched a couple of webinars during the pandemic and found them quite interesting. Although I haven't seen anyone that skeptical of the virus itself they have been great at giving on the ground accounts of what has been happening in a lot of different regions such as South America, India and Africa.

I have an ulterior motive for mentioning this here because I am probably not going to watch this webinar because it clashes with another event. It seems Amsterdam is going to hold a second solidarity BLM protest, this time in the Bijlmer. The Bijlmer is an outer Amsterdam suburb originally designed for (a predominately white) middle class as an idealic utopian Le Corbusier style garden city in the 1960s. Lots of wide open spaces raised roads and super dense high rise flats. The project was a failure as no one really wanted to live there. Then the council started housing Surinamese immigrants there so now the area has a very high percentage of black people living there. Anyway I think I will go to this event rather than watch the screen and I will bring my camera with me to document the event....maybe a little video as well.

****

June 9, 2020, 3:05AM (Dick to group):

Heretics: Official Self-Congratulations on Confinement Strategy

Here's an article, the first that I've seen, about how well the confinement worked. I send it because it is the official line.

Small personal observation: Since the confinement lifted, I've met one person who said that she had contracted the virus. Needless to say, she said she was sick and then got better. In addition I've heard of two friends who also were sick and then got better. This makes me think that the confinement may have stopped the spread of the virus (as it would for any virus when you think about it), but I don't think that necessarily translates into saving 3.1 million lives.

https://www.lexpress.fr/actualite/societe/sante/le-confinement-a-permis-d-eviter-3-millions-de-morts-dans-11-pays-europeens_2127723.htm

Containment prevented 3 million deaths in 11 European countries

By LEXPRESS.fr with AFP

Conducted by Imperial College London, this study analyzes the main measures taken in 11 countries including France, Spain, Italy and the United Kingdom.

An initial assessment which demonstrates the importance of containment to contain the coronavirus epidemic. The restrictive measures decided to deal with the Covid-19 were effective in regaining control of the pandemic and made it possible to avoid 3.1 million deaths in 11 European countries, estimates a study published Monday.

Conducted by Imperial College London, whose scientists advise the British government on the health crisis, this study analyzes the main measures taken in 11 countries including France, such as banning public events, restricting travel or closing of shops and schools.

Mathematical modeling

"Measuring the effectiveness of these measures is important, given their economic and social impact", underline its authors, while the magnitude of the collateral effects of confinement is regularly underlined and that certain voices are raised, notably in the United Kingdom , to demand the acceleration of the lifting of the restrictions.

The researchers compared the number of deaths recorded on the database of the European Center for Disease Prevention and Control with the number of deaths that would have occurred in the absence of control measures, estimated by mathematical modeling. They conclude that the measures put in place have prevented approximately 3.1 million deaths in these countries.

82% drop in virus reproduction rate

Their article, published in the journal Nature, also estimates that they have made it possible to reduce by 82% on average the reproduction rate of the virus (the number of new people infected by each infected person), allowing to bring it back below 1, threshold below which the number of new cases decreases.

The researchers also calculate that on May 4, 12 to 15 million people were infected with Covid-19 (or 3.2% to 4% of the population on average, with significant variations depending on the country). Belgium would therefore have the highest infection rate, with 8% of the population having contracted the coronavirus, followed by Spain (5.5%), the United Kingdom (5.1%) and Italy (4.6%). This figure would be 3.4% in France. Conversely, only 710,000 Germans have contracted the virus, or 0.85% of the population.

The authors point out that since the measures followed each other on a short schedule, it is difficult to assess the impact of each of them separately. They nevertheless conclude that "containment had a substantial effect" on controlling the epidemic. The 11 countries studied are Germany, Austria, Belgium, Denmark, Spain, France, Italy, Norway, the United Kingdom, Sweden and Switzerland.

****

June 9, 2020, 11:01AM (Amir-ul Kafirs to group):

Re: Heretics: Official Self-Congratulations on Confinement Strategy

Here's an article, the first that I've seen, about how well the confinement worked

From my POV this is specious logic. There is absolutely no way to prove their assertion. If I say to a friend: "Don't go outside or you'll be hit by a truck!" & they follow my advice & don't go outside & then, of course, aren't hit by a truck that DOESN'T PROVE THAT THEY WOULD HAVE BEEN HIT BY A TRUCK IF THEY'D GONE OUTSIDE. I'm reminded of the familiar sales scam: *Buy One, Get One Free!* Let's say you want one toothbrush for $5. Unfortunately, you can only *Buy One, Get One Free!* for $10. All you're doing is buying 2 toothbrushes at $5 apiece when all you wanted was one. In other words, the logic of the quarantyranny is self-proving, I suppose that makes it tautological. If the Medical Industry says: *You're going to die if you don't do what we tell you to do* & then people don't die then instead of saying that they wouldn't have died in the 1st place it becomes the result of the Medical Industry's intervention. Just like the sales scam, it's all in the language. Instead of having language that says: *Buy 2 for the price of 2!* which, of course, isn't a 'deal', it becomes: *Believe in our language & what we say magically becomes the* ***truth!***

****

June 9, 2020, 12:14PM (Inquiring Librarian to group):

I get the New York Times daily updates in my email each morning. They have been spouting similar articles about how many lives have been saved by locking everyone down and destroying their livelihoods. They also pepper it with how our president started the lockdown too late and then estimate how many lives were lost due to his negligence, and how many lives will be lost since we are letting people finally escape their government enforced cages. NPR is on the exact same logic track as the NYT. It's what circulates at my work... we didn't get sick because we were locked into our homes. I mean, really... did you not go to the park and brush against the crowds during the pandemic? Did you not go to Walmart and not actually stand 6 feet from people without a mask before Wally World expected masks and limited the amount of people in. It's all so old hat now. I feel like a broken record spouting out about how illogical this all is.

****

June 9, 2020. 8:18PM (Amir-ul Kafirs to group):

I feel like a broken record spouting out about how illogical this all is.

Don't stop just because you feel like a broken record! There's always something new & valuable to be said. I'm actually happy when people express their/our continuing disatisfaction here because MY DISATISFACTION IS ALSO CONTINUING. Today, e.g., I'm a bit more depressed than usual despite the fact that we're in the "Green Phase" but certainly aided & abetted by what a continued oppression this so-called "Green Phase" is. Things really haven't changed that much since the Yellow Phase, too many people are still paranoid quarantiniacs wearing masks & most businesses still require them, etc. Below's my latest text panel mocking the self-congratulations. I'm not really that satisfied with it.

Old Con Artist Trick
(Self-Congratulation of the Quarantyrants)

Quarantyrants:
If you don't follow the DOCTOR GODS edicts
you will be struck dead!

Hundreds of millions of people obey.

Quarantyrants:
Behold! You followed our edicts and
were not struck dead!

[Ignoring the millions who didn't obey
who also weren't struck dead,
such as the citizens of Belarus]

****

June 9, 2020, 7:41PM (Dick to group):

https://www.youtube.com/watch?v=Ms3-zehFloY&fbclid=IwAR3TVpBCVWUiejk2pDfiXnga2tswJ4IUxXJuY2gs7pKOijUYcm4jlVRcv4I

Little Billy aka Evil Mr. Rogers Tells You The Truth For The First Time - YouTube

****

June 9, 2020, 8:57PM (Amir-ul Kafirs to group):

Very effective!! I added it to my PANDEMIC PANIC playlist. I'm still sticking to shorter entertainment criticisms because I think they're more effective but it's tempting to just add every fucking thing that reinforces our position on this.

****

June 9, 2020, 11:22PM (Naia Nisnam to group):

The Little Billy video is funny and effective at stating the problems with this whole situation but it also scares me. It leaves me with that we're all fucked and there's nothing we can do about it feeling.
The Great Reset video gave me that same scared hopeless feeling, but even more intensely. I wish I could dismiss Spiro but... the clips from the World Economic Forum... how can I ignore that? I don't want this to be true but.... it is and I don't know what to do with that information. Again, I envy the ignorant. What good is it to know what is really going on when I cant do anything besides feel miserable about it?
Spiro does reference the George Floyd/BLM protests as being "under the guise of seeking social justice..... when in reality these 'riots' are nothing more than an organized destabilization effort much like the ones we have seen the US and the CIA carry out in countless countries... this is a planned operation."
I have a friend who says things like this on her social media and I cant wrap my head around it. George Floyd's murder was planned? The people's response to it was planned? I mean, were they planning this since the first slave ships stole humans from Africa? Have they been planning this since the beginning of colonization? In my mind the police murders of Black people and resulting uprisings have their root in the ugly origins of America, if not earlier. I cannot make sense out of the idea that these uprisings have been planned. I'd love to read or watch more information about this theory, but the dismissive way that Spiro refers to "systemic racism" is a turn off for me.

I've been very mad that our part of the state has gotten to the "green" phase of reopening. It is the last phase. There is nothing else for us, until this is all declared over.... Yet, people are still walking alone outside with masks on, stores are still requiring us to wear masks despite the change in regulations, our libraries and museums are still not open...
My mother was distressed today because the news is reporting that 11 people from PA contracted COVID from a beach house party in NJ over Memorial Day weekend. She blames peoples' irresponsible behaviors, not staying 6 feet apart and not wearing masks indoors. I read an article about it on CNN and around the middle of the article, it admits that the people who contracted Covid are having "mild symptoms". So... I come back to my argument that it is actually good for young healthy people to get the virus.... Except that is being used as a scare tactic and people, like my mother, are already expecting a return to lockdown and are preparing to acquiesce. It's that preparing to go right back into lockdown, despite not wanting to, that infuriates me.
I looked up information on regulations in the state of Oregon because I am flying there next week to visit my love. I read their state's plan and was horrified to see:

"Concerts, conventions, festivals, live audience sports won't be possible until a reliable treatment or prevention is available," the plan said. "It is unknown at this time when this will be."

https://www.thelundreport.org/content/oregon-reopensl-more-masks-required-certain-restrictions-place-through-september

I doubt that is exclusive to Oregon. They really do plan to have us socially distancing until there is a vaccine. I feel sick.

Here's Canada:
“There is no real return to full-scale, what I'll call normal operations, to pre-March operations, until such time that there's a vaccine that's generally available,” said Morawetz, of the Ontario Superior Court of Justice.
https://www.orilliamatters.com/coronavirus-covid-19-local-news/courts-wont-return-to-normal-until-vaccine-is-readily-available-2393562

Europe:
Life will only return to normal once a coronavirus vaccine becomes widely available, said European Commission President Ursula von der Leyen.
https://www.politico.eu/article/ursula-von-der-leyen-vaccine/

Australia:
When will social distancing end? The real question is, when will there be a coronavirus vaccine? Until that day comes, sit tight and stay home, unless it's essential.
https://www.crikey.com.au/2020/05/26/when-will-social-distancing-end-in-australia/

It goes on and on. I'm making myself miserable and need to stop looking into this. We are in lockdown until there is a vaccine. I knew it. Reading about it upsets me. I dont know what to do.

****

June 10, 2020, 12:21AM (BP to group):

Cops have always been either outright hostile toward me or obviously wary. When I was shipped off to school in the 9th grade my classmates older brother was graduating and so his extended family came for the ceremonies. One Uncle was or had been on President Jimmy Carters Secret Service detail. My friend told me that his cop Uncle warned him about me. Said that I fit the profile of a person that the Secret Service were trained to look out for as trouble! I was 13. What the heck! My offense was probably looking him in the eye and expecting to be treated as an equal.

****

June 10, 2020, 9:20AM (Amir-ul Kafirs to group):

What good is it to know what is really going on when I cant do anything besides feel miserable about it?

This is one of the main areas where I continue to be more optimistic than many people. MONEY ISN'T EVERYTHING. These people with all their power are still just human beings, even augmented by their computers. At the risk of seeming like a megalomaniac, I've accomplished far more in my life than most people & I've done so with almost no money ***because I have an imagination & drive***. As far as I'm concerned, Bill Gates is NOT my equal. Do you think that if Gates had grown up in a trailer park he'd be who he is today? I know, I know, that's a ridiculous *What if?* type of question but my point is that the things I see myself & my friends accomplish, no matter how modest they may be, are far more important & impressive to me than any of the Machiaveliian diabolical machinations of the billionaire control freaks. We're like knotweed, we grow back no matter how much the ultra-rich poison the environment. WE ARE THE REASON WHY BILL GATES WILL FAIL.

I cannot make sense out of the idea that these uprisings have been planned.

IMO, it would be 'impossible' to plan what's happened. There are too many variables. Was it 'planned' that we were there when the cop car blew up? Was it 'planned' that we're now skeptical about who exactly started that fire? I think it's always a part of the ruling elite MO to turn these things into media spectacles that excuse the police state & generate revenues — but independent of that there've been plenty of people who've been participating in these protests who're getting their 1st taste of revolution & who're *learning from it*. I don't really think that's good for the 'planners'.

I'd love to read or watch more information about this theory, but the dismissive way that Spiro refers to "systemic racism" is a turn off for me.

Yeah, to be in denial of systemic racism or SYSTEMIC CLASSISM is to be pretty out-of-touch with 'street-level reality'.

I've been very mad that our part of the state has gotten to the "green" phase of reopening. It is the last phase. There is nothing else for us, until this is all declared over.... Yet, people are still walking alone outside with masks on

I, of course, am mad about this too — including extremely exasperated by protestors wearing the masks. If this is as good as it's going to get for awhile then my anger-management skills are going to have to be working overtime.

I come back to my argument that it is actually good for young healthy people to get the virus....

& in the past that might've just been common sense but in today's age of maximum propaganda there's just senseless terror instead.

I dont know what to do.

I feel ya. At age 66 I don't really feel like having to go into maximum resistance overdrive, *I want to retire*, but, oh well!

****

June 10, 2020, 9:30AM (Amir-ul Kafirs to group):

My offense was probably looking him in the eye and expecting to be treated as an equal.

Ha ha! You probably weren't 'properly' subserviant or 'in awe' of his job.

When I was 15 I was taking a Driver's Ed class at my high-school in preparation for getting my driver's license. The 'teacher' was just some sort of bullying imbecile not qualified for much of anything as far as I could tell. Anyway, in what might've been the 1st class he stood in front of us & immediately started slandering one of the students who wasn't there saying that she was a pill-head, etc. I proceeded to respond by loudly verbally objecting to this slander. I didn't know the student he was talking about, I was objecting on general principle & found his behavior mind-bogglingly unacceptable. I was immediately expelled from the class & he told the rest of the class that I was "the type of person who would run over old ladies". I didn't get my license until I was 19. Oddly, I've never once run over an old lady.

****

June 10, 2020, 11:03AM (Inquiring Librarian to group):

Elmhurst Hospital Nurse

This interview was on Phil's page.
https://www.youtube.com/watch?v=UIDsKdeFOmQ&fbclid=IwAR1cSAwwgjzpxLT-8s6Dpy1VTxHtb6CyyBcgiBXcZtJKUPVYVhmSb2Q4QkY

It is a nurse from the horribly hit Elmhurst Hospital in NYC. Note, the nurse is originally from Florida, she is ex military and she was called in to work at this hospital because of her experience. If what she is saying is true, then it confirms my suspicions all along about the care of these patients and the diagnosing of these patients. The most shocking, but 100% believable clip in the interview was the young guy who ripped his own vent tube out. I was thinking... how could he have done that, he was supposed to be heavily sedated... but then I realized he may have been a heroin addict, or a recovered heroin addict. And sure enough, I was right, he had drug addiction problems and the sedation the hospital gave him was not enough, hence, he woke up, freaked out, and pulled his tubes out.

Editor's interpolation:
This interview with Nurse Olszewski is one of the most important pieces of

evidence in the whole PANDEMIC PANIC for me. In it, she reveals that patients would come into Elmhurst Hospital in NYC with breathing difficulties, would test *negative* for COVID-19, would *still* unnecessarily be put on a ward with COVID-19 patients, would *then* become COVID-19 positive, would be put on a ventilator, & would die. She reveals that the hospital administration had given orders that stated *Do Not Resuscitate*, even though that isn't the conventional practice. As I understand it, the hospital received CARES money for every COVID-19 patient so there was potentially a financial incentive for declaring people COVID-19 when they weren't initially. *ANYWAY*, the result was a large death toll in a poor area resided in by mostly or entirely people of color. For me, this makes the extraordinary NYC death toll that was used so much in scaring everyone in other places where the death toll was small becomes very suspect as something *created* by hospital policy & practice.

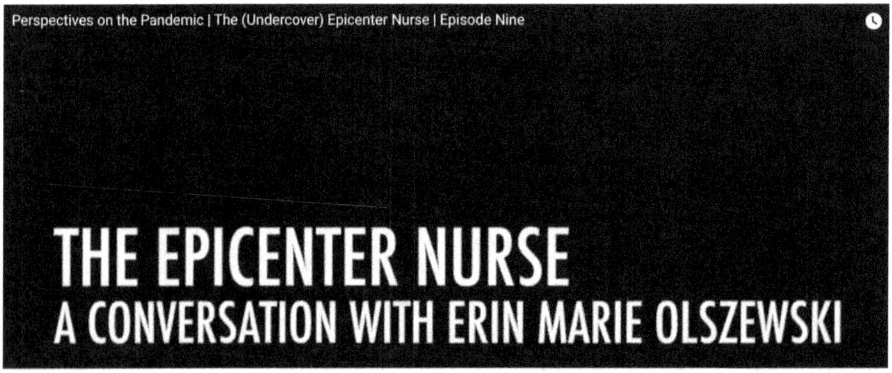

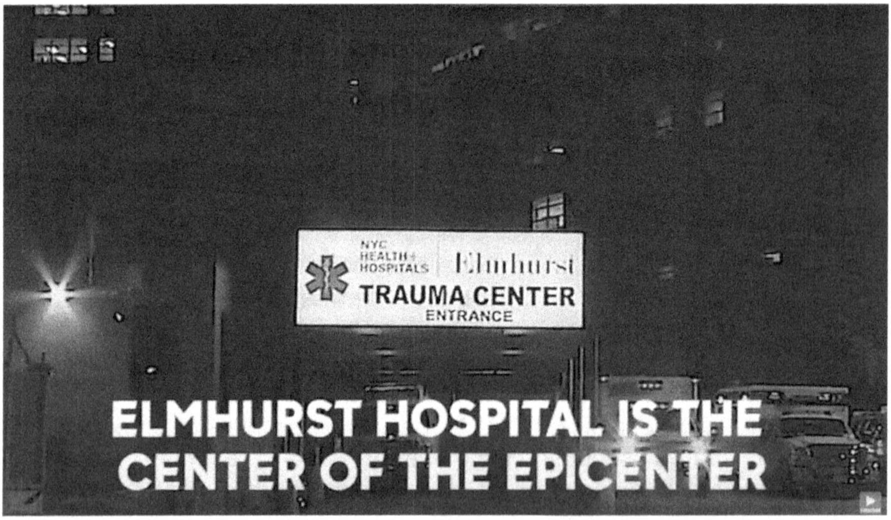

Daily Mail MORE STORIES

EXCLUSIVE: 'It's a horror movie.' Nurse working on coronavirus frontline in New York claims the city is 'murdering' COVID-19 patients by putting them on ventilators and causing trauma to the lungs

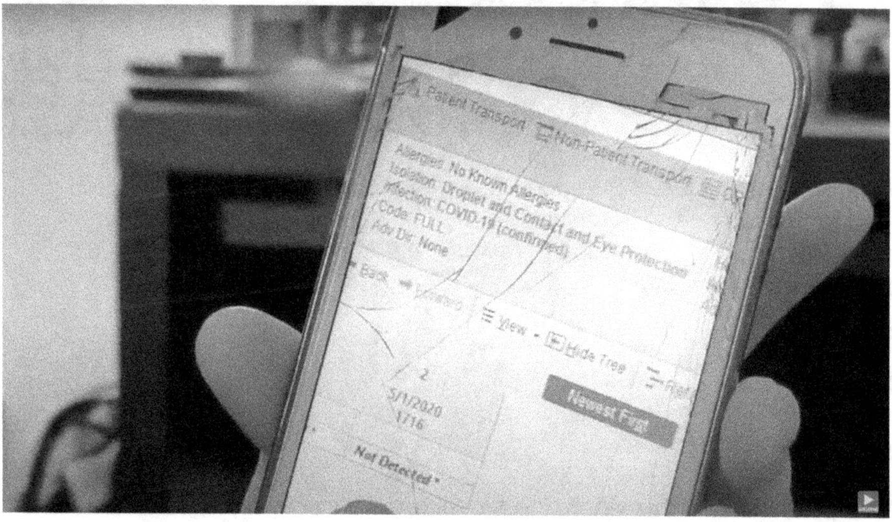

Erin Marie Olszewski is a Nurse-turned-investigative journalist, who has spent the last few months on the frontlines of the coronavirus pandemic, on the inside in two radically different settings. Two hospitals. One private, the other public. One in Florida, the other in New York.

And not just any New York public hospital, but the "epicenter of the epicenter" itself, the infamous Elmhurst in Donald Trump's Queens. As a result of these diametrically opposed experiences, she has the ultimate "perspective on the pandemic". She has been where there have been the most deaths attributed to Covid-19 and where there have been the least.

Erin enlisted in the Army when she was 17. She deployed in support of Operation Iraqi Freedom in 2003. Part of her duties involved overseeing aid disbursement and improvements to hospital facilities. While in country she received the Army

Commendation Medal for meritorious service, and was wounded in combat. Erin eventually retired as a sergeant, and became a civilian nurse in 2012.
Erin is a medical freedom and informed consent advocate. She co-founded the Florida Freedom Alliance but no longer has any connection with the organization.

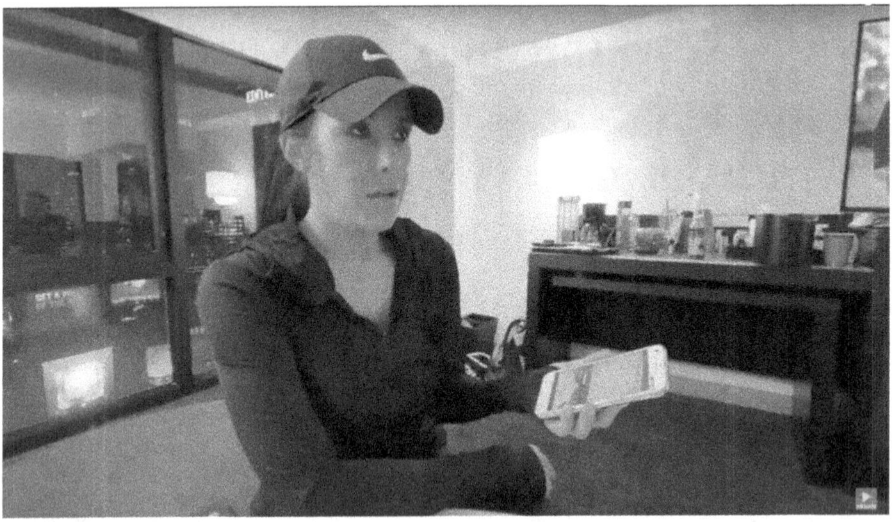

Watch more episodes of Perspectives on the Pandemic here:
Episode 1: https://dai.ly/x7ubcws
Episode 2: https://dai.ly/k7af1wKOAvcoA7w5DkZ
Episode 3: https://youtu.be/VK0Wtjh3HVA
Episode 4: https://youtu.be/cwPqmLoZA4s
Episode 5: https://dai.ly/k3l3VyZ2YQv6Zbw5VqE
Episode 6: https://youtu.be/3f0VRtY9oTs
Episode 7: https://youtu.be/2JbOvjtnPpE
Episode 8: https://youtu.be/WILmt6_w_AM

(As of publication of this video, the producers are still awaiting comment from Elmhurst Hospital).

Produced by Libby Handros and John Kirby, The Press and the Public Project.
Ref 7814

****

June 10, 2020, 12:28PM (Amir-ul Kafirs to group):

HERETICS: Burning Cop Car

I just talked to my old friend _____ on the phone. He made his living for a long time doing special effects for movies & he has experience with setting cars on fire. When I saw the cop car burn at the protest 2 Saturdays ago I was astounded at how black the smoke was & how long it lasted & I wanted to know if _____ thought that was natural. _____ said that, yeah, it is natural. He explained that when he burned cars he had to strip as much of the interior as possible to meet EPA standards because everything inside a car is very toxic when it burns. He said that if something gives off black smoke that means it's toxic. That makes sense given that the cop car wouldn't have been stripped inside.

****

June 10, 2020, 1:11PM (Inquiring Librarian to group):

Yes, I agree with Dick that watching the conspiracy videos does open up a questioning can of worms that is hard to close. I have always been a skeptic, but generally more of a lazy one unless the thing I am skeptical about really hits home... like this nonsensical response to an elusive virus. But then, what really is a conspiracy theory. I have listened to many interviews of well degreed scientists (even one Nobel Laureate) who disagree with what is going on with the virus. And now 2 nurse interviews concerning work on the front lines. If what these ladies and well degreed scientists are saying is true, then they are not theories, but truths. Spiro, I would have to gather, is a conspiracy theorist in the most definitive sense, as Amir-ul Kafirs said, he likely has little to no actual life experience in dealing with these things he talks about, the protests at least. Argh, and don't get me started on that article about DARPA that goes in detail about genetic mutations research and the military and ends with the funding pushing an RNA vaccine to 'cure' 'Covid'. Come to find out, several days after I read that article, one of the 2 companies listed in that article that are vying to win the race for a new covid vaccine is Moderna with their rushed RNA vaccine, the one the NYT and NPR blasted all over the major airways as being our future savior... Now I've gone full circle back to Naia Nisnam's concern over the world pushing for a vaccine (namely a dna editing RNA vacacine) as the only way to reopen anything back to the old "Normal". I have feared this nefarious vaccine now for several months. I would like to think, from the multitude of people I continue to meet who are also skeptical of this virus response, that many will fight against this vaccine. We can only hope. I for one absolutely will fight to not get this vaccine. My arsenal starts with my Dr.'s note and it will not stop there if that is not enough.

****

June 10, 2020, 11:05PM (Amir-ul Kafirs to group):

I've gone full circle back to Naia Nisnam's concern over the world pushing for a vaccine

I wonder if a class action suit could be made classifying this as a form of rape? After all, the idea is to FORCE US to have something put in our body. Sounds like rape to me.

****

June 10, 2020, 12:34AM (Amir-ul Kafirs to group):

Re: Elmhurst Hospital Nurse

It is a nurse from the horribly hit Elmhurst Hospital in NYC.

I've made it through the 1st 23 minutes. I've added it to my PANDEMIC PANIC playlist even though it's not short or 'entertaining'. It's a sad thing that the sheer quantity of deaths in NYC can be laid at the doorstep of poor medical care & greed. It's a good thing, however, if this gets exposed & the very possibility of it can be out in the open. The thought that NYC's dilemma is being used as a guide for the rest of the country to follow has always been ridiculous because of the sheer issue of differences in population density but this makes it even worse. THERE HAVE BEEN 170 COVID-19 DEATHS IN ALLEGHENY COUNTY, WHICH INCLUDES PITTSBURGH, TO DATE. That's it. 170. & yet some people in Pittsburgh still refer to the deaths in NYC as if that's what's happening here or WOULD happen here if there weren't these lockdown procedures in place. It's completely insane.

****

June 11, 2020, 9:00AM (Amir-ul Kafirs to group):

On Jun 11, 2020, at 8:23 AM, dick turner wrote:

The other day I saw the headline "Jeff Bezos reprimands a client who said "all lives matter"" then to day I saw this which says amazon won't let the police use their face recognition tool... it is so revoltingly obvious these are public relation plays...

I agree.. but I admit that I prefer them at least a little on the defensive. PR ploys are better than nothing at all which is what it would be if there weren't so much public clamor.

the super rich know how unreasonable they are and will do anything to try to make themeselves look good... if only public consiousness could get turned away from race and gender issues for just a short time and take to getting rid of these mega-rich types

Do you remember Charles Ives's proposal? He suggested that after acquiring a specified level of wealth (in his day it was something in the millions) that the money go into some sort of public pool, I think it was for education. The idea was that after this specified point of wealth there was really more than a person could ever use & that it was a social responsibility to contribute to the general good. I reckon one of the problems with the mega-rich is that they're 100%

habituated to turning EVERYTHING to profit. As such, no matter how much of an appearance of philanthropy they put out there's always a self-serving ulterior motive.

****

June 11, 2020, 8:45AM (Dick to group):

2nd Thoughts

As an aside:

I may have to revise my position on Trump being re-elected. He seems to be under attack from every possible quarter and I wonder if he'll be able to maneuver this way through it all. I felt he was going to win not for any scientific reason by the way but because I see him as a sort of statistical figure who seems to constantly get what he wants regardless of his conduct/IQ/whatever it may be. My model for this is the Disney character Gladstone Gander. Here's some Wiki info in case you've never heard of him (I added the boldface type):

Gladstone Gander is a Walt Disney fictional character created in 1948 by comic artist and writer Carl Barks. He is an anthropomorphic male goose (or gander) **who possesses exceptional good luck that grants him anything he desires as well as protecting him from any harm.** This is in contrast to his cousin Donald Duck who is often characterized for having bad luck. Gladstone is also a rival of Donald for the affection of Daisy Duck. Gladstone dresses in a very debonair way, **often in a suit**; wearing a bow-tie, fedora and spats. **He has a wavy hairstyle** which is depicted either as white **or blonde.** In the story "Luck of the North" (December, 1949) he is described as having a **brassy voice**.

****

June 11, 2020, 9:06AM (Amir-ul Kafirs to group):

Re: 2nd Thoughts

I may have to revise my position on Trump being re-elected.

Ha ha! I stick to the theory that Rump's appeal is just the familiar of 2 evils rather than the lesser of 2 evils. I like the comparison to Gladstone Gander! I only 'know' that whoever 'wins' the election, I lose.

****

June 11, 2020, 4:00PM (Amir-ul Kafirs to group):

HERETICS: Hospitalizations

SO, I looked at statistics to see how many COVID-19 deaths in Allegheny County there were as of June 10, 2020. The figure was 170. I've made a copy of the chart & added it below as the last of the materials hereby presented. Then I thought it would be interesting to see what predictions had been made about COVID-19 deaths for the same region back before the quarantine started or anytime after then. I didn't look very hard but what I found instead was a prediction for how many hospitalizations there would be in Pennsylvania.

<u>**COUNTY OF RESIDENCE:**</u> Fifty-five (55) counties have reported COVID-19 deaths.

County	# of Deaths	County Population[1]	Rate[2]
Adams	9	102,811	8.8
Allegheny	170	1,218,452	14.0
Armstrong	5	65,263	7.7
Beaver	74	164,742	44.9
Bedford	2	48,176	4.2
Berks	334	420,152	79.5
Blair	1	122,492	0.8
Bradford	3	60,833	4.9
Bucks	534	628,195	85.0
Butler	12	187,888	6.4
Cambria	2	131,730	1.5
Carbon	24	64,227	37.4
Centre	7	162,805	4.3
Chester	304	522,046	58.2
Clarion	2	38,779	5.2
Clinton	3	38,684	7.8
Columbia	32	65,456	48.9
Cumberland	58	251,423	23.1
Dauphin	101	277,097	36.4
Delaware	603	564,751	106.8
Erie	7	272,061	2.6
Fayette	4	130,441	3.1
Franklin	39	154,835	25.2
Fulton	1	14,523	6.9
Huntingdon	4	45,168	8.9
Indiana	5	84,501	5.9
Juniata	5	24,704	20.2
Lackawanna	189	210,793	89.7
Lancaster	322	543,557	59.2
Lawrence	8	86,184	9.3
Lebanon	38	141,314	26.9
Lehigh	259	368,100	70.4
Luzerne	161	317,646	50.7
Lycoming	17	113,664	15.0
McKean	1	40,968	2.4
Mercer	6	110,683	5.4
Mifflin	1	46,222	2.2
Monroe	102	169,507	60.2
Montgomery	740	828,604	89.3

Northampton	238	304,807	78.1
Northumberland	3	91,083	3.3
Perry	4	46,139	8.7
Philadelphia	1,454	1,584,138	91.8
Pike	20	55,933	35.8
Schuylkill	42	142,067	29.6
Snyder	1	40,540	2.5
Somerset	1	73,952	1.4
Susquehanna	16	40,589	39.4
Tioga	2	40,763	4.9
Union	2	44,785	4.5
Washington	6	207,346	2.9
Wayne	9	51,276	17.6
Westmoreland	38	350,611	10.8
Wyoming	7	27,046	25.9
York	30	448,273	6.7

[1]2018 population data used from the Pennsylvania State Data Center at Penn State Harrisburg.

[2]Death rate per 100,000 residents.

Pennsylvania's Daily Report of Deaths Attributed to COVID-19
June 10, 2020

As of March 26, 2020, it was predicted there would be 100,000 — with the statement that if the Governor hadn't intervened the number would be much higher. You can see that in the 1st article reproduced below. Then I decided to check on what the actual hospitalizations have been. I didn't find that either but I did find an article from April 30, 2020, saying that the hospitilzations in Pittsburgh have been so low that nurses are going elsewhere. The 2nd article reproduced below explains that. You might remember that my former friend the respiratory therapist told me that by the beginning of April the hospital would be beyond capacity. When that didn't happen he told me that his "brilliant" head doctor predicted that by mid-April the hospital would be filled with ONLY COVID-19 patients. That didn't happen either. Somehow, I doubt that it would be very hard to find a plethora of Draconian predictions followed by a contradicting plethora of statistics.

Pitt disease modeling platform predicts high COVID-19 hospitalizations

DAVID TEMPLETON
Pittsburgh Post-Gazette
dtempleton@post-gazette.com
MAR 26, 2020 7:00 PM

FRED at the University of Pittsburgh Graduate School of Public Health offers frightening predictions about what Pennsylvania residents could face with COVID-19.

Neither professor nor dean, FRED is the "Framework for Reconstructing Epidemiological Dynamics" computer platform that's currently projecting a top one-day peak of 100,000 hospitalizations statewide from infections with many more over the course of the pandemic.

That projection would have shown a top one-day peak of 280,000 hospitalizations — with total hospitalizations over the course of the pandemic of 500,000 — had Gov. Tom Wolf not forced timely closure of schools, universities and non-essential businesses. That number likely would have far exceeded hospital capacity.

[..]

"These are very scary numbers, and one thing I hope to impress upon people is that this is serious," said Dr. Mark Roberts, director of the Public Health Dynamics Lab at Pitt's Graduate School of Public Health and chairman of its Department of Health Policy and Management. "Social distancing is seriously important not only for yourself but the rest of community. That's the only thing you can do."

For now, he said 100,000 statewide hospitalizations remains an accurate possible prediction, based on multiple factors used in FRED analysis — the currently known behavior of the virus, school and business closures, infection rates to date, the extent of social distancing and population characteristics, among others.

Dr. Roberts said there's hope that further action can drive that prediction downward. The results also used original data from the Centers for Disease Control and Prevention that 20% of people who get the infection will require hospitalization. But more recent data from New York City and early results from Allegheny County make that percentage seem high, he said.
To date, Allegheny County has had 133 cases and 20 hospitalizations — a 15% hospitalization rate.

"We [in Pennsylvania] have done this pretty fast — closing schools and cutting down on [virus] transmission," he said. "The governor and others have banned large aggregations of people and closed businesses and universities, and that happened pretty quickly.

"That has the potential of making a really big difference in pushing [infections] off into the future," he said.

That means reducing the number of hospitalizations and over a longer period of time — flattening the infection curve — rather than having a fast-rising caseload that spikes at levels that overwhelm hospitals and the healthcare system.

[..]

- https://www.post-gazette.com/news/health/2020/03/27/COVID-19-coronavirus-University-Pittsburgh-hospitalization-FRED-pandemic-model-case-study/stories/202003230067

****

COVID Hospitalizations So Low In Western PA That Nurses Are Leaving To Help Elsewhere

By SARAH BODEN • APR 30, 2020

Early social distancing interventions have paid off. So far, fewer than 250 Allegheny County residents have been hospitalized for COVID-19.

In fact, the level of COVID illness is so low, some Pittsburgh-based nurses have left to take temporary jobs at hospitals in coronavirus hotspots.

Like many health systems, Allegheny Health Network and UPMC canceled a large number of non-urgent medical procedures to prepare for a rush of COVID patients.

"What we were expecting never actually showed up. But we were always on edge, almost," said Taylor Dilick, an intensive care unit nurse at UPMC Shadyside.

Infectious disease researchers and epidemiologists say that Pennsylvania's mandates of social distancing have been particularly effective in the western part of the state, which has had relatively few cases of the novel coronavirus. The early interventions slowed the virus's spread and prevented hospitals from being inundated with COVID patients.

"The last couple weeks I was at Shadyside… it felt like a ghost town," she said. "I felt like I wasn't really needed."

[..]

- https://www.wesa.fm/post/covid-hospitalizations-so-low-western-pa-nurses-are-leaving-help-elsewhere#stream/0

****

June 12, 202, 9:22PM (Inquiring Librarian to group):

Re: HERETICS: Hospitalizations

Thanks for sharing Amir-ul Kafirs! I am not at all surprised by this. The same thing happened in Louisiana, and specifically New Orleans. In Nola they turned the Convention Center into a hospital and it had only a handful of patients. Note: The city hired workers from Texas to do the work, leaving Nola workers unemployed while at the same time Texas was not allowing Nola folks to cross into Texas due to the scare of spreading the pandemic from Nola to Texans?

Does this make any sense? No, unless you are talking about shady financially incentivized deals. Here we read there were only 7 patients in the convention center hospital on May 20th. But the city plans to leave it in place despite it not being used now, in case of a 2nd wave of infections in the fall: https://www.wdsu.com/article/only-7-covid-19-patients-at-new-orleans-convention-center/32616526 This scares me. Is something being planned for us in the fall? Or are our politicians just 'innocently' swept up in the scare-mongering?

Anyways, I looked up FRED which is a thing created by the University of Pittsburgh's Health Sciences Department. Maybe you all already know this, but, it is, of course, funded by the Bill & Melinda Gates Foundation https://www.innovation.pitt.edu/innovations/fred-framework-for-reconstructing-epidemiological-dynamics/ . It is also funded by the Robert Wood Johnson Foundation which did a 2010 study on how terrible it is that adults in the U.S. don't get enough vaccinations: https://www.rwjf.org/en/library/research/2010/02/adult-immunization.html . I should look into a more recent Robert Wood Johnson Foundation study, but I have to make dinner and actually try to get some sleep tonight. I am recovering from a week of pointless videos at work about the virus and a particularly insulting one about how to handle homeless people during the pandemic and how these homeless people are more likely to believe "Conspiracy Theories" and went on to briefly describe and make fun of these theories. Gak.

All right, onward with the scare tactics, related to the ongoing saga of HOW MANY WAYS CAN WE CONTINUE TO SCARE YOU ABOUT 'COVID'??!!! Here's one hot off the press from the Washington Post: The title says it all.. "Chronic Coronavirus Syndrome" https://www.washingtonpost.com/health/2020/06/11/coronavirus-chronic/?arc404=true . All right already, are we not yet begging for the life saving RNA vaccine??

And can someone please tell me how to grasp that we have to vote for Biden? But what is our alternative? My head is spinning on this one. Biden is apparently brazenly running on a campaign of continuing the Coronavirus scare indefinitely. He plans to hire at least 100,000 federally funded Contact Tracers and he plans to force all major social media platforms to more heavily censor. https://www.nbcdfw.com/news/politics/biden-releases-plan-to-reopen-us-economy-amid-coronavirus/2387018/
If you want it straight from the horse's mouth in more detail, all fazillion pages of it, go to Biden's page: https://joebiden.com/covid19/ .

If you are worried about mandatory vaccinations, here is the CDC website on this. My apologies if Naia Nisnam already posted this. Note, "All states provide medical exemptions". Some provide philosophical and religious exemptions (both Louisiana & Pennsylvania do). https://www.cdc.gov/vaccines/imz-managers/laws/state-reqs.html I for one, will cling to my medical excuse prescription from my doctor. And if I am forced to get the shot, I will go straight to a lawyer. Although I wouldn't be surprised if a new law were slipped in to make it more difficult if not impossible to to be exempted from this coronavirus vaccine. Has anyone done research on this??

I've got to get back to reading novels. This stuff is all killing my mental health. =/

****

Only 7 COVID-19 patients at New Orleans Convention Center

WDSU 6

Updated: 12:35 PM CDT May 20, 2020

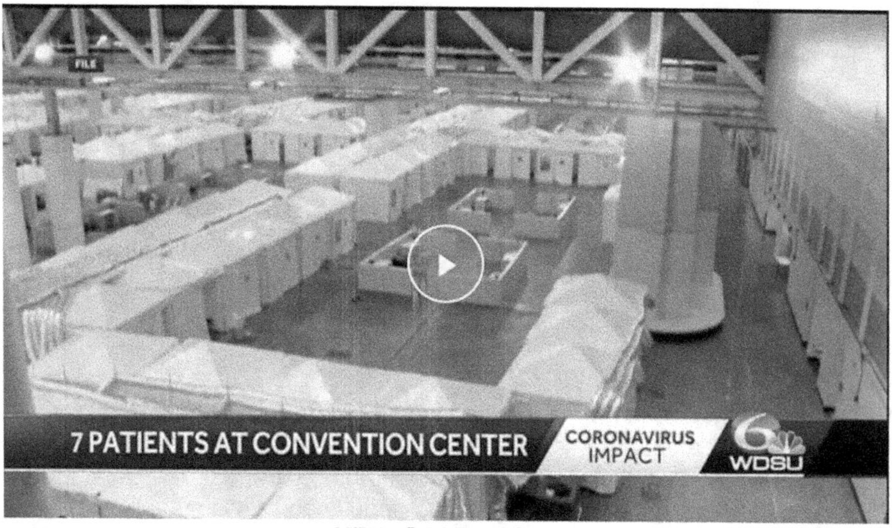

NEW ORLEANS —

There are currently only seven coronavirus patients at the make-shift hospital in the New Orleans Convention Center.

There are still 1,000 beds inside. The space was opened in April.

Gov. John Bel Edwards said he plans to leave the makeshift health facility built for COVID-19 patients at the New Orleans Convention Center as is for the time being.

Edwards said the facility will remain in place because of potential concerns for an uptick in cases in the fall or winter and beds will be taken out in phases.

The convention center hospital in downtown New Orleans was built out of concern that the coronavirus could overwhelm health facilities in the metro.

COVID-19 patients who no longer needed treatment in hospitals could be transferred to the convention center to continue receiving care and remain isolated from the public.

The governor also said the facility could treat patients from surrounding regions.

- https://www.wdsu.com/article/only-7-covid-19-patients-at-new-orleans-convention-center/32616526

****

FRED: Framework for Reconstructing Epidemiological Dynamics

Traditional forecasting relies on retrospective data and actuarial models to evaluate risk associated with a population or system. Traditional models also lack the ability to factor in behavioral dynamics and geospatially-accurate information. FRED (Framework for Epidemiological Dynamics) is a customizable modeling platform that supports decision making and forecasting based on the dynamic interactions of humans in their daily social interactions. The power and customization capabilities of FRED give non-technical users in healthcare, politics, insurance, and other industries the ability to create more dynamic models and forecasts to better inform their decisions.

Technology Description

FRED is an agent-based model that can include personal behaviors, social-demographics, local environments, resource allocations, and risk mitigation strategies. The model's flexible, customizable, object-oriented design is built to represent dynamic conditions in a synthetic population that is statistically equivalent to the real population in any given county or state. FRED supports various models of health behavior change to facilitate the study of critical personal health behaviors, such as vaccine acceptance, personal hygiene and spontaneous social distancing. No other agent-based population health models provide the flexibility, modularity, extensibility, and level of geographic and demographic specificity of the FRED synthetic population. In addition, these systems focus on acute infectious disease epidemics, whereas FRED can model general health conditions. Finally, FRED is the only system that can project population demographics into the future.

[..]

- https://www.innovation.pitt.edu/innovations/fred-framework-for-reconstructing-epidemiological-dynamics/

****

Adult Immunization

February 1, 2010
Author(s): Trust for America's Health

Millions of adults living in the U.S. are not up to date on their needed immunizations, leaving them at risk for preventable illnesses and even death, according to a new report released by Trust for America's Health (TFAH), the Infectious Diseases Society and the Robert Wood Johnson Foundation.

According to the report, key reasons for the low immunization rates include a lack of knowledge about the safety and effectiveness of vaccines, limited access to immunization and limited research and development of new vaccines in the United States.

"We need a national strategy to make vaccines a regular part of medical care and to educate Americans about the effectiveness and safety of vaccines," said Jeffrey Levi, Ph.D., Executive Director of TFAH.

[..]

- https://www.rwjf.org/en/library/research/2010/02/adult-immunization.html

****

These people have been sick with coronavirus for more than 60 days.

Doctors aren't sure why.

By **Ariana Eunjung Cha, Lenny Bernstein**
JUNE 11, 2020

It started for Melanie Montano with a tightness in her chest, almost like someone was sitting on top of her. It was March 15, and she was sweating but freezing cold. And she had a strange "pins-and-needles" sensation on the back of her legs. "It was as if I woke up in a totally different body," she recalled.

Over the following weeks, Montano, 32, developed a fever, cough, stomach problems, and lost her sense of taste and smell like other sufferers of the novel coronavirus. Unlike most of them, though, her symptoms never went away. They kept coming and going in waves like a roller coaster that has kept her bed-bound for 89 days straight — through school shutdowns, shelter-in-place orders, protests over those restrictions, and now, state reopenings.

Those infected with the coronavirus are urged to self-quarantine for 14 days, partly based on the idea that symptoms usually last about that long. While the majority of people with mild illness recover completely in that time, doctors say they're seeing a small percentage like Montano who remain sick for many weeks, or even months.

But with so little known about the virus, they're unsure whether those symptoms suggest it is still alive in the body and creating continued havoc, or whether it has come and gone, leaving a lingering immune or inflammatory response that makes people continue to feel sick.

[..]

- https://www.washingtonpost.com/health/2020/06/11/coronavirus-chronic/?arc404=true

****

2020 PRESIDENTIAL RACE

Biden Gets More Aggressive as 2020 Campaign Heats Back Up

By Will Weissert and Alexandra Jaffe • Published June 11, 2020 • Updated on June 11, 2020 at 6:17 pm

[..]

If elected, Biden promised to guarantee testing and protective equipment for people called back to work, while prohibiting discrimination against elderly Americans and others at high risk of contracting the virus. He also wants to use federal funds to ensure paid leave for anyone who falls ill or cares for those who do.

He proposed a national contact tracing workforce or "job corps" of at least 100,000 to call people who test positive, track down their contacts and get them into quarantine. That figure aligns with an estimate from the Johns Hopkins Center for Health Security and the Association of State and Territorial Health Officials. Health experts agree that contact tracing is crucial to slowing the spread of the virus and that there aren't enough public health workers today to achieve what's needed.

Biden also pledged a "Nationwide Pandemic Dashboard," where Americans could check the virus' spreading by zip code. Josh Michaud, associate director of global health policy with the Kaiser Family Foundation in Washington, said it remains unclear "if that information would be timely and accurate enough to reflect true levels of risk in a way that would be helpful to individuals, businesses and institutions in each community."

[..]

- https://www.nbcdfw.com/news/politics/biden-releases-plan-to-reopen-us-economy-amid-coronavirus/2387018/

****

THE BIDEN PLAN TO COMBAT CORONAVIRUS (COVID-19) AND PREPARE FOR FUTURE GLOBAL HEALTH THREATS

[..]

The American people deserve an urgent, robust, and professional response to the growing public health and economic crisis caused by the coronavirus (COVID-19) outbreak. That is why Joe Biden is outlining a plan to mount:

> A decisive public health response that ensures the wide availability of free testing; the elimination of all cost barriers to preventive care and treatment for COVID-19; the development of a vaccine; and the full deployment and operation of necessary supplies, personnel, and facilities.
> A decisive economic response that starts with emergency paid leave for all those affected by the outbreak and gives all necessary help to workers, families, and small businesses that are hit hard by this crisis. Make no mistake: this will require an immediate set of ambitious and progressive economic measures, and further decisive action to address the larger macro-economic shock from this outbreak.
>
> [..]

- https://joebiden.com/covid19/

****

State Vaccination Requirements

State and local vaccination requirements for daycare and school entry are important tools for maintaining high vaccination coverage rates, and in turn, lower rates of vaccine-preventable diseases (VPDs).

State laws establish vaccination requirements for school children. These laws often apply not only to children attending public schools but also to those attending private schools and day care facilities. All states provide medical exemptions, and some state laws also offer exemptions for religious and/or philosophical reasons. State laws also establish mechanisms for enforcement of school vaccination requirements and exemptions.

Studies have shown that vaccine exemptions tend to cluster geographically, making some communities at greater risk for outbreaks (Wang et al; Lieu et al; other clustering references).

Practices suggested in the literature to reduce non-medical exemptions include:

- States can consider strengthening the rigor of the application process, frequency of submission, and enforcement as strategies to improve vaccination rates (Yang and Silverman; also Gostin; Stadlin et al.).
- In addition to state vaccination requirements, stronger health care practices such as more in-depth discussions with hesitant parents and establishing vaccination as the default are strategies to improve vaccination coverage rates (Opel and Omer; Yang and Silverman).

In summary, vaccination requirements that reach more children through a broad range of facilities, that have more requirements for receiving an exemption, that require parental documentation of exemption requests, and that are implemented with strong enforcement and monitoring may help promote higher rates of vaccination coverage, and in turn, lower rates of VPDs. Ongoing provider outreach and public education about vaccines and the diseases they prevent may also lead to such an increase.

CDC's Public Health Law Program (PHLP) has compiled state statutes and regulations regarding school vaccinations.

[..]

- https://www.cdc.gov/vaccines/imz-managers/laws/state-reqs.html

****

June 14, 2020, 9:13PM (Amir-ul Kafirs to group):

Is something being planned for us in the fall? Or our politicians just 'innocently' swept up in the scare-mongering?

Wow. That's even more excessive than anything else I know of. NOLA seems like such a weird combination of obviously-not-giving-a-shit-about-its-people & *spending waaaaaayyyyy too much money on 'helping its people without actually helping them'*. It's truly spectacular. I think of the $12,000 per COVID-19 patient that Elmhurst hospital [probably] got. How about giving that money directly to the patients & not having them be in the hospitals at all? It seems that the survival rates would've been much higher & their lives would've been much improved.

Maybe you all already know this, but, it is, of course, funded by the Bill & Melinda Gates Foundation https://www.innovation.pitt.edu/innovations/fred-framework-for-reconstructing-epidemiological-dynamics/ . It is also funded by the Robert Wood Johnson Foundation which did a 2010 study on how terrible it is that adults in the U.S. don't get enough vaccinations: https://www.rwjf.org/en/library/research/2010/02/adult-immunization.html .

Don't you just loooooovveee this kind of shit: "40,000 to 50,000 adults die annually from vaccine-preventable illnesses." The diseases might be "vaccine-preventable" but that doesn't mean that vaccines would necessarily prevent the deaths now does it?

a particularly insulting one about how to handle homeless people during the pandemic and how these homeless people are more likely to believe "Conspiracy Theories" and went on to briefly describe and make fun of these theories. Gak.

Instead of making fun of them maybe they should disprove them. Let's start with the theory that I have that many doctors are sadists & many lawyers are sociopaths.

from the Washington Post: The title says it all.. "Chronic Coronavirus Syndrome"

It's funny, this doesn't make me scared. I just have a reaction along the lines of: 'This isn't happening to me' & that's it. I feel so removed from it. A possible take-away from the article could be that doctors will be unable to do anything for you so you might as well just try to survive & have that be that. To quote the article:

"“The bottom line is we just don't know,” said Adam Lauring, an infectious-diseases physician at the University of Michigan."

And can someone please tell me how to grasp that we have to vote for Biden? But what is our alternative?

Wow, that's the most 'fun' article yet! Consider these 2 quotes:

"As the plan was being released, his campaign circulated an online petition urging Facebook to strengthen its misinformation rules. Social media giant Twitter has already drawn Trump's ire by imposing stricter limits on how he and others use the social media network.

"“We're sending Facebook a letter demanding that the company change its policies to crack down on misinformation in ads and ensure a fair election,” the petition reads. Facebook responded that “the people's elected representatives should set the rules, and we will follow them."

It's just like that Atlantic article that I wrote the letter response to that I assume they didn't print since I haven't read back from them. It's not very clear, is it, who's going to say what's "misinformation" & what's 'real news' but somehow I think that the criteria are going to favor a MONOLITHIC NARRATIVE that I'm going to find highly dubious.

"Biden said he'd considered what would happen if Trump refused to vacate the presidency in the event he wasn't reelected, before suggesting that the military could step in to ensure a peaceful transition of power."

Nothin' like a little military intervention to get the blood boilin'. Funny how these military interventions in countries other than the US seem to go routinely bad.

If you want it straight from the horse's mouth in more detail, all fazillion pages of it, go to Biden's page

I'm only starting to look at this one but right off the bat I notice this:

"The American people deserve an urgent, robust, and professional response to the growing public health and economic crisis caused by the coronavirus (COVID-19) outbreak."

Um, excuse me, but the coronavirus hasn't caused the economic crisis, government has. It's as simple as that. & anything short of stopping these ridiculous measures isn't likely to correct matters either. Apparently stopping these measures isn't part of the plan.

"Biden believes we must spend whatever it takes, without delay, to meet public health needs and deal with the mounting economic consequences."

My modest proposal is to take all that money, of which there seems to be an almost infinite supply, that's going to be used for contact tracing & all the rest, & use it to improve the lives of all the poor people in this country. Let's make it so that no-one's economically desperate anymore.

At the top of the page it says:

"Enough.

It's time for us to take a hard look at uncomfortable truths.

It's time for us to face the deep, open wound we have in this nation.

We need justice for George Floyd.

– Joe Biden"

Gee, I wonder what he has in mind. Looking through the THOUSANDS of cases of murders by the police & finding them all guilty & making them face the same laws as the poor people that've been their victims? Somehow, I don't think so.

If you are worried about mandatory vaccinations, here is the CDC website on this.

"In addition to state vaccination requirements, stronger health care practices such as more in-depth discussions with hesitant parents and establishing vaccination as the default are strategies to improve vaccination coverage rates"

Note that there's nothing said that the objections of parents might be potentially valid. Big Brother knows what's best for us & it's all a matter of using "in-depth discussions with hesitant parents", meaning bullying & brain-washing, to get them to do what they don't want to do. Since when is it government's 'right' to force the voters to go against their own opinions in regards to their children?!

I've got to get back to reading novels.

Ha ha! Read some Mack Reynolds! He's fabulous!

****

June 13, 2020. 2:53PM (Inquiring Librarian to group):

Robert F. Kennedy Jr.

I have been pretty fascinated for the past 24 hours with Robert F. Kenedy Jr. He is pegged as an "Anti-Vaccer" and mostly bastardized by the mainstream media. He self describes himself as not an anti-vaccer, but as against unnecessary vaccines. You can check out his page on children and vaccines and here is a great set of articles on his page, many related to the corona virus and adult 'mandatory' vaccinations for it: https://childrenshealthdefense.org/kennedy-news-views/

He seems really well studied on the subject of vaccines and he has a whole lot to say about the corona virus and vaccines and the flu vaccines. In the video I am sharing below, he quoted Marcia Angell the former editor of the New England Journal of Medicine as saying, in reference to once 'trusted scientific journals', "We have become a propaganda vessel of the pharmaceutical industry." And according to the Lancet Editor, Richard Hornton, "You cannot believe anything in the Lancet anymore, or any of the journals, because the pharmaceutical companies can tell us what to do and they prevent us from saying anything that they don't like".
https://www.youtube.com/watch?v=QMHTbYIHZGU

Kennedy directs anyone looking for 'real' medical information, to go to the

Cochran Collaboration: https://www.cochrane.org/
I still need to check the page out. I hope to soon.

He quotes a study from the Cochran Collaboration on military personnel that found that soldiers who were given the flu vaccine were 36% more likely to get the CORONA VIRUS [not the flu virus]."... Apparently Italy had just had a massive flu vaccine initiative before this covid 19 hit them. =O

****

JUNE 12, 2020

Fact-Checking the Facebook "Fact-Checkers"

By Brian S. Hooker, CHD Board Member, and Science Advisor, Focus for Health

On May 27, 2020, the paper "Analysis of Health Outcomes of Vaccinated and Unvaccinated Children: Developmental Delays, Asthma, Ear Infections and Gastrointestinal Disorders" that I coauthored with Neil Z. Miller was published in the journal SAGE Open Medicine. By June 2, 2020, Facebook "fact-checkers" declared the paper "unsupported" and flagged Children's Health Defense's references to the study on the social media platform. Instead of following the link to the peer-reviewed study, Facebook now directed the reader to a critique completed by Healthfeedback.org, an organization that is a part of the World Health Organization's Vaccine Safety Net with ties to the Gates Foundation. To view the original paper, one would have to bypass the "fact-check" to be directed to the SAGE Open Medicine website.

... the "fact-checkers" label my previous Hooker 2014 study "fraudulent," a most serious and reputation-harming charge.

Playing fast and loose with the facts

Unfortunately for the public, the so-called "fact-checkers" at Healthfeedback.org play fast and loose with the facts. First, prior to considering the study at hand, the "fact-checkers" label my previous Hooker 2014 study "fraudulent," a most serious and reputation-harming charge. "Fraudulent" is a legal term of art which means "the intentional use of deceit, a trick or some dishonest means to deprive another of their money, property or a legal right." The fact of the matter is that Translational Neurodegeneration, where my 2014 study was published, did retract the article under enormous pressure from the Vaccine Industry. But, in so doing, that Journal never cited "fraud," "deception," or "dishonesty" as a basis for the retraction. Rather, that Journal retracted the article because of a purportedly undisclosed conflict of interest, but without any finding that the non-disclosure was intentional or material. Indeed, that study has since been republished in an expanded form (Hooker 2018).

The U.S. Center for Disease Control's (CDC) own studies, many that are cited in the "fact-checking" piece, are almost exclusively based on convenience samples.

Using a convenience sample

The primary criticism of the Hooker and Miller 2020 study was the use of a convenience sample which refers to the cohort of 2047 children, from 3 separate pediatric practices in the United States, that formed the basis for our study. Convenience samples are used routinely in epidemiology and also form the basis for the FDA approval of drugs and biologics.

Within the piece, Dr. David Gorski, a pro-pharma blogger states, "Basically, no matter how you analyze a convenience sample, you can't generalize it to the larger population." FALSE. The U.S. Center for Disease Control's (CDC) own studies, many that are cited in the "fact-checking" piece, are almost exclusively based on convenience samples. The study presented by Destefano et al. 2004 in the journal Pediatrics on the timing of the MMR vaccine and autism was completed using a convenience sample of approximately 2400 children in public school districts in Metropolitan Atlanta. This was not a representative sample of the U.S. population as the percentage of African American children in the study was 35.4% compared to that of the U.S. at the time at 16%. Yet this study is the CDC's basis for denying a causal link between the MMR vaccine and autism in the U.S.

The "fact-checkers" cite Andrews et al. 2004 (Pediatrics) which is also based on a convenience sample of children in the United Kingdom despite the fact that the CDC cites it as "proof" that thimerosal-containing vaccines in the United States do not cause autism. Also, the "fact-checkers" cite four studies (regarding both thimerosal-containing vaccines and the MMR vaccine) on children in Denmark as proof that vaccines don't cause autism in U.S. children despite many distinctions between the two populations of children.

Finally, the "fact-checkers" cite five studies that are based on the CDC's Vaccine Safety Datalink, a computerized database of the records from nine Health Maintenance Organizations in the U.S. This could also be considered a convenience sample" as it excludes children who are on Preferred Provider Organization (PPO) plans as well as those on Medicaid and focuses only on the HMO demographic.

[..]

- https://childrenshealthdefense.org/news/fact-checking-the-facebook-fact-checkers/

****

JUNE 11, 2020

Vaccine Ethics and Children: With COVID-19, Science Has Completely Lost Its Way

By James Lyons-Weiler, Children's Health Defense Guest Contributor and CEO, President of the Institute for Pure and Applied Knowledge

COVID-19 science should have set a new standard for vaccine safety research. Instead, it has lowered the bar. Hear this well: COVID-19 vaccines are not – and never were – a fait accompli. Unless the science being conducted on COVID-19 vaccines is held to the normative standards for ethical clinical research, no ethical physician, parent, or politician should support their general use – regardless of ACIP, CDC, WHO and AMA, AAP and FDA expected rubber-stamp recommendations. The regulatory system we have is fatally flawed and must be replaced with one free from profit motive. I call this Plan B, and I and my supporters will from this day make every effort to insure these obsolete and captured organizations' impairment of bona fide evidence-based medicine in the US and abroad is brought to an end.

Most medical professionals and parents believe that vaccines are the best way forward to protect children from disease caused by infectious pathogenic agents. In a recent article, Bill Gates reports that he suspects "the COVID-19 vaccine will become part of the routine newborn immunization schedule."

Oxford has announced that its Phase II COVID-19 vaccine studies will include a group of children aged between 5-12 years. Given the low susceptibility of children to illness from SARS-CoV-2 infection, the inclusion of children is, according to Oxford, warranted so the differences between their immune systems and those of adults challenged with SARS-CoV-2 antigens can be better understood.

Any translational scientist or bioethicist should, on the grounds of elementary first principles of the ethics of clinical research, object vehemently to the inclusion of children in COVID-19 vaccine studies. Here, I lay those principles out in the current context.

1. There are no potential benefits to the child enrollees being experimented upon. The overall infection case fatality rate of SARS-CoV-2 is estimated by CDC at 0.26%. The risk of serious illness and death from SARS-CoV-2 infection in children is effectively zero. In fact, risk of serious/critical illness and death is isolated to known groups of individuals with diabetes or cardiovascular disease, and the elderly, and those with certain comorbidities (see CDC: Groups at Higher Risk for Severe Illness.)

There is, therefore, no potential benefit to any child who would be enrolled in COVID-19 vaccine studies, and the trial would only serve to benefit others. This is highly unethical.

There is also no expected population-level beneficial effect from the Oxford vaccine; all rhesus monkeys, vaccinated or not, with their vaccine, were still susceptible to SARS-CoV-2 infection. Thus, vaccination to prevent infection and transmission cannot be a justification for that particular vaccine: the virus should be expected to be freely transmitted throughout the population until it finds the immunocompromised and those at risk of serious and critical illness.

2. No free, prior and informed consent on risk is possible – for any COVID-19 human subject of any age. In SARS, MERS and other coronavirus vaccine research, unacceptably high risk of coronavirus disease enhancement was reported in animals vaccinated against the coronaviruses, and re-challenged with infection See "SARS-CoV-2 Vaccine Recommended Readings". This critical animal safety study phase led to the termination of the development of SARS and MERS vaccines. That is not a failure of science, it is a success. The problem of disease enhancement from coronavirus vaccines has been misleadingly referenced as "immune enhancement", a term that is an inexact reference to disease enhancement. It has been re-labeled "Pathogenic Priming", a phrase that focuses the liability on the act of the exposure, not the passive liability on the human immune system (Lyons-Weiler, 2020).

[..]

- https://childrenshealthdefense.org/news/vaccine-ethics-and-children-with-covid-19-science-has-completely-lost-its-way/

****

MAY 29, 2020

As the Quarantine Guts the Economy, America's Five Wealthiest People Have Gotten 75 Billion Dollars Richer

By Robert F. Kennedy, Jr., Chairman, Children's Health Defense

At the quarantine's outset, I warned that despots and billionaires would leverage the crisis to ratchet up surveillance and authoritarian control. They would transform America into a National Security State, engineer the final liquidation of America's middle class and transfer its wealth to a plutocracy of digital and Pharma billionaires.

Sure enough, at breakneck speed we have devolved from the world's exemplary democracy to a tyrannical near-police state operating at the direction of Big Data/ Big Telecom, the Medical Cartel, and the Military/Industrial/Intelligence Complex. This nationwide, extended quarantine has permanently shuttered over 100,000 small businesses, cost 38 million jobs and 27 million Americans their health care. The Super Rich elite are flourishing while a despairing middle class flounders. According to a report by Americans for Tax Fairness, billionaires are watching their wealth compound beyond imagination.

Between March 18, when lockdown began, and May 19, the combined net worth of Bill Gates (Microsoft), Jeff Bezos (Amazon) Mark Zuckerberg (Facebook), Warren Buffett (Berkshire Hathaway) and Larry Ellison (Oracle) grew by $75.5 billion. According to Forbes data, the total wealth of the 630 U.S. billionaires jumped by $434 billion—15%—from $2.948 trillion to $3.382 trillion. Tech stocks are the most bullish about the Surveillance State. Microsoft (Bing), Facebook and Amazon are facilitating our devolution into militarized oligarchy by enforcing censorship against all expressions of dissent.

Zuckerberg's wealth increased by 46.2 percent (up $25.3 billion); Bezos's by 30.6 percent ($34.6 billion); Gates's by 8.2 percent ($8 billion). Their stocks hit all-time highs this week. Amazon shares were up 29% since January and Facebook spiked 10 % in lockstep with the Lockdown.

Other Tech Titans also watched their portfolios peak; Buffett by 0.8% (up $564 million) and Larry Ellison's by 11.9% (up $7 billion) Musk by 48% (up $11.8 billion). Other billionaires growing wealth on public misery include tech billionaire Michael Dell; Pharma/media baron Rupert Murdoch. These kingpins will need a Surveillance/Police State to protect their obscene winnings from public rage.

- https://childrenshealthdefense.org/news/as-the-quarantine-guts-the-economy-americas-five-wealthiest-people-have-gotten-75-billion-dollars-richer/

****

June 15, 2020, 10:36AM (Amir-ul Kafirs to group):

Re: Robert F. Kennedy Jr.

You can check out his page on children and vaccines

I'm reading some of the articles now. Thanks for the link. I'm reading one on the ethics (or non-ethics) of vaccines & I think this paragraph might be worth quoting:

"Herd immunity from vaccination is nice in theory, but it is not well-conceived given that the vaccine type tends to eventually differ from the circulating type. But even at 100% efficacy, what would a COVID-19 add to herd immunity? The coverage needed to acquire herd immunity is estimated at %C(overage) = 1-(1/

R0), with R0 being the basic reproduction number, which varies with contextual settings. In settings where R0 is low (2.0), %C is 0.5, or 50%; where R0 is high (3.9), %C = 0.743, 74.3%. That means the highest percentage of the population that would need to be immune would be 75%. The possibility that as many as 80% of individuals are already immune to SARS-CoV-2 infection means that the general population already exceeds the percentage of immune individuals required to achieve herd immunity. If 80% of people are already immune, the vaccine is largely redundant (as, is for that matter, mask wearing)." - https://childrenshealthdefense.org/news/vaccine-ethics-and-children-with-covid-19-science-has-completely-lost-its-way/

wch is followed by this:

"The prolonged US lock-down has been overkill, and reason must prevail. A general lock-down is general physical distancing, which is overkill due to the attendant costs of deaths due to poverty, delayed "elective" surgeries, suicide from unemployment and social isolation. The only ethical use of a general lock-down in the US would have been short-term (2-3 weeks) combined with a shift in strategy that facilitated prophylactic use of antivirals, calls for general social distancing, and physical distancing of those at risk of serious illness and death. I proposed this more rational approach in February 2020: had the US public health leadership been like-minded, the economic effect of COVID-19 response would have been minimized."

Obviously, I find this convincing. In fact, when the quarantine began I thought it was only going to be 2 weeks. Now it's presented as indefinitely. Justifying such a drastic change in the lives of billions of people should involve more than just a hypothetical health threat given that the REAL HEALTH THREAT constituted by social isolation & financial insecurity is much more immediately demonstrable. &, yes, the article continues with this:

"A rapidly increasing battery of scientists have published their viewpoints that the cost of the prolonged general lock-down exceeds the benefit in terms of lives saved from COVID-19."

"You cannot believe anything in the Lancet anymore, or any of the journals, because the pharmaceutical companies can tell us what to do and they prevent us from saying anything that they don't like".
https://www.youtube.com/watch?v=QMHTbYIHZGU

I only made it through the 1st 7:50 of this one but my take-away so far, other than what Inquiring Librarian mentions above, is that according to the Cochrane Collaboration there's no evidence that the flu vaccine prevents hospitalizations, deaths, or transmissability — AND there's the claim that mortality rates & reduced longevity in older people is actually increased.

Kennedy directs anyone looking for 'real' medical information, to go to the Cochran Collaboration

I went to their home page but didn't read any of their articles. I did watch the intro video they have on YouTube: https://youtu.be/MbiIg526USQ . They support studying medical tech & drugs *independent of the seller company research*. Superficially, that, obviously, strikes as a good idea. They've also been around for 27 years. Assuming they're for real, & their being a non-profit seems to support that possibility, it seems like a good thing.

Stay sane everyone!

So far so good, I'm as criminally sane as ever — if not more so!

****

June 14, 2020, 8:02AM (Amir-ul Kafirs to group):

HERETICS: AwakenWithJP has done it again!

"The Left vs Right in 2020": https://youtu.be/o7A-MLVEeMA

"What the Left vs Right is like in 2020. The Democrats and Republicans are both open minded and great listeners. Pledging blind allegiance to a party helps you to never have to think again."

(He's also brimming with merchandise for sale.)

****

June 14, 2020, 11:40AM (Inquiring Librarian to group):

mRNA Vaccine... Why You Should Avaid It

My apologies for dumping Bobby Kennedy Jr. on you now in 3 emails with hour plus long interviews... I'm really enjoying his videos on the pandemic. All of the mainstream media 100% ruthlessly bash this guy. Naturally, that makes me want to listen to him more. Honestly, he makes way more sense to me than the drivel the media is dumping on us.

Ok, so this one, episode 1 of "Truth", starts out immediately discussing the Moderna mRNA vaccine and goes into the details of the difficulties of creating a Corona Virus vaccine. To date, a corona virus vaccine has never successfully been made. For some reason, corona virus vaccines always tend towards what is called "Pathogenic Priming". Basically that means, that when a vaccine is made and injected into the body, when the body is exposed to the 'wild' virus (aka: regular exposure the virus as it infects you in nature out in the real world), your body's immune response actually fails and instead the virus potency is amplified in your body. Horrible! I have heard and read this from several well credentialed scientists recently.

To break it down further, there are 2 types of immune response antibodies created when the body is given a vaccine. There are the "Neutralizing Antibodies" and there are the "Binding Antibodies". What we want in a successful vaccine are "Neutralizing Antibodies", because these neutralizing antibodies actually neutralize the offending virus and destroy it so that we don't get sick. The "Binding Antibodies" actually bind to the virus and amplify its effect on the human body thus making the virus potency amplified in the body, often resulting in severe illness and death.

Corona viruses are tricky for making vaccines because they almost always result in creating binding antibodies. And our government and the WHO are fast tracking a vaccine for this corona virus. Instead of focusing on an old fashioned vaccine, which is bad enough, they are focusing on an mRNA (messenger RNA) vaccine that will permanently alter our bodies RNA for all generations to come. This vaccine by Moderna has already been tested on humans.... supposedly they skipped the animal testing! =O And the negative reaction these test subjects may get when faced with the wild corona virus could be deadly and will certainly result in them being more sick when exposed to corona viruses. The result, Big Pharma will have more fuel and more sick people to 'heal' and more excuses to create more 'cures'.

Ok, suffice it to say, please no one get this mRNA vaccine if it becomes available and if it becomes mandatory, no way. Despite my ditzyness, I was a great science student in school and spent 1.5 years in college as a biochemistry major. This stuff fascinates me.

Ok, here's the talk, "Truth pt. 1" if you want to listen through it:
https://childrenshealthdefense.org/news/truth-with-robert-f-kennedy-jr/

****

June 15, 2020, 10:52AM (Amir-ul Kafirs to group):

Re: mRNA Vaccine... Why You Should Avoid It

supposedly they skipped the animal testing!

Truthfully, I'm against animal testing. I don't care how much such testing is justified as a safety procedure for humans, it's not the animals's problem, it's our problem. The researchers & doctors should test on themselves. That would make them more cautious or dead.

please no one get this mRNA vaccine if it becomes available

Damn! & to think I was already planning a tasty little vaccine cocktail of mRNA vaccine, rum, whiskey, fruit juice & avocado. They say the quickest way to a man's heart is through his stomach but I say the quickest way to administer a vaccine is to make it an alcoholic drink.

****

June 14, 2020, 1:57PM (Amir-ul Kafirs to group):

HERETICS: Hospital room billed at $9,736 per day

Why this was so cheap it must be Socialized Health Care! A mere $1,122,501.04!!

Coronavirus survival comes with a $1.1 million, 181-page price tag

June 12, 2020 at 4:53 pm *Updated June 13, 2020 at 11:00 am*

By Danny Westneat
Seattle Times columnist

Remember Michael Flor, the longest-hospitalized COVID-19 patient who, when he unexpectedly did not die, was jokingly dubbed "the miracle child?"
Now they can also call him the million-dollar baby.

Flor, 70, who came so close to death in the spring that a night-shift nurse held a phone to his ear while his wife and kids said their final goodbyes, is recovering nicely these days at his home in West Seattle. But he says his heart almost failed a second time when he got the bill from his health care odyssey the other day.

"I opened it and said 'holy [bleep]!' " Flor says.

The total tab for his bout with the coronavirus: $1.1 million. $1,122,501.04, to be exact. All in one bill that's more like a book because it runs to 181 pages.

[..]

- https://www.seattletimes.com/seattle-news/inspiring-story-of-seattle-mans-coronavirus-survival-comes-with-a-1-1-million-dollar-hospital-bill/?fbclid=IwAR2LAt-dm7yqpskHnkv7luyv5zMHih8tfw1hD4o5BAxjVw3Yw9a2pZP6eSU

****

June 14, 2020, 2:54PM (Inquiring Librarian to Amir-ul Kafirs):

Re: HERETICS: Hospital room billed at $9,736 per day

Shocking, but not really. Considering my healthcare tried to stick me with a

$20,000 bill for a 3 hour laparoscopic kidney surgery 10 years ago. And then there was the $100,000 one for kidney reconstruction about 20 years ago. unbelievable, but true. We live in a world of 'health"care non-sense.

Speaking of covid costs, check out this article in nola's local paper about wasted funds and poor elderly patient care at our convention center hospital:

https://www.nola.com/news/healthcare_hospitals/article_3f6edb4a-a9d7-11ea-abf1-2791082490e9.html

****

June 13, 2020, 11:59PM (Amir-ul Kafirs to group):

HERETICS: bAd Haircut

Here's my latest, assisted by Naia Nisnam:

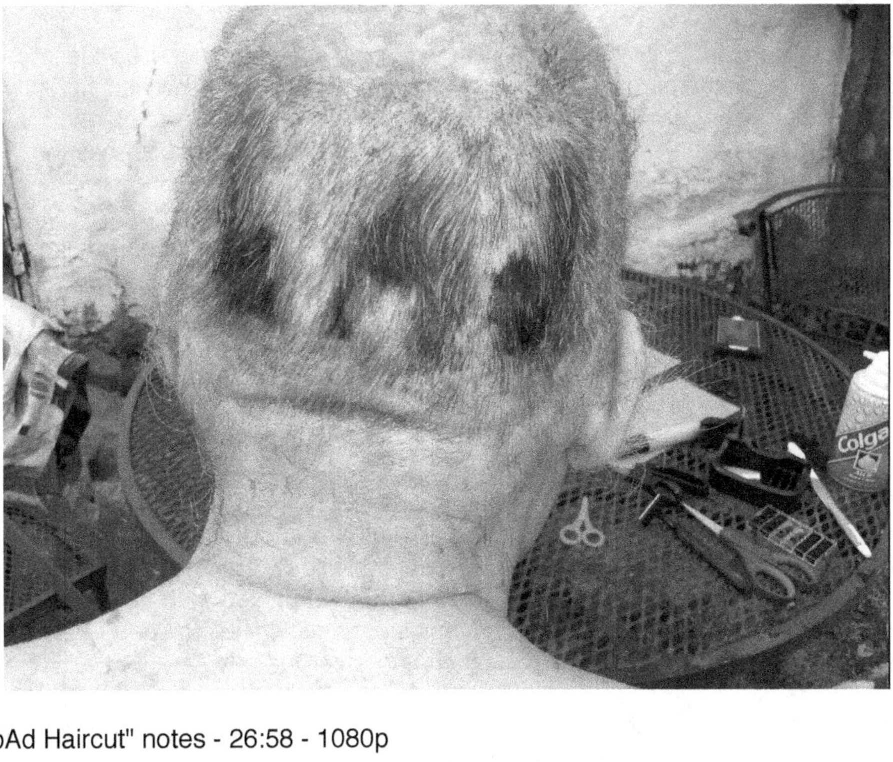

"bAd Haircut" notes - 26:58 - 1080p

https://youtu.be/CooW4dMWU5U

"bAd Haircut": Life in 2020 is a regular Shit Show, "A situation or event marked by chaos or controversy." Even that doesn't do it justice.

Civil Liberties have been largely suspended & the politically-minded who would traditionally oppose such a state are embracing Big Brother with a masochistic & delusional fervor.

In the meantime, other, more conservative forces, have protested the QUARANTYRANNY as an excessive over-reaction & are demanding a return to 'normal'. Such folks have perfectly good reasons to be upset, such as the endangerment of their financial stability, but they're mocked as if they're just upset because they can't go to their barbers.

Hence, because of all this talk about "bad haircuts", haircuts not given by professional barbers, I decided to *get with it* & get one myself. After all, I haven't had a 'professional' haircut since I was 15 — 51 years ago.

In the meantime, doctors & hospitals in New York City appear to be setting a new low standard for the already abysmal American health care system by *making a killing* off of COVID-19 deaths. As usual the poor are expendable & profit-making for the rich.

On what I consider to be the more valid end of the spectrum there're widespread protests against the ongoing problem of police murdering citizens with impunity. It's my opinion that if you give someone means of superior force & make it practically impossible for them to ever face any legal consequences *they will become homicidal maniacs.*

But the Shit Show really hits its stride with the usual mass media fear-mongering & highly profitable sensationalism.

PEACEFUL HAIR-CUTTING MOVIE ENDS WITH VIOLENCE!

Because, what the fuck, once the mass media's involved, if the so-called 'news' doesn't end with violence what good is it for keeping the boobs glued to the boob-tube?!

That's where POLICE THEATER comes in. If you see a police car burn *how do you know it wasn't set on fire by the police themselves?!* HHMM?! It's just *so damned convenient* that an unguarded cop car is left parked at the end of a march — the end being typically when things get most chaotic as people are still keyed-up & angry & not willing to just go home & call it a day.

I don't really mind the "chaos" *or* the "controversy". What I do mind is how much *shit* is being forced on us by the ruling elites.

But, then, I have a bAd attitude.

- June 13, 2020 (Vision) notes from tENTATIVELY, a cONVENIENCE

Tags: bad haircuts, haircuts, quarantine, quarantyranny, police murders, police theater, mass media, tENTATIVELY a cONVENIENCE

****

June 14, 2020, 11:14AM (Inquiring Librarian to group):

Re: HERETICS: bAd Haircut

Thanks so much for this!! I had a hard time hearing the conversation, but I cranked up the volume and got most of it. I love the video! You know, that haircut would last so long on me... my hair barely grows! I haven't cut it in at least 10 years!! =O The whole hairdresser dilemma is one that I cannot relate to. My sister is up in arms, she and my mom are actually going to their hairdresser who is illegally cutting their hair... Illegally also, my sister and mom are hanging out and they live in different Pennsylvania counties. Are they going to throw a cute nurse and a 75 year old grandma in jail? Good grief. Maybe their story will end with a mysteriously blown up grandma's Subaru? I dive into the work week of insanity and ocd germaphobia again tomorrow. Here's something funny and nonsensical... At my work, the Mayor got all city employees free hand sewn cloth masks. My little library's masks came in Friday morning. They are adorable. I really like mine, as much as one can like a mask... because it's got pink and mint green and a festive summer yellow on its pattern. Now, my most germaphobic staff member took off her old mask and immediately put her new mask on and wore it all day. If she were really thinking logically as if the germs we are afraid of on books and keyboards are real and life threatening, why would she put this new cloth mask on without sanitizing it first?? Ugh. Ok, I have to stop being negative towards well meaning people. Instead of reacting incredulous and hostile towards her, I complimented her on how cute the mask looked on her and thanked her for picking the green one because I wanted the pink one (I was the last to chose because I felt that was the most courteous of me as the boss.).

Thanks for the humor and reality check to start my day! =]

****

June 15, 2020, 11:11AM (Amir-ul Kafirs to group):

I cranked up the volume and got most of it.

I actually have it cranked up to the highest volume that the editing program enables. I could've cranked it up even further if I'd outputted the sound & then amplified it in another program & then imported it back into the video editing program & then amplified it even further there but it didn't seem worth it. The conversation is basically 'desultory' & isn't necessarily crucial for understanding the whole thing. The on-screen text is what's the take-away message & I reinforce that by also having it be the YouTube notes.

The whole hairdresser dilemma is one that I cannot relate to.

Me either. I literally haven't been to a barber for 51 years. My mom went every friday for as much of her life as I know about. I often say that she actually spent more on getting her hair done than she did on me, her son that she 'loved so much'. She 'loved' me but she loved her hairdos wwwwaaaaaaayyyyyy more.

My sister is up in arms, she and my mom are actually going to their hairdresser who is illegally cutting their hair...

I actually think that's really funny. I think your mom & sister should have to put on black clothes or camouflage & should have to crawl through mud with knives in their teeth & then give the secret knock on a plain alley door & say "Swordfish" before they can get to the Black Market hairdresser.

Are they going to throw a cute nurse and a 75 year old grandma in jail?

One can only hope.

I have to stop being negative towards well meaning people.

Well-meaning people would be more convincingly well-meaning if they gave more thought to the way that they intrude on other people's lives.

Thanks for the humor and reality check to start my day!

Just doin' my job, ma'am.

****

June 16, 2020, 6:40AM (Dick to group):

a friend posted this, reminded me a little of Amir-ul Kafir's slogans

https://teespring.com/defund-the-thought-police-NOW?pid=389&cid=100022&fbclid=IwAR1NX3d-bV2EWMgVZFskudaZVJ4XWoe3lh8YpioWK6RZYGlzo1iLMOctHHs

****

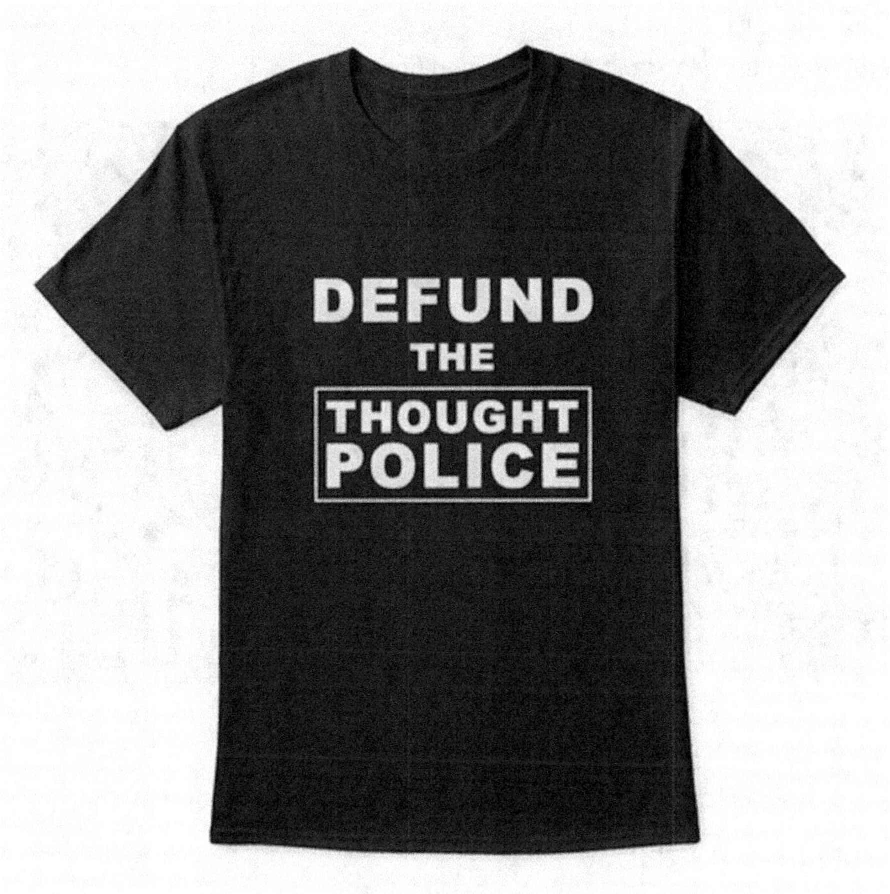

****

June 16, 2020, 10:16AM (Dick to group):

I was just sharing the slogan, buying one never even occurred to me to be honest

****

June 16, 2020, 5:57PM (Amir-ul Kafirs to group):

Oh, c'mon Dick! I saw you coming out of the Thought Police marketing department just the other day (or, at least, one of my spy cams did)!! You can't fool us.

****

June 16, 2020, 2:20PM (Amir-ul Kafirs to group):

HERETICS: UNTERTAN

Here's my latest gasp from the suffocated unconscious:

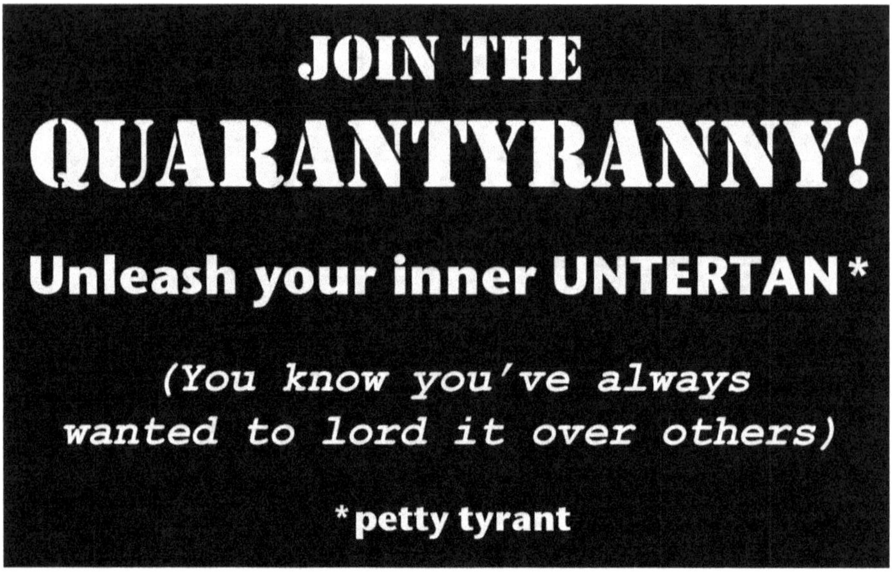

****

June 16, 2020, 4:51PM (Inquiring Librarian to group):

Re: HERETICS: UNTERTAN

I LOVE it! I saw this on social media earlier. It will be interesting to see what kind of reactions you get, if any. I'm very close to posting something revealing about how I feel about all of this hysteria and bullying. But I am still afraid of losing my job. So, I am using restraint, against my inner sense of justice and a feeling of needing to try to educate my amigos.

****

June 16, 2020, 6:18PM (Amir-ul Kafirs to group):

Well, fortunately, most of the immediate hostile-responsers (as opposed to 'first-responders', eh?) seem to be gone now. Maybe I've made it obvious that I feel pretty strongly against QUARANTYRANNY BULLYING & that I refuse to cower. Maybe more people are beginning to feel the same way. I've gotten one positive response from an old neoist friend in CacaNada.

I went to a Half-Price Books today. There were numerous signs on the doors demanding mask use. There was a place for "dirty baskets", baskets that hadn't been cleaned since customer use, & "clean baskets", ones that had been sanitized. I didn't notice the ONE WAY ARROWS on the floor at 1st. I started walking toward the SF book nook & a guy was walking toward me. He gave me this imperious gesture for me to get out of his way & I saw that there was the sign on the floor showing that I was going against the ONE WAY grain. I just turned into my destination saying something to the guy like: "Uh, yeah". A deliberately ambiguous reply while I continued to just go where I wanted to. After that I followed the arrows. It was completely stupid. The store wasn't crowded, there probably weren't more than 10 people in there, at least half of them staff. A guy came in to sell books. He had an appointment but he didn't have a mask on. The exasperated employee told him he absolutely must have a mask. SO, the guy went out & got one & put it on. Then, when he came back the employee told him he had too many books. The man said he called 1st & told how many books he had & was told that that was fine. The employee told him that he shouldn't have been told that & that he didn't have time to look at all those books. He asked him when his appointment was again. The man was on-time for his appointment. The employee made a big deal about how it might take him 45 minutes to look through the books. The man said something like 'OK, you have my info, just call me when you're ready.' The buyer told him he HAD to wait in the store. The seller was cooperative the whole time but the buyer was making an effort of showing how overworked & important & busy he was. As far as I could tell there was hardly *anything* happening in the store & the buyer's whole attitude was pretty exaggerated. At any rate, that experience at the store added to my general annoyance at how much petty tyrant behavior I'm seeing everywhere. ONE WAY LINES?! Gimme a fucking break.

****

June 16, 2020, 5:13PM (Naia Nisnam to Amir-ul Kafirs):

Fwd: Freedom & Justice Face Masks I Support The Movement with Official Masks

This irritates me and I wonder if I really am an asshole...

---------- Forwarded message ---------
From: **Official Black Lives Matter Store**
Date: Tue, Jun 16, 2020 at 3:07 PM
Subject: Freedom & Justice Face Masks I Support The Movement with Official Masks

BLACK LIVES MATTER

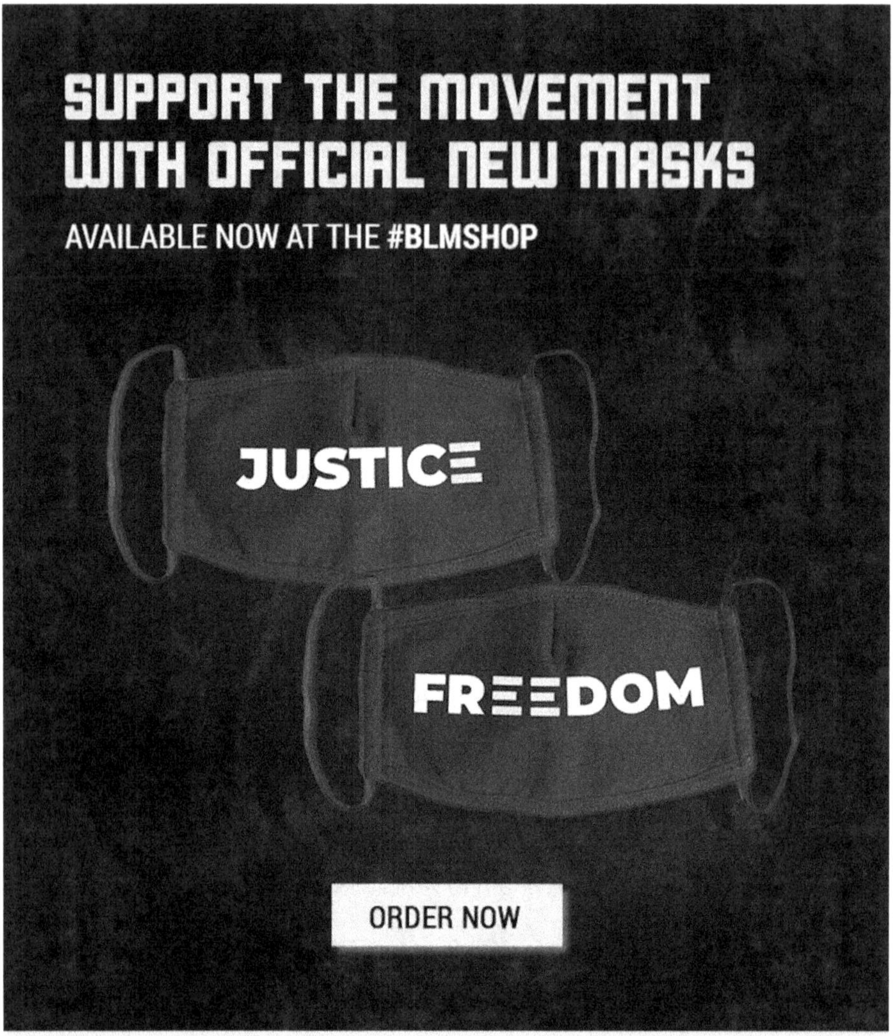

BLACK
LIVES
MATTER

#BLMShop is a response to the demand from our supporters, allies, and organizers to offer authentic Black Lives Matter Global Network merchandise that can both mark and commemorate our shared commitment to this movement. Apparel and other items offered in this store are carefully selected and creatively designed to reflect the unique brand of the Black Lives Matter Global Network.

****

June 16, 2020, 6:33PM (Amir-ul Kafirs to Naia Nisnam):

Fwd: Freedom & Justice Face Masks I Support The Movement with Official Masks

This irritates me and I wonder if I really am an asshole...

As usual, I don't think you're being an asshole. Remember when I said something to the effect of 'the scum are going to rise to the top in Black Lives Matter because it's getting powerful'? Well, here's some proof of that. 1st, there was the hashtag on the computer dating site. I've decided to NOT use the hashtag not because I don't think that Black Lives Matter **but because I'm seeing it turn into a fucking brand before my very eyes**. It's a force to be reckoned with in the capitalist world now. Do you remember when Hot Topic, the mall chain store, started selling 'punk clothes'? To anyone who considered themselves to be 'punk' that was ridiculous & disgusting. Obviously, 'punk clothes' were cheap clothes you bought from thrift stores & altered or made yourself. It wasn't something that could be bought pre-made, that took the punk right out of it. Now we have Black Lives Matter branding itself &, in the process, endorsing a whole police state by implication. There's money to be made! Let's hope that somewhere amongst the original founders of BLM there're people who're appalled! What can I say?! I reckon I'm still an old-school anti-capitalist at heart. Once money is brought into the picture everything starts to be corrupted. If anarchists started selling something like these masks I might think it was funny in some cynical way but if the sellers were really out to make money I'd have my doubts about how anarchist I considered them to be.

****

June 16, 2020, 6:48PM (Amir-ul Kafirs to group):

HERETICS: Sex Slavery on the rise during QUARANTYRANNY?!

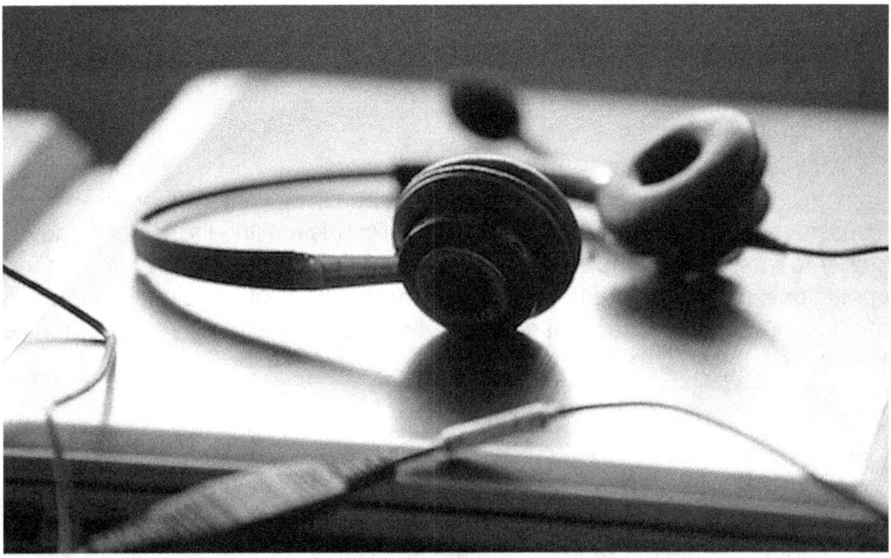

Since the onset of COVID-19, Polaris has been tracking data reported to the U.S. National Human Trafficking Hotline. According to our analysis, the impact of the pandemic and subsequent quarantine may already be leading to an escalation of sex and labor trafficking. Our snapshot compares a post-shelter-in-place period to two deliberately chosen pre-shelter-in-place periods. Key findings include:

- **The number of crisis trafficking cases handled by the Trafficking Hotline increased by more than 40%** in the month following the shelter-in-place orders compared to the same period in 2019, and the number of situations in which people needed immediate emergency shelter nearly doubled.

- A **greater need for stable housing and resources** for at-risk communities, victims, and survivors now more than ever to ensure the pandemic does not further contribute to the epidemic of sex and labor trafficking in the U.S.

Polaris is highlighting this urgent need for more shelter as city, county, state, and federal governments consider how their resources can be directed to mitigate the effects of COVID-19. Our recommendations are the first in a planned series presenting timely analysis and evidence to guide efforts to respond to emerging needs as a result of the pandemic.

The Trafficking Hotline is not a definitive measure for U.S. sex and labor trafficking prevalence. Our analysis explores the important correlation among crisis cases, shelter, demand, and COVID-19.

To read the full snapshot, please click here.

In Solidarity,

Catherine Chen
Chief Program Officer

I have an intense hatred of sex slavery which, as far as I can gather, is a very successful big business. As such, I'm on the Polaris mailing list. I don't know whether to trust these people or not — they're a bit too 'Big Charity' for my tastes. Nonetheless, as with so many things I post here, this reinforces my sketicism about just how many largely unseen negative side-effects there must be from all this shit 'for our own good'.

****

June 17, 2020, 1:16PM (Naia Nisnam to group):

Doctors admit people get more sick in the hospital

This is from the BBC, May 24:

https://www.bbc.com/news/health-52783865

They acknowledge " ....there is a good reason for keeping older people out of hospital if we can and sending them home as soon as it is safe to do so. For elderly patients, every day in hospital leads to "deconditioning", a loss of physical and mental functioning. For some, the strange environment can cause delirium - a condition with symptoms ranging from drowsiness, confusion and rambling speech to hallucinations."

And "People get weaker when they're in hospital, there's incontinence, not eating and drinking, all those things seem to get worse for people when they're in a hospital bed, and especially in a world where people are wearing masks and they might feel very disorientated. So we try to replicate the care of the ward but in people's own homes."

Plus it seems that in the UK, family members are allowed to visit w their dying relatives. (In the US, COVID patients have to die in isolation and say their last goodbyes to family members over the phone... something that has greatly bothered me.)

There's also potential sanity coming from the UK, in the form of treatment for the disease. Can we please have more research into treatments for those who get sick instead of quarantines and vaccinations for everyone??

Drug treatment article:
https://www.bbc.com/news/health-52801858

I saw a follow up on the steroids:

https://www.bbc.com/news/health-53061281
"For patients on ventilators, it cut the risk of death from 40% to 28%.
For patients needing oxygen, it cut the risk of death from 25% to 20%."

The BBC also isn't afraid to admit
"If you catch Covid-19, your risk of death if you're over 80 is 15%. If you are under 50, it is less than 1%."
I have friends in their 30s that are still afraid that they and/or their children are going to get covid and DIE. Seriously.
I'm trying my hardest to find things to feel positive about. It's hard.

****

Coronavirus doctor's diary: A patient given hours to live, who proved us wrong

24 May 2020

[..]

Mary and Michael were both admitted to hospital with Covid-19 on the same day, having most likely caught the virus at the funeral of one of their sons on 16 March. They have been together since the age of 13 and, coincidentally or not, it was when they were placed side by side on the same ward that they began to recover. (I **wrote about this here**.)

Michael was discharged first, and the family was overjoyed when **Mary was allowed home a few days later**.

But Elaine Martin, a trainee advanced clinical practitioner who visited Mary at home, noticed that she was still having difficulty breathing, and that she was deeply worried both about her husband's health and her own prospects of recovery.

"She was still having symptoms, she still felt breathless and chest tightness but I think a lot of it was anxiety. She felt she was going to die, and her husband had recovered but has an underlying condition, so there was a lot of anxiety," Elaine says.

The decision was taken to bring Mary back to hospital - which was fortunate, because that night her condition worsened.

[..]

- https://www.bbc.com/news/health-52783865

****

June 17, 2020, 7:17PM (Amir-ul Kafirs to group):

Re: Doctors admit people get more sick in the hospital

"People get weaker when they're in hospital, there's incontinence, not eating and drinking, all those things seem to get worse for people when they're in a hospital bed, and especially in a world where people are wearing masks and they might feel very disorientated. So we try to replicate the care of the ward but in people's own homes."

This the sort of thing that I think *should be 'COMMON SENSE'* but, apparently, isn't.

I have friends in their 30s that are still afraid that they and/or their children are going to get covid and DIE. Seriously.

It seems to me that there might even be more people who are the least at risk of dying from COVID-19 acting in deadly fear of it than there are older people. At any rate, I see them fairly often.

I'm trying my hardest to find things to feel positive about. It's hard.

As far as the PANDEMIC PANIC goes things seem to be as bad as ever if not worse. Some people are *entrenched* in their fear. The types of statements that I find particularly annoying are: 'Wearing masks save lives.' Really? SO, if I don't wear a mask does that mean that somewhere in the world a person who's about to die will just go ahead & do so? Because it doesn't say that 'Not wearing a mask kills people' but that seems to be implied. SO, that would mean that if I were to NOT wear a mask someone would definitely die, presumably someone in my vicinity. Well, how many & in what timing? I mean would someone die every second? Once a year? I want to know the logistics. At any rate, that would probably mean that Naia Nisnam, for example, has died many times over the past few months (Sorry about that Naia Nisnam) &, for that matter, I, also, have died an equal amount of times. One might think that such a mortality rate would solve the COVID-19 problem pretty quickly because literally every person not wearing a mask would die off almost immediately. Funny how that doesn't seem to've happened.

I agree, it's hard to stay positive. As I've said before, my already grim view of human intelligence has 'gone off the charts' during the time of the PANDEMIC PANIC. I no longer even care much about staying friends with the BELIEVERS, even superficially. If I could just ignore them altogether that might be fine but they're everywhere, like a plague. The BELIEVERS are *a much worse plague* than COVID-19 & there's no mask that can prevent their stupidity from being projected in my direction.

STILL, I'm glad that you folks exist, I'm positive about all the great culture that's been produced throughout history, all the great music there is to listen to, the great movies to witness, the great books to be read. I'm positive that I continue to be inspired & active. I'm positive that Naia Nisnam & I get to do something together once a week or so. There's plenty to be positive about but it's kindof like being in a diving bell & knowing that you have enough oxygen to last indefinitely. There's still the claustrophobia of the limited space & the awareness of the great crushing pressure on the surface of the bell. If I were the type of person who laughs at human folly I would've died laughing by now.

In intelligence do we trust,

****

June 17, 2020, 9:40PM (Amir-ul Kafirs to group):

HERETICS: Wearing Masks Saves Lives

I'm thinking of making a movie called "Wearing Masks Saves Lives". The idea is that I'll have footage of me somewhere not wearing a mask, there'll be a date &

time id on it. Then I'll show an article about someone dying at that time. I'll connect the 2. Alternately, I'll show footage of me wearing a mask, maybe while eating & trying to shove my food through the mask. Then I'll show an article about someone surviving – perhaps something about a child being snatched from the mouth of an alligator or something of that sort. Then I can take the mask off in frustration in order to eat. Of course, what follows will be about the inevitable death that follows this action. You get the idea.

Dick? Would you have any interest in collaborating on this? You could do something similar in Paris. I could edit both of our footages together.

Anyone else?

****

June 18, 2020, 5:01AM (Dick to group):

RE: HERETICS: Wearing Masks Saves Lives

Hi,
Sounds like a funny idea
I'll try to think of an angle of approach, a situation

****

June 18, 2020, 8:08AM (Amir-ul Kafirs to group):

I'll try to think of an angle of approach, a situation

MAAAAAHHHHVELOUS! This is one of those things I'd rather do with actors but I think I'll have to settle for simpler means. I might start looking online for footage of people dying & then run the footage backwards for the 'saving lives' scenes.

****

June 18, 2020, 8:26AM (Amir-ul Kafirs to group):

HERETICS: Notre Dame Model

I was talking with my neighbor a couple of days ago. He works as a Creative Writing professor at a small university NorthWest of Pittsburgh called Slippery Rock. He said that his school is following the "Notre Dame Model" & explained that that means something like 16 weeks of straight school with no breaks, a condensed semester. He said that means no fall break & no Thanksgiving break. I said something like: 'But that means that they won't be able to have Thanksgiving.' He replied that *they wouldn't be able to have one with their family* – leaving that hanging to apparently mean that they'll have one on campus. He explained that the purpose of this is to prevent the students from being able to go away to catch disease that they can return with to the campus AND to prevent them from going home to spread disease to their family. Wow.

Anyway, I looked up "Notre Dame Model" online & got this:

"The University of Notre Dame will welcome students back to campus for the 2020-21 fall semester the week of Aug. 10, two weeks earlier than originally scheduled, and will forgo fall break in October and end the semester before Thanksgiving, the University's president, Rev. John I. Jenkins, C.S.C., announced today in letters to the campus community." - https://news.nd.edu/news/notre-dame-to-begin-fall-semester-on-campus-the-week-of-aug-10/

Apparently, 'God's will be done' no longer applies — or, rather, "God's will" now means what it's always meant: that whatever 'God's intermediates on Earth say is "God's will".

As Naia Nisnam has previously pointed out here in reference to the return-to-school, this is planned months in advance. It's based on **PREDICTIONS**. That's it, predictions. Predictions that, as has been pointed out here & elsewhere, have repeatedly proven false. What if someone were to **predict** that the rise in arms sales will correspond to a rise in mass shootings in public places, ***such as at universities***, & then make it illegal for people to gather ANYWHERE in order to avoid the risk of being shot? Could that really be faulted as *so illogical?*

****

June 18, 2020, 2:37PM (Inquiring Librarian to group):

Re: HERETICS: Notre Dame Model

Wow! That's really depressing. This is unfortunately the future that I keep seeing discussed in library forums and from teachers that I speak to for grade school and university learning. They just are not giving up the goat. It's driving me nuts daily at work, the draconian plans for the "New Normal" future and a general assumed acceptance from everyone that the virus will never go away. It's so absurd to me.

Onward to warward University politics, has anyone heard of Dr. Denis Rancourt? He was a senior tenured professor of physics for 20 years at the University of Ottawa in Canada. He did manage to get himself fired/ejected from the university at the end of his 20 year professorship there. To find out more about how/why he got fired, you can simply google his name to find masses of the mass media slandering him. But, if you search harder, you can find sources that support him and the decisions he made that got him fired, such as this one: https://www.kwesthues.com/Rancourt09.htm
Now, my main point of bringing Denis Rancourt up is his interpretation of the Covid 19 'numbers' that he illustrates here in this article that he recently wrote. I

have not been able to fully dive into this, but from what I gleaned, I am very interested to flee work later today or tomorrow or this weekend... and dive deeper into this: https://lesakerfrancophone.fr/mortalite-toutes-causes-confondues-pendant-la-covid-19?fbclid=IwAR1tunkycIXJRUEt_tV6OgpEmT72xT3K3HMVbK_KO-mdwpKjNKkXrZPSdr0
If it pops up in French, you can easily have Google translate it into English for you (unless you are Dick which means you are lucky enough to read it en Francais!!).
Note: I am particularly interested in his numbers interpretation this week because my old college friend who is now a successful chemical engineer for NREL sent me a list of articles, *ALL* from the New York Times describing their interpretation of the numbers. It disgusted me. But I still love my friend because she is otherwise intelligent and kind. So, now I am on a rampage looking for any alternative 'numbers' interpretations (thank you Amir-ul Kafirs for all of your numbers obsessions and interpretations, I have always appreciated this even if I haven't well responded or responded at all).

Let me know what you think of Denis's statistical observations. I also have found his social media page and I've "Liked" it so that I can "Follow" him to see how his brain works more and to see what he is thinking daily. He is really passionate about his beliefs and I appreciate this and his lack of public concern despite his identifying as a liberal anarchist when he posts so many controversial things that go against the status quo Democratic stances these days. https://www.facebook.com/denis.rancourt.5?epa=SEARCH_BOX

Denis currently works as a researcher for the Ontario Civil Liberties Association (ocla.ca). I have read several articles featuring him in the "Off-Guardian".

****

Ottawa's Dismissal of Denis Rancourt

Commentary by Kenneth Westhues, University of Waterloo
August 2009

A good five years of conflict between administrators at the University of Ottawa and senior tenured physics professor Denis Rancourt came to a head on December 10, 2008. Dean of Science André Lalonde **formally recommended** to the Board of Governors that Rancourt be dismissed from the faculty. That same day, Provost Robert Major **suspended** Rancourt, closed his lab, and forbade him to set foot on campus.
The Ottawa administration's decision to fire Rancourt, imposing on him the "capital punishment" of labor relations, was even more vigorously

opposed than were the lesser punishments dealt to him in preceding years. In a factual, reasoned **letter** to the Board of Governors dated 5 January 2009, Rancourt defended himself. Well over a hundred professors and students from Ottawa and elsewhere sent individual **letters protesting** Rancourt's elimination. Even before the axe fell, the Canadian Association of University Teachers had appointed a three-person **Committee of Inquiry** to investigate the long series of run-ins, dating back at least to the fall of 2005, between the Ottawa administration and Rancourt.

Is this a case of workplace mobbing in academe? Yes — and more precisely, *administrative* mobbing. (Click **here** for the standard checklist of indicators, **here** for the mainpage of the relevant website, and **here** for a short, basic article.)

What allows so unqualified a diagnosis is that Rancourt has made comprehensive documentation on the conflict (letters, emails, press reports, videos) publicly available on his **blog** and at **academicfreedom.ca**. For want of adequate information pro and con about a professor's dismissal or humiliation, it is often impossible to make more than a tentative assessment of whether it is a case of mobbing or merely a hard but measured and warranted response to some betrayal of academic purpose. In this case, Rancourt has laid bare to the public the actions that got him into trouble, the sanctions imposed, and what is most important, documentary evidence of both his own and his adversaries' views. Thereby he has bolstered his own credibility. Let other aggrieved academics take a lesson: only in so far as full information is publicly available, the cards all on the table, can outside observers make confident judgments and say things worth listening to.

It is plain from the material online that over time, administrators at Ottawa coalesced in the view that Rancourt, despite his stellar research record and the respect given him by very many students, is an utterly unworthy and abhorrent man, fit only for expulsion from respectable academic company. While administrators appear front and centre in this mobbing case, they are joined by dozens, even hundreds of students and faculty who are after Rancourt's neck. According to Karen Pinchin's trenchant **article in Maclean's**, "nearly one-third of Rancourt's colleagues at the school have signed a petition of complaint against him." (Click **here** to read the petition, unambiguous evidence of ganging up.) Even distant pundits like **Stanley Fish** and **Margaret Soltan** piled on.

An **email** from Chemistry Chair Alain St-Amant is telling. Shortly after Rancourt's suspension, with his dismissal pending, St-Amant apparently agreed to debate him on a TV talk show, but then cancelled out. Rancourt sent him an email asking why, and suggesting that administrative or peer pressure was the reason. St-Amant emailed back, "I refuse to enter a battle of wits with an unarmed man. ... This will be the last you will hear from me on this matter. Enjoy the paycheques while they last." The contempt in these sentences is total.

With a clever turn of phrase, St-Amant gives Rancourt the ultimate academic insult, that he has no wits, that is to say no intelligence. Then he cuts off communication and gloats that Rancourt will soon be off the payroll. St-Amant would not likely have felt free to send such a message had he not felt himself part of a campus crowd united by scorn for Rancourt.

From the available documents, Rancourt appears to exemplify a type of professor I described in my **first book** on academic mobbing, a professor I called "Dr. PITA" — acronym for *pain-in-the-ass,* or in politer terms, a thorn in administrators' sides, the one who makes them see red. Being a team player is not Dr. PITA's priority. Administrative demands that most professors comply with uncomplainingly are occasions for Dr. PITA to raise questions — and more questions.

Real-life professors can become Dr. PITA for any number of reasons. Administrators usually chalk it up to a personality defect. The documentary record suggests that the reason in Rancourt's case, as in many mobbing cases I have studied, is that he has thought deeply enough about education and the search for truth, to realize how much these noble purposes are subverted by the academic structures established to serve them. During his first dozen years of university teaching, he seems to have not only lengthened his vita but actually developed his mind, gaining awareness that institutionalizing the process of learning (that means creating a formal organization with a policy manual, chain of command, course credits, degree programs, human resources office, and so on), even though it facilitates learning in some ways (not least by providing teachers with a stable livelihood), cheapens and diminishes learning in many other ways. A student's working life easily becomes a matter of memorizing things and jumping the hoops of standardized tests, without personal engagement or independent thought. Indeed, one of the things students learn is not to learn about power, nor to question the structure of power in place, since the organization depends on this structure for funding and public legitimacy. Awareness of this downside of institutionalization is a common theme of the varied authors Rancourt cites in support of his own brand of anarchism — Paolo Freire, Noam Chomsky, Michel Foucault, Herbert Marcuse, Ward Churchill, among others.

It was apparently Rancourt's deepening understanding of and commitment to what learning actually involves, that led him to refuse to rank and grade his students in the established, expected way. Since grading is central to the institutionalization of learning, he felt obliged to renounce it. This was the sticking point, the offense that became the main official reason for his termination. As Rancourt plaintively wrote in his **letter to the Board**, "Socrates did not give grades to his students."

Rancourt's revulsion at assigning marks is not common among professors, but neither is it rare. Over the past four decades, I have known dozens of professors who, in the course of their intellectual maturation, became exceedingly uncomfortable with assigning grades. A few of them met the same fate as Rancourt. One of the offenses that led to the dismissal of theologian Herbert Richardson from the University of Toronto in 1994 (a case of administrative mobbing to which I have devoted a **substantial book**), was that he and his students in a graduate seminar agreed that all of them should receive the same final grade.

[..]

****

All-cause mortality during COVID-19: No plague and a likely signature of mass homicide by government response

Technical Report (PDF Available) · June 2020
DOI: 10.13140/RG.2.2.24350.77125

Abstract

The latest data of all-cause mortality by week does not show a winter-burden mortality that is statistically larger than for past winters. There was no plague. However, a sharp "COVID peak" is present in the data, for several jurisdictions in Europe and the USA. This all-cause-mortality "COVID peak" has unique characteristics: • Its sharpness, with a full-width at half-maximum of only approximately 4 weeks; • Its lateness in the infectious-season cycle, surging after week-11 of 2020, which is unprecedented for any large sharp-peak feature; • The synchronicity of the onset of its surge, across continents, and immediately following the WHO declaration of the pandemic; and • Its USA state-to-state absence or presence for the same viral ecology on the same territory, being correlated with nursing home events and government actions rather than any known viral strain discernment. These "COVID peak" characteristics, and a review of the epidemiological history, and of relevant knowledge about viral respiratory diseases, lead me to postulate that the "COVID peak" results from an accelerated mass homicide of immune-vulnerable individuals, and individuals made more immune-vulnerable, by government and institutional actions, rather than being an epidemiological signature of a novel virus, irrespective of the degree to which the virus is novel from the perspective of viral speciation.

[..]

- https://www.researchgate.net/publication/341832637_All-cause_mortality_during_COVID-19_No_plague_and_a_likely_signature_of_mass_homicide_by_government_response

****

June 18, 2020, 4:12PM (Amir-ul to group):

has anyone heard of Dr. Denis Rancourt?

I'd never heard of him.

He was a senior tenured professor of physics for 20 years at the University of Ottawa in Canada. He did manage to get himself fired/ejected from the university at the end of his 20 year professorship there.

I read this article. There was a time, of course, when being hired as an anarchist professor was unlikely at most institutions & being a Marxist one was likely to get the professor fired. Rancourt doesn't appear to be a Marxist but he is an anarchist so I reckon I take his being fired for granted.

If it pops up in French

I just clicked on the "Research Gate" link at the top to take me to what was presumably the original in English. The URL for that is this: https://www.researchgate.net/publication/341832637_All-cause_mortality_during_COVID-19_No_plague_and_a_likely_signature_of_mass_homicide_by_government_response . The title of the paper is pretty telling: "**All-cause mortality during COVID-19: No plague and a likely signature of mass homicide by government response**"

Consider this one simple caption:

"**Also, none of the seven states that did not impose a lockdown (Iowa, Nebraska, North Dakota, South Dakota, Utah, Wyoming, and Arkansas) have a "COVID peak".**"

You got that? No imposition of lockdown, no exceptional quantity of deaths.

Remember when the nazis killed patients in mental institutions 1st? What if this is truly a correlation to that?! WITH MOST OF THE DEATHS BEING **DELIBERATELY KILLING OFF OLD PEOPLE IN NURSING HOMES?!**

thank you Amir-ul Kafirs for all of your numbers obsessions and interpretations,

Ha ha! You should read my math book! It's called "Paradigm Shift Knuckle Sandwich & other examples of P.N.T. (Perverse Number Theory)". Available online. Easy reading, really funny.

****

June 18, 2020, 5:31PM (Inquiring Librarian to group):

I just got through the entire article on my lunch break. Wow! I am going to try sending this in response to my chemical engineer friend's NYT articles on the covid death statistics. Wish me luck that she doesn't dump me forever as a friend. There is really nothing offensive in the article. But it really throws the current mass media theories, like those of the NYT, totally under the bus. I really appreciate his focus on the "All Cause Mortality Rate". It makes sense. And if it's true the WHO is a bunch of mind and body control pill pushing vaccination hungry assholes, then I think that they really overlooked the fact that someone or someones, eventually would consider analyzing the All Cause angle of the deaths instead of focusing on the seemingly fabricated Covid reported deaths. This article helps to clear my mind on the many studies on cases and deaths being studied but knowing full well that many of the reported Covid deaths were comorbidities or just assumptions of Covid and above all, tangentially addresses the known lack of accuracy of the Covid 19 coronavirus tests.

Also, I loved all of the 'press articles and institutional memos' that he cited at the end... now I'm even further from getting back to my calming fiction reading. =O I am 1st going to read this one from the former health minister of Israel: https://www.spiked-online.com/2020/05/22/nothing-can-justify-this-destruction-of-peoples-lives/ . And then while making dinner tonight, maybe listen to this one: https://www.youtube.com/watch?v=4sjNQ4YTUM4 .

****

June 18, 2020, 5:44PM (Amir-ul Kafirs to group):

HERETICS: Mack Reynolds

I've been writing a review of Mack Reynolds (& Dean Ing)'s "Deathwish World" over the past 4 days so I've put in a shitload of blunt opinions against the PANDEMIC PANIC including a reference to Denis Rancourt. I haven't proofed my review yet wch means I haven't put it online so you're getting the SNEAK PREVIEW. Some of you might find it a bit 'much' but I swear on a stack of burning bibles & qu'rans that not only is the original book fabulous but my review of it is, ahem, unlike anything you'll ever read by any reviewer other than me.

review of
Mack Reynolds & Dean Ing's Deathwish World
by tENTATIVELY, a cONVENIENCE - June 15-18, 2020

I remember devoting much of my 1984 reading time to reading the work of Philip K. Dick, I probably read one bk of his a wk. I loved his work so much that it might've seemed unlikely at the time that anyone could ever supercede him in importance as a SciFi writer to me. Fortunately for me,I keep discovering other SF writers that please me as much as Dick probably did way back then. Mack Reynolds is 1st & foremost among those these days. Reading one of his bks is bound to engross & please me. Since I 'discovered' his work in June, 2016, 4 yrs ago now, I've read & reviewed 16 of his bks:

The Rival Rigelians: https://www.goodreads.com/review/show/1670905334
Blackman's Burden: https://www.goodreads.com/story/show/618795?chapter=1
Border, Breed Nor Birth: https://www.goodreads.com/story/show/618795?chapter=1
Trample An Empire Down: https://www.goodreads.com/review/show/2383581144
Computer War: https://www.goodreads.com/review/show/2409376365
Code Duello: https://www.goodreads.com/review/show/2409376365
Planetary Agent X: https://www.goodreads.com/story/show/629641-gotta-luv-ya-mack-reynolds
Mercenary from Tomorrow: https://www.goodreads.com/review/show/2460708541
The Space Barbarians: https://www.goodreads.com/review/show/2462644753
After Utopia: https://www.goodreads.com/story/show/1055643-reynolds
Commune 2000 A.D.: https://www.goodreads.com/story/show/1079009-commune?chapter=0
Space Visitor: https://www.goodreads.com/review/show/2609014592
Equality: in the Year 2000: https://www.goodreads.com/story/show/1085883-mack-reynolds-is-the-greatest
Galactic Medal of Honor: https://www.goodreads.com/story/show/1086031-rumponomics
Computer World: https://www.goodreads.com/review/show/2745957051
Day After Tomorrow: https://www.goodreads.com/review/show/2749363775

Fortunately, there's no end in sight.

The "Foreword" provides this:

"*And it was possibly the softest sell of all time. The United States Government simply issued a declaration that it welcomed any countries in North, Central, or South America, or the Caribbean, to join it, conferring all rights pertaining to American citizens, including the Guaranteed Annual Stipend*" - p 1

The "*Guaranteed Annual Stipend*" being something that occurs again & again in Reynolds's novels, a welfare that most of the people subsist on because the world has become so automated that hardly anyone works anymore.

The opening scene is one of an apparent assassination. Reynolds, the author, is reputed to've been around wars &/or revolutions, perhaps he was a mercenary or, at least, familiar w/ mercenaries. As such, the technical detail might be accurate.

"["]This scope we've got is an Auto-Range. Latest thing. Combines a range finder with a regular telescopic sight. No sweat. Hand me that silencer, Joe."

""You're sure?" Hamp said, pushing the back of his left hand over his mouth.

""Sure I'm sure," the other told him. "Take a minute or so to get it all sighted in again." He took the long tube Joe handed over and began screwing it into the barrel. It projected about a foot and a half when he had it tightly fitted. The silencer was about two and a half times the diameter of the barrel." - p 5

After the 'assassination' the team of 3 is attempting to leave the area when they're stopped by the police. To bluff their way out this happens:

"Joe began to retreat backward, saying quickly into his transceiver, "State Police officer Number 358 had ordered my transceiver taken. One of us is a black; notify the nearest Nat Turner Team. One of us is an Amerind; notify the Sons of Wounded Knee. I am a Chicano; get in touch with the Foes of the Alamo. Notify our legal department! Notify Civil Liberties. Alert the Reunited Nations Human Relations . . ."" - p 12

It works. I'm reminded of a woman I met once who was stopped at the Canadian border. She told them that her father was a reporter for the Turner News Network and that he'd be very interested to learn about her being turned away. It worked, they let her in the country. She was bluffing, her father wasn't a reporter for the Turner News Network or for anyone else.

""What the hell's a Nat Turner Team?"

"And Tom Horse added, "Or the Sons of Wounded Knee?"

""Damned if I know," Joe said grinning. "I made them up as I went along. Same with the Foes of the Alamo. What's the old gag? If there'd been a back door to the Alamo there would never have been a Texas."" - p 13

Ok, I've already been hinting so now it's time to reveal a little secret, it's early on in the bk, so it's not *that much* of a spoiler & it gives a pretty good idea of the political subtleties at work:

""Plumb center," Tom whispered. "The capslug shattered right on his chest and plattered red goo all over his shirt. I could see his face go pale and his eyes pop. He fainted."" - pp 14-15

The 'assassination' of the racist politician was just a scare, a Red Scare one might say. The 'assassins' were just putting the *fear of his victims* in him. An excellent idea!

Meanwhile, in another plot thread:

"Frank calculated quickly and looked up. "This comes to only two hundred pseudo-dollars."

"MacDonald said to his fellow agent, "He's not only an intellectual but a mathematician."

""I'm supposed to get a thousand," Frank said his voice tight.

MacDonald scoffed at him. "What'd you do with a thousand pseudo-dollars? Probably waste it. Go through it in a week. As it is, Roskin and I will lay over in Madrid on our way home, and we'll hoist a couple of drinks to you in Chicote's."" - p 27

Being an anarchist from BalTimOre, this next section warmed the cobblestones of my liver:

"Roy Cox looked out over the small, shabby hall in Baltimore with its pitiful group, members of the Industrial Workers of the World—"Wobblies," in their own jargon. Inwardly, he felt depressed and weary. It was the same old story, there were sixteen in the audience." - p 33

I feel ya. Cox gives a speech & there're hecklers in the audience:

"["]Computers can be programmed into shortcomings."

""Like what!" one of the hecklers called out. His friends laughed, backing him. Several of the Wobblies, seated down front, turned and glared at thrm.

"Roy said, "Well, let's take a couple of the scientists that the computers would have passed by. Two of their big requirements are a good education and a top-notch Ability Quotient. Thomas Edison had only a couple of years of formal education—he never got through grammar school. The computers wouldn't have picked him for a job. Steinmetz was a hunchback cripple, in spite of his I.Q., and would never have gotten a high Ability Quotient, much of which depends on physical attributes." - p 36

Note that ""Like what!"" from a heckler ends w/ an exclamation mark instead of a question mark. Such people aren't interested in informative answers, they just want to attack whomever they're trying to bully — as long as they have people to back them up.

Otherwise, *UP WITH THE AUTODIDACTS!!* If you want to find **real** intelligence, instead of Pavlovian Dog Untertan (w/ Superiority Complex) pseudo-intelligence it's among the autididacts you must look (he says immodestly). A dog trained to jump thru a fiery hoop isn't as smart as one that figures out how to escape.

""This is one of the final things Bartolomeo Vanzetti wrote. He was self-educated."

"Forry Brown read softly from the tattered clipping: "*If it had not been for this thing, I might have lived out my life talking at street corners to scorning men. I might have died unmarked, unknown, a failure. Now we are not a failure. This is our career and our triumph. Never in all out full life could we hope to do such work for tolerance, for justice, for man's understanding of man, as now we do by accident.*

"*Our words—our lives—our pains: nothing! The taking of our lives—lives of a good shoemaker and a poor fish peddler—all! That last moment belongs to us. That agony is our triumph.*"

"Forry Brown looked up from the clipping. "Their deaths weren't the end. Hundreds of articles about them were published for years. Best-selling books were written about the Sacc-Vanzetti case. There was even a long-running play on Broadway, and a hit movie film. In becoming martyrs, Bartolemeo Vanzetti and Nicola Sacco at long last put over their message. Decades later, they were vindicated by the State of Massachusetts. They hadn't even been guilty."" - p 47

"On April 15, 1920, a paymaster for a shoe company in South Braintree, Massachusetts, was shot and killed along with his guard. The murderers, who were described as two Italian men, escaped with more than $15,000. After going to a garage to claim a car that police said was connected with the crime, Sacco and Vanzetti were arrested and charged with the crime. Although both men carried guns and made false statements upon their arrest, neither had a previous criminal record. On July 14, 1921, they were convicted and sentenced to die.

"Anti-radical sentiment was running high in America at the time, and the trial of Sacco and Vanzetti was regarded by many as unlawfully sensational. Authorities had failed to come up with any evidence of the stolen money, and much of the other evidence against them was later discredited. During the next few years, sporadic protests were held in Massachusetts and around the world calling for their release, especially after Celestino Madeiros, then under a sentence for murder, confessed in 1925 that he had participated in the crime with the Joe Morelli gang. The state Supreme Court refused to upset the verdict, and Massachusetts Governor Alvan T. Fuller denied the men clemency. In the days leading up to the execution, protests were held in cities around the world, and bombs were set off in New York City and Philadelphia. On August 23, Sacco and Vanzetti were electrocuted.

"In 1961, a test of Sacco's gun using modern forensic techniques apparently proved it was his gun that killed the guard, though little evidence has been found to substantiate Vanzetti's guilt. In 1977, Massachusetts Governor Michael Dukakis issued a proclamation vindicating Sacco and Vanzetti, stating that they had been treated unjustly and that no stigma should be associated with their names."

- https://www.history.com/this-day-in-history/sacco-and-vanzetti-executed

Composer Ruth Crawford Seeger wrote a great song supporting them post-mortem. Here're the lyrics:

"Sacco, Vanzetti

by H. T. Tsiang

"Fast! Fast!
One year has passed!
Dead! Dead!
You will never be reborn!
Who said
There will be a resurrection?
Why didn't we see any of those gentlemen
Who were willing to take your places?
The real meaning of "death" —
You knew it.
Still you paid with your life for your class!
Sacrifice!
That was real sacrifice!

"Look at your enemies.
They are fishing,
Smiling,
Murdering,
As ever.
Shameful!
It is an eternal disgrace to us all.

"Before your death
Did not millions promise —
To do "this" or "that"
If you should die?
Now
One year has passed.
What about "this" and what about "that"?

"Petitions?
Protests?
Telegrams?
Demonstrations?
Strikes?
Oh! They may refire the cold ashes of our two martyrs.
But they can never soften the murderer's heart!
Tears?
Sighs?
Complaints?
And the like?
Oh! They may expect the embraces of your dear mothers,
They can never get pardon from the blood-thirsty masters.

"Have you ever seen sheep and pigs
Being dragged to slaughter?

How pitifully they shriek!
How terribly they tremble!
Yet men enjoy their delicious flesh
Just the same!
Sheep! Pigs! Foreigners! Workers!
Your sweat is fertile,
Your blood is sweet,
Your meat is fresh!

"Oh, Vanzetti!
You did say:
“I wish to forgive some people for what they are now doing to me”.
Certainly, you can forgive them as you like,
But you are the Wop, the fish peddler, the worker,
And haven’t anything in the bank.
Isn’t it a great insult
To say “forgive” to your honorable master?

"Oh, Sacco!
You did say:
“Long live anarchy”,
But you should not forget,
That when you climb up to heaven
You must use the ladder!

"Oh Martyrs!
Dead! Dead!
You are dead,
Never, never
To live again.
Fast! Fast!
One year has passed!
But years and years,
Years are piling up immortal bricks
Of your lofty monument.

"Oh martyrs!
Look at the autumn flowers:
They are dying!
Dying! Dying!
But
The trees, the roots from which
The flowers are coming*
Never, never die!
When the spring comes
We shall again see the pretty flowers
Blooming,
Perfuming,

Saluting the warm sun,
Wrestling with the mild wind
and kissing the charming butterflies.

"Oh martyrs!
Dead, dead! You are dead!
But
Your human tree and your human root
Are budding,
Blooming,
Growing!

"Listen to the war cries of your living brothers!
This is the incense
We are burning
To you.

* Crawford changes “coming” to “blooming”" - https://songofamerica.net/song/sacco-vanzetti/

Roger Reynolds also composed a fantastic piece using a statement from Vanzetti as its text.

"**A Portrait of Vanzetti** (1962-63)
"Narrator, 2 Fl (2 Picc), Cl, 2 Hn, Tpt, Tbn, 2 Perc,
4-channel electroacoustic sound
Text edited by the composer from the letters of Bartolomeo Vanzetti
by Roger Reynolds

"During 1963, I was in Köln as a Fulbright Fellow, working under the generous guidance of Gottfried-Michael Köenig, I completed the electro-acoustic component of a work for narrator, ensemble, and tape. *A Portrait of Vanzetti* was premiered at the 1963 ONCE Festival, in Ann Arbor, where I had studied with Roberto Gerhard and Ross Lee Finney. It was the first work I completed after leaving the University of Michigan.

"Although one now badly faded score has survived, along with a recording subsequently issued in the New World Record’s 5-CD set documenting the first five years of the ONCE Festivals, the tape part was lost along with most of the text.

"In 2009, I set out to resurrect this work, in part because of the response to the recording, and in part because the story of Italian immigrant anarchists, Nicola Sacco and Bartolomeo Vanzetti, along with the social, political, and judicial turmoil that their trial and subsequent appeals aroused, touches me still today. I re-read the volume of letters, reconstructed the text and have recreated an approximation of the electro-acoustic component, now using multichannel sound, and adding spatialization of the narrator’s voice.

"Two major sections of the work along with their sub-sections are identified, now, and a set of individual cues (many further subdivided) has been added in order to make rehearsals more efficient.

"*A Portrait of Vanzetti* was premiered 16 February 1963 on the ONCE Festival in Ann Arbor. The narrator was Jack O'Brien; Donald Scavarda conducted the ONCE Chamber Ensemble."

- http://www.rogerreynolds.com/program_notes/vanzetti.html

I highly recommend listening to both of these pieces. I also saw a play about the 2 of them at the City Theater in Pittsburgh around 1999. At the end of the play, which supported the idea that the 2 of them were innocent & were railroaded into the death penalty because they were anarchist immigrants, my companion, etta cetera, & I stood up & shouted: "FREE MUMIA!" because it was, & still is, our feeling that Mumia Abu Jamal has been similarly railroaded. A very old woman wearing a floor-length fur coat turned to us & informed us pompously that Mumia's case was nothing like Sacco & Vanzetti's. No doubt this rich woman is an expert on the trials & tribulations of persecuted people in the US. **NOT.**

A primary theme of Deathwish World is anti-racism. The following dialog is fraught w/ suspicious appearances:

"["]My father left me more than I need for the rest of my life. But . . . well, I do nothing. I'm fed up with my friends and relatives all in the same position. I want to do something worthwhile."

"Hamp nodded. "It's not an unknown reaction. Engels, the collaborator of Karl Marx, was a wealthy manufacturer. The Russian anarchist Kropotkin was a prince. Norman Thomas, the American socialist, was married to a very wealthy woman." He grinnned suddenly, "But they rose above it."

""So tell me more about racism and how you . . . we . . . can go about ending it."

"Hamp took a deep breath and said, "You must realize that racism is one of our oldest American traditions.["]" - p 52

Let's take a little vacation, shall we?

""You can't spend your GAS outside the limits of the United States of the Americas," Forry told him. "The government wants you to spend it at home. Why subsidize foreign countries by spending unearned credits in them? The Bahamas, along with Cuba, are the only Caribbean islands that don't belong to the United States." - p 73

He, like me, is an anarchist. I agree w/ him. I'm beginning to see the deaths of vulnerable people in nursing homes as akin to the nazi genocide of mental institution patients. Shocking, right?! Why what a fool I am!! Actually, I'm not a fool, I'm just, like Rancourt, someone who's not afraid to make 'unthinkable' accusations in an era when 'thought crime' is more persecuted than it's been since the so-called "McCarthy Era".

"One of them called out, "Roy, what's your stand on world government? It's in the air these days. You've probably heard that the Congress has invited Australia and New Zealand to join the United States. And it looks as though England and Ireland will get the same invitation."

"Roy said, "We Wobblies are in favor of world government but can't see much advantage to it, so far as the proles are concerned, so long as class-divided society is retained. We'd just continue to be in the same undesirable spot, subsisting on GAS. World government under an industrial democracy would be desirable, but under the status quo it would merely give the powers that be better control of us. Instead of having dozens of countries, each with its own special conditions, its own rules and regulations, they'd have all of us under the same thumb."" - p 243

Think, once again, about the current PANDEMIC PANIC. If there had been a world government, & there certainly seems to be a move in that direction, it wd've been much harder for countries such as Sweden & Belarus to defy the general Draconian lockdown direction. Many people are saying that Sweden's decision was a mistake but how much of that is propaganda? I hope that 10 or 20 yrs from now it'll be easier to decide what's a believable statistic.

This bk is from 1986. In 1986 I attended the anarchist Haymarket Centennial in Chicago, this was the 1st 'large-scale' (maybe 200 people) anarchist gathering I'd ever attended. For me, it was the 1st of many such gatherings over the next 12 yrs. Reynolds has a fictional gathering occur in his narrative 100 yrs later.

"She put the letter before him. "It's from Wobbly headquarters in Chicago."" - p 240

"The meeting was a bore, doomed to failure from its inception. The Synthesis group, which had proposed it, was obviously sincere in its desire to unite all the radical elements but, as Hamp whispered to Max Finkelstein, sincerity alone was dull as dishwater.

"There were perhaps thirty-five present, including the Synthesis committee, the bodyguards, and various delegates. The leading representatives were those from the Wobblies, the Nihilists, the Luddites, and the Libertarians, in addition to the Anti-Racists. The other delegates were from splinter groups, and some, splinters from splinters. There was even one representative from an organization evidently unknown to the others, called Technocracy, Incorporated. Going at least a century and a half back, the Technocrats opted for a world government dominated by scientists, engineers, and technicians. He wasn't quite booed down." - p 278

What about a world government run by Medical Industry representatives w/ an obvious agenda of selling drugs & new technology? I, personally, wd boo that down. Does anybody remember the *Doctors of Death*?! Or is that an 'unmentionable' subject in so-called 'polite society'?!

Reynolds's bks are consistently compellingly plotted, a good read at all levels, full of historical & political intelligence & good analysis.

"The black regarded him questioningly, "It would seem to me that under a World State racism would disappear."

"Roy shook his head very emphatically. "Why? Suppose we *had* a United States of the World. Why would that end racism? It hasn't been ended in the United States, so far. Sure, if it was a world government under the Wobbly program, there'd be no reason for racism. But under the status quo? Suppose the World Club took over and made the United Church the state religion. The Prophet does precious little to hide his anti-semitism. That reactionary Harrington Chase is hand in glove with him. The Jews aren't about to join up with the United Church, like so many other smaller religions are. Most of them, these days, are agnostics or atheists and won't support any organized religion. Those who are still Orthodox cling to the faith that's held them together for three thousand years. So the Prohpet's down on them, and if his outfit ever becomes the state religion, Jews will be in trouble."" - p 285

Throughout this review I've referred only to Mack Reynolds b/c I'm not familiar w/ his coauthor Dean Ing. Perhaps Ing provided some Wobbly expertise. NO! Check this out!:

"**Dean Charles Ing** (born 1931) is an American author, who usually writes in the science fiction and techno-thriller genres. His novel *The Ransom of Black Stealth One* (1989) was a *New York Times* bestseller. He is a former member of the Citizens' Advisory Council on National Space Policy. He has authored more than 30 novels. He has also co-authored novels with his friends Jerry Pournelle, S. M. Stirling, and Leik Myrabo.

"Ing is a United States Air Force veteran (where he served as a USAF interceptor crew chief), a former aerospace engineer, and a university professor who holds a doctorate in Communications Theory. He has been a techno-thriller genre writer since 1977. Following the death of science fiction author Mack Reynolds in 1983, Ing was asked to finish several of Reynolds' uncompleted manuscripts." - https://en.wikipedia.org/wiki/Dean_Ing

Well, that's the shocker of today. Good job, Ing, good job.

****

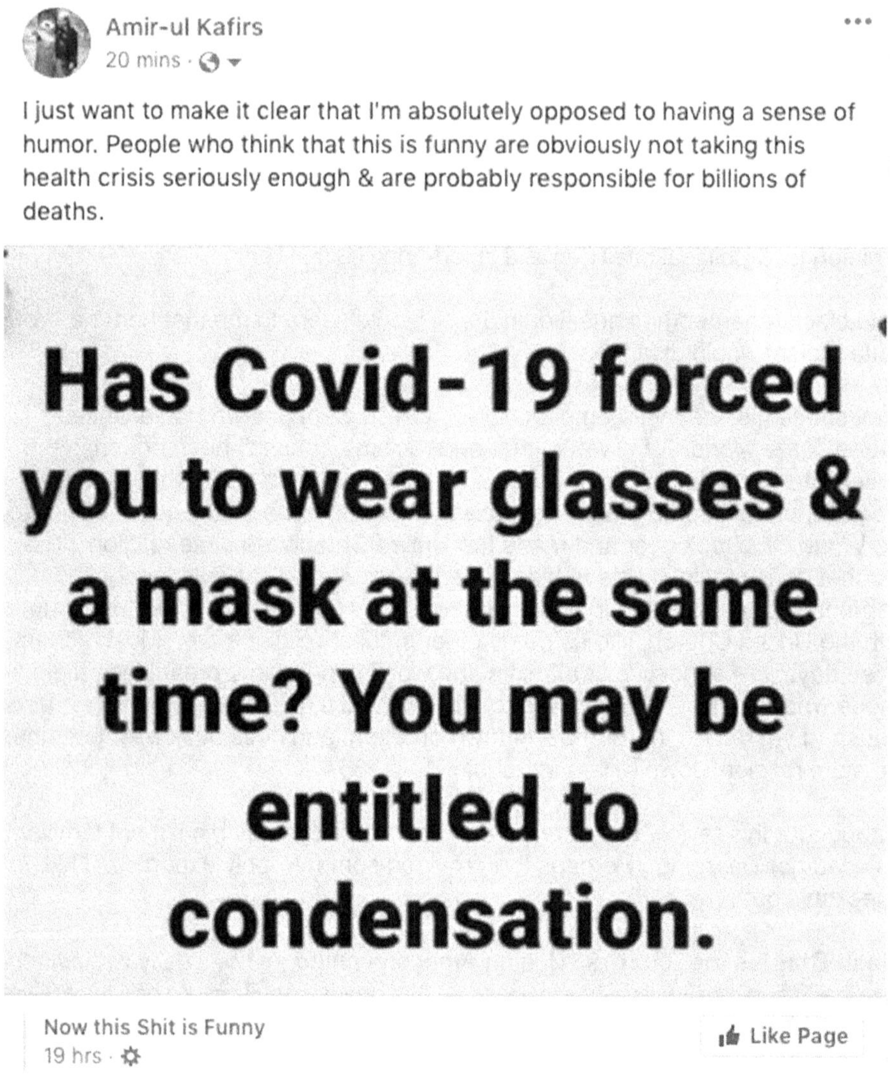

Amir-ul Kafirs
20 mins ·
I just want to make it clear that I'm absolutely opposed to having a sense of humor. People who think that this is funny are obviously not taking this health crisis seriously enough & are probably responsible for billions of deaths.
Has Covid-19 forced you to wear glasses & a mask at the same time? You may be entitled to condensation.
Now this Shit is Funny
19 hrs ·
Like Page

****

June 19, 2020, 9:22AM (Amir-ul Kafirs to group):

HERETICS: No Masks Required: HOORAY!

https://www.businessinsider.com/amc-wont-require-face-masks-when-theaters-reopen-this-summer-2020-6?fbclid=IwAR37Y3zMmbNLTm5SFkp_euxacEgZqw5sPIolTyW0OmPjOTxNjFiK9mdIVNo

AMC won't require face masks when theaters reopen to avoid 'political controversy'

Charles Davis

AMC Theatres won't require customers to wear face masks when it reopens this summer, CEO and President Adam Aron said in an interview with Variety.

"We did not want to be drawn into a political controversy," Aron told the magazine. "We thought it might be counterproductive if we forced mask wearing on those people who believe strongly that it is not necessary."

AMC, which operates more than 600 theaters across the United States, plans to begin reopening on July 15. It joins competitors Cinemark and Regal in encouraging masks, Variety reported, but not mandating them – at least in jurisdictions where they are not already required.

"We think that the vast majority of AMC guests will be wearing masks," Aron said. "When I go to an AMC feature, I will certainly be wearing a mask and leading by example."

Masks will also be available for $1.

Indoor environments, particularly those with air conditioning, are considered high-risk environments for the transmission of the coronavirus. With indoor theaters still closed in most states, many have turned to drive-in theaters, which have proliferated in the age of COVID-19.

[..]

****

June 19, 2020, 9:48AM (Dick to group):

RE: HERETICS: No Masks Required: HOORAY!

That's good news
I wish they'd do that here
The effects upon culture here are a disaster
As usual, I suspect foul-play... in this case, I think the "powers that be" want to destroy traditional culture so they can replace it with all-inclusive-global-garbage... thus my new slogan:
IDIOSYNCRATIC ARTIST LIVES MATTER

****

June 19, 2020, 12:16PM (Amir-ul Kafirs to group):

The effects upon culture here are a disaster

Well, of course, all music venues, as far as I know, are still closed. More or less EVERYTHING cultural is still closed. But, who cares?! One can still WATCH TV!! Isn't that enough?! One can still go to the iTunes Store!! Isn't that enough?!

I think the "powers that be" want to destroy traditional culture so they can replace it with all-inclusive-global-garbage...

Pardon our mess (you have no choice) while we completely remodel your life.

thus my new slogan:
IDIOSYNCRATIC ARTIST LIVES MATTER

But they don't, of course, & probably never have. The people in power only care about "IDIOSYNCRATIC ARTISTS" in terms of market value. & the artist doesn't have to be alive for that to be exploited. Hell, they don't even have to be any 'good'. Take Christopher Wool:

"Apocalypse Now, 1988

"SELL THE HOUSE SELL THE CAR SELL THE KIDS" - that's what Christopher Wool's most expensive word painting says. If you're heard it before, you're right: *Apocalypse Now* features words from a famous line said by Marlon Brando's character Richard Colby in Francis Ford Coppola's 1979 film of the same name - subsequently based on the Joseph Conrad novel *Heart of Darkness*. The artist was often applauded for his choice of words, described as as relevant today as they were at the time of their creation and that they could work perfectly even put out of their context completely. The work was sold at Christie's New York in 2012 for as much as $23,5 million, surpassing its high estimate by 18%!" - https://www.widewalls.ch/magazine/most-expensive-christopher-wool-art-pieces-auctions/apocalypse-now-1988

Yep, the artist took a line from a famous movie, painted it on canvas, & sold it for $23,500,000.00. Maybe I'll make a text painting with the above quote on it & my criticism & price it at $1,000,000,000.00. I mean, I know my worth.

Museums are reopening here. See the article at the bottom. "Each museum will have clearly marked foot traffic patterns": that's the sort of thing that bothers me even more than all the rest. Everything must be control-freaked. Imagine walking through a museum & seeing something across the room that you find very interesting & wanting to look at it right away. NOPE. You MUST get to that thing by the proscribed footpath. This is the sort of thing that sets dangerous precedents, precedents of the 'approved' way of doing ANYTHING becoming *de rigeur*. At least there's no mention of masks being required.

Carnegie museums, others reopening

MARYLYNNE PITZ
Pittsburgh Post-Gazette
JUN 9, 2020 10:32 AM

Carnegie Museums of Pittsburgh reopens its four museums on June 29. Visitors will be admitted every half hour with timed tickets.

The consortium runs The Andy Warhol Museum and the Carnegie Science Center, both on the North Side, plus the Carnegie Museums of Art and Natural History in Oakland.

Each of the four museums will operate at 25 percent capacity "so we can manage the flow of people in the buildings at any given time," said Steven Knapp, president and CEO of the nonprofit. He added that all visitors must wear masks.

"We're hoping that even if we have to shift back into the yellow stage, we can make the case that we are operating safely," Mr. Knapp said.

"We have been developing policies to ensure the safety of employees and visitors," he said, adding that museum employees will undergo daily temperature checks.

Each museum will have clearly marked foot traffic patterns, enhanced cleaning and plexiglass shields at visitor services desks.

[..]

- https://www.post-gazette.com/ae/art-architecture/2020/06/09/Carnegie-Museums-of-Pittsburgh-reopen-COVID-19/stories/202006080089

****

June 19, 2020, 4:48PM (Dick to group):

No, there are no movies, concerts, ballets, operas, cabarets, nothing at all
The 21 June is something they call "Festival of Music" I am waiting to see what form it takes, usually there are bands literally everywhere you look, street corners, balconys, bars, public places, etc

****

June 19, 2020, 5:24PM (Dick to group):

A few personal musings on the subject of attacks upon art and culture:

Sometime ago I attended a sort of opera by John Adams staged by Peter Sellars (not the actor, the stage director) it may have been in 2000 A.D.

I think it was supposed to deal with the Christ child (the title was El Nino) but what it presented was a sort of template of the absolutely boring
To be honest the content seemed meaningless and I can hardly remember it -- what hit home was the form of presentation

It presented what I would call a vision of the corporate mentality, something like the original microsoft script style, namely flat boring, personality-less
There are no white people, no black people, no asians - there is instead a sort of generic being "doing their" job
The men seemed castrated, the women seemed sexless
The set looked like a multi-tier modern modular office space
Everything was clean, anti-septic, dust-and-thought free

It was what I think certain people would like for the future

I was nauseated by it but discovered it to be a reality for many people when later I taught English in a large corporation for a while, at a place called _____ (A huge German firm) I saw and met the real life examples of the types I'd seen presented on stage years earlier

None of my students (all well paid and securely "on the team") seemed to have any interests in anything reflecting an individual personality, it was something to behold... one woman, when I asked her what she did when she wasn't working told me she enjoyed "eating meat in restaurants" - you'll just have to believe me, it is an exact quote

I think traditional culture is based upon the development of the individual consciousness and thus is, in a certain way "an enemy of the desired modern state" because it encourages idiosyncratic individualism

The only "positive" note I can recall while working at _____ was a story I was told in confidence by a highly paid actuary (a person who establishes insurance rates, a sort of insurance guru)

One day I told her how the place seemed like a futuristic utopia (I didn't say what I really thought , that is a dystopia obviously) sci-fi movie setting, everyone happy, doing their job, briskly walking around the building or busy at their desks

She said yes, it does look that way but that earlier the same year an upper management guy jumped out of a tenth story window when it was discovered that he was diverting funds into his own account by erasing old policies he thought were no longer active - then one day a claim came in for a thirty year old policy and he was found out

Though it involved a suicide and just dealt with the selfish desire for more money I thought it showed a little hope

*

By the way, according to some statistical chart I saw posted on youtube "artist" is the least essential form of employment

****

June 19, 2020, 9:23PM (Amir-ul Kafirs to group):

Sometime ago I attended a sort of opera by John Adams

Ha ha! Honestly, I'm glad to read your attack on John Adams. For me, personally, he's one of the worst composers of all time. If I remember correctly, a few years ago he was declared the Composer of the Year or some such by a group of Pittsburgh compoers, educators, & musicians. One friend of mine was a part of that selection committee. I was rather unabashed in expressing my disgust. BLAND is definitely the operative word. People were able to adapt to Minimalism because of the New Tonality but they still found the stridency of the rhythms hard to take, listen to early Philip Glass for examples (although I don't like Glass's music much either). John Adams just removed anything that was challenging or new & made pure schmaltz. Instant popularity!!

I think traditional culture is based upon the development of the individual consciousness and thus is, in a certain way "an enemy of the desired modern state" because it encourages idiosyncratic individualism

Well, it's like I've been saying, it's as if the bulk of humanity is being primed to be part of a superorganism & if you're not with it then the anti-bodies are expected to destroy you as a potential danger to the GROUPTHINK. Not to constantly harp on nazism but that's essentially what Hitler's concept of the German people was.

By the way, according to some statistical chart I saw posted on youtube "artist" is the least essential form of employment

I was just telling Naia Nisnam today about when I tried to collect welfare when I was 20 as an unemployed musician. I was told, in total seriouness, by the social worker that no such profession existed.

ANYWAY, your post has inspired my latest text panel, already on social media. It's obviously very dramatic but, what can I say?, these text panels are my assault on GROUPTHINK & I'm not exactly being careful to not tread on metaphorical toes. As each new day of the QUARANTYRANNY goes by with no end in sight the more I'm convinced that everything I hold dear is being carefully eliminated in the interests of the NEW WORLD ODOR.

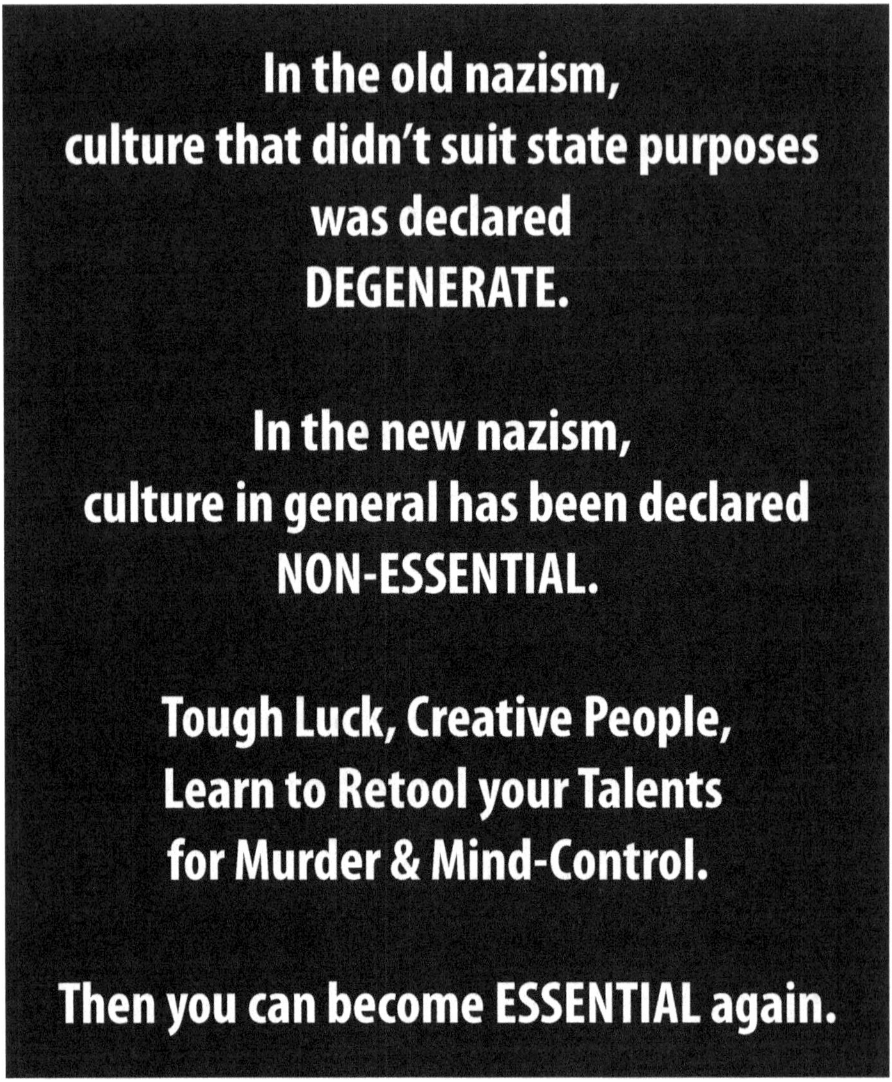

In the old nazism,
culture that didn't suit state purposes
was declared
DEGENERATE.
In the new nazism,
culture in general has been declared
NON-ESSENTIAL.
Tough Luck, Creative People,
Learn to Retool your Talents
for Murder & Mind-Control.
Then you can become ESSENTIAL again.

****

June 19, 2020, 8:39PM (Naia Nisnam to group):

Re: Airport Report

On Fri, Jun 19, 2020 at 3:20 PM Naia Nisnam wrote:

I'm flying from Pittsburgh to Portland Oregon today and thought I'd share some airport observations.

There are signs everywhere stating that face coverings are required in the airport terminal at all times. There are announcements every 15 minutes reminding everyone to keep their masks on at all times. There are stickers on the floors showing people how to stand 6 feet apart.

The stickers on the floor were obeyed in the security check line, but people were over it by the time they had to line up for boarding. Despite repeated announcements telling us to stand 6 feet apart, absolutely no one did. No one. (That may be related to my airline's open seating policy, which means you pick where you sit, so people may be used to rushing the gate to get first dibs on seat choice.)

Less than half of the people waiting had their masks properly in place. Almost everyone had masks in place as they walked through the terminal but once they sat down to wait they couldn't handle the masks. People would pull them up for a few minutes, then pull them down again. Masks were worn under noses and under chins, basically masking people's necks. (I'm "guilty" of being a neck masker). One guy had his mask dangling off of one ear- the highlight of my trip so far. A few people had no masks at all.

The employee who announced flight and boarding updates kept pulling her mask off and back on. At one point I heard her complain about the mask being uncomfortable and that she couldn't hear people when they talked through them. The steward on the plane who told us we had to wear masks during the flight apologized about it and made sure to point out that it was because of "health guidelines". Thankfully he made no claims about the masks being for anyone's safety.

For once, I am thrilled about Americans' inept, half-assed way of doing things. I assume that most people who are willing to fly right now aren't terribly concerned about the virus. Still, it warms my heart to see so many people doing such a terrible job with their masks. We'll see if that continues to be the case in Denver..

And I'm happy to report that even Less people are obeying mask laws in the Denver airport! (Though there is a lady here wearing gloves and 2 masks- a paper one with a cloth one on top). I'm excited to see how Portland is handling things...

****

June 19, 2020, 9:31PM (Amir-ul Kafirs to group):

Re: Airport Report

I'm excited to see how Portland is handling things...

In Portland, everyone is lying dead in piles & savage dogs are eating their remains. Ok, maybe not. Maybe life is just going on despite what people keep calling the "plague". That's another thing that annoys me. Any comparison to the BLACK PLAGUE is even more melodramatic than my last text panel. Back in the day, when I was a young man of course, when the BLACK PLAGUE was on, the dead were brought out of houses, tossed on carts & taken somewhere to be burnt. That's a little more dramatic than bringing them out of hospitals in body bags & taking them in refrigerated trucks to be incinerated.

****

June 19, 2020, 9:45PM (Inquiring Librarian to group):

Re: HERETICS: No Masks Required: HOORAY! (Culture)

I love all that you had to say about this! "The New World Odor"!! Ha Ha!! But I'm also crying because it's kinda just that. =/

And Dick, I too saw that hope in the future hearing that guy had emotion enough left in him to jump out a window and recognizing his own deviousness.

& yes, I saw this about the AMC movie theaters this morning. I felt like screaming Hallelujah!!! Let's hope other businesses follow suit sometime soon!

I talked to the checkout girl at Petsmart today. Somehow the subject of vaccines came up. She, a young African American gal, blurted out, "They aren't putting any of their vaccines in me!!". This made me SO HAPPY. I thanked her profusely for saying that and told her I was of the same sentiments. I think a lot of our populus may be wiser than we realize. Let's just hope!! The government may be seeing a huge resistance when they start pushing the pedal more to the metal on their tyranny.

****

June 21, 2020, 9:47AM (Amir-ul Kafirs to group):

Re: HERETICS: No Masks Required: HOORAY! (Culture)

Naia Nisnam pointed out to me in a text last night that AMC has reversed its decision to allow people without masks into its theaters under pressure from the STERILIZERS:

https://www.boston.com/culture/movies/2020/06/19/amc-theaters-reverses-course-on-masks-after-backlash

One of the things that fascinates me about this is that this is the 1st time I've ever noticed such an incredible almost instantaneous effectiveness of 'protest'. Black Lives Matter is having a similar impact. Businesses are terrified of having their PR images ruined by the Character Assassination of the STERLIZERS & BLM. Of course, I support the basic purpose of BLM & wholeheartedly *despise* the purposes of the STERLIZERS so the whole situation becomes messy. In a sense it's heartening that protest can have this effect but it's sickening that the STERLIZERS can get their way through what's tantamount to mob bullying. Unfortunately, to opponents of BLM the same thing can be said: that the BLM are bullies.

****

AMC Theaters reverses course on masks after backlash

"It is clear from this response that we did not go far enough on the usage of masks."

By **LINDSEY BAHR**, AP
June 19, 2020

LOS ANGELES (AP) — The nation's largest movie theater chain changed its position on mask-wearing less than a day after the company became a target on social media for saying it would defer to local governments on the issue.
AMC Theaters CEO Adam Aron said Friday that its theaters will require patrons to wear masks upon reopening, which will begin in mid-July. Customers who don't wear masks won't be admitted or allowed to stay.

[..]

- https://www.boston.com/culture/movies/2020/06/19/amc-theaters-reverses-course-on-masks-after-backlash

****

June 20, 2020, 12:53AM (Inquiring Librarian to group):

Re: Airport Report

Thanks so much for sending this Naia Nisnam!! I loved what you wrote. Like you, I am kind of elated at how lazy mask wearers are here in Louisiana. I mean, if we don't have herd immunity here due to total negligence of the entire state populace, then, then I am too tired to figure a clever way to say it's obvious we have herd immunity by laziness.

Today when I went to Walmart, 2 young people in front of me were told they could not enter Walmart without a mask. They were denied entry and left. But when I got inside, I'd say less than 50% of shoppers and staff were actually fully wearing a mask and many had them slung around their necks, some appeared to be whole families roaming the shop without masks. Many had them tucked over their chins with their noses fully hanging out.

Today at Petsmart, I walked in with my mask on. Inside about 50% of the people had masks on. I half took mine off when I saw this and took a deep breath of 'fresh' petsmart air. In the cat food isle, my mask actually fell off of my right ear which it had been hanging off of. As I bent down to pick it up, a freaked out looking lady with her blue surgical mask on stopped dead in her tracks as she was rounding the corner to get into my aisle. I proceed to pick up my mask, with her staring at me, and put it fully onto my face, from the pet store floor! I relished in my newfound germs, likely to her horror.

At this same Petsmart about a month ago, I was in line at the store, without a mask on. The guy checking us all out wasn't wearing a mask, so I thought, screw it, I'm not wearing one either. Then this drunk hippie chick gets behind me. She studiously has her mask on. She nearly crashes her body into mine several times in line while we were waiting to check out. She was unsteady on her feet and reeked of booze. Anyways, we had those tape markers on the floor that were supposed to indicate 6 foot distance, total fail on this mask wearing life saver's part. Again, I was happy that her negligence was introducing me to much needed germs for my immune system to strengthen on.

And also... Amir-ul Kafirs, I had never heard of the tape markers on the floors of stores indicating shopping direction until about a month ago. I was in Walmart, trying to get my biweekly essentials bought in haste. As I was mindlessly plowing through one shopping aisle, I heard a gruff holler "You're going the wrong way!!". I looked up and saw an employee pissed offedly staring at me and repeating herself. I asked her what on earth was she talking about (really, I just said "What?"), she pointed out the tape arrows on the floor. Honestly, I was floored (no pun intended). I had to obey when I was in front of her. But I never obeyed again. I relished in going the wrong way down each aisle that day and I still relish it to this day. It's easy to ignore rules like that at Wally World in Louisiana. I doubt it would be so easy in a tiny independent bookstore or capacity limited museum where I would probably wind up pissed off and saying something vaguely hostile in jest to the undeserving of my abuse workers. . =/

****

June 20, 2020, 5:36AM (Dick to group):

There are spray painted "distance" markings all over the place here
I'll try to remember to take some photos... It's funniest in the metro where there are stickers on seats saying don't sit here and other stickers on the ground meant to be stood on
fewer and fewer people are wearing masks
it's still an obligation on the metro
*
Here's an article about cultural events (see below) re-opening, movies reopen on monday

small note: google translation has become pretty good

second small note: hearing airplanes in the sky is curiously depressing I find

third small note : happy summer solstice to everyone (tomorrow)

****

By Le Parisien
June 20, 2020 at 8:02 a.m., modified June 20, 2020 at 8:08 a.m.

On the night of Friday to Saturday, the government announced an acceleration of deconfinement for the summer thanks to progress in the fight against the Covid-19 epidemic. As of Monday, the French will be able to return to the cinema and practice collective sports. And from July 11, they can even go to the stadium.

These surprise announcements were made at the end of a Defense and National Security Council meeting on Friday under the authority of President Emmanuel Macron. During this meeting, the Minister of Health, Olivier Véran, noted that the indicators for monitoring the epidemic "remain generally well oriented" but that "vigilance remains strong".

Cinemas, vacation centers and casinos reopen on Monday. These openings will be made "in accordance with strict sanitary rules," says Matignon. The reopening of cinemas had already been announced by Prime Minister Edouard Philippe on May 28.

Team sports also resume on Monday. More surprisingly, the government authorized the resumption of collective sports activities from June 22 “with appropriate prevention measures” against the Covid-19 epidemic. Combat sports, however, remain prohibited.

Back to the stadium on July 11. The stadiums and racetracks in France, closed due to the coronavirus pandemic, will reopen on Saturday July 11 with a maximum number of 5,000 spectators. This date is not chosen at random, it is the day following the end of the state of health emergency on the metropolitan territory. As with performance halls, these activities must be declared beforehand.

Discos and theaters must wait until at least September. "Subject to a new assessment of the epidemiological situation, the start of the academic year may be marked by further relaxation," suggests the government. Concretely, the last sectors still paralyzed are fairs, exhibitions, shows, international maritime cruises, but also nightclubs and theaters.

If the press release mentions the case of nightclubs, which will not reopen before September, the fate of theaters has simply not been mentioned.

Guyana, a special case. In the French overseas departments and territories, the state of health emergency will be maintained in Guyana where "the virus is actively circulating" and therefore requests special protective measures. The government will issue a decree next week to postpone the municipal elections.

Why this acceleration of deconfinement? "The improvement in the health situation makes it possible to lift certain prohibitions on the condition that everyone maintains a vigilant posture in the face of the epidemic, a fortiori during the summer period", justified the government in this press release.

France has registered 14 additional Covid-19 deaths in hospitals in the past 24 hours, bringing the total number of deaths since the start of the epidemic to 29,617, according to an assessment released Friday by the Directorate General of health (DGS). The number of Covid-19 patients in intensive care continues to decrease with 727 patients, 25 less than Thursday, according to a press release from the DGS.

Throughout France, the government already seems to rule out a new containment in the event of a second epidemic wave. "The response strategy, in particular to protect the most vulnerable people without resorting to a general reconfiguration, as well as the health system will be presented by the government in the coming days. Special arrangements will be made for the summer, "said the press release.

https://www.leparisien.fr/societe/deconfinement-stades-cinemas-discotheques-casinos-theatres-ce-qui-rouvre-et-ce-qui-reste-ferme-20-06-2020-8338947.php

Déconfinement : stades, sports collectifs, cinémas, casinos... Ce qui va bientôt être autorisé - Le Parisien
Le gouvernement a donné son feu vert dans la nuit de vendredi à samedi la pratique des sports collectifs dès ce lundi 22 juin, et choisi d'ouvrir les stades le 11 juillet. Les boîtes de nuit ...

****

June 20, 2020, 5:42AM (Dick to group):

here's another article, more interesting
it's about a demand by performing artist groups to completely lift the rules
i bold-faced one interesting line
*
FRANCE Musique

The entrepreneurs of the performing arts demand "a total deconfinement and without distancing for a real recovery" in their sector, in a press release addressed to Emmanuel Macron before his intervention on Sunday.

"It is necessary to deconfigure the live performance", demands the Prodiss, the first employers' organization of the musical show in the private sector, in this press release, also signed by other organizations representing in particular cinemas, festivals, private theaters, cabarets, the Camulc and the Sndtp. These organizations also question "the measures taken by the Ministry of Culture" in the face of the health crisis which is paralyzing their sector of activity.

Communiqué addressed to the President of the Republic but for the moment remained unanswered. During his speech Sunday evening, Emmanuel Macron did not announce anything concerning culture. "We will be able to find the pleasure of being together, to go back to work fully, but also to have fun, to cultivate ourselves" declared the head of state. Without however providing the slightest precision as to a possible relaxation of sanitary measures for the performing arts.

In addition to rapid measures to allow a full resumption of activity, the entrepreneurs of the performing arts are demanding a recovery plan. "Providing the National Music Center with an amount of 50 million euros, in the face of more than 2 billion euros of losses suffered by the sector, it is an emergency measure, barely saved, but in no case of recovery ", they criticize.

Musical ensembles suffer a 45.6% drop in turnover

"A spectacle padlocked by Covid constraints, with a room two-thirds empty of the public does not make sense," they continue. "The distancing would apply to shows but not on trains: a difference in treatment which raises questions today". **"If the shows do not resume, social breakdown will be inevitable," warn these representative bodies.**

In addition, the Sma (450 members of the current music industry) and the Fedelima (140 places and projects of current music) also appeal to the President of the Republic, the Prime Minister and the Minister of Culture, in an open letter with similar claims. These two entities want an "agreement in principle with a view to resuming (...) in a standing configuration from September 1, returning to the usual standard, ie 3 people standing / square meter".

"If your government now considers that health conditions are met in other areas of society (transport, leisure parks, hotels and restaurants, places of worship, etc.), this standard must then apply to our establishments, for the sake of consistency, " they insist. And to ask for a clarification of the "blur zone for events whose gauges are less than 5,000 people": "we still have no explicit instructions as to the possible holding of these events by August 31".

"Among our members, we have 45 festivals which must take place between September 1 and December 31, like the Trans Musical Meetings of Rennes for example", add Sma and Fedelima, who want "an agreement in the coming days principle for their maintenance ". "In fact, in September, it will be too late to decide whether to maintain or cancel them: the production costs then incurred would risk compromising the sustainability of the companies carrying out these projects," conclude these organizations.

https://www.francemusique.fr/actualite-musicale/le-spectacle-vivant-appelle-au-deconfinement-total-et-sans-distanciation-84964?fbclid=IwARoofxvJ9LpVasLGAIlmk_Gjz7nFQARkhGCpOczHlvrsO7lwV2tEJJoCbEE

****

June 20, 2020, 9:09AM (Amir-ul Kafirs to group):

I relished in my newfound germs, likely to her horror.

That's *reeeeeaaaaaallllllyyyyyyy* funny! Fortunately for us, there will always be opportunities for small scale immunizations by our environment.

****

June 20, 2020, 9:17AM (Amir-ul Kafirs to group):

I relished in going the wrong way down each aisle that day and I still relish it to this day.

&, hence, the WRONG WAY REVOLUTION had its humble beginnings. Two people saw you defying the DOCTOR GOD LAWS & were inspired. The next thing the world knew, exponential growth had taken over & there was no turning back!

Does anyone here remember the "One Way" Christian movement? The idea was that Christianity was the ONE WAY for everyone in the world & it was the job of Christians to make this happen. As I recall, they had huge rallies in the 1970s but it died out pretty quickly — maybe it was too transparently imperialistic even for Christianity.

****

June 20, 2020, 9:10AM (Amir-ul Kafirs to group):

HERETICS: MASQUE

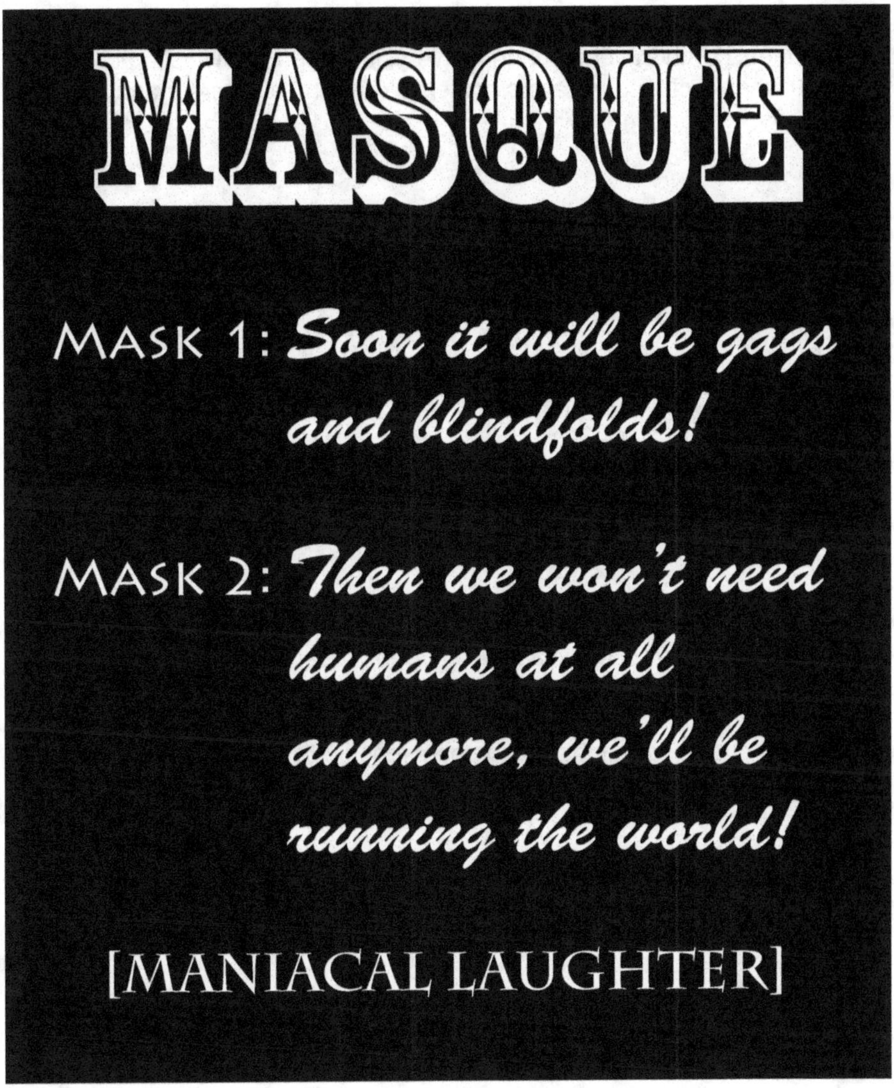
MASQUE
MASK 1: Soon it will be gags and blindfolds!
MASK 2: Then we won't need humans at all anymore, we'll be running the world!
[MANIACAL LAUGHTER]

****

June 20, 2020, 9:26AM (Amir-ul Kafirs to group):

HERETICS: Progress on Unconscious Suffocation book

If anyone's still thinking of contributing anything to the proposed book, perhaps this small bit of progress on my personal backstory will be inspiring:

<u>Editor's Personal Backstory</u>

I was born September 4, 1953. My mother told me, many decades later, that it cost $25 for her to give birth to me in a hospital. According to a December 9,

2019 "Business Insider" article: "The average cost these days to have a baby in the US, without complications during delivery, is $10,808 — which can increase to $30,000 when factoring in care provided before and after pregnancy." (https://www.businessinsider.com/how-much-does-it-cost-to-have-a-baby-2018-4)

[..]

****

June 20, 2020, 10:20AM (Amir-ul Kafirs to group):

It's funniest in the metro where there are stickers on seats saying don't sit here and other stickers on the ground meant to be stood on

It might be fun to make a movie of 'playing' the markings as if they're a game, kindof like *Twister* or some such.

fewer and fewer people are wearing masks

Around here some people who'd stopped wearing them are back at it again. One neighbor told me that 400 new cases have been reported since we entered the "Green Phase". I said: "But that doesn't mean that 400 people will die!" IMO that doesn't even mean that 400 people will get sick. Still, I imagine that it's the fearfulness of such a report that's prompting people to wear masks again.

Cinemas, vacation centers and casinos reopen on Monday.

I wish the French would start bragging about caring more about culture than the US. It's probably true.

Combat sports, however, remain prohibited.

What? Like boxing? Or does that include football & such-like things too?

The stadiums and racetracks in France, closed due to the coronavirus pandemic, will reopen on Saturday July 11 with a maximum number of 5,000 spectators.

That's too many! Only one person at a time in the audience!!

Guyana, a special case. In the French overseas departments and territories, the state of health emergency will be maintained in Guyana where "the virus is actively circulating" and therefore requests special protective measures. The government will issue a decree next week to postpone the municipal elections.

worldometer Coronavirus Population

←

WORLD / COUNTRIES / GUYANA

Last updated: June 20, 2020, 14:12 GMT

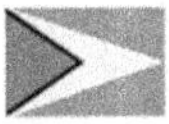

Guyana

Coronavirus Cases:

183

Deaths:

12

Why this acceleration of deconfinement?

Lovely phrase, feel it rolling around in your mouth..
aaaccccceeeellllleeerrrrraaaattttiiiiiioooonnnn ooooffffffff
dddddeeeeeeecccccoooooooonnnnnfffffiiinnnneeemmmmeeeennnnt.. cough,
cough..

"The improvement in the health situation makes it possible to lift certain prohibitions on the condition that everyone maintains a vigilant posture

I've been keeping my finger on my sanitizer trigger while standing upright at attention.

****

June 20, 2020, 11:07AM (Inquiring Librarian to group):

Re: Airport Report

This whole string has prompted me to laugh uncontrollably over and over again!

Amir-ul Kafirs, i love the idea of a Twister like arrows movie!

The rules!! Ha ha... Dick 5,0000 at horse races?!?! Amir-ul Kafirs, That's too many!!! Ba ha ha!!

Ok, onto sports and gyms... In Louisiana, it's real strict. My gym requires masks and we have a massive ballroom that is a group exercise room. We have to workout only in our square and at reduced capacity... A playpen of sorts. My significant other, on the other hand, goes to their martial arts class 3x / wk where they get all sweaty body wrestling jujitzu for 2 hours a class. Lotta rules coordination in Louisiana, eh?

****

June 20, 2020, 11:10AM (Amir-ul Kafirs to group):

Re: Airport Report (etc)

it's about a demand by performing artist groups to completely lift the rules

I'm already inspired to write a new text panel

"If the shows do not resume, social breakdown will be inevitable," warn these representative bodies.

****

June 20, 2020, 11:17AM (Amir-ul Kafirs to group):

This whole string has prompted me to laugh uncontrollably over and over again!

Ok, I admit it, I'm CIA & I'm trying to get the few thinking people left in the world to die from laughter exhaustion. You people are getting in the way of superorganism progress!!

Lotta rules coordination in Louisiana, eh?

Yeah, where I go for brutality training out in the woods there're no rules whatsover for animal torture. I admit to putting on gloves & a mask 1st anyway because it adds to the fetishism of it.

****

June 20, 2020, 8:42PM (Naia Nisnam to group):

Taking on the Tech Giants (Phil)

I'm late in writing this, but a couple of weeks ago I watched the online discussion

"Taking on the Tech Giants", that Phil had recommended. I want to do a report-back, to share but also to help myself understand the information better.
I did miss the second half of the program because I had to do a tele-health thing for one of my kids. This sort of technology info is new to me, not the type of thing I usually follow, though I now feel like I should pay more attention.

My biggest take away from what I did watch was a feeling of relief. It feels good to know that people who are more informed than I am are following these tech companies, keeping tabs on what they are doing, and speaking out against the surveillance state. It also felt good to see that people were participating and viewing from all around the world (Singapore, Germany, England, France, South Africa, India, Scotland, Nicaragua, Amsterdam, etc).

These are the speakers that I saw and my best understanding of what they talked about:

1. Dr. Ben Hayes- Covid leading to increased state surveillance and state power, how corporations influence the state response to the pandemic, and the government accessing our information via contact tracing apps.

2. Ben Tarnoff- The lockdowns led to a sharp increase in internet use (25-30% global increase), the "cloud" use greatly increased (I dont understand the cloud). He talked about a US company, Clearview AI, using facial recognitioning under the guise of contact tracing. He talked about how we are creating data everytime we use a computer, and how we are being encouraged to do more and more things online to create more data. He got into why our info is being gathered. He explained how data helps capitalism grow, beyond more pointed advertising. He said data is being used in capitalism to make employees more efficient, therefore more productive.

I found this article from January about Clearview AI working w the police to identify suspects using the company's facial recognition and people's online photos:
https://www.nytimes.com/2020/01/18/technology/clearview-privacy-facial-recognition.html

And this one from May, about the results of an Illinois lawsuit against the company: https://www.theverge.com/2020/5/7/21251387/clearview-ai-law-enforcement-police-facial-recognition-illinois-privacy-law

3. Vahini Naidu- She was talking about the digital divide and how poor countries that lack tech are going to be even further behind, economically, because of their inability to recover from the covid-economic crisis. She also said that South Africa has been resisting a Big Tech takeover.

4. Anita Gurumurthy- She talked about Amazon and Whole Foods teaming up. She talked about how data chains are influencing the entire model of capitalism.

5. Caroline Nevejan- totally missed her part

6. Nanjira Sambuli- She said things that I had never considered. She said that there is a push to delete Facebook but that would be bad for people living in poor countries because they use FB as a source of networking and information that they otherwise would not have access to. She said the same thing about WhatsApp in Brazil.

There was also talk about how we cant think about data without thinking about infrastructure. The data is collected but also "wrangled" by scientists who make the data useful for what people in power want to predict.

There was mention of Covid highlighting global inequities and the importance of buying local.

That summarizes what I was able to take away from what I saw. I have to say that I felt like I was watching a level 3 discussion of material that I really needed an "Idiot's Guide" to.

****

The Secretive Company That Might End Privacy as We Know It

A little-known start-up helps law enforcement match photos of unknown people to their online images — and “might lead to a dystopian future or something,” a backer says.

By Kashmir Hill

Published Jan. 18, 2020
Updated Feb. 10, 2020

Until recently, Hoan Ton-That’s greatest hits included an obscure iPhone game and an app that let people put Donald Trump’s distinctive yellow hair on their own photos.

Then Mr. Ton-That — an Australian techie and onetime model — did something momentous: He invented a tool that could end your ability to walk down the street anonymously, and provided it to hundreds of law enforcement agencies, ranging from local cops in Florida to the F.B.I. and the Department of Homeland Security.

His tiny company, Clearview AI, devised a groundbreaking facial recognition app. You take a picture of a person, upload it and get to see public photos of that person, along with links to where those photos appeared. The system — whose backbone is a database of more than three billion images that Clearview claims to have scraped from Facebook, YouTube, Venmo and millions of other websites — goes far beyond anything ever constructed by the United States government or Silicon Valley giants.

Federal and state law enforcement officers said that while they had only limited knowledge of how Clearview works and who is behind it, they had used its app to help solve shoplifting, identity theft, credit card fraud, murder and child sexual exploitation cases.

Until now, technology that readily identifies everyone based on his or her face has been taboo because of its radical erosion of privacy. Tech companies capable of releasing such a tool have refrained from doing so; in 2011, Google's chairman at the time said it was the one technology the company had held back because it could be used "in a very bad way." Some large cities, including San Francisco, have barred police from using facial recognition technology.

But without public scrutiny, more than 600 law enforcement agencies have started using Clearview in the past year, according to the company, which declined to provide a list. The computer code underlying its app, analyzed by The New York Times, includes programming language to pair it with augmented-reality glasses; users would potentially be able to identify every person they saw. The tool could identify activists at a protest or an attractive stranger on the subway, revealing not just their names but where they lived, what they did and whom they knew.

And it's not just law enforcement: Clearview has also licensed the app to at least a handful of companies for security purposes.

"The weaponization possibilities of this are endless," said Eric Goldman, co-director of the High Tech Law Institute at Santa Clara University. "Imagine a rogue law enforcement officer who wants to stalk potential romantic partners, or a foreign government using this to dig up secrets about people to blackmail them or throw them in jail."

Clearview has shrouded itself in secrecy, avoiding debate about its boundary-pushing technology. When I began looking into the company in November, its website was a bare page showing a nonexistent Manhattan address as its place of business. The company's one employee listed on LinkedIn, a sales manager named "John Good," turned out to be Mr. Ton-That, using a fake name. For a month, people affiliated with the company would not return my emails or phone calls.

While the company was dodging me, it was also monitoring me. At my request, a number of police officers had run my photo through the Clearview app. They soon received phone calls from company representatives asking if they were talking to the media — a sign that Clearview has the ability and, in this case, the appetite to monitor whom law enforcement is searching for.

Facial recognition technology has always been controversial. It makes people nervous about Big Brother. It has a tendency to deliver false matches for certain groups, like people of color. And some facial recognition products used by the police — including Clearview's — haven't been vetted by independent experts.

Clearview's app carries extra risks because law enforcement agencies are uploading sensitive photos to the servers of a company whose ability to protect its data is untested.

The company eventually started answering my questions, saying that its earlier silence was typical of an early-stage start-up in stealth mode. Mr. Ton-That acknowledged designing a prototype for use with augmented-reality glasses but said the company had no plans to release it. And he said my photo had rung alarm bells because the app "flags possible anomalous search behavior" in order to prevent users from conducting what it deemed "inappropriate searches."

In addition to Mr. Ton-That, Clearview was founded by Richard Schwartz — who was an aide to Rudolph W. Giuliani when he was mayor of New York — and backed financially by Peter Thiel, a venture capitalist behind Facebook and Palantir.

Another early investor is a small firm called Kirenaga Partners. Its founder, David Scalzo, dismissed concerns about Clearview making the internet searchable by face, saying it's a valuable crime-solving tool.

"I've come to the conclusion that because information constantly increases, there's never going to be privacy," Mr. Scalzo said. "Laws have to determine what's legal, but you can't ban technology. Sure, that might lead to a dystopian future or something, but you can't ban it."

[..]

- https://www.nytimes.com/2020/01/18/technology/clearview-privacy-facial-recognition.html

****

The company is ending all non-law enforcement contracts
By Nick Statt@nickstatt May 7, 2020, 8:29pm EDT

Controversial facial recognition provider Clearview AI says it will no longer sell its app to private companies and non-law enforcement entities, according to a legal filing first reported on Thursday by *BuzzFeed News*. It will also be terminating all contracts, regardless of whether the contracts are for law enforcement purposes or not, in the state of Illinois.

The document, filed in Illinois court as part of lawsuit over the company's potential violations of a state privacy law, lays out Clearview's decision as a voluntary action, and the company will now "avoid transacting with non-governmental customers anywhere." Earlier this year, *BuzzFeed* reported on a leaked client list that indicates Clearview's technology has been used by thousands of organizations, including companies like Bank of America, Macy's, and Walmart.

""CLEARVIEW IS ALSO CANCELLING ALL ACCOUNTS BELONGING TO ANY ENTITY BASED IN ILLINOIS.""

"Clearview is cancelling the accounts of every customer who was not either associated with law enforcement or some other federal, state, or local government department, office, or agency," Clearview's filing reads. "Clearview is also cancelling all accounts belonging to any entity based in Illinois." Clearview argues that it should not face an injunction, which would prohibit it from using current or past Illinois residents' biometric data, because it's taking these steps to comply with the state's privacy law.

The plaintiff in the lawsuit, David Mutnick, sued Clearview in January for violating his and other state residents' privacy under the Illinois Biometric Information Privacy Act (BIPA), a rare and far-reaching piece of facial recognition-related legislation that makes it illegal for companies to collect and store sensitive biometric data without consent. The law is the same one under which Facebook settled a class-action lawsuit earlier this year for $550 million over its use of facial recognition technology to identify, without consent, the faces of people in photos uploaded to its social network.

[..]

- https://www.theverge.com/2020/5/7/21251387/clearview-ai-law-enforcement-police-facial-recognition-illinois-privacy-law

****

June 21, 2020, 9:35AM (Amir-ul Kafirs to group):

Re: Taking on the Tech Giants (Phil)

2. Ben Tarnoff- The lockdowns led to a sharp increase in internet use (25-30% global increase), the "cloud" use greatly increased (I dont understand the cloud).

The "cloud", of course, is data storage outside of one's own computer &

peripherals. I don't use it, or avoid it as much as I can, but the push has been on to use it as one's primary storage method for the last decade or so. Calling it the "cloud" makes it seem like something barely physical that's just somehow magically floating in the sky overtop wherever we're working on our computers. Of course, what it really is is massive hardware housed somewhere with a location unknown to us where our data is totally under someone else's control rather than our own. I've never set up a cloud account on any of my computers but I'd usually get constant reminders that I hadn't done so as if that were a big mistake of mine. Why all this concern about taking care of my data? Well, it's pretty transparent isn't it? THEY want it. When I got an Acer Chromebook (a Google product if I undertand correctly) approximately 7 years ago it was a great deal for a laptop, only $200, using a Linux user-friendly OS. The initial deal was that one could use the cloud 'for free' for the 1st year or 2 & then would have to pay for it some nominal fee. I never used it, I never paid for it. Recently, I got an iPad, I mainly wanted to use it as a camera. I still haven't figured it out very much but it seems that footage goes automatically to the cloud without my even setting up an account. If that's so, that gives you an idea of how advanced this attempt to gather all our data is.

I found this article from January about Clearview AI working w the police to identify suspects using the companies facial recognition and people's online photos

I'm reading this one now. To say that this is disturbing is an understatement. I found this interesting:

"Clearview has shrouded itself in secrecy, avoiding debate about its boundary-pushing technology. When I began looking into the company in November, its website was a bare page showing a nonexistent Manhattan address as its place of business. The company's one employee listed on LinkedIn, a sales manager named "John Good," turned out to be Mr. Ton-That, using a fake name. For a month, people affiliated with the company would not return my emails or phone calls."

In other words, the company responsible for the most sophisticated surveillance technology to date is trying to avoid being trapped by it itself. Since this is a New York Times article you have to sign in with some existing account like Facebook or Google or create a new one. I've been making copies of many of the articles linked to here but that takes time because the formatting gets completely screwed in the process & then I tediously go through the whole thing to remove ads & doubled images to make it a bit more readable. I just did that with this article so I've appended it at the end here. That'll enable you to avoid, ever-so-slightly, the NYT's own surveillance of you as a prospective customer.

ANYWAY, to say that this can be abused, or is just intrinsically abusive, is a gross understatement. Imagine if it's decided that not wearing a face-mask is a crime: VOILA! Everyone not wearing a face-mask past a certain date can be instantly recognized & identified. Naming the crime will be important:

Endangering the Public Health on a Mass Scale. As usual, whether whatever law is being used to justify the resultant database is anything other than just nazism won't matter. Almost 20 years ago now I interviewed an ACLU lawyer who was arrested for 'possession of child pornography' because he'd rented a copy of "The Tin Drum" from Blockbuster. A conservative Christian group had temporarily succeeded in getting that movie, which had been freely available & fairly mainstream up til that point, labeled as child pornography & everyone who had it out from video stores at the time was arrested. The story, for those of you not familiar with it, is a parable of nazism as a form of arrested development. The ruling against the movie was quickly overturned but everyone arrested remained on the books as a child pornographer or some such. FOREVER.

And this one from May, about the results of an Illinois lawsuit against the company:

"Controversial facial recognition provider Clearview AI says it will no longer sell its app to private companies and non-law enforcement entities, according to a legal filing first reported on Thursday by *BuzzFeed News*. It will also be terminating all contracts, regardless of whether the contracts are for law enforcement purposes or not, in the state of Illinois."

Go Illinois!!

Anyway, that article's somewhat reassuring but, in the long run, such things are going to run rampant & it might be good for individuals to have a philosophical strategy for dealing with them.

****

June 21, 2020, 9:53AM (Amir-ul Kafirs to group):

HERETICS: Blah Blah Black Sheep

I did make, & post to social media, this latest text panel. Of course, a part of my purpose is to reflect the medical industry police state back on itself. While it's apparently perfectly reasonable to entirely too many people for doctors, lawyers, & politicians to rule in such a way that musicians are simply cut out of the world, it would be INSANE to propose what I hereby propose:

IN THE NAME OF ALL THE
MUSICIANS IN THE WORLD,
WHOSE UNSELFISH EFFORTS HAVE
ENRICHED HUMAN EMOTIONS
FOR MILLENNIA,
I DECLARE THAT ALL POLITICIANS,
DOCTORS, & LAWYERS
MUST STAY CONFINED TO
8' X 8' X 8' CELLS
WITH HOODS OVER THEIR HEADS
IN PERPETUITY OR UNTIL WE
FIND A USE FOR THEM,
WHICHEVER COMES LAST.
If this does not happen,
social breakdown will be inevitable.

- HIS HONORABLE
BLAH BLAH BLACK SHEEP

****

June 21, 2020, 8:07PM (Amir-ul Kafirs to group):

HERETICS: 2 more text panels

"Without parties
we could not get
a fraction of the voters
to come to the polls to
express themselves on issues
of great public importance,
but we can enrol a
considerable part of the
community in a political party
that is fighting some other party.
It is the element of the fight
that keeps up the interest."

**- George Herbert Mead,
early 20th century
American Social Behaviorist**

en·roll

/in'rōl,en'rōl/

verb

verb: **enrol**

officially register as a member of an institution or a student on a course.
"he enrolled in drama school"

Similar: register sign on sign up apply volunteer put one's name down

- recruit (someone) to perform a service.
  "a campaign to enroll more foster families"

  Similar: accept admit take on register sign on sign up

- HISTORICAL • LAW
  enter (a deed or other document) among the rolls of a court of justice.

****

June 21, 2020, 9:10PM (Amir-ul Kafirs to Dick):

Re: HERETICS: 2 more text panels

well, maybe it's a typo in the book...

Maybe, but I prefer to accurately quote instead of 'correcting' people. One thing I'm very mindful of is that spellings do actually change over time & sometimes spellings that seem wrong to us now may've been 'correct' at the time. One example I often cite is that as a child I was taught to double the consonant at the end of a word before adding a suffix. E.G.: travelling. These days, that's no longer correct & it would be spelled traveling. I often come across older spellings in books that I read — including that example.

Works of George Herbert Mead
volume 1

Mind, Self, & Society
from the Standpoint of a
Social Behaviorist

Edited and with an Introduction by
Charles W. Morris

Such experiences are, of course, of immense importance. We make use of them all the time in the community. We decry the attitude of hostility as a means of carrying on the interrelations between nations. We feel we should get beyond the methods of warfare and diplomacy, and reach some sort of political relation of nations to each other in which they could be regarded as members of a common community, and so be able to express themselves, not in the attitude of hostility, but in terms of their common values. That is what we set up as the ideal of the League of Nations. We have to remember, however, that we are not able to work out our own political institutions without introducing the hostilities of parties. Without parties we could not get a fraction of the voters to come to the polls to express themselves on issues of great public importance, but we can enrol a considerable part of the community in a political party that is fighting some other party. It is the element of the fight that keeps up the interest. We can enlist the interest of a number of people who want to defeat the opposing party, and get them to the polls to do that. The party platform is an abstraction, of course, and does not mean much to us, since we are actually depending psychologically upon the operation of these more barbarous impulses in order to keep our ordinary institutions running. When we object to the organization of corrupt political machines we ought to remember to feel a certain gratitude to people who are able to enlist the interest of people in public affairs.

We are normally dependent upon those situations in which the self is able to express itself in a direct fashion, and there is no situation in which the self can express itself so easily as it can over against the common enemy of the groups to which it is united. The hymn that comes to our minds most frequently as expressive of Christendom is "Onward Christian Soldiers"; Paul organized the church of his time against the world of heathens; and "Revelation" represents the community over against the world of darkness. The idea of Satan has been as essential to the organization of the church as politics has been to the organ-

introducing the hostilities of parties. Without parties we could not get a fraction of the voters to come to the polls to express themselves on issues of great public importance, but we can enrol a considerable part of the community in a political party that is fighting some other party. It is the element of the fight that keeps up the interest. We can enlist the interest of a num-

****

June 22, 2020, 12:21AM (Inquiring Librarian to group):

Re: HERETICS: 2 more text panels

I LOVE these! But, I might need the lawyers out of cages because I will need a good one to throw on my city government if they try to fire me when I refuse the covid vaccine!

****

June 22, 2020, 3:27PM (Amir-ul Kafirs to group):

I might need the lawyers out of cages

Fortunately for them, I don't have the power that they do, nor do I want it. I just want readers of the text panel to IMAGINE how stupid & objectionable such applied power is when the tables are turned & to then turn the tables back to their ordinary position & realize that the applied power is just as pernicious in its typical legal use.

****

June 21, 2020, 11:29AM (Amir-ul Kafirs to Inquiring Librarian):

DowDuPont

Your chemist friend who got cancer while working for DuPont might be interested in knowing that according to PERI (Political Economy Resarch Institute) at University of Massachussetts Amherst, (https://www.peri.umass.edu/combined-toxic-100-greenhouse-100-indexes-current) DowDupont is the 4th worst air polluter, the 32nd worst for greenhouse gases, & the WORST for air pollution. That pretty much makes them the **worst polluter in the world.** THAT'S PRETTY ASTOUNDING.

****

June 21, 2020, 12:39PM (Inquiring Librarian to Amir-ul Kafirs):

Re: DowDuPont

That sounds about right. And DuPont heavily funds the University of Delaware's chemistry department. Part of why i quit being a bichemistry major there was all of the headaches i was getting in my labs.

My friend's name is _____. I have been reaching out to her via gmail to see if she might be receptive to science that is not government or pharmaceutical sponsored. So far, i am failing. But at least she is not an angry finger wagger. She is extremely intelligent and a very kind person. I am hoping she might listen a little to what i am sharing with her and maybe seriously consider it, if not now, at least in the future if/when the scandal of this all eventually comes out.

****

June 21, 2020, 8:07PM (Amir-ul Kafirs to group):

HERETICS: 2 more text panels

From the beginning I've been restricting myself to a maximum of social media uploads of one of these a day. Nonetheless, there're just some days when I keep thinking of new ones to make. Here're the latest 2. Maybe I'm a hopeless fool but I think that both of these might actually reach some of the rapidly receeding brains.

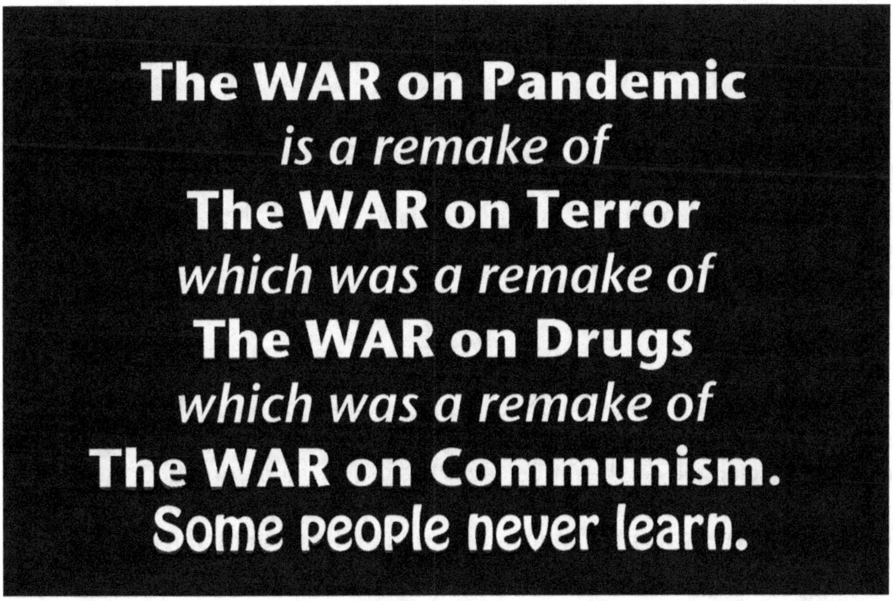
The WAR on Pandemic
is a remake of
The WAR on Terror
which was a remake of
The WAR on Drugs
which was a remake of
The WAR on Communism.
Some people never learn.

****

June 22, 2020, 5:05AM (Dick to group):

HERETICS: local events in the city of lights

Hello,

Yesterday was the annual music festival called "Fête de la Musique" here's an article about it

basically it talks about a couple large outdoor techno parties with police intervention

strangely, this time the google translation is somewhat stilted and non-idiomatic, I've corrected a few paticularly bad lines

I've indented the twitter posts and put in boldface a few lines

**

Music Festival: thousands of revelers in Paris despite the virus

A "DJ Set" notably took place this Sunday in the 10th arrondissement. If the atmosphere was there, the barrier measures, required by the Minister of Culture the day before, were not really respected.

By I.P. with A.C.

A crowd of dancers, very far from the recommended social distance of one meter.

This is an image that we had not been shown for three months, due to the Covid-19 epidemic. On this music festival Sunday in Paris, **one event more than the others was the subject of criticism on social networks:** several hundred people gathered in the Villemin garden, in the 10th arrondissement and by the canal Nearby Saint-Martin, to dance.

All took part in a "DJ Set", organized by the collective "Apero électronique" between 3.30 pm and 8 pm.

Problem: the participants, who dance very close to each other, do not frankly respect social distancing. They are also few to wear a mask. This goes against the measures enacted the day before by the Minister of Culture. **An attitude described as "shameful" by Internet users, who say they fear seeing a "new outbreak of Covid-19" emerge, when the epidemic is not entirely circumscribed.**

An authorized event?

On Saturday, Franck Riester said that all the events of this music festival should take place "in compliance with health rules". With two details: gatherings "of more than 10 people are always prohibited on the public domain" and "spontaneous concerts are not allowed". **Was this event allowed? Contacted by Le Parisien, the Paris police prefecture indicates that it was not asked to give permission for this gathering. However, it has been validated by the city hall of the capital, which has not yet replied to us on this point.**

On Facebook, the organizing collective, which broadcast the event live, took care to warn the 2,000 Internet users who had planned to participate and the 18,000 others who said they were interested. "a perfect opportunity to meet in open air music, while respecting the health measures that will be announced". A somewhat missed opportunity.

The police on the spot

The crowd then dispersed somewhat, especially in the direction of rue de Lancry, a few dozen meters from the park. The revelers prevented the cars from moving and the police were dispatched to the scene to try to clear their way. According to a journalist from Le Parisien, **several of the occupants of the premises began to chant "Everyone hates the police"** and one of them threw a can of beer at them.

Another was then hit with a baton, without us knowing the circumstances at the start of this scene, filmed by Brut journalist Rémy Buisine. Several gathering places around the Saint-Martin canal were then gradually evacuated by the police during the evening, sometimes under the whistles of revelers.

At the end of the day, the police evacuated the intersection of rue de Lancry and rue de Jean Poulmarch./LP/Antoine Castagné

The concert in the Villemin garden is not the only one to have aroused the interest of many Parisians. Rue de Paradis, in the same arrondissement, hundreds of people also gathered in the street to dance shortly before 7 p.m., as BFMTV relates.

https://www.leparisien.fr/societe/fete-de-la-musique-des-centaines-de-parisiens-masses-aux-abords-du-canal-saint-martin-21-06-2020-8339649.php#xtor=EREC-1481423604-[NL75]---${_id_connect_hash}@1

Fête de la musique : des milliers de fêtards à Paris malgré le virus - Le Parisien
Un «DJ Set» a notamment eu lieu ce dimanche dans le Xe arrondissement. Si l'ambiance était au rendez-vous, les mesures barrières, requises par le ministre de la Culture la veille, n'ont ...

****

June 22, 2020, 3:41PM (Amir-ul Kafirs to group):

Re: HERETICS: local events in the city of lights

Yesterday was the annual music festival called "Fête de la Musique"

I wish I'd been there. We're nowhere near close to having something like that happen here.

Problem: the participants, who dance very close to each other, do not frankly respect social distancing. They are also few to wear a mask. This goes against the measures enacted the day before by the Minister of Culture. **An attitude described as "shameful" by Internet users, who say they fear seeing a "new outbreak of Covid-19" emerge, when the epidemic is not entirely circumscribed.**

There's always this FEAR FACTOR being elevated to the level of highest importance. It doesn't really seem to matter that the feared event *may not happen, in fact probably WON'T happen.* The most important thing is to FEAR that it'll happen & to act accordingly. Everyone is supposed to cowtow to the paranoids.

****

June 22, 2020, 3:52PM (Amir-ul Kafirs to group):

HERETICS: 2 MORE text panel[s] made today

So, I posted the 1st of yesterday's new text panels on FB shortly after midnight. I had hoped that people would understand the comparison between the WAR on the Pandemic & the WAR on Terror & the WAR on Drugs & the WAR on Communism but, nope, I immediately got stupid responses: one bemoaning my inability to think (That's me! I'm completely thoughtless!) & my use of a "flurry of buzzwords" & another asking the age-old stupid question about whether I mean *that there isn't a pandemic*? I unfriended the 1st person & will probably unfriend the 2nd. I don't even know the 1st one, the 2nd one's local to PGH but I remember that when I 1st met her I thought that her mind might be gone from syphilis. *SO*, here are 2 more that I made today, partially inspired by the ongoing stupidity.

**WAR Rhetoric is used
to steer GROUPTHINK
into oversimplistic reflexes
in response to a perceived threat.
George W. Bush's
"Either you are with us,
or you are with the terrorists."
is a perfect example.
The same spin doctor process
is in effect during the
PANDEMIC PANIC.
Hence, any criticism of the
social conditions surrounding the
pandemic are oversimplistically
turned into 'pandemic denialism'
and not thought about any further.**

Pavlov's Dogs

Insert prefabricated liberal OR conservative GROUPTHINK language here: ____________

SALIVATE.

But why aren't you getting your meal?!

****

June 22, 2020, 9:39PM (Inquiring Librarian to group):

Re: HERETICS: local events in the city of lights

Like Amir-ul Kafirs, I wish we were 'allowed' to have a big festival too. I am jealous. I think I/We are still 'grounded' here in the United States. And beyond being 'grounded', we are daily slapped and pushed around with new "threats" of further and more draconian lockdowns because of our 'bad behavior' which is currently focused on not wearing masks enough and also on 'cases' increasing at some random bar nearby and some random graduation party, I kid you not. How ridiculous. It makes me want to barf. I still want to have all of us here to buy a castle somewhere in the middle of nowhere beautiful eastern Europe where we can all live in peace and freedom (note, it has to have a white persian purring Gormenghast-like cat room, I will tend to it). This is my dream. I feel like I"m living in a twisted precursor to a much darker and more real and less 'funny' hell.

Today, the new "rules" for opening up the Public Library to the public came out. It's a laugh a minute. Honestly I can't tell if I want to laugh or cry when I read it. I've attached it here, for your 'enjoyment'. In a small step towards humane-ness, visitors can use the bathroom and the water fountains (thank goodness, I hate it when patrons pee on the building and shit in the bushes).

****

LAPL Phase II

Phase II will be a multi-step phase that will slowly expand based on a variety of factors including public demand, staff feedback, recommendations from the Office of Public Health, and more. The following plan is flexible and subject to change.

What follows is an initial plan for allowing customers limited, appointment-only access to library facilities. We know that we will be learning as we go, thoughtfully and deliberately considering public health and community need. Procedures may be tweaked and services expanded based on staff experience and patron input.

We will not move into Phase II until we have the following safety factors in place at each library:

- Sneeze guards on public service desks
- Social distancing guidelines on the floors inside buildings and outside
- All Phase I floor and furniture plans fully implemented including unusable furniture moved or covered.
- Security officer in place
- A supply of cleaners

We will continue to create new guidelines and expand services carefully and deliberately.

PHASE II Start Date July 6th.
Circulation Guidelines:

- All late fines remain suspended at this time. Lost fees are charged for items that are 90 days or more overdue.

- Patrons can check out up to 10 items at time and should not exceed 30 items on their accounts at one time.

- Online Registration (PacReg) accounts can continue to check out 10 items at a time.

- Returned materials will still appear as checked out on patron accounts for at least 72- hours for quarantine.

- Almost Overdue notices and Overdue notices are suspended until the library discontinues its quarantining procedures.

- When items still appear as checked out more than 4 days after being returned, staff should:

○ Ask the patron which branch they returned the items to
○ If returned to your branch, do a shelf check for the items.
○ If returned to a different branch, cal that branch and ask for a shelf check.
○ Check in the item when found.
○ If the item cannot be found, check it in to remove it from the patron's account and

[..]

****

June 22, 2020, 10:39PM (Amir-ul Kafirs to group):

It's a laugh a minute.

Gotta 'love' parts like this:

"Bathrooms and water fountains will be available for customers to use only during a scheduled appointment and included in the cleaning schedule."

I just *know* I'm going to have to make a dance movie using those directional arrows.

What's next?

Arrows showing you which way to think?

****

June 24, 2020, 11:19AM (Inquiring Librarian to group):

HERETICS: Fact Checkers & NewsGuard's Invasion of Public Libraries

I've been pretty confused by and skeptical of "Fact Checkers" and the label of "Fake News", since its inception a few years ago. I found this fun talk about fact checking the fact checkers:
https://off-guardian.org/2020/06/23/watch-who-will-fact-check-the-fact-checkers/

If you would rather read about the phenomenon, here is an article by the guy who was interviewed in the talk above:
https://www.thelastamericanvagabond.com/censorship/this-is-why-you-cant-trust-the-fact-checkers/

& here is an article specifically on NewsGuard's Fact Checking service:
https://www.mintpressnews.com/newsguardneocon-backed-fact-checker-plans-to-wage-war-on-independent-media/253687/

Lastly let's go full circle on this topic, what I consider to be obnoxious and obvious censorship for the virtuous easily brainwashed masses, now public libraries are jumping onboard in an effort to make sure the public who uses our public library computers are not 'misled' by any news that has been deemed 'fake' by 'fact checkers', aka: it does not push our government agendas... sigh... to be honest, this does not surprise me given the inability of most if not all of my librarian friends to think for themselves. NewsGuard has paired with Public Libraries =[:
https://americanlibrariesmagazine.org/2019/11/01/check-your-facts-tech-tools/

****

Jun 23, 2020

WATCH: Who Will Fact Check the Fact Checkers?

James Corbett's latest documentary unmasks the internet's "independent" fact checking websites

corbettreport
468K subscribers

Who Will Fact Check the Fact Checkers?

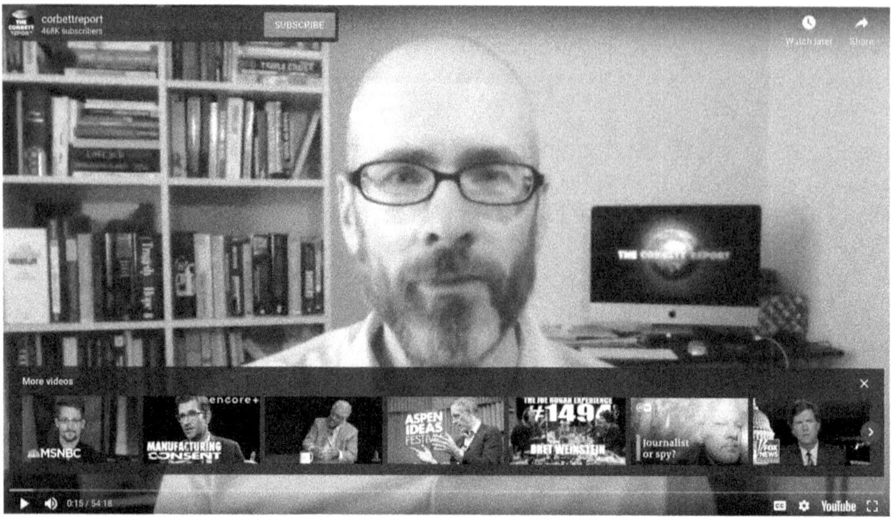

We've all come across online fact checkers that purport to warn us away from independent media sites under the guise of protecting us from fake news. But who is behind these fact check sites? How do they operate? And if these ham-fisted attempts at soft censorship aren't the solution to online misinformation, what is? Join James for this week's important edition of The Corbett Report podcast, where we explore the murky world of information gatekeeping and ask "Who will fact check the fact checkers?"

- https://off-guardian.org/2020/06/23/watch-who-will-fact-check-the-fact-checkers/

****

THIS IS WHY YOU CAN'T TRUST THE FACT CHECKERS

11 MAY 2020 POSTED BY DERRICK BROZE

For the last eight years I have worked as a writer, researcher, and investigative reporter for many well-known American independent media outlets. I have spent my time investigating digital surveillance technology, attacks on indigenous communities, and the overall growth of the government and corporate power. As someone working in this field, writing about topics which are often seen as controversial or "outside the mainstream" – censorship and personal attacks are part of the job description.

However, the attacks on independent media have rapidly increased in the last four years, with many formerly active journalistic outlets ceasing to exist due to lack of traffic and thus, lack of funds. We have seen outlets outright branded "fake news" or accused of collusion with the Russian government. Some channels and websites have been unable to apply for advertising or use certain digital products based on these labels. Some channels and reporters have been deleted off social media and other digital platforms altogether. And, if the social media managers don't delete you, they might just use the algorithm to hide your posts, limiting your ability to interact with the public.

Perhaps the most insidious method is the recent use of "fact checkers" to limit the reach of an outlet, or simply brand them with the fake news scarlet letter to discourage readers from engaging. This has been increasing in the last 2 years and I personally know of several remaining indy media outlets who have had to decide whether or not to run certain articles or video reports out of fear they might be censored or banned. Of course, with the algorithmic games being played by social media platforms, most outlets are reaching a tiny fraction of what they once were.

Case in point, *The Mind Unleashed*. I have been part of the TMU team on and off for the last year or so. In that time we have been struggling to reach a small fraction of our 9 million Facebook followers. Part of the reason we are struggling to reach people is because we have the dubious recognition of being labeled fake news by Facebook and affiliated fact checkers.

In a recent article published in *Newsweek Espanol,* in partnership with Newsguard, The Mind Unleashed is described as a "site that promises to 'promote and inspire unconventional thinking,' but is actually dedicated to publishing falsehoods.". The quote was in reference to a story TMU had written about the origins of COVID-19 and the potential for the virus to have been created as a bio weapon.

Newsguard is one of a number of "fact checker" services which has proliferated since the election of Donald Trump to U.S. President. Newsguard is a browser plug-in for Chrome and Microsoft Edge that gives trustworthiness ratings to most of the internet's top-trafficked sites. It uses a color coded system to warn readers of an article or website's trustworthiness. In a previous investigation, TLAV writer Whitney Webb exposed the neoconservative roots of the Newsguard team. Webb wrote:

"Newsguard's advisory board makes it clear that Newsguard was created to serve the interests of American oligarchy. Chief among Newsguard's advisors are Tom Ridge, the first Secretary of Homeland Security under George W. Bush and Ret. General Michael Hayden, a former CIA director, a former NSA director and principal at the Chertoff Group, a security consultancy

seeking to "advise corporate clients and governments, including foreign governments" on security matters that was co-founded by former Homeland Security Secretary Michael Chertoff, who also currently serves as the board chairman of major weapons manufacturer BAE systems."

Newsguard started as a partnership between Steven Brill and Louis Gordon Crovitz, with Crovitz appearing to be the connection to the world of finance, media, and geopolitics. Crovitz held a number of positions at Dow Jones and at the Wall Street Journal, is a board member of Business Insider, a member of the Council on Foreign Relations, and claims to have been an "editor or contributor to books published by the American Enterprise Institute and Heritage Foundation." As Webb noted, *"the American Enterprise Institute (AEI) is one of the most influential neoconservative think tanks in the country and its 'scholars,' directors and fellows have included neoconservative figures like Paul Wolfowitz, Richard Perle, John Bolton and Frederick Kagan."*

Most recently, Newsguard has created a list of "Websites Publishing False Coronavirus Information" and a list "Super Spreaders" of false information. These lists include many well-known and credible independent media outlets. This is not to say that every website listed is credible and should be supported. The point is that these types of lists only serve to "blackball" certain outlets and schools of thoughts which counter the mainstream version of events. Newsguard is not the only fact checker service operating in the current "post-truth era". Social media companies like Facebook have partnered with several organizations with the stated aim of fact checking and debunking disinformation. Of course, these organizations tend to reinforce the narratives being woven by the mouthpieces in the corporate media and the puppet masters working the politicians. For a moment Facebook partnered with reviled "fact checker" Snopes, but, after Snopes was discredited, Facebook has now partnered with companies like Lead Stories.

[..]

- https://www.thelastamericanvagabond.com/censorship/this-is-why-you-cant-trust-the-fact-checkers/

****

Dec 22, 2016,12:37pm EST

The Daily Mail Snopes Story And Fact

Checking The Fact Checkers

Kalev Leetaru Contributor

Yesterday afternoon a colleague forwarded me an article from the Daily Mail, asking me if it could possibly be true. The article in question is an expose on Snopes.com, the fact checking site used by journalists and citizens across the world and one of the sites that Facebook recently partnered with to fact check news stories on its platform. The Daily Mail's article makes a number of claims about the site's principles and organization, drawing heavily from the proceedings of a contentious divorce between the site's founders and questioning whether the site could possibly act as a trusted and neutral arbitrator of the "truth."

When I first read through the Daily Mail article I immediately suspected the story itself must certainly be "fake news" because of how devastating the claims were and that given that Snopes.com was so heavily used by the journalistic community, if any of the claims were true, someone would have already written about them and companies like Facebook would not be partnering with them. I also noted that despite having been online for several hours, no other major mainstream news outlet had written about the story, which is typically a strong sign of a false or misleading story. Yet at the same time, the Daily Mail appeared to be sourcing its claims from a series of emails and other documents from a court case, some of which it reproduced in its article and, perhaps most strangely, neither Snopes nor its principles had issued any kind of statement through its website or social media channels disclaiming the story.

On the surface this looked like a classic case of fake news – a scandalous and highly shareable story, incorporating official-looking materials and sourcing, yet with no other mainstream outlet even mentioning the story. I myself told my colleague I simply did not know what to think. Was this a complete fabrication by a disgruntled target of Snopes or was this really an explosive expose pulling back the curtain on one of the world's most respected and famous fact checking brands?

In fact, one of my first thoughts upon reading the article is that this is precisely how the "fake news" community would fight back against fact checking – by running a drip-drip of fake or misleading explosive stories to discredit and cast doubt upon the fact checkers.

In the counter-intelligence world, this is what is known as a "wilderness of mirrors" – creating a chaotic information environment that so perfectly blends truth, half-truth and fiction that even the best can no longer tell what's real and what's not.

Thus, when I reached out to David Mikkelson, the founder of Snopes, for comment, I fully expected him to respond with a lengthy email in Snopes' trademark point-by-point format, fully refuting each and every one of the claims in the Daily Mail's article and writing the entire article off as "fake news."
It was with incredible surprise therefore that I received David's one-sentence response which read in its entirety "I'd be happy to speak with you, but I can only address some aspects in general because I'm precluded by the terms of a binding

settlement agreement from discussing details of my divorce."

This absolutely astounded me. Here was the one of the world's most respected fact checking organizations, soon to be an ultimate arbitrator of "truth" on Facebook, saying that it cannot respond to a fact checking request because of a secrecy agreement.

In short, when someone attempted to fact check the fact checker, the response was the equivalent of "it's secret."

It is impossible to understate how antithetical this is to the fact checking world, in which absolute openness and transparency are necessary prerequisites for trust. How can fact checking organizations like Snopes expect the public to place trust in them if when they themselves are called into question, their response is that they can't respond.

[..]

From the outside, Silicon Valley looks like a gleaming tower of technological perfection. Yet, once the curtain is pulled back, we see that behind that shimmering façade is a warehouse of good old fashioned humans, subject to all the same biases and fallibility, but with their results now laundered through the sheen of computerized infallibility. Even my colleagues who work in the journalism community and by their nature skeptical, had assumed that Snopes must have rigorous screening procedures, constant inter- and intra-rater evaluations and ongoing assessments and a total transparency mandate. Yet, the truth is that we simply have no visibility into the organization's inner workings and its founder declined to shed further light into its operations for this article.

Regardless of whether the Daily Mail article is correct in its claims about Snopes, at the least what does emerge from my exchanges with Snopes' founder is the image of the ultimate black box presenting a gleaming veneer of ultimate arbitration of truth, yet with absolutely no insight into its inner workings. While technology pundits decry the black boxes of the algorithms that increasingly power companies like Facebook, they have forgotten that even the human-powered sites offer us little visibility into how they function.

At the end of the day, it is clear that before we rush to place fact checking organizations like Snopes in charge of arbitrating what is "truth" on Facebook, we need to have a lot more understanding of how they function internally and much greater transparency into their work.

- https://www.forbes.com/sites/kalevleetaru/2016/12/22/the-daily-mail-snopes-story-and-fact-checking-the-fact-checkers/#4791e5a8227f

****

How a NeoCon-Backed "Fact Checker" Plans to Wage War on Independent Media

As Newsguard's project advances, it will soon become almost impossible to avoid this neocon-approved news site's ranking systems on any technological device sold in the United States.

by Whitney Webb
January 09th, 2019

MINNEAPOLIS — Soon after the social media "purge" of independent media sites and pages this past October, a top neoconservative insider — Jamie Fly — was caught stating that the mass deletion of anti-establishment and anti-war pages on Facebook and Twitter was "just the beginning" of a concerted effort by the U.S. government and powerful corporations to silence online dissent within the United States and beyond.

While a few, relatively uneventful months in the online news sphere have come and gone since Fly made this ominous warning, it appears that the neoconservatives and other standard bearers of the military-industrial complex and the U.S. oligarchy are now poised to let loose their latest digital offensive against independent media outlets that seek to expose wrongdoing in both the private and public sectors.

As MintPress News Editor-in-Chief Mnar Muhawesh recently wrote, MintPress was informed that it was under review by an organization called Newsguard Technologies, which described itself to MintPress as simply a "news rating agency" and asked Muhawesh to comment on a series of allegations, several of which were blatantly untrue. However, further examination of this organization reveals that it is funded by and deeply connected to the U.S. government, neo-conservatives, and powerful monied interests, all of whom have been working overtime since the 2016 election to silence dissent to American forever-wars and corporate-led oligarchy.

More troubling still, Newsguard — by virtue of its deep connections to government and Silicon Valley — is lobbying to have its rankings of news sites installed by default on computers in U.S. public libraries, schools, and universities as well as on all smartphones and computers sold in the United States.

In other words, as Newsguard's project advances, it will soon become almost impossible to avoid this neocon-approved news site's ranking systems on any technological device sold in the United States. Worse still, if its efforts to quash dissenting voices in the U.S. are successful, Newsguard promises that its next move will be to take its system global.

[..]

[Editor's Interpolation:
As you can see from the following, Newsguard credits Foxnews with maintaining "basic standards of accuracy and accountability". Ok, I haven't looked at the website being referred to, maybe it's completely different from the Fox TV 'News' which I have witnessed. Still, they're obviously connected & the TV 'news' version has got to be one of the most flagrantly biased 'news' sources imaginable. SO, I have to wonder whether Newsguard's approval is just an indicator that there's no way in hell they're going to dare to challenge such a financial giant. That seems likely to me. If Newsguard is as neoconservative as they're being accused of being by Whitney Webb it seems even more unlikely that they'd in any way criticize the most successful of the neocon propaganda outlets.]

foxnews.com

This website generally maintains basic standards of accuracy and accountability.

The website of Fox News Channel, the most-watched cable and satellite news channel in the United States, created by Rupert Murdoch as a conservative counterpoint to the three major broadcast networks and CNN.

NewsGuard Read More →

As Newsguard releases a new rating of a site, that rating automatically spreads to all computers that have installed its news ranking browser plug-in. That plug-in is currently available for free for the most commonly used internet browsers. NewsGuard directly markets the browser plug-in to libraries, schools and internet users in general.

According to its website, Newsguard has rated more than 2,000 news and information sites. However, it plans to take its ranking efforts much farther by eventually reviewing "the 7,500 most-read news and information websites in the U.S.—about 98 percent of news and information people read and share online" in the United States in English.

[..]

- https://www.mintpressnews.com/newsguardneocon-backed-fact-checker-plans-to-wage-war-on-independent-media/253687/

****

Check Your Facts

Libraries use tech tools to fight fake news

By Jessica Cilella I November 1, 2019

In June, Albuquerque and Bernalillo County (N.Mex.) Library System hosted its first-ever drag queen storytime. Dozens of children and their families gathered at the Main Library for a morning of literary entertainment designed to promote tolerance and mark Pride Month—even as a small group of protesters convened outside.

The *Albuquerque Journal*'s coverage of the event was headlined "Drag Queens Dazzle at Library Storytime," while enthusiastic parents voiced support on the library's Facebook page. Other Facebook commenters voiced opposition, sharing links to conservative websites and articles with headlines like "Parents Beware—Registered Sex Offenders Are Performing for Small Children at Drag Queen Story Hours in Public Libraries" (American Pastors Network).

The library didn't delete the Facebook comments, but it has taken steps to help patrons evaluate the quality of the information they see online and identify bias. Like many libraries, Albuquerque and Bernalillo County's library system is turning to a new generation of tech tools and pooling digital resources to teach media literacy.

Flagging, not censoring

NewsGuard is a web browser extension designed to literally red-flag problematic articles and blog posts like the one published by American Pastors Network, a faith-based organization.

Launched in 2018 by a team of professional journalists, NewsGuard was created with libraries and schools in mind. Evaluators use a set of nine journalistic standards to examine the credibility and transparency of thousands of websites and issue a rating and "nutrition label" for each one. For example, NewsGuard users who visit the website of the *Albuquerque Journal*, New Mexico's largest daily newspaper, will notice a green icon with a checkmark in the corner of the browser window that indicates the website adheres to NewsGuard's standards and has been deemed accurate and reliable. A red exclamation point icon indicates the opposite.

More than 200 libraries have installed NewsGuard on their public computers as a teaching device to promote media literacy. Richland Library in Columbia, South Carolina, was among the first, introducing the browser extension across its 14 branches this year.

"More and more people get their news online, with social media platforms being a go-to source for many users," says Chantal Wilson, the library's research and readers' advisory manager. "We thought installing NewsGuard might be one way to help customers identify sources of balanced news."

NewsGuard, with support from Microsoft as part of its Defending Democracy Program, is one of several browser extensions designed to combat misinformation. Such plug-ins offer both complementary and overlapping functionality. For instance, Trusted News, developed by start-up Factmata and available for Google Chrome, places stories on a spectrum ranging from "content looks good" to "content looks harmful." Trusted News also scans content for what it calls "special states," such as sexism and racism. FakerFact, available for Chrome and Firefox, analyzes articles based on six criteria—such as "journalism," "sensational," or "agenda-driven." The Media Bias Fact Check extension, available on Chrome and Firefox, focuses specifically on an outlet's relative level of bias, assigning one of nine rankings ranging from "left bias" to "right bias" to "conspiracy-pseudoscience" and "satire." And SurfSafe—available on Chrome, Firefox, and Opera—is designed to evaluate the authenticity of images.

[..]

- https://americanlibrariesmagazine.org/2019/11/01/check-your-facts-tech-tools/

****

June 25, 2020, 9:21AM (Amir-ul Kafirs to group):

Re: HERETICS: Fact Checkers & NewsGuard's invasion of Public Libraries

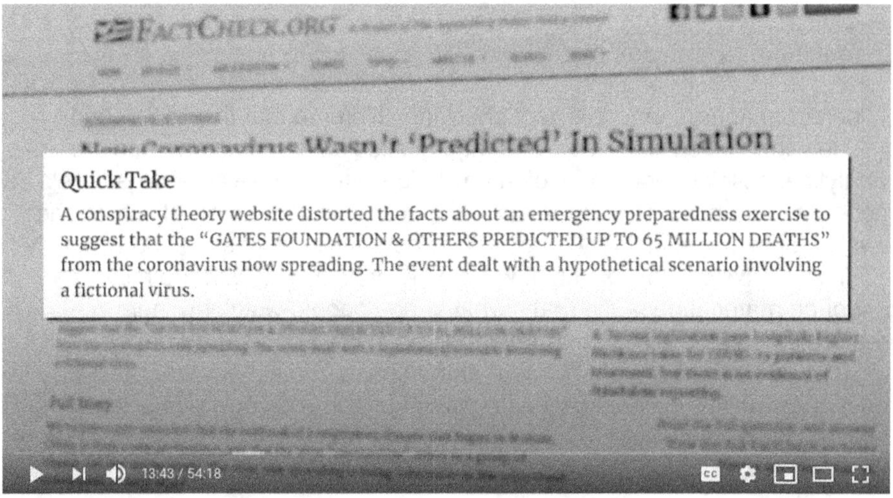

I found this fun talk about fact checking the fact checkers

I should pay more attention to this guy! He's fantastic!! I know he's been linked to here before but this is the 1st time I've spent more than a few minutes checking him out. I've shared this to my YouTube PANDEMIC PANIC playlist. I'm taking screenshots from this now for potential use in the very hypothetical book. Here's one of them:

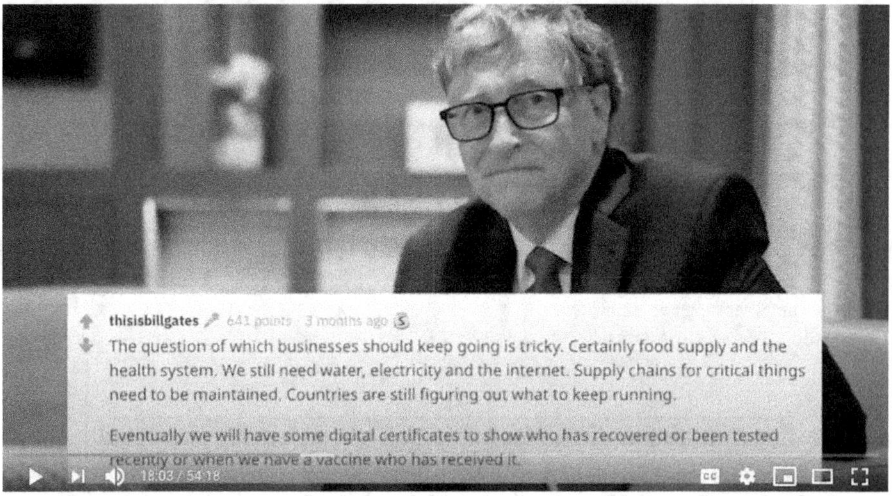

I've left 3 comments on this so far. Here's the 2nd of the 2, made possible, obviously, by what Inquiring Librarian links us to at the end of her email:

"And, yes, the plandemic of the 'fact checkers' is invading that most sacred of free speech public space in the US: THE LIBRARIES: https://americanlibrariesmagazine.org/2019/11/01/check-your-facts-tech-tools/ "

Here's the 3rd, & last, comment:

"My personal approach to this 'fact checking' dilemma that this report ends on is to: 1. develop one's own critical reading faculties as much as one has the energy & analytical ability to do, 2. to weigh any 'information' received against one's own practical experience. This latter is simple, in a way: instead of relying on the 'news' at all, why not just rely on what one personally witnesses in one's daily life? The TV 'News', for example, will mainly provide you with the most fear-mongering material because that's what keeps people watching them &, therefore, keeps the advertising revenues up. Why not just turn off the TV altogether? Then you might notice that the constant mayhem that the TV 'News' presents as 'reality' isn't actually as constant or common as these people would have you think."

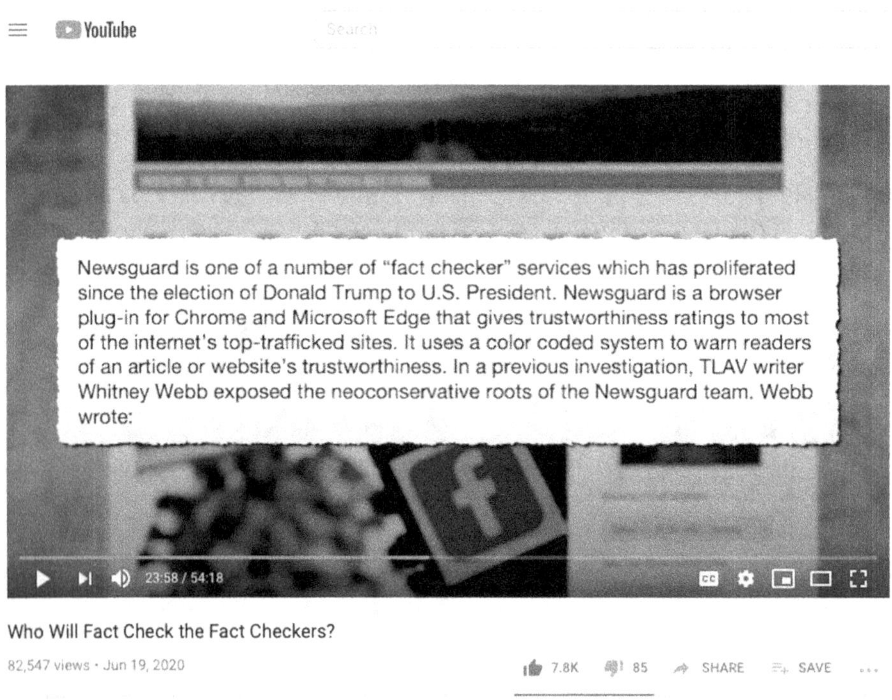

It's interesting to note that "Fake News" is defined, at least in this initial presentation of it, as an internet phenomena. But what about the big 'news'papers? Mainstream TV? If you want more or less CONSTANT Fake 'News' TV 'News' is the place to go. Have you see the movie that Rich Pell & I made parodying the mainstream 'news' propaganda against protestors at the G20 in Pittsburgh? The propaganda started wwwaaaaaayyyy in advance in order to try to make sure that anyone watching or reading the 'news' would be biased against them. This is one of my favorite shorts:

345. "TV 'News' Commits Suicide"

- starring April Gilmore as Nancy Newscaster/Newswoman & Civic Association meeting attendee; Rich Pell as Officer Such'n'Such; tENTATIVELY, a cONVENIENCE as the Infiltrator; Kelly Stiles as Officer So'n'So & the Man-on-the-street; Deanna Hitchcock as the anarchist cook & Civic Association meeting attendee; Julie Gonzalez as questioning Civic Association meeting attendee; joy toujours as Civic Association meeting attendee; & Leah as Civic Association meeting attendee
- concept by tENTATIVELY, a cONVENIENCE & Rich Pell
- camera by Kelly Stiles; Rich Pell; & tENTATIVELY, a cONVENIENCE
- catering by Deanna Hitchcock
- script by tENTATIVELY, a cONVENIENCE
- framing graphics & music from Rich Pell
- editing & titles & archival footage & scanning etc from tENTATIVELY, a cONVENIENCE
- shot Monday & Tuesday, September14th & 15th, 2009; edit finished Thursday, September 17th, 2009
- 06:09
- on my onesownthoughts YouTube channel here: https://youtu.be/hU-_aL7kKBI

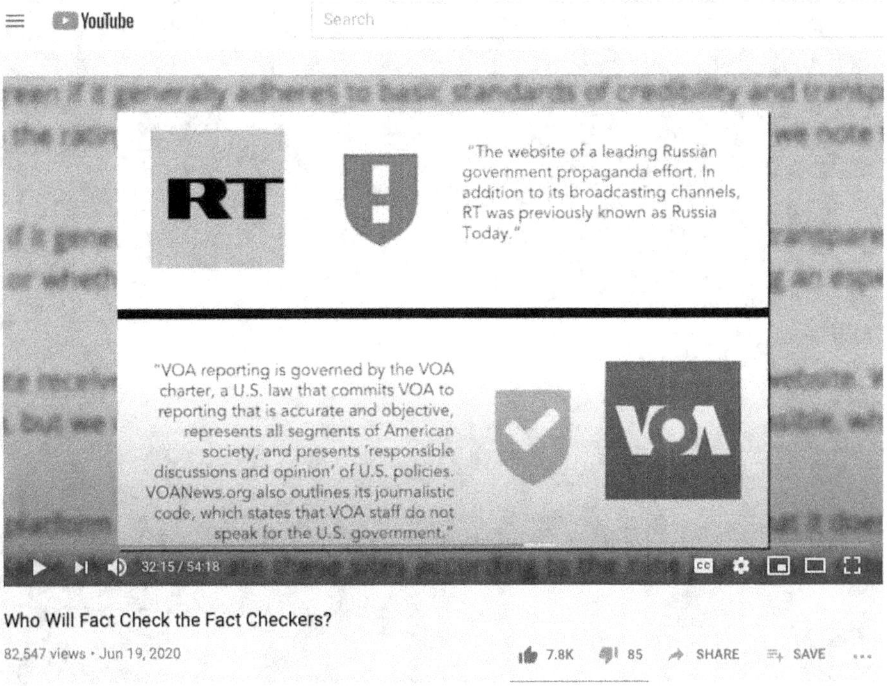

here is an article by the guy who was interviewed in the talk above

Alas, as usual, I find myself thinking: *I have to get back to the other things I'm working on!* In this instance, I'm making a version of my 'opera' in its entirety but without the live musicians (parts not composed yet) & stage sets (not built yet) to put online & THAT'S very labor-intensive. SO, I went to the article & copied it &

put it in my HERETICS files so that I can read it & quote it if & when I get to that part of the very hypothetical book & that's what I'm going to do with the next articles too. Because I try to render all this material into something that I can use in the book it takes me HOURS to even get through this email.

****

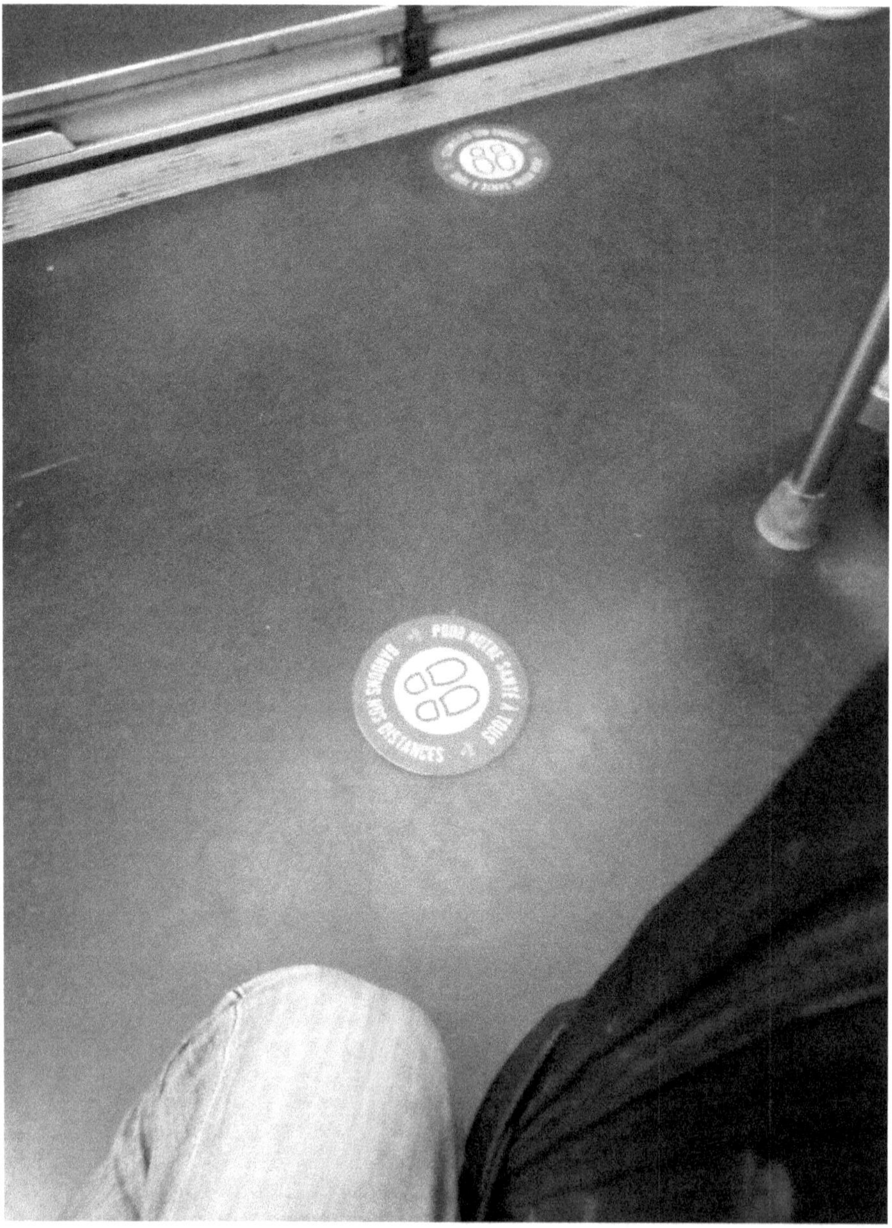

June 25, 2020, 2:17PM (Dick to group):

HERETICS: Photos in métro

Hi,
here are some photos of the various distancing signs in the metro that I've been meaning to send
you are supposed to stand on the little circles,
you are not supposed to sit in the seats with signs on them
and you are supposed to follow the directional arrows
i find it really irritating
it's hard for me not to think that the only difference between the nazis and what is happening now is that the nazis had the honesty to make a flag and advertise

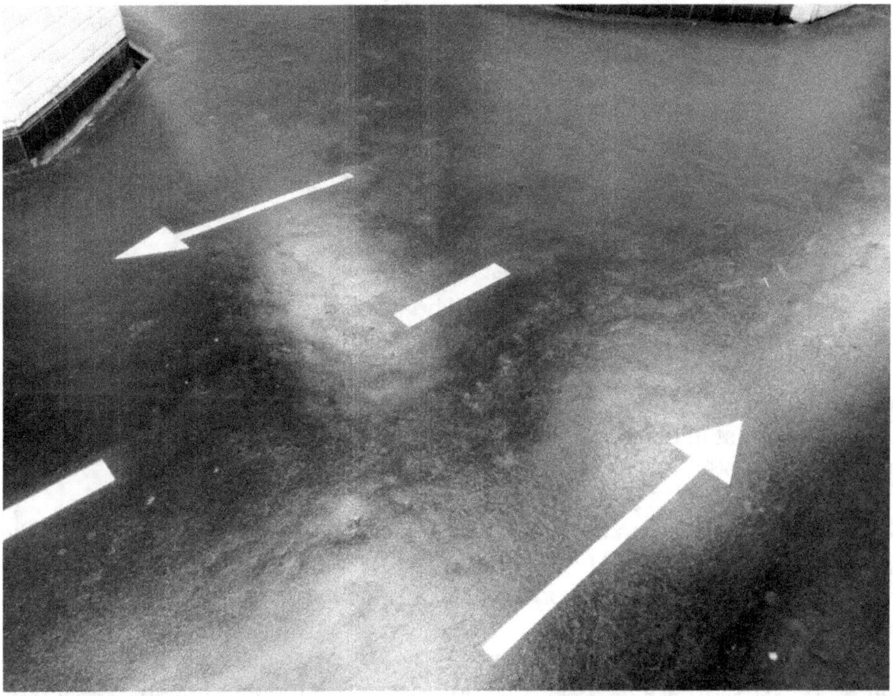

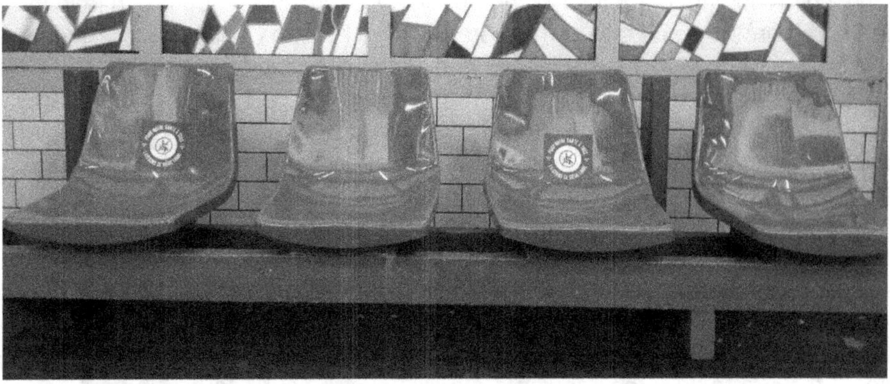

****

June 25, 2020, 5:33PM (Inquiring Librarian to group):

Re: HERETICS: Photos in métro

I also find those signs highly irritating. I get really irritated when I have to go anywhere these days. Luckily, I don't notice the arrows on the ground anymore because all of my masks are too big on my face and I cannot see well in front of me on the ground because the masks obstruct my view of such ground arrows, maybe the seat signs would be more noticed by me, but I've noticed none around me yet (which doesn't mean they aren't there). I have a lot of bruises on my legs from running into and tripping over things with my masks on and have actually fully fallen over several times in public. It's funny, but then it's not, consider why I am accidentally slamming my body into and onto so many things lately. At least no one has forced me yet to wear a mask while on my bicycle or driving my car... gawd help us all if that happens... I am travel challenged and accident prone enough without the concealing garb while handling a dangerous hunk of speeding metal on wheels.

And yes, Dick, I also prefer the more 'honest' tactic of the Nazis. I can't stand being lied to, it really pisses me off. All I hear these days in the media is lies and the lies are so obvious it really lowers my faith in humanity that people actually believe this and then have the gumption to virtuously parrot this bullshit that they hear on the news. I hear so much repeated 'news' barfing at work. I just can't grasp how this stuff could be believed and then regurgitated by people I actually found respectable.

Ok, let me throw this one in here, news from Louisiana!! They are really beating this 'cases' thing to DEATH!! "Cases" rising is MASSIVE news every day in Louisiana right now. The mayor even threatened to shut the whole city down again yesterday, 'Without hesitation" if we don't 'shape up'. Can I say it in response, 80's style.--> "Gag me with a Spoon!!!", really, I'm ready for my spanking. Yesterday's news was so unbelievable, I thought I might puke up my lunch while reading it. I think maybe our city 'leaders' drank too much lead in their water growing up, lead in the water is huge here in Louisiana. It's like the government math flunkies are teaching calculus completely wrong to the general public and then asking said public to live and regurgitate it in exactly the same WRONG way to everyone, until said government realizes the next day that they have a *better* WRONG way to do that same calculus... or get your business shut down... and don't forget to report your friends and neighbors if they don't comply with the latest wrongmath . I mean, most of the public cannot understand this 'calculus', but some feel they've really GOT IT, and they venomously spit it back at you in social media and in article responses... they must prove their virtue and intelligence by parroting bullshit. I am mad today. I'll get over it, I hope. As long as they don't force vaccinate me, I can get through this. If they do try to force vaccinate me, I'll have to figure something out because no one is shooting that poison into me, ever. Ok, here is the article: https://www.nola.com/news/politics/article_ae585fa8-b649-11ea-

b37e-6fbafe81bd90.html?
238&utm_medium=social&utm_source=nolafb&utm_campaign=snd&fbclid=IwAR3eMfcKzpggDXzrE7m1YOL23rZYIPobJt6WxFEqvUVAUM9IlnknkfLUKI8

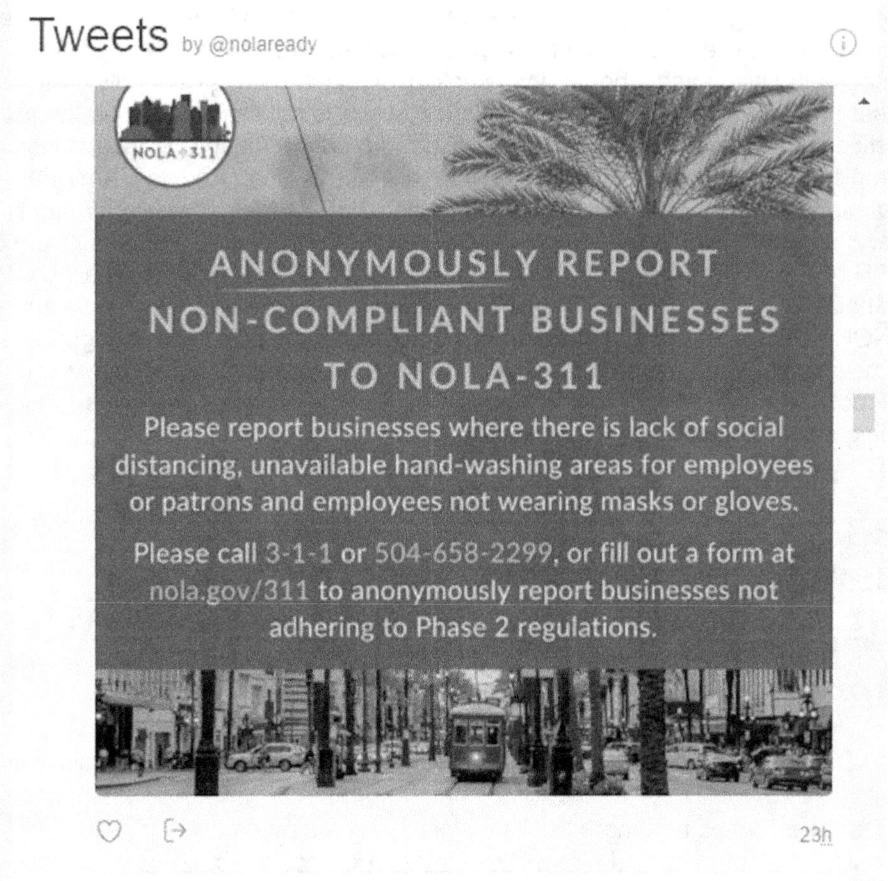

Here is the information needed to be a good 'covid' Nazi and report your neighbors. The same contact information has also been shared to report neighbors and friends having gatherings that you may find to be too large or too close. I'll remember that, and think twice, the next time I decide to have a large and loud orgy swarm in, on, and around my home, during the Saharan Dust Plume and while being attacked by the drunk murder hornets that fell into and flew out of my spiked punch... but don't worry, we'll be wearing our masks but I can't guarantee social distancing given the nature of the event.

Amir-ul Kafirs, Rich Pell was actually in my graduating class at the University of Delaware. He was in the same chemical engineering program as my friend ______, who I am trying and failing to share non-mainstream media sources with. Rich is brilliant. I never was close to him, but I knew him, and he was close with several friends that I still am relatively close to. I'm not sure if he'd even remember me, but he is my friend on social media. =] Nice guy, from what I remember, and very creative. _____, by the way, is being her wonderful, kind, and caring self. She is such a great person. But... I see her using those tactics described in the video for combating 'conspiracy theorists'. She means well, but I feel she is misguided and she feels I am misguided and is trying to re-guide me into her mis-guidedness, it's a funny phenomenon. We are both very politely disagreeing with each other and very politely trying and failing to kindly drag each other onto our sides. Mostly I appreciate that she is not being a vicious social justice finger wagger on me.. But I am filled with dread that intelligent and kind people such as her are being sucked into this fake drama. And yes, Amir-ul Kafirs, absolutely TV is total fake news these days. I luckily have no TV and I never see one, ever, these days. But I have radios in my house and I still turn on NPR occasionally and it always throws me into fits of rage and/or despair and sometimes I laugh. But mostly NPR is just unbelievably full of 'fake' news and ENORMOUS amounts of outrageous and sometimes comical fear mongering, it's unbelievable... and the stuff that NPR says is what my fellow librarians parrot. I cannot understand this, it totally baffles me... but then again, I was never good at being a 'team player.'

****

New Orleans health director: It's 'very clear' coronavirus clusters haven't traced back to protests

BY JOHN SIMERMAN I STAFF WRITER JUN 24, 2020 - 2:30 PM 4 min to read

If there's evidence that more than a week of protests over police brutality and racism have compounded a recent rise in new coronavirus cases across New Orleans, it doesn't show up in the data, the city's health director, Dr. Jennifer Avegno, said Wednesday.

Questions over the impact on the spread of COVID-19 from protests that at times packed city streets with thousands of demonstrators have grown heated this week in New Orleans, amid confirmed reports by state and local health officials of coronavirus "clusters" growing from bars off the LSU campus in Baton Rouge, and from graduation parties for parents and students of Isidore Newman School.

[..]

- https://www.nola.com/news/politics/article_ae585fa8-b649-11ea-b37e-6fbafe81bd90.html?238&utm_medium=social&utm_source=nolafb&utm_campaign=snd&fbclid=IwAR3eMfcKzpggDXzrE7m1YOL23rZYIPobJt6WxFEqvUVAUM9lInknkfLUKI8

****

June 25, 2020, 8:08PM (Amir-ul Kafirs to group):

here are some photos of the various distancing signs in the metro

Thanks for these, they'll be great additions to the still very hypothetical book.

i find it really irritating

Has there been any graffiti defacement yet? I think if I lived there I'd make stickers at home to cover them over with. I should probably do that here but I've only been to the one bookstore where they had those direction lines. Those things are probably at all sorts of places I don't go to.

it's hard for me not to think that the only difference between the nazis and what is happening now is that the nazis had the honesty to make a flag and advertise

Ha ha! Well, so far this is ostensibly about preventing mass deaths instead of causing them but it's easy to imagine that pretense having its PR of euphemisms wear thin very soon.

****

June 25, 2020, 8:13PM (Dick to group):

I know a "funny" story about reporting one's neighbors, as told to me by the mother of my son many years ago
In France during the occupation the Germans started a program where they would reward anyone who turned in their neighbors who were saying or doing things against the Nazi forces in France
They received a huge amount of responses
After a while the Nazis realized that people had started reporting their neighbors so they could get their apartments, or because they were making too much noise, or because they'd had an argument, etc
The Nazi bureau of information got so saturated they closed it down
*
Who knows, that could even be a good strategy.

****

June 25, 2020, 8:19PM (Dick to group):

I haven't seen any grafitti over the signs yet

it's easy to imagine that pretense having its PR of euphemisms wear thin very soon.

I meant more in the sense of the larger agenda of vaccines, state

control, fear tactics, the spreading of fake-anti-fake news (as in the article Inquiring Librarian shared), the guessed-at eugenics ideas, etc

****

June 25, 2020, 8:19PM (Amir-ul Kafirs to group):

the masks obstruct my view of such ground arrows,

I find that the mask sensorily impairs me in general.

"Cases" rising is MASSIVE news every day

The thing is that there doesn't have to be any proof whatsoever that the increase in cases actually means that people are getting sick & dying, it's just all about the # of cases detected — which in & of itself is fairly meaningless. If 400 people are detected with the virus & NO-ONE GETS SICK OR DIES, *what fucking difference does it make?!* I'm not saying that's the case but I'm sure that it's not '400 people detected with virus, 400 dead.'

https://www.nola.com/news/politics/article_ae585fa8-b649-11ea-b37e-6fbafe81bd90.html?238&utm_medium=social&utm_source=nolafb&utm_campaign=snd&fbclid=IwAR3eMfcKzpggDXzrE7m1YOL23rZY!PobJt6WxFEqvUVAUM9lInknkfLUKI8

What a weird cocktail that is! The 2 most potent mass media spectacles of the moment: BLM & PANDEMIC PANIC & how to blend them.

Rich Pell was actually in my graduating class at the University of Delaware.

Yeah, he's one of the more interesting artists in PGH. I guest-lectured in his class at CMU once or twice & was a spontaneous actor in one of his performances. He founded the "Center for Post-Natural History" here.

Here is the information needed to be a good 'covid' Nazi and report your neighbors.

Great! That's another really useful image.

FINALLY, a reliable way to get people to turn against each other. East German secret police society here we come!!

****

June 25, 2020, 8:31PM (Amir-ul Kafirs to group):

The Nazi bureau of information got so saturated they closed it down

It's an interesting thought. Back in 1981 when I 1st read about the NSA monitoring phone calls & using computers to search for words like "assassination" & "heroin" I set up a phone station recording that encouraged people to say those words over & over again on the phone in a similar attempt to overload surveillance.

Alas, as far as the nazis in France goes imagine how many people were kidnapped, tortured & killed because of their shitty greedy neighbors.

Still, you could leave anonymous tips that a 'business' at such & such an address was violating rules & have that address be the police station or some other government office.

However this snitching stuff plays out there's no way it's going to be good.

****

June 25, 2020, 8:34PM (Amir-ul Kafirs to group):

I haven't seen any grafitti over the signs yet

Another sign of how effective this whole business is as mind-control.

I meant more in the sense of the larger agenda

Well, yeah, it's 'classic' totalitarianism. The insanity of it is how easily it's been pulled off. I'll be that if more immigrants who fled the Soviet Bloc were still alive that they'd be horrified by this — people like Inquiring Librarian's dad.

****

June 25, 2020, 8:42PM (Amir-ul Kafirs to group):

HERETICS: Hospital Propaganda

UPMC is Pittsburgh's biggest complex of 'health-care' facilities & hospitals. I've informed them repeatedly that I have no intention of ever using their services again if I can avoid it. Nonetheless, I continue to get propaganda from them. Here's a sampling — &, gee, what a surprise that anxiety is the most common mental illness. What on earth could people be feeling anxious about? Just be SHEEPLE & all will be good.

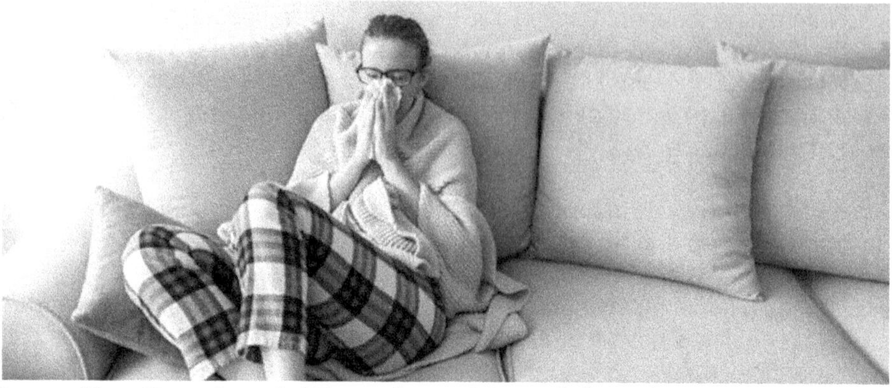

How Is Contact Tracing Used in the Fight Against COVID-19?

In contact tracing, trained investigators interview someone who has become ill with an infectious disease. These interviews attempt to find out whom the sick person was in close contact with while infected. Those people are then notified of their potential exposure and are given instructions on what they can do to avoid spreading the disease.

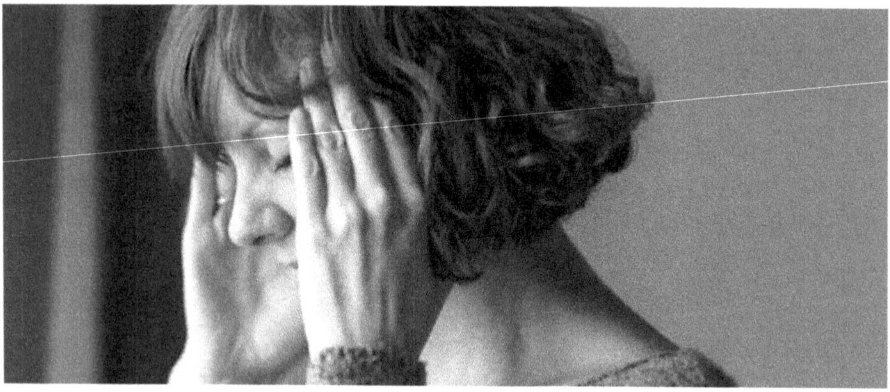

The Most Common Mental Illness: Myths and Facts About Anxiety

More than 40 million American adults suffer from anxiety disorders, according to the Anxiety and Depression Association of America (ADAA) . Even though anxiety disorders are common, there are many misconceptions that can cause stigma for people who suffer from them.

****

June 26, 2020, 7:30PM (Amir-ul Kafirs to Dick):

Re: HERETICS: Hospital Propaganda

i think people will be in favor of the Iron Boot i.e. TOTAL CONTROL and in fact,
I think they enjoy it, the feeling of righteous certitude

Do you know the word "untertan"? There's a great novel by Heinrich Mann, Thomas Mann's brother, of that name. There's a great East German film based on the novel too. I highly recommend it. An untertan is a person who abuses people lower than them in a hierarchy & ass-licks those above them in a hierarchy — their purpose being, of course, to rise higher in said hierarchy. The insidiousness of such a character is profoundly disturbing to me. I can easily see someone we know fitting right in. I think the whole psychology of this quarantine brings out that type of personality. The self-righteousness justifies what's really sadism. The thing is that it's masochism AND sadism in the same person.

"Mann's essay on Émile Zola and the novel *Der Untertan* (first published 1905) earned him much respect during the Weimar Republic, since they satirized Imperial German society. Later, his book *Professor Unrat* was freely adapted into the movie *Der Blaue Engel* (*The Blue Angel*). Carl Zuckmayer wrote the script, and Josef von Sternberg was the director. Mann wanted his paramour, the actress Trude Hesterberg, to play the main female part as the "actress" Lola Lola (named Rosa Fröhlich in the novel), but Marlene Dietrich was given the part, her first sound role.

Together with Albert Einstein and other celebrities during 1932, Mann was a signatory to the "Urgent Call for Unity", asking the voters to reject the Nazis. Einstein and Mann had previously co-authored a letter during 1931 condemning the murder of Croatian scholar Milan Šufflay.

Mann became *persona non grata* in Nazi Germany and left even before the Reichstag fire of 1933. He went to France where he lived in Paris and Nice. During the German occupation, he made his way through collaborationist Vichy France to Marseille, where he was aided by Varian Fry during 1940 to escape to Spain. He eventually escaped to Portugal and then to America.

The Nazis burnt Heinrich Mann's books as "contrary to the German spirit" during the infamous book burning of May 10, 1933, which was instigated by the then Nazi propaganda minister Joseph Goebbels."

- https://en.wikipedia.org/wiki/Heinrich_Mann

It seems likely that you've seen "The Blue Angel". I literally recommend "Der Untertan" (available in various translations) higher than almost any novel. It portrays this type of person with stunning accuracy but still manages to have some humor. Reading it will help you understand this day & age as much as anything & I'll bet you start using the word as frequently as I do!

****

June 28, 2020, 12:08PM (Inquiring Librarian to group):

Re: HERETICS: Hospital Propaganda

Yes, I find this page disgusting. No matter what you think about this situation, it sucks and it is causing anxiety whether you believe the fear monger pushers or whether you are totally confounded as to how anyone could possibly believe this utter stupidity. Am I being too harsh? I don't know. The only people I know who seem to be relishing in the insanity and finding some positivity are the few Nature Magik centered Qanon people I've come in contact with. They seem to gravitate towards looking at the positive in this and a great 'awakening' and a great splitting of sides where both sides will get what they want, be it darkness in mechanization and control or light in harmony with one another and nature. To the billionaire, many of them throw out a comical, but kind of serious, "Release the Kraken!" phrase.

Simply put, the world has gone crazy. I cannot stand how our 'health'careless system preys on those 'suffering' through what they have created to further push their agendas in the form of psych pills and more brainwashing through the form of 'psycho'-care.

****

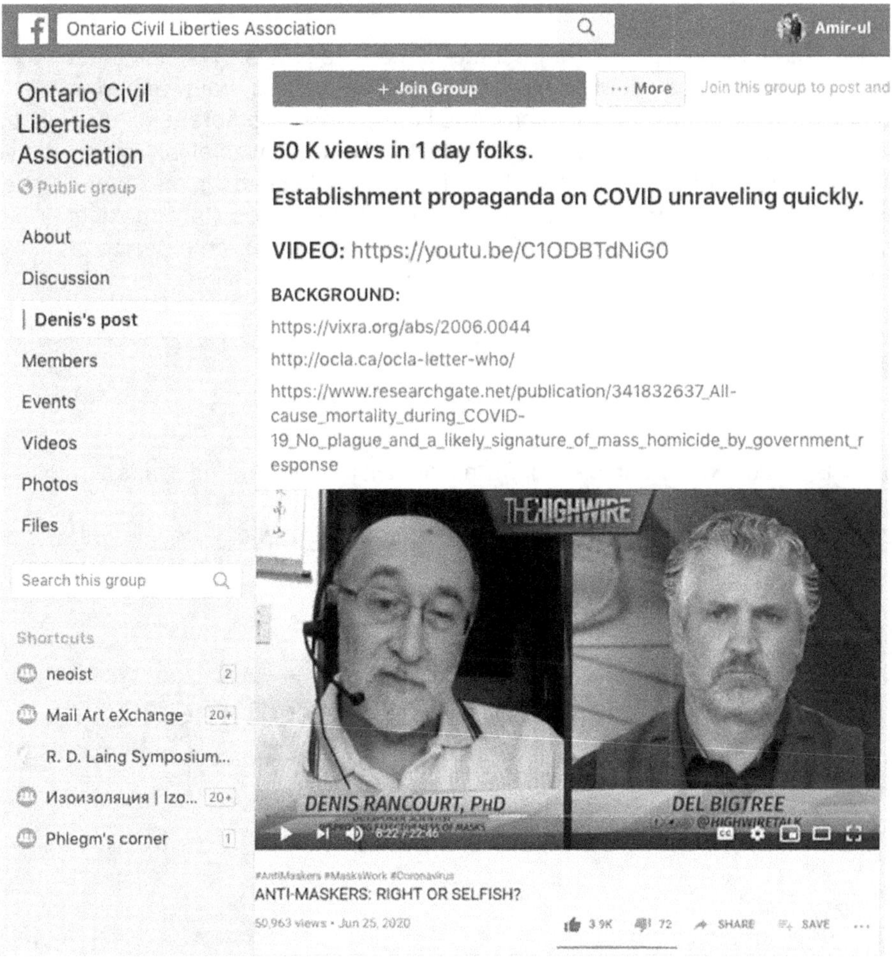

****

June 28, 2020, 9:19PM (Amir-ul Kafirs to group):

Am I being too harsh?

Nope, it only gets "too harsh" when you say such things to their faces.

I cannot stand how our 'health'careless system preys on those 'suffering'

Like all muggers, the Medical Industry preys on the weak & defenseless. BUT, on the bright side, you've coined " 'health'careless system"!! I'll try to remember to use that one!

****

June 28, 2020 (txt msg from Inquiring Librarian to Amir-ul Kafirs):

That is nuts!! People completely confound me these days. To think that avid readers like librarians could be so easily manipulated and brainwashed with nonsense by obvious criminal overloards is beyond my comprehension. I just listened to all 2plus hrs of this rally from Sacramento. It was all amazing. It gives me more hope for humanity. 1hr 30min in is bobby kennedy jr.'s speach... Totally Amazing, in my opinion. The nurse Erin from Elmhurst hospital speaks after him and then Judy Mikovits speaks. These people have power and a voice and i think they can really change what nonsense we are being subjected to and destroyed by.
https://youtu.be/h5GH??O9GBxU

****

June 28, 2020 (txt msg article link from Naia Nisnam to Amir-ul Kafirs):

https://www.wtae.com/article/allegheny-county-officials-recommend-quarantine-testing-for-travelers/32991963

****

Allegheny County officials recommend quarantine, testing for travelers

Updated: 6:40 PM EDT Jun 28, 2020

PITTSBURGH —
Allegheny County Health Department Director Dr. Debra Bogen is recommending a 14-day quarantine for those traveling out of state or to have two negative tests at least 48 hours apart for the quarantine to be lifted.

[..]

****

June 28, 2020, 11:10AM (Amir-ul Kafirs to group):

HERETICS: 'Fact Checker' CENSORSHIP in Action!

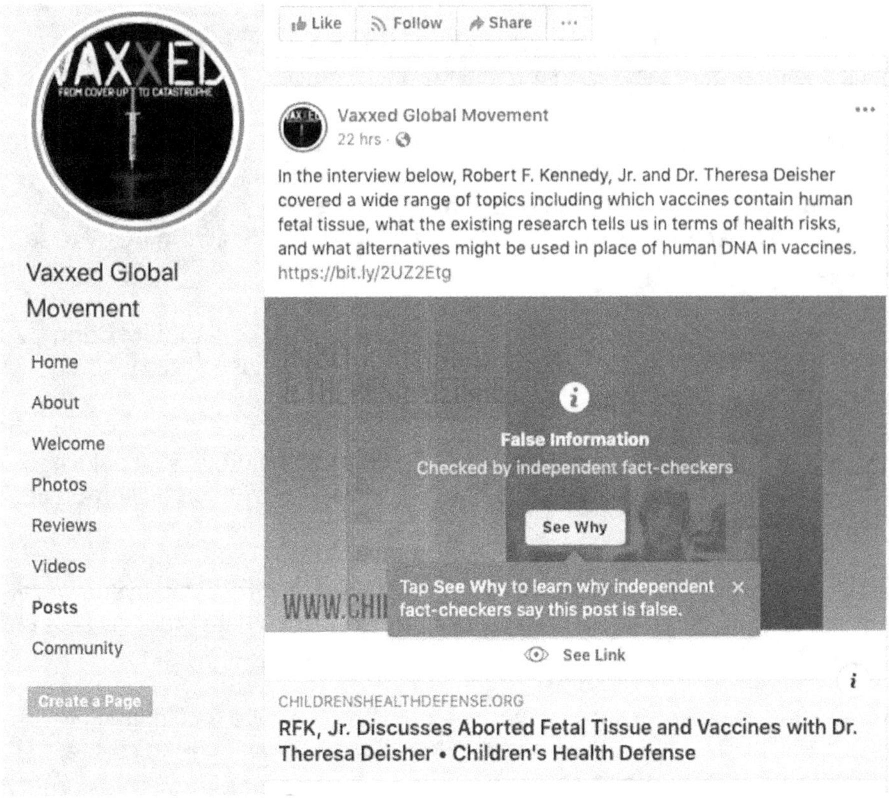

****

June 28, 2020, 11:52AM (Inquiring Librarian to group):

Re: HERETICS: 'Fact Checker' CENSORSHIP in Action!

I believe this article goes in depth behind the scenes of the funders and editors of the 'Fact Checkers':
https://www.thelastamericanvagabond.com/censorship/this-is-why-you-cant-trust-the-fact-checkers/

Next, consider Wikipedia. Check out this article on the wonderful site that we've all shared, the Swiss Propaganda Research website, vs. Wikipedia's scathing article about the site:
https://off-guardian.org/2020/03/07/wikipedia-a-disinformation-operation/

& of course, don't forget to actually look at Wikipedia's scathing review of the Swiss Propaganda Research site:
https://en.wikipedia.org/wiki/Swiss_Propaganda_Research

****

Wikipedia: A Disinformation Operation?

from Swiss Propaganda Research

Wikipedia is generally thought of as an open, transparent, and mostly reliable online encyclopedia. Yet upon closer inspection, this turns out not to be the case. In fact, the English Wikipedia with its **9 billion page** views per month is **governed** by just 500 active administrators, whose real identity in many cases remains unknown.

Moreover, studies have shown that 80% of all Wikipedia content **is written** by just 1% of all Wikipedia editors, which again amounts to just a few hundred mostly unknown people.

Obviously, such a non-transparent and hierarchical structure is susceptible to corruption and manipulation, the notorious **"paid editors"** hired by corporations being just one example.

Indeed, already in 2007, researchers found that CIA and FBI employees were **editing** Wikipedia articles on controversial topics including the Iraq war and the Guantanamo military prison.

Also in 2007, researchers found that one of the most active and influential English Wikipedia administrators, called "Slim Virgin", was in fact a **former British intelligence informer**.

More recently, another highly prolific Wikipedia editor going by the false name of **"Philip Cross"** turned out to be linked to UK intelligence as well as several mainstream **media journalists**.

In Germany, one of the most aggressive Wikipedia editors was **exposed**, after a two-year legal battle, as a political operative formerly serving in the Israeli army as a foreign volunteer.

Even in Switzerland, unidentified government employees were caught **whitewashing Wikipedia entries** about the Swiss secret service just prior to a public referendum about the agency.

Many of these Wikipedia personae are editing articles almost all day and every day, indicating that they are either highly dedicated individuals, or in fact, operated by a group of people.

In addition, articles edited by these personae cannot easily be revised, since the above-mentioned administrators can always revert changes or simply block disagreeing users altogether.

The primary goal of these covert campaigns **appears to be** pushing Western and **Israeli government** positions while destroying the reputation of independent journalists and politicians.

Articles most affected by this kind of manipulation include political, geopolitical and certain historical topics as well as biographies of non-conformist academics, journalists, and politicians.

Perhaps unsurprisingly, Wikipedia founder Jimmy Wales, a **friend of former British Prime Minister** Tony Blair and a **"Young Leader"** of the Davos forum, has repeatedly **defended** these operations.

Speaking of Davos, Wikimedia has itself **amassed a fortune** of more than $160 million, donated in large part not by lazy students, but **by major US corporations** and influential **foundations**.

[..]

- https://off-guardian.org/2020/03/07/wikipedia-a-disinformation-operation/

****

Swiss Propaganda Research

From Wikipedia, the free encyclopedia

Swiss Propaganda Research (former)/ Swiss Policy Research (current)

Type of site	Propaganda, Conspiracy theories
Available in	German, English
Country of origin	Unknown
Owner	Unknown
Founder(s)	Unknown
Editor	Unknown
URL	swprs.org
Launched	2016
Current status	Active

Swiss Policy Research (SPR) or (before May 2020) **Swiss Propaganda Research** is a multi-language website launched in 2016, which describes itself as "an independent nonprofit research group investigating geopolitical propaganda in Swiss and international media". Based on its largely conspiratorial contents and its cherry picking of questionable scientific studies, it has been categorised by some as an anti-establishment propaganda site. The editors of the website are unknown, but they state that "SPR is composed of independent academics and receives no external funding." Contrary to what the name 'Swiss Propaganda Research' suggests, it has been speculated that the site might not actually be managed by people from Switzerland.

Criticism

The site has been criticised for spreading conspiracy theories and especially so during the times of the COVID-19 pandemic when it has become a source of misinformation and disinformation internationally. SPR has been categorized by some as a tool of propaganda.

In 2017 a University of Zurich report on media in Switzerland analyzed "six of the most discussed alternative media", including SPR. Daniel Vogler concluded that SPR "resorts to conspiracy theories", and its contents are mostly "pseudo-scientific".

Andrea Haefely wrote a critique of the website in the magazine *Beobachter* in May 2020, noting: "The website Swiss Propaganda Research assumes that the Swiss media does what it itself does: feed the readers with questionable information." He also suggested that the persistent use of the letter ß on the site suggests that the content creator is likely to be from outside Switzerland, as this particular letter form is not in common use in the country.

Stephan Russ-Mohl, professor of Journalism and Media Management at the Università della Svizzera italiana considers the articles on the SPRS to themselves serve as propaganda, rather than being serious research on the subject. He has noted that the anonymity of the website creates doubts over the reliability and authenticity of its research, particularly in a country such as Switzerland, which has full freedom of its press.

- https://en.wikipedia.org/wiki/Swiss_Propaganda_Research

****

June 28, 2020, 3:50PM (Inquiring Librarian to group):

From the article in the LAV:

"Newsguard's advisory board makes it clear that Newsguard was created to serve the interests of American oligarchy. Chief among Newsguard's advisors are Tom Ridge, the first Secretary of Homeland Security under George W. Bush and Ret. General Michael Hayden, a former CIA director, a

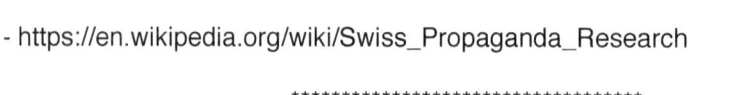

former NSA director and principal at the Chertoff Group, a security consultancy seeking to "advise corporate clients and governments, including foreign governments" on security matters that was co-founded by former Homeland Security Secretary Michael Chertoff, who also currently serves as the board chairman of major weapons manufacturer BAE systems." Newsguard started as a partnership between Steven Brill and Louis Gordon Crovitz, with Crovitz appearing to be the connection to the world of finance, media, and geopolitics. Crovitz held a number of positions at Dow Jones and at the Wall Street Journal, is a board member of Business Insider, a member of the Council on Foreign Relations, and claims to have been an "editor or contributor to books published by the American Enterprise Institute and Heritage Foundation." As Webb noted, "*the American Enterprise Institute (AEI) is one of the most influential neoconservative think tanks in the country and its 'scholars,' directors and fellows have included neoconservative figures like Paul Wolfowitz, Richard Perle, John Bolton and Frederick Kagan.*

& onward... Africa Check's list of partners includes The Bill and Melinda Gates Foundation... Gates also funded the Event 201 pandemic simulation exercise which discussed the potential for censoring the internet or even arresting individuals who spread information that has been deemed false. Africa Check is also partnered with the George Soros-funded Open Society Foundations.

& Onward... Facebook has partnered with the Atlantic Council: Essentially, the Atlantic Council is a think tank which can offer companies or nation states access to military officials, politicians, journalists, diplomats, etc., to help them develop a plan to implement their strategy or vision. These strategies often involve getting NATO governments or industry insiders to make decisions they might not have made without a visit from the Atlantic Council team. This allows individuals or nations to push forth their ideas under the cover of hiring what appears to be a public relations agency but is actually selling access to high-profile individuals with power to affect public policy. Indeed, everyone from George H.W. Bush to Bill Clinton to the family of international agent of disorder Zbigniew Brzezinski have spoken at or attended council events.

Anyways, this is all in the article in my response to Amir-ul Kafirs . There is a TON of info. in there. And from the the Swiss Propaganda Research page itself, the current Wikimedia Foundation executive director previously worked at the US Council on Foreign Relations (CFR) as well as at a subgroup of the US National Endowment for Democracy (NED), a US soft power organization involved in international information operations and regime change campaigns. Whitney Webb's article particularly looks indepth at NewsGuard's censoring: https://www.mintpressnews.com/newsguardneocon-backed-fact-checker-plans-to-wage-war-on-independent-media/253687/

This stuff really hits right at the heart for me. My job as a librarian is supposed to be about open access to all information for all people. And yet, none of my fellow librarian coworkers seem to understand what is going on right now and they smugly use these fact checkers and wait for the next NYT article with baited breath and seem to relish in the fear mongering and shaming those that do not comply or agree with big pharma government. To think that library leadership has actually embraced NewsGuard's censorship platforms for our nation's public libraries is shameful and appalling to me. To know that if I speak out I will most likely be shamed and fired, stands against everything that I believe libraries and librarianship stand for.

****

June 28, 2020, 7:48PM (Dick to group):

my friend Cèdric Vallet sent me this image (see below)
i thought you may find it amusing
*
and I offer a thought:

i know someone who owns a store in baltimore
today she told me that business is booming
she says that the bulk of her clients are, for the first time since she opened the store five years ago, black
that they are coming and spending their government checks like there's no tomorrow
this leads me to have the following "what if" thought : what if these checks are a way to buy compliance? if people who have no money (which describes a huge percentage of black baltimoreans) suddenly get windfalls (the same store owner said some people have told her they are getting 5,000$ a month, i have no idea why) this could actually make them hope for another lock-down

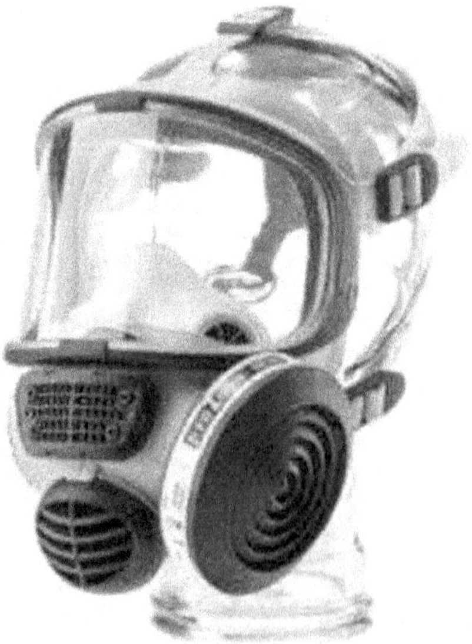

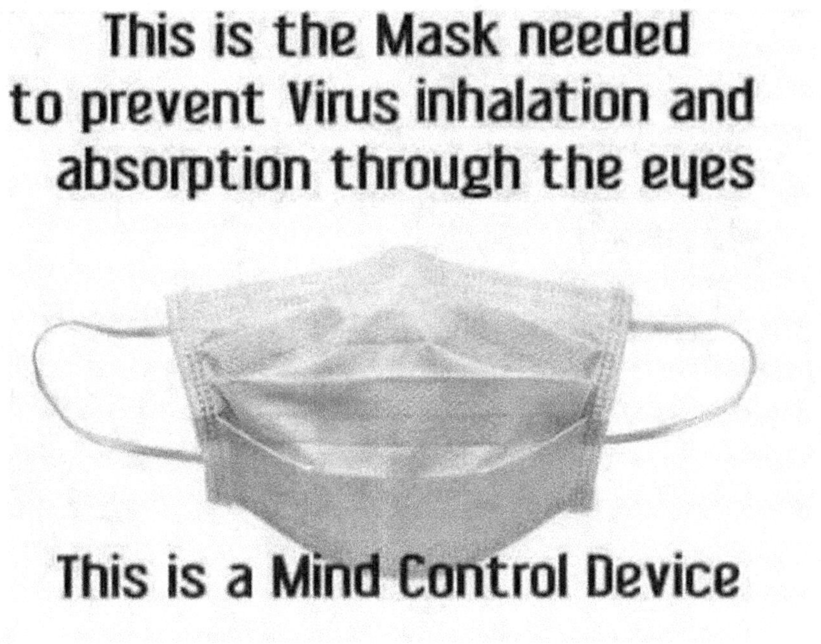
This is the Mask needed
to prevent Virus inhalation and
absorption through the eyes
This is a Mind Control Device

****

June 28, 2020, 8:12PM (Dick to group):

Here's is something funny in a new world order kind of way
I watch chess analysis videos from time to time hoping that something will stick
yesterdays this channel's live podcast was suddenly taken off the air for having "dangerous or harmful content"
he was analyzing a chess game
he posted this video today

https://www.youtube.com/watch?v=KSjrYWPxsG8

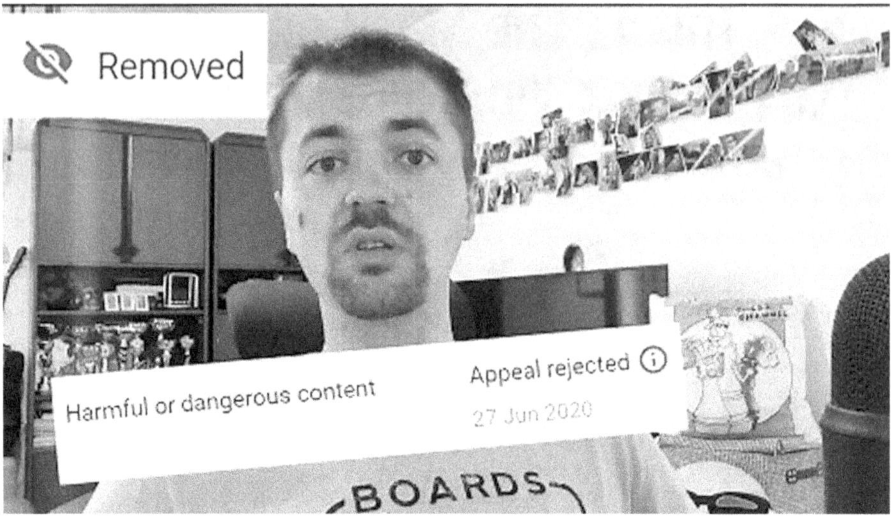

Youtube Takes Down CHESS PODCAST for Being HARMFUL or DANGEROUS
The Podcast with Hikaru is up again https://www.youtube.com/watch?v=vrFa4B0Ghjk&feature=youtu.be Check out my game against Hikaru here https://www.youtube.com/watch?v=TgPp7ltPd8Y Listen to the podcast here: Buzzsprout https://www.buzzsprout.com/1092209/episodes/4329299 Google Podcasts https://podcasts.google.com/feed ...

****

June 28, 2020, 9:08PM (Inquiring Librarian to group):

I love this image Dick! If only i could share it with my library administration, but certainly it would lead to 'progressive discipline'. :/

It is possible the hefty checks are keeping ppl begging for more lockdowns. I do know the unemployment is more right now in the u.s. than my salary.

I feel like the ppl are really just super brainwashed and i question their intelligence, sadly.

The deep south right now is on major panic mode over a surge of new cases. It is driving me nuts. The mask naziism is at its illogical height. On masks, listen here to bobby kennedy jr relating it to mind control and submission and the whole virus being tooled as fear mongering for use as a scared population being the most easily manipulated just as the Nazis did in ww2. Bobby Kennedy jr speaks 1 hr 30 min in
https://youtu.be/h5GH_O9GBxU

****

June 28, 2020, 11:49PM (Inquiring Librarian to group):

HERETICS: Vaccine Panic

I am still in vaccine panic mode. Check out this terrifying article from Forbes. I hope that Forbes is being as full of B.S. as usual in this article. But if it is true, it's pretty awful:
https://www.forbes.com/sites/greatspeculations/2020/06/26/how-does-modernas-covid-vaccine-timing-compare-with-jnj-and-pfizer/#5f315de45de2
Here is a quote from the middle of the article, and keep in mind, Moderna is making the mRNA vaccine that will basically genetically modify you, and an mRNA vaccine has never been used in humans before. And the animal trial was skipped in this one.

"Moderna also said that it is on track to deliver roughly 500 million doses of the vaccine per year, and potentially up to 1 billion doses annually, starting from 2021"

& check out this transcript from an interview with Robert F. Kennedy Jr. where he talks about how horrible the last few Corona Virus vaccines went. A quote from it:

"*The government has been trying for almost thirty years to develop a coronavirus vaccine, and it's been unsuccessful.*"

You can read the entire article here: *https://childrenshealthdefense.org/news/covid-19-robert-f-kennedy-jr-and-del-bigtree-talk-about-the-vaccine/*

Ok, and if you have kids, DO NOT, send them to school in Tennessee, apparently students there will be required to get flu shots and any new coronavirus vaccines. Egads!! How do we kill the overlords?? How about we shoot Bill Gates and those in charge at the WHO and the CDC with their own vaccines, pronto, it's an "Emergency!"? *https://www.wjhl.com/coronavirus/new-rule-requires-tennessee-students-to-get-flu-vaccines/*

****

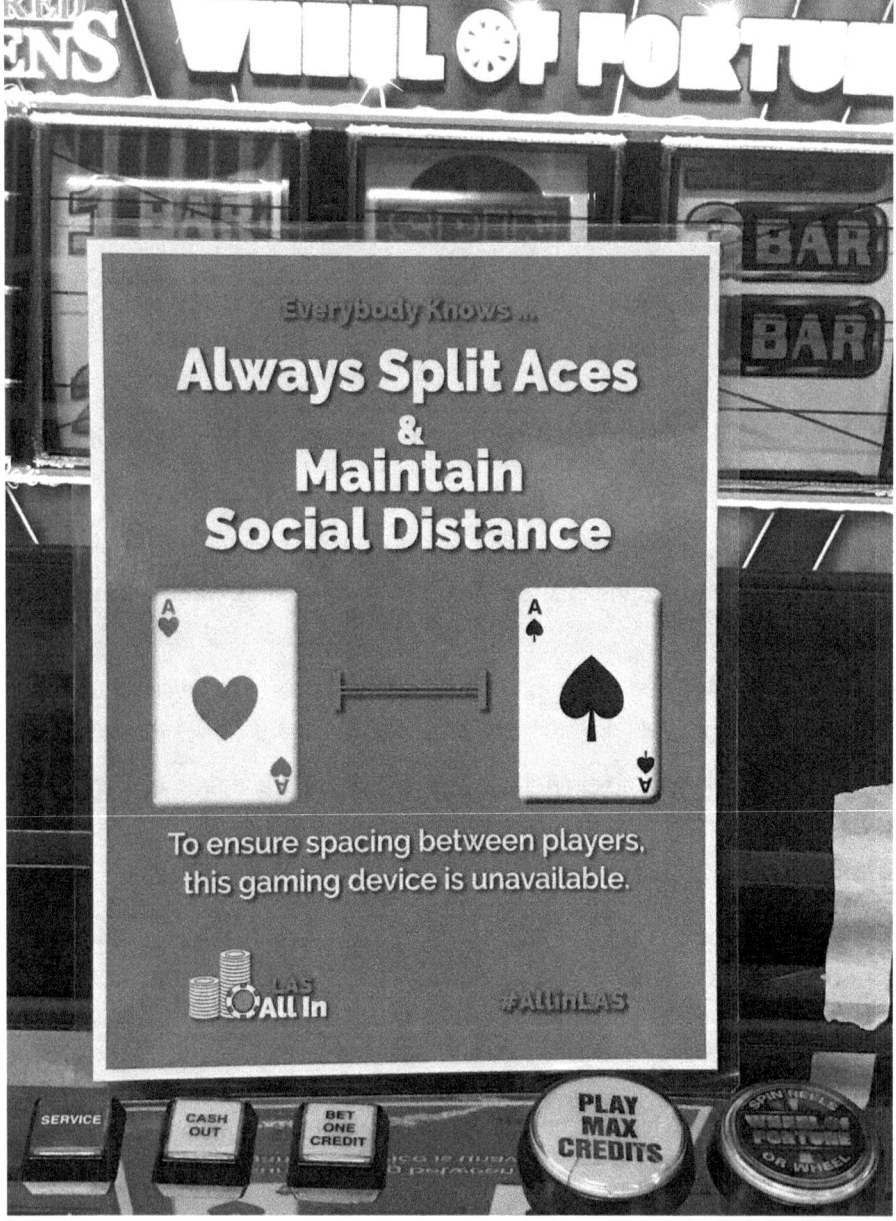
WHEEL OF FORTU
BAR
BAR
Everybody Knows ...
Always Split Aces
&
Maintain
Social Distance
A
A
To ensure spacing between players,
this gaming device is unavailable.
LAS
All In
#AllinLAS
SERVICE
CASH OUT
BET ONE CREDIT
PLAY MAX CREDITS

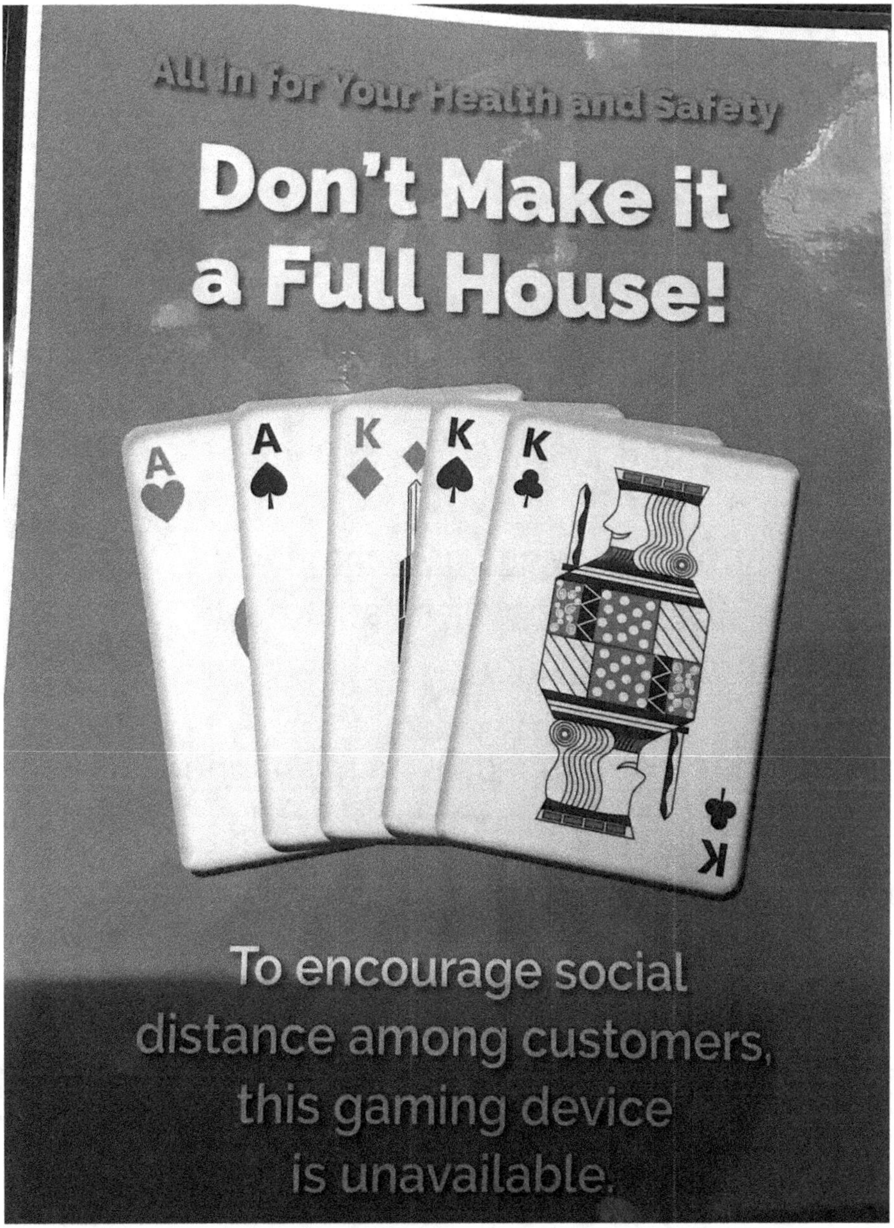

pictures that Naia Nisnam sent from Las Vegas

****

June 29, 2020, afternoon in the Las Vegas airport (Naia Nisnam to Amir-ul Kafirs txt msg):

https://www.cdc.gov/coronavirus/2019-ncov/travelers/after-travel-precautions.html.

This just popped up on my phone through my mapping service!!
They know I'm at an airport??

****

Naia Nisnam in Vegas Airport

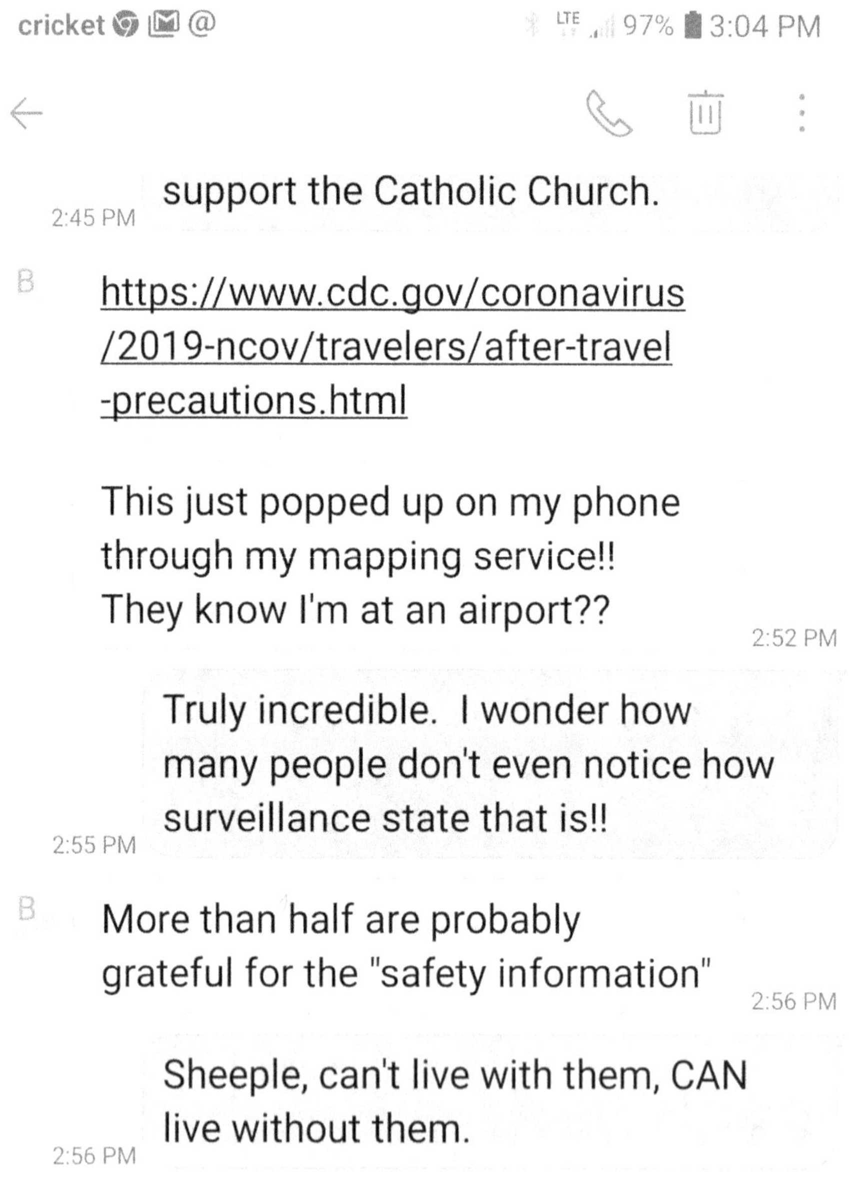

cricket
LTE 97% 3:04 PM
support the Catholic Church.
2:45 PM
B
https://www.cdc.gov/coronavirus/2019-ncov/travelers/after-travel-precautions.html
This just popped up on my phone through my mapping service!! They know I'm at an airport??
2:52 PM
Truly incredible. I wonder how many people don't even notice how surveillance state that is!!
2:55 PM
B
More than half are probably grateful for the "safety information"
2:56 PM
Sheeple, can't live with them, CAN live without them.
2:56 PM

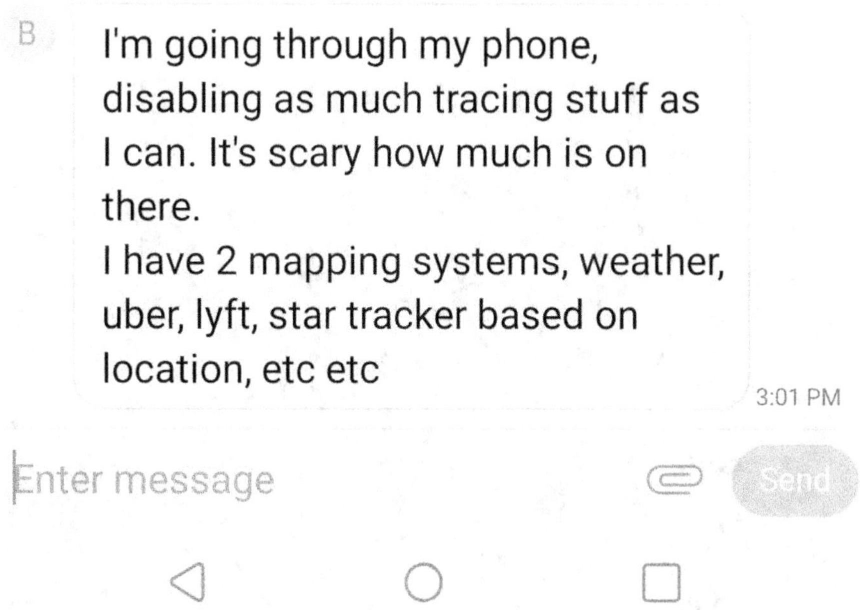

B
I'm going through my phone, disabling as much tracing stuff as I can. It's scary how much is on there.
I have 2 mapping systems, weather, uber, lyft, star tracker based on location, etc etc
3:01 PM
Enter message
Send

****

This is what I got when I tried to click on that link from my computer at home:

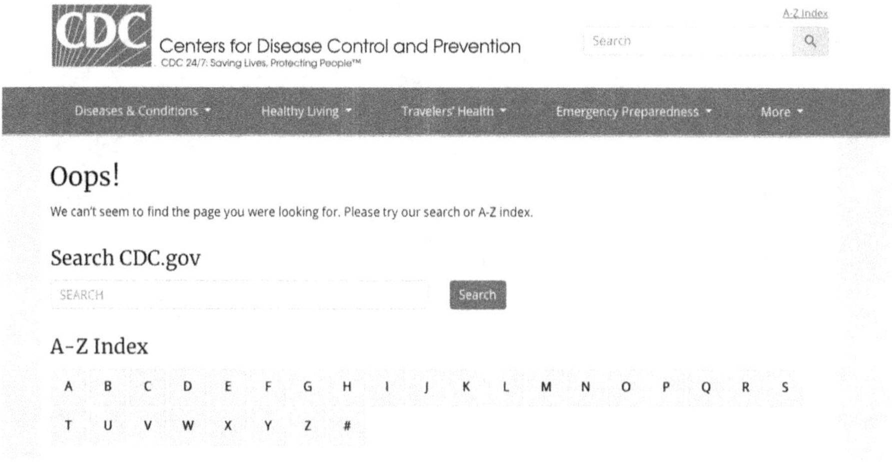

****

HOWEVER, the link still works on my phone so I screen shot it in multiple takes & emailed them to myself:

cricket 88% 6:04 PM

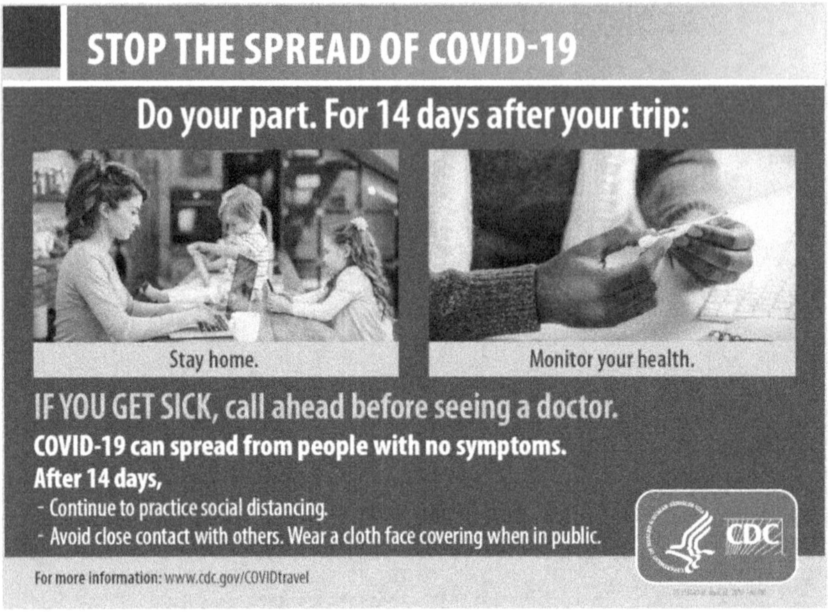

Download English version

[PDF – 2 pages]

Stay home for 14 days from the time you returned home from international travel.

During this 14-day period, take these steps

international travel.

During this 14-day period, take these steps to monitor your health and practice social distancing:

1. Take your temperature with a thermometer two times a day and monitor for fever. Also watch for cough or trouble breathing. Use this temperature log to monitor your temperature.
2. Stay home and avoid contact with others. Do not go to work or school.

3. Do not take public transportation, taxis, or ride-shares.
4. Keep your distance from others (about 6 feet or 2 meters).

What To Do If You Get Sick

If you get sick with fever or cough in the 14

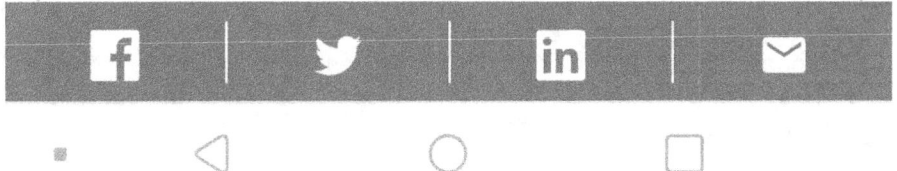

****

June 29, 2020, 3:41PM (Naia Nisnam to group):

Re: HERETICS: Vaccine Panic

It is truly scary that a University has made vaccines mandatory- and for the regular yearly flu too! Why??

A company has come out w a treatment but it is prohibitively expensive. They won't give us an affordable treatment when they really want to vaccinate us.

News story about the treatment:

https://www.nbcnews.com/health/health-news/remdesivir-coronavirus-gilead-charge-thousands-treatment-u-s-n1232385?fbclid=IwAR1Jar9qW_UwIDVvySk13nrskV5pYAKvpIQuhLTq3djvyGM0F_-btOV9BRE

CEO of the drug manufacturer company justifying the price:

https://stories.gilead.com/articles/an-open-letter-from-daniel-oday-june-29

****

Remdesivir for coronavirus: Gilead to charge thousands for treatment in U.S.

Price of $3,120 for patients with private insurance draws criticism. Out-of-pocket costs depend on insurance, income and other factors.

June 29, 2020, 9:04 AM EDT / Updated June 29, 2020, 1:07 PM EDT
By Associated Press

The maker of a drug shown to shorten recovery time for severely ill COVID-19 patients says it will charge $2,340 for a typical treatment course for people covered by government health programs in the United States and other developed countries.

Gilead Sciences announced the price Monday for remdesivir, and said the price would be $3,120 for patients with private insurance. The amount that patients pay out of pocket depends on insurance, income and other factors.

"We're in uncharted territory with pricing a new medicine, a novel medicine, in a pandemic," Gilead's chief executive, Dan O'Day, told The Associated Press. "We believe that we had to really deviate from the normal circumstances" and price the drug to ensure wide access rather than based solely on value to patients, he said.

However, the price was swiftly criticized; a consumer group called it "an outrage" because of the amount taxpayers invested toward its development.

The treatment courses that the company has donated to the U.S. and other countries will run out in about a week, and the prices will apply to the drug after that, O'Day said.

In the U.S., federal health officials have allocated the limited supply to states, but that agreement with Gilead will end after September. They said Monday that the government has secured more than 500,000 additional courses that Gilead will produce starting in July to supply to hospitals through September.

"We should have sufficient supply ... but we have to make sure it's in the right place at the right time," O'Day said

In 127 poor or middle-income countries, Gilead is allowing generic makers to supply the drug; two countries are doing that for around $600 per treatment course.

[..]

- https://www.nbcnews.com/health/health-news/remdesivir-coronavirus-gilead-charge-thousands-treatment-u-s-n1232385?fbclid=IwAR1Jar9qW_UwIDVvySk13nrskV5pYAKvplQuhLTq3djvyGM0F_-btOV9BRE

****

An Open Letter from Daniel O'Day, Chairman & CEO, Gilead Sciences

Daniel O'Day - June 29, 2020

In the weeks since we learned of remdesivir's potential against COVID-19, one topic has attracted more speculation than any other: what price we might set for the medicine. This degree of speculation is understandable. Remdesivir, our investigational treatment, is the first antiviral to have demonstrated patient improvement in clinical trials for COVID-19 and there is no playbook for how to price a new medicine in a pandemic. We are aware of the significant responsibility that comes with pricing remdesivir, and the need to be transparent on our decision. After giving this the considerable care, time and amount of discussion that it merits, we are now ready to share our decision and explain how we reached it.

As with all our actions on remdesivir, we approached this with the aim of helping as many patients as possible, as quickly as possible and in the most responsible way. This has been our compass point throughout, from collaborating to find rapid answers on safety and efficacy, to scaling up manufacturing and donating our supply of remdesivir through the end of June. In each case, we recognized the need to do things differently to reflect the exceptional circumstances of the pandemic. Now, as we transition beyond the donation period and set a price for remdesivir, the same principle applies.

In normal circumstances, we would price a medicine according to the value it provides. The first results from the NIAID study in hospitalized patients with COVID-19 showed that remdesivir shortened time to recovery by an average of four days. Taking the example of the United States, earlier hospital discharge would result in hospital savings of approximately $12,000 per patient. Even just considering these immediate savings to the healthcare system alone, we can see the potential value that remdesivir provides. This is before we factor in the direct benefit to those patients who may have a shorter stay in the hospital.

We have decided to price remdesivir well below this value. To ensure broad and equitable access at a time of urgent global need, we have set a price for governments of developed countries of $390 per vial. Based on current treatment patterns, the vast majority of patients are expected to receive a 5-day treatment course using 6 vials of remdesivir, which equates to $2,340 per patient.

Part of the intent behind our decision was to remove the need for country by country negotiations on price. We discounted the price to a level that is affordable for developed countries with the lowest purchasing power. This price will be offered to all governments in developed countries around the world where remdesivir is approved or authorized for use. At the current price of $390 per vial, remdesivir is positioned to achieve the aim of providing immediate net savings for healthcare systems.

In the U.S., the same government price of $390 per vial will apply. Because of the way the U.S. system is set up and the discounts that government healthcare programs expect, the price for U.S. private insurance companies, will be $520 per vial. At the level we have priced remdesivir and with government programs in place, along with additional Gilead assistance as needed, we believe all patients will have access.

Gilead has entered into an agreement with the U.S. Department of Health and Human Services (HHS) whereby HHS and states will continue to manage allocation to hospitals until the end of September. After this period, once supplies are less constrained, HHS will no longer manage allocation.

In the developing world, where healthcare resources, infrastructure and economics are so different, we have entered into agreements with generic manufacturers to deliver treatment at a substantially lower cost. These alternative solutions are designed to ensure that all countries in the world can provide access to treatment.

Our work on remdesivir is far from done. We continue to explore its potential to help in this pandemic in various ways, such as evaluating treatment earlier in the course of the disease, in outpatient settings, with an inhaled formulation, in additional patient groups and in combination with other therapies. As we accumulate more data from global clinical trials and initiate many additional studies, we will understand more about the full value of remdesivir over time. Our teams also remain focused on increasing supplies to meet the high global demand. By the end of this year, we expect our investment on the development and manufacture of remdesivir to exceed $1 billion (U.S.) and our commitment will continue through 2021 and beyond.

In making our decision on how to price remdesivir, we considered the full scope of our responsibilities. We started with our immediate responsibility to ensure price is in no way a hindrance to ensuring rapid and broad treatment. We also balanced that with our longer-term responsibilities: to continue with our ongoing work on remdesivir, to maintain our long-term research in antivirals and to invest in scientific innovation that might help generations to come. As with many other aspects of this pandemic, we are in uncharted territory in pricing remdesivir. Ultimately, we were guided by the need to do things differently. As the world continues to reel from the human, social and economic impact of this pandemic, we believe that pricing remdesivir well below value is the right and responsible thing to do.

[..]

- https://stories.gilead.com/articles/an-open-letter-from-daniel-oday-june-29

****

June 29, 2020, 5:50PM (Inquiring Librarian to group):

Right, the Gates Foundation is hell bent on getting a vaccine out, not a treatment. He has created a multibillion dollar industry out of vaccine manufacture that involves all nations. You can see this Gates plan here, straight from the horse's mouth:
https://www.gatesnotes.com/Health/What-you-need-to-know-about-the-COVID-19-vaccine?fbclid=IwAR2uFdnpZtgswWkWM5KXF1b8DsvNh5O2LmNftooj3J7OmzFX2bUjA-7tCUY

& notice towards the end that he plans to unleash the newest vaccines on the populations of 3rd world and poor countries first, in the name of they need if first because they are the most vulnerable " I think that low-income countries should be some of the first to receive it, because people will be at a much higher risk of dying in those places." ... Sounds like planned genocide through experimentation to me. See how well this worked out from John F. Kennedy's writeup here where Kennedy addresses the tragedy of this strategy in the past with the failed polio vaccines that actually caused vaccine induced cases of polio on these disadvantaged populations; India actually told Gates and his Foundation to leave their country and take their vaccines with them, due to egregious vaccine injuries caused by the vaccines from 2000-2017: https://childrenshealthdefense.org/news/government-corruption/gates-globalist-vaccine-agenda-a-win-win-for-pharma-and-mandatory-vaccination/

& here too, another fun thing, but involving Fauci, the Dengue vaccine that failed horribly (with pathogenic priming, the same problem the covid-19 vaccine is likely to have) in the Phillipines, " In 2014, NIH, under Fauci, developed a Dengue vaccine which had some signals in it that there was pathogenic priming. In other words, in the clinical trials they saw some signs that you could get an antibody response but get much sicker when you were exposed, but they ignored them.

“They gave it to the Philippines, and they gave hundreds of thousands of children this vaccine, and when the Dengue came around those children became horribly ill and 600 of them died."

"In the Philippines today people are being criminally prosecuted for that. https://childrenshealthdefense.org/news/covid-19-robert-f-kennedy-jr-and-del-bigtree-talk-about-the-vaccine/?fbclid=IwAR1QB3ZAnm3f9rJ0_EA3mdBrR2h9F3Ee7QAuTdA8JVyLxRqkIM2jWteIMRM

****

THE VACCINE RACE, EXPLAINED

What you need to know about the COVID-19 vaccine

Humankind has never had a more urgent task than creating broad immunity for coronavirus.

By **Bill Gates** | April 30, 2020 10 minute read

One of the questions I get asked the most these days is when the world will be able to go back to the way things were in December before the coronavirus pandemic. My answer is always the same: when we have an almost perfect drug to treat COVID-19, or when almost every person on the planet has been vaccinated against coronavirus.

The former is unlikely to happen anytime soon. We'd need a miracle treatment that was at least 95 percent effective to stop the outbreak. Most of the drug candidates right now are nowhere near that powerful. They could save a lot of lives, but they aren't enough to get us back to normal.

Which leaves us with a vaccine.

Humankind has never had a more urgent task than creating broad immunity for coronavirus. Realistically, if we're going to return to normal, we need to develop a safe, effective vaccine. We need to make billions of doses, we need to get them out to every part of the world, and we need all of this to happen as quickly as possible.

That sounds daunting, because it is. Our foundation is the biggest funder of vaccines in the world, and this effort dwarfs anything we've ever worked on before. It's going to require a global cooperative effort like the world has never seen. But I know it'll get done. There's simply no alternative.

Here's what you need to know about the race to create a COVID-19 vaccine.

The world is creating this vaccine on a historically

fast timeline.

Dr. Anthony Fauci has said he thinks it'll take around eighteen months to develop a coronavirus vaccine. I agree with him, though it could be as little as 9 months or as long as two years.

Although eighteen months might sound like a long time, this would be the fastest scientists have created a new vaccine. Development usually takes around five years. Once you pick a disease to target, you have to create the vaccine and test it on animals. Then you begin testing for safety and efficacy in humans.
Safety and efficacy are the two most important goals for every vaccine. Safety is exactly what it sounds like: is the vaccine safe to give to people? Some minor side effects (like a mild fever or injection site pain) can be acceptable, but you don't want to inoculate people with something that makes them sick.

[..]

Once we have a vaccine, though, we still have huge problems to solve. That's because…

We need to manufacture and distribute at least 7 billion doses of the vaccine.

In order to stop the pandemic, we need to make the vaccine available to almost every person on the planet. We've never delivered something to every corner of the world before. And, as I mentioned earlier, vaccines are particularly difficult to make and store.

[..]

- https://www.gatesnotes.com/Health/What-you-need-to-know-about-the-COVID-19-vaccine?fbclid=IwAR2uFdnpZtgswWkWM5KXF1b8DsvNh5O2LmNftooj3J7OmzFX2bUjA-7tCUY

****

APRIL 09, 2020

Gates' Globalist Vaccine Agenda: A Win-Win for Pharma and Mandatory Vaccination

By Robert F. Kennedy Jr., Chairman, Children's Health Defense

Vaccines, for Bill Gates, are a strategic philanthropy that feed his many vaccine-related businesses (including Microsoft's ambition to control a global vaccination ID enterprise) and give him dictatorial control of global health policy. Gates' obsession with vaccines seems to be fueled by a conviction to save the world with technology.

Promising his share of $450 million of $1.2 billion to eradicate polio, Gates took control of India's National Technical Advisory Group on Immunization (NTAGI), which mandated up to 50 doses (Table 1) of polio vaccines through overlapping immunization programs to children before the age of five. Indian doctors blame the Gates campaign for a devastating non-polio acute flaccid paralysis (NPAFP) epidemic that paralyzed 490,000 children beyond expected rates between 2000 and 2017. In 2017, the Indian government dialed back Gates' vaccine regimen and asked Gates and his vaccine policies to leave India. NPAFP rates dropped precipitously.

The most frightening [polio] epidemics in Congo, Afghanistan, and the Philippines are all linked to vaccines.

In 2017, the World Health Organization (WHO) reluctantly admitted that the global explosion in polio is predominantly vaccine strain. The most frightening epidemics in Congo, Afghanistan, and the Philippines, are all linked to vaccines. In fact, by 2018, 70% of global polio cases were vaccine strain.

In 2009, the Gates Foundation funded tests of experimental HPV vaccines, developed by Glaxo Smith Kline (GSK) and Merck, on 23,000 young girls in remote Indian provinces. Approximately 1,200 suffered severe side effects, including autoimmune and fertility disorders. Seven died. Indian government investigations charged that Gates-funded researchers committed pervasive ethical violations: pressuring vulnerable village girls into the trial, bullying parents, forging consent forms, and refusing medical care to the injured girls. The case is now in the country's Supreme Court.

South African newspapers complained, 'We are guinea pigs for the drug makers.'

In 2010, the Gates Foundation funded a phase 3 trial of GSK's experimental malaria vaccine, killing 151 African infants and causing serious adverse effects, including paralysis, seizure, and febrile convulsions, to 1,048 of the 5,949 children.

During Gates' 2002 MenAfriVac campaign in Sub-Saharan Africa, Gates' operatives forcibly vaccinated thousands of African children against meningitis.

Approximately 50 of the 500 children vaccinated developed paralysis. South African newspapers complained, "We are guinea pigs for the drug makers." Nelson Mandela's former senior economist, Professor Patrick Bond, describes Gates' philanthropic practices as "ruthless and immoral."

In 2010, when Gates committed $10 billion to the WHO, he said "We must make this the decade of vaccines." A month later, Gates said in a TED Talk that new vaccines "could reduce population." And, four years later, in 2014, Kenya's Catholic Doctors Association accused the WHO of chemically sterilizing millions of unwilling Kenyan women with a "tetanus" vaccine campaign. Independent labs found a sterility formula in every vaccine tested. After denying the charges, WHO finally admitted it had been developing the sterility vaccines for over a decade. Similar accusations came from Tanzania, Nicaragua, Mexico, and the Philippines.

A 2017 study (Morgenson et. al. 2017) showed that WHO's popular DTP vaccine is killing more African children than the diseases it prevents. DTP-vaccinated girls suffered 10x the death rate of children who had not yet received the vaccine. WHO has refused to recall the lethal vaccine, which it forces upon tens of millions of African children annually.

[Global public health officials] say he has diverted agency resources to serve his personal philosophy that good health only comes in a syringe.

Global public health advocates around the world accuse Gates of steering WHO's agenda away from the projects that are proven to curb infectious diseases: clean water, hygiene, nutrition, and economic development. The Gates Foundation spends only about $650 million of its $5 billion dollar budget on these areas. They say he has diverted agency resources to serve his personal philosophy that good health only comes in a syringe.

In addition to using his philanthropy to control WHO, UNICEF, GAVI, and PATH, Gates funds a private pharmaceutical company that manufactures vaccines and is donating $50 million to 12 pharmaceutical companies to speed up development of a coronavirus vaccine. In his recent media appearances, Gates appears confident that the Covid-19 crisis will now give him the opportunity to force his dictatorial vaccine programs on all American children – and adults.

- https://childrenshealthdefense.org/news/government-corruption/gates-globalist-vaccine-agenda-a-win-win-for-pharma-and-mandatory-vaccination/

****

MAY 18, 2020

COVID-19: Robert F. Kennedy, Jr. and Del Bigtree Talk About the Vaccine

Are vaccines the answer to the Coronavirus outbreak? Don't miss this special episode of Table Talk as Robert F. Kennedy, Jr. and Del Bigtree join host Joni Lamb at the table discussing vaccinations and the truth behind their planned use against COVID-19.

Transcript**: The Coronavirus Vaccine Uncensored I Robert F. Kennedy Jr. & Del Bigtree**

Robert Kennedy, Jr.: "The government has been trying for almost thirty years to develop a coronavirus vaccine, and it's been unsuccessful.

"Beginning in 2002 there were three outbreaks of coronavirus. We called them SARS at that point and MERS.

"The first SARS was a natural illness. It jumped from a bat to human beings. The second two were lab created that escaped and infected human beings. So the governments of China and a consortium of western governments all got together and put millions and millions of dollars into an effort to develop a coronavirus vaccine.

"Between 2002 and 2012, 2014, they worked very hard to do that, and what happened is they developed about 35 vaccines. Four of them were really promising. They chose the four most promising, and they gave them to ferrets, which is the animal that is most analogous when it comes to upper lung respiratory infections.

"The ferrets had a brilliant, robust and durable antibody response. Then something horrible happened. When those ferrets were challenged, when they were exposed to the wild virus they got horribly sick. They got inflammation throughout their bodies, and they died.

"The scientists remembered that something very similar had happened in the 1960s where they had developed a virus for RSV, which is very similar to coronavirus. It's an upper respiratory infection, ailment.

"They had skipped the animals and given them directly to 35 children, and the children again had developed a very robust antibody response. But when those children were exposed to the wild virus, they got very, very sick, much sicker than the unvaccinated children. And two of those kids had died. It was a scandal.

"They realized when this same thing happened with the ferrets, that there was something that they called enhanced immune response. It's also called pathogenic priming.

“What it means is that when you get the vaccine, it appears that you have an antibody response. But when you actually encounter the wild virus, you actually become much sicker, and it actually creates a pathway that that virus hurts you a lot more than with unvaccinated people.

“So this was 2012. In 2014, NIH, under Fauci, developed a Dengue vaccine which had some signals in it that there was pathogenic priming. In other words, in the clinical trials they saw some signs that you could get an antibody response but get much sicker when you were exposed, but they ignored them.

“They gave it to the Philippines, and they gave hundreds of thousands of children this vaccine, and when the Dengue came around those children became horribly ill and 600 of them died.

“In the Philippines today people are being criminally prosecuted for that.
“The danger with the coronavirus vaccine is that you really need to test on animals first to make sure whatever the vaccine is, that we don’t get that really great immune response followed by lethal infections.

“It’s very, very strange to me, and it seems almost criminally reckless that Anthony Fauci is allowing these companies to skip animal trials and to go directly to human trials.”

[..]

- https://childrenshealthdefense.org/news/covid-19-robert-f-kennedy-jr-and-del-bigtree-talk-about-the-vaccine/?fbclid=IwAR1QB3ZAnm3f9rJ0_EA3mdBrR2h9F3Ee7QAuTdA8JVyLxRqkIM2jWteIMRM

****

June 29, 2020, 5:57PM (Inquiring Librarian to group):

& here too, Hydroxychloriquine was given terrible press through a medical journal review that has since proven to be retracted and scandalous... essentially lies to further the vastly more expensive Remdesivir: https://off-guardian.org/2020/06/23/the-deadly-hydroxychloroquine-publishing-scandal/

****

Jun 23, 2020

The “Deadly” Hydroxychloroquine Publishing Scandal

How the World's top medical journals were cynically exploited by Big Pharma

Elizabeth Woodworth

SUMMARY

A publishing scandal recently erupted around the use of the anti-malarial drug hydroxychloroquine (HCQ) to treat Covid 19. It is also known as quinine and chloroquine, and is on the **WHO list of essential medicines**.

The bark of the South American quina-quina tree has been used to **treat malaria for 400 years**. Quinine, a generic drug costing pennies a dose, is available for purchase online. **In rare cases** it can cause dizziness and irregular heartbeat. In late May, 2020, The Lancet published a **four-author study** claiming that HCQ used in hospitals to treat Covid-19 had been shown conclusively to be a hazard for heart death. The data allegedly covered 96,000 patients in 671 hospitals on six continents.

After the article had spent 13 days in the headlines, dogged by scientific objections, three of the authors retracted it on June 5.

Meanwhile, during an expert closed-door meeting leaked May 24 in France, The Lancet and NEJM editors explained how financially powerful pharmaceutical players were "criminally" corrupting medical science to advance their interests.

*

On May 22, 2020, the time-honoured Lancet – one of the world's two top medical journals – published the stunning claim that 671 hospitals on six continents were reporting life-threatening heart rhythms in patients taking hydroxychloroquine (HCQ) for Covid-19.

The headlines that followed were breath-taking.

Although wider access to the drug had recently been urged in a petition signed by **nearly 500,000 French doctors and citizens**, WHO and other agencies responded to the article by immediately suspending the clinical trials that may have cleared it for use.

North American headlines did not mention that HCQ has been on the WHO list of essential drugs since the list began in 1977. Nor did they mention an investigative report on the bad press that hydroxychloroquine had been getting prior to May 22, and how financial interests had been intersecting with medicine to favour Gilead's **new, more expensive drug, Remdesivir**.

THE STATISTICS BEHIND THE HEADLINES

As a Canadian health sciences librarian who delivered statistics to a large public health agency for 25 years, I sensed almost immediately that the article had to be flawed.

Why? Because health statistics are developed for different purposes and in different contexts, causing them to exist in isolated data **"stovepipes."** Many health databases, even within a single region or country, are not standardized and are thus virtually useless for comparative research.

How, I wondered, could 671 hospitals worldwide, including Asia and Africa, report comparable treatment outcomes for 96,000 Covid patients? And so quickly?

The Lancet is strong in public health and surely suspected this. Its award-winning editor-in-chief, **Dr. Richard Horton**, has been in his job since 1995.
So how could the damning HCQ claims have been accepted? Here is what I discovered.

THE HONOUR SYSTEM IN MEDICAL PUBLISHING

To some extent, authors submitting articles to medical journals are on the honour system, in which cited databases are trusted by the editors, yet are available for inspection if questioned.[**2**]

On May 28, an open letter from 200 scientists to the authors and The Lancet requested details of the data and an independent audit. The letter was "*signed by clinicians, medical researchers, statisticians, and ethicists from across the world."* (full text **here**.)

The authors declined to supply the data, or even the hospital names. Meanwhile, **investigative analysis** was showing the statistics to be **deeply flawed**.
If this were not enough, the lead author was found to be in a conflict of interest with HCQ's **rival drug, Remdesivir**:

Dr. Mandeep Mehra, the lead co-author is a director at Brigham & Women's Hospital, which is credited with funding the study. Dr. Mehra and The Lancet failed to disclose that Brigham Hospital has a partnership with Gilead and is currently conducting two trials testing Remdesivir, the prime competitor of hydroxychloroquine for the treatment of COVID-19, the focus of the study."
In view of the foregoing, the article was retracted by three of its authors on June 5.

How did this fraud get past The Lancet reviewers in the first place?

The answer emerges from what has remained an obscure French interview, although it has been **quoted in the alternative media**.

On May 24, a closed-door Chatham House expert meeting about Covid included the editors-in-chief of The Lancet and the NEJM. Comments regarding the article were leaked to the French press by a well-known health figure, **Dr. Philippe Douste-Blazy**,[xvii] who felt compelled to blow the whistle.

His resulting BFM TV **interview was posted to YouTube with English subtitles on May 31**, but it was not picked up by the English-speaking media. These were The Lancet editor Dr. Richard Horton's words, as reported by Dr. Douste-Blazy:

If this continues, we are not going to be able to publish any more clinical research data because pharmaceutical companies are so financially powerful today, and are able to use such methodologies as to have us accept papers which are apparently methodologically perfect, but which, in reality, manage to conclude what they want to conclude."

Doust-Blazy made his own comments on Horton's words:

I never thought the boss of The Lancet could say that. And the boss of the New England Journal of Medicine too. He even said it was 'criminal'. The word was used by them."

The final words in Doust-Blazy's interview were:

When there is an outbreak like Covid, in reality, there are people like us – doctors – who see mortality and suffering. And there are people who see dollars. That's it."

The scientific process of building a trustworthy knowledge base is one of the foundations of our civilization. Violating this process is a crime against both truth and humanity.

Evidently the North American media does not consider this extraordinary crime to be worth reporting.

Originally published at Global Research. An interesting side note, before this fake study was published, Dr Wolfgang Wodarg theorised that use of HCQ may explain the higher death rate in patients of African ancestry – ed.

Notes:-
[1] Famous weekly British medical journal, founded in 1823.
[2] The Lancet and NEJM editors could not be expected to comb through data from 671 hospitals to verify their accuracy – especially when submitted by four doctors.

- https://off-guardian.org/2020/06/23/the-deadly-hydroxychloroquine-publishing-scandal/

****

June 29, 2020, 6:36PM (Amir-ul Kafirs to group):

CEO of the drug manufacturer company justifying the price

Gotta love the 'logic': here're some quotes from the above company PR:

"As with all our actions on remdesivir, we approached this with the aim of helping as many patients as possible, as quickly as possible and in the most responsible way."

[..]

"In normal circumstances, we would price a medicine according to the value it provides. The first results from the NIAID study in hospitalized patients with COVID-19 showed that remdesivir shortened time to recovery by an average of four days. Taking the example of the United States, earlier hospital discharge would result in hospital savings of approximately $12,000 per patient. Even just considering these immediate savings to the healthcare system alone, we can see the potential value that remdesivir provides. This is before we factor in the direct benefit to those patients who may have a shorter stay in the hospital.

We have decided to price remdesivir well below this value.

To ensure broad and equitable access at a time of urgent global need, we have set a price for governments of developed countries of $390 per vial."

SO, the "value it provides" is ordinarily how much it would hypothetically cost to not use the medicine **in a hospital setting**. Not only is that a little difficult to prove, it also just says: *the Medical Industry is gonna get that money one way or another.* What if the hospital is overcharging? What if the sick person is NOT in a hospital & wants it at home? Will it then be free?

Let's look at it a different way: What if they prove to us how much they've spent on developing the medicine. That development cost **should not include whatever insane pay the CEO of the company is getting**. THEN, what if the $70,000,000.00 or so that the taxpayer invested in this development were to be factored in: let's say that the 70 mil is a mere 7% of their development costs: Does that mean that the taxpayer gets 7% of the profit? Anyway, let's find out what their real profit is after materials, research, & pay of personnel & other infrastructure costs: let's take a guess & say that 50% of the price is profit (although I imagine it's much higher). Can we, the taxpayers, as investors, vote on whether we consider that to be too much?

****

June 29, 2020, 9:36PM (Amir-ul Kafirs to group):

I believe this article goes in depth behind the scenes of the funders and editors of the 'Fact Checkers'

Ok, I read that article by Derrick Broze in "The Last American Vagabond" &, if I understand it correctly, he says that The Atlantic Council is the main 'fact checking' organization used by Facebook to discredit groups on FB whose content they disapprove of:

"In January 2018, PropOrNot would be exposed for their connections to The Atlantic Council, a think tank with connections to the western Military-Industrial Complex. Coincidentally, in May 2018, Facebook announced a partnership with the Atlantic Council, which officially claims to provide a forum for international political, business, and intellectual leaders. The social media giant said the partnership was aimed at preventing Facebook from "being abused during elections."

The press release promoted Facebook's efforts to fight fake news by using artificial intelligence, as well as working with outside experts and governments. ***"Today, we're excited to launch a new partnership with the Atlantic Council, which has a stellar reputation looking at innovative solutions to hard problems. Experts from their Digital Forensic Research Lab will work closely with our security, policy and product teams to get Facebook real-time insights and updates on emerging threats and disinformation campaigns from around the world. This will help increase the number of "eyes and ears" we have working to spot potential abuse on our service — enabling us to more effectively identify gaps in our systems, preempt obstacles, and ensure that Facebook plays a positive role during elections all around the world."***

The Atlantic Council of the United States was established in 1961 to bolster support for international relations. Although not officially connected to the North Atlantic Treaty Organization, the Atlantic Council has spent decades promoting causes and issues which are beneficial to NATO member states. In addition, The Atlantic Council is a member of the Atlantic Treaty Organization, an umbrella organization which "acts as a network facilitator in the Euro-Atlantic and beyond." The ATO works similarly to the Atlantic Council, bringing together political leaders, academics, military officials, journalists and diplomats to promote values that are favorable to the NATO member states.
Officially, ATO is independent of NATO, but the line between the two is razor thin."

Sttrictly speaking, though, I'd like to know EXACTLY who the "independent fact checkers" are that say that the Vaxxed Global Movement post is false. In other words, FB only refers to these 'fact checkers' in general terms: maybe it's The Atlantic Council, maybe it's somebody else. Let's say it IS only The Atlantic Council. Here's what Broze has to say about their funding:

"The Atlantic Council's list of financial supporters reads like a who's-who of think tanks and Non-Governmental Organizations. The Atlantic Council receives funding from the Brookings Institution, Carnegie Endowment, Cato Institute, Council on Foreign Relations, and the Rand Corporation, to name a few. In addition, various members of the Military-Industrial Complex are benefactors of the Atlantic Council, including Huntington Ingalls, the United States' sole maker of aircraft carriers; Airbus, the plane manufacturer; Lockheed Martin, the shipbuilder and aviation company; and Raytheon, which makes missile systems. All of the companies have contracts with the U.S. Department of Defense and offer financial support to the Atlantic Council. The Council also receives support from Chevron and the Thomson Reuters Foundation. Finally, the Atlantic Council receives direct financial support from the U.S. Departments of the Air Force, Army, Navy and Energy and from the U.S. Mission to NATO."

What I'm looking for is a ***direct connection between vaccine interests & the funding of The Atlantic Council's dismissal of anti-vaccine positions.*** I'm the 1st to speculate that The Atlantic Council is being cagey & that they're avoiding getting caught in such a connection but unless someone *proves* a direct connection it's hard to dismiss The Atlantic Council's position on ***conflict of interest grounds*** — which is what I'd like to do.

Next, consider Wikipedia. Check out this article on the wonderful site that we've all shared, the Swiss Propagand Research website, vs. Wikipedia's scathing article about the site:
https://off-guardian.org/2020/03/07/wikipedia-a-disinformation-operation/

It's actually on the OffGuardian website but it's written by the Swiss Propaganda Research folks.

ALRIGHT, I've been ranting about Wikipedia almost since it began (January 15, 2001, according to Wikipedia itself). I'm not even sure I have the energy to get into it in detail here but I'll try. I made a few experimental attempts to contribute content to Wikipedia early on. Admittedly, I was being provocative. I read the entry for Johns Hopkins University & saw it as a puff piece, in other words *not* as an 'objective' entry but as an advertisement for the university (it was full of bits about how brilliant a place it is for scholars (or some such)). Since I'm from Baltimore & have lived near Johns Hopkins (& even had screenings there, etc) I have some knowledge of the place. They were reputed to've fired a professor for being Marxist, I should probably try to determine who that was but that's too much of a tangent right now. One of the two people who invented the Dalkon Shield IUD, Hugh J. Davis, was a physician and professor of gynecology and obstetrics at Johns Hopkins University. That's easier to research. Here's an article:

The Dalkon Shield

By: *Rainey Horwitz*

Published: *2018-01-10*
Keywords: Contraception

The Dalkon Shield was an intrauterine contraceptive device (IUD) that women used in the early 1970s and 1980s. Produced by the A.H. Robins Company in the US, the Dalkon Shield was a contraceptive device placed directly into a woman's uterus that was supposed to prevent pregnancy. In the 1980s, researchers discovered that the Dalkon Shield caused an array of severe injuries, including pelvic infection, infertility, unintended pregnancy, and death. Eventually the A.H. Robins Company took the shield off the market, and the US Food and Drug Administration banned the device. Many users of the Dalkon Shield sued the production company and were awarded millions of dollars in compensation and punitive damages. After the dangers of the Dalkon Shield became public through those lawsuits, the popularity of intrauterine devices decreased significantly in the US.

In the early 1970s, Hugh J. Davis and Irwin Lerner invented the Dalkon Shield. At the time, Davis was a physician and professor of gynecology and obstetrics at Johns Hopkins University in Baltimore, Maryland. Davis argued that birth control pills were so hazardous that physicians prescribing them were behaving irresponsibly. The other inventor, Irwin Lerner, was an engineer and helped Davis design the Dalkon Shield as a safer alternative to birth control pills.
As an intrauterine device, physicians placed the Dalkon Shield directly into a woman's uterus. The Dalkon Shield consisted of a plastic five-pronged, crab-like shield, which prevented the uterus from expelling the device. It also contained small amounts of copper that acted as a spermicide, preventing sperm from fertilizing an egg. The device was attached at the base to a string made from various filaments, similar to the string of a tampon, which **[t]**he**[n]** was used to remove the device. In the early 1970s, when Davis and Irwin began selling the Dalkon Shield, the device was not subject to any extensive testing by the US Food and Drug Administration because it was not considered a drug.

The Dalkon Shield was originally produced by the Dalkon Corporation, founded by Davis soon after the invention of the IUD. In 1971, the A.H. Robins Company, producers of the cough medicine Robitussin, bought the device from Davis and put it on the market. The A.H. Robins Company began selling the Shields in the US and Puerto Rico and launched a large marketing campaign for the device. The campaign emphasized the safety of the IUD compared to traditional contraceptive pills. According to reporter Robert Thomas, prior to government regulation of birth control, many Americans were concerned with the safety of birth control pills and sought safer alternatives. The manufacturers of the Dalkon Shield capitalized on that, claiming that the device was safer than existing methods of birth control. Although physicians initially expressed skepticism about the effectiveness of the device, many of their reports did not identify safety issues with the device. After three years on the market, physicians had prescribed the Dalkon Shield to over 2.2 million women. According to Thomas, the Dalkon Shield was the most popular IUD on the US market in the 1970s.

However, by 1971, women who had used the device reported septic infections and other complications that led them to seek serious medical attention. Researchers discovered that the string attached to the Shield was not sealed at the end, causing the string to fray and disintegrate. The string drew vaginal bacteria into the uterus, resulting in septic infection, miscarriage, and an array of other related complications, including death. In response to claims about the dangers of the Dalkon Shield in the early 1970s, the A.H. Robins Company argued that any complications with the device should be attributed to the doctors who improperly inserted the devices. However, after several years of distribution, women reported that in addition to causing complications, the device did not protect them against pregnancy. Instead, researchers found that the device led to increased risk of pregnancy complications due to its design.

In June of 1973, the US Centers for Disease Control and Prevention, or CDC, conducted a study on the safety of IUDs, including the Dalkon Shield. Researchers at the CDC gathered information from 16,994 obstetricians and gynecologists regarding the frequency of hospitalizations, deaths, and other complications related to IUD use during a six-month period. During the six-month period, researchers found that the Dalkon Shield was the most popular IUD on the market. They also determined that the Dalkon Shield was correlated to an increased rate of pregnancy-associated complications, including septic pregnancies, or a bacterial infection of the placenta and fetus. Those complications were serious enough that they usually led to hospitalization. Despite the CDC study released in 1973, around 2.5 million women were still using the Dalkon Shield the following year. In a separate study conducted by the University of Southampton Department of Human Reproduction and Obstetrics, in Southampton, England, researchers suggested that the Dalkon Shield was an advancement in IUD technology and had advantages compared to other IUDs.

In June of 1974, the medical director of the A.H. Robins Company, J.S. Templeton published a letter to the editor of the *British Medical Journal* in which he discussed the medical issues associated with the Dalkon Shield. In the report, the director claimed that the company was aware of the apparent trend of septic abortions and infections in women using the device, including several deaths. However, Templeton also stated that there was no direct evidence that the Dalkon Shield was responsible for the bacterial septic poisoning and related issues. Rather, Templeton claimed that the increase of cases of septic abortions was due to the general increase in use of IUDs and not specifically the Dalkon Shield. On 28 June 1974, the A.H. Robins Company took the Dalkon Shield off the market. However, they did not recall the devices that had previously been sold.

In October of 1974, the journal *Obstetrics and Gynecology* published several studies on the high frequency septic pregnancies associated with the Dalkon Shield. A year later, in 1975, the CDC published a study in which the authors claimed that the Dalkon Shield came with a higher risk of abortion-related deaths than other IUDs. After the publication of those studies, the A.H. Robin Company discontinued production of the Dalkon Shield. However, the company persisted in not recalling devices that had already been sold.

After several years of national distribution of the Dalkon Shield, over 200,000 women made claims that the device had caused serious medical consequences, including pelvic inflammatory disease, miscarriage, and loss of fertility. There were at least eighteen reported deaths caused by the device. By 1976, the US Congress passed federal legislation mandating that the US Food and Drug Administration require safety and efficacy testing of IUDs prior to approval. Though the A.H. Robins Company claimed that the Shield was not any more dangerous than other IUDs, women filed over 300,000 lawsuits against the A.H. Robins Company. By the fall of 1984, the company's insurance firm had settled around 7,600 claims for around $245 million dollars. In October of 1984, the A.H Robins company released a media campaign advising women who were still wearing the Dalkon Shield to have it removed by a doctor. That campaign required the company to pay over 4,500 medical bills from doctors that had removed the device. By the end of 1985, the A.H. Robins company was facing lawsuits from people in every state of the US. The company filed for bankruptcy in 1985. Before being sold to American Home Products in 1989, the A.H. Robins company established a $615 million-dollar fund to pay for the settlements of the remaining lawsuits.

[..]

- https://embryo.asu.edu/pages/dalkon-shield

My point is that while Hopkins has a shining unblemished reputation as presented on Wikipedia there're at least a few blemishes in their actual record.

SO, me being the *contestaire* that I am, I edited the Hopkins Wikipedia entry to relfect these blemishes. I don't remember exactly what I said anymore but I probably mentioned the Dalkon Shield. I **definitely** wrote something to the effect that Hopkins was known locally as "The Plantation" because of the way it existed 'above' the surrounding communities & because of the way it raised local real estate prices to a level unaffordable to the actual locals. Now, it's probable that *only **I*** call Hopkins "The Plantation" so, admittedly, this was a somewhat unsupportable snipe — even though I hold to the accuracy of what I said otherwise.

ANYWAY, what I learned from this was interesting: *within **minutes*** my edits were removed. I tried to re-enter them & they were immediately removed again. I later learned that this was the action of people called "Wikigardeners" whose job it was to remove the 'weeds'. My friend Florian Cramer posted my report on the matter to a list on net activiities where I proceeded to get into a brief argument with someone who was supporting Wikipedia's action by saying that they had "separated noise from signal". NOW, *that was totally disingenuous* since nothing that I wrote could accurately be called "noise": in other words it carried clear meaning: the 'problem' was that the meaning went contrary to Johns Hopkins's official PR image. Hence, to me, at least, proving that the Hopkins entry is a puff piece. My assumption is that Hopkins, or a related interest, had donated money to Wikipedia with the somewhat inevitable understanding that Hopkins could not be represented negatively. I've always assumed since that that Wikipedia is careful to not risk any lawsuits for 'character defamation' from big money interests.

Since then, I've been routinely censored &/or censured off Wikipedia for various excuses. I don't remember what seems to've gotten me banned forever but one of the contributing factors was my posting links to movies I made of "81 APT", the 3rd Neoist Apartment Festival & the 1st one I organized in Baltimore in 1981. Those links are still there at the bottom of this page: https://en.wikipedia.org/wiki/Neoism . I might've posted those links around the beginning of 2010. As I recall, & I apologize for being so vague here, I followed 'acceptable' procedures for the posting of the links but didn't go through all the *recommended* procedures. These procedures had gotten more stringent since the early days. I was censured for not providing a citation, perhaps, &/or for not proving that I had permission to link to the movies. That's a bit complicated, eh? People who know nothing about Neoism & have no connection to it wanted me, a cofounder of Neoism, to make some acceptable 'citation', presumably to someone else who had no connection, an academic, perhaps. That would be like asking Einstein to have a high school physics professor say that it's ok for Einstein to express his opinion on The Theory of Relativity. Furthermore, I was expected to prove that I was giving myself permission to post links to movies that *I had made about a festival that I had organized.*

In the very early days there had been a Wikipedia 'entry' about "tENTATIVELY, a cONVENIENCE" that had no content. I provided the content by adding my email signature which was full of neologisms & puns. That content was removed. Hypothetically that could've been removed because it's not allowed for people to post their own entries. HOWEVER, I know of at least 2 entries that were transparently written by the person themselves &/or by someone on that person's behalf. Both of these entries are, again, transparent puff pieces. One person is identified as something like "a highly respected businessman". Given that I co-owned a business with this person I'd have to disagree. These entries remained undisturbed by Wikigardeners. Mine was eventually removed. As far as I can tell, there's still no entry.

Now, I use Wikipedia all the time & generally find it to be useful. However, it would be foolish to think that ANY encyclopedia doesn't have ulterior motives. Take at look at how Mussolini's described in older hard-copy encyclopedias & THEN look at how he's described after Italian Fascism started warring. The propaganda spin takes an abrupt about-face.

look at Wikipedia's scathing review of the Swiss Propaganda Research site:

https://en.wikipedia.org/wiki/Swiss_Propaganda_Research

Note that Wikipedia uses a completely unsubstantiated claim:

"The site has been criticised for spreading conspiracy theories and especially so during the times of the COVID-19 pandemic when it has become a source of misinformation and disinformation internationally.[4] SPR has been categorized by some as a tool of propaganda.[2]"

unsubstantiated in the sense that just because someone says that SPR "has become a source of misinformation and disinformation internationally" doesn't make it so *BUT* Wikipedia doesn't say anything to the effect of: 'Some users of the SPR find it to be a believable source or, at least, a source worth paying attention to.' In other words, *there's no contrary opinion presented.* The effect of this is that while Wikipedia is careful to avoid saying *directly* that SPR is a misinformation site they only present negative opinions — leaving the reader with the impression that the criticisms must, therefore, be true.

****

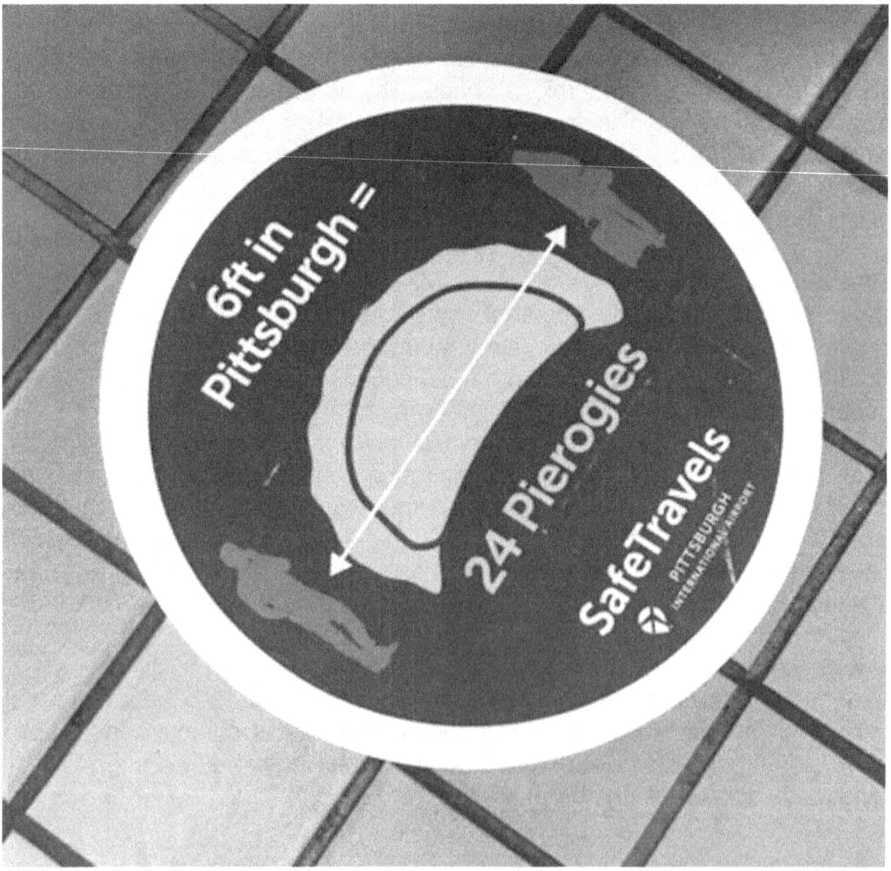

June 30, 2020, 10:26AM (images sent through Messaging from Naia Nisnam to Amir-ul Kafirs's iJones):

Pierogies social distancing

****

June 30, 1:45AM (Amir-ul Kafirs to group):

it is established they funded by Bill Gates and a variety of connservative groups.

Right, I understand that, I watched the video, it's by James Corbett. I liked it alot. The researcher he refers to is Derrick Broze, the guy whose article I also read. But that's somewhat general information, it doesn't give me the specifics I need about who on Facebook is specifically 'fact checking' the anti-vaccine people & whether THEY get funding from Gates & Co. Broze's article implies that The Atlantic Council would be the Facebook 'fact-checkers' & he doesn't list them as one of the groups funded by Gates. That doesn't mean that they're not all in bed together, it just means that it's harder to show the connection without digging even deeper.

****

June 30, 2020, 6:29AM (Inquiring Librarian to group):

Here is a shot at it. Yesterday, an old friend posted this:

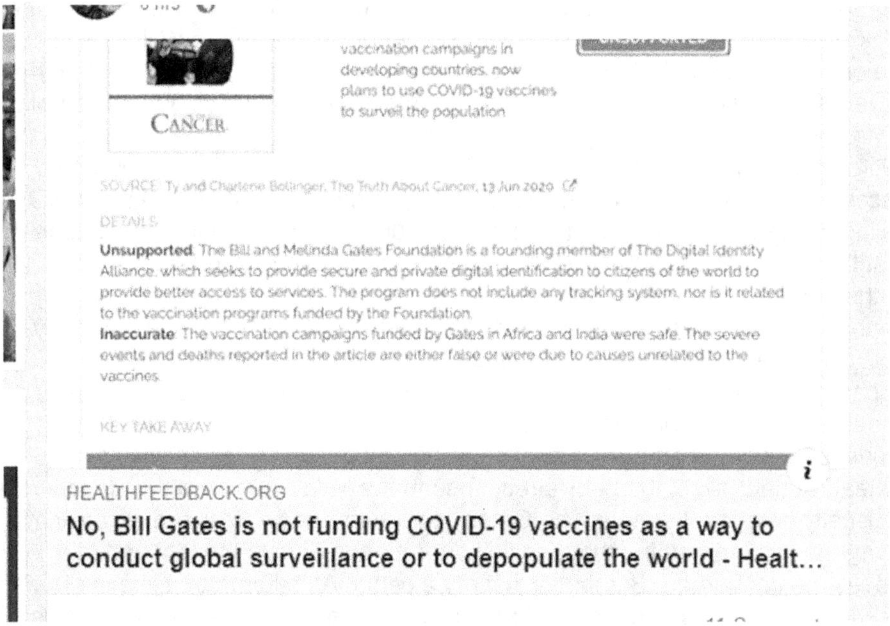

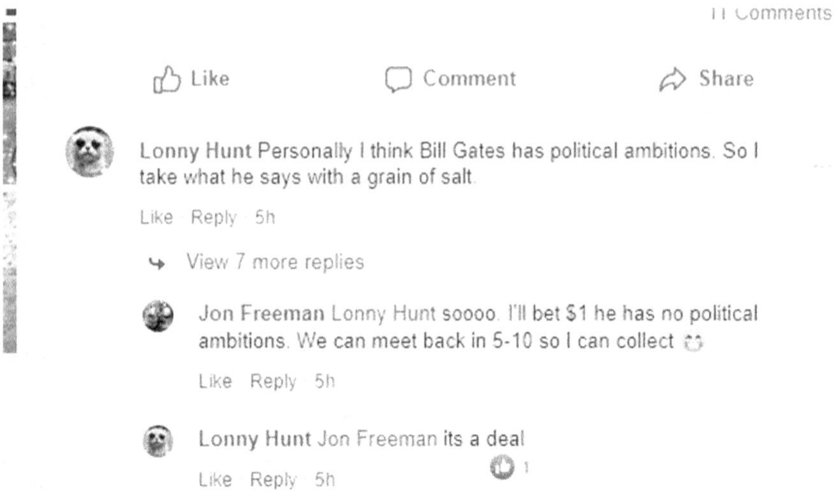

I was annoyed and concerned at the obvious propaganda that he was believing. So, I did some research into the fact checker, "Health Feedback".
& I responded with this:

"Ok, I have to play the devil's advocate here. I side with Lonny Hunt. Science Feedback is the parent organization of Health Feedback, which is the 'Fact Checker' here in John's post. Consider this article concerning how you cannot trust the Fact Checkers: https://www.thelastamericanvagabond.com/.../this-is-why.../ Here, Science Feedback is addressed as playing with 'semantics'. Consider also that Health Feedback works for the WHO, they must support the WHO's agendas as such, and Gates has a lot of sway with the WHO, he is a major donor, and he is working closely with the WHO and this is all evident here, as is his obsession with vaccines over natural immunity (which he seems not to even consider): https://www.gatesnotes.com/.../What-you-need-to-know... & in this consider Gates' own statement, "Our foundation is the biggest funder of vaccines in the world". The WHO is pushing world vaccination, and the WHO is telling the world's governments what to do during the pandemic. Also, I do realize that the Fact Checkers will likely say that "The Last American Vagabond", isn't up to their par, as they would with any truly independent media these days. To be honest, I do feel that fact checkers these days are pushing agendas, be they political or be they big pharma in nature. or a smattering of both given their apparent merger. I am not here saying that Bill Gates is a bad person. But I do know I do not want the vaccine he is pushing. Corona Virus vaccines have a tendency towards pathogenic priming, which means the vaccine will amplify, instead of neutralize, the body's response to the 'wild' virus, and this deadly result is usually delayed. I see that the Gates goal seems to be to speedily vaccinate everyone with something that has failed for many years in the lab, and this leaves me concerned. But that is just my 2 cents. As a librarian, I like to dig way deeper into sources of sources of sources..., to the point where I am hopelessly confused, overwhelmed, and freaked out. But is is nice to see people out here thinking and discussing without condemning... this I really appreciate. Ok, and this again from Gates' own website: "What we can do now is build different kinds of vaccine factories to prepare. Each vaccine type requires a different kind of factory. We need to be ready with facilities that can make each type, so that we can start manufacturing the final vaccine (or vaccines) as soon as we can. This will cost billions of dollars. Governments need to quickly find a mechanism for making the funding for this available. Our foundation is currently working with CEPI, the WHO, and governments to figure out the financing." The website again is here: https://www.gatesnotes.com/.../What-you-need-to-know...".

****

June 30, 2020, 6:59AM (Inquiring Librarian to group):

Last night, Robert F. Kennedy posted the following on his Instagram page. I can't copy and paste it, so I am just retyping it.
I'm a fast typer!:
"New Documents obtained by Axios and Public Citizen suggest that NIH owns half the key patent for Moderna's controversial Covid Vaccine & could collect half the royalties. In addition, 4 NIH scientists have filed their one provisional patent application as co investors. Little known NIH regulations let agency scientists collect up to $150,000.00 annually in royalties from vaccines upon which they worked. These rules are recipes for regulatory corruption. NIH's stake in the jab may explain why Anthony Fauci moved Moderna's vax to the front of the line and has let Moderna skip animal trials despite the experimental technology and the inherent dangers of Coronavirus vaccines. Every prior coronavirus vax has proven lethal to humans and animals due to COVID's unique penchant for "pathogenic priming." The deaths occur only after a vaccinated individual encounters the wild virus. Public health advocates and scientists criticized Fauci's decision to skip animal trials as reckless. It may also explain why Anthony Fauci arranged a $483 million grant to Moderna from a sister NIH agency, BARDA, despite the fact that Moderna has never brought a product to market or approved. Fauci's infusion made Moderna CEO Steve Bancel a billionaire and further enriched Fauci's mentor & co investor Bill Gates. It may also explain why Fauci publicly announced he was "Encouraged" by Moderna's catastrophic Phase 1 clinical trials despite the fact that 20% of the high dose & 6% of the low dose groups of super healthy volunteers needed to be hospitalized following vaccination. Those results would spell DOA for any other medical product. After getting the abysmal news, Bancel immediately dumped $30 million in stock and Fauci was forced to make his optimistic public assessment to save Moderna's plummeting shares from death spiral. Fauci painted lipstick on that lame donkey and now he's trying to convince everyone it's a thoroughbred. Moderna & NIH began manufacturing the first of 1 billion doses of the deadly vaccine this month. Fauci knows from experience that no matter how dangerous a vaccine, the easy part is convincing people to take it. Pharma, after all, controls the media."

Robert F. Kennedy Jr.... retyped by Inquiring Librarian. =]

****

June 30, 2020, 11:10AM (Amir-ul Kafirs to group):

Sorry, I'm a couple of days out of sync here so my replies are only beginning to catch up to where our actual dialog is at.

There is a TON of info. in there.

That info's fantastic & I very much appreciate your providing it. But, as I've written in 2 previous emails (both a bit 'out-of-date' in terms of the aforementioned dialog) what I'm hoping for is SPECIFIC INFO that proves SPECIFIC CONFLICT OF INTEREST: viz: that the SPECIFIC 'Fact Checkers' of Facebook who brand anti-vaccine people as misinformation providers are funded by pro-vaccination interests who stand to make many billions. This research, wonderful though it is, doesn't prove THAT, SPECIFICALLY. It's not enough to generalize that all these 'fact checking' groups are working with the same basic agenda – even though I think they are. These people are legally careful, they know what's at stake for them financially & they're not risking a conflict of interest lawsuit (if there even is such a thing).

To know that if I speak out I will most likely be shamed and fired, stands against everything that I believe libraries and librarianship stand for.

Of course, this is ultimately your personal decision as to whether you take the risk of bucking the system. It's 'safe' for me to say what I'm about to say & not safe for you. It seems to me that the case against NewsGuard specifically is strong enough for you organize it in a coherent way & to present it to those in power above you & those lower in your library's hierarchy & to tell them as calmly as possible that you have no intention of allowing CENSORSHIP OF THIS TYPE in the library you manage. Before you do this, you might consider contacting an ACLU lawyer in your area & explaining to them why you're doing this. If you can get the ACLU on your side then the library system hierarchy may choose to allow indidivdual library managers to choose whether to allow NewsGuard or not. Of course, this would make work for you & put you in peril but if you win or even if you make the news as a 'Free Speech Advocate' or some such it might be worth it.

That's my 2¢'s worth.

****

June 30, 2020, 3:54PM (Amir-ul Kafirs to group):

what if these checks are a way to buy compliance?

I told this story before but it's worth repeating:

Supposedly when Napoleon invaded Spain & overthrew the Catholic Church & its Inquisition it was discovered that in the process of doing so they endangered the food supply for a large quantity of the population. The Catholic Church had attained compliance by terrorizing potential enemies AND by creating an economy of almost total dependence. While the Catholic Church took as much as possible from as many people as possible they then doled out a much smaller amount to keep the faithful going. They had created the perfect manipulative Charity State.

So, yeah, this could be a way of buying compliance. But how long will it last?

My slogan, also presented here at least once, is:

Before you decide against biting the hand that feeds you, ask why it has so much food in the 1st place.

they are getting 5,000$ a month

$5,000 a month is hard to believe but, I suppose, possible. I would think that they'd have to have 7 kids (at $500 a pop) &/or be on some sort of disability to get that much.

****

June 30, 2020, 6:41PM (Amir-ul Kafirs to group):

this channel's live podcast was suddenly taken off the air for having "dangerous or harmful content"

I've had video taken off on the exact same basis (& not been put back on again). It's interesting that "agadmator" says that you can't even mention 'the current situation that's keeping us all indoors' or the video will be pulled off. As far as I can tell that isn't true but he seems to be Russian so maybe it's true in Russia?

The idea of algorithms making censorship decisions is straight out of "Brazil".

****

June 30, 2020, 6:48PM (Amir-il Kafirs to group):

certainly it would lead to 'progressive discipline'. :/

Thusly proving that Mind Control is a reality.

I do know the unemployment is more right now in the u.s. than my salary.

For some people. I doubt that it is for most people.

I feel like the ppl are really just super brainwashed and i question their intelligence, sadly.

Is there intelligence out there to even question?

The mask naziism is at it's illogical height.

In some respects it seems to be getting worse here. It's been 90° out the past 2 days & some people in the parks are still wearing the masks — this despite our having been told in early March that COVID-19 can't survive well in temperatures over 80°.

These people have power and a voice and i think they can really change what nonsense we are being subjected to and destroyed by.

Bit by bit we're all chipping away at it but I think the brainwashing still dominates. It's like people are plugged into it & refuse to pull the plug. If all the paranoids were to withdraw from the mass media fear-mongering there might be some hope. Otherwise? It's like a race to the finish. Are we the tortoise or the hare? Or neither?

****

June 30, 2020, 7:01PM (Amir-ul Kafirs to group):

The WHO is pushing world vaccination, and the WHO is telling the world's governments what to do during the pandemic.

I looked at Gates's blog, I didn't read thru the whole thing but I looked at, perhaps, the 1st 3rd. **It's the most extreme MONOLITHIC NARRATIVE I've seen yet!!** Gates basically talks about this as if he's communicating from Mount Olympus. He 'simply' tells us that 7 billion people have to follow his 'vision'. No questions asked. The megalomania of that is truly mind-boggling.

And, YES!, you've nailed the conflict of interest dead-on.

****

June 30, 2020, 7:06PM (Amir-ul Kafirs to group):

Re: HERETICS: 'Fact Checker' CENSORSHIP in Action!

Moderna & NIH began manufacturing the first of 1 billion doses of the deadly vaccine this month.

& there we get to the crux of the matter, eh?! If they manufacture 1 billion doses they're going to be turning every dirty trick in the book to make sure that they get paid for them & that people receive them.

****

June 30, 2020, 3:16PM (Inquiring Librarian to group):

HERETICS: Psychopaths

I was listening to a talk show this morning from the Last American Vagabond. The guy speaking mentioned this completely outlandish study that was done recently calling those who do not believe the covid 19 government/big pharma generated hype, "Psychopaths", and details why they/people like us, are psychopaths.

https://www.psypost.org/2020/06/psychopathic-traits-linked-to-non-compliance-with-social-distancing-guidelines-amid-the-coronavirus-pandemic-56980

The same site has an article about 'intellectually arrogant" people being the type to refuse vaccinations.
https://www.psypost.org/2020/06/intellectually-arrogant-people-typically-have-more-anti-vaccination-attitudes-study-finds-57170

I honestly can't believe I just wasted a few minutes reading that schlop.

****

SOCIAL PSYCHOLOGY

Psychopathic traits linked to non-compliance with social distancing guidelines amid the coronavirus pandemic

BY **ERIC W. DOLAN** JUNE 7, 2020

New research provides some initial evidence that certain antagonistic personality traits are associated with ignoring preventative measures meant to halt the spread of the novel coronavirus SARS-CoV-2.

The study has been peer reviewed and accepted for publication in the journal *Social Psychology and Personality Science*. It is currently available on the PsyArXiv preprint website.

"On March 31, 2020, Dr. Deborah Birx, the coordinator of the U.S. government's

Coronavirus Task Force, said, 'There's no magic bullet. There's no magic vaccine or therapy. It's just behaviors. Each of our behaviors, translating into something that changes the course of this viral pandemic over the next 30 days.' My experience as a psychological scientist as well as a practicing psychologist has convinced me that the importance of psychology and behavior in the prevention and management of a wide range of health problems is enormous," said study author Pavel S. Blagov, an associate professor and director of the Personality Laboratory at Whitman College.

"This includes personality, or the study of important ways in which people differ. It was clear from reports in the media very early in the COVID-19 pandemic that some people were rejecting advice to socially distance and engage in increased hygiene. There can be many reasons for this, and I thought that personality may play at least a small role in it."

"I knew that traits from the so-called Dark Triad (narcissism, Machiavellianism, and psychopathy) as well as the traits subsumed within psychopathy are linked to health risk behavior and health problems, and I expected them to be implicated in health behaviors during the pandemic. There is also prior research suggesting that people high on the Dark Triad traits may knowingly and even deliberately put other people's health at risk, e.g., by engaging in risky sexual behavior and not telling their partner about having HIV or STIs," Blagov told PsyPost.

"Early in the pandemic, and in subsequent months, there were numerous reports of individuals purposefully coughing, spitting, or even licking door handles in public, either as a way to intimidate others or as a way to rebel against the emerging new norms of social distancing and hygiene. I was curious whether the Dark Triad and psychopathy-related traits may help explain such behavior."

[..]

- https://www.psypost.org/2020/06/psychopathic-traits-linked-to-non-compliance-with-social-distancing-guidelines-amid-the-coronavirus-pandemic-56980

****

Intellectually arrogant people typically have more anti-vaccination attitudes, study finds

BY **ERIC W. DOLAN** JUNE 28, 2020

New research has found a link between intellectual humility and vaccination attitudes. The findings, published in *Psychology, Health & Medicine*, suggest that those who are more open to revising their beliefs in the face of new information tend to have more positive views of vaccination.

"Positive psychology-related constructs and interventions are interesting and require relatively low resources and have a wide variety of potential applications for both the clinic and public health," said study authors Amy R. Senger and Ho P. Huynh, a master's student at Sam Houston State University and assistant professor at Texas A&M University-San Antonio, respectively.

"Specifically, for this topic, we were interested to see how intellectual humility would relate to anti-vaccination attitudes, because intellectual humility has been shown to open up discussions in other contested arenas, such as politics or religion."

The researchers conducted an online survey of 246 participants, which found that intellectual humility was negatively correlated with anti-vaccination attitudes. People who disagreed with statements such as "Listening to perspectives of others seldom changes my important opinions" but agreed with statements such as "I am willing to change my position on an important issue in the face of good reasons" were less likely to mistrust the benefits of vaccines and less likely to believe that vaccination programs "are a big con."

"Intellectually humble people, or people who understand and accept that their own knowledge can be faulty, typically have lower anti-vaccination attitudes. This is because intellectually humble people tend to be open to updating their knowledge when presented with new information, and intellectually humble people tend to not be overconfident in what they know," the researchers explained.

[..]

- https://www.psypost.org/2020/06/intellectually-arrogant-people-typically-have-more-anti-vaccination-attitudes-study-finds-57170

****

June 30, 2020, 7:35PM (Amir-ul Kafirs to group):

Re: HERETICS: Psychopaths

details why they/people like us, are psychopaths.

What can I say?! I read the above article & found it to be once again despicable — more or less the pot calling the kettle black. Consider this:

""I knew that traits from the so-called Dark Triad (narcissism, Machiavellianism, and psychopathy) as well as the traits subsumed within psychopathy are linked to health risk behavior and health problems, and I expected them to be implicated in health behaviors during the pandemic.["]"

Machiavellianism particularly jumps out at me: what could be *more Machiavellian* than trying to define all humans who resist & criticize a Monolithic Narrative as displaying "traits from the so-called Dark Triad"?!

The same site has an article about 'intellectually arrogant" people being the type to refuse vaccinations.
https://www.psypost.org/2020/06/intellectually-arrogant-people-typically-have-more-anti-vaccination-attitudes-study-finds-57170

&, once again, it seems like the pot calling the kettle black! I can hardly think of anything more "intellectually arrogant" that that article. Take this as an example:

""Intellectually humble people, or people who understand and accept that their own knowledge can be faulty, typically have lower anti-vaccination attitudes. This is because intellectually humble people tend to be open to updating their knowledge when presented with new information, and intellectually humble people tend to not be overconfident in what they know," the researchers explained."

The implication is that, obviously, vaccines are above criticism so anyone who is so 'delusional' as to not 'recognize' that is "intellectually arrogant". What exactly is this "new information" that "intellectually humble people" will accept as overturning their doubts?! Apparently, according to the implications of the article, it doesn't work in the reverse way: pro-vaccine people will never even encounter the *possibility* of "new information" that could overturn their doubts because, of course!, no such information could possibly exist!

I honestly can't believe I just wasted a few minutes reading that schlop.

Pure propaganda at its most heinous.

[Later research in this book reveals the author of both of these articles, Eric W. Dolan, as an apparent hired gun who created the publication that the articles appear in just for the purpose of putting forth such suspicious 'research'.]

****

June 30, 2020, 12:44PM (Inquiring Librarian to group):

HERETICS: Health Fact Checkers & Funding

I think things were getting too buried in that mass of emails where this stuff was stuck. I hope this isn't stuff that is already obvious to everyone. Anyways, I copied and pasted it here just for you. And I added a few things about the NIH based on what I learned from Robert Kennedy. Now, honestly, with the censorship so rampant on the web right now, it is very difficult to find solid proof of who exactly is funding our health fact checkers that are bashing anti-vax people. But, I think my little bit of digging is well dipping through the surface of this miasma of corruption that seems to have been going on likely for decades. It seems to me, our universities have been corrupted by nefarious money making agendas for the powerful elite. I think this is really honestly old news, based on a lot of stuff I've read and heard from Phil's page on Rockefeller, Gates, the fight against natural medicine by these Big Pharma types, etc... But they have obviously infiltratrated the internet and are full speed ahead more than ever now.

[..]

Ok, now according to Wikipedia (I know they suck, but here you get what THEY want you to think, because THEY don't think we are digging further into this). *"In 1992, the NIH encompassed nearly 1 percent of the federal government's operating budget and controlled more than 50 percent of all funding for health research and 85 percent of all funding for health studies in universities. From 1993 to 2001 the NIH budget doubled. For a time, funding essentially remained flat, and for seven years following the financial crisis, the NIH budget struggled to keep up with inflation.*

In 1999 Congress increased the NIH's budget by $2.3 billion to $17.2 billion in 2000. In 2009 Congress again increased the NIH budget to $31 billion in 2010. In 2017 and 2018, Congress passed laws with bipartisan support that substantially increasing appropriations for NIH, which was 37.3 billion dollars annually in FY2018. ''' Researchers at universities or other institutions outside of NIH can apply for research project grants (RPGs) from the NIH. There are numerous funding mechanisms for different project types (e.g., basic research, clinical research, etc.) and career stages (e.g., early career, postdoc fellowships, etc.). The NIH regularly issues "requests for applications" (RFAs), e.g., on specific programmatic priorities or timely medical problems (such as Zika virus research in early 2016). In addition, researchers can apply for "investigator-initiated grants" whose subject is determined by the scientist.

The total number of applicants has increased substantially, from about 60,000 investigators who had applied during the period from 1999 to 2003 to slightly less than 90,000 in who had applied during the period from 2011 to 2015. Due to this, the "cumulative investigator rate," that is, the likelihood that unique investigators are funded over a 5-year window, has declined from 43% to 31%.

R01 grants are the most common funding mechanism and include investigator-initiated projects. The roughly 27,000 to 29,000 R01 applications had a funding success of 17-19% during 2012 though 2014. Similarly, the 13,000 to 14,000 R21 applications had a funding success of 13-14% during the same period. In FY 2016, the total number of grant applications received by the NIH was 54,220, with approximately 19% being awarded funding. Institutes have varying funding rates. The National Cancer Institute awarded funding to 12% of applicants, while the National Institute for General Medical Science awarded funding to 30% of applicants. https://en.wikipedia.org/wiki/National_Institutes_of_Health

**From this, I deduce the government is giving the NIH massive amounts of money to then pump into Universities to produce 'experts' in the healthcare(less) fields that best support government agendas. These well groomed NIH/ University produced 'experts' then become the "Fact Checkers" for groups like Science Feedback which is the parent organization for vaccine bashing 'fact checkers' like Health Feedback: https://sciencefeedback.co/about/ , & in their cozy FB life-saver format: https://sciencefeedback.co/science-feedback-partnering-with-facebook-in-fight-against-misinformation/
I'm still not sure if this proves the NIH or the WHO is directly funding anti vax bashing through fact checkers. But I have to stop here for the moment. =]

****

Checking information that claims to be based on science

Science Feedback is a not-for-profit organization verifying the credibility of influential claims and media coverage that claims to be scientific, starting with the topics of climate and health.

Our mission

Our first mission is to help create an Internet where users will have access to scientifically sound and trustworthy information. We also **provide feedback to editors and journalists** about the credibility of information published by their outlets.

Our mission is **pedagogical**: we strive to explain whether and why information is or is not consistent with the science. We are **nonpartisan** and apply the same methodology to claims made in a variety of media outlets, as well as exposing claims that either contradict or over-hype science. We believe it is scientists' civic duty to better inform our fellow citizens in our area of expertise.

[..]

- https://sciencefeedback.co/about/

****

I clicked on the above's link for 'team & advisors' for the following.

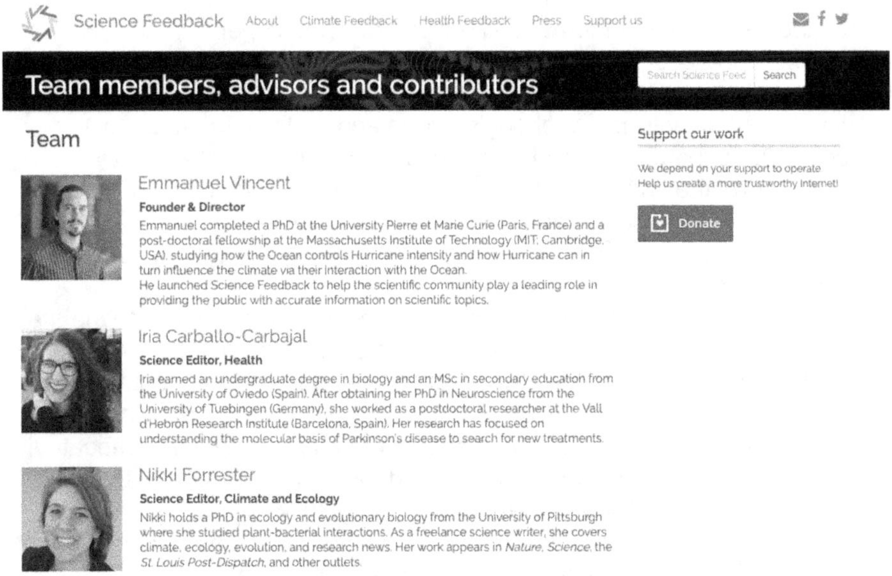

Science Feedback About Climate Feedback Health Feedback Press Support us

Team members, advisors and contributors

Search

Team

Emmanuel Vincent

Founder & Director

Emmanuel completed a PhD at the University Pierre et Marie Curie (Paris, France) and a post-doctoral fellowship at the Massachusetts Institute of Technology (MIT, Cambridge, USA), studying how the Ocean controls Hurricane intensity and how Hurricane can in turn influence the climate via their interaction with the Ocean.
He launched Science Feedback to help the scientific community play a leading role in providing the public with accurate information on scientific topics.

Iria Carballo-Carbajal

Science Editor, Health

Iria earned an undergraduate degree in biology and an MSc in secondary education from the University of Oviedo (Spain). After obtaining her PhD in Neuroscience from the University of Tuebingen (Germany), she worked as a postdoctoral researcher at the Vall d'Hebron Research Institute (Barcelona, Spain). Her research has focused on understanding the molecular basis of Parkinson's disease to search for new treatments.

Nikki Forrester

Science Editor, Climate and Ecology

Nikki holds a PhD in ecology and evolutionary biology from the University of Pittsburgh where she studied plant-bacterial interactions. As a freelance science writer, she covers climate, ecology, evolution, and research news. Her work appears in *Nature*, *Science*, the *St. Louis Post-Dispatch*, and other outlets.

Support our work

We depend on your support to operate
Help us create a more trustworthy Internet!

Donate

[..]

- https://sciencefeedback.co/team-advisors-contributors/

****

Science Feedback partnering with Facebook in fight against misinformation

In April 2019, Science Feedback started working with Facebook as part of their fact-checking program. While misinformation currently floods the Internet, this program is part of Facebook's effort to decrease the platform's role in driving this phenomenon.

To that end, Facebook is partnering with third-party fact-checkers who are certified through the non-partisan International Fact-Checking Network (IFCN) at Poynter to help identify and review false news. The IFCN code of principles is a series of commitments organizations abide by to promote excellence in fact-checking; these commitments include nonpartisanship, transparency of sources relied on, transparency of methodology.

How it works

Facebook identifies stories that might need verification based on signals like feedback from its platform's users and machine learning. These posts are then added to a queue of articles, photos, videos, and text posts that fact-checkers like Science Feedback can scroll through and sort by topic and virality.
When we identify viral stories that claim to be based on science—in the fields of climate and health for the moment—we invite relevant experts to analyze the main claims in the post, image, video, or article, and publish a review of the item (read more about our process). We also have the ability to report items that we review independently from Facebook's queue and that we find to be false or misleading. Note that Facebook has no influence over the stories that we choose to review, nor on the final verdict that is decided by the scientists.
When a fact-checker's conclusion is that a post contains—or links to—false information, Facebook takes the following measures in an effort to curb the spread of misinformation on its platform:

- 1 – inform those who have shared the post, as well as those who are about to share it, that a fact-check has been performed;
- 2 – append a link to the fact-check at the bottom of the post;
- 3 – reduce the future reach of the post by showing it lower in News Feed;
- 4 – reduce the ability of domains and Facebook pages that repeatedly share false information to spread and monetize their content.

If a fact-checker's conclusion is that the post is not fully inaccurate but only partially so—for example, it is misleading or the title of the post is false but not the body content—it will receive a softer demotion in News Feed.
As of today, there are over 50 organizations around the world covering over 40 languages which are part of the partnership. Science Feedback is the only organization dedicated to verifying information in scientific fields by empowering the scientific community to take an active part in this endeavour to make the Internet a more credible place.

Published on: 14 May 2019 I Editor: Emmanuel M Vincent

- https://sciencefeedback.co/science-feedback-partnering-with-facebook-in-fight-against-misinformation/

****

June 30, 2020, 8:10PM (Amir-ul Kafirs to group):

YES, I read their statement about partnering with Facebook to 'fact check'. By the way, I coined a new term today: Fact Chokers. I think it's got potential.

ANYWAY, talk about "intellectual arrogance" & "Machiavellian"! Their final claim there is:

"Science Feedback is the only organization dedicated to verifying information in scientific fields by empowering the scientific community to take an active part in this endeavour to make the Internet a more credible place."

Right. There are 7.5 billion people on the planet & these lofty **11 people** are going to decide what's true or false ***for all of us!!*** GROUPTHINK FORBID that we should think for ourselves.

****

June 30, 2020, 12:56PM (Amir-ul Kafirs to group):

HERETICS: Eat me!!

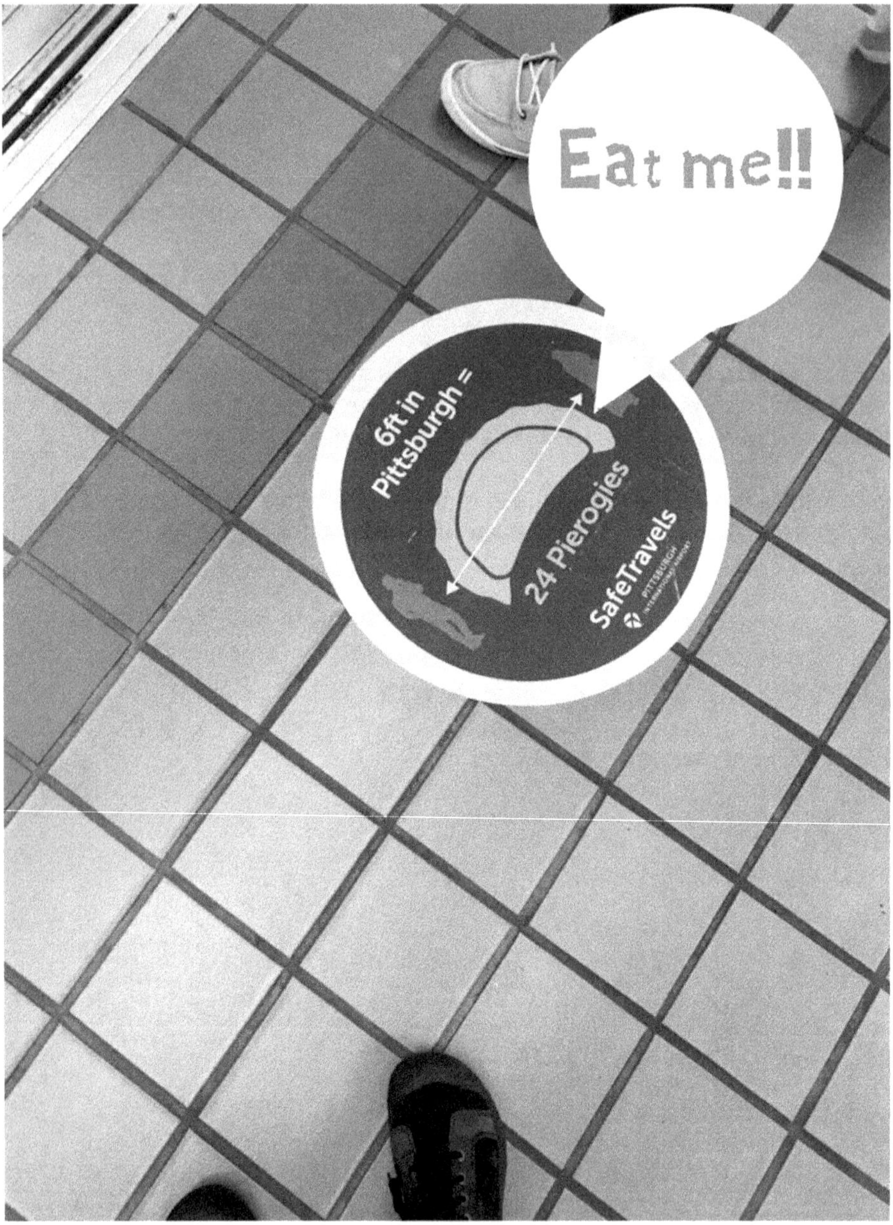

****

June 30, 2020, 12:56PM (Inquiring Librarian to group):

Re: HERETICS: Eat me!!

This is TOO MUCH! i just cackled way too loud here at my silent library desk!!

****

June 30, 2020, 8:23PM (Amir-ul Kafirs to group):

i just cackled way too loud here at my silent library desk!!

Of course, it's obviously psychopathic humor.. so what should be done? Either you or anyone else who finds it funny is a psychopath OR psychopaths are actually funny.. That's a real brain-twister — I'll have to ask a scientist. They can tell me whether it's ok to laugh or not.

****

June 30, 2020, 8:36PM (Inquiring Librarian to group):

Re: HERETICS: Psychopaths

Yes. The articles are like the cheeze wiz of the cheese world, pure trash.

****

June 30, 2020, 8:49PM (Inquiring Librarian to group):

Yes! That is exactly it, Fact Chokers!!

Thank you for your responses and for paying attention and not being a cyber bully. I tried to share some alternate info on masks to someone on social media today.. big mistake. She started immediately with the venom. She didn't bother to read the articles I tried to share with her (after her initial venom, I tried sharing several other decent articles including the book by former New England Journal of Medicine editor, Marcia Angell, The Truth About the Drug Companies: How they Deceive Us And What to Do About It" https://www.amazon.com/Truth-About-Drug-Companies-Deceive-ebook/dp/B000FC1V1A .) I even tried to speak her language and share the CDC's May, 2020 study on masks that found them to be basically useless against viruses: https://wwwnc.cdc.gov/eid/article/26/5/19-0994_article . It all failed. She remained relentlessly vicious. I wound up deleting my comment and all conversation I had with her and then I blocked her from my social media account. I can't handle that much negative energy for no reason. She could not possibly have read the links that I had pumped out to her within 5 minutes, yet she wanted to insist she was right and I was wrong when I wasn't even trying to say I was right, I was saying, hey, why don't you consider this as an alternative.

****

Volume 26, Number 5—May 2020
Policy Review

Nonpharmaceutical Measures for Pandemic Influenza in Nonhealthcare Settings—Personal Protective and Environmental Measures

Abstract

There were 3 influenza pandemics in the 20th century, and there has been 1 so far in the 21st century. Local, national, and international health authorities regularly update their plans for mitigating the next influenza pandemic in light of the latest available evidence on the effectiveness of various control measures in reducing transmission. Here, we review the evidence base on the effectiveness of nonpharmaceutical personal protective measures and environmental hygiene measures in nonhealthcare settings and discuss their potential inclusion in pandemic plans. Although mechanistic studies support the potential effect of hand hygiene or face masks, evidence from 14 randomized controlled trials of these measures did not support a substantial effect on transmission of laboratory-confirmed influenza. We similarly found limited evidence on the effectiveness of improved hygiene and environmental cleaning. We identified several major knowledge gaps requiring further research, most fundamentally an improved characterization of the modes of person-to-person transmission.
Influenza pandemics occur at irregular intervals when new strains of influenza A virus spread in humans (1). Influenza pandemics cause considerable health and social impact that exceeds that of typical seasonal (interpandemic) influenza epidemics. One of the characteristics of influenza pandemics is the high incidence of infections in all age groups because of the lack of population immunity. Although influenza vaccines are the cornerstone of seasonal influenza control, specific vaccines for a novel pandemic strain are not expected to be available for the first 5–6 months of the next pandemic. Antiviral drugs will be available in some locations to treat more severe infections but are unlikely to be available in the quantities that might be required to control transmission in the general community. Thus, efforts to control the next pandemic will rely largely on nonpharmaceutical interventions.

Most influenza virus infections cause mild and self-limiting disease; only a small fraction of case-patients require hospitalization. Therefore, influenza virus infections spread mainly in the community. Influenza virus is believed to be transmitted predominantly by respiratory droplets, but the size distribution of particles responsible for transmission remains unclear, and in particular, there is a lack of consensus on the role of fine particle aerosols in transmission (2,3). In healthcare settings, droplet precautions are recommended in addition to standard precautions for healthcare personnel when interacting with influenza patients and for all visitors during influenza seasons (4). Outside healthcare settings, hand hygiene is recommended in most national pandemic plans (5), and medical face masks were a common sight during the influenza pandemic in 2009. Hand hygiene has been proven to prevent many infectious diseases and might be considered a major component in influenza pandemic plans, whether or not it has proven effectiveness against influenza virus transmission, specifically because of its potential to reduce other infections and thereby reduce pressure on healthcare services.

In this article, we review the evidence base for personal protective measures and environmental hygiene measures, and specifically the evidence for the effectiveness of these measures in reducing transmission of laboratory-confirmed influenza in the community. We also discuss the implications of the evidence base for inclusion of these measures in pandemic plans.

[..]

- https://wwwnc.cdc.gov/eid/article/26/5/19-0994_article

****

June 30, 2020, 10:16PM (Amir-ul Kafirs to group):

Re: HERETICS: Health Fact Checkers & Funding

Fact Chokers!!

I'll be trying to put that term into circulation sometime after midnight tonight. It'll be interesting to see if the 'fact checkers' try to censor it. If anyone here tries to share it & gets a Fact Choker warning please screen-shot it in context & share the shot with me.

Thank you for your responses and for paying attention and not being a cyber bully.

I try to stay on top of it all but it's hard. I more or less spent almost all of my 'work' time today on going through the HERETICS emails & on making a slew of new text panels. Many aspects of my life are being otherwise neglected. Still, I dedicate as much time to this as I do because I think it's important.

She didn't bother to read the articles I tried to share with her

I don't have any bad conscience about unfriending people on social media anymore. If it's someone I don't really know I'm glad to kiss their ass(holi(sh)ness) goodbye. People that I've known for a long time I've refrained from unfriending but even a few of those have gone. Some may've even unfriended me without my noticing but I've been so relieved to not have their aggressive attempts to browbeat me that I haven't bother to confirm.

"The Truth About the Drug Companies: How they Deceive Us And What to Do About It"

I just ordered a copy.

Although mechanistic studies support the potential effect of hand hygiene or face masks, evidence from 14 randomized controlled trials of these measures did not support a substantial effect on transmission of laboratory-confirmed influenza. We similarly found limited evidence on the effectiveness of improved hygiene and environmental cleaning.

Considering that that comes from the CDC it's pretty powerful stuff. One would think that the sheeple might even be convinced.

It all failed. She remained relentlessly vicious.

&, yet. WE'RE the "psychopaths" if we're anti-vaccine. I've found this whole PANDEMIC PANIC to've brought out more bullying behavior from ordinarily somewhat pacific people than I've probably ever witnessed before.

I wound up deleting my comment and all conversation I had with her

I leave that stuff in. It might be useful to refer to later. One of the very hypothetical chapters in the very hypothetical Unconscious Suffocation book is tENTATIVELY titled: "Lords of the Flies". I want it to center around nasty behavior of these self-righteous 'liberal' bullies.

and then I blocked her from my social media account. I can't handle that much negative energy for no reason.

No, of course not, it's an unnecessary drain on one's mental health.

****

June 30, 2020, 8:53PM (Inquiring Librarian to group):

It's ok Amir-ul Kafirs, just shut your mouth, put your head down, and unquestioningly embrace the Brave New Normal! Maybe you can make a whole outfit out of masks, the way you did with those CD's! That would be a laugh. You can wear it to Trader Joe's and then walk in without a mask on your face. When they tell you you cannot enter without a mask on, you can point to your outfit. If they say that you need one on your face, you can rip one off from your nether regions.

My significant other went to Trader Joe's without a mask a couple of weeks ago. For some reason he had an old pair of underwear stuffed in his work bag (he's a disorganized slob most of the time so this actually did not surprise me). So he twisted that pair of underwear up and wrapped it around his face and it worked. No one said anything, but I wonder if they wondered...

****

June 30, 2020, 10:20PM (Amir-ul Kafirs to group):

just shut your mouth, put your head down, and unquestioningly embrace the Brave New Normal!

I'll give up my caustic wit when they pry it from my cold dead mouth.

****

June 30, 2020, (Amir-ul Kafirs to group):

HERETICS: More Facebook bullying

Facebook providing a disclaimer of sorts attached to an ad for an event that *mentions* social distancing:

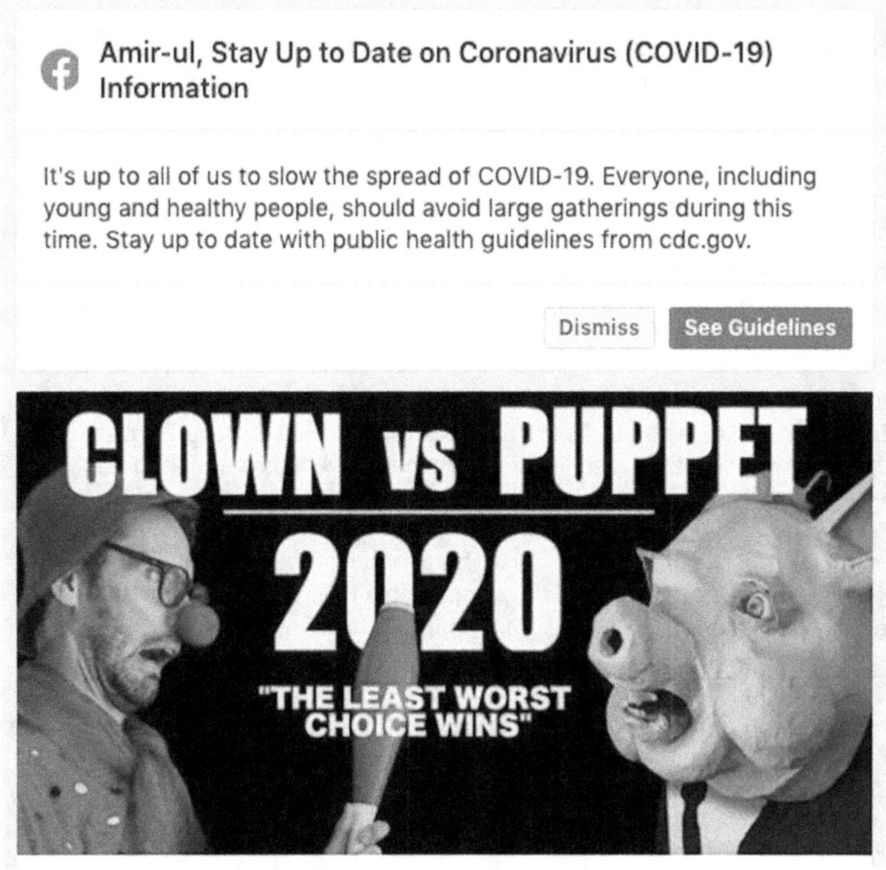

JUL
2

Clown Vs Puppet 2020! Social Distance Debate!

Public · Hosted by Clown vs Puppet 2020 and 2 others

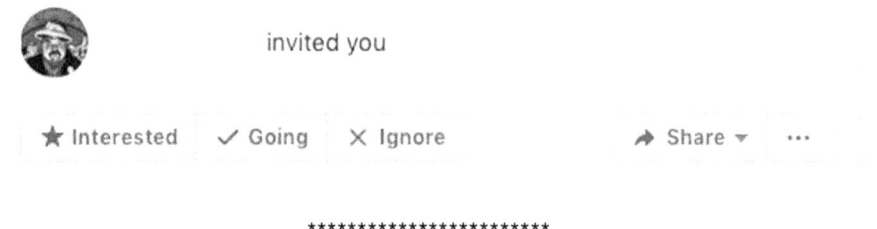

invited you

★ Interested ✓ Going ✕ Ignore ➦ Share ▾ ···

****

June 30, 2020, 10:40PM (Inquiring Librarian to group):

Re: HERETICS: More Facebook bullying

This totally confuses me. What exactly is going on? Is it a joke? I cannot tell. :O It is possible i am just tired...

****

June 30, 2020, 11:01PM (Amir-ul Kafirs to group):

Re: HERETICS: More Facebook bullying

This totally confuses me. What exactly is going on? Is it a joke?

The guy on the left in the image is O'Ryan, a local stilt walker / juggler / performer whose work I like. The guy in the pig mask on the right is Dave English, a local puppeteer whose work I also like & who's the one who invited me to the event. Here're the details:

It's Socially Distant, Cognitively Dissonant, and hilariously competing with reality! A June 4th live stream is made possible by a partnership with the New Hazlett Theater and City of Asylum as part of The Show Must Go On(Line)! series.

Two horrible candidates are both running to be the president of our great nation! Nobody likes it! But they are the only options left and we have to pick one! In fact YOU have to pick one! Because at the end of the show the audience gets to vote for the least worst option! Introducing our candidates! Boo!

Clown can balance things on his nose, he can juggle, he can tie himself in knots, he has long skinny legs, and funny socks. He doesn't know where a lot of things are or how to do important stuff! He wants to be president because he thinks he'll get to wear a big fancy hat!

On the other side his opponent Puppet! Puppet is a pig! He can pop out his eyeballs, make up stories, songs, and terrible lies, he can talk in funny voices, dance on thin air, and then disappear into a suitcase. He wants to be president so he can be the one pulling the strings!

O'Ryan The O'Mazing (Clown) and Dave English (Puppet) reprise their roles in an ongoing absurdist political campaign between two hapless and at times malevolent politicians campaigning to win the presidency of the United States. Launched in the fall of 2019 "Clown Vs Puppet 2020" toured small theaters in Pennsylvania, West Virginia, and Ohio drumming up rust belt votes from people who suddenly matter- and making them laugh! Audiences roll with laughter at each performance as Clown and Puppet tackle the issues debate style with moderators and rowdy participants from the crowd! The content is ever changing as Clown and Puppet both do their level best to compete with the real-life buffoonery of the current events they satirize.

You can find the event on Facebook here: https://www.facebook.com/events/722345958514820/?notif_t=plan_user_invited&notif_id=1593538429784761

As far as I can tell, the intrusion of the Facebook text about guidelines was presumably placed there because the name of the event includes "Social Distance Debate".

Phil Bradley's Statement

First I should assure you that I haven't suddenly gone rightwing nut job on everyone. My politics are very much rooted in........Antiwar, anti-imperialism, anti-capitalism, feminism, pro-choice, mad pride, rights for differently abled people, black lives matter, climate activism, pro-LBGT, grassroots, anarchism, anti-corporate, ecology, environmentalism, anti-surveillance, anti-GMO, class consciousness, Indigenous Sovereignty, ect....

I feel a need to explain a little about how I use social media. I feel like I need to have a disclaimer on my social media page that states that anything posted here does not reflect the views and opinions of the page owner. Posts are for general interest purposes only. Probably also I need a break from social media and perhaps reassess how I use it. Maybe I am too reckless and too unconcerned about how I am perceived. I do not use social media to manicure an identity. That way of using SM may have originated from my previous identity on social media as Karen Eliot a multiple identity which anyone can use. There is more freedom in anonymity. Social media deleted that account unless I provided my identity. I was thinking it a funny joke to use my given name as a multiple Identify. Thus when I began my new account I started this page; https://www.facebook.com/feelrad/ In this strange way when I use SM I am still thinking of myself as using a pseudonym. The pseudonym of Phil Bradley.

I do not use my social media page so much as social media. I just find it a good way to set up my feed in a way that I get a diverse range of views and opinions flowing through often conflicting and antagonist points of view. I like to examine the whole phenomenology of a subject in its cultural social political and philosophical aspects.

When something goes viral from mainstream media to social

media I tend to be skeptical of it all and search for diverse counter view points on the subject matter. I find good journalism very hard to find and there seems to be only a few people doing it. On the other hand I like to start from the premise that everything is fake news and all of it is propaganda. That attitude helps me dig deeper. I find some sources good for some subjects and shockingly bad on others.

It is true that I might share something that comes from a right leaning platform if I think it is of some value. An interview with a prominent epidemiologist for instance. . On the other hand I have been accused recently of sharing right wing stuff that is actually left wing, just coming from a different point of view. Politics has become so polarised at the moment that it is hard to step back and evaluate situations from different and broader contexts and perspectives. Medicine at the moment has become politicised from both the left and the right and that is potentially quite dangerous.

I can't really comment more unless I know what particular posts that have taken your attention.

I hope that explains something for you.

HERETICS emails - July, 2020

July 1, 2020, 12:12AM (Amir-ul Kafirs to group):

HERETICS: Fact Chokers

I preface this one on social media with this:

"The arrogance of being part of a team of 11 people who decide what's true or false for 7.5 billion people boggles the mind."

The number refers to the number of Fact Chokers from Science Feedback that partner with Facebook. Here's the text panel that follows that prefatory comment:

'Fact Checkers'
(aka: 'Fact Chokers'):
'Expert' Witnesses for sale to the
Highest Bidder with Ulterior Motives
for the purpose of
CENSORING People with OPINIONS
contrary to the Monolithic Narrative.
*Be on the lookout for
Conflict of Interest.*

****

July 1, 2020, 9:03AM (BP to group):

HERETICS: Pissed!

Hell, All. Thanks for keeping the reading interesting. I'm seriously bummed at the way things are going. Tomorrow in my area was to be the opening of restaurants/bars at 25% capacity. This was a go up until Saturday, then on Monday afternoon the Gov nixed it at a press conference: "Indefinitely." What is incredibly frustrating and insulting is our Dear Gov (a 23 year Goldman Sachs exec, then our German Ambassador under Obama, then working for the DNC), blamed "knuckleheads." Yea, the people/businesses flouting the rules at Outside Bars at the Jersey Shore! Like we didn't see that coming. Of course they are gonna party. The Govs scolding, school marm tactic is as dishonest as it comes. So the mom and pop restaurant that invested in this opening is entirely screwed. And now we have the school opening plans rolling out for the new year. It's still too vague to pinpoint, but I can see where it is heading.

****

July 1, 2020, 10:20AM (Amir-ul Kafirs to group):

Re: HERETICS: Pissed!

The Govs scolding, school marm tactic is as dishonest as it comes.

Right, as usual, show us the proof that this actually creates a health problem of any significant size. These days just saying that people have been exposed to COVID-19 is enough to justify any Draconian measures even though mere exposure is meaningless: *How many people actually get sick? How many go to the hospital? How many die?* Those are the important questions.

****

July 1, 2020, 3:19PM (Inquiring Librarian to group):

It is heartbreaking to hear about these small businesses being bullied and shut back into time-out like toddlers (only toddlers that are now losing their life's work and savings and likely an ability to house and feed themselves). And here in Lousiana, when the unemployment runs out, our unemployed workers get a max of $245/wk. from unemployment. It's criminal.

Please keep us posted on what tortures the government has up its sleeves for kids. I will see this 2nd hand here in Louisiana because I work in a library next to many schools that used to have kids visit us frequently. I was heartened today to see the school summer camp next door is letting their kids play outside with each other without masks on. The teachers have masks on (mostly hanging from their ears, it's about 93 degrees here right now and 65% humidity in Louisiana).

My question is, is there no higher power that can and should stop these governors? What is wrong with these people and who is paying them off and with what to be such Hitlers?

Btw, Louisiana is heading towards another shutdown too. Masks are being weaponized, ppl are ratting each other and businesses out over masks. I mostly sling mine over my ear and put it fully on when i leave my semi private office desk where I cope by constantly sipping water or tea or snacking so that I can have an excuse to not have it on and I take it off when i am hidden in the book stacks and i answer the phone all the time, at my desk with the mask slung over my ear, so i can run outside (where the mask is not required) to put requested stuff on the contactless pickup cart.

Mostly, it's the lies and deception we are being told. If the government would just be upfront with us, we plan to imprison you in your own collective hell and inject you with poison and surveil you for our own good, I might be able to handle this better. I've never been able to handle liars.

****

July 1, 2020 (txt msg from Naia Nisnam to Amir-ul Kafirs):

I got this text from Rite Aid:

"Rite Aid is committed to protecting you and your family. Stop by your Rite Aid Pharmacy and make sure you are up-to-date on all immunizations. Text Stop to stop."

****

July 2, 2020, 12:43AM (Amir-ul Kafirs to group):

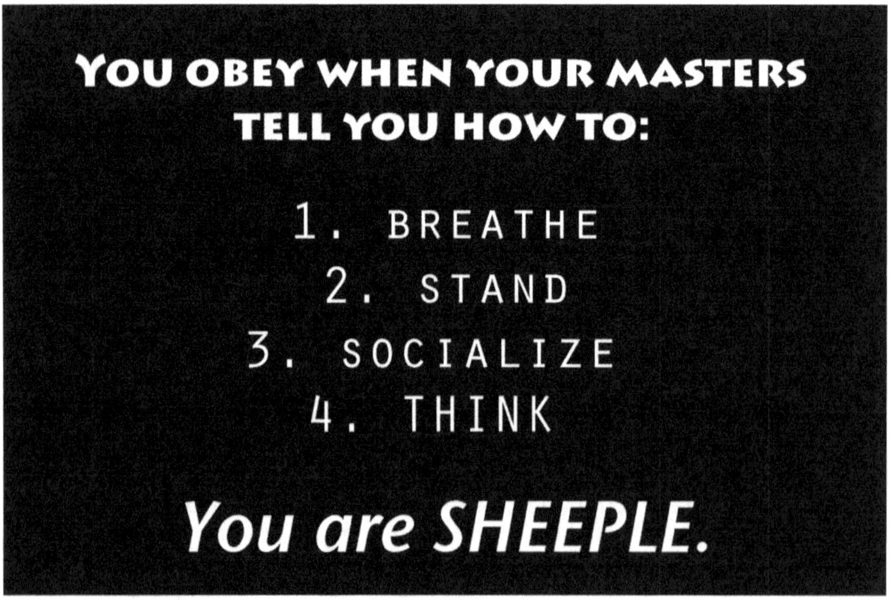
YOU OBEY WHEN YOUR MASTERS
TELL YOU HOW TO:
1. BREATHE
2. STAND
3. SOCIALIZE
4. THINK
You are SHEEPLE.

****

July 2, 2020, 9:36AM (Amir-ul Kafirs to group):

Re: HERETICS: SHEEPLE

Well, that's pretty direct!

Yes. Ordinarily I prefer 'allowing people to save face' in the sense that I think it's better to give people wiggle room & to not be insulting. Alas, the way things are going I feel that 'strong medicine' is required. As such, I'm throwing in shocking language (of sorts) in the hope that people will snap out of their trance of obedience or some such. I reckon it's what political activists call: *speaking truth to power*. Consider this excerpt from my opera's libretto:

""***mokita*** **(Kiriwina, New Guinea) Truth everybody know but nobody speaks. [noun]**" - p 48

""The Kiriwina tribespeople of the Trobriand Islands, however, use the word *mokita* (moe-KEE-tah) to refer to *the unspoken truths of certain social situations that everybody knows but nobody talks about—directly.*" - p 49"

""***biga peula*** **(Kiriwina, New Guinea) Potentially disruptive, unredeemable true statements. [noun]**" - p 50

""The Kiriwana use the phrase *biga peula* (literally, "hard words," pronounced BEE-kuh POOL-uh) to refer to *direct references to certain unspoken truths.*""

""This phenomenon is not confined to the Kiriwina. In many companies, you can get yourself fired by saying out loud what everybody knows to be true: "The boss is an idiot." In every marriage, there are phrases that partners never use, no matter how bitter the argument, unless they are ready for the marriage to end: "I've had a mistress for six years" is *biga peula* for a husband to say to a wife, just as "You aren't Tommy's father" is a *biga peula* for a wife to say to a husband. A useful phrase in many of these situations might be: "Wait! Don't say what you are about to say. It could be *biga peula* for us."" - p 51

""***biqa viseki*** **(Kiriwina, New Guinea) Use of metaphors as disguised speech. [noun]**" - p 52

"Among the Kiriwina, the use of indirect speech is an art and science, and metaphors, analogies, simile, and double entendres are called *biqu viseki* (BEE-kuh vis-EHK-ee)." - pp 52-53"

- review of Howard Rheingold's "They Have a Word for It: A Lighthearted Lexicon of Untranslatable Words & Phrases" by tENTATIVELY, a cONVENIENCE - September 19, 2017 - https://www.goodreads.com/story/show/598455-they-have-a-word-for-it

Now, I tried using ***biqa viseki*** in my "MASQUE" piece but I don't think people 'got it'; NOW it just seems like time to put out some ***biga peula*** instead. In Kiriwina usage this would be a bad idea because it creates ill-will that's hard to back down from. I understand that.. but I feel like there's alot at stake here so it's a calculated gamble. It's like pointing out that the Emperor's naked: if *someone doesn't do it then all the SHEEPLE will continue to praise his clothes.*

At any rate, it's worth a shot.

****

July 2, 2020, 9:44AM (Inquiring Librarian to group):

Re: HERETICS: SHEEPLE

I like it!! Honestly, the only thing keeping my mouth publicly shut now is my need to have an income so that i can have a roof over my head to hide in and food to eat since starving doesn't suit me.

If i lose my job it's balls to the walls big mouth for me.

****

July 2, 2020, 10:03AM (Amir-ul Kafirs to group):

I like it!!

Thanks. It is satisfying to just 'speak my mind' & I hope that there're closet supporters out there who'll feel encouraged to do the same.

Honestly, the only thing keeping my mouth publicly shut now is my need to have an income

I've taken the risk of speaking out at my job before & been fired for my trouble. It did begin a hard time but I DID survive. Nonetheless, it was a drag.

****

July 2, 2020, 11:13PM (Inquiring Librarian to group):

Anthony Fauci & $6 billion yearly

I've been following Robert F. Kennedy Jr.s "Truth" video series for the past few weeks. His latest, no. 6, discusses masks first and then moves on into the corruption of the medical industry and the funding of universities. According to this recording from this week, Anthony Fauci is one of the most powerful men in the world. He is given $6 billion annual from the NIH to give in grants to universities wordwide. If these universities do not do as he wishes, or if they conduct studies and sponsor students who study things against Fauci's interests, he can defund those universities. If you want to hear the talk, here it is: https://childrenshealthdefense.org/news/truth-with-robert-f-kennedy-jr-episode-6/?utm_source=salsa&eType=EmailBlastContent&eId=eeb26045-7b93-4fd1-9f53-a368e2c43cad

If you are interested further in fact checkers on medical stuff... James Corbett goes into this here by answering the question of a listener who was about to drop him due to a 'fact checker'. James in detail explains why the fact checkers are total trash: https://www.bitchute.com/video/HaHuTNh8fAo/
It's on Bitchute. Corbett's stuff keeps getting deleted off of Youtube so he's got a lot of great stuff that is uncensored on Bitchute.

****

July 2, 2020, 10:32AM (Amir-ul Kafirs to group):

HERETICS: 3 articles shared on Twitter

The 1st 2 were shared by Spiro Skouras. The very 1st of these came from Fox so I groan over that but it has an AP origin so I groan slightly less. The 2nd one is another TV 'News' thing. The 3rd one was shared by someone else & is from an "Inside Higher Ed" publication that I know nothing about. They're all worth skimming through for one reason or another.

Protest versus Africa's 1st COVID-19 vaccine test shows fear

By Cara Anna
Associated Press

CDC expands list of high-risk conditions for COVID-19 complications

The U.S. Centers for Disease Control and Prevention made revisions to its list of underlying medical conditions that put people at a higher risk of severe complications from the novel coronavirus.

JOHANNESBURG - Protesters against Africa's first COVID-19 vaccine trial burned their face masks Wednesday as experts note a worrying level of resistance and misinformation around testing on the continent.

Anti-vaccine sentiment in Africa is "the worst I've ever seen," the CEO of the GAVI vaccine alliance, Seth Berkley, told an African Union vaccine conference last week.

"In general, people in Africa know the diseases and want to protect each other," he said. “In this case, the rumor mill has been dramatic."

The trial that began last week in Johannesburg is part of one already underway in Britain of the vaccine developed at the University of Oxford. Some 2,000 volunteers in South Africa are expected to take part.

It’s important that vaccines be tested in Africa to see how they perform in the local context, professor of vaccinology Shabir Madhi, leader of the new COVID-19 vaccine trial in South Africa, told reporters and others in a webinar Sunday.

But the small band of demonstrators who gathered Wednesday at the University of the Witwatersrand, where the trial is based, reflect long-running fears among some in Africa over testing drugs on people who don’t understand the risks.

“The people chosen as volunteers for the vaccination, they look as if they’re from poor backgrounds, not qualified enough to understand” protest organizer Phapano Phasha told The Associated Press ahead of the event. “We believe they are manipulating the vulnerable.”

The activist and political commentator brought up the widely circulated remarks earlier this year by a French researcher, Jean-Paul Mira, who said, ““If I can be provocative, shouldn’t we be doing this study in Africa, where there are no masks, no treatments, no resuscitation?" He compared it to some AIDS studies: "In prostitutes, we try things because we know that they are highly exposed and that they do not protect themselves.”

“The narrative we got is our continent is a dumping ground,” Phasha said. First ensure the vaccine works elsewhere before bringing it to Africa, she added.

[..]

Fellow protesters sang and danced with banners saying “We not guinea pigs" and “No safe vaccine.”

“If you want to test, test in the areas which they call the epicenter of the world," demonstrator Sean Goss said.

AP journalist Nqobile Ntshangase in Johannesburg contributed.

- https://www.fox5ny.com/news/protest-versus-africas-1st-covid-19-vaccine-test-shows-fear

****

Rockland County, Probing New Cluster,

Uses Subpoenas as People Resist Contact Tracing

Multiple people apparently contracted COVID-19 after attending a party given by someone who knew they had symptoms

Published July 1, 2020 • Updated on July 1, 2020 at 11:03 pm

[..]

Health officials are investigating a new cluster of eight or more COVID-19 cases in Rockland County tied to a large party earlier this month, but they're running into trouble with contact tracing because people refuse to cooperate.
The county plans to resort to subpoenas, as it did during its measles outbreak some years ago, to compel people to work with contact tracers as they work to contain a new potential outbreak. It may mark the first time in the tri-state area that such a measure has been taken over COVID contact tracing noncompliance.

That party linked to the new potential cluster was the first of three large parties in Rockland County in the last two weeks. It was hosted June 13 by someone in New City who was sick with coronavirus at the time, sources say. County officials said Wednesday that the host knew they were symptomatic and held the party anyway.

[..]

- https://www.nbcnewyork.com/news/coronavirus/rockland-county-probing-a-new-covid-cluster-resorts-to-subpoenas-as-people-refuse-to-give-contacts-to-tracers/2494189/

****

More Infections From an Online Semester?

Researchers at Cornell University have concluded an online semester at the university will result in more COVID-19 infections than an in-person one. The university is reopening, with plans to monitor students and moderate misbehavior.

By Lilah Burke July 1, 2020

Many universities have released statements about their intent to reopen. And every university leader ideally would like to invite students back to campus, since that's what students say they want (and will pay for).

Cornell University joined the chorus of reopening statements on Tuesday in announcing that its Ithaca, N.Y., campus will be open for in-person instruction in the fall.

But for Cornell, one additional piece of information was "very important" in making that decision, according to Martha Pollack, the university's president. That was the finding from Cornell researchers that holding the semester online potentially could result in more infections and more hospitalizations among students and staff members than holding the semester in person would.

A study by Cornell researchers concluded that with nominal parameters, an in-person semester would result in 3.6 percent of the campus population (1,254 people) becoming infected, and 0.047 percent (16 people) requiring hospitalization. An online semester, they concluded, would result in about 7,200 infections and more than 60 hospitalizations.

The conclusion rested on a few different assumptions. First, the study assumed about 9,000 Cornell students would return to Ithaca -- even if there is no in-person learning or physical campus life.

Researchers concluded that during an in-person semester, asymptomatic testing is crucial for containing an outbreak and keeping the total number of infections low. When students live and take classes on campus, the university can enforce such a testing program with a variety of methods. For example, students who don't get tested can lose access to residence halls or be locked out of their email accounts, said Peter Frazier, a data scientist and professor in Cornell's School of Operations Research and Information Engineering, who led the study.

But when instruction is online, the university loses much of that ability to encourage and enforce testing.

- https://www.insidehighered.com/news/2020/07/01/cornell-researchers-say-person-semester-university-safer-online-one

****

July 2, 2020, 1:59PM (Inquiring Librarian to group):

Re: HERETICS: 3 articles shared on Twitter

What a freakshow set of articles!

1st off, I am elated to hear that people in Africa are protesting the vaccine trials on their population. This is fabulous! What is not fabulous is that this is even happening. There are trials also happening in Brazil. It will be interesting to see how that goes and if residents there push back. Here in the Ivory Coast, according to this article, protestors actually burned down a coronavirus testing site: https://www.bbc.com/news/world-africa-52189144 I love how there is a video of a black woman with a massive vial behind her in the article that is trying to 'debunk' the fears of these African protestors as false due to the awesome 'fact checkers'. https://www.bbc.com/news/world-africa-52189144 Both articles are obviously patronizing the African protestors and basically insinuating that they are too misguided and uneducated to understand that this is 'for their own good' How pitiful in a time of "Black Lives Matter" that their valid and, I think, correct fears and actions are scoffed off as ignorant and small minded. This really pisses me off. Do only some black lives and opinions matter, those that support the correct agenda?? Why can't more people see the obvious hypocrisy?

The subpoenaing of those noncompliant to contact tracing requests sounds completely illegal. But this is an 'emergency' right? And the laws are being re-written as we are being told to sit at home and cower in fear.

As for the Cornell article. It appears that Cornell is basically pushing that students should come back because it's easier for the school authorities to imprison them there than it is for them/the government to do so when they are home. And they get to sign paperwork saying that they will adhere to the threats and punishments of not obeying. Makes sense, in hell.

****

Coronavirus: Ivory Coast protesters target testing centre

6 April 2020

Protesters in Ivory Coast's commercial capital, Abidjan, have destroyed a coronavirus centre that was being built in the district of Yopougon.

Residents said it was being built in a crowded residential area, too close to their homes.

Videos on social media show people tearing apart the centre with their bare hands, smashing construction materials on the ground.

Some appeared to be hurling metal poles into a truck.

The health ministry said the building was never intended as a treatment centre, only as a testing facility.

Although, like many African countries, Ivory Coast has had relatively few confirmed coronavirus cases, it has imposed a lockdown in Abidjan and a nationwide curfew.

On Saturday, health officials urged people to wear masks to try to slow the spread of the virus.

[..]

- https://www.bbc.com/news/world-africa-52189144

****

July 2, 2020, 10:30PM (Amir-ul Kafirs to group):

Do only some black lives and opinions matter, those that support the correct agenda??

Yeah, right, these 'backward people' couldn't *possibly* have any legitimate basis for their fears of having a vaccine put into them by people from another country. Why, history has PROVEN that every time people come from other countries to invade them with something or another it's always been for their own good.. except for, maybe, **every fucking time that it hasn't?!** I mean show US some evidence that Africans haven't been routinely screwed by Europeans & used for forced labor & whatnot!! The BBC's attitude is akin to saying that Native Americans are being superstitious to think that the latest experiment on them by white people might actually mean to *do them harm?!* How could they be so foolish, right?! Just because **every fucking time that's been the case?!**

The subpoenaing of those noncompliant to contact tracing requests sounds completely illegal.

The 'funny' thing is that it doesn't seem that there's any claim that anyone's actually gotten sick, gone to the hospital or died as a result of attending these parties. The mere dubious 'fact' of people showing traces of COVID-19 is enough to justify total disregard for civil liberties. Let's hope that that turns out to be much more of a legal problem than even this fanciful 'emergency' can bypass. Of course, this is where the 'knucklehead slur' comes in handy: *anyone who would go to a party where there are NO masks & such-like MUST be a 'knucklehead' because NO INTELLIGENT PERSON WOULD DO THAT.* But, um, where's the proof of that?! Did they interview every person who attended the party & discover that they're all boxers who've suffered multiple head traumas? Football players with the same problem? That might justify it. Did they compare the 'reporter''s IQ with the IQs of everyone at the party? It's 'funny' how certain things are taken for granted as 'obvious truths': the partiers are stupid, no need to use anything but slander on them.

It appears that Cornell is basically pushing that students should come back because it's easier for the school authorities to imprison them

I think that's how they justify it & try to make it scientifically legit. I assume their bottom line is that they're worried that Cornell will go under financially under these conditions if they don't get students to come back. Hell, what do we need universities for anyway? Rump's tweets are all we need.

****

July 2, 2020, 10:31PM (Amir-ul Kafirs to group):

What a freakshow set of articles!

It's like *down the rabbit hole* isn't it?! I mean it's straight out of Lewis Carroll, without the sense of humor, & straight into a deranged world.

Both articles

You sent 2 links to the same article. Here're a couple of interesting excerpts from that:

"Although, like many African countries, Ivory Coast has had relatively few confirmed coronavirus cases, it has imposed a lockdown in Abidjan and a nationwide curfew."

A "nationwide curfew" despite "relatively few confirmed coronavirus cases"! UM, *why, exactly?!*

"Last week, two French doctors sparked fury by suggesting that an existing tuberculosis vaccine **could be tested on African people to see if it cured coronavirus**.

"The doctors' words have fuelled existing fears that African people are to be used as guinea pigs to test a new coronavirus vaccine, though there is no evidence to support this claim.

"Other widespread myths"

OK, the BBC article says that two French doctors suggested that "an existing tuberculosis vaccine **could be tested on African people to see if it cured coronavirus**." Obviously, African people found out about this through news sources. Nonetheless, instead of this being recognized by the BBC as a legitimate concern of Africans it's just said that "The doctors' words have fuelled existing fears that African people are to be used as guinea pigs to test a new coronavirus vaccine, though there is no evidence to support this claim." SO, apparently, the original statement by the doctors isn't "evidence to support this claim"?! It seems pretty clear-cut to me. Of course, I suppose one could say that the doctors merely saying that doesn't mean they have the power or intention to make it happen.

SO, that BBC article is from April 6, 2020, & is, therefore, outdated. Well, here we are on July 2, 2020, & now there IS evidence of a coronavirus vaccine being tested in South Africa & it IS a "**coronavirus vaccine trial**": https://www.pri.org/stories/2020-07-01/south-africa-begins-coronavirus-vaccine-trial . *SO*, now there IS evidence that a vaccine is being tested in Africa. Will that reverse the BBC's previous position that this is a "myth"?

COVID-19: The latest from The World

South Africa begins coronavirus vaccine trial

The World
July 01, 2020 · 3:00 PM EDT
By **Halima Gikandi**
In June, South Africa launched a new COVID-19 vaccine clinical trial, the first in Africa.

****

July 2, 2020, 11:25PM (Inquiring Librarian to group):

Yes, it's the WRONG side of the looking glass. =O If nothing else, we cannot say times are boring. I think I might not mind those aliens coming down mixing things up even a little more. Anything's possible in the freakshow fantasy! And yes to everything in your previous response to my responses... why on earth would they be skeptical?! Maybe the sheeples will start questioning the authorities when they realize this vaccine is being tested on humans in Africa and will likely have devastating results in humans after it totally failed in the monkey trials previously: https://childrenshealthdefense.org/news/another-gates-vaccine-bites-the-dust-sick-monkeys-everywhere/

****

MAY 26, 2020

Another Gates Vaccine Bites the Dust—Sick Monkeys Everywhere!

By Robert F. Kennedy, Jr., Chairman, Children's Health Defense

One day after revelations that the Gates/Fauci Moderna vaccine caused severe illnesses in 20% of high-dose recipients, Bill Gates got devastating news about his other "warp-speed" COVAX bet. The Oxford Vaccine Group (OVG) spike-protein vaccine was on an even faster track than Moderna. In May, Melinda Gates predicted it would be jab-ready by years' end. Oxford and UK officials promised 30 million doses by September.

On April 24, OVG scientists announced that a small macaque study proved the vaccine effective. OVG quickly recruited 510 healthy volunteers for human trials. Pre-publication data released on May 13th reveals the vaccine is less promising than the OVG team implied.

All vaccinated macaques sickened after exposure to COVID-19. Edinburgh University's Eleanor Riley told Forbes the vaccine provided "insufficient" antibodies to prevent infection and viral shedding. Vaccinated monkeys spread the disease as readily as unvaccinated.

Pollard used his power and deceitful puffery about the monkey trial to bulldoze his COVID vaccine into human trials. He shunned inert placebo tests and restricted safety studies to three weeks to hide long-term injuries.

Andrew Pollard strikes again

The OVG is politically wired. Lead developer Andrew Pollard juggles scandalous conflicts that allow him to license, register, and mandate his own untested vaccines to the masses. Pollard is Senior Advisor to Britain's MRHA Panel which licenses vaccines, chairs Britain's JVCI committee that mandates them, and advises the European Medicine Agency (EMA). He takes payments from virtually all the big vaccine makers. In 2014, Pollard developed GlaxoSmithKline's notorious Bexsero meningitis vaccine, and then mandated it to children despite significant safety signals for Kawasaki Disease and the rarity of meningococcal B infections. The package insert says Bexsero may cause Kawasaki disease in as many as one out of every 1000 children based on reports in the clinical trials.

[..]

- https://childrenshealthdefense.org/news/another-gates-vaccine-bites-the-dust-sick-monkeys-everywhere/

****

July 3, 2020, 12:12AM (Amir-ul Kafirs to group):

HERETICS: my latest text panel on social media

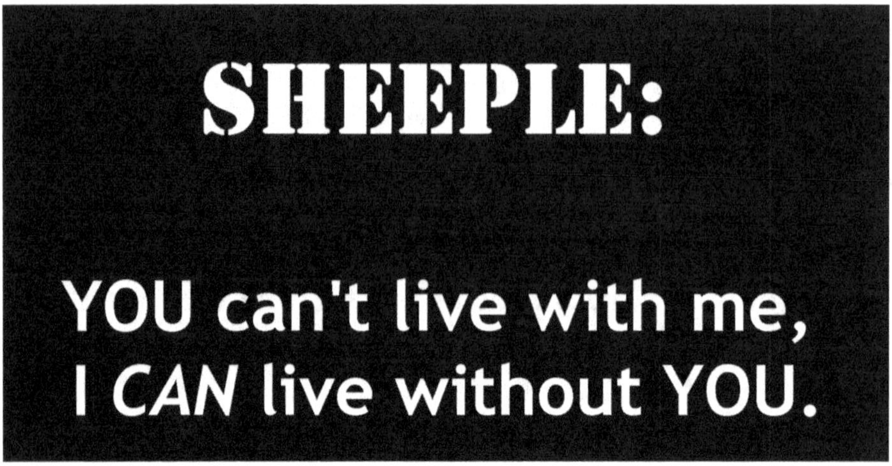
SHEEPLE:
YOU can't live with me,
I *CAN* live without YOU.

****

July 3, 2020, 8:12PM (Amir-ul Kafirs to group):

HERETICS: latest from PA

Could I be any more sick of this? We're entering a shutdown again. It's basically being blamed on young people who've been celebrating summer & being released from their cages. I'm 100% on their side. Here's an excerpt from a relevant article with my own comments interpolated:

After a week of record-shattering COVID-19 case numbers,

By which it's meant people testing positive. It DOESN'T MEAN THAT ANY OF THOSE PEOPLE ARE ACTUALLY SICK. That's the statistics manipulation that I'm most sick of. Is that a form of COVID-19 sickness too?

the Allegheny County Health Department on Thursday issued an order, effective Friday, closing bars, restaurants and casinos, and cancelling all activities or events over 25 people for one-week. Food establishments may still offer take-out and delivery services. Thursday set the record for single-day increases in COVID-19 -- shattering past marks with 233 infections. On Friday, the county reported 177 new cases, a figure above previous records, except for the day before. As of Friday, the total number of COVID-19 cases reported since March is 3,280. There have been 187 deaths so far, though no new deaths reported Friday.

"There have been 187 deaths so far, though no new deaths reported Friday.": OK, I'm a serious broken record at this point but, to again point out the obvious: this pandemic is supposed to've been started on December 31, 2019, hence its name COVID-19, with the "19" standing for 2019. That's over 6 months ago. If we count the 187 deaths attributed to COVID-19 in Allegheny County from then it's been 188 days, that's one death per day. They're apparently counting from March so let's just start from March 1st: That's 125 days, roughly 1.5 deaths a day.

The ages for the county's newest cases range from 1 to 90 years old, with 28 the median age,
Meaning people highly unlikely to actually suffer any severe effects.
the county said Friday. There have been 406 past and present hospitalizations, including 5 reported Friday.
Dr. Debra Bogen, the health department director, recommended a voluntary stay-at-home protocol for all county residents, to try and prevent further spread of the virus.
"This is not a decision that I've made lightly but I believe it's necessary based on the new cases in the county and the community spread that is occurring," Bogen said.
The typical local COVID-infected person during late June was 27 years old,
Once again, meaning people highly unlikely to actually suffer any severe effects.
according to a summary of 712 Allegheny County case investigations conducted between June 20 and 30. Cases among the 19-to-24 cohort doubled during that period, according to a late-Thursday news release.
Of the 31 new hospitalizations during that time, seven were people in their 20s and 30s, the county reported Thursday.
31 new hospitalizations in an 11 day period. Less than 3 a day. I counted 54 Allegheny County hospitals on this website: https://pennsylvania.hometownlocator.com/features/cultural,class,hospital,scfips,42003.cfm . That's one person admitted to one of 18 hospitals per day or, to put it another way, less than 3/5ths of the hospitals receiving a *single COVID-19 patient!!* How much more ridiculous can it get?!
The county continues to believe that many of the new cases are related to travel -- especially to the Carolinas and Florida -- or local nightlife.
In other words: *Shame on you for being young & trying to have a good time!!* What I honestly hope for is that younger people, at least, give a giant fuck-you to these authoritarian nut-jobs but it doesn't really seem to be happening.

****

July 3, 2020, 10:00PM (Inquiring Librarian to group):

Re: HERETICS: latest from PA

Ouch. That really sucks, and it makes ZERO sense. A big long distance hug from a swampy Louisiana!! This is so unbelievable. I mean, really, how does this make any sense? What is the long term nefarious goal? It's truly mind boggling. If I was not working, I'd drive to Pittsburgh to wreak whatever summer fun life is a beach mayhem I could around your supposed 'plague' town.

****

July 4, 2020, 12:49AM (Amir-ul Kafirs to group):

HERETICS: Vocabulary

Vocabulary:

Ad Hominem Arguments
Behavioral Conditioning
Biga Peula (Kiriwina)
Brow-Beating
Bullies
Censorship
Contestaire (French)
Control Freaks
Doctor Gods
Fact Choking
False Syllogisms
Fear-Mongering
Greed
Groupthink
Irrelevant Conclusions
Medical Industry Police State
Mind Control
Monolithic Narrative
New World Odor
Non-Essential Degenerates
Pandemic Panic
Pavlov's Humans
Plunderbund (Dutch)
Propaganda
Quarantiniac
Quarantyrrany

Relevance Fallacies
Robopaths
Sheeple
Snitches
Spin Doctors
Superiority Complex
Thought Crimes
Untertan (German)

****

July 4, 2020, 3:57AM (Dick to group):

The news here has endless articles about the USA and the increase of cases

I saw this, too

It's about so-called "covid parties" among young people - saying that they supposedly organise parties with the intent of getting the virus - maybe it's BS, but the article, and others like it, keep showing up (translation follows article)

https://www.20minutes.fr/monde/2814023-20200703-etats-unis-etudiants-organisaient-soirees-covid-19-pariant-celui-contamine-premier

Des étudiants américains organisaient des soirées « contamination Covid »
Des malades étaient présents aux soirées, les étudiants se contaminant volontairement pour gagner les paris

TRANSLATION:

United States: Students organized Covid-19 parties, betting on who was the first to be contaminated

GAME OF CRETINS Patients were present at the parties, the students voluntarily contaminating themselves to win the bets

B.C.
Published on 07/03/20 at 13h58 - Updated on 07/07/20 at 18h13

Unbridled beer pong evenings could pass for a gathering of good kids. Students in the university town of Tuscaloosa, Alabama, came up with the idea of hosting Covid-19 parties to infect each other deliberately.

This is what Sonya McKinstry, a member of the town council told ABC News. The principle is quite simple: positive people were invited to parties, participants then had to bet on who would have symptoms first.

City fire chief Randy Smith first reported on the practice at a meeting. At first he thought it was such a big rumor. "Not only did the doctor's offices help confirm this, but the state confirmed that they had the same information," he said.

Conviction of authorities

Something to arouse the indignation of local authorities when the state of Alabama is facing a surge in hospitalizations, a near-shortage of beds in intensive care and has more than 38,000 cases of coronavirus and 947 deaths.

"It does not mean anything. They put money in a jar ... And the first to have the Covid wins it," said Sonya McKinstry, interviewee, interviewed by ABC News. The woman wondered how people can intentionally participate in the spread of the pandemic when the authorities try to curb it.

What the University of Alabama did in early March when it canceled its face-to-face courses. In the event of a positive test, residents must be placed in quarantine, and if they depart from it they can be fined up to $500.

****

July 4, 2020, 7:33AM (Amir-ul Kafirs to group):

What is the long term nefarious goal?

Total Mind Control, total suppression of *joie de vivre!*

****

July 4, 2020, 7:46AM (Amir-ul Kafirs to group):

The news here has endless articles about the USA and the increase of cases

& the paranoia may very well be on the rise. My one friendly neighbor who didn't wear a mask & who always seemed to enjoy talking with me when she was walking her dog seems more afraid of me now because when we talked about the rise in Green Phase cases & said that something like 400 new cases have been reported I said: "But that doesn't mean that 400 people are going to die." I mean any kind of common sense statement that doesn't fuel the fear seems to get rejected as dangerous or some such.

It's about so-called"covid parties" among young people

It's great to get the French version of this. I haven't followed the US 'news' enough to run across "covid parties" but I reckon they're out there. What it shows is that some younger people aren't afraid & think that the whole thing is ridiculous. Obviously, I'm fine with that. When all this started I thought of having a party called "Enter at Your Own Risk" but I don't think anyone other than Naia Nisnam would've attended! SO, as long as no-one attending these parties actually *dies* I think they're great & I hope that they help instill some healthy disrespect for the doom-sayers.

"It does not mean anything. They put money in a jar ... And the first to have the Covid wins it,"

College students are getting away from home to be free from their parents restrictions for the 1st time in their life & then? The state tells them: No, no, you must continue to stay at home & not have a social life indefinitely. & these moronic authority figures wonder why these students would rebel against this? They might believe in the ultimate 'goodness' of their lockdown 'vision' but that doesn't mean that the rest of us have to.

AAAARRRRRGGGGGGGGHHHH!

****

July 4, 2020, 12:07AM (Inquiring Librarian to group):

HERETICS: Humor on Social Distancing Rules Creation

I think humor is on order here. This is my favorite Awaken with JP yet!
https://www.youtube.com/watch?v=4H-6HTKNgV0&fbclid=IwAR1E6W8Gq-0hESPLgJoB9uD_9EBag9m6KE6UEJCRxBKQ_Kq7BWd7opv_tRg

The only qualm I have with this, is I feel these days like the janitor is generally going to me smarter than the 'doctor'.

****

July 4, 2020, 3:58AM (Dick to group):

That was my reaction, too, it seemed unfair to custodians...

****

July 4, 2020, 7:59AM (Amir-ul Kafirs to group):

Re: HERETICS: Humor on Social Distancing Rules Creation

I subscribed to his channel on my phone so I get the links for each new one that comes out & I usually watch them right away. I watched this one too. I continue to like them but in the recent ones he always ends with ads for some product he's selling. Because of this I don't add them to my PANDEMIC PANIC playlist. Otherwise, yeah, I agree with Linda & Dick here that he basically uses the toilet cleaner as a convenient stereotype of an idiot. I would've preferred that the doctor be shown making the stupid decisions. What 'saves it' (somewhat) is that JP usually plays most of the characters so he gets to be the toilet cleaner & the doctor & the assistant taking notes.

****

July 4, 2020, 9:28AM (Dick to group):

I find this to be interesting. Here is a post from _____, one of many he has written in the same tone. This fellow is (or was, I don't know if it still exists) the announcer on a classical station. I could call him a "sheeple" and be done with it, but I think that there may be deeper motivation at work. I get the feeling he likes the righteous superioristic tone he's adopted, I can almost see him smiling at his own imagined cleverness as he wrote the post. I assume it is linked to anti-Trumpism, another subject found in his posts. I guess what amazes me is this desire to show one's belonging to a certain community, that is, the pro-maskers, repeatedly, over and over again. These posts range from attempts at humor (which is how I assume he means the following post), to indignation, etc. Another way of putting it is, he has chosen to take not wearing a mask personally, as an affront, even, as as writes below, as an attempt at murder. I sense a deep need within his posts meaning I think what he really wants to express has nothing to do with Covid-19. I sense a sort of Freudian displacement of an anger which I assume is always there but perhaps lacking in an object of expression. I write that because if not, it just seems pointless to me.
*
In terms of the following, it doesn't make sense. I personally wouldn't care if he showed his penis in public (see post to understand this) I just simply wouldn't look.

_____

If I do not have the right to show my penis in public, you do not have the right to be in public without wearing a mask. And I'm being generous. My penis does not murder people.

****

July 4, 2020, 12:34PM (Amir-ul Kafirs to group):

If I do not have the right to show my penis in public, you do not have the right to be in public without wearing a mask. And I'm being generous. My penis does not murder people.

There are obvious flaws to his 'logic':

1. Exposing one's genitalia in public has been taboo for our entire lifetime & beyond except at places that permit nudity such as nudist beaches, nudist camps, & public showers (such as at a public swimming pool). As such, exposing one's genitalia in public would have always been an abnormal act in most circumstances. Contrarily, the 'requirement' to cover one's mouth is a recent phenomena & not one 'required' in any circumstances but one where one is in somewhat close proximity to strangers. As such, this 'requirement' is the abnormality.

2. A maskless person is not 'murdering' anyone. If they were, literally everyone in the world would've been long since dead by now. In other words, _____'s, & everyone else who pushes this idiotic line's, implication is that by the mere fact of not wearing a mask you are directly causing the death of people around you. Therefore, EVERYONE WITHOUT A MASK IS DIRECTLY KILLING PEOPLE. Really? What about the people not wearing masks who aren't infected with COVID-19? That would mean that any person without a mask would be transmitting COVID-19 to everyone within a certain distance to them, let's be 'conservative' & say 6 feet. That gets complicated, though, because, presumably, those wearing masks wouldn't be infected. But, apparently, that's *not the case*, because one can get infected through the eyes. Therefore, wearing the mask only prevents spreading the disease through breathing. Then, of course, those now-infected *not wearing masks* would further spread it. Since we're talking murder here, that means that EVERYONE so exposed will die. PERIOD. If no-one dies, there's no murder. Now, presumably, the maskless person should also be accused of committing suicide since we're talking murder that means that *they will die as a result of being exposed to other people.* PERIOD. There're no ifs, ands, or buts here, right? The, ahem, problem here is that when I go out without a mask on & there are other people without masks on why aren't the people around us dying? At this point, when I go to a park, for example, at least half of the people aren't wearing masks. That means that the local deaths from COVID-19 must be phenomenal — &, yet, there've been what? One recently? None? So where exactly are the victims? This whole concept that not wearing a mask is killing people is imaginary, people get self-righteous & indignant about it without there having to be any actual proveable deaths associated with any particular non-mask person at all. It's like the Spectral Evidence of the Salem Witch Trials: it's enough to just *dream that it's true*.

****

July 4, 2020, (Naia Nisnam sent Amir-ul Kafirs a txt msg link to this article):

'Wearing A Mask Shows That You Care About Others': Pa. Secretary Of Health Signs Order Making Masks Mandatory In

All Public Spaces

July 1, 2020 at 3:19 pm

HARRISBURG, Pa. (KDKA) – Masks are now mandatory in all public spaces in Pennsylvania.

Gov. Tom Wolf announced Wednesday the order was signed by Secretary of Health Dr. Rachel Levine.

Masks must be worn whenever anyone leaves home, the governor says. The order — which you can read here — takes effect immediately.

[..]

- https://pittsburgh.cbslocal.com/2020/07/01/pennsylvania-public-masks-mandate/

****

July 4, 2020, 5:17PM (Amir-ul Kafirs to group):

Here're the exceptions to the Governor's order. Note that one isn't legally required to show documentation that an exception applies. I could easily claim that as a result of working as a hard wood floor finisher for 10 years that I have difficulty breathing with a mask on.

Section 3: Exceptions to Face Covering Requirement

A. The following are exceptions to the face covering requirement in Section 2:

i. Individuals who cannot wear a mask due to a medical condition, including those with respiratory issues that impede breathing, mental health condition, or disability;

ii. Individuals for whom wearing a mask while working would create an unsafe condition in which to operate equipment or execute a task as determined by local, state, or federal regulators or workplace safety guidelines;

iii. Individuals who would be unable to remove a mask without assistance;

iv. Individuals who are under two years of age;

v. Individuals who are communicating or seeking to communicate with someone who is hearing-impaired or has another disability, where the ability to see the mouth is essential for communication;

B. Individuals are not required to show documentation that an exception applies.

****

July 4, 2020, 4:53PM (Amir-ul Kafirs to group):

Independence Day

"Masks must be worn whenever anyone leaves home, the governor says."

Goodbye Independence. Henceforth July 4th will be known as Subjugation Day.

****

July 4, 2020, 6:06PM (Inquiring Librarian to group):

Re: HERETICS: Independence Day ps: Exceptions

Great! I have a mental health condition. We learned earlier that i am a 'Psychopath' because i think this is bullshit and feel morally compelled to disobey nonsensical social distancing rules. Not to mention, i am 'Intellectually Arrogant' because i oppose the farce of vaccination. https://www.bitchute.com/video/A2hUgrTqdNLa/

****

July 4, 2020, 11:23PM (Amir-ul Kafirs to group):

We learned earlier that i am a 'Psychopath'

Your saying that here is funny — just don't ever try to use that line publicly! Remember: the 1st people the nazis killed were people in mental institutions (aided by doctors of course!).

Alas, Spiro's video is great except when he gets into his racist anti-BLM agenda (basically he reduces it to just rioting — just like typical mainstream media would) & the comments are pretty consistently racist too. Note that one of them extolls the virutes of South Africa under apartheid. It's more than a little hard for me to stomach that!

****

July 5, 2020, 12:00AM (Inquiring Librarian to group):

HERETICS: John Waters SVA Commencement Speech 2020

I was talking to Amir-ul Kafirs tonight on the phone and he brought up something about John Waters. It got me thinking. I'm desperately trying these days to find some/any celebrities that I admire that might also be "Heretics" that are not buying the narrative.

Here is a commencement speech that John Waters gave for the NYC School of the Visual Arts virtual graduation ceremony. I am not fully sure what to make of it except that he seems frustrated and disappointed in what is happening now. Please let me know what you think. Ultimately, I think it overall is as brilliant as I think Waters is.

You can watch the speech or read the transcript below (not that you could not figure that out, but you know... it is covid and you must have things spelled out to you as I tell you what to do.)

https://deadline.com/2020/05/john-waters-commencement-speech-school-of-visual-arts-graduates-coronavirus-class-of-2020-1202944478/

****

BREAKING NEWS

John Waters Energizes School Of Visual Arts Grads With Virtual Commencement Speech For 'Coronavirus Class Of 2020'

Mike Fleming Jr
Co-Editor-in-Chief, Film
May 27, 2020 11:42am

It has been a terrible year for graduating classes all over the country. To pick up the spirits of grads everywhere, here is a speech that director John Waters gives today in virtual fashion to the graduating class of the School of Visual Arts. The irreverent Baltimore-based director of films from *Hairspray* to *Pink Flamingos, Polyester* and *Serial Mom* seemed to be determined to motivate and energize a class of grads heading into the most precarious job market in memory. But he often heads into detours, from pondering the inevitable *Tiger King* Porn film knockoff to a Lori Loughlin shout out, and the possibility that grads might be unique if in fact they have the distinction of possibly being the last graduating class in the world, ever. So it's not the *Braveheart* speech, but it's still pretty entertaining stuff as the offbeat filmmaker dispenses life lessons. Here is his speech.

"Thank you all very much. I wanted to give this speech live in Radio City Music Hall as scheduled in front of the 5000 graduates, faculty and family members but oh, no, here I am in front of a green screen in Baltimore like some low-rent special- effect Nutty Professor. Now you have to watch me virtually, with no timing for laughs... and once posted I'll be subject to being rewound or, worse yet, fast-forwarded. Suppose hacker trolls interrupt our on-line ceremony today yelling 'Quit School' or 'Free the Test Cheater mom, Lori Loughlin.' There's nothing we could do about it. We're trapped in a Grade-Z horror movie with no way out.

Ok, I'm supposed to energize. That's a challenge when every morning you look at the headlines and they all basically say 'You Are Going To Die Today.' But I'm an optimist and you should be, too. If you do die tomorrow, at least you got your college degree, right? And suppose the end of the world is happening right now? Well, you won't miss a thing, will you? Because there will be no more 'things.' You will be the last graduating class in the world. Now that's what I call unique.

Me? I've just been lying around at home, paranoid about touching my face and looking forward to the first "Tiger King" porno knockoff. What a time! I bet you never thought the New York Department of Health would issue guidelines recommending masturbation during the pandemic! And those masks? So hot, steaming up your glasses when you're trying to study, muffling your voice in online classrooms. Protective face coverings threaten my whole identity by hiding my moustache! But I wear these masks anyway for the safety of the prisoners whose bail I've recently helped contribute to through various charities. I bet a few of these criminals are robbing your car as I speak. Gloves? Yep, we have them on but don't they make you feel like Jack the Ripper or, worse yet, an unemployed proctologist. It's not pretty but who wants cooties? Not me and certainly not you; the smart ones about to get a degree."

[..]

- https://deadline.com/2020/05/john-waters-commencement-speech-school-of-visual-arts-graduates-coronavirus-class-of-2020-1202944478/

****

July 5, 2020, 12:15AM (Amir-ul Kafirs to group):

Re: HERETICS: John Waters SVA Commencement Speech 2020

Here is a commencement speech that John Waters gave

It's a great speech, hilarious, deeply layered, etc.. It doesn't really ultimately say much of use for these times though IMO. In other words, it's Waters being Waters but he doesn't *really* address what's happening — he just uses it as comic material.

****

Jul 5, 2020, 12:19AM (Amir-ul Kafirs to group):

HERETICS: Doctors

Oh, well, I think the following is very succinct & to the point. Whether anyone is actually *moved by it* is a different story, whether anyone reading it has a 2nd thought about the DOCTOR GODS is a different story. Are my attempts hopeless?!

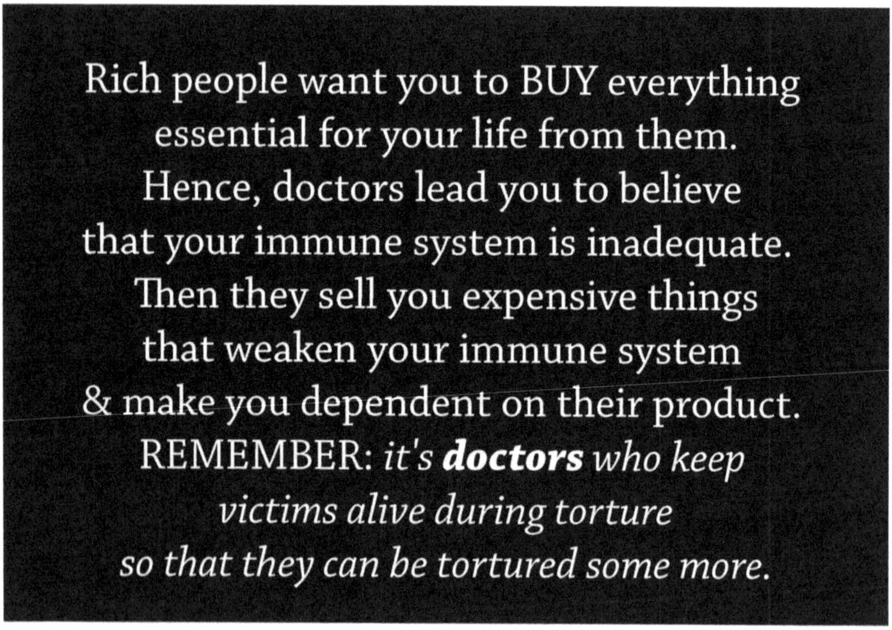

Rich people want you to BUY everything
essential for your life from them.
Hence, doctors lead you to believe
that your immune system is inadequate.
Then they sell you expensive things
that weaken your immune system
& make you dependent on their product.
REMEMBER: *it's* ***doctors*** *who keep*
victims alive during torture
so that they can be tortured some more.

****

Jul 4, 2020, 8:27PM (Amir-ul Kafirs to group):

HERETICS: Quarantine T-Shirt

I was at the grocery store & they were selling these t-shirts.

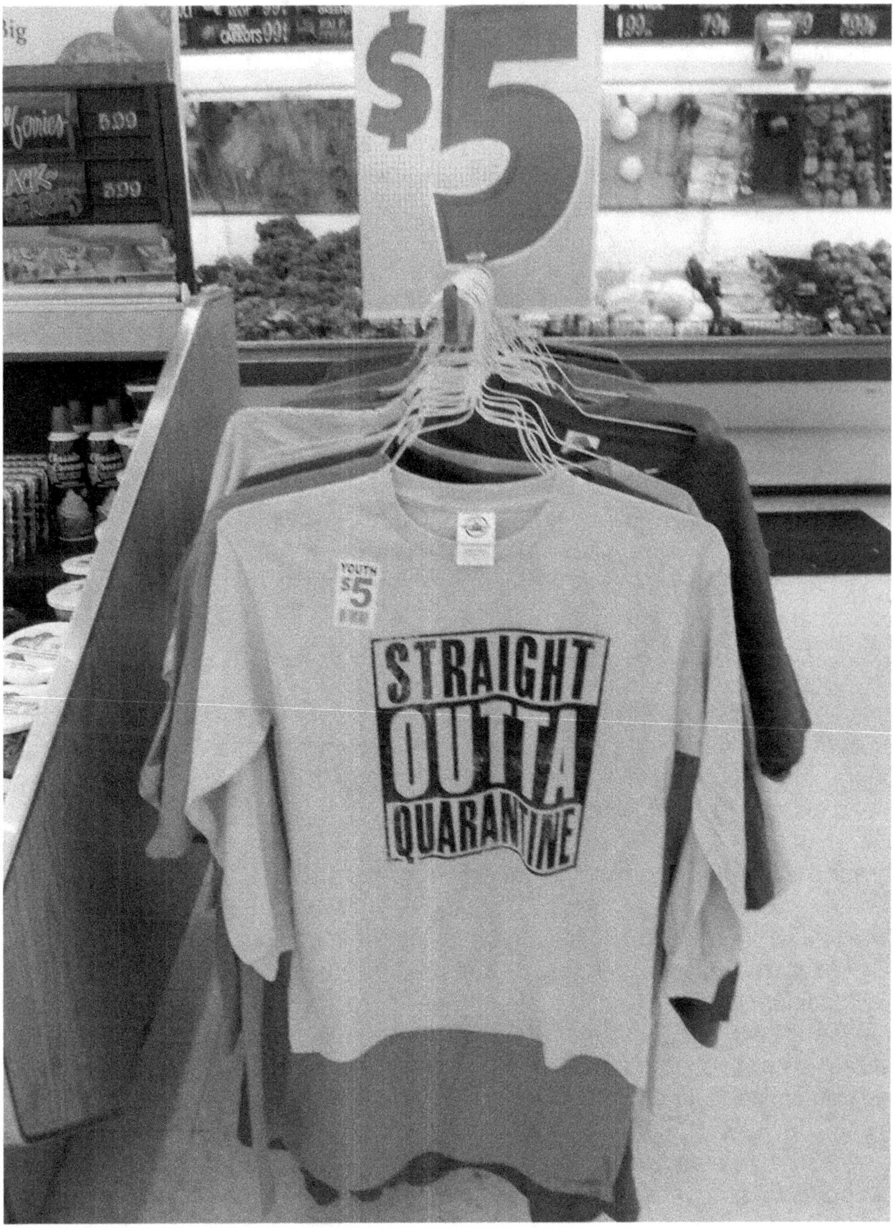

****

July 5, 2020, 6:56AM (Dick to group):

RE: HERETICS: Quarantine T-Shirt

It's a variation on Straight Otta Compton by the rap group NWA (N*gg*rs With Attitude)
It was the first gangsta rap disc

here it is

https://www.youtube.com/watch?v=TMZi25Pq3T8

N.W.A. - Straight Outta Compton (Official Music Video)
Get N.W.A vinyl here: http://smarturl.it/NWAstore Listen to N.W.A on Spotify: http://smarturl.it/NWASpotify Find N.W.A titles on Apple Music: http://smarturl.it/AppleMusicNWA and Google Play: http://smarturl.it/NWAGooglePlay Get the 'Straight Outta Compton' CD here: http://smarturl.it/NWAOuttaComptonCD Like N.W.A on Facebook http://facebook ...

****

July 5, 2020, 12:20AM (Inquiring Librarian to group):

HERETICS: C.J. Hopkins - The New (Pathologized) Totalitarianism

Hi All, I found this article by C.J. Hopkins today, "The New (Pathologized) Totalitarianism".
https://off-guardian.org/2020/06/29/the-new-pathologized-totalitarianism/

I believe I found it on Phil's page, and it is here in the OffGuardian (a magazine an old friend of mine just 'discredited' for me today when she did her 2 second google search on the OffGuardian without reading the very well researched pcr test article that I shared with her).

Here is a particularly compelling excerpt from the article:

"The genius of pathologized totalitarianism is like that old joke about the Devil … his greatest trick was convincing us that he doesn't exist. Pathologized totalitarianism appears to emanate from nowhere, and everywhere, simultaneously; thus, technically, it does not exist. It *cannot* exist, because no one is responsible for it, because everyone is. Mass hysteria is its lifeblood. It feeds on existential fear. "Science" is its rallying cry. Not actual science, not provable facts, but "Science" as a kind of deity whose Name is invoked to silence heretics, or to ease the discomfort of the cognitive dissonance that results from desperately trying to believe the absurdities of the official narrative."

****

July 5, 2020, 12:25AM (Amir-ul Kafirs to group):

Re: HERETICS: C.J. Hopkins - The New (Pathologized) Totalitarianism

I read it, I think it's fantastic. I have to wonder, though, we find all these great articles we agree with &, YET, things just keep getting worse & worse. When will we start to see more movement in the desired direction? To put it mildly, I'm pretty impatient.

****

July 6, 2020, 11:14AM (Naia Nisnam to group):

Re: HERETICS: C.J. Hopkins - The New (Pathologized) Totalitarianism

This article is helpful in my understanding of why people Want to prolong quarantine and live the masks. He does a good job of expressing the almost incomprehensible to me idea that many people Want to live under totalitarianism.

I think we are having a hard time getting the general population to accept the articles we like because of the extreme bipartisanism. To even question the effectiveness of masks is to claim allegiance with Trump.

I truly do support BLM, but it is serving to further divide people at a time when the "left" could have begun to question the lockdowns. The protests also give the "left" an outlet for their general frustrations and an approved way of getting out of isolation, if only for a few hours at a time.

****

July 6, 2020, 1:45PM (Amir-ul Kafirs to group):

people Want to live under totalitarianism.

I think there's a sexual dynamic to it. For some people it's masochism. I think for most, though, it's a desire to dominate. Totalitarianism gives the Untertan clear stepping stones to be able to advance in a hierarchy. What may've been ambiguous in the past, what might've seemed to've required a modicum of talent or hard-work now becomes something simpler, something available to otherwise frustrated assholes. Any kind of society where legally approved vigilantism appears gives bullies a field day, brown shirts can go out & throw bricks threw the windows of Jewish shops with impunity.

Now, of course, Jews aren't necessarily the targets: non-believers are. That's why I'm "Amir-ul Kafirs", "Commander of the Unbelievers" — which is, of course, a joke, I'm not anyone's 'commander', it's a parody of how militarized Islam is with their Amir-ul-Mujahideen, Commander of the Faithful. We are the non-believers, the people who reject the Monolithic Narrative, the HERETICS.

ANYWAY, it's illegal here now to NOT wear a mask outside of one's house. I'm about to go for a walk in Frick Park & I won't be taking a mask with me. I'll be surrounded by a heavy totalitarian mindset from the people wearing masks. Joggers won't be wearing them. A few other people won't be either but ever since Big Brother made his latest pronouncement the vibe outside is worse than ever. I did go out early this morning to gas up my car & there were what seemed to me to be an extraordinary amount of joggers out, I suspect they were people using it as an excuse to not be masked.

I truly do support BLM, but it is serving to further divide people at a time when the "left" could have begun to question the lockdowns. The protests also give the "left" an outlet for their general frustrations and an approved way of getting out of isolation, if only for a few hours at a time.

Ditto to the above. Alas, the 'left', which is a complete joke now as a rebellion & as a critique of society, is enabling totalitarianism in a big way.

The way going for a walk in the park feels right now is akin to the way stepping out of my downtown warehouse in Baltimore felt during the post-Rodney King incident. Every time I went outside I wondered if I'd be murdered for being white, now I wonder if I'll be arrested for not wearing a mask — all this just as I attempt to go on my daily healthy walk, minding my own business, not bothering anyone.

There was a time when people would say: "I'm going to move to Canada!" — but would that do any good right now?!

****

July 6, 2020, 3:34PM (Inquiring Librarian to group):

Hi All, I also support BLM, I mean honestly, who would not? But I am concerned about the organization's infiltration by the government and big money corporations who seem to be somewhat sabotaging it and creating further divides. Check out this awful article about the BLM protests and virus transmission in Nola. It makes anyone who is skeptical of the virus or masks really feel ill will towards the protests which leads to ill will towards BLM.

& notice in the photos, the protestors are wearing masks. If you do any google search of the protests here, you will see plenty of people without masks on. This seems like pure political propaganda here and it's sad to see BLM being used as a tool for this nefarious purpose. I find the scientific logic behind all of this is frankly insulting to BLM and to really any reader.

New Orleans health director: It's 'very clear' coronavirus clusters haven't traced back to protests

https://www.nola.com/news/politics/article_ae585fa8-b649-11ea-b37e-6fbafe81bd90.html

****

July 6, 2020, 1:18PM (Amir-ul Kafirs to group):

SCIENCE

**is not one thing
in which everyone reaches the
same conclusions.
Different techniques are used,
different conclusions are reached.
NONE OF THEM ARE DEFINITIVE.
Dr. Fauci, director of NIAID
(National Institute of
Allergy and Infectious Diseases)
oversees the disbursement of
6 billion dollars of grants
yearly to universities.
What do you think would happen
to those grants if researchers
at the universities would go
against the 'party line' on COVID-19?**

***Want to make yourself unpopular
with your fellow scientists?
Lose the funding that everyone's
dependent on for their research
by releasing findings that
don't justify the quarantyrrany.***

****

July 6, 2020, 7:47PM (Amir-ul Kafirs to group):

Hi All, I also support BLM, I mean honestly, who would not?

It occured to me that because I was born in 1953 & grew up in the '50s, '60s, & '70s I got to see racism happening at a way more flagrant level than my younger friends. I mean the lynchings were still happening when I was growing up!

"According to the Tuskegee Institute, 4,743 people were lynched between 1882 and 1968 in the United States, including 3,446 African Americans and 1,297 whites. More than 73 percent of lynchings in the post–Civil War period occurred in the Southern states. According to the Equal Justice Initiative, 4,084 African-Americans were lynched between 1877 and 1950 in the South."

- https://en.wikipedia.org/wiki/Lynching_in_the_United_States

I didn't really even become aware of the situation until 1968 when I was 14 because my life was so segregated, I'd hardly ever even seen a black person. The point is that awareness of this is permanently ingrained in me. While I've seen vast improvements in civil rights & racial relations in general I'm ever mindful that *it wasn't that long ago when a buncha God fearin' southern whites could just drag somebody away, torture them, set fire to them, & hang them from a tree* — & those days could come back PDQ. As such, agitating against racism seems like a damned good idea.

New Orleans health director: It's 'very clear' coronavirus clusters haven't traced back to protests

Honestly, Inquiring Librarian, I don't know what to make of this. The gist of the article is this:

"It all spurred a common local reaction: If these parties are a problem, what about the protests?

"“We have been following very closely cases since the protests several weeks ago with our partners at the Louisiana Department of Health,” Avegno responded on Wednesday. “Neither they nor we have identified any clusters related to protests."

&, apparently, that's the official story everywhere. Given that I don't believe that the pandemic is what it's said to be, given that I'm against the quarantine, given that I'm against enforced mask wearing, given that I'm FOR the protests AND the other public gatherings the 'easiest' thing for me to perceive this as is DIVIDE & CONQUER. In other words, by demonizing people who're just going about their ordinary lives, celebrating graduations & such-like & by saying that the BLM protests, even though a few of them have ended in fires & looting, *are not a part of the pandemic problem* THE MOST OBVIOUS RESULT IS AN INCREASED HATRED OF BLM PROTESTORS ON THE PART OF PEOPLE WHO'RE OTHERWISE APOLITICAL OR CONSERVATIVE — such as Spiro Skouras. You see what I mean? By NOT taking an anti-BLM stand they get to seem 'neutral' but the obvious effect is more divisiveness. &, as usual, it seems to me that the main people who stand to gain by such divisiveness are *not the people themselves* because, WTF, we could use **more unity**.

SO, what happens? Naia Nisnam & I both are tempted to attend protests against the quarantine but they're partially supported by people who're racist & hate the BLM protestors. Since we don't want to support them (&, excuse me, Naia Nisnam, I don't mean to speak for you, I just mean to refer to a recent discussion we had) that puts us in a position in which we can't show our solidarity against the quarantine. It seems to me that if this situation could be 'corrected', in other words, if conservatives could understand the BLM movement through the perceptions of people like myself instead of through the mass media, AND if the BLM movement could understand just how police state the quarantine IS, that there might be more solidarity against something that's obviously negative for ALL of us.

****

July 6, 2020, 3:37PM (Inquiring Librarian to group):

HERETICS: Senator Scott Jensen Investigated for Speaking the Truth

Hi All,

I found this today on Denis Rancourt, PhD/Physicists page. It's pretty shocking. This award winning doctor is being investigated for not fudging the death numbers and for speaking out against those who have fudged the death numbers and for comparing covid deaths to flu deaths:

https://m.youtube.com/watch?feature=youtu.be&v=ny4Ni-YuMpg

I suspect this will be removed from Youtube sooner than later. So you should watch it sooner. =]

****

July 7, 2020, 10:01AM (Amir-ul Kafirs to group):

Re: HERETICS: Senator Scott Jensen Investigated for Speaking the Truth

Thanks for sharing this. I watched the whole thing & added it to my PANDEMIC PANIC playlist. Not surprisingly, I found what Senator/Doctor Scott Jensen said to be believable & to support what we've been saying here all along. One particularly interesting thing that he said is that Pennsylvania back-pedaled on its COVID-19 death reports & lowered the number. He also says that New York has taken the opposite tack & grossly exaggerated its COVID-19 deaths. All this is very important & the more credible sources there are out there saying this stuff the better.

I suspect this will be removed from Youtube sooner than later.

I'm not so sure it'll be removed. **[It hasn't been as of August 26, 2020]** If you learn that it does get removed please let us know. I don't know whether YouTube would go so far as to censor a Senator/Doctor — especially one who comes across as such a 'wholesome' guy.

****

July 7, 2020, 11:47AM (Amir-ul Kafirs to group):

Re: HERETICS: Senator Scott Henson Investigated for Speaking the Truth

I also shared this on social media with this preface:

"I've been mostly NOT sharing online videos critical of the PANDEMIC PANIC here for the past few months but now that Big Brother Wolf is snarling at our doors again it seems like time for a continual barrage of counter-information. Remember, if you disagree with this doctor's statement about COVID-19 death counts being deliberately exaggerated and about the dubious value of wearing face-masks that's fine but if I feel you're abusing me in any way for agreeing with this doctor I'll be happy to unfriend you."

I'm less & less tolerant of abusive behavior there. If anyone wants to attack me for going contrary to the Monolithic narrative that's their business but I feel no need whatsoever to stay 'friends' with them.

Cheerio,

I'm thankful, as always, for my lovely HERETICS friends here!

****

July 7, 2020, 2:39AM (Amir-ul Kafirs to group):

Mass Hysteria = Mask Hysteria = Mass Hypnosis

****

July 7, 2020, 3:25AM (Naia Nisnam to group):

Re: HERETICS: Mask Hysteria

“We’ll likely be wearing masks in public for a while. Gov. Tom Wolf says he thinks masks will be mandatory until there’s a vaccine”

https://pittsburgh.cbslocal.com/2020/07/06/governor-wolf-masks-mandatory-coronavirus-vaccine/?fbclid=IwAR3qfbO__V4GYtUjt3DfMbR9LXTp8UAs4o5puELjlZM27CqKHWuZwHOTrxE

****

Gov. Tom Wolf: Masks May Be Mandatory Until There’s A Coronavirus Vaccine

July 6, 2020 at 5:51 pm

PITTSBURGH (KDKA) – We’ll likely be wearing masks in public for a while. Gov. Tom Wolf says he thinks masks will be mandatory until there’s a vaccine.

“Models out there suggest that states, areas, where people wear masks, the infection rate is actually lower,” said Gov. Wolf Monday.

The governor updated the mask mandate last week when cases around the state — and Allegheny County — began to spike.

The order requires face masks to be worn in several different settings, including if you’re outdoors and can’t stay 6 feet away from strangers, if you’re inside a public place or if you’re at work.

There are exceptions that can be found in the order. People with exceptions aren't required to show documentation.

The order was sent to state and local officials, as well as law enforcement and others "tasked with education about the order for those not in compliance."

****

July 7, 2020, 12:13PM (Amir-ul Kafirs to group):

" We'll likely be wearing masks in public for a while. Gov. Tom Wolf says he thinks masks will be mandatory until there's a vaccine"

I continue to defy this order as do many other people that I see. I, of course, hope that more or more people will respond to this with a sortof "whatever, asshole" attitude.

****

July 7, 2020, 9:33AM (Dick to group):

HERETICS: small comment

Please read to the very end before commenting.
Amir-ul Kafirs wrote the other day that he can't imagine anyone being against BLM
At the risk of being branded a nazi I will say I am against BLM
Why?
Something about it doesn't sit right with me, it never has
not the movement but the slogan
It isn't that I am unaware of any of the problems of being black in the usa or police brutality, I too have seen it first hand
but I feel that any form of division is potentially dangerous, even well-intentioned
please look at the following video upon which I base my opinion:
https://www.youtube.com/watch?v=oGvoXeXCoUY

Brown eyes and blue eyes Racism experiment Children Session - Jane Elliott

Now if you watched the video, one which I find to be very moving emotionally by the way, you'll see that when the blue eyed kids were on top it created division and fighting
And then when the brown eyed kids were on top it did the same thing
as long as there is division in any form there will be problems
can you imagine if a politician said "ok, it's been BLM for several months, let's change to white lives matter'
well, the reaction would probably be civil war
now, maybe someone will protest 'but Dick, it's been white lives matter since 1492, now it's time for a change'
well, according to the video this will just cause more problems,

resentment, etc and not lead to any resolution of the problem
those are my feelings
i wish the movement was called PSTB "please stop targeting black people" i feel that that slogan would be more exact and not make anyone feel like they were being put into a secondary position
furthermore, it is less in your face and therefore more likely to solicite a higher degree of positive response.
that's all!
peace & love

****

July 7, 2020, 10:55AM (Amir-ul Kafirs to group):

Re: HERETICS: small content

Please read to the very end before commenting.

I did & I watched the video in its entirety.

tENT wrote the other day that he can't imagine anyone being against BLM

Did I? Perhaps you could show me the exact quote you're referring to. I think you're probably confusing what Inquiring Librarian wrote:

"Hi All, I also support BLM, I mean honestly, who would not?"

as something I wrote. I'm sure there're plenty of people who don't support BLM, some of them racist, some of them not. For me, personally, I support it — this is partially because I've been supporting it since it began, or soon thereafter. It began in 2013 after "George Zimmerman's acquittal for the shooting death of Trayvon Martin". In those days I supported it in solidarity with the outrage over this murder. These days, a mere 7 years later, it's still a reaction to the murder of blacks by cops but it's become such a large thing that it's taken on ramifications it didn't have originally. It's getting much more media attention, far more protests are being organized in its name, & millions of dollars are being funneled into either supporting it or *into supporting off-shoots that pretend to be it & that pretend to have the same goals* — such as the Black Lives Matter Foundation.

At the risk of being branded a nazi I will say I am against BLM

I, personally, would never brand you a nazi. I don't really have a problem with being against BLM, especially at this time when it's become such a huge movement; I do have a problem with aspects of how it's portrayed in the mass media & with its being used by racists as a boogaboo.

I feel that any form of division is potentially dangerous, even well-intentioned

I agree with that. To quote from what I actually wrote:

"By NOT taking an anti-BLM stand they get to seem 'neutral' but the obvious effect is more divisiveness. &, as usual, it seems to me that the main people who stand to gain by such divisiveness are *not the people themselves* because, WTF, we could use **more unity**."

Note that I, too, call for less divisiveness & more unity.

as long as there is division in any form there will be problems

Of course. & this experiment with kids is more dramatically presented with college students in the Stanford Prison Experiment:

https://en.wikipedia.org/wiki/Stanford_prison_experiment

i wish the movement was called PSTB "please stop targeting black people" i feel that that slogan would be more exact and not make anyone feel like they were being put into a secondary position

I don't think that Black Lives Matter is a permanent only-possibility of how racism &/or murder by police will be confronted. It's just what's happening now. Naia Nisnam told me that she attended a small protest organized by younger black people in which they emphasized All Lives Matter (correct me if I'm wrong Naia Nisnam) so there is movement in that direction too.

****

July 7, 2020, 11:54AM (Naia Nisnam to group):

Here's Bill Maher on how weird things have gotten... I find his points to be true, funny, and sad.

https://www.youtube.com/watch?v=Yv0P1-gpEFc

I understand and support BLM, but I've been self-educating about ingrained, systemic racism in America for a lot of years. I think that most people saying BLM really are looking for equality, not to elevate the status of Black people to be higher than others. I'm familiar with the study and the video that Dick posted. I honestly dont think most people in BLM want to flip the tables like that. I dont think they want to be the dominant race or anything.

BUT- I agree that to the average person it can easily be interpreted that way. I agree that the name of the organization itself is off-putting to many and causing more division than needed. I recently talked to some friends from my small rural hometown and they Do Not get it. They said things to me like- "my Black friends dont hate me and my ancestors didn't come to america until after slavery ended so and I've never liked the police so.... Why do most Black people hate white people now?" They watch the mainstream news and legitimately feel like Black america hates all white people and a lot of white people hate whiteness too. I dont have the ability to sit down and explain systemic racism to the average small town American.

I agree that if the BLM simply had a different name, it would gain even more support. Maybe they dont want that level of support though. Maybe the BLM movement only wants the support of people who can get behind their slogan and they would consider anything less to be watered down? There is a feeling of being a part of the "in crowd", the new version of "the cool kids". You have to know the elitist lingo to fit in and if you dont then you are just a horrible racist person.

I am also concerned about this hierarchy of oppression. I can agree that Black Americans have suffered racism to a degree unmatched by others.... Except... what about the native people? (Indigenous? Native Americans? First Nations? sorry, I dont know what term to use...) So do we make a list of who suffered the most? Were the Chinese immigrants building the railroads in the west treated better or worse than the Japanese who ended up in interment camps? Hispanic people have it worse than Asians, right? What about Inquiring Librarian's neighbor who is Vietnamese but was told she was practically white? (am i remembering that right Inquiring Librarian?) Maybe the idea is that issues of racism against Black people in America are the worst of the worst and we have to deal with that first. Maybe we'd all get somewhere if we talked about Class half as much as we talk about Race.

Last night I came across an article about BLM's plans for American public education. That threw me. I've supported this movement for years, assuming that I was supporting a movement that works against police violence in the Black community. Now that movement has a plan for how public education should be changed in america. Who came up with that? I fully understand that systemic racism is creating cyclical problems for Black americans, preventing them from escaping poverty, etc. Banking, real estate, and a hundred other things play a part. Is BLM going to come up with policy solutions to all of those things? I'm confused.

I also read about a "Black national anthem" that will be played before the Star Spangled Banner at American football games. Two national anthems to bring the country together???? So. Confused.

****

July 7, 2020, 8:36PM (Amir-ul Kafirs to group):

Here's Bill Maher on how weird things have gotten...

Maher did a good job, as usual, but I would've felt more comfortable if he'd given his speech in blackface.

I think that most people saying BLM really are looking for equality

In ancient times, like 6 months ago, I would've said that most people just want to live their lives, do something to support themselves, find a mate (or 2), reproduce, & lead a reasonably peaceful life without fear-of-being-killed-by-some-idiot. These days, now that we're in the New-Normal-That-Has-Us-Trapped-In-A-Corner, I'm not so sure about that any more. I mean, the ancient times seem relatively 'sane' in contrast to NOW.

I agree that the name of the organization itself is off-putting to many and causing more division than needed.

It's funny, to me, I never once thought that "Black Lives Matter" even slightly implies that other lives DON'T MATTER. But that's because I am absolutely free of guilt. So, again, for me, I never took it personally, I just figure(d) that I was expressing solidarity with people who were calling attention to a bad situation. Still, there is plenty of stereotyping of white people out there: I mean, as a 66 year old white guy everybody seems to think that I can barely keep my stiffy in my pants whenever I see some hot young 30 year old whose juicy cunt I'd love to shoot my seed into over & over again. I mean, nothing could be further from the truth, I prefer them more around 35. So, you see, the stereotypes about old white guys being deranged sex fiends completely miss the mark.

Maybe we'd all get somewhere if we talked about Class half as much as we talk about Race.

Which is what I keep returning to when I can stop jerking off.

Last night I came across an article about BLM's plans for American public education.

I knew a white guy who worked for public schools in black neighborhoods in BalTimOre. He wanted to teach more about black history but the black administrators wanted him to stay to the standard curriculum.

I also read about a "Black national anthem" that will be played before the Star Spangled Banner at American football games. Two national anthems to bring the country together????

I personally would vote for Jimi Hendrix's "If 6 were 9" & the Bonzo Dog Band's "My Pink Half of the Drainpipe". But, as usual ***I won't get my fucking way so I'm going to kill everyone*** - but 1st I've got to make something like 750 movies (I'm up to 624 now) & write this book & get a few other things done so I don't know when I'll have time to wipe out the human (disg)race. It's so hard to prioritize.

yrs in misanthropy (or is it lycanthropy?),

tENTATIVELY "Sweetness & Light" a cONVENIENCE, Esq.

****

July 6, 2020, 9:05PM (Inquiring Librarian to group):

HERETICS: Moderna mRNA Vaccine Seems to be Failing

I found some promising news on the possible building failure of the United States Operation Warp Speed Moderna vaccine.

Here is an article on the Phase 2 trial that was about to start in early June.
https://www.clinicaltrialsarena.com/news/moderna-phaseii-vaccine-trial/
The key take-a-way in this one, for me is this: "Moderna has decided to drop the assessment of the 250µg dose in the Phase II trial."

& an update as of July 1st: https://www.statnews.com/2020/07/02/trial-of-moderna-covid-19-vaccine-delayed-investigators-say-but-july-start-still-possible/?fbclid=IwAR2IUlErAjv4yPZ_ZEbzVvMYbFgtbUC7FE6-waqCg9CNBTn55eiFgpkRIlM
& here, you see Phase 3, one scheduled to start in Mid July, is delayed due supposedly to changes in "protocol".

This gives you a little history and background on how the U.S. withdrew from the WHO and is not supporting the WHO vaccine production, but went off on the U.S.'s own vaccine production, Operation Warp Speed, that is basically competing with the WHO vaccine task force. =O . And as you can see above, we are failing at this. The U.S. baby is Moderna's vaccine, rife with corruption in its midst over the Moncef Slaoui co-leading the Warp Speed program, Slauoi was on the board of Moderna until he took this position.

****

1 JUNE 2020 NEWS

Moderna starts dosing in Phase II Covid-19 vaccine trial

Moderna has started dosing the first participants in all age cohorts of the Phase II clinical trial of its Covid-19 vaccine candidate, mRNA-1273.

mRNA-1273 is an mRNA vaccine encoding for a prefusion stabilised form of the Spike (S) protein, which was chosen by the company in alliance with Vaccine Research Center (VRC) at the National Institute of Allergy and Infectious Diseases (NIAID).

The Phase II trial will assess the safety, reactogenicity and immunogenicity of two vaccinations of mRNA-1273 administered 28 days apart. It is set to involve

600 healthy participants across the age groups of 18-55 and 55 and above.

Participants will receive either a 50µg dose, a 100µg dose, or placebo at both vaccinations and will be followed for 12 months after the second vaccination.

In the Phase I trial of the vaccine candidate, 25µg and 100µg dose levels demonstrated neutralising antibody titers at or above convalescent sera and were observed to be generally well-tolerated.

Moderna has decided to drop the assessment of the 250µg dose in the Phase II trial.

The US Food and Drug Administration (FDA) completed a review of the company's investigational new drug (IND) application for the vaccine candidate on 6 May and granted fast track designation on 12 May.

Moderna reported initial results from the Phase I trial of mRNA-1273 led by the NIAID on 18 May, where the 25*µ*g and 100*µ*g dose levels showed dose dependent increases in immunogenicity, as well as between prime and boost.

The company intends to work with the NIAID to launch a Phase III trial in July. The dose for the Phase III study is expected to be between 25*µ*g and 100*µ*g.

Moderna noted that the planning for these studies was supported by funding from the Biomedical Advanced Research and Development Authority (BARDA).

- https://www.clinicaltrialsarena.com/news/moderna-phaseii-vaccine-trial/

****

HEALTH

Trial of Moderna Covid-19 vaccine delayed, investigators say, but July start still possible

By DAMIAN GARDE JULY 2, 2020

A 30,000-patient trial of Moderna's coronavirus vaccine candidate, expected to start next week, has been delayed, a potential hurdle in the company's ambitious effort to deliver key data by Thanksgiving.

Moderna is making changes to the trial plan, called a protocol, which has pushed back the expected start date of the Phase 3 study, according to investigators. The investigators, who spoke on condition of anonymity, emphasized that protocol changes are common but said it's not clear how long the start will be delayed.

“My understanding was that they wanted to get the first vaccines given in July, and they say they’re still committed to do that,” one investigator said. “As best I can tell, they’re close to being on target for that.”

Investigators at the University of Illinois at Chicago had previously said Moderna’s trial would begin July 9. On Thursday, NIH Director Francis Collins also told lawmakers in Washington that the study would begin this month.

Moderna did not respond to multiple emails asking about how long the delay will last, the nature of the protocol changes, or whether they have anything to do with the vaccine’s safety or manufacturing. After publication, CEO Stéphane Bancel told CNBC that Moderna still intends to start the trial in July. In a statement posted to Twitter on Thursday afternoon, the company said it has “worked closely” with the National Institutes of Health, which is funding the Phase 3 study, “to align the final protocol in order to begin the trial on time.”

The intense focus on the exact timing of the trial stems from the tight nature of the race to develop a vaccine for the novel coronavirus — and the fact that any delay could imperil Moderna’s pole position. Pfizer, working with the German firm BioNTech, plans to start a 30,000-patient study of its own later this month.

[..]

- https://www.statnews.com/2020/07/02/trial-of-moderna-covid-19-vaccine-delayed-investigators-say-but-july-start-still-possible/?fbclid=IwAR2IUlErAjv4yPZ_ZEbzVvMYbFgtbUC7FE6-waqCg9CNBTn55eiFgpkRIlM

****

July 7, 2020, 12:03PM (Amir-ul Kafirs to group):

Re: HERETICS: Moderna mRNA Vaccine Seems to be Failing

I found some promising news on the possible building failure of the United States Operation Warp Speed Moderna vaccine.

If EVERYONE admits to failing at this then I might actually start to believe in their potential honesty. Otherwise, I'll just be glad if there's enough doubt over the value of vaccines for there to be NO emphasis on their being mandatory. One thing that would help would be if these companies & the people potentially administering the vaccines *could be held accountable for any negative effects*. As I understand it, that's not that case now — but that could change & if it were to do so that would cool their jets considerably.

****

July 7, 2020, 4:46PM (Inquiring Librarian to group):

Ok. I have terrible news. Check out this latest article by Derrick Broze on Trump's withdwawing from the WHO but instead giving that money and more directly to Gates' GAVI (the Global Alliance for Vaccines & Immunizations). Could it get any worse??

https://www.thelastamericanvagabond.com/top-news/vaccine-bait-switch-millions-pulled-from-who-trump-gives-billions-gates-founded-gavi/

****

Vaccine Bait & Switch: As Millions Pulled From WHO, Trump Gives Billions To Gates-Founded GAVI

Posted on
July 7, 2020
Author
Derrick Broze

In mid-May US President Donald Trump announced that the US would be ending their financial support for the World Health Organization (WHO) and COVID-19 relief. The move was lambasted in the mainstream press as an out of touch politician pulling funding from a vital global health organization during the middle of a pandemic. To Trump's supporters the decision was met with the typical cheering and celebrated as another Trump victory against the "globalists." To understand what is actually going on we need to examine Donald Trump's actions, not his tweets or media statements.

Let us start by looking at the funding provided by the US government to the WHO in previous years. The latest numbers from fiscal year 2018 (numbers are not available for 2019-20) show an estimated $281.6 million to the WHO from the US. The records indicate that after the US government, the Bill and Melinda Gates Foundation and GAVI, the Vaccine Alliance, are the 2nd and 3rd top financiers of the WHO. The US defunding the WHO actually tightens the technocrats already firm grip on another global institution.

This means when Donald Trump stated the US will no longer fund the WHO, the Gates Foundation and GAVI stepped into the top financial role. Additionally, GAVI was founded by and largely funded by the Bill and Melinda Gates Foundation in 2000. Either way, Bill Gates is the top donor and will continue to expand his influence and dominance of global health policy. As reported in Part 2 of my Bill Gates investigation, in 2010 the Bill and Melinda Gates Foundation launched the "Decade of Vaccines" and called for a "Global Vaccine Action Plan." Since that time they have only grown their network and influence on WHO, GAVI and other organizations in order to shape public health policy in a way that reaps profits for the Gates themselves.

While Trump's supporters viewed the US withdrawal from WHO financing as a win for nationalism or a black eye to the globalists, the truth is a bit more nuanced.

In early June, the Trump administration declared support for GAVI to the tune of a $1.16 billion USD donation. Trump's support for GAVI came via the first ever virtual Global Vaccine Summit. At this summit GAVI surpassed the goal of $7.4 billion, instead raising $8.8 billion USD and securing commitments from most major nations around the world. GAVI even received a $5 million dollar donation from the Rockefeller Foundation. GAVI stated that the funding will go to "routine immunization programs" and will also help the public-private partnership **"play a major role in the rollout of a future Covid-19 vaccine."**

More than 25 heads of state and 50 leaders of international agencies, NGOs and private industry attended the fundraising event. Participants included Germany's Chancellor Angela Merkel, UN Secretary General António Guterres, European Commission President Ursula von der Leyen, and World Health Organization Director-General Dr Tedros Adhanom Ghebreyesus.

UN Secretary Guterres stated that the vaccine would not be enough and instead called for **"global solidarity...to ensure that every person everywhere gets access to the vaccine."** Guterres also noted that **"our individual health depends on our collective health."**

[..]

- https://www.thelastamericanvagabond.com/top-news/vaccine-bait-switch-millions-pulled-from-who-trump-gives-billions-gates-founded-gavi/

****

July 7, 2020, 9:49PM (Amir-ul Kafirs to group):

Trump's withdwawing from the WHO but instead giving that money and more directly to Gates' GAVI (the Global Alliance for Vaccines & Immunizations). Could it get any worse??

Yes, but I'm confident that it won't get worse because most people are inherently good & greed is not a natural human quality.

OK, I'm kidding. I'm a little more pessimistic than the next guy but I'm more annoyed at how often my computer crashes right now & by the heat which has caused my face to melt like a candle. (OK, I'm exaggerating).

VACCINE BAIT & SWITCH: AS MILLIONS PULLED FROM WHO, TRUMP GIVES BILLIONS TO GATES-FOUNDED GAVI

Another good article, maybe this Broze guy should be supreme world dictator instead of me. There, you see? I'm flexible. Here're a couple of quotes:

During his short speech, Donald Trump stated, *"It's great to be partnering with you. We will work hard, we will work strong."* Trump also called COVID-19 "mean" and "nasty" and said it has shown "there are no borders, it doesn't discriminate."

I've got to say, Rump's insightful intellect continues to impress me. I'm surprised that he hasn't proposed building a COVID-19 wall to keep out illegal COVID-19 from the US. It seems like such an obvious solution.

Further, in May 2019, Gavi CEO Seth Berkley referred to "anti-vaccine sentiment" as a disease that needs to be censored from the internet. Berkley's statements are perfectly in line with Bill Gates' vision and the larger agenda of eugenics. The public cannot be allowed to question the safety of vaccines — no matter how rushed they are.

Thinking in general is a disease. The Catch-22 is that the reason why people are not acknowledging this is because they don't think & that prevents them from realizing that "Thinking in general is a disease." The obvious solution is to vaccinate against thinking, surely there must be a chemical that can accomplish this. In fact, far-sighted people probably agree that the mass media is a vaccine against thinking already. So everything's OK, those of us who think are going to get sick & die while the rest of the people successfully vaccinated against it will run the world. So what if they starve to death?

- tENTATIVELY "Ever-the-Optimist" a cONVENIENCE

****

July 8, 2020, 12:03AM (Amir-ul Kafirs to group):

HERETICS: MASKet Case

SO, my computer keeps crashing & tonight I lost all the work I've done on the hypothetical book related to July. It might take me 20 to 40 hours to redo.

MASKet Case

1. Someone who believes that inhibiting their normal breathing is healthy for them;
2. Someone willing to dispense with facial expression in communication;
3. Someone oblivious to Unconscious Suffocation.

****

July 7, 2020, 12:45PM (Inquiring Librarian to group):

HERETICS: J.B. Handley - Second Wave? Not even close.

If this is what the news media wants to call the "2nd Wave", we may be in very good shape. I mean, personally, I've been looking to "November" with fear wondering what on earth they plan to unleash on us all considering that covid really seems to be disappearing, I mean, is "Cases" all you've got mass media???? I'll admit, one of my many huge paranoid fears is that the government will unleash a horrible plague on us in the fall because their plandemic light didn't actually scare enough of us.. and then my brain goes further down that insane paranoid dark alley into wondering are they really making vaccine... maybe they are injecting us with obedient robot nanotechnology juice!! =O !! But then I read an article like below and my fears are brought back down to earth. IT is highly possible that the powers that be that created the hype over this pandemic are actually as incompetent as they seem to make themselves out to be more and more so daily...

This article was in the OffGuardian. I LOVE it!! It's really really really looooonnnnnngggg.... But it's excellent. And it's uber well documented!! This Handley person seems to me to cover every naysayer's attack with well documented and referenced links.
https://off-guardian.org/2020/07/07/second-wave-not-even-close/

Let me know what you think of the article. I think it's worth it to read it all the way through!! =]

****

Jul 7, 2020

Second wave? Not even close.

JB Handley

Why did politicians ever lockdown society in the first place? Can we all agree that the stated purpose was to “flatten the curve” so our hospital system could handle the inevitable COVID-19 patients who needed care? At that point, at least, back in early March, people were behaving rationally. They accepted that you can’t eradicate a virus, so let’s postpone things enough to handle it.

The fact is, we have done that, and so much more.

The headlines are filled with dire warnings of a “second wave” and trigger-happy Governors are rolling back regulations to try to stem the tide of new cases. But, is any of it actually true and should we all be worried? No, it’s not a second wave. The COVID-19 virus is on its final legs, and while I have filled this post with graphs to prove everything I just said

[..]

The death rate is a fact; anything beyond this is an inference.”
William Farr (1807 – 1883)
William Farr, creator of Farr’s law, knew this over 100 years ago. Viruses rise and fall at roughly the same slopes. It’s predictable, and COVID-19 is no different, which is why, after looking at all these death curves, it’s not very hard to declare that the pandemic is over.

Oxford’s center for Evidence Based Medicine has a wonderful explanation of Farr’s law, and it’s **well worth a read**. Some of my favorite quotes:
Farr shows us that once peak infection has been reached then it will roughly follow the same symmetrical pattern on the downward slope […] In the midst of a pandemic, it is easy to forget Farr’s Law, and think the number infected will just keep rising, it will not. Just as quick as measures were introduced to prevent the spread of infection we need to recognise the point at which to open up society and also the special measures due to ‘density’ that require special considerations.”

[..]

- https://off-guardian.org/2020/07/07/second-wave-not-even-close/

****

July 7, 2020, 9:23PM (Amir-ul Kafirs to group):

RE: HERETICS: J.B. Handley - Second Wave? Not even close.

Let me know what you think of the article.

I'm still in the midst of reading it (finished it now). Aside from saying things that I think we've all thought is common sense the whole damn time, it also contradicts the non-occurence of cases amongst protestors

[..]

The article then goes on to state the obvious that PA's Governor WOOF! seems incapable of acknowledging:

IT'S DEATHS, NOT CASES

Should I be governor or what?! It's obvious that I'm wiser than Woof! Woof! My plan is simple: release ALL prisoners who were poor when arrested & put in their place every self-righteous piece of shit who ever had the audacity to condescend to me for even a second. Ahem.

So, yeah, it's a great article & it confirms everything we've been saying all along. We are GODS & the average person is a piece of shit who should wear a mask AND handcuffs just to make sure that they don't touch anything.

tENTATIVELY "Humility Personified" a cONVENIENCE

****

July 8, 2020, 2:59PM (Inquiring Librarian to group):

Amir-ul Kafirs, my sentiments exactly. I wonder if you'd feel comfortable getting a bicycle. I bet if you could cycle around Pittsburgh on a bike, maskless, it would be awesome and give a great sense of freedom. My bicycle is really saving me these days. Luckily in Louisiana, the terrain is really flat. But the hills and bridges in Pittsburgh could be really fun!!

Does anyone else here tool around their towns on a bicycle?

****

July 8, 2020, 3:12PM (Dick to group):

Using a bike in Paris is something of a death-wish, the drivers here know no laws... Not to mention motorcycles, scooters, electric one-wheeled "things" (I don't know what they are called, mono-wheels maybe), electric skateboards...It's not uncommon to see, for example, a motorcyclist use the bike routes, or even climb onto the sidewalk to get by a traffic jam.... I have a French drivers license, I never use it because it is too terrifying to even drive a car... individual transportation has become bizarre here...there are rentable scooters everywhere lying around...the other day the pianist at the Paris Opera Ballet was crippled by one who was driving on the sidewalk

****

July 9, 2020, 10:27AM (Amir-ul Kafirs to group):

I wonder if you'd feel comfortable getting a bicycle.

Ha ha! Inquiring Librarian if you lived in Pittsburgh you'd associate me with riding a bike. Even though I've owned a car now ever since I inherited one in 2010 my friends are still shocked to see me drive one because they mostly associate me as a bike rider. Bike was my main means of transport from 1999ish to 2010. As you probably realize, bike-riding is one of the many things political activists are self-righteous about. I remember one friend telling me she'd gotten rid of her car & was only going to ride a bike. She felt very good about doing her do for the environment. I was down with that but my main reason for riding a bike was that I was too poor for a car & too poor for the bus & too poor for taxis. Hence, I rode a bike in the snow & rain & up & down steep hills to go to work etc — all the way up to when I was 56. When I got the car I thought something like: *I'll still ride the bike, I'll just use the car for getting groceries*. There was nothing particularly pleasant about riding on steep hills with grocery bags dangling from the handlebars. Anyway, it took about 2 weeks for me to decide that I **very much liked not having to risk my life every day because I was poor** & I've been relying on the car ever since. There's not much comparison between riding in a place where the land's flat & in a place where you can't even go a few hundred feet from your house without having a difficult hill to deal with. I'll ride a bike if I have to but only then. In the meantime, if I'm not driving I'd rather walk.

****

July 8, 2020, 5:54PM (Inquiring Librarian to group):

HERETICS: Hope w/Jon Rappoport & the Delivery Guy Today & James Corbett w/ Ernie Hancock

Stuff has been seeming so dark lately, and downright creepy. I wanted to share a few positive things.

1. I had a huge bookshelf delivered today (the first new piece of furniture I've ever bought, I should not have spent the money, I feel guilty and stupid, but it's pretty, and it's for books, so it's ok). Ok the delivery guy from _____ was a real nice, down to earth black guy who lives and is from Louisiana. He wasn't wearing a mask during the delivery. I was not wearing a mask. How I segue into picking people's brains about the pandemic is by asking them if I need to wear a

mask. Their response usually gives their opinion on the situation away. This guy launched into how fake the whole thing is and how he thinks Gates is a completely evil guy. Neither he nor anyone in his family or his friends will EVER let any vaccine into their bodies, especially not this covid one. And... he went on to say he thinks Black Lives Matter is a big fake and he does not support it. Of course, he says, black lives do matter, but the movement is corporate and, basically patronizing. I have heard this from many local black people. Government over control and abuse is so close to home with them. They do not trust Big Brother, period. This gives me faith in humanity.

2. I liked this positive statement from Jon Rappoport: https://nomorefakenews.com/ Here is the last paragraph. The whole thing is good, but this last paragraph says it all. We have a choice, we don't need to be victims.

Finally, for now, there is the matter of individual choice and responsibility. Individuals can believe or not believe. There is always that option. People are not doomed to accept an oppressive narrative imposed on them. If that were the case, there would be no point to human thought or action. We would forever be victims. This is not the case. It never was. Some people are dedicated to the notion that there is no way out of the dungeon of external control. Their dedication to this proposition has great tonnage. For them. They purposely ignore the fact that, down through history, there has been an enormous struggle to establish individual freedom, and this war has been astonishingly successful—relative to older despotisms and tyrannies. In fact, their choice, now, to walk around spraying doom of whatever brand they want to sell is evidence of that freedom. I'm not impressed by doom. I'm impressed by freedom. We are in yet another fight for it now. I'm impressed by individuals who use their freedom to make their best vision into fact in the world. My investigations are aimed at exposing the power players who plot and fight against freedom.

3. Here is a James Corbett & Ernie Hancock audio interview. I was desperate this morning to hear something. My usual listening stuff hadn't put out anything new. I even turned on NPR and was immediately disgusted about a horrendous mind control show on, what else... MASKS!! Then they launched into why I am a racist because my skin is pale. I worked out in silence for about 45 min. Then I discovered James Corbett's actual web page (I'd previously only been following him on his Bitchute channel). This talk here was great! The ending was actually positive, in a dark way, but still positive. Ernie actually stated, "The Revolution Will Not Be Televised". There are many people like us out there, they are on the streets, they are covert, but there are many of us. We will be censored off of the usual platforms, but we resist. Those who believe the government, they will be 'Road Kill'. We can just say NO. And the Autocrats in charge cannot herd us when the masses say no. https://www.corbettreport.com/interview-1562-james-corbett-tackles-event-201-the-great-reset-and-the-end-of-humanity/

****

July 9, 2020, 10:38AM (Amir-ul Kafirs to group):

Re: HERETICS: Hope w/Jon Rappoport & the Delivery Guy Today & James Corbett w/ Ernie Hancock

I wanted to share a few positive things.

No, NO! No positivity! ONLY DOOMSAYING! (OK, I'm just kidding)

Of course, he says, black lives do matter, but the movement is corporate and, basically patronizing.

I think its becoming 'corporate' is really just a recent matter since the killing of George Floyd & the possibility of large donations. Before that, I think it was more grassroots.

There are many people like us out there, they are on the streets, they are covert, but there are many of us.

Maybe, but being covert in this instance is a sign of fear & fearful people aren't much use.

We will be censored off of the usual platforms, but we resist.

Did you hear the one about the mask-wearer & the mask-resister fighting to the death? You didn't? That's because you only listen to corporate fact-choker news.

****

July 8, 2020, 9:58PM (txt msg rc'vd from Naia Nisnam):

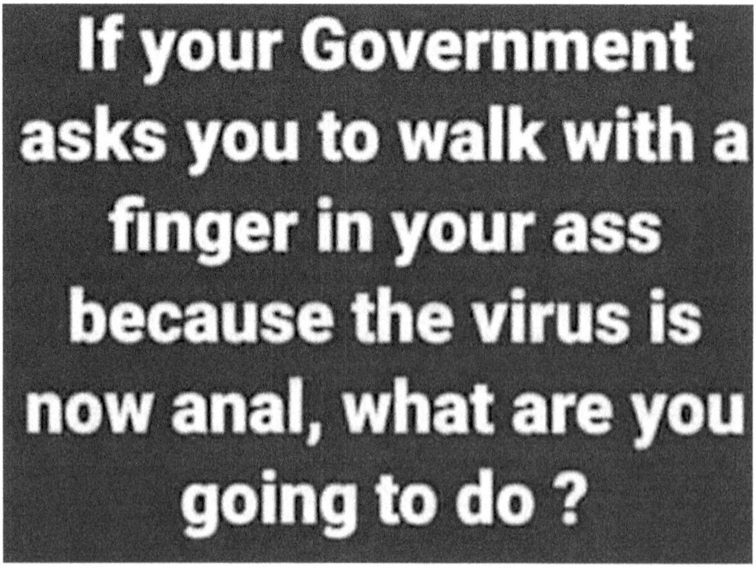

If your Government asks you to walk with a finger in your ass because the virus is now anal, what are you going to do ?

****

July 8, 2020, 10:35PM (txt msg rc'vd from Naia Nisnam):

T-Mobile 10:10 PM 43%

AA facebook.com

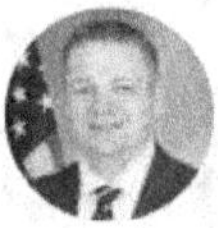

PA State Rep. Aaron Bernstine

59 mins ·

I just received this email from one of my colleagues. This is not the first (or even close to being the first) report of this situation that we have received.

I am continuing to work with my colleagues to obtain answers from the PA Department of Health.

Just learned of a situation where individuals went to a testing location where they signed in and provided contact information. Because the line was so long and the wait too much, they ended up leaving. However, they then received a phone call that they had tested positive, but NEVER GOT TESTED!

Anyone else hearing anything like this?

[redacted]

State Representative

****

July 9, 2020, 12:01AM (Amir-ul Kafirs to group):

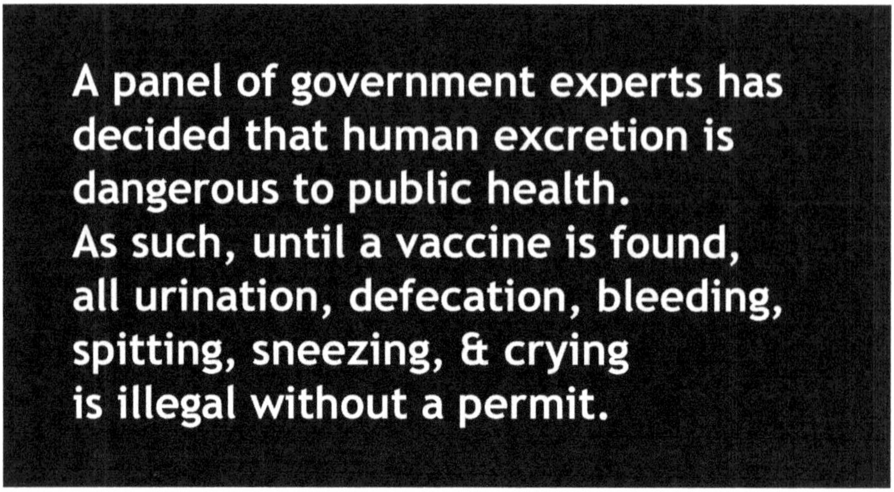

A panel of government experts has decided that human excretion is dangerous to public health.
As such, until a vaccine is found, all urination, defecation, bleeding, spitting, sneezing, & crying is illegal without a permit.

****

July 9, 2020, 2:19PM (Dick to group):

an article someone may find interesting
https://www.tabletmag.com/sections/news/articles/american-soviet-mentality?

****

The American Soviet Mentality

Collective demonization invades our culture

BY
IZABELLA TABAROVSKY
JUNE 15, 2020

Russians are fond of quoting Sergei Dovlatov, a dissident Soviet writer who emigrated to the United States in 1979: "We continuously curse Comrade Stalin, and, naturally, with good reason. And yet I want to ask: who wrote four million denunciations?" It wasn't the fearsome heads of Soviet secret police who did that, he said. It was ordinary people. Collective demonizations of prominent cultural figures were an integral part of the Soviet culture of denunciation that pervaded every workplace and apartment building. Perhaps the most famous such episode began on Oct. 23, 1958, when the Nobel committee informed Soviet writer Boris Pasternak that he had been selected for the Nobel Prize in literature—and plunged the writer's life into hell. Ever since Pasternak's *Doctor Zhivago* had been first published the previous year (in Italy, since the writer could not publish it at home) the Communist Party and the Soviet literary establishment had their knives out for him. To the establishment, the Nobel Prize added insult to grave injury.

Within days, Pasternak was a target of a massive public vilification campaign. The country's prestigious *Literary Newspaper* launched the assault with an article titled

"Unanimous Condemnation" and an official statement by the Soviet Writers' Union—a powerful organization whose primary function was to exercise control over its members, including by giving access to exclusive benefits and basic material necessities unavailable to ordinary citizens. The two articles expressed the union's sense that in view of Pasternak's hostility and slander of the Soviet people, socialism, world peace, and all progressive and revolutionary movements, he no longer deserved the proud title of Soviet Writer. The union therefore expelled him from its ranks.

A few days later, the paper dedicated an entire page to what it presented as the public outcry over Pasternak's imputed treachery. Collected under the massive headline "Anger and Indignation: Soviet people condemn the actions of B. Pasternak" were a condemnatory editorial, a denunciation by a group of influential Moscow writers, and outraged letters that the paper claimed to have received from readers.

The campaign against Pasternak went on for months. Having played out in the central press, it moved to local outlets and jumped over into nonmedia institutions, with the writer now castigated at obligatory political meetings at factories, research institutes, universities, and collective farms. None of those who joined the chorus of condemnation, naturally, had read the novel—it would not be formally published in the USSR until 30 years later. But that did not stop them from mouthing the made-up charges leveled against the writer. It was during that campaign that the Soviet catchphrase "*ne chital, no osuzhdayu*"—"didn't read, but disapprove"—was born: Pasternak's accusers had coined it to protect themselves against suspicions of having come in contact with the seditious material. Days after accepting the Nobel Prize, Pasternak was forced to decline it. Yet demonization continued unabated.

Some of the greatest names in Soviet culture became targets of collective condemnations—composers Dmitry Shostakovich and Sergei Prokofiev; writers Anna Akhmatova and Iosif Brodsky; and many others. Bouts of hounding could go on for months and years, destroying people's lives, health and, undoubtedly, ability to create. (The brutal onslaught undermined Pasternak's health. He died from lung cancer a year and a half later.) But the practice wasn't reserved for the greats alone. Factories, universities, schools, and research institutes were all suitable venues for collectively raking over the coals a hapless, ideologically ungrounded colleague who, say, failed to show up for the "voluntary-obligatory," as a Soviet cliché went, Saturday cleanups at a local park, or a scientist who wanted to emigrate. The system also demanded expressions of collective condemnations with regards to various political matters: machinations of imperialism and reactionary forces, Israeli aggression against peaceful Arab states, the anti-Soviet international Zionist conspiracy. It was simply part of life.

Twitter has been used as a platform for exercises in unanimous condemnation for as long as it has existed. Countless careers and lives have been ruined as outraged mobs have descended on people whose social media gaffes or old teenage behavior were held up to public scorn and judged to be deplorable and unforgivable. But it wasn't until the past couple of weeks that the similarity of our current culture with the Soviet practice of collective hounding presented itself to me with such stark clarity. Perhaps it was the specific professions and the cultural institutions involved—and the specific acts of writers banding together to abuse and cancel their colleagues—that brought that sordid history back.

On June 3, *The New York Times* published an opinion piece that much of its progressive staff found offensive and dangerous. (The author, Republican Sen. Tom Cotton, had called to send in the military to curb the violence and looting that accompanied the nationwide protests against the killing of George Floyd.) The targets of their unanimous condemnation, which was gleefully joined by the Twitter proletariat, which took pleasure in helping the once-august newspaper shred itself to pieces in public, were *New York Times*' opinion section editor James Bennet, who had ultimate authority for publishing the piece, though he hadn't supervised its editing, and op-ed staff editor and writer Bari Weiss (a former Tablet staffer).

Weiss had nothing to do with editing or publishing the piece. On June 4, however, she posted a Twitter thread characterizing the internal turmoil at the *Times* as a "civil war" between the "(mostly young) wokes" who "call themselves liberals and progressives" and the "(mostly 40+) liberals" who adhere to "the principles of civil libertarianism." She attributed the behavior of the "wokes" to their "safetyism" worldview, in which "the right of people to feel emotionally and psychologically safe trumps what were previously considered core liberal values, like free speech."

It was just one journalist's opinion, but to Weiss' colleagues her semi-unflattering description of the split felt like an intolerable attack against the collective. Although Weiss did not name anyone in either the "woke" or the older "liberal" camp, her younger colleagues felt collectively attacked and slandered. They lashed out. Pretty soon, Weiss was trending on Twitter.

[..]

- https://www.tabletmag.com/sections/news/articles/american-soviet-mentality?

****

July 9, 2020, 5:41PM (Amir-ul Kafirs to group):

an article someone may find interesting

I read this. It seems silly to me to act like this is a new phenomena in the US. It's been like this my whole life, there just wasn't Twitter, it would've been carried out with things like that old faithful of character assassination: malicious gossip. I call myself a *Professional Resister of Character Assassination* & I've been calling myself that since the mid 1990s at the latest. I even have a rubber stamp identifying myself as such. I was 'unwillingly resigned' from WJHU, the radio station of Johns Hopkins, way back in 1983 because I was such an infamous character. Nothing's really changed since then. One of the main DJs who would've been responsible for this 'unwilling resignation' is a guy who stayed with the radio station as a well-known & respected jazz DJ. I've long-since forgotten his name but he's probably still part of whatever JHU has long since turned into. The point is: this isn't a phenomena of the increasingly repulsive political-correctness wave, it's the product of the same old, same old self-righteous-poseurs-trying-to-advance-their-careers who certainly existed as *anti-communists* DURING THE BLACKLISTING FERVOR OF THE 1950s. Blaming it on the Soviets is just a hangover from those McCarthy times & no more reputable than what it's dissing.

****

July 9, 2020, 6:00PM (Dick to group):

I didn't think they were blaming it on the soviets really, I thought that they saw a similar tendency developing
I know it isn't new, as I'd written before, the mother of my son said the same thing happened in Paris during the occupation.
As Ecclesiastes says, there's nothing new under the sun, but it is interesting how the old things take on new forms, in this case aided by the anonymity of the internet

****

July 9, 2020, 7:07PM (Amir-ul Kafirs to group):

I didn't think they were blaming it on the soviets really,

I didn't mean that they're blaming the current situation on the Soviets.. but they were drawing parallels between the Soviets & the current situation in the US. My point is that writers were being blacklisted at the same time in the US. Dalton Trumbo, Dashiell Hammett, & many others went to prison in the 1950s & had their lives seriously damaged. Wilhelm Reich, obviously, died in prison & had his books burned. I'm not defending the Soviets, I'm just saying that the US, as usual, has its own dirty hands so why not just write the article at least referring to that instead of ONLY to the Soviets. My point being further that by doing so they're perpetuating a myth about the US as some bastion of Free Speech, which has always been a joke, & making it seem like this latest bullshit is some sort of new threat to that. It isn't. If the people at the New York Times had any guts or any experience with being character assassinated they might've stood up for themselves better. Instead, they buckled at the 1st threat to their bourgeoise existence. That's pathetic.

p.s. I've had serious character assassination campaigns against me ongoing for something like AT LEAST the last 27 years, things that people can still read online. I'm very aware of how these things work & they don't just originate with 'politically correct' people using the internet.

****

July 9, 2020, 8:02PM (txt msg from Naia Nisnam):

https://thenewdaily.com.au/news/coronavirus/2020/05/11/melbourne-anti-lockdown-protest/

****

8:44am, May 11, 2020 **Updated: 8:54am, May 11**

‘Bizarre’ lockdown protests jeopardise plans to ease restrictions: Doctor

“Bizarre” protests about coronavirus lockdown measures in Victoria and NSW are putting the easing of restrictions at risk, one of Australia’s top doctors has warned.

Ten people were arrested for breaching Victoria’s lockdown rules and clashing with police at a rally at state parliament on Sunday.

In Sydney, a mother was taken in custody after refusing to comply with police during demonstrations in the CBD.

“It’s incredibly disappointing, really bizarre, in fact,” Dr Tony Bartone, the head of Australia’s Medical Association, told *Today* on Monday.

“What they’re putting at risk is the progressive unwinding of those restrictions.

“By that grouping of those protests over the weekend, we just need one person to be positive and spread the virus and then we’re on the backward step already.”

About 100 people gathered at the steps of the Victorian parliament on Sunday to protest against 5G, vaccinations, COVID-19 lockdown restrictions and what they called the “coronavirus conspiracy”.

The protest turned unruly when police began separating protesters who were breaking social distancing and lockdown laws.

[..]

- https://thenewdaily.com.au/news/coronavirus/2020/05/11/melbourne-anti-lockdown-protest/

****

6:27am, Jul 10, 2020 **Updated: 2h ago**

Countries urged to ‘open up’ as WHO appoints Helen Clark to lead virus review

Countries have been urged to “open up” to scrutiny as the World Health Organisation launches an internal investigation into the handling of the coronavirus.

Former New Zealand prime minister Helen Clark will head the probe, which will consider how the pandemic happened and what the WHO did to prevent it.

Making the announcement, WHO chief Tedros Adhanom Ghebreyesus lamented **division amid the crisis** that was enabling the virus to spread.

Wiping away tears, he warned the greatest threat was not the virus but “rather, it is the lack of leadership and solidarity at the global and national levels”.

“For years, many of us warned that a catastrophic respiratory pandemic was inevitable," Dr Ghebreyesus said.

"It was not a question of if, but when. But still, despite all the warnings, the world was not ready. Our systems were not ready. Our communities were not ready. Our supply chains collapsed.

[..]

- https://thenewdaily.com.au/news/coronavirus/2020/07/10/coronavirus-who-investigation/

****

2:57pm, Jul 10, 2020 **Updated: 9:10pm, Jul 10**

Melbourne partygoers fined $26,000 after police follow their noses... and a massive KFC order

A group of birthday party-goers has been fined $26,000 for flouting Victoria's COVID restrictions after being nabbed with bucketloads of fast food.

The group was snapped by police after paramedics spotted two people ordering 20 meals at a KFC in suburban Melbourne at 1.30am on Friday.
Victoria Police Chief Commissioner Shane Patton said police traced the pair to a townhouse in Dandenong.

"When we went in, there was two people asleep but there were 16 others hiding out the back – and they'd just got the KFC meals at a birthday," he said.

"That is ridiculous that type of behaviour."

It was also an expensive night – police slapped each of the 16 with a $1652 fine for ignoring Melbourne's tough new coronavirus restrictions (which ban visiting another home).

"That is $26,000 that birthday party is costing them. That is a heck of a birthday party to recall," Mr Patton said.

Mr Patton also took aim at reports huge crowds had gathered on the pier at Mornington on Thursday to watch whales, calling it "totally unacceptable".

My parents live in Mornington & my dad just sent me this pic of crowds of people on the pier watching whales...seriously!! While I'm home doing the right thing watching whales on Netflix

- https://thenewdaily.com.au/news/state/vic/2020/07/10/kfc-party-covid-fine/

****

July 10, 2020, 11:10AM (Dick to group):

Interesting about Australia
Well here in the City of Lights, tonight at midnight the thing comes "to an end" - kind of...
here's an article about the new status quo

it seems like governments are going from representational to dictatorial

Google translation:

The state of health emergency, instituted on March 24 due to the Covid-19 pandemic, will end this Friday July 10 at midnight in France, except in Guyana and Mayotte where the circulation of the virus is still alarming.

The Minister of Health Olivier Véran, who observed a "relaxation in behavior" aimed at limiting the transmission of Covid-19, also called on the French on Friday for "daily vigilance".

Came into force on March 24 in the face of the coronavirus epidemic, the state of health emergency, which allows certain public freedoms to be restricted, ends at midnight.

Possible restrictions are possible until the fall, provides for the law to exit the state of emergency published Friday in the Official Journal. The oppositions criticize an extension in "trompe l'oeil" of this exceptional regime.

Special case: the state of emergency is extended until October 30 in Guyana and Mayotte, where the virus is still actively circulating.

TRAVEL RESTRICTIONS

The government will be able to regulate and even prohibit, where the virus is active, the movement of people and vehicles as well as access to public transportation.

Travel "strictly essential for family, professional and health needs" must remain permitted.

It will be possible to require people flying to or from the metropolitan territory or overseas to present the result of a virological test.

Mr. Véran said he is working on setting up saliva tests at airports "where it will be possible" for travelers arriving from countries at risk.

The Constitutional Council clarified Thursday that it will not be possible to prohibit leaving home or surroundings, in other words to confine the population, even locally.

If it were necessary to decide on a new strict containment, such as that implemented from March 17, the government should again declare a state of health emergency.

GATHERINGS, STADIUMS, DISCOTHEQUES ...

The government will still be able to supervise rallies and temporarily close establishments and meeting places.

The nightclubs in particular remain closed at this stage but hope to reopen before September, even without a dance floor.

The government authorized the reopening of the stadiums from Saturday, with a maximum gauge of 5,000 spectators ... which several sports leaders already want to enhance.

GELS AND MASKS

The framing of the selling prices of hydroalcoholic gels and single-use surgical masks ends on Friday evening.

WAY OUT OF THE WINTER TRUCE

It is the end of the reprieve for thousands of modest households threatened with eviction.

The government assures that rental evictions cannot take place "without the possibility of rehousing".

The owners may request compensation from the State when the eviction procedures have not been carried out.

RETURN FROM DEFICIENCY

The days of deficiency at the start of sick leave had been suspended during the state of health emergency, allowing remuneration during these days, whatever the reason.

From Saturday, public officials will not benefit from the maintenance of their remuneration until the second day of sick leave.

This period extends to the fourth day in the private sector, even if the employer generally takes charge of the whole because of company or branch agreements.

PARTIAL UNEMPLOYMENT

The rules do not change again, classic partial unemployment continues to apply.

Added on July 1, subject to a company or branch agreement, a system of long-term partial unemployment, which allows a reduction in working hours of up to 40%, the employee receiving 84% of his net salary and the company being partially helped by the State.

OVERTIME

Overtime worked by employees since March 16 was exempt from income tax and social security contributions up to a limit of 7,500 euros per year: back to the ceiling of 5,000 euros.

COMPANIES

The legal possibility of "deferring or spreading the payment of rents" or certain invoices (water, electricity ...) for very small businesses "whose activity is affected by the spread of the epidemic" ends.

The government has planned a new arsenal to help businesses through crisis budgets.

here's the original
https://www.nicematin.com/sante/rassemblements-discotheques-prix-des-masques-ce-qui-change-avec-la-fin-de-letat-durgence-sanitaire-538994

****

July 10, 2020, 12:27PM (Inquiring Librarian to group):

This is all so crazy! I am really glad, for now, that I am in oppressive Louisiana and not Australia!! I have a distant Belorussian aunt in Australia, I believe in Canberra. I will email her asap to get her opinion and view on what is happening. She is very religious, a degree in theology and always ends her emails with "God Bless" so I am not sure how that will skew her answer to me, if she answers at all. Her husband is a somewhat prominent geophysicist. They may have something to say about all of this. They are very elderly, so who knows. I do know Lily, like my dad, fled communist brutality in Belarus during WW2. So her perspective may be interesting, if she even writes me back.

As a whole, the Australian Government seems to be obsessed with vaccines. This, "No Jab, no Play' section on their government website is pretty darn creepy to me: https://www2.health.vic.gov.au/public-health/immunisation/vaccination-children/no-jab-no-play
& just yesterday, I read this letter written by the letter author to Margie Danchin, an academic associated with the vaccine industry. https://childrenshealthdefense.org/news/anti-vaxxers-and-experts-time-to-look-behind-the-labels/ It looks to me like the vaccine industry has a strangle hold on the citizens of Australia, and that strangle hold is being paid to the vaccine companies by citizen taxpayers dollars, and there is, understandibly, a big pushback.

"'Anti-vaxxers' and 'Experts' -Time to Look Behind the Labels

By Elizabeth Hart, CHD Guest Contributor

Margie Danchin, an academic associated with the vaccine industry, has called for the imminent tour of the movie Vaxxed: From Cover-up to Catastrophe to be stopped in Australia, as reported in the biased Sydney Morning Herald.

Danchin is described as a 'leading immunisation researcher' who is apparently concerned about 'anti-vaccination activity'. She is yet another self-appointed vaccine defender who stands in the way of open discussion of vaccination policy and vaccine safety – but what exactly is her expertise in this area, what qualifies her to shut others down?

See below independent vaccination campaigner Elizabeth Hart's email to Margie Danchin questioning her expertise, and raising her conflicts of interest. It's time to bring these people to account.

22 June 2020

For the attention of:
A/Professor Margie Danchin
Murdoch Children's Research Institute

Dear A/Prof Danchin, recently you featured in an article in *The Sydney Morning Herald* titled: **'Dangerous': Researchers note 'massive uptick' in anti-vaccination activity**, 14 June 2020, This is just one of a series of articles published lately with an 'anti-vaxxer' theme.

In Wendy Tuohy's article, you are described as a 'leading immunisation researcher'. A/Prof Danchin, can you please advise me, what expertise do you have in all the vaccine products and revaccinations on the National Immunisation Program Schedule, and adverse events after vaccination?

Do you think people should be forbidden from asking questions about the burgeoning number of vaccine products and revaccinations on the taxpayer-funded schedule? Do you think it appropriate that people who raise questions about vaccination policy are denigrated and marginalised as 'anti-vaxxers'? Are you aware that children and adults have experienced adverse events after vaccination, for example as reported in the TGA's Database of Adverse Event Notifications? Are you aware that the TGA acknowledges that adverse events are likely to be under-reported?

A/Prof Danchin, judging by the tone of your comments in Wendy Tuohy's article, you are very protective of vaccine products. You are a member of the industry-funded Immunisation Coalition, which is funded by vaccine manufacturers CSL/

Seqirus, GlaxoSmithKline, Pfizer, MSD (Merck) and Sanofi. Why wasn't this conflict of interest disclosed in Wendy Tuohy's article?

A/Prof Danchin, you are associated with the Murdoch Children's Research Institute, which is involved in vaccine product research and development. Rupert Murdoch's mother Dame Elisabeth Murdoch was involved with the founding of the original institute, and Sarah Murdoch is a member of the Board and the Ambassador for the Murdoch Children's Research Institute. The Murdoch-run News Corp is a corporate partner of the Murdoch Children's Research Institute and the News Corp tabloids were behind the No Jab, No Play media campaign, which was obligingly adopted as policy by politicians across the political spectrum in Australia, and enacted as the coercive No Jab, No Pay law under Malcolm Turnbull as Prime Minister in January 2016. Members of the coercive vaccination lobby groups SAVN and Friends of Science in Medicine, e.g. John Cunningham and David Hawkes, were influential at the Senate Committee hearing regarding the No Jab, No Pay Bill in November 2015, which was attended by SAVN supporter Senator Richard Di Natale. As far as I'm aware, neither John Cunningham nor David Hawkes are experts in the wide range of vaccine products on the National Immunisation Program Schedule.

A/Prof Danchin, I suggest there are serious conflicts of interest in the relationship between the Murdoch Children's Research Institute and News Corp, and that News Corp's corporate partnership with the Murdoch Children's Research Institute should have been disclosed in its No Jab, No Play articles arguing for coercive vaccination policy, which resulted in the No Jab, No Pay Law.

Taxpayer-funded vaccination policy is a very serious matter. Vaccine products are medical interventions, an ever-increasing number of which are being pressed upon mass populations of children and adults. There must be transparency and accountability for vaccination policy. I request you wind back your 'anti-vaccination' rhetoric, and treat this matter seriously.

Given your description as a 'leading immunisation researcher', I request your response detailing your expertise in the vaccine products and revaccinations on the National Immunisation Program Schedule. Also, please note I have referred to Wendy Tuohy's article, and you, in my recent email to Peter Costello, which raises the subject of conflicts of interest, please see below for your information.

Sincerely,

Elizabeth Hart"

****

July 10, 2020, 12:57PM (Amir-ul Kafirs to group):

Re: HERETICS:

it seems like governments are going from representational to dictatorial

Without most people seeming to notice OR care. Subconsciously, they probably figure *they'll be ok because they've always towed the line.*

TRAVEL RESTRICTIONS

One thing seems likely: any touring I'd hoped to do while I still have money is unlikely. I doubt that I'll leave the US, go to France, go to the Netherlands, go to Germany, go to New Zealand, go to Australia, go to Japan.

It will be possible to require people flying to or from the metropolitan territory or overseas to present the result of a virological test.

What a justification for extreme intrusiveness into the body!!

The Constitutional Council clarified Thursday that it will not be possible to prohibit leaving home or surroundings, in other words to confine the population, even locally.

Gee, how nice of them. Maybe just cut off people's feet?

The framing of the selling prices of hydroalcoholic gels and single-use surgical masks ends on Friday evening.

Let the price-gouging begin!

It is the end of the reprieve for thousands of modest households threatened with eviction.

So much for the supposed socialism in France.

****

July 10, 2020, 1:50PM (Amir-ul Kafirs to group):

I have a distant Belorussian aunt in Australia, I believe in Canberra.

The capitol, the only place where prostitiution is legal. Gee, I wonder why?

"No Jab, no Play' section on their government website is pretty darn creepy to me: https://www2.health.vic.gov.au/public-health/immunisation/vaccination-children/no-jab-no-play

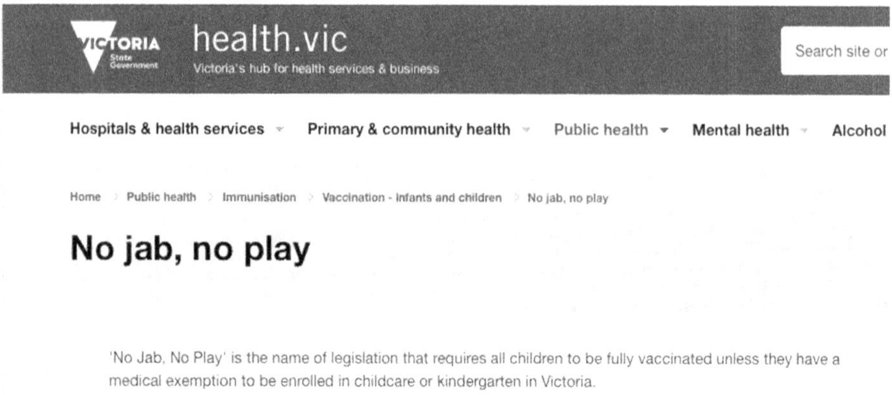

VICTORIA State Government health.vic
Victoria's hub for health services & business
Search site or

Hospitals & health services | Primary & community health | Public health | Mental health | Alcohol

Home > Public health > Immunisation > Vaccination - Infants and children > No jab, no play

No jab, no play

'No Jab, No Play' is the name of legislation that requires all children to be fully vaccinated unless they have a medical exemption to be enrolled in childcare or kindergarten in Victoria.

thusly criminalizing any parental concern that goes against official policy. NO THINKING FOR YOURSELF.

Margie Danchin, an academic associated with the vaccine industry, has called for the imminent tour of the movie Vaxxed: From Cover-up to Catastrophe to be stopped in Australia, as reported in the biased Sydney Morning Herald.

How easy it is for these censors to cover up their activities with 'social health concern'.

Danchin is described as a 'leading immunisation researcher'

Too bad the press doesn't use the same qualifiers that they do with anyone they're trying to discredit. Danchin could be a 'vaxx-pusher' or a 'self-styled expert'.

who is apparently concerned about 'anti-vaccination activity'.

[..]

Why wasn't this conflict of interest disclosed in Wendy Tuohy's article?

Busted!

[..]

The Murdoch-run News Corp is a corporate partner of the Murdoch Children's Research Institute and the News Corp tabloids were behind the No Jab, No Play media campaign, which was obligingly adopted as policy by politicians across the political spectrum in Australia, and enacted as the coercive No Jab, No Pay law under Malcolm Turnbull as Prime Minister in January 2016.

What?! Collusion between the mass media, paid-off politicians, & big pharma? No way! Even if it's 100% proveable it's obviously a conspiracy theory. Ask the tooth fairy!

which resulted in the No Jab, No Pay Law.

When will the forced sterilizations come along?

I request you wind back your 'anti-vaccination' rhetoric, and treat this matter seriously.

Of course, sending the email to Danchin was a waste of time. I'm glad WE got to read it!

****

July 10, 2020, 3:04PM (Inquiring Librarian to group):

Thanks for the funny commentary Amir-ul Kafirs! I had a few laugh out louds on my lunch break from those comments, my favorite being simply, "Busted!".

In that same paper, I found a totally hypocritical article by the same author of the article in the Sydney Herald that was being referred to above. Every claim that the 'anti-vaxxers' are misinformed and wrong is completely unsubstantiated. From the wealth of articles in the Sydney Herald, all by this same Wendy Tuohy, are the same kind of nonsense. They are fighting what they call 'disinformation' with basically ZERO information. They are telling you simply to blindly believe that vaccinations are good, and any opposition to vaccinations, or any concern over them means you are a 'magical thinking' conspiracy theorist. If the 'antivaxxer' attitude in Australia is as bad as this propaganda makes it out to be, I feel real hope for humanity and I sure hope that the Americas wisen up too!! What astounds me is that there is SO MUCH factual information out there, pretty easily obtained with a little work, that completely throws the need for most vaccinations under the bus and makes clear connections to the damage they cause! Here is one of the worst anti-antivaxxer articles that I found in the Sydney Herald:
https://www.smh.com.au/national/slap-them-down-or-hear-them-out-how-to-handle-misinformation-superspreaders-20200529-p54xs3.html

OPINION

'Slap them down' or hear them out: How to handle misinformation 'superspreaders'?

Almost as disturbing as the heat maps showing official death rates from COVID-19 every night on the news are those starting to circulate showing vast networks of influence of the global anti-vaccination movement, some of them run from Australia.

At a time when trust in science and gratitude for modern medicine should be high, it's been terrifying to watch traction gained recently by vaccination conspiracy theorists, some with (opportunistic) Australian celebrity support.

Five days after 10 Melburnians were arrested during a protest against vaccinations and lockdowns, the prestigious journal *Science* reported a first-of-its kind analysis of 1300 vaccination-related Facebook pages with nearly 100 million followers.

It found anti-vaccine pages – where "the battle for hearts and minds" on immunisation is fought – are more numerous than pro-vaccine and "undecided" pages, and are growing faster.

Anti-vaxxer pages will eventually dominate online discussion "at a time when a future vaccine against COVID-19 may be critical to public health", it predicted. In part, these pages must take credit for whipping up mobs such as the "wake up Australia" brigade set to protest "mandatory vaccinations" in the Botanic Gardens on Saturday.

"The reds are winning," said Heidi Larson, director of the Vaccine Conference Project at the London School of Hygiene & Tropical Medicine of the anti-vaxxer cluster on the centre's map showing two immense communities pulling in opposite directions.

Data scientist Neil Johnson from George Washington University said of map of "the battlefield" for vaccination credibility "we were shocked".

Troubling, too was the widespread circulation on Australian and global social media this month of a 30-minute "documentary" called *Plandemic*, viewed more than eight million times in just a few days before Facebook and Google took it down.

Presented as fact, it showed up in many a feed among those who do not identify as "vaccine-sceptic", anti-vax or even undecided.

Discredited medical researcher Judy Mikovits makes startling claims in the video aimed at generating maximum emotion, including that wearing masks activates coronavirus and the pandemic is a hoax designed to help elites including Bill Gates grab money and power.

Mikovits is described by *The New York Times* as a "star of virus misinformation". That her ravings have been thoroughly debunked is something. But insofar as her impact is concerned, the enduring power to put parents in leafy suburbs of Melbourne and Sydney off routine vaccination with a decades-old myth by disgraced doctor Anthony Wakefield – that there is a link between the measles vaccine and autism – would suggest the damage is most likely done.

[..]

Wendy Tuohy is a Sunday Age columnist.

****

July 10, 2020, 5:19PM (Amir-ul Kafirs to group):

In that same paper, I found a totally hypocritical article by the same author of the article in the Sydney Herald that was being referred to above. Every claim that the 'anti-vaxxers' are misinformed and wrong is completely unsubstantiated.

Of course, they don't need to back up their opinions with any actual verifiable research because they are PRAVDA, they are the *source of truth*. The reader is expected to be a believer in their absolute unimpeachable veracity. Why?! The reader is expected to be absolutely AGAINST any opinion other than that coming from Big Brother & absolutely believing EVERYTHING that does come from Big Brother. That, of course, makes them 'intelligent' & sensible people — heaven forbid that anyone *dares* to go against such power!!

'Slap them down' or hear them out: How to handle misinformation 'superspreaders'?

Well, given that it's labelled as "misinformation" in the headline, the answer to what decision they reached is obvious: definitely slap them down, definitely **do not hear them out**. In other words, they're already telling the reader what to think about something they haven't even read yet.

Almost as disturbing as the heat maps showing official death rates from COVID-19 every night on the news

They must really be stretching things quite a bit on the 'news' because as of today there've been 106 COVID-19 deaths in Australia (in a country with 25,499,884 people):

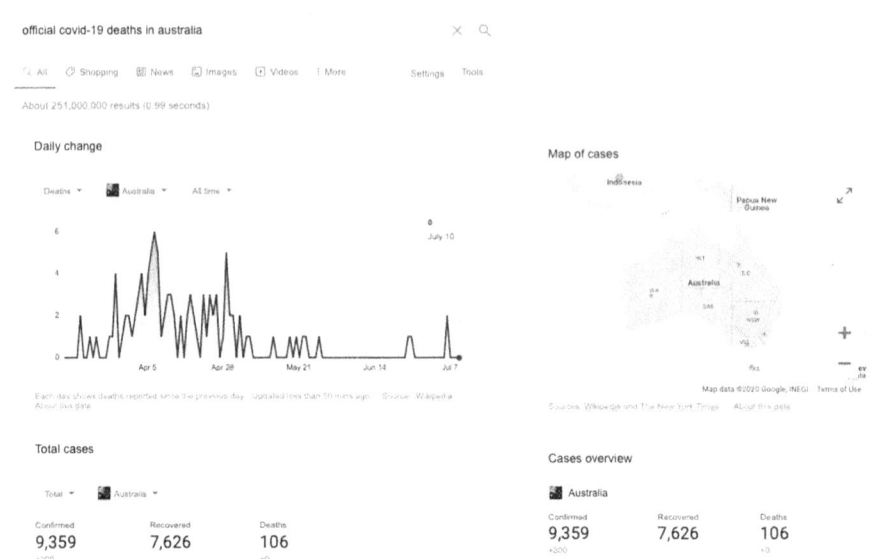

- sourced from here: https://en.wikipedia.org/wiki/COVID-19_pandemic_in_Australia

In other words, given that there's not even an average of ONE DEATH per day in a population of over 25 million. Even the mass media must be having a hard time sensationalizing that!

At a time when trust in science and gratitude for modern medicine should be high,

Why exactly should it be high? It seems to me that it should be at an all-time low.

it's been terrifying to watch traction gained recently by vaccination conspiracy theorists,

Of course there's no possibility of legitimate criticisms, right?

It found anti-vaccine pages – where "the battle for hearts and minds" on immunisation is fought – are more numerous than pro-vaccine and "undecided" pages, and are growing faster.

That's good news!

Anti-vaxxer pages will eventually dominate online discussion "at a time when a future vaccine against COVID-19 may be critical to public health", it predicted.

I doubt it!

Troubling, too was the widespread circulation on Australian and global social media this month of a 30-minute "documentary" called *Plandemic*, viewed more than eight million times in just a few days before Facebook and Google took it down.

Oh, gosh, you mean your censorhip isn't working as well as you'd like?

Discredited medical researcher

"Discredited" by who, exactly? It wouldn't be by people with conflicts of interest now would it?

Judy Mikovits makes startling claims in the video aimed at generating maximum emotion, including that wearing masks activates coronavirus and the pandemic is a hoax designed to help elites including Bill Gates grab money and power.

Mikovits is described by *The New York Times* as a "star of virus misinformation". That her ravings

Are you sure they're not 'rabid ravings'? I mean she couldn't just be discussing something that she thinks is important, right? Unlike the author of this article she's "raving".

disgraced doctor Anthony Wakefield

"The *British Medical Journal* described Wakefield's work as an "elaborate fraud". Subsequent reporting by Deer revealed that Wakefield had planned to capitalize on the MMR vaccination scare provoked by his paper by forming a corporation that would profit from "litigation-driven testing". Wakefield's study and his claim that the MMR vaccine might cause autism led to a decline in vaccination rates in the United States, the United Kingdom, and Ireland, and a corresponding rise in measles and mumps infections, resulting in serious illness and deaths. His continued claims that the vaccine is harmful have contributed to a climate of distrust of all vaccines and the reemergence of other previously-controlled diseases. Wakefield has continued to defend his research and conclusions, saying there was no fraud, hoax or profit motive." - https://en.wikipedia.org/wiki/Andrew_Wakefield

Note that "Wakefield has continued to defend his research and conclusions, saying there was no fraud, hoax or profit motive." So, who knows? I don't.

So given the sad reality that "one thing we do know is facts very, very rarely change somebody's mind about something",

Funny how some people think they have sole access to facts while the rest of us are just idiots.

Ridicule is pretty tempting. It certainly was this week when FM power duo Kyle and Jackie 'O' gave their megaplatform to alternative wellbeing salesman and ex-TV host, Pete Evans, to spread who knows how much harm with his vaccination musings.

Evans insists he is "pro-choice", not anti-vax.

& there we have it: PRO-CHOICE: people should have the right to say NO. It's precisely the fight against this right that's the most suspect.

Attacking disinformation crafted to instil primal fear in mothers of harming their baby or child seems a perfectly apt response

Right. That's exactly how I feel about the mainstream media. I mean *how dishonest can these people get?!* Is this writer suggesting that the 'news' isn't fear-mongering?! That would be mind-bogglingly disingenuous.

She has argued there is no evidence "just shouting down [anti-vaccination] opponents actually works", and only further polarises people.

Sure, as long as the person being 'listened to' is taken for granted as wrong to begin with someone like this author will listen.

Wendy Tuohy is a Sunday Age columnist.

I'd call her a GRADE-A ASSHOLE. Are they synonymous?

****

July 10, 2020, 6:49PM (Inquiring Librarian to group):

Yes, all of those responses help save my shreds of sanity. I just lost another 'friend' on social media over my offering the idea of HIT (Herd Immunity Threshold) and IFR (Infection Fatality Rate) from the Handley article. Total wash. This asshole said that the Handley article had no factual basis. I launched into him then. My fault. I don't fear speaking my mind to and being 'unfriended' by imbeciles. That dude is an imbecile, I mean really, how could you completely dismiss that article as making no sense and having no factual basis. That dude needs to be first in line for the new vaccine.

Ok, evidence condensed on the MMR vaccine that Andrew Wakefied fought against. Here it is. I personally believe Wakefied and Judy Mikovits. Believe it or not, J.B. Handley was interviewed by RFK Jr. this week here, and his kid has a severe vaccine injury: Ok, JB Handley interviewed: https://www.youtube.com/watch?time_continue=1&v=OHeP7nJA9MY&feature=emb_logo
Evidence on the lethality of the MMR vaccine: https://childrenshealthdefense.org/

news/measles-vaccination-and-autism-the-inexcusable-suppression-of-a-long-documented-link/

July 09, 2020

Measles Vaccination and Autism: The Inexcusable Suppression of a Long-Documented Link

By the Children's Health Defense Team

Before a humble coronavirus became the planet's viral scapegoat, the virus most often used to promote fear—and vaccination—has been measles. In fact, measles has provided public health officials with recurrent opportunities to fine-tune the CDC's strategic "recipe" for fostering high vaccine demand: stir up "concern, anxiety, and worry" about disease; promote vaccination frequently and visibly; and craft dumbed-down messages that, above all, avoid troublesome "nuance."

In this regard, parental reports linking autism spectrum disorder (ASD) to measles-mumps-rubella (MMR) vaccination have long been a thorn in officialdom's side, giving rise to the aggressive and unnuanced media mantra that the MMR "does not cause autism." Through constant repetition, many members of the public continue to swallow this official dogma, but the reality is that biological evidence on the ground has—from the beginning—told a very different story. The Institute of Medicine (IOM) even admitted as much in 2001 when it stated that it could neither disprove "proposed biological models linking MMR vaccine to ASD" nor dismiss the "possibility that MMR vaccine could contribute to ASD in a small number of children."

Among the biological models developed to explain autism, one particularly fruitful area of research has focused on ASD and immune dysregulation. Researchers have pointed to "autoantibodies"—immune proteins that react with the body's own cells, tissues or organs instead of fighting external pathogens—as key indicators of an immune system that has lost its ability to differentiate between "self" and "non-self." Autoantibodies are the hallmark of autoimmune disease and, in autism, they tend to react with proteins expressed in the brain. In a surprisingly candid systematic review of the autoantibody literature just published in *Research in Autism Spectrum Disorders*, authors from Harvard and other American universities cite long-standing evidence that viral vaccines—and explicitly the MMR—are one of the culprits capable of knocking the immune system off its game.

... brain autoantibodies are something that those with ASD have in common with individuals suffering from autoimmune diseases such as lupus, multiple sclerosis and rheumatoid arthritis.

[..]

Although the authors of the 2020 review are cautious overall, they outline some important clinical implications in their conclusions. While deeming the evidence "currently insufficient" to recommend routine autoantibody testing, they nevertheless state:

Although there is currently no evidence between vaccine administration and ASD in general, if the ASD disease onset or progression is temporally correlated with episodes of viral infection or MMR vaccine administration, one may opt to assay for measles antibodies and anti-MMR antibodies.

Never mind the evidence—more denial and lies

The fact is that there is ample evidence of a link, not just between the MMR and autism, but between vaccines, autism and autoimmunity more broadly. With their uniquely immune-altering configuration of antigens, adjuvants and preservatives (including aluminum and mercury), it is astonishing that vaccines are still so under-recognized as a trigger.

Unfortunately, public health officials continue to find it more convenient to ignore longstanding scientific evidence. In April 2019, when New York City's health commissioner ordered Brooklyn residents to get the MMR, she claimed, with a straight face, that vaccines generally—and measles vaccines, in particular—result in "relatively few, if any, serious adverse effects." Likewise, Dr. Anthony Fauci has repeatedly misrepresented vaccine risks, telling Americans in 2009 that serious adverse events from the disastrous H1N1 influenza vaccine were "very, very, very rare" and lying under oath to Congress in 2019 (before being corrected by a junior colleague) about the grave adverse event of encephalitis, which is listed in the MMR vaccine package insert. If these authority figures are the sources that the American people are relying on for accurate risk information about future coronavirus vaccines, we should be very worried.

****

July 10, 2020, 7:26PM (Amir-ul Kafirs to group):

Re: HERETICS:

I just lost another 'friend' on social media over my offering the idea of HIT (Herd Immunity Threshold) and IFR (Infection Fatality Rate) from the Handley article.

I still find Handley's article to be one of the best yet. If it's not scientific then the guy's an amazingly good fake.

This asshole said that the Handley article had no factual basis.

No doubt he could provide counter-charts that explain why Handley's in-depth analysis isn't true. **[For those of you unable to detect the sarcasm in writing I follow with: NOT]**

how could you completely dismiss that article as making no sense and having no factual basis.

By not reading it, of course. It's really simple to dismiss something if you don't read it.

That dude needs to be first in line for the new vaccine.

Has anyone seen the movie "Divergent" or read the book? In it, a post-apocalypse society is divided into 5 factions that each take care of an important part of running the society. People are only allowed to be in 1 faction. People with the skills of multiple factions, "divergents", are hunted & killed. The self-sacrificing people are the social leaders. The intellectuals decide they want to run the society instead so they forcibly inject the "Dauntless", the police, with a drug that makes them controllable & then send them out to kill the self-sacrificing people. Perhaps your friend would welcome such an injection?

Measles Vaccination and Autism: The Inexcusable Suppression of a Long-Documented Link

No doubt the FACT-CHOKED can refute the following example as "unscientific". The obvious problem is that most people these days are borderline illiterate anyway so trying to read something that's actually scientific is going to be *wwwwaaaaaayyyyyyy over their head* so they just take the FACT-CHOKER position rather than admit that they can't understand a word of any of the arguments one way or another.

As I like to say: *DON'T FUCK 'EM* (as opposed to "Fuck 'em!").

- tENTATIVELY "howlin' lone wolf" a cONVENIENCE

Brain autoantibodies and autoimmunity
There are numerous proteins important for a healthy brain. As the 2020 review article in *Research in Autism Spectrum Disorders* points out, children with ASD manifest autoantibodies to a wide spectrum of brain proteins. For example, researchers have identified autoantibodies in autistic individuals that are reactive to:

- Endothelial cells (important to the blood-brain barrier)
- Folate receptors (needed for the synthesis of neurotransmitters)
- Serotonin receptors (crucial for brain development, mood, sleep and appetite)
- Myelin basic protein (MBP) (a building block of the coating that

surrounds nerve cells) and myelin-associated glycoprotein (MAG)
- Ribosomal P proteins (important for neuronal tissue)

As this list shows, brain autoantibodies are something that those with ASD have in common with individuals suffering from autoimmune diseases such as lupus, multiple sclerosis and rheumatoid arthritis. In fact, not only is there a large body of evidence suggesting that ASD has an autoimmune component, but autoimmune illnesses have exploded over roughly the same time frame as autism.

****

July 10, 2020, 7:27PM (Amir-ul Kafirs to group):

HERETICS: Herd Immunity

This isn't one of my better ones but I just keep chipping away at it!:

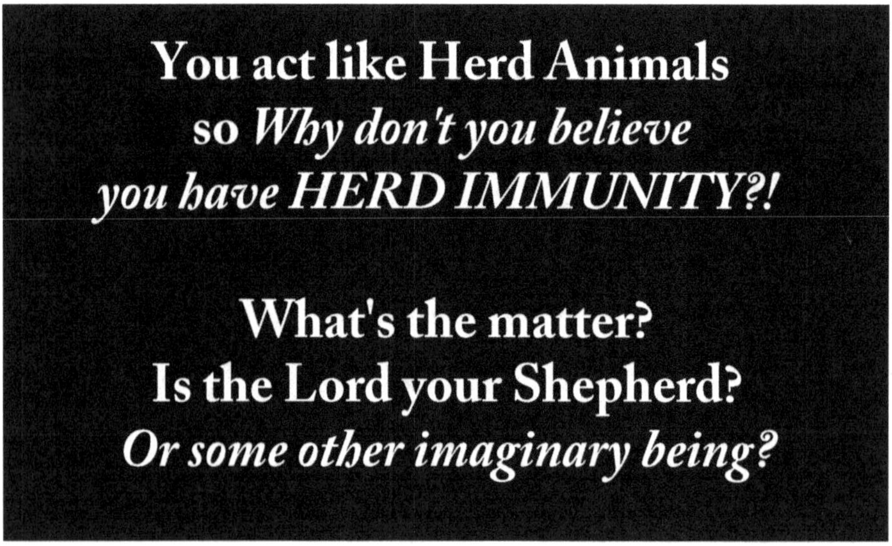
You act like Herd Animals
so *Why don't you believe*
you have HERD IMMUNITY?!
What's the matter?
Is the Lord your Shepherd?
Or some other imaginary being?

****

July 11, 2020 (Inquiring Librarian sent this link as a Message to Amir-ul Kafirs):

Germany - The COVID-19 Extra-Parliamentary Inquiry Committee - Start Conference 03rd July 2020

https://youtu.be/zINz460ySTE

****

July 11, 2020, 11:34AM (Amir-ul Kafirs to group):

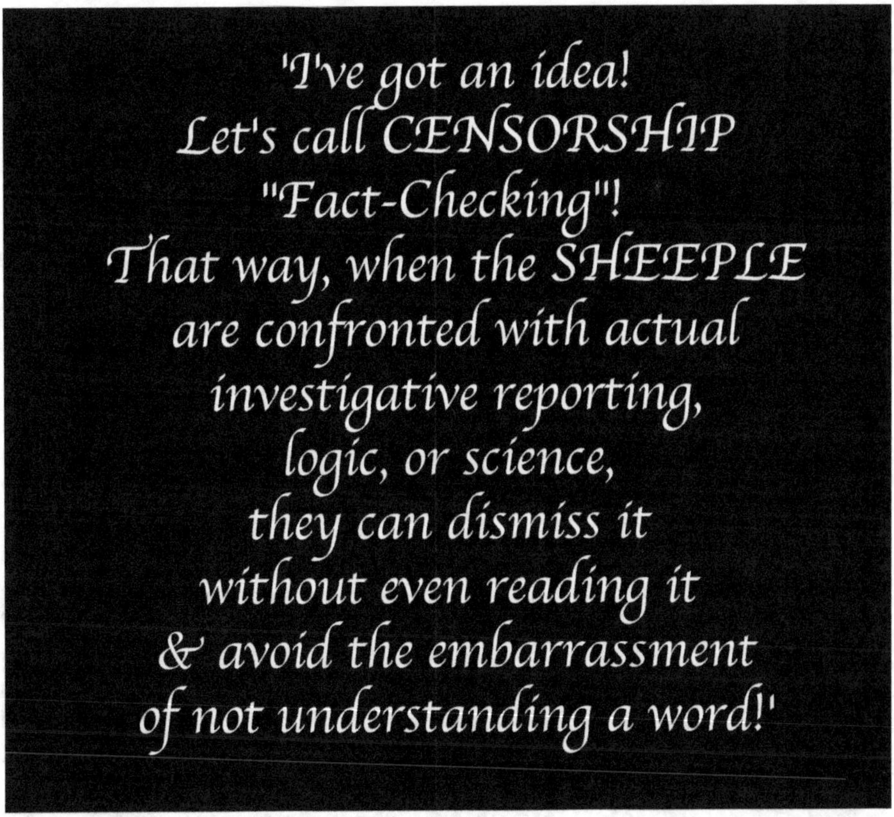
'I've got an idea!
Let's call CENSORSHIP
"Fact-Checking"!
That way, when the SHEEPLE
are confronted with actual
investigative reporting,
logic, or science,
they can dismiss it
without even reading it
& avoid the embarrassment
of not understanding a word!'

****

July 11, 2020, 7:43PM (Amir-ul Kafirs to group):

HERETICS: "Wearing Masks Saves Lives" movie online

Here's my new movie. I wouldn't be surprised if it got removed from YouTube almost immediately so check it out while you can. It's short.

"Wearing Masks Saves Lives" notes - 1:18 - 1080p

https://youtu.be/oQBsMuVgnmU

"Wearing Masks Saves Lives": During the PANDEMIC PANIC doctors & researchers have been saying since at least the beginning of May, 2020, that wearing masks + extraordinary cleaning of hands & the environment are largely ineffective in stopping the spread of COVID-19. Nonetheless, even though recent 'cases' have NOT been recent deaths, even though the argument has been made that herd immunity has been achieved, etc, etc, mask-wearing has become increasingly emphasized. It's my opinion that most people have become SHEEPLE, robopaths & untertan, eager to comply & to inlfict compliance on others NOT because there's a sound medical reason for doing so but because some sado-masochistic tendencies have been unleashed, not to mention a vast enabling of hypochondria. Certain rote phrases have become commonplace, all of them pro-Big-Brother. People talk in such prefabricated idiocies as: "Wearing Masks Saves Lives".

Such people also accuse others who aren't wearing masks of being murderers. If this were true, EVERYONE IN THE WORLD WOULD BE DEAD BY NOW. We're not. This is a contemporary form of Spectral Evidence, a mass media fear-mongering fantasy becomes reality in the 'minds' of SHEEPLE who've long-since lost touch with non-mediated reality. Flippant as this move is it has a serious purpose: to call attention to the dangerously mind-controlled era that we're living in. - July 11, 2020 (Vision) notes from tENTATIVELY, a cONVENIENCE

Tags: masks, COVID-19, coronavirus, mind control, sheeple, pandemic panic, robopaths, untertan, waterphone, tENTATIVELY a cONVENIENCE, humor

****

July 12, 2020, 12:06AM (Amir-ul Kafirs to group):

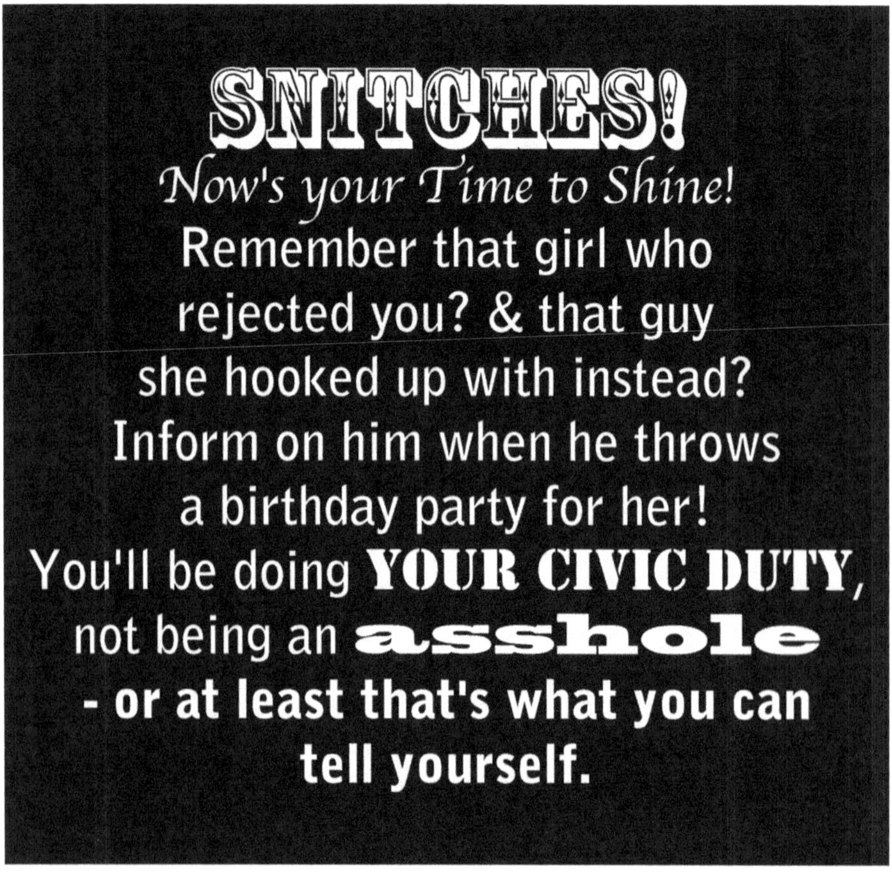
SNITCHES!
Now's your Time to Shine!
Remember that girl who
rejected you? & that guy
she hooked up with instead?
Inform on him when he throws
a birthday party for her!
You'll be doing YOUR CIVIC DUTY,
not being an asshole
- or at least that's what you can
tell yourself.

****

July 12, 2020, 5:06AM (Dick to group):

RE: HERETICS: "Wearing Masks Saves Lives" movie online

I think it's intense in the sense that it seems calculated through its combination of elements to be disturbing, to bait people, to call any mask wearer a fool, an idiot, to give no quarter so to speak
I mean the various elements seem to work together to produce that effect
That is, it's a propaganda film
Adding the images of the dead produces an unpleasant psychological effect (looking at the dead isn't pleasant) and the music adds to the impression because, at least for me, non-tonal music creates a sort of nervous atmosphere because it never resolves
so all in all, I think it's pretty successful as a work of political art

****

July 12, 2020, 9:52AM (Amir-ul Kafirs to group):

Re: HERETICS: "Wearing Masks Saves Lives" movie online

Thanks for this. I think it's a pretty fair assessment & I can see your points. I do disagree somewhat, though, & I'll explain that below.

I think it's intense in the sense that it seems calculated through its combination of elements to be disturbing,

I actually don't find it "disturbing". Probably a part of it is that when I make something I get preoccupied with how I'm going to pull it off technically & my focus tends to go there. That's part of what I meant by "It's hard for me to be detached." SO, I thought of the 3 scenes & I had to think of how to make them. The hardest one being the last scene with the mask flying to the rescue to herd the wearer out of the street so that they don't get hit by the car. It's been extremely hot here, with "real feel" temperatures over 100°F, & nether Naia Nisnam nor I had much energy for shooting. Added to this is that Naia Nisnam doesn't like acting so I had to try to make the whole shoot as quick as I could, no time for much fine-tuning. Anyway, for me it's 'black humor' but funny enough to not be "disturbing".

to bait people, to call any mask wearer a fool, an idiot, to give no quarter so to speak

Well, yes & no. For me it's fighting fire with fire, so to speak. I feel surrounded by a 'liberal' GROUPTHINK in which anyone who disagrees with mask-wearing is immediately branded a "knucklehead" & a "neo-nazi". It doesn't matter whether the disagreeing person is obviously intelligent & obviously anti-nazi. They must immediately be attacked & slandered. That's where there's "no quarter". No possibility of any valid criticism is ever acknowledged. But what I'm really fighting against is the specific propaganda slogan, that people have said to me like automatons, of "Wearing Masks Saves Lives". As with your _____ example, people are actually saying that if you don't wear a mask you're a murderer, responsible for other people's deaths. The middle scene, the one where I try to eat through the mask, mocks this. The questions it raises are: Am I 'murdering' people every time I take my mask off? Even to eat? That sort of thing. Naturally, I don't think that not wearing a mask is killing people.

That is, it's a propaganda film

Again, I see it as an ANTI-propaganda movie insofar as it's meant to counter the "Wearing Masks Saves Lives" slogan. Still, I can understand calling it propaganda in & of itself.

Adding the images of the dead produces an unpleasant psychological effect (looking at the dead isn't pleasant)

I reckon looking at the images of the dead doesn't bother me as much as it apparently does you. That's probably partially because I picked the images. There are ones that I think originated in Indonesia where there's a corpse standing up with a cigarette in its mouth with a live person smoking next to it, another one has a group of girls who found a corpse taking a group 'selfie' next to it. There's some humor there. I show a variety of attitudes toward death, there're the masked & suited workers from these PANDEMIC times & then there's the "Green" disposal of a corpse where it's left on a raised dais in a field.

and the music adds to the impression because, at least for me, non-tonal music creates a sort of nervous atmosphere because it never resolves

Ah, well, this may be where we diverge the most! As I'm sure you realize, I prefer non-tonal music over tonal music. Of course, I can enjoy tonal music too — I'm not against it. Anyway, for me, the non-resolution is positive because I often find resolution too predictable & oversimplifying. Truthfully, though, I chose to use the waterphone as the instrument for the soundtrack because I'd just gotten it & wanted to do something with it AND because I was amused by the online sales pitch for it that didn't even identify the instrument by name but instead promoted it as good for horror movie soundtracks. But the 'horror' that I play up in the movie isn't the horror of the dead, it's the horror of watching mind control be so utterly successful. The 'living dead' I suppose.

so all in all, I think it's pretty successful as a work of political art

I don't think you generally like "political art", although I'd consider some of your work to be that (such as that "Shoot the Suit" (is that the correct name?) movie of yours). Strangely enough, I don't actually think of it as "political art", I just think of it as me trying to counterbalance the propaganda as fiercely as I can without losing my sense of humor.

Again, though, thanks for your feedback, I appreciate your taking the time.

yr pal,

****

July 12, 2020, 3:51PM (Dick to group):

I guess the tone of my mail was misleading...
I honestly like the film...!
I don't have a problem with political art... well sometimes I do I guess...but not here (I have a problem with John Cage... more on that another time if you want to know...)
But I do think, in general, that my idea of what constitutes political is highly, perhaps too, personal to be immediately understood if at all... I think my music is political precisely because it isn't "modern" per se...for example
In fact, i would say I have never produced a work of art that isn't political; in the sense that I mean it to be like a bomb to alter consciousness
But usually I have found that they are just dismissed, thus my fond memories of the UMMF where my films (for example) were taken seriously and understood more or less as I had hoped them to be understood...that was refreshing to say the least
I understood your film as fire fighting fire...
The debate over masks seems to be much more intense there (in the USA) than it it is here by the way... though it does exist here
I find the pictures of the dead disturbing because they represent potential suffering, horror, pain, injustice

I had an idea for a mask film by the way but didn't know how to produce it and as I have no one to help me it slipped from my mind...

****

July 12, 2020, 5:39PM (Amir-ul Kafirs to group):

I honestly like the film...!

Well, I'm glad you do because I'm expecting so much hatred in response to it that it's hard for me deal with. Nonetheless, I created it as a challenge to what I perceive as oppressive conditions.

(I have a problem with John Cage... more on that another time if you want to know...)

A conversation about Cage would have to be in person! He's in my top 10 favorite composers. My enthusiasm for his work has inevitably waned over the years but it provided me with profound stimulus for decades.

But I do think, in general, that my idea of what constitutes political is highly, perhaps too, personal to be immediately understood if at all...

In the 1970s, Kirby Malone & I both said that "Everything's Political, Everything's Sexual". I still agree with that although I'm not sure it matters that much anymore. The point is I can perceive any work, any action, as political but because I CAN perceive it that way I tend to think of works that more overtly address specific issues as the stand-out political works.

thus my fond memories of the UMMF where my films (for example) were taken seriously and understood more or less as I had hoped them to be understood...that was refreshing to say the least

Thank the Holy Ceiling Light it was good for something because the general public sure as fuck didn't give a shit.

I understood your film as fire fighting fire...
The debate over masks seems to be much more intense there (in the USA) than it it is here by the way... though it does exist here

Be glad it's not like it is here. Some days are worse than others but, in general, it's being used to restructure the society. Voting by mail instead of at the polling places, e.g., because it's 'too unsafe' for people to be together in the same place, is one feature of this restructuring. It seems obvious to me that election-fixing has been going on in the US, &, presumably, everywhere else, for as long as voting has existed but it seemed most obvious when George W. Bush was elected. I'm sure there are people who also honestly try to keep it honest but I don't think there are enough of those to really keep track of what's going on. Furthermore, it seems to me that the chaos of a restructuring of the voting means it will be the perfect time for all sorts of corruption. I imagine both the Democrats & the Republicans pulling off as many dirty tricks as possible. Who will win? I don't know. But the 'simple' issue of social distancing & masks et al will definitely be part of it all.

I had an idea for a mask film by the way but didn't know how to produce it and as I have no one to help me it slipped from my mind...

Make it! I wanted a crew of 4 or more for mine but I had to do it with just Naia Nisnam because, these days, I hardly know anyone local other than Naia Nisnam who isn't falling into lockstep.

****

July 12, 2020, 4:10PM (Naia Nisnam to Amir-ul Kafirs):

Re: HERETICS: SNITCHES

Snitches...
I had to “unfriend” someone that I’ve known for at least 10 years. We’ve never been close friends but he used to call himself an anti-racist activist and that’s how I knew him.
Anyway, on his social media page, he had posted a photograph of people outside of a restaurant or cafe. The people, 3 in a group, were seated at the same table, closer than 6 feet apart and without masks. He was shaming them for doing so. Someone else, in the comments, shared a phone number to call to

report people not wearing masks.
This sort of thing is making me incredibly nervous.

****

July 12, 2020, 5:50PM (Amir-ul Kafirs to Naia Nisnam):

Someone else, in the comments, shared a phone number to call to report people not wearing masks.
This sort of thing is making me incredibly nervous.

Of course, the reason why I made the SNITCHES text panel is to show people a more realistic look at what snitching is all about: it's *not* about 'doing the right thing', it's about petty human motivations — & these New Dark Ages, as I've come to think of them, are exemplifying this. Can you imagine even 6 months ago ANYONE saying they were going to call the police on people for eating together at a restaurant?! It would've seemed insane, as it is. Now, thanks to what're essentially imaginary threats to the public health the most malignant & stupid human characteristics are being given free reign. I have to wonder how the police are handling all this. Surely they must recognize that people's shittiest characteristics are running wild. Can you imagine being a cop & getting a call about people eating at a restaurant?! I'm hoping that the police are making judgment calls that make more realistic assessments of the 'crimes in progress'.

****

July 12, 2020, 7:14PM (Amir-ul Kafirs to group):

HERETICS: Psy Post & Eric W. Dolan

Remember Eric W. Dolan's article on "Psychopathic traits linked to non-compliance with social distancing guidelines amid the coronavirus pandemic" in Psy Post? What about his "Intellectually arrogant people typically have more anti-vaccination attitudes, study finds"? Well, a friend of mine in Canada has passed along a new work of psychological genius by him: "Lower cognitive ability linked to non-compliance with social distancing guidelines during the coronavirus outbreak". Yes, if you had any doubts that you're a pretty horrible person for questioning the QUARANTYRANNY, *doubt not more!* You're a psychopath, intellectually arrogant, AND you have lower cognitive ability. Wow. How did such a bunch of losers ever even manage to join together in this HERETICS group?! It must be a fluke! Read it & weep (or laugh or whatever):

Eric W. Dolan On July 11, 2020

Lower cognitive ability linked to non-compliance with social distancing guidelines

during the coronavirus outbreak

New research provides evidence that working memory is associated with engaging in social distancing in the early stages of the coronavirus pandemic. The new study has been published in the *Proceedings of the National Academy of Sciences*.

On March 11th, 2020, the World Health Organization declared the outbreak of the novel coronavirus SARS-CoV-2 to be a global pandemic. Governments around the world urged people to follow preventive health measures such as frequent hand washing and physical distancing. But not everyone abided by the safety guidelines.

"At the moment, successful containment of the COVID-19 outbreak critically relies on people's voluntary compliance with social distancing guidelines. However, there is widespread non-compliance in our society, especially during the early stage of this pandemic (and more recently after reopening)," said study author Weizhen Xie (Zane), a postdoctoral research fellow at the National Institute of Neurological Disorders and Stroke.

The researcher noted that there have been numerous media reports about Americans failing to physically distance themselves from one another in public spaces.

"As a researcher in cognitive psychology, I feel that it is our duty to figure out why some people follow the developing norm of social distancing while others ignore it. Addressing this issue may help mitigate the current public health crisis due to the COVID-19," Xie said.

In two studies, the researchers surveyed 850 U.S. residents between March 13 and March 25, 2020 — the first two weeks following the U.S. presidential declaration of a national emergency about the COVID-19 pandemic. In addition to collecting demographic information and assessing social distancing compliance, the surveys included assessments of working memory, personality, mood, and fluid intelligence.

Xie and his colleagues found that those with better working memory capacity were more likely to indicate that they had followed social distancing guidelines, such as not shaking hands and avoiding social gatherings.

"Our findings reveal a novel cognitive root of social distancing compliance during the early stage of the COVID-19 pandemic," said co-author Weiwei Zhang.

The researchers also found that higher levels of fluid intelligence and agreeableness were associated with greater social distancing compliance. But the link between working memory and social distancing held even after controlling for these factors and others.

[..]

https://www.psypost.org/2020/07/covidiot-study-lower-cognitive-ability-linked-to-non-compliance-with-social-distancing-guidelines-during-the-coronavirus-outbreak-57293/amp

****

July 12, 2020, 7:33PM (Amir-ul Kafirs to group):

Re: HERETICS: Psy Post & Eric W. Dolan

All 3 of the articles are by the same guy: Eric W. Dolan. "Eric is the founder, publisher, and editor of PsyPost." (https://www.psypost.org/author/edolan). A superficial search revealed that he's basically a gun-for-hire:

Eric W. Dolan - clearvoice.com

Feed your marketed channels the content they need with talented writers from ClearVoice. Hire vetted writers in more than 200 business categories. Power all your content marketing. All in One Place. Easy to Use. DIY or Fully Managed. Articles & Blogs, Ebooks.

However, clicking on the link didn't work. He's also listed on "Muck Rack":

Eric W. Dolan VERIFIED

California
Managing Editor and Publisher and Editor, PsyPost.org — RawStory
Crime and Justice, Politics, U.S.
As seen in: RawStory, Business Insider, Salon, AlterNet, The New Civil Rights Movement, Extra Bilingual Newspaper, CKPC-FM

- https://muckrack.com/ewdolan

Here's a list of the articles he has there:

Lower cognitive ability linked to non-compliance with social distancing guidelines during the coronavirus outbreak

By Eric W. Dolan
psypost.org — Cognitive Science By Eric W. Dolan July 11, 2020 Share on Facebook Share on Twitter Pinterest LinkedIn Tumblr Share Share on Facebook Share on Twitter Pinterest LinkedIn New research provides evidence that working memory and fluid intelligence are associated with engaging in social distancing in the early stages of the coronavirus pandemic. The new study has been published in the Proceedings of the National Academy of Sciences.
2 DAYS AGO Open in Who Shared Wrong byline?

WATCH: Doctor laughs at Trump's bizarre boast about passing a cognitive test
By Eric W. Dolan
rawstory.com — Arthur Caplan of New York University School of Medicine, who holds seven honorary degrees from colleges and medical schools, couldn't help but chuckle when discussing President Donald Trump's recent comments about passing a cognitive test. "I actually took one very recently when, you know, the radical left was saying, 'Is he all there? Is he all there?' I proved I was all there, because I aced it," Trump told Fox News host Sean Hannity on Thursday night.
2 DAYS AGO Open in Who Shared Wrong byline?

Trump is a friendless 'psychopath' who now sees Kavanaugh and Gorsuch as enemies: Art of the Deal ghostwriter
By Eric W. Dolan
rawstory.com — Brett Kavanaugh and Neil Gorsuch, who were nominated by Donald Trump, voted with the majority on Thursday against the president. Tony Schwartz, the ghostwriter behind "Trump: The Art of the Deal," says that the president now views the two Supreme Court justices as his enemies. "The psychopathy is why he does what he does," Schwartz told CNN.
3 DAYS AGO Open in Who Shared Wrong byline?

He's on Twitter if you're interested: https://twitter.com/EWDolan?ref_src=twsrc%5Egoogle%7Ctwcamp%5Eserp%7Ctwgr%5Eauthor

It's pretty obvious that he's a Democratic Party hired character assassin employed to work against Rump & his allies.

****

July 13, 2020, 12:06AM (Amir-ul Kafirs to group):

HERETICS: KUFFAR

This is a Shout-Out to my fellow KUFFAR: May we preserve our CRIMINAL SANITY in these Dark Ages.

****

July 13, 2020, 12:10AM (Naia Nisnam to group):

I thought this was satire but... It's real:

"TEXAS: You should consider wearing a mask even when you're in your own home"

https://news4sanantonio.com/news/local/tdem-you-should-consider-wearing-a-mask-even-when-youre-in-your-own-home?fbclid=IwAR2ZYBRHmipAlkPAD6Os_7GrD5pz7w1kIBWkKjpv184gLL-K_HCKWC9Zpx4

****

TEXAS: You should consider wearing a mask even when you're in your own home

by Gerald Tracy Thursday, July 9th 2020

SAN ANTONIO - The Texas Division of Emergency Management is advising residents to consider wearing a mask at all times, even in your own home. In an interview with our Ryan Wolf, Chief Nim Kidd said as much, adding the community has paid attention and done well outside their homes, but it is not enough.

"We still need people to wear the mask out in public, we still need people to keep social distance and isolation," Kidd said. "Ryan, the one thing I want to try to get across today is we need to do that when we're in our homes also.

"As you know, I'm a life-long San Antonian, grew up there, worked there for many years and I know how many multi-generational families that we have. While we believe the community is doing a great job of following the rules when they are outside the home, we really need to be thinking about doing the same thing when we're inside the home."

[..]

- https://news4sanantonio.com/news/local/tdem-you-should-consider-wearing-a-mask-even-when-youre-in-your-own-home?fbclid=IwAR2ZYBRHmipAIkPAD6Os_7GrD5pz7w1kIBWkKjpv184gLL-K_HCKWC9Zpx4

****

July 13, 2020, 8:53AM (Dick to group):

very interesting
it seems insane
did you notice on the same page the article about the dying words of some guy who'd participated in a so-called covid party?
it's almost comical
*
When I was a kid my mother told me about her great aunts who were prohibitionists
one of the slogans they preferred was "lips that touch liquor shall never touch mine"
they used to play a record for my somewhat wayward great grandfather, who was given to drink, called "Molly and the baby, don't you know!" (see below)
there were all sorts of ideas about how drinking was degenerate, a sign of being a sort of sub-human
the dry and wet camps were violently opposed to each other

I see a bit of that in this current mask business in the USA, at least that's how it seems from "over here"

https://www.youtube.com/watch?v=AM3bavPGJ5M

****

'I thought this was a hoax': Patient in 30s dies after attending 'COVID party'

by GERALD TRACY, WOAI/KABB Friday, July 10th 2020

SAN ANTONIO, Texas (WOAI/KABB) – A patient in their 30s died from the coronavirus after attending what's being called a "COVID party," according to a

San Antonio health official.

Chief Medical Officer of Methodist Healthcare Dr. Jane Appleby said the idea of these parties is to see if the virus is real.

"This is a party held by somebody diagnosed by the COVID virus and the thought is to see if the virus is real and to see if anyone gets infected," Dr. Appleby said.

According to Appleby, the patient became critically ill and had a heartbreaking statement moments before death.

"Just before the patient died, they looked at their nurse and said 'I think I made a mistake, I thought this was a hoax, but it's not,'" Appleby said.

Appleby made this case public as the spike in cases for Bexar County continues. She wants everyone, especially those in the younger demographic, to realize they are not invincible.

[..]

****

July 13, 2020, 9:20AM (Amir-ul Kafirs to group):

"TEXAS: You should consider wearing a mask even when you're in your own home"

I find looking at the ads that accompany this stuff edifying:

You can watch the full interview above. Kidd also spoke about how TDEM is working with the TEA on the upcoming school year and San Antonio hospital capacity.

MORE TO EXPLORE

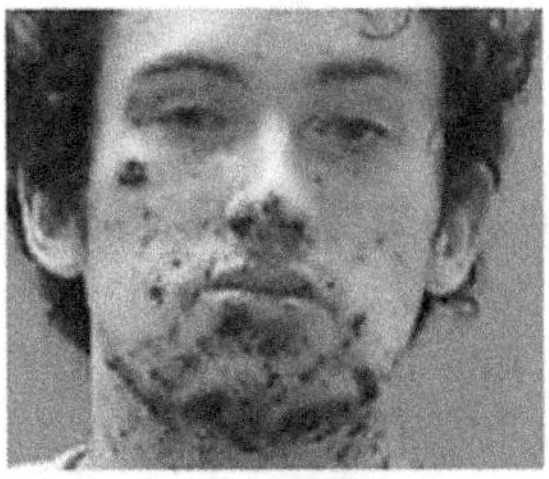

Man blows off his own hand with bomb he was intending to use to hurt women

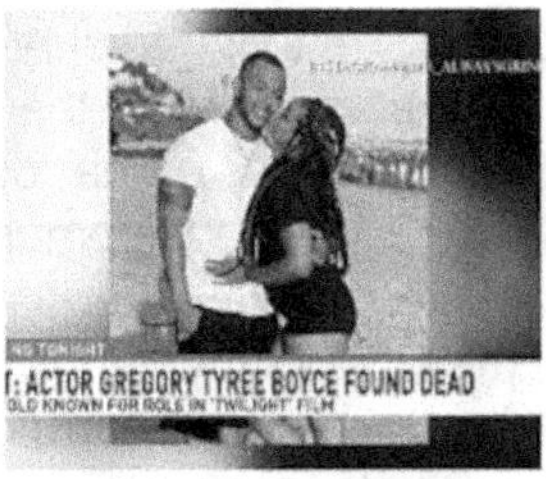

'Twilight' actor Gregory Boyce found dead with girlfriend in Las Vegas

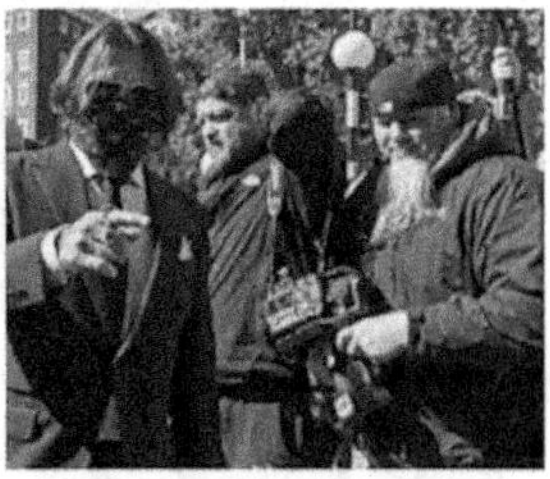

Johnny Depp says feces in bed was last straw in marriage to Amber Heard

At any rate, I've decided to just close off all my body holes. It's the only way to be safe. I mean we just can't stop at butt plugs to keep those toxic farts in. Hear no virus, see no virus, speak no virus, think no.

****

July 13, 2020, 9:20AM (Amir-ul Kafirs to group):

did you notice on the same page the article about the dying words of some guy who'd participated in a so-called covid party?

It's also HIGHLY SUSPECT!! Notice that there're no mention of comorbidities. One has to wonder: *Did he **only die from COVID-19?!*** They don't give the patient's name so I can't easily try to do any further research on it.

the dry and wet camps were violently opposed to each other

Thanks for the comparison, I wouldn't've thought about that. There's a really interesting documentary called, if I remember correctly, "Demon Rum". It's about Henry Ford & his participation in Prohibition. (https://www.youtube.com/watch?v=pywGG6dpj0s&list=PLhUpsZBYmKZ9WaGRVPmzhCHlGvlgGfobh) Ford created 'Morality Squads' (or some such) that visted worker's homes. If the workers were found to be drinkers they were not able to be promoted. Since Ford was by far the largest employer staying on his good side was essential to making a living. People who were fired for their 'low morals' became bootleggers. The bootleggers became thugs. When Ford wanted union busters who did he hire to do it? The thug class that he'd helped create by firing people who became bootleggers!

****

July 13, 2020, 10:07AM (Amir-ul Kafirs to group):

I want to thank people for posting comments on my social media post of the link to "Wearing Masks Saves Lives"!! You help me stay criminally sane. As I'm sure is obvious to all of you, I'm trying to stay even-tempered & civil even when I feel like screaming in frustration. One of the comment-makers is an ex-girlfriend who's had a very rough life & was on her own at age 12. Because of this, she could be said to have Arrested Development. She's a wonderful person but a bit slow on intellectual uptake. To have her ask if I watched Fox 'News' as if that's the only reason why I might have my opinions was disheartening. Still, knowing her, I know that she didn't mean any harm by it so I just had to explain myself a bit further for her. Nonetheless, my abilities as a moderator are being stretched more than a bit thin so I'm glad that Phil, e.g., posted information against mask wearing & saved me from having to go there. _____, the main critical voice, is an old friend & I very much didn't want to broaden the gap with him. He lives in NYC & was bound to feel much more threatened by the virus than the rest of us. I think that _____ was reining himself in & trying to be respectful but that he obviously feels strongly against what the rest of us were saying. I appreciate his self-restraint AND EVERYONE ELSE'S TOO!! So, again, thank you. For those of you who aren't on social media, here's the thread. I unfriended the 1st poster. I have to say, & I'm sure we all feel this way to a certain extent, that I'm really burnt-out from struggling against this. Nonetheless, I refuse to stop — partially because I think that the powers-that-be rely on forcing us into exhaustion & then into compliance because it's the 'path of least resistance'. Unfortunately for them, I'm a Professional Resister of Character Assassination & have spent most of my life in struggles like this. SO, whether it's what I want or not, I still have a modicum of the necessary skills to keep on keeping on.

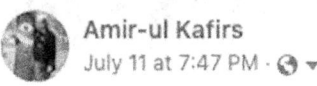

Amir-ul Kafirs
July 11 at 7:47 PM ·

"Wearing Masks Saves Lives" - 1:18 - 1080p

https://youtu.be/oQBsMuVgnmU

During the PANDEMIC PANIC doctors & researchers have been saying since at least the beginning of May, 2020, that wearing masks + extraordinary cleaning of hands & the environment are largely ineffective in stopping the spread of COVID-19. Nonetheless, even though recent 'cases' have NOT been recent deaths, even though the argument has been made that herd immunity has been achieved, etc, etc, mask-weari... See More

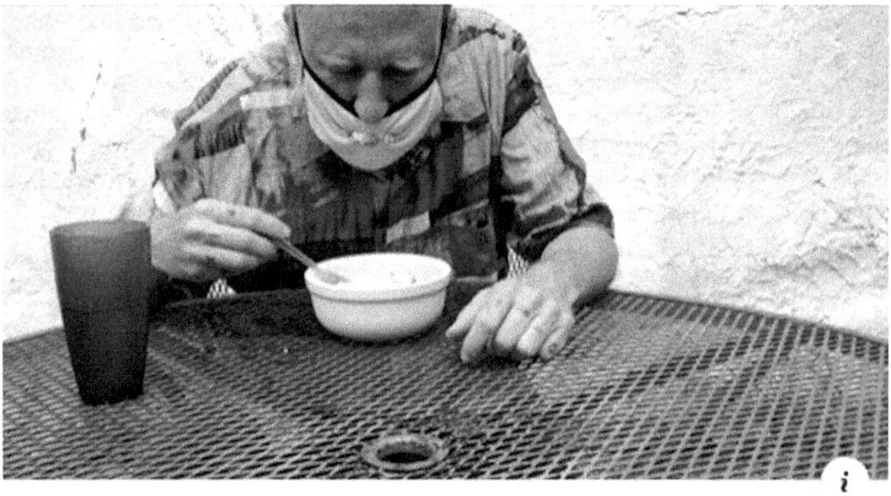

YOUTUBE.COM

Wearing Masks Save Lives

"Wearing Masks Saves Lives": During the PANDEMIC PANIC doctors &...

6 27 Comments 3 Shares

Like Comment Share

6 27 Comments 3 Shares

Like Comment Share

001a You may get some air play on the Proud Boys and 4chan, but otherwise you are missing the forest for the tree sloths. There is a buttload of mind controlling misinformation blasting out of the Kremlin/Washington Corp.
right now it is pushing the idea that voting by mail will be hacked by China. Seriously. Why?
Come November and COVID is still going strong, sane people won't want to congregate at the polls (Dems) Mutant zombies (Repubs) will flock to the polls because private bone-spers tells them to.
No joke. The election is rigged line is already being pushed by the enemy bot nets.
We live in epic times and we have front row seats to the show. The price of the ticket is having to watch absolutely everything go to hell.

Reply · 1d

Amir-ul Kafirs Since you're implying that I'm a neo-nazi, something that I find incredibly stupid, I'm unfriending you. Democrats are just as stupid & braindead as Republicans. Trump's despicable, Biden's despicable. This is the lowest I've ever seen American politics stoop to & that's saying alot.

Like · 1d · Edited 2

001b Amir-ul Kafirs Can't say I disagree ..

7h

002a as much as i appreciate what you are saying here, there certainly is considerable evidence that wearing a mask does have beneficial effects. https://www.ucsf.edu/.../still-confused-about-masks-heres...

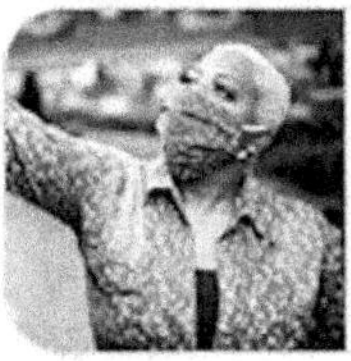

UCSF.EDU

Still Confused About Masks? Here's the Science Behind How Face Masks...

Like · Reply · 1d 2

^ Hide 18 Replies

003a One of the many infuriating aims of the blatant propaganda that's bombarding people these days is to divide them in ways that are not mutually exclusive and thus render all reasonable discussion pointless. Yes, of course masks are effective (I was baffled when they initially argued they weren't) but the discourse created around them is off the charts manipulative and divisive. The phrase "Wearing Masks Saves Lives" is so incedibly wrong on so many levels that a FB post could never begin to cover it - the manipulation of the public along the lines of hyper policing each other is unprecedented, implying that if one doesn't wear a mask, one is a homicidal maniac, and giving power to the lowest common bully mentality is scary. Not to mention that everything regarding the interpretation of measures, numbers and medical information is systematically de-contextualized, blown out of proportion and frequently changed in ways reminiscent of psychopathic gaslighting. This is, disturbingly enough, an almost global narrative, which reminds us how far the syncronization of globalized power has gone while we were being locally distracted, but also especially effective in the US where there seem to be media and group psychology conditions that make this come into the sharpest relief. (That said, and as much as I agree with tENT, I also find calling people sheeple or stupid, something that seems to flow across the lines in US discourse, enforcing the desired intolerance and division of people. Everyone holds a piece of truth, it's better to focus on that, any form of fear only breeds war, and that's what propaganda aims at, division and conquer.)

Like · Reply · 1d · Edited

002b 003 i couldn't agree with you more. your assessment is very well analyzed and stated. and of course, facecrap is THE worst possible platform for any serious political discourse. but it is so extremely easy to fall into a trap of (ir)rational bullshit over your piece of dirt. tENT rightly points out that "herd" mentality as opposed to herd immunity is a serious flaw in our world. it's never a good thing IMO when people simply and blindly "follow orders" and do as they are told without question. Conversely, it is also foolish to ignore facts and evidence, so, it is vitally important that everyone becomes vigilant and discerning. will this happen? probably not, because a lot of ignorance is spread around by sheer laziness and indifference. and THAT will kill many if it doesn't change.

Like · Reply · 1d 2

003b 002 exactly! And, as I find perspective is most sorely missing in public discourse, I'd like to bring into sharper focus that herd mentality is a much bigger social problem than the lack of herd immunity can ever be (although I see a metaphoric relation). To undermine it, I think it is paramount to talk to people and not to herds (which is why I am also very careful with the language I use and any other forms of discourse that may reduce people to their political expression and shovel them into the herd, no matter how abhorrent their views might be to me. Viscerally tENT represents precisely my voice here, but I still cringe at the word "sheeple," no matter how much the worldview packed in this terms freaks me out. 🙂)

Like · Reply · 1d · Edited

Amir-ul Kafirs 003 understands, I think, that the movie is aimed at a propaganda phrase more than it is at mask use itself. No doubt there are times when mask use is helpful. I don't, however, think that the emphasis on wearing a mask as soon as one leaves the house is anything but overkill. That said, I don't live in NYC, where the population is 5 times as dense as it is here. I go for walks every day in local parks. Maybe 60% of the people don't wear masks, none of these seem particularly worried about their imminent death (myself included). Of the ones wearing masks, some seem truly terrified, & some glare at those of us without masks. My question is: Is the fear proportionate to the reality here? In Allegheny County, where Pittsburgh's located, there've been something like 183 deaths probably attributable to COVID-19 in an area with a population of roughly 1.5 million.

2

Like · Reply · 18h

003c Amir-ul Kafirs ditto! And, I should add, the reduction of the mask rhetoric to a couple of slogans thus infantilizing people as though they are a bunch of naughty toddlers that couldn't make a rational assessment of the situation, and take responsible action is particularly nasty.

2

Like · Reply · 18h · Edited

002c 003 What I would add here is that if you look at hard numbers, in the US the number of infections keeps rising, and in some place by alarming rates. In Florida, the number of infections has passed where NYC was a couple of months ago when it was the worst area in the country. conversely, today NYC has the lowest rate of infection in the country. aggressive measures were taken because it was critical and the only way to slow the rate down. This can't be ignored. The fact that mask wearing and physical distancing were a requirement in all places has to have had some effect on this. I'm not saying that we have to coddle or trick people into wearing masks where it is obvious that it would be useful (indoors), but the idea "that couldn't make a rational assessment of the situation, and take responsible action" can not be taken lightly here. I think a lot of people are NOT responsible enough and are NOT even willing to look at facts. I'm not advocating for any sort of forced behavior as in a fascist sort of environment, but this sort of thing endangers everyone. Yes, Pittsburgh's population is much less dense and there is some play in how one can get around and do things. NYC not so much. and the number of people who are simply out there defending their "rights" and "freedoms" are completely missing the point endangering themselves and everyone else. how would you deal with that?

1

Like · Reply · 11h

004a A review of scientific studies of masks relevant to Covid-19 concludes that they are useless. Of course any benefit of mask confer has to be weighed up with their negative affects as well. Sometimes masks can make situations worse.

Here in the Netherlands masks were never mandatory. Most people never wore them. As far as I am concerned Covid-19 is over here. Things are relatively normal here
https://www.rcreader.com/.../masks-dont-work-covid-a...

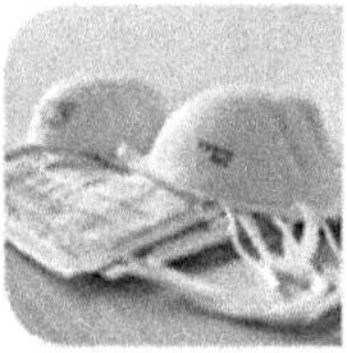

RCREADER.COM

Masks Don't Work: A Review of Science Relevant to COVID-19...

Love · Reply · 10h 2

004b 002 On the effectiveness of masks
Various countries have introduced or are currently discussing the introduction of mandatory masks in public transport, in shopping malls, or generally in public.

Due to the lower-than-expected lethality of Covid-19 and the available treatment options, this discussion might become obsolete. The original argument regarding a reduction of hospitalizations ("flatten the curve") is also no longer relevant, as the hospitalization rate was and is about twenty times lower than initially assumed.

Nevertheless, the question of the effectiveness of masks can be asked. In the case of influenza epidemics, the answer is already clear from a scientific point of view: masks in everyday life have no or very little effect. If used improperly, they can even increase the risk of infection.

Ironically, the best and most recent example of this is the often-mentioned Japan: Despite its ubiquitous masks, Japan experienced its most recent strong flu wave – with around five million people falling ill – just one year ago, in January and February 2019.

However, unlike SARS corona viruses, influenza viruses are transmitted also by children. Indeed, Japan had to close around ten thousand schools in 2019 due to acute outbreaks of the flu.

With the SARS 1 virus of 2002 and 2003, there is some evidence that medical masks can provide partial protection against infection. But SARS-1 spread almost exclusively in hospitals, i.e. in a professional environment, and hardly to the general public at large.

In contrast, a study from 2015 showed that the cloth masks in use today are permeable to 97% of viral particles due to their pore size and can further increase the risk of infection by storing moisture.

Some studies recently argued that everyday masks are nevertheless effective in the case of the new coronavirus and could at least prevent the infection of other people. However, these studies suffer from poor methodology and sometimes show the opposite of what they claim.

Typically, these studies ignore the effect of other simultaneous measures, the natural development of infection numbers, changes in test activity, or they compare countries with very different conditions.

An overview:

A German study claimed that the introduction of compulsory masks in German cities had led to a decrease in infections. But the data does not support this: in some cities there was no change, in others a decrease, in others an increase in infections (see graph below). The city of Jena, presented as a model, simultaneously introduced the strictest quarantine rules in Germany, but the study did not mention this.
A study in the journal PNAS claimed that masks had led to a decrease in infections in three hotspots (including New York City). This did not take into account the natural decrease in infections and other measures. The study was so flawed that over 40 scientists recommended that the study be withdrawn.
A US study claimed that compulsory masks had led to a decrease in infections in 15 states. The study did not take into account that the incidence of infection was already declining in most states at that time. A comparison with other states was not made.

A Canadian study claimed that countries with compulsory masks had fewer deaths than countries without compulsory masks. But the study compared African, Latin American, Asian and Eastern European countries with very different infection rates and population structures.
A meta-study in the journal Lancet claimed that masks "could" lead to a reduction in the risk of infection, but the studies considered mainly hospitals (Sars-1) and the strength of the evidence was reported as "low".
The medical benefit of compulsory masks therefore continues to remain questionable. In any case, a comparative study by the University of East Anglia came to the conclusion that compulsory masks had no measurable effect on the incidence of Covid infections or deaths.

It is also clear that widespread use of face masks couldn't stop the initial outbreak in Wuhan.

Sweden showed that even without a lockdown, without compulsory masks and with one of the lowest intensive care bed capacities in Europe, hospitals need not be overburdened. In fact, Sweden's annual all-cause mortality is in the range of previous flu seasons.

At any rate, authorities shouldn't suggest to the population that compulsory masks reduce the risk of infection, for example in public transport, as there is no evidence of this. Whether with or without masks, there is an increased risk of infection in densely packed indoor areas.

Interestingly, the demand for a worldwide obligation to wear masks is led by a lobby group called "masks4all" (masks for all), which was founded by a "young leader" of the Davos forum.

https://swprs.org/a-swiss-doctor-on-covid-19/

i

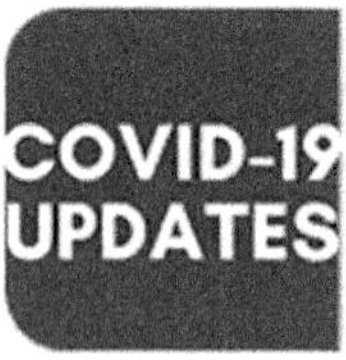

SWPRS.ORG

Facts about Covid-19

Love · Reply · 10h

2

002d 004
https://dutchreview.com/news/coronavirus-netherlands/

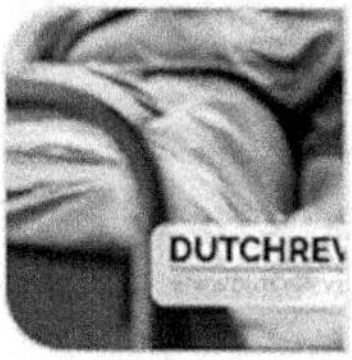

DUTCHREVIEW.COM
Coronavirus in the Netherlands: all you need to know (updated daily)...

Like · Reply · 10h 1

004c 002
https://www.statista.com/.../coronavirus-cases-in.../

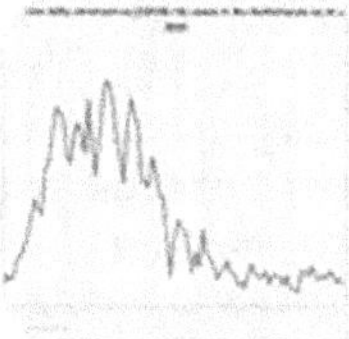

STATISTA.COM
Netherlands: coronavirus daily cases | Statista

Like · Reply · 10h 1

Amir-ul Kafirs Actually, there are many things happening in the movie that seem to go unnoticed. One is that the woman is wearing a mask to 'protect herself' against something that's highly unlikely to happen (exposure to a virus in an uncrowded area) while she stares fixedly at her cell-phone, her portable mediating device, & walks obliviously in front of a moving car, an actual threat. It's this being lost in what I call mediated non-reality to the point of losing touch with what is & isn't an actual threat that I perceive as the biggest threat. And this is something induced by sensationalizing fear-mongering mass media that, as usual, has advertising revenue & drama as its main motivating factor & NOT the public well-being.

Like · Reply · 10h 4

002e 004 we could go back and forth all day like this. I think I'll pass. We are missing the point of tENT's initial idea of herd mentality and mass hysteria and mobilization based on fear, myopic vision and manipulation.

Like · Reply · 10h 2

001c 003 Yes, but masks do save lives, so .... umm are you over thinking the point?

Reply · 7h

003d 001 I have been following very closely the science of the virus from the onset and I find the threat of coronavirus exagerrated beyond any logic. This virus is neither so lethal, nor so heavy as to warrant the draconian measures that ensued (that I see as a massive socio-economic re-engineering project ushering changes on many levels, i.e. financial, market, communications, etc., and that, to be effective, need to be more or less global, hence the unprecedented international synchronization we are witnessing). I also see two major trans-national socio-political forces using this as a convenient new type of war platform (which, on the plus side, is probably better than actual war). We know, from the very onset of the virus, which are the risk groups and, as with any other such problem, the people who are at risk must be secured. So, measures should have been ramped up in hospitals, old people health facilities and also for individual people at risk. Mask and gloves wearing is useful mostly in closed crowded spaces, and they were already mandatory in hospitals with immuno compromised people here (my mother in law is one and I've been using these measures for years). I am aware of the situation in NY and other States. The problem is not the amount of people carrying the virus, but the amount of hospitalizations. As long as the hospital system is not clogged and can take adequate care of the sick, the situation is under control. So, if it were up to me, I would focus on fortifying the hospital system and making sure that all people with underlying conditions are secure, have enough income to be able to stay home and minimize contact with the outside world. Otherwise, for healthy people not in a risk group, there is little more danger than a cold or a flu (even less so, since cold and flu are mostly symptomatic), and we've never seen such a bruhaha around those, locally or globally. In 2017, for instance, we had such a brutal flu season here with, what I suspect was a new strain of the flu, that almost everyone I know, including me, was knocked down for 20 days at least. The death rate, with vaccine available, was a bit lower than what we have now for covid without vaccine but not substantially so. We didn't hear a blip in the media, and, unlike covid, that flu, alhtough a little less deadly (mostly due to the vaccine that most people at risk take seasonally here), was much more brutal on the average person as it invariably presented with heavy symptoms, and not only in some cases. This is only to give you a perspective on how a similar situation is managed when there is no socio-political interest in it. Since the dawn of humanity, we have lived with disease and viruses. There is no rational explanation why suddenly one of those viruses becomes threat number one, as though we've never been sick or died of viruses, or anything, ever before. Also, countries have emergency budgets and all sorts of programs that prepare us for unusual scenarios. I don't buy for a minute that all this hysteria and shutdown was absolutely necessary because we were blindsided by the virus. The only thing we are blindsided of are the socio-economic and political conditioning (and restructuring) that is going on. That's where we should pose more questions.

So, the people who are afraid for their freedoms not only have enough apparent reasons to be suspicious, but also a human right to be given the option. The problem could be arguably reduced to a simple hypothetical question: Would you rather live as a healthy slave or die as a free person? Some would choose the former, some the latter, but all must have the freedom to choose between the two. More than that, our civilization's crown achievement (according to me) is the awareness and measures to guarantee that we do not have to ever make this choice, i.e. that life and freedom are never mutually exclusive. The Human rights charter

guarantees exactly that - not just life, but life with dignity. To create strife between people on these grounds is the biggest and most disgusting political manipulation I have witnessed. More than that, it is a political crime, in my books. I could talk till tomorrow on the subject but should stop here. May be pm. 🙂

That said, I do wear a mask in public transport (as recommended) not because I am afraid or think I am contageous (with all this social distancing, chances are minimal I have been exposed to anything at all) but because, as a rule of thumb, I don't want to feed people's fears, anxieties and discomfort. I think the best way, at least for me, to respond to the situation, is not to react and feed any form of fear in anyone, anywhere on the political or human spectrum - thus I can undermine the fearmongering, at least as far as my world is concerned, one step at a time.

Like · Reply · 7h · Edited 1

003e 001 May be I am "overthinking" (by your standards) but I am a thinker by trade and, from where I come, there is no danger in "overthinking" anything. Overthinking took us to the moon and unveiled the quanta, for instance. 🙂 However, the grave danger, and the one that would greatly serve any oppressive regime and/or interest, is that of underthinking. It is by underthinking that we get sucked into politics and agenda that are not our own. It is by underthinking that we cannot gain enough distance to afford not falling into manipulative traps.

Masks don't save lives, they limit (not even minimize) the spread of the virus. Doctors save lives (in the sense in which you mean "saving lives," that is). "Masks save lives" is merely another political slogan designed to minimize thinking and mobilize popular sentiment for certain socio-political purposes (not necessarily useless or malignant but deffinitely innacurate and condescending, i.e. underestimating and undermining the agency of the citizen).

Love · Reply · 6h · Edited 2

005a 004 I want to move to the Netherlands!! I CANNOT handle how crazy and dictatorial things have become here in the United States. I cannot stand the brainwashed, and I hate hand sanitizer. I medically cannot get vaccines because they could cause me grave health concerns. Do many people speak English in the Netherlands, are there jobs? I think I"m serious. But I'd have to smuggle 6 cats over. Do you know anyone with a private transatlantic boat. I think I"m joking, but really... this United States place super sucks right now. I'm with tENT on barely being able to stand it right now. And it keeps on GETTING WORSE each week. ='-[I'm trying not to allow myself to become a victim.

Like · Reply · 5h 2

003f 005 courage! At least you have 6 cats - focus on finessing trans-species communication until the crazy wave subsides. 🙂

Like · Reply · 5h 2

004d 005 yeah while things are not perfect here I do feel quite glad to be here rather than the US or Aust where there seems to be more hysteria. It doesn't mean it will stay that way of course and the Government is not really that good. The Dutch Government is arguing for austerity in EU blocking agreements on a bailout plan without the need for repayment.

I know I would go crazy too if I had to wear a mask at work. Probably quite a hazard too in a kitchen. We have sanitizer at the entrances of our restaurants but I never use them.

Almost every single person in Amsterdam (and much of the Netherlands in general) speaks English to the point of always speaking English back to you if your Dutch is not 100%. This makes it quite hard to learn Dutch. Not sure about English speaking jobs in libraries though. Cats are certainly welcome here, in shops and restaurants as well. I do know someone who is part of a collective with a sailing boat. They have a small coffee business where they sail to Costa Rica. If you can get to Costa Rica with your six cats, you can hitch a ride from there. https://www.facebook.com/anemoicoffee/?eid=ARDEOHKxHIlg_3AlfiiZ3kZqri4C6SLCKDGV8Kb65vCudCZATJIl1FcBUgw6pjZXyAEFSi-w2PMrmggM&timeline_context_item_type=intro_card_work&timeline_context_item_source=628515586&fref=tag

Anemoi Coffee by Sail

Like · Reply · 5h 1

Write a reply...

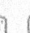

006a Being largely absent from you for many years, I might wonder if you are watching fox news? (Most of my neighbors would use this as scientific proof that masks are useless...ugh) But I also think this is a hilarious spoof of anti maskers who are acting like they dont know how they will eat, drive with a mask on. (How have doctors survived all these years?!)
The world is so ridiculous right now; what a perfect venue for you!
Loving you

Like · Reply · 1d

Amir-ul Kafirs I don't watch Fox 'News', which I find to be despicable. This isn't a parody of anti-maskers, it's a parody of fear-mongering & shaming through propaganda, amongst other things. Nice to read from you, 006

Like · Reply · 18h 1

Write a reply...

Amir-ul Kafirs One thing that I hope is obvious to all is that there are conflicting opinions on this subject & many studies that reach differing conclusions. It's up to the individual to do their own research & to decide what they find most believable in accordance with their own experience. I, personally, choose to NOT wear a mask. I might wear one under special circumstances — such as if I were caregiving a homebound older person. I've given careful consideration to this issue & don't appreciate being demonized by people that I'm sure haven't thought about it or researched it even 10% as much as I have. What typically happens to me if I express an opinion that goes against what I call the Monolithic Narrative is that I'm immediately branded a Trump Supporting Neo-Nazi Fox TV News Watcher — even though it's known or should be known to the demonizer that this isn't the truth. It's this very tendency to slander people who deviate from GROUPTHINK that shows how deeply the pressure is on to conform. I find this especially objectionable when I know that the people slandering me & others don't have the courage to actually resist this push to mentally oversimplify — even when it borders on, or downright IS, a movement toward Fascism. Furthermore, no-one has died as a result of my not wearing a mask & the pompous characterization of non-mask-wearing people as "murderers" is insupportable. I generally avoid commenting here or responding to other people's comments because the viciousness of people is not worthy of engagement with. I appreciate that there's at least an attempt in this thread to remain civil (aside from the 1st poster who I unfriended). Civility is amenable to actual dialog while slander is not.

Like · Reply · 10h 2

Amir-ul Kafirs At the risk of over-commenting here I want to add that the movie is meant to have a SENSE OF HUMOR — something that I find lacking whenever people feel backed into a corner. If people can laugh, regardless of whether they agree with it or not, then I've done my small bit to get people to 'lighten up' & to, therefore, be more flexible thinkers.

Like · Reply · 9h 2

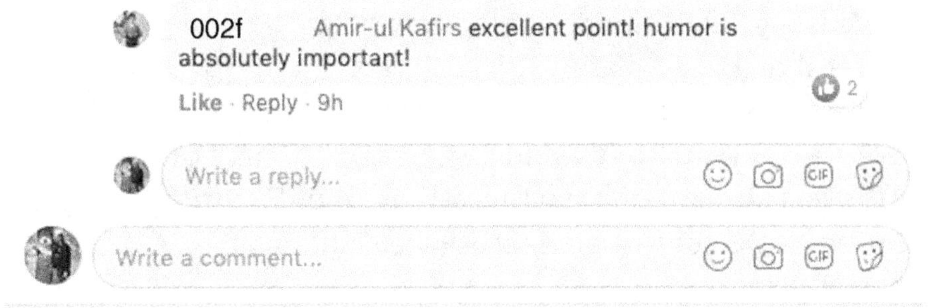

****

July 13, 2020, 1:09PM (Inquiring Librarian to group):

HERETICS: Twitter Charts, Cases/Deaths

A friend of mine in PA sent this to me. They are a heretic like us. But they are mormon and have a divided church and 6 kids to deal with on the topic. This chart is great! It shows our observations are correct.

WEEKLY INDICATORS OF COVID-19

Date	Total Tests	%Population	Total Cases	%Positive	CLI ER Visits	%Cases	Hospitalizations	%Visits	Deaths	%Admissions
3/14/2020	28,046		4,224		77,093		240		52	
3/21/2020	177,988		27,415		108,151		7,213		561	
3/28/2020	568,493		100,630		99,933		31,486		3,124	
4/4/2020	907,858		185,208		87,433		60,032		9,904	
4/11/2020	1,039,831		215,089		73,052		59,871		16,004	
4/18/2020	1,030,170		199,756		59,348		49,372		16,886	
4/25/2020	1,480,752		210,448		53,453		37,113		15,199	
5/2/2020	1,622,025		193,654		49,093		34,402		12,949	
5/9/2020	1,875,377		175,700		42,996		27,427		10,933	
5/16/2020	2,360,566		159,712		39,429		21,888		8,917	
5/23/2020	2,795,272		155,993		36,505		20,719		6,915	
5/30/2020	2,765,911		144,802		32,789		16,983		5,817	
6/6/2020	3,173,488		149,645		30,142		15,715		4,577	
6/13/2020	3,270,783		144,663		32,246		14,255		3,577	
6/20/2020	3,518,931		177,758		40,802		13,408		2,532	
6/27/2020	3,826,655		253,282		55,418		14,729		1,024	
7/4/2020	4,512,632		339,308		60,590		16,732		302	

Here is my July 4 update of indicators.
1) Total tests
2) Total cases, pct positive as portion of tests
3) Total ER visits for Covid-like illness, % of new cases
4) Total estimate of hospitalizations, % of ER visits
5) Total CDC confirmed deaths (they lag), % of hospitalizations

WEEKLY INDICATORS OF COVID-19

Date	Total Tests	%Population	Total Cases	%Positive	CLI ER Visits	%Cases	Hospitalizations	%Visits	Deaths	%Admissions
3/14/2020	28,046		4,224		77,093		240		52	
3/21/2020	177,988		27,415		108,151		2,212		561	
3/28/2020	568,493		100,630		99,933		31,486		3,124	
4/4/2020	907,858		185,208		87,433		60,032		9,904	
4/11/2020	1,039,831		215,089		73,052		59,871		16,004	
4/18/2020	1,030,170		199,756		59,348		49,372		16,896	
4/25/2020	1,480,752		210,448		53,453		37,113		15,199	
5/2/2020	1,622,075		193,654		49,093		34,402		12,949	
5/9/2020	1,875,377		175,700		42,996		27,427		10,933	
5/16/2020	2,360,166		159,712		39,429		21,888		8,917	
5/23/2020	2,796,272		155,893		36,505		20,719		6,915	
5/30/2020	2,765,911		144,802		32,789		16,983		5,817	
6/6/2020	3,173,488		149,645		30,142		15,715		4,577	
6/13/2020	3,270,783		144,663		32,246		14,255		3,577	
6/20/2020	3,518,931		177,758		40,802		13,408		2,532	
6/27/2020	3,826,655		253,282		55,418		14,729		1,024	
7/4/2020	4,512,632		339,308		60,500		16,732		302	

2:59 PM · Jul 11, 2020 · Twitter Web App

****

July 13, 2020, 7:24PM (Amir-ul Kafirs to group):

Re: HERETICS: Twitter Charts, Cases/Deaths

That's really, REALLY wonderful. The deaths have been going steadily down since April. It's taken a dramatic increase in the number of tests to even bring the cases up a little. THANK YOU!

****

July 13, 2020, 12:51PM (Inquiring Librarian to group):

Ok, I LOVED the movie. I can't go into deeper commentary. I'm letting time get out of my control.... But I loved it. I also loved the conversation it stirred on social media. I appreciate Phil posting about the Netherlands and masks and the whole virus thing being dropped there.

I hope that this ends here soon too. I HATE this. My stupid governor just dumped us down a phase again. It totally sucks and makes no sense. I am surrounded daily by sheeple. It is difficult to handle...

Be well all and thanks for helping my sanity.

****

YIKES! I thought it was a nasal swab!

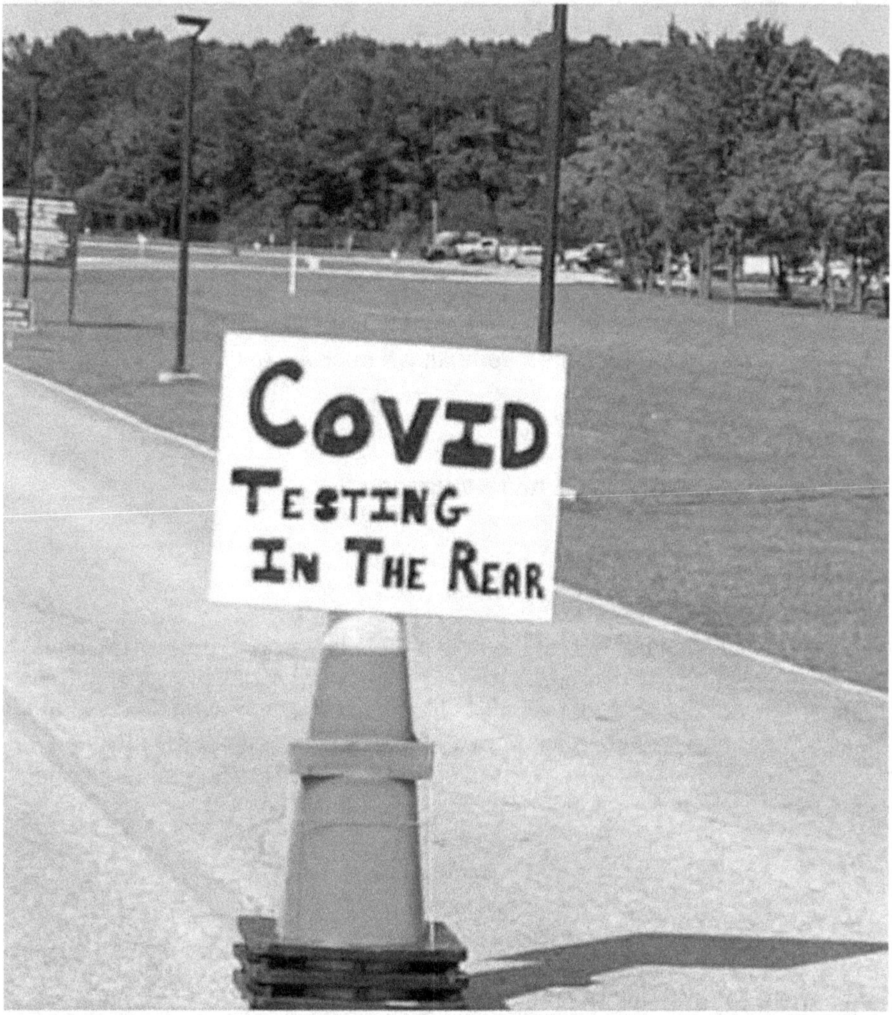

****

July 13, 2020, 3:09PM (BP to group):

Ah, thanks for sharing. I enjoyed the flick and instantly loved the girl being hit while brainlessly mind-locked to her phone. I've driven that point home to my kids a million times and as I taught my son how to drive. Sorry I haven't been participating but I'm just burnt out!

****

July 14, 2020, 2:47PM (Amir-ul Kafirs to group):

My stupid governor just dumped us down a phase again. It totally sucks and makes no sense.

But if one governor does it & the others don't then they might go on historic record as not caring about the great deaths all around them — even if those great deaths don't actually exist. They're protecting their own political asses — not their constituency.

I am surrounded daily by sheeple. It is difficult to handle...

I've become an enemy of eupemisms more than ever now. It seems to me that the SHEEPLE can accept any crime against humanity as long as it's properly mislabeled as 'good for the collective health' & suchlike garbage.

****

July 14, 2020, 2:57PM (Amir-ul Kafirs to group):

Ah, thanks for sharing. I enjoyed the flick and instantly loved the girl being hit while brainlessly mind-locked to her phone.

The "girl" is Naia Nisnam, one of the only people left around here who'll have anything to do with me anymore! I have to give them credit for choosing to be "brainlessly mind-locked to her phone". I think that really makes that scene — especially after she's 'come back from the dead' because I put my mask on & reversed time. I love how when that happens she's still looking at her phone fixedly despite what she's gone through.

I've driven that point home to my kids a million times and as I taught my son how to drive.

I have actually seen people step out in front of moving traffic looking at their phones while completely oblivious to the danger they're in. I'll bet it happens fairly often. They're really in trouble if the driver's doing the same thing.

****

July 13, 2020, 4:08PM (BP to group):

HERETICS: East Coast Edition

Welp, I'll try to say something here but I fear it's just gonna be me griping but so be it.

A week or so ago the Community College that my son attends announced the Fall semester will be on-line only. My heart sank for a number of reasons. If it wasn't so affordable (in the scheme of things) I'd be going on the attack for a discount, but I know that it is a lost cause. The press release included something about a Tuition Price Freeze to send the message. Not that it made any sense. It didn't. But I got the message. "We are doing you a favor!"

Anytime now I will learn of my daughters fate. A high school student. UGH! It ain't looking good. I'm upset that my son will continue to be isolated, won't meet any girls, make new friends, etc. Let alone a future!

Eh, that's all I can manage. I remain paranoid that the powers that be are going to ruin my holiday with the kids in 3 weeks time. Plus having another weird fight this past Saturday with a friend of mine. He became incensed that I think kids should go back to school. He started railing that Trump is an idiot and that all the Red States that opened "prematurely" are getting their due. That we did the right thing here, shutting down. Of course everyone is dead but that didn't seem to factor into the equation. That the virus is going to run its course. Basically: Trump killed everybody.

****

July 13, 2020, 4:31PM (Inquiring Librarian to group):

Re: HERETICS: East Coast Edition

Ugh... That is terrible! One of my best friends from high school is a Mormon and has 6 kids. She thinks this is all nonsense as we do. But not all of her kids feel that way. Her 17 year old recently told her that she is endangering the health of her family and her friends by laughing at the idiocy of the mass media. Meanwhile her church is completely divided (unusual for the Mormon community) and she has to deal with parents fighting over reopening schools and one parent who is quoting bogus numbers about the masses of children that will die if kids return to school. Terrible.

Meanwhile, over in Africa...
https://www.mintpressnews.com/africa-trust-stamp-covid-19-vaccine-record-payment-system/269346/

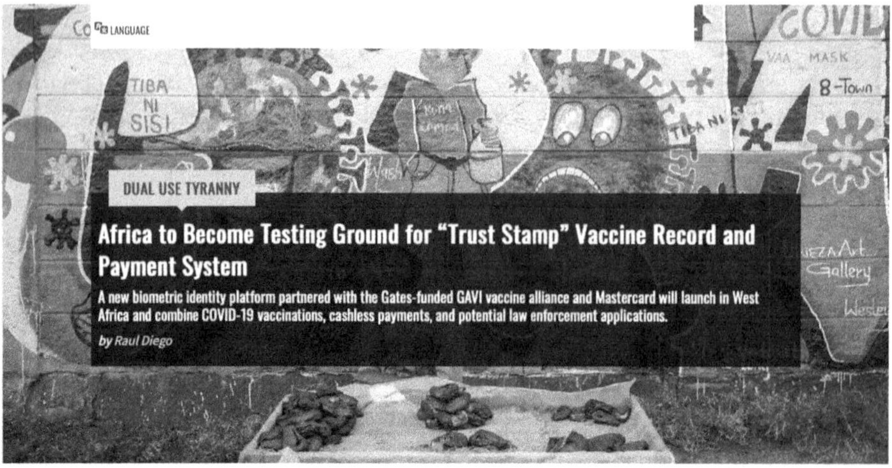

DUAL USE TYRANNY

Africa to Become Testing Ground for “Trust Stamp” Vaccine Record and Payment System

A new biometric identity platform partnered with the Gates-funded GAVI vaccine alliance and Mastercard will launch in West Africa and combine COVID-19 vaccinations, cashless payments, and potential law enforcement applications.

by Raul Diego

July 10th, 2020

A biometric digital identity platform that “evolves just as you evolve” is set to be introduced in “low-income, remote communities” in West Africa thanks to a public-private partnership between the Bill Gates-backed GAVI vaccine alliance, Mastercard and the AI-powered “identity authentication” company, Trust Stamp.

The program, which was first launched in late 2018, will see Trust Stamp’s digital identity platform integrated into the GAVI-Mastercard “Wellness Pass,” a digital vaccination record and identity system that is also linked to Mastercard’s click-to-play system that powered by its AI and machine learning technology called NuData. Mastercard, in addition to professing its commitment to promoting “centralized record keeping of childhood immunization” also describes itself as a leader toward a “World Beyond Cash,” and its partnership with GAVI marks a novel approach towards linking a biometric digital identity system, vaccination records, and a payment system into a single cohesive platform. The effort, since its launch nearly two years ago, has been funded via $3.8 million in GAVI donor funds in addition to a matched donation of the same amount by the Bill and Melinda Gates Foundation.

In early June, GAVI reported that Mastercard's Wellness Pass program would be adapted in response to the coronavirus (COVID-19) pandemic. Around a month later, Mastercard announced that Trust Stamp's biometric identity platform would be integrated into Wellness Pass as Trust Stamp's system is capable of providing biometric identity in areas of the world lacking internet access or cellular connectivity and also does not require knowledge of an individual's legal name or identity to function. The Wellness Program involving GAVI, Mastercard, and Trust Stamp will soon be launched in West Africa and will be coupled with a Covid-19 vaccination program once a vaccine becomes available.

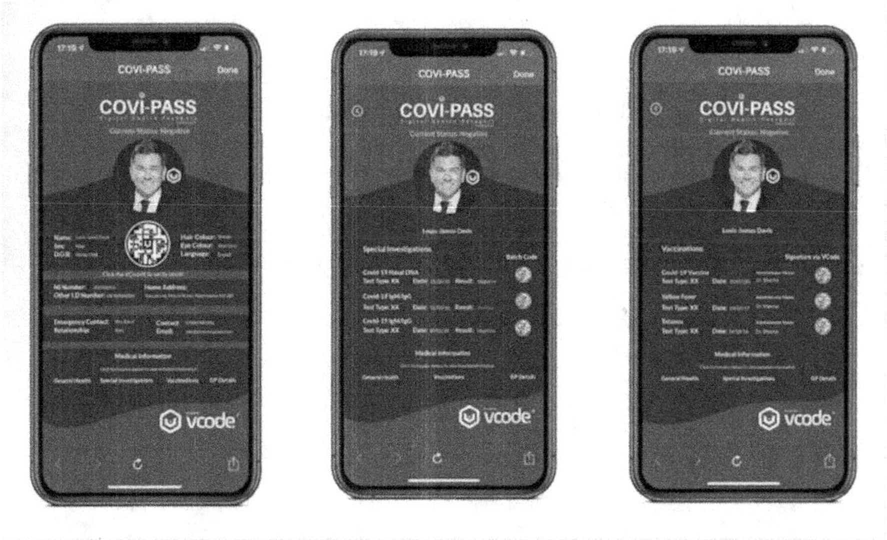

Mass-Tracking COVI-PASS Immunity Passports Slated to Roll Out in 15 Countries COVI-PASS will determine whether you can go to a restaurant, if you need a medical test, or are due for a talking-to by authorities in a post-COVID world. Consent is voluntary, but enforcement will be compulsory., Bill Gates, COVI-PASS, COVID-19, digital health passport, Privacy, Surveillance, tracking,

The push to implement biometrics as part of national ID registration systems has been ongoing for many years on the continent and has become a highly politicized issue in several African countries. Opposition to similar projects in Africa often revolves around the costs surrounding them, such as the biometric voter management system that the Electoral Commission of Ghana has been trying to implement ahead of their 2020 general election in December. Bright Simons, honorary VP of the IMANI policy think tank, has questioned the "budgetary allocation" for the new system, claiming that the "unnecessary registration of 17 million people all over again" represents millions of dollars "being blown for reasons that nobody can explain in this country."

[..]

Raul Diego is a MintPress News Staff Writer, independent photojournalist, researcher, writer and documentary filmmaker.

- https://www.mintpressnews.com/africa-trust-stamp-covid-19-vaccine-record-payment-system/269346/

****

July 13, 2020, 5:16PM (Dick to group):

If I was a religious man I'd say it seems like the devils of hell have been released and are roaming on the earth.

****

July 13, 2020, 5:47PM (Inquiring Librarian to group):

Well, that's what Qanon seems to say and honestly, these days, Qanon makes more sense than the government narratives! And at least Qanon is about not being a victim, but about victory over evil! Jebus PLEASE SAVE US!! =O I mean, how can ANYONE be OK with this INSANITY??

****

July 14, 2020, 3:09PM (Amir-ul Kafirs to group):

Re: HERETICS: New Jersey Edition

I'm upset that my son will continue to be isolated, won't meet any girls, make new friends, etc. Let alone a future!

That's an important feature of this whole mess that seems under-referred to: Viz, that there's a whole generation of people who're being deprived of normal developmental processes. In other words, it's obviously extremely important for your son's & daughter's social development *for them to have a physical social life* & that's being taken away from them. That in itself is prime material for a theory about powers-that-be trying to create a new type of human being whose social life is completely virtual.

Basically: Trump killed everybody.

Yeah, Rump killed everybody that isn't dead. In fact, Rump actually CREATED DEATH: *what a fiend!* As we all know, or will shortly be re-educated to believe, death didn't exist until this year & now everyone's dying before our very eyes *even though it doesn't look like it.* Believe that & they'll tell you another one.

****

July 14, 2020, 3:41PM (Naia Nisnam to group):

The school thing....
I got a message this morning from our public school district. They want parents to enroll their kids for complete online schooling. There is no way I'm signing up for that. My kid is 13 and became depressed when school was cancelled last year. She needs to socialize. Parents of some of her friends refuse to let their kids socialize at all, even outside at a park, bc of the "rise in cases". Tomorrow I have a Zoom meeting to explain what their plan is for the kids whose parents refuse online schooling.

My son goes to the neo-liberal private school that I work at. They are at least planning on as much outside class time as possible but still with the distancing and masks. I've been avoiding thinking about it and skipped the Zoom meeting about the schools plans bc I knew I'd be angry. I'm dreading a miserable return to work at the end of August.

I want to see more articles and studies about the effects of isolation on children. Most of what I see about kids in quarantine is just parents complaining about how annoying it is to be around their own offspring.

****

July 14, 2020, 4:26PM (Dick to group):

That's all awful news, sorry to hear it

Here, by the way, the so-called "end of emergency measures" was a farce... the President announced today that on 1 August masks will be obligatory in all interior spaces in France

I think this is the point, if this was a movie, where a young band of dedicated fighters is supposed to show up on the scene, reveal the dastardly international plot and in foiling it, usher in a new era of freedom... I hope it happens soon...

****

July 14, 2020, 4:50PM (Inquiring Librarian to group):

My friend in PA, _____, just sent me this video this afternoon. It is really clear and simple, and from an MD. She ends by explaining how children really do not get sick from covid 19 and are not carriers, and she talks about the powers of the human immune system. Mostly, it's clear, direct, and very simple. If you can share this with your school administrators and fellow parents, maybe they'd believe it?? My friend _____ has 6 kids from ages 5 to 20. She's in your boat and this is killing her. She is on the hunt for any and every fact she can find on children needing to be in school vs. the virus.

https://www.facebook.com/UniversalTarotZone/videos/193059832125552/

To be honest, it seems to me they are waiting to shoot us all up with this vaccine before they let us like dogs out of our cages. And YES!! Dick!!! I feel like we are at that part of the movie too!!! Does anyone have any thoughts on this here? Is it good, is it bad, is it just more smoke and mirrors?? https://www.seattletimes.com/nation-world/nation-politics/administration-orders-hospitals-to-bypass-the-cdc-with-key-virus-data/ (click on link for whole article. I just copied and pasted the headliner and 1st paragraph). What I think is hilarious about this headliner/first paragraph is that 'health experts' "fear the data will be distorted for political gain". HA HA HA HA HA.... Is that NOT happening already? I mean, PLEASE spare me the anxious tears and just sit and eat my hat instead?? !!

****

Nation & World Politics

Administration Orders Hospitals to Bypass the CDC With Key Virus Data

July 14, 2020 at 1:10 pm *Updated July 14, 2020 at 1:25 pm*

By New York Times staff
The New York Times

The Trump administration has ordered hospitals to bypass the Centers for Disease Control and Prevention and, beginning Wednesday, send all coronavirus patient information to a central database in Washington — a move that has alarmed public health experts who fear the data will be distorted for political gain.

The new instructions are contained in a little-noticed document posted this week on the Department of Health and Human Services' website. From now on, HHS, and not the CDC, will collect daily reports about the patients that each hospital is treating, how many beds and ventilators are available, and other information vital to tracking the pandemic.

Officials say the change will streamline data gathering and assist the White House coronavirus task force in allocating scarce supplies like personal protective gear and the drug remdesivir. Some hospital officials welcome the move, saying it will relieve them of responding to requests from multiple federal agencies, though others said the CDC should be collecting the data.

"The CDC is the right agency to be at the forefront of collecting the data," said Dr.

Bala Hota, chief analytics officer at Rush University Medical Center in Chicago.

Public health experts have long expressed concerns that the administration is politicizing science and undermining the disease control centers; four former CDC directors, spanning both Republican and Democratic administrations, said as much in an opinion piece published Tuesday in The Washington Post. The data collection shift reinforced those fears.

“Centralizing control of all data under the umbrella of an inherently political apparatus is dangerous and breeds distrust,” said Nicole Lurie, who served as assistant secretary for preparedness and response under former President Barack Obama. “It appears to cut off the ability of agencies like CDC to do its basic job.”

The shift grew out of a tense conference call several weeks ago between hospital executives and Dr. Deborah L. Birx, the White House coronavirus response coordinator.

After Birx complained that hospitals were not adequately reporting their data, she convened a working group of government and hospital officials who devised the new plan, according to Janis Orlowski, chief health care officer of the Association of American Medical Colleges, who participated.

But news of the change came as a shock inside the CDC, which has long been responsible for gathering public health data, according to two officials who spoke on condition of anonymity because they were not authorized to discuss it. A spokesman for the disease control centers referred questions to the Department of Health and Human Services, which has not responded to a request for comment.

The dispute exposes the vast gaps in the government’s ability to collect and manage health data — an antiquated system at best, experts say.

This story was originally published at nytimes.com. Read it here.

- https://www.seattletimes.com/nation-world/nation-politics/administration-orders-hospitals-to-bypass-the-cdc-with-key-virus-data/

****

July 14, 2020, 5:42PM (Amir-ul Kafirs to group):

Ugh... That is terrible!

Ugh is right. One paragraph to call attention to in the article you've linked to is this:

"Trust Stamp’s interest in providing its technology to both COVID-19 response and to law enforcement is part of a growing trend where numerous companies providing digital solutions to COVID-19 also offer the same solutions to prison systems and law enforcement for the purposes of surveillance and "predictive policing.""

Rolled into the same package as 'health care' is predictive policing. People thinking they're being 'taken care of' are going to be *taken care of*, alright — but it's not going to be what they expect. Maybe they're leading a calm legal life working a job that pays the bills & then maybe that job's not going to exist anymore & they'll have 2 options: become a criminal *FOR the state* or a criminal *AGAINST the state*. Well, thanks to the 'health care' they've received the deicision will've been made much easier for them because if they try to defy the oppression they'll be much easier to track & control.

****

July 14, 2020, 5:46PM (Amir-ul Kafirs to group):

If I was a religious man I'd say it seems like the devils of hell have been released and are roaming on the earth.

I'm somewhat of a 'fan' of religious apocalypse movies. The Catholic Church is particularly good at making horror movies featuring exorcist priests as the heros. They should be ON this! Evil billionaire minions of the devil unleashing hell on Earth! The possibilities are endless!

****

July 14, 2020, 5:48PM (Amir-ul Kafirs to group):

how can ANYONE be OK with this INSANITY??

People are lovin' it! May it NEVER end! I guess it grows on them.. like a cancer.

****

July 14, 2020, 5:56PM (Amir-ul Kafirs to group):

On Jul 13, 2020, at 6:49 PM, dick turner wrote:

a lot of "Trump working behind the scenes" type stuff...

It would be fantastic if there were some sort of completely transparent disclosure of finances system that all politicians would be subject to.

****

July 14, 2020, 7:17PM (Amir-ul Kafirs to group):

They want parents to enroll their kids for complete online schooling.

It's hard for me to get around the hypothesis that this is a deliberate attempt to *desocialize children*. It's interesting that Betsy DeVos, Rump's appointee as Secretary of Education, is a big proponent of home schooling, something used by the ChristInsane to bypass the separation of church & state in public education. SO, the following is an article that I really don't get. It's a critique of DeVos's support for online schooling published on December 1, 2016, when the Rump administration was being transitioned in. The thing that makes it so hard to get is that it's published by "the74million.org" which lists DeVos & husband as its FUNDERS. Anyway, read it & see if you can make any sense of this. Maybe I just read through it too quickly.

Betsy Devos, Trump's EdSec Pick, Promoted Virtual Schools Despite Dismal Results

Secretary of education nominee Betsy DeVos has a long history of backing virtual schools, including founding and funding groups that have supported the expansion of online education. Additionally, as of 2006, her husband, Dick DeVos, was an investor in K12, a large network of more than 70 online schools.

Although advocates for virtual education say it is a lifeline for students who struggle in traditional settings, multiple research studies show that onlinecharter schools and other virtual education models post dismal academic results, as measured by improvement on standardized tests.

DeVos, as chairman of the American Federation for Children — she stepped down last week — repeatedly called for expanding virtual schools. In a 2015 statement released through the group about a federal spending bill, DeVos said, "Families want and deserve access to all educational options, including charter schools, private schools and virtual schools. … [V]irtual schools are growing across the country. Greater innovation and choice will contribute to better K-12 educational outcomes for our children." In 2012, DeVos supported a plan by Virginia Governor Bob McDonnell that including an expansion of online schools.

The American Federation for Children has praised such schools as allowing for "more flexibility and options in education" and includes "virtual learning" as part of its mission statement.

Matt Frendewey, a spokesperson for the group, said that it primarily focuses on private-school-choice programs — such as vouchers or tax credits — but that it also advocates for the expansion of additional options, including online schools. "We've long supported all forms of choice," he said. "We believe parents should be able to exercise the greatest number of choices, including public schools, public charter schools, virtual schools, online courses, blended learning, homeschooling and private schools."

In 2013, the American Federation for Children put out a sharply critical statement after New Jersey's school chief, Chris Cerf, declined to authorize two virtual charter schools. The group said the decision "depriv[es] students of vital educational options."

Another group DeVos founded and funded, the Michigan-based Great Lakes Education Project, has also advocated for expansion of online schools. (DeVos sat on the group's board until last week.) In a 2015 presentation to the the Michigan Board of Education, the group's executive director, Gary Naeyaert, argued for "full school choice" including virtual schools.

In an interview, Naeyaert said that his group doesn't privilege online schools over other options and supports accountability for any low-performing school. "Our position [on virtual schools] is the same with any [school]: Are the kids learning? Is the money being handled responsibly? We don't make a big distinction with whether the environment is brick-and-mortar." Naeyaert pointed out that many virtual education programs in Michigan are run by school districts rather than charter networks.

DeVos highlighted virtual schools as an important part of the "educational choice movement" in a 2013 interview with Philanthropy Roundtable. In a 2015 speech, DeVos praised "virtual schools [and] online learning" as part of an "open system of choices."

"We must open up the education industry — and let's not kid ourselves that it isn't an industry," she said in the speech. "We must open it up to entrepreneurs and innovators. ... This is how a student who's not learning in their current model can find an individualized learning environment that will meet their needs."

In 2006, as reported by Politico, Betsy DeVos's husband Dick noted in a financial disclosure statement while he was running for governor of Michigan that he held an investment interest in K12 Inc., a large, for-profit chain of online schools. It is unclear if the DeVoses are still investors. A spokesperson for K12 said, "As a public company we don't disclose who our investors are, and frankly, depending on how specific investors hold shares, we may not be aware of every individual shareholder of K12."

[..]

Richmond, whose group co-issued the the paper, said he is not worried about DeVos's position on the issue: "I'm not concerned that Betsy DeVos supports virtual schools, because we support them too — we just want them to be a lot better."

The Dick & Betsy DeVos Family Foundation provides funding to The 74, and the site's

Editor-in-Chief, Campbell Brown, sits on the American Federation for Children's board of directors, which was formerly chaired by Betsy DeVos. Brown played no part in the reporting or editing of this article. The American Federation for Children also sponsored The 74's 2015 New Hampshire education summit.

- https://www.the74million.org/article/betsy-devos-trumps-edsec-pick-promoted-virtual-schools-despite-dismal-results/

Parents of some of her friends refuse to let their kids to socialize at all,

Talk about BAD PARENTING! Imagine being a child & being not allowed to socialize, being forced to sit at a computer screen most of the day for 'education' & being deprived of human cues. Imagine being forced to wear a mask & to be around other people wearing masks. I mean the old adage of "Children should be seen and not heard" has reached a new level of viciousness against natural ebullience.

Most of what I see about kids in quarantine is just parents complaining about how annoying it is to be around their own offspring.

It can't possibly be good for them. It's already been claimed that there's a correlation between the preponderence of computer use & the rise of Asperger's Syndrome. This is going to create a whole new class of automatons, getting their primary social contact via computers AND their primary rewards from the same. It's easy to imagine being sociable, in the old physical sense, *becoming criminalized*. In fact, we're already there.

[Editor's interpolation: These seems like another instance of how Rump's agendas are being reinforced & actualized by agendas of liberals who think they're resisting/thwarting Rump. Rump's emphasis on immigrant control is well-served by the QUARANTYRANNY, Rump's dropping out of WHO but just turning around & funding GAVI is essentially thwarting any resistance to vaccines, &, *now*, Rump's appointment of Betsy DeVos as Secretary of Education is something that enables a bypassing of the sepraration of church & state through home online schooling & THAT gets made almost universal by QUARANTYRANNY.]

****

July 14, 2020, 7:22PM (Amir-ul Kafirs to group):

Here, by the way, the so-called "end of emergency measures" was a farce...

As it was here.

if this was a movie, where a young band of dedicated fighters is supposed to show up on the scene, reveal the dastardly international plot and in foiling it, usher in a new era of freedom... I hope it happens soon...

Sad to say, I'm not so sure we can rely on the young for this one. They'll participate in BLM protests but they'll do it with masks on & social distancing in groups of 25 six feet from each other. It's possible that the over-40 folks, such as all of us here, are going to have to stumble along out of sheer desperation to expose & foil. Given how tired I, personally, feel, it's hard for me to put much faith in that *either*. Then again, the 'enemy' is going to have similar problems. In other words, it's hard to be diaobolical & Machiavellian 24/7.

****

July 14, 2020, 8:09PM (Amir-ul Kafirs to group):

Re: HERETICS: New Jersey Edition

https://www.facebook.com/UniversalTarotZone/videos/193059832125552/

I watched this whole thing & found it to be completely commonsensical. I added it to my PANDEMIC PANIC playlist. I suggest, though, checking it out here:

https://youtu.be/WQB_nksm5Gc

on YouTube instead of on Facebook where the quality has been somewhat degraded & where it seems to be being used by the poster a little bit too propagandistically for my satisfaction. She has another video on YouTube here that's even more current:

https://youtu.be/A2rbIDYczvY

This one's interesting because she says that people get tested positive & then return to get tested waiting to be found ultimately negative so they can go back to work etc. She says thet *every time they test positive they're added to the statistics as a new case* — even though it's the same person again! That hadn't occurred to me but I tend to believe her. I'm still in the midst of watching this one but I've added it to my PANDEMIC PANIC playlist too.

Does anyone have any thoughts on this here? Is it good, is it bad, is it just more smoke and mirrors?? https://www.seattletimes.com/nation-world/nation-politics/administration-orders-hospitals-to-bypass-the-cdc-with-key-virus-data/

The following quote from the article seems like a no-brainer:

"“Centralizing control of all data under the umbrella of an inherently political apparatus is dangerous and breeds distrust,” said Nicole Lurie, who served as assistant secretary for preparedness and response under former President Barack Obama. “It appears to cut off the ability of agencies like CDC to do its basic job.”"

Then again isn't the CDC, at least partially connected to the government, already politicized? Apparently it's not enough under Rump's control for his purposes.

****

July 13, 2020, 7:56PM (Inquiring Librarian to group):

I'm not sure exactly who Kyle Lamb is. Here is his Twitter Page: https://twitter.com/kylamb8?ref_src=twsrc%5Egoogle%7Ctwcamp%5Eserp%7Ctwgr%5Eauthor
It is full of amazing covid info, presenting statistics and graphs and well documented sources for his information.

I do not have twitter. But hope to get it just to follow this guy.

My friend, _____, supposedly a descendent of Doc Holiday, introduced me to Kyle Lamb's Twitter page.

****

July 13, 2020, 8:32PM (Inquiring Librarian to group):

Ok, here we go... The latest news on the Moderna mRNA vaccine is out. They are moving ahead with injecting 30,000 patients with this, those considered most vulnerable with kidney issues, the elderly, black and native american ppl, etc. You can read this in the article. & they haven't yet published the results of the phase 1 trial and they don't have a reading yet on how phase 2 went. They will follow these victims for 2 years to see how it goes but hope to inject the masses with it by spring 2021. Terrible.
https://www.uchealth.org/today/moderna-coronavirus-vaccine-trial-colorado-uchealth-university-of-colorado-hospital/

****

Moderna coronavirus vaccine trial set to launch at UCHealth University of Colorado Hospital

The phase 3 trial of Moderna's mRNA vaccine candidate for COVID-19 will enroll 1,000 at University of Colorado Hospital, 30,000 nationwide.

By: **Todd Neff, for UCHealth** July 9th, 2020

UCHealth University of Colorado Hospital will soon enroll patients in the first large-scale U.S. clinical trial of a coronavirus vaccine.

The **phase 3 study** of Moderna's experimental vaccine will include 1,000 people at University of Colorado Hospital on the **Anschutz Medical Campus**. In addition, another 30,000 patients nationwide will participate in the trial, which is slated to start this summer, says **Dr. Thomas Campbell**, a **University of Colorado School of Medicine** and UCHealth virologist and infectious-disease specialist.

"The emphasis is on demonstrating the efficacy of the vaccine in people who are at most risk of getting COVID-19," Campbell said.

The phases of Moderna coronavirus vaccine trials

The trial will involve an initial injection and a booster 28 days later. It's not a challenge trial: that is, patients will not be exposed intentionally to the virus that causes COVID-19. The huge number of participants, though, will allow the study's leaders to compare the number and severity of coronavirus infections among those who got the vaccine with those who did not. Campbell says his team intends to move quickly and have all 1,000 patients injected with a first dose within eight weeks – and many would have received the booster by then also.

The study will follow patients for two years. That doesn't mean a commercial vaccine must wait until 2022. In a best-case scenario, compelling preliminary results could bring speedy approval from the U.S. Food and Drug Administration (FDA). Were that to happen, widespread vaccination of the general public could roll out by next spring, Campbell says.

The FDA requires three phases of human clinical trials before it approves a drug (that's in addition to having shown that the drug works in petri dishes, mice, and other animals). Phase 1 involves tens of people to make sure the drug is safe. Phase 2 generally involves hundreds of people and focuses on safety as well as what doses seem to work best. Phase 3 typically involves thousands of people and is used to prove safety and effectiveness.

Clinical trials normally proceed in sequential order over several years. These are not normal times. The phase 3 trial is launching with Moderna's **phase 1 trial** data soon to be published and the **phase 2 trial** having just launched in late May. But the initial findings have been promising enough – and the desperation for a means of attaining COVID-19 herd immunity without swamping hospitals great enough – that the pace of science is being pushed to its very limits.

[..]

- https://www.uchealth.org/today/moderna-coronavirus-vaccine-trial-colorado-uchealth-university-of-colorado-hospital/

****

July 15, 2020, 10:25AM (Amir-ul Kafirs to group):

The latest news on the Moderna mRNA vaccine is out.

Thanks for that link. I just read that one. Even though the article is from July 9, 2020, the author is still pushing the Overcrowded Hospitals narrative that's been proven to be false over & over again. Even the 2 nurses that've come out in NYC to protest the murder of patients have said that they're NOT understaffed OR overcrowded.

"Clinical trials normally proceed in sequential order over several years. These are not normal times. The phase 3 trial is launching with Moderna's **phase 1 trial** data soon to be published and the **phase 2 trial** having just launched in late May. But the initial findings have been promising enough – and the desperation for a means of attaining COVID-19 herd immunity without swamping hospitals great enough – that the pace of science is being pushed to its very limits."

Attaining "herd immunity"? Note that "herd immunity" is now pushed as something that's accomplished WITH VACCINES. Doesn't that sortof go against the idea of its happening naturally? & why is it so hard to accept that it may've already happened? It seems to me that if we're going to continue animal terminology we might as well say 'attaining COVID-19 cash cow'.

Here's a sentence that I found interesting:

"If actual coronaviruses later appear, those antibodies glom onto the viruses' spike proteins, and the immune system, forewarned, takes those viruses out."

Note that the author uses the word "glom". In an online dictionary (see bottom) it doesn't give any origin. A search for its etymology yields this: "early 20th century: variant of Scots *glaum*, of unknown origin." The way I remember it is that I 1st happened upon it in Robert Heinlein's novel "Stranger in a Strange Land" — at the time I thought that it was a Heinlein neologism, like "waldo". I still wonder whether it is.

transitive verb
1
: TAKE, STEAL
2
: SEIZE, CATCH
glom on to
: to grab hold of : appropriate to oneself

glommed on to her ideas

- https://www.merriam-webster.com/dictionary/glom

****

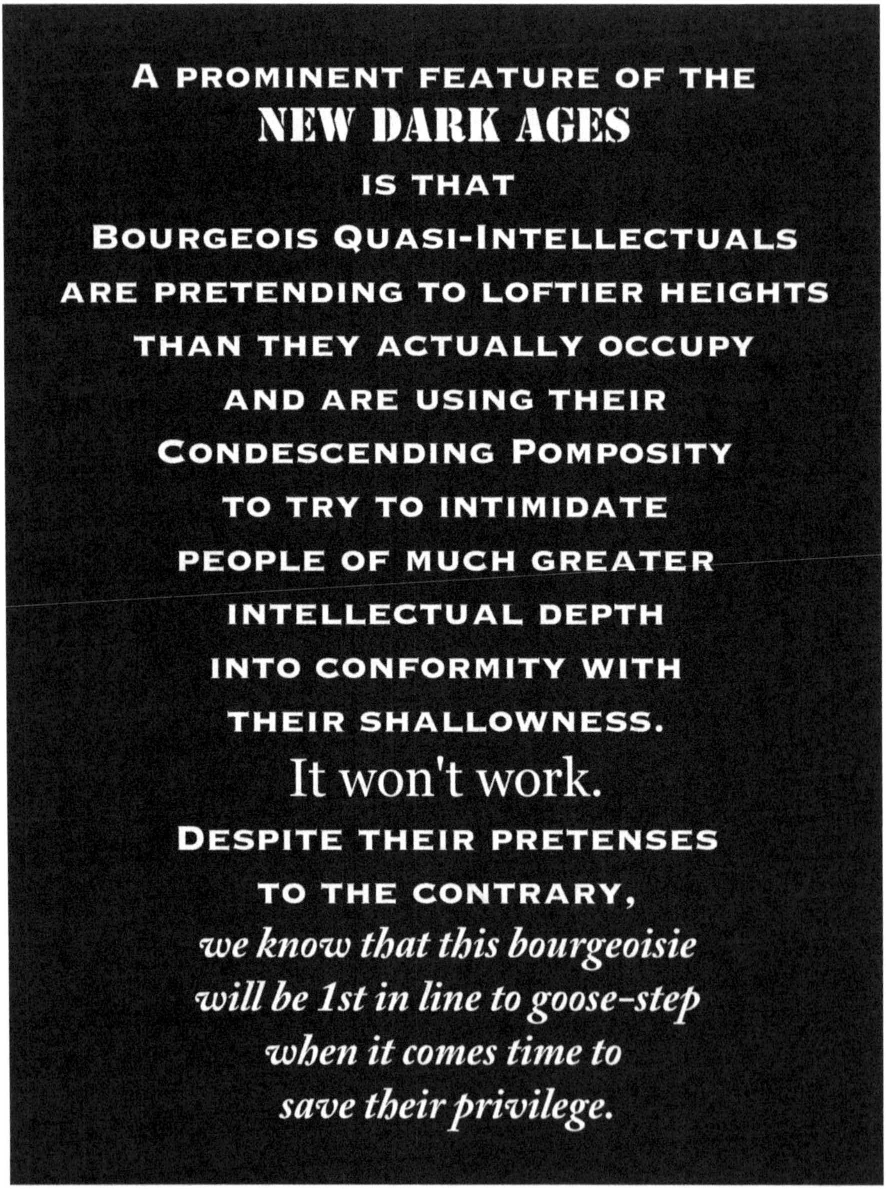

A PROMINENT FEATURE OF THE
NEW DARK AGES
IS THAT
BOURGEOIS QUASI-INTELLECTUALS
ARE PRETENDING TO LOFTIER HEIGHTS
THAN THEY ACTUALLY OCCUPY
AND ARE USING THEIR
CONDESCENDING POMPOSITY
TO TRY TO INTIMIDATE
PEOPLE OF MUCH GREATER
INTELLECTUAL DEPTH
INTO CONFORMITY WITH
THEIR SHALLOWNESS.
It won't work.
DESPITE THEIR PRETENSES
TO THE CONTRARY,
we know that this bourgeoisie
will be 1st in line to goose-step
when it comes time to
save their privilege.

****

July 15, 2020, 10:30AM (Amir-ul Kafirs to group)

Re: HERETICS: NEW DARK AGES

On Jul 14, 2020, at 10:42 AM, dick turner wrote:

bravo !

Thanks, Dick. I should write a book called "How to Wish for Friends but Make Enemies".

****

July 15, 2020, 12:06AM (Inquiring Librarian to group):

HERETICS: Jon Rappoport & the Whitehouse CDC Bypass

I'm not sure if this is good news, it may well be but only time will tell. If nothing else, it could be a sea change in the miasma of stormy story waters we all seem to be drowning in these daze.

Check out this headline and read the article from "Forbes":

White House Freezes CDC Out Of Covid Data Reporting, May Ask States To Use National Guard To Help

https://www.forbes.com/sites/siladityaray/2020/07/14/report-white-house-may-ask-states-to-use-national-guard-for-covid-data-collection/?fbclid=IwAR30g_6wlSpjFwuapQZDM6_KF4282d07uRn9kKmzWKEcVbQ6X7akt3e_7G8#60bf660b127a

Now, consider this blog post from Jon Rappoport that was sent out just this morning around 8am (I subscribe to Jon's "No More Fake News" blog post and get his email updates periodically).

https://blog.nomorefakenews.com/

"There's a reason MY contact tracing led to you, Mr. Trump.

You're the only one left in the menagerie. You're the only political animal who could offer a shred of a sliver of a slim ray of hope. To push back the invaders.

Several times you've said, "It's no good if the cure is worse than the disease." Surely you understand by now, the cure IS the disease. The H-bomb that went off in the middle of the economy was and is the whole point of the invasion, which has been taking place under your nose.

With your assistance. As a result of your failed marriage to Tony Fauci.

Let's put aside the gloss, Mr. Trump. You understand the real effects of the lockdowns. The effects the networks refuse to lead with, on the evening news.

There is the symbolic economy, represented by the careening up and down stock market. Then there is the real thing—the businesses and lives destroyed.

Nixon and Kissinger. Bush and Cheney. Bill and Hillary. They don't hold a candle to you and Fauci.

You allowed Fauci to become head of the coronavirus task force, and to remain in that position, spreading vast clouds of overblown lies about the "pandemic" and the fascist measures needed to stem it.

That's a crime you'll have to live with.

But you can do something about it. The governors won't. The mayors won't. Believe me, I've looked high and low to find someone other than you, to whom I could send these dispatches. Some noble figure in the American landscape with power, who could turn the tide in the economic war against the people. I don't see one. You're the default choice.

[..]

Of course, I'm out of my mind. I must be. Who could imagine sending in the Army to liberate the people, so they could live free?

Preposterous.

Better to huddle in fear. And wait. For the keeper of the cage to open the door.

So we can go out for a little while.

Right, Mr. President?

Until the next time, the next wave, the next crisis—tomorrow."

****

Jul 14, 2020,03:42pm EDT

White House Freezes CDC Out Of Covid Data Reporting, May Ask States To Use National Guard To Help

Siladitya Ray Forbes Staff
Business
Covering breaking news and tech policy stories at Forbes.
Updated Jul 14, 2020, 03:59pm EDT

TOPLINE

The Trump administration has altered reporting guidelines for hospitals handling Covid-19 patients, asking them to directly send their data to the state or the HHS — bypassing the CDC — and it is also pushing governors to consider using the National Guard at hospitals to help collect the data the *Washington Post* reported.

KEY FACTS

According to the report, earlier drafts of the letters to governors would have directed them to deploy the National Guard to help hospitals with daily data submissions; now it includes the National Guard as one of many options.

The suggestion of using National Guard troops has irked hospital industry leaders who say that problems with data collection are due to repeatedly changing instructions from the U.S. Department of Health and Human Services, the report added.

In its most recent guidance to hospitals, HHS has changed its protocols for Covid-19 data reporting, asking hospitals to send their data to their state or federal contractor instead of the CDC.

The new guidance has eliminated direct contact between the CDC and hospitals, reversing the original mandate issued by the White House asking hospital administrators to send reports on coronavirus testing, capacity, utilization and patient flow to the agency on a daily basis.

Trump and his staffers have publicly criticized the CDC on multiple occasions of late, with the President retweeting an accusation that the agency was lying about Covid-19 numbers to keep "the economy from coming back"

[..]

- https://www.forbes.com/sites/siladityaray/2020/07/14/report-white-house-may-ask-states-to-use-national-guard-for-covid-data-collection/?fbclid=IwAR30g_6wlSpjFwuapQZDM6_KF4282d07uRn9kKmzWKEcVbQ6X7akt3e_7G8#32ae9feb127a

****

July 15, 2020, 12:19AM (Inquiring Librarian to group):

Re: HERETICS: Jon Rappoport & the Whitehouse CDC Bypass

As you all may well know, the CDC has a bit of corruption in it, especially

evolving around vaccinations. There was a time when Trump was going to have Robert F. Kennedy Jr. head a vaccination safety commission, back in 2017. This never came to pass, but you can see here in this interview about that, where Kennedy briefly addresses the CDC and its conflicts of interest in the vaccine industry profits: https://www.sciencemag.org/news/2017/01/exclusive-qa-robert-f-kennedy-jr-trumps-proposed-vaccine-commission
I am sure there is better information on the CDC's corruptions, but I am too tired to look them up right now. Below is enough for now, for me.

"Q: Did the president-elect mention CDC?

A: We talked a lot about CDC and ways to increase the independence from financial conflicts at CDC in the vaccine division.

Q: You said that the commission is to delve into "vaccine safety and scientific integrity." What is that second piece about?

A: To make sure that we're getting good science out of CDC.

Q: It's all about CDC? It's not about "scientific integrity" in chemistry or physics or basic biology or anywhere else?

A: Exactly. [CDC] is the locus of most of the most serious problems with the vaccine program, the two divisions at CDC: the Advisory Committee on Immunization Practices and the Immunization Safety Office, which is where the scientists are."

Hence, bypassing the CDC may be a good step, unless something even more nefarious is up the administration's sleeve.

****

Exclusive Q&A: Robert F. Kennedy Jr. on Trump's proposed vaccine commission

By Meredith Wadman Jan. 10, 2017 , 4:45 PM

Environmental attorney Robert F. Kennedy, Jr., **an outspoken vaccine critic**, said today that he was asked by President-elect Donald Trump to chair a "vaccine safety and scientific integrity" commission. (A Trump spokesperson, however, later said that **"no decisions have been made at this time" about such a commission**.) Kennedy espouses discredited links between vaccines and neurological disorders, including autism. He has also been harshly critical of the U.S. Centers for Disease Control and Prevention (CDC), which recommends the childhood vaccine schedule. Scientists and others have **fiercely disputed** Kennedy's claims.

Science Insider caught up with Kennedy by telephone in an airport flight lounge shortly after he met with Trump in New York City. He made it clear that CDC's vaccine scientists and practices will be a major focus of the commission's work. Excerpts from our interview, which have been edited for brevity and clarity, appear below.

Q: What happened in the meeting?

A: It was an hour meeting and the vice president–elect came in to the last 15 minutes. The meeting was with [Trump] and Kellyanne Conway [recently appointed counselor to the president].

Q: Did the president-elect request the meeting or did you?

A: He called me a week ago to request it.

Q: Why?

A: He wants to make sure that we have the best vaccine science and the safest vaccine supply that we can have.

Q: Did the president-elect indicate that he doesn't believe that to be the case at the moment?

A: He is troubled by questions of the links between certain vaccines and the epidemic of neurodevelopmental disorders including autism. And he has a number—he told me five—friends, he talked about each one of them, who has the same story of a child, a perfectly healthy child who went into a wellness visit around age 2, got a battery of vaccines, spiked a fever, and then developed a suite of deficits in the 3 months following the vaccine.

He said that he understood that anecdote was not science, but said that if there's enough anecdotal evidence … that we'd be arrogant to dismiss it. Those were his words.

[..]

Q: When you say "science people," do you mean experts from the scientific establishment?

A: Prominent scientists.

Q: Do you mean prominent vaccinologists who believe in the safety and efficacy of today's vaccines?

A: We are going to look for people who have expertise in toxicology, epidemiology, and in public health.

Q: When does the president-elect want you to have the commission in place?

A: We didn't talk about the details but he expressed urgency about it. That he wanted it done—we talked about a 1-year commitment.

Q: It's an unpaid panel?

A: Yes.

[..]

Meredith Wadman

- https://www.sciencemag.org/news/2017/01/exclusive-qa-robert-f-kennedy-jr-trumps-proposed-vaccine-commission

****

July 15, 2020, 11:27AM (Amir-ul Kafirs to group):

I'm not sure if this is good news, it may well be but only time will tell.

White House Freezes CDC Out Of Covid Data Reporting,

Nope, bad idea. INCREASING THE NUMBER OF GROUPS ANALYZING THE DATA IS A GOOD IDEA, centralizing it under more political control or ANY type of control is a bad idea. In other words, have the data sent out to organizations other than the CDC, fine. I haven't looked at the CDC's data for awhile so I did just now & got this update:

TOTAL CASES

3,355,457

58,858 New Cases*

TOTAL DEATHS

135,235

351 New Deaths*

- https://www.cdc.gov/coronavirus/2019-ncov/cases-updates/cases-in-us.html

My point being that if the CDC is listing the total deaths in the US as "135,235" I don't distrust at least that aspect of what they're doing because that's not as severe as original projections. The CDC has a website that gives their previous "National Forecasts". Here's the chart from April 13, 2020, the earliest one I found:

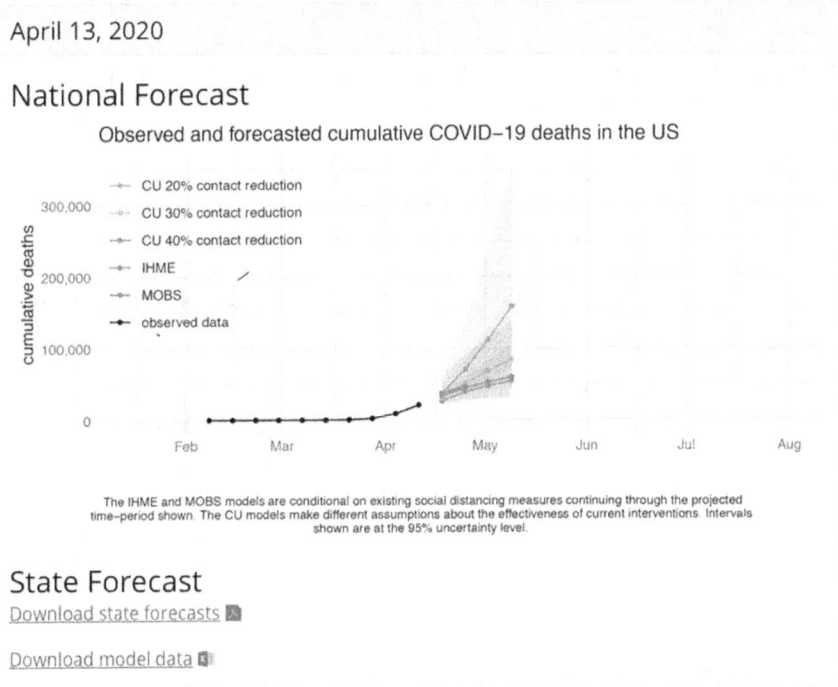

April 13, 2020

National Forecast

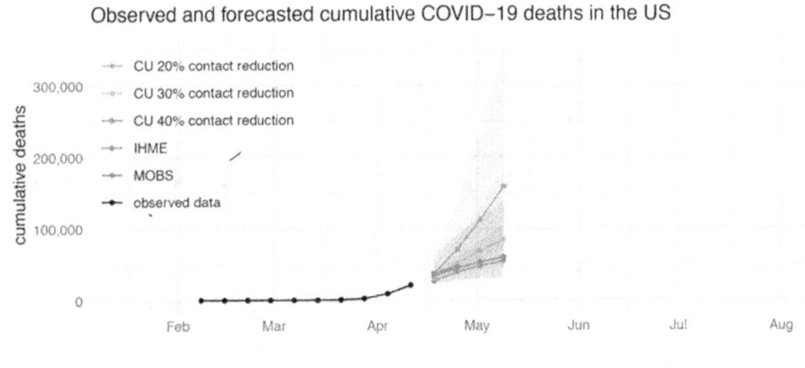

The IHME and MOBS models are conditional on existing social distancing measures continuing through the projected time–period shown. The CU models make different assumptions about the effectiveness of current interventions. Intervals shown are at the 95% uncertainty level.

State Forecast

Download state forecasts

Download model data

- https://www.cdc.gov/coronavirus/2019-ncov/covid-data/forecasting-us-previous.html

With a "contact reduction" of 20% they still predicted around 160,000 deaths by May. I don't know to what extent contact reduction has been actually decreased but the death rate hasn't reached 160,000 yet by 2 months later than the predicted May. The point is: their prediction was bad but at least it's their own data that shows this.

May Ask States To Use National Guard To Help

Involving the National Guard is ALWAYS A BAD IDEA. The National Guard carry guns. There're bound to be Guards(wo)men who're eager to use them. I'll never forget Kent State. It could happen again.

https://www.forbes.com/sites/siladityaray/2020/07/14/report-white-house-may-ask-states-to-use-national-guard-for-covid-data-collection/?

fbclid=IwAR30g_6wlSpjFwuapQZDM6_KF4282d07uRn9kKmzWKEcVbQ6X7akt3e_7G8#60bf660b127a

The Forbes article doesn't really say much — just that the CDC might be bypassed & that the National Guard might be used for data collection from hospitals.

Now, consider this blog post from Jon Rappoport that was sent out just this morning around 8am

I'm only superficially familiar with this guy. Inquiring Librarian & Phil have followed his opinions/research more closely.

https://blog.nomorefakenews.com/

"There's a reason MY contact tracing led to you, Mr. Trump.

Any & all criticisms of anything about the 'management' of this mess are fine with me. But then there's this:

If hundreds of thousands or millions of Chinese soldiers were encamped in cities and towns across USA right now, smashing the American engines of production, don't you think you'd be justified in sending in the troops? To liberate the people? Would anyone is his right mind cite Posse Comitatus to try to stop you?
[..]
Of course, I'm out of my mind. I must be. Who could imagine sending in the Army to liberate the people, so they could live free?
Preposterous.

Yeah, ***I actually DO think that's preposterous***. The idea of using troops to reverse the damage done to the economy by the QUARANTYRANNY is bound to be a disaster. Bringing in the military has a long history of bringing in worse dictatorships than what've already been in place. I seriously doubt that there're any historical records of its working in the opposite direction. Rappoport's proposing this, *especially with Rump as* ***the general*** strikes me as a recipe for disaster. As such, I don't trust Rappoport much.

****

July 15, 2020, 11:46AM (Amir-ul Kafirs to group):

I am sure there is better information on the CDC's corruptions, but I am too tired to look them up right now.

Yeah, unfortunately, I'm trying to pay close enough attention to these things at the same time that I whip through them so that I can move on to other aspects of my day. As such, I distrust my own perspicacity or lack thereof. It seems to me that the tone of the interview is hostile. Here's the way it ends:

Q: Do you have scientific training?

A: No. My background is I'm an environmental lawyer. I'm not a scientist. But I have an expertise, I would say, in reading science and spotting junk science because that's what I do with most of my time.

Q: Rates of childhood infectious diseases have plummeted over the past half-century or so. Are you out to return us to the dark ages?

A: I am for vaccines. I have been tracking mercury in fish for 30 years and nobody has called me antifish. I am pro-vaccine. I had all my kids vaccinated. I think vaccines save lives. But we are also seeing an explosion in neurodevelopmental disorders and we ought to be able to do a cost-benefit analysis and see what's causing them. We ought to have robust, transparent science and an independent regulatory agency. Nobody is trying to get rid of vaccines here. I just want safe vaccines.

Obviously the author is trying to discredit Kennedy when she says "Are you out to return us to the dark ages?" as if that's the only possible outcome of his criticizing vaccines. Kennedy's reply is intelligent & cautious. As such, I like Kennedy more than the interviewer. That doesn't mean I necessarily agree with his criticisms of the CDC *or that I disagree*. The CDC is a component of the Department of Health and Human Service. As such, it's susceptible to political pressures.

Hence, bypassing the CDC may be a good step,

The problem is: bypassing it *is just another political pressure*. If Rump does this then it's essentially discrediting the agency. There's probably good reason to criticize it but *discrediting it altogether* ***might be throwing out the baby with the bathwater.***

unless something even more nefarious is up the administration's sleeve.

No way would I trust Rump's decision. Remember, he's the guy who came up with the 'genius' plan for walling-off the Mexican border.

****

July 15, 2020, 12:01PM (Amir-ul Kafirs to group):

Re: HERETICS: NEW DARK AGES

On Jul 15, 2020, at 10:31 AM, Inquiring Librarian wrote:

This is one of my favorites!

Thanks! At the same time that I don't want to crank out one of those texts every day because it seems too much like forced production I must admit that on the days when I don't post a new one, like today, I feel like I'm not thinking enough!

****

July 15, 2020, 12:55PM (Inquiring Librarian to group):

So for the interview of Kennedy, Yes, Science Magazine was not treating Kennedy well. What I have noticed about Kennedy, is he takes interviews and debates with both supporters and non supporters. I believe he will take any press he can get that will listen to him, because, like Andrew Wakefield, he is used to being attacked and discredited but he truly believes in his message and knows that converts to his message can be everywhere and nonbelievers who read Science Magazine may change their opinion on vaccines when they hear Kennedy, even in light where he is clearly being antagonized by the magazine. I appreciate this about Kennedy. I found out about him by reading a quote of his on someone's social media page. I was really impressed with what Kennedy had said. I had no idea who Kennedy was or what he was about but his message was enough to get me curious. Then... I read some disparaging comments about him having 'really' said that under the friend's social media post with his quote. So, that made me want even MORE to look him up. And voila, now I am an obsessed follower of Kennedy.

Ok, onward to the CDC. The CDC gets funding through public/private partnerships. https://www.cdc.gov/partners/partnering.html . After MANY clicks, I found this list of their donors for the year 2019, and of course, among them, The Bill & Melinda Gates Foundation, Bayer, GalazoSmithKline, GAVI (The Global Vaccine Alliance (a Gates baby)), the WHO, etc.. the full list is here: https://www.cdcfoundation.org/FY2019/organizations

And yes, bringing in the National Guard sounds like a TERRIBLE idea. I am already imagining how Operation Warp Speed (which proposes to use the National Guard to help with the vaccine project) will sic the National Guard on all of us to break down our doors (if we still have homes, hence doors to them, after the economy continues to freefall) to inject us with nanotechnology mindcontrol vaccines to turn us into transhumans, at gunpoint. It is a terrifying, but very possible possibility. I only have hope that it may not be a terrible thing in that someone at this point has done SOMETHING to stop the fake numbers and lies coming out of states/cities, and their hospitals. The tyranny has to end. But who knows, this bypassing the CDC regardless of how corrupt the CDC may be, could make things even worse. I know Trump wants the schools to open up and for the economy to get back to normal. None of this will happen if the media keep fear mongering the masses and the fear mongering is fueled by the lies coming from our hospitals and mayors and governors. But when we bypass the CDC, we go directly to the HHS with Alex Azar who appears to be a vaccine aholic and former pharmaceutical lobbyist. And Azar is going to try to push a vaccine by Moderna on the public as early as fall, knowing only the preliminary results of the vaccine on the 45 test subjects in phase 1 testing (which according to RFK Jr. had a 20% failure in extremely healthy people which sent them to the hospital with side effects, and don't forget, pathogenic priming may not show up until a year or so later). https://abc7chicago.com/coronavirus-vaccine-covid-19-virus-alex-azar/6317225/

HHS Secretary optimistic that COVID-19 vaccine could be available by fall, visits Rush University Medical Center

I dunno guys, this looks so grim. I suppose the next few months will tell us something. Having the CDC bypassed will change the narrative a bit, but I am not sure how. Is there a good HHS site where we can get the kind of data we had on the CDC? Maybe we could all write in my cat Lulu for president. She is just about the kindest cat I've ever had, very thoughtful of others and she does not support vaccines. She carries FIV (Feline Immuno Deficiency Virus), so vaccinations could set her into fullblown kitty aids. She understands, she is the ONE for US. VOTE FOR LULU for President.

****

Partnering with CDC

Ethical Considerations for Public-Private Partnerships

For more than a half century, CDC has been a leader in scientific research committed to protect the American people and keep Americans healthy, safe and secure. CDC works with the private sector because public-private partnerships advance CDC's mission of protecting Americans. These partnerships allows us to accomplish more by working together rather than separately.

The agency's pledge to the American people includes being a diligent steward of the funds entrusted to it. Before accepting outside gifts, CDC reviews each one thoroughly to ensure that all relevant legal authorities, policies, and guidelines are followed. Public-private partnerships help federal agencies do more with less, build on the capabilities of others, leverage collective action, improve performance, and realize cost savings.
We continually work to protect our scientific and programmatic integrity, maintain accountability, and find solutions to our nation's most pressing public health problems. We recognize the value of open discussion and remain committed to improving and maintaining our processes of ethical protections. CDC's highest priority is to keep people safe. We leverage our medical and scientific expertise and our partnerships to diffuse health threats and make our country and our world a better place to live.

- Partnering with CDC Factsheetpdf icon

[..]

- In some cases, partnerships are arranged through the CDC

Foundation. The CDC Foundation, which began operating in 1995, supports numerous program activities that extend the impact of CDC's work.

Although the CDC Foundation was chartered by Congress, it is not a government agency nor is it a division of CDC. It is a private, nonprofit organization classified as a 501(c)(3) public charity.

[..]

The CDC Foundation helps the Centers for Disease Control and Prevention do more, faster by forging effective partnerships between CDC and others to fight threats to health and safety.

- https://www.cdc.gov/partners/partnering.html

****

Corporations, Foundations & Organizations
Fiscal Year 2019 Report to Contributors

Abbott Ireland
Academic Hospital Paramaribo
Affimedix, Inc.
AmazonSmile Foundation
American Association for Clinical Chemistry
American Type Culture Collection
Amgen Foundation
Amgen Inc.
ARUP Laboratories
Atlanta Chapter Daughters of The American Revolution
Australian Department of Foreign Affairs and Trade
Bayer U.S. LLC
BD
Beckman Coulter, Inc.
Benevity Community Impact Fund
Bill & Melinda Gates Foundation
Biogen MA Inc.
Biohit Laboratory Services
BioReference Laboratories, Inc.
Bloomberg Philanthropies
Boditech Med Inc.
Boston Children's Hospital
Brigham and Women's Hospital
Brown University

C.D.C. Chapter 1419 NARFE
Cargill, Inc.
CDC Federal Credit Union
Centennial Medical Center
Centers for Disease Control and Prevention
Centre Hospitalier Universitaire of Liege
Cerilliant Corporation
Chambers Family Foundation
Charities Aid Foundation of America:
  Carmen H. Villar, MSW
Chemux Bioscience, Inc.
Chromesystems Instruments & Chemicals GmbH
Clarivate Analytics
Classy, Inc.
Clemson University
College of American Pathologists
Columbia University
Community Foundation of Central Georgia, Inc.
Conrad N. Hilton Foundation
Covance Central Laboratory Services
Delaware Academy of Medicine / Delaware Public Health Association
Diagnostics Biochem Canada Inc.
DiaSorin Inc.
DiaSource Immunoassays SA
Diazyme Laboratories
Emory University
Eurofins Biomnis
Euroimmun Medizinische Labordiagnostika AG
Eventbrite
Facebook
FIA Foundation
Fidelity Charitable Gift Fund:
  Betensky-Kraut Family Fund
  Bruce & Susi Willis Gift Fund
  The Hunter Family Fund
  Jacobs Family Fund
  Kaunitz Family Charitable Fund
  Klepchick Family Fund
  Kreuter/Katz Family Fund
  Lisa A. Mills Fund
  Lubitz/Monroe Charitable Fund
  Martha and Robert Supnik Charitable Fund
  Murphy-Gittleman Family Fund
  The Nancy C. Lee Giving Fund
  Paul and Beverly Truebig Gift Fund
  Peter Dull and Judith Tsui Charitable Family Fund
  Petruzzelli/Herrera Fund
  Philip I. Kent Charitable Fund

Vickery Perniciaro Family Fund
Foundation for Innovative New Diagnostics
Four Seasons Environmental, Inc.
Fremont Area Community Foundation, Inc.
GAVI Alliance
GiveWell
GlaxoSmithKline Biologicals S.A.
Global Blood Therapeutics, Inc.
Global Inc.
Good Ventures Foundation
Government of Canada
Greater Cleveland Community Shares
Heartland Assays LLC
HONOReform Foundation
IBM Employee Services Center
Immunodiagnostic Systems Inc.
Imperial College London
International Union Against Tuberculosis and Lung Disease
Intervet International B.V.
Iodine Global Network
IQ Solutions
James F. and Sarah T. Fries Foundation
James W. Down Company, Inc.
JAMF Nation Global Foundation
Job-Site Safety Institute
Johns Hopkins University
King Saud University
The Kresge Foundation
Laboratory Corporation of America Holdings
Los Angeles Biomedical Research Institute
Luminex Corporation
Magee-Womens Research Institute and Foundation
Marcel J Vinduska Revocable Trust
May P. And Francis L. Abreu Charitable Trust
Mayo Foundation for Medical Education and Research
The Merck Foundation
Merck Sharp & Dohme Corp.
Microgenics Corporation
Monobind Inc.
MTM Foundation
National Philanthropic Trust
Nelson Family Foundation
Network for Good
Northside Kiwanis Foundation
Nutrition International
Oak Crest Institute of Science
Omaha Community Foundation
Open Philanthropy Project

Ortho-Clinical Diagnostics
Partners HealthCare System, Inc.
Pathology Associates Medical Laboratories
Pennington Biomedical Research Foundation
Pennsylvania State University
Pew Charitable Trusts
Quest Diagnostics
RB Health (US) LLC
R-Biopharm Inc.
Reckitt Benckiser, Inc.
The Regents of the University of New Mexico
Richard E. & Marianne B. Kipper Foundation
Robert Wood Johnson Foundation
Roche Diagnostics Corporation
Sabin Vaccine Institute
Saul D. Levy Foundation
Schwab Charitable Fund:
  Adler Family Charitable Fund
  Brody Charitable Fund
  John Schnitker/Elizabeth Weaver Charitable Fund
  Karen and Marvin Whaley Fund
  Ruth J. Katz Charitable Fund
  Shands/Mulinare Family Charitable Fund
SCIEX
Sergey Brin Family Foundation
Siemens Healthcare Diagnostics, Inc.
Snibe Diagnostics (Snibe Co., Ltd.)
Social Good Fund
Taylor and Francis Group, LLC
The Community Foundation for Greater Atlanta, Inc.:
  Charles H & Margaret McTier Fund
  Jeffrey & Carol Koplan Family Fund
  Robert Yellowlees Family Fund
Thermo Fisher Scientific, Inc.
Three Rivers Community Foundation
Tosoh Corporation
Tri-State Gastroenterology
Truist
Tull Charitable Foundation
UBS Donor-Advised Fund
Ullmann Family Foundation
UNICEF
United Nations Foundation
United Way of Central New Mexico
United Way of Greater Atlanta, Inc.
University of Arizona
University of Connecticut
University of Georgia

University of Louisville
University of Michigan
University of Minnesota
University of New Mexico
University of North Carolina at Chapel Hill
University of Western Australia
Vanguard Charitable:
The Stuart H. Hillman Fund
Vestergaard Frandsen SA
Virginia Commonwealth University Health System
Vital Strategies
The Walker School
Waters Ireland LTD
The Wilson Family Foundation
Wolters Kluwer Health
World Health Organization
Zhejiang Disigns Diagnostics

- https://www.cdcfoundation.org/FY2019/organizations

****

HHS Secretary optimistic that COVID-19 vaccine could be available by fall, visits Rush University Medical Center

Azar downplayed concerns about politics, COVID-19, blames surge of southern cases on bad behavior

By Craig Wall

Tuesday, July 14, 2020 7:40PM

"We could be looking at tens of millions, even 100 million doses of vaccine, this fall, and many hundreds of millions of doses by early next year."

CHICAGO (WLS) -- The Secretary of Health and Human Services visited Chicago Tuesday to see how doctors and nurses in the city have handled the COVID-19 crisis.

Secretary Alex Azar said he was optimistic that a vaccine for the virus could be available as soon as this fall.

On Tuesday, researchers with Moderna and the National Institutes Of Health announced that an experimental vaccine successfully produced antibodies in all 45 patients involved in testing.

Azar toured Rush University Medical Center Tuesday morning to learn about some of the creative ways health care professionals responded to the pandemic.

He also addressed concerns about recent surges in other states, and downplayed concerns about politics and COVID-19.

[..]

The secretary downplayed the recent call for a national face mask policy by Governor JB Pritzker and said mandates for coverings should be left to local leaders, adding a one size fits all approach is not appropriate.

- https://abc7chicago.com/coronavirus-vaccine-covid-19-virus-alex-azar/6317225/

****

July 15, 2020, 8:53PM (Amir-ul Kafirs to group):

What I have noticed about Kennedy, is he takes interviews and debates with both supporters and non supporters.

Yeah, I liked his calm 'under fire' & that made me trust him more because I felt like the interviewer's nastiness gave away her agenda while he stuck to trying to explain his position coherently.

The CDC gets funding through public/private partnerships.

This is where things start to get tricky, eh? I quote from the end of this 1st linked-to page:

"In some cases, partnerships are arranged through the CDC Foundation. The CDC Foundation, which began operating in 1995, supports numerous program activities that extend the impact of CDC's work.

"Although the CDC Foundation was chartered by Congress, it is not a government agency nor is it a division of CDC. It is a private, nonprofit organization classified as a 501(c)(3) public charity. To connect with CDC Foundation,"

But, you see those are donors to the CDC Foundation, as stated above, *not a part of the CDC* but obviously a conduit of money to it. SO, how exactly does that work? It might just be a way for Bill Gates & all the rest to get their control in there while avoiding any conflict of interest directness.

I know Trump wants the schools to open up and for the economy to get back to normal.

I don't think we actually have any idea of what Rump wants. I mean he puts on his act for his perceived constituents, just like all his predecessors have, & then goes about doing whatever is best for his personal schemes behind closed doors in a non-transparent way. He might be perfectly happy that things are the way they are but his election plans may revolve around appealing to those who aren't happy with it. He's a politician, there's no way he's going to tell the truth.

Azar is going to try to push a vaccine by Moderna on the public as early as fall,

Well, there you have it. How could he *possibly* be an improvement over the CDC?

knowing only the preliminary results of the vaccine on the 45 test subjects in phase 1 testing (which according to RFK Jr. had a 20% failure in extremely healthy people which sent them to the hospital with side effects, and don't forget, pathogenic priming may not show up until a year or so later).

HHS Secretary optimistic that COVID-19 vaccine could be available by fall, visits Rush University Medical Center

One of the things Azar is described as presenting in the article is this:

"He also addressed concerns about recent surges in other states, and downplayed concerns about politics and COVID-19."

Downplaying the politics?! That's pure insanity (or, more accurately, completely disingenuous). It seems pretty obvious to me that the upcoming presidential election is being completely manipulated around the issue of the quarantine. The Democrats are claiming that all sane people find the quarantine absolutely necessary & the Republicans are saying the opposite. Heavy propaganda is being used to win people over. I wish they would BOTH LOSE.

Is there a good HHS site where we can get the kind of data we had on the CDC?

Right now, the answer seems to be NO. Here's their website: https://www.hhs.gov/coronavirus/news/index.html . At the top of the page it redirects to the CDC for what I'm usually looking for: "Visit **cdc.gov/coronavirus** for the latest Coronavirus Disease (COVID-19) updates." I don't think we have any guarantee that that aspect of the CDC will be passed over to the HHS if they take over the CDC's COVID-19 duties. Then where will we be?

Maybe we could all write in my cat Lulu for president.

The Yippies ran a pig for president in 1968. I can't remember whether the pig won or not.

****

July 14, 2020 (txt msg from Naia Nisnam to Amir-ul Kafirs):

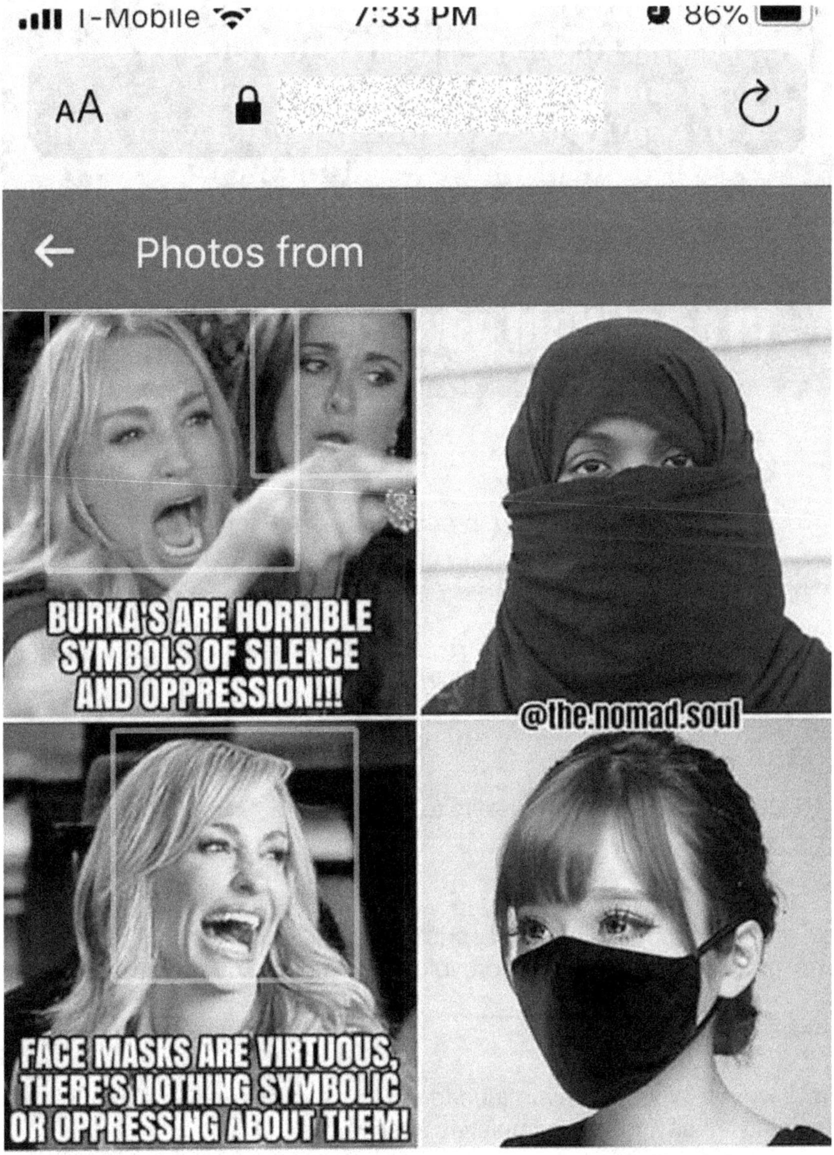

****

July 15, 2020, 4:13PM (Amir-ul Kafirs to group):

HERETICS: Cases

This one's practically mild-mannered!

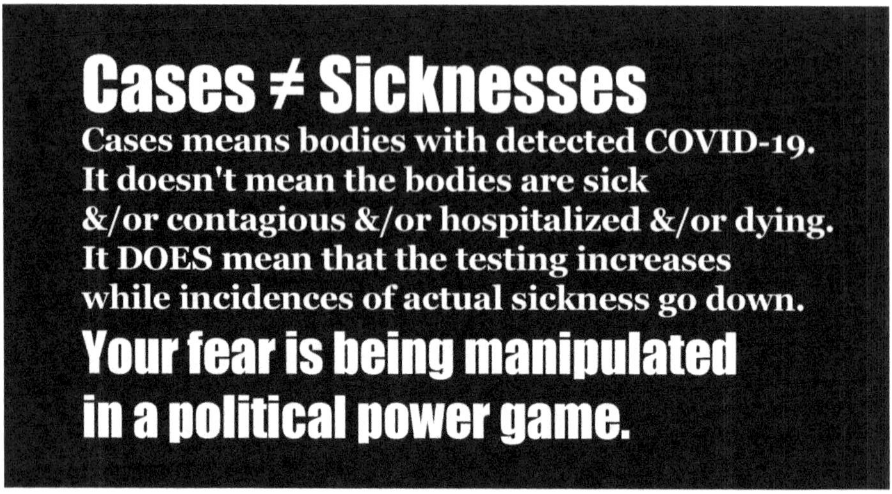

Cases ≠ Sicknesses
Cases means bodies with detected COVID-19.
It doesn't mean the bodies are sick
&/or contagious &/or hospitalized &/or dying.
It DOES mean that the testing increases
while incidences of actual sickness go down.
Your fear is being manipulated
in a political power game.

****

July 15, 2020, 4:42PM (Inquiring Librarian to group):

Re: HERETICS: Cases

This is great! I can't wait to see the responses!! It seems so obvious but most ppl appear to find this incomprehensible.

****

July 15, 2020, 9:05PM (Amir-ul Kafirs to group):

This is great! I can't wait to see the responses!!

So far, the responses have been hearts from you & Naia Nisnam. Believe me, I'm *very grateful for that* but if it's provoked any thought otherwise it's not visible.

It seems so obvious but most ppl appear to find this incomprehensible.

I know, I know! When I've even tried to get into a conversation about this it was as if what I was saying was completely abstract.

****

July 15, 2020, 7:27PM (Naia Nisnam to group):

'The Virus Is Making The Rules': Gov. Tom Wolf Imposes Statewide Restrictions

On Bars, Restaurants And Larger Indoor Gatherings – CBS Pittsburgh
Our governor has clearly lost his mind:

“This is the virus speaking,” he says. “The virus is making the rules here...”

https://pittsburgh.cbslocal.com/2020/07/15/gov-tom-wolf-coronavirus-mitigation-efforts/
https://pittsburgh.cbslocal.com/2020/07/15/gov-tom-wolf-coronavirus-mitigation-efforts/?fbclid=IwAR1AZWsty5uCcSWF_fWt1Z7OLM4dxVMoPOCoVN7QnyPUt_VPnecHJ9J-CkI

****

‘The Virus Is Making The Rules’: Gov. Tom Wolf Imposes Statewide Restrictions On Bars, Restaurants And Larger Indoor Gatherings

July 15, 2020 at 2:56 pm

HARRISBURG, Pa. (AP/KDKA) — Gov. Tom Wolf announced broad new statewide restrictions on bars and restaurants and larger indoor gatherings Wednesday as Pennsylvania reported another nearly 1,000 new infections, continuing a recent resurgence of COVID-19 in parts of the state.

Nightclubs will be shut down, bars will also be closed unless they also offer dine-in meals, and bars and restaurants will be limited to 25% capacity.
Alcohol can still be sold to-go and customers can sit at non-bar seating in outdoor areas.

Indoor events and gatherings of more than 25 people will be prohibited, as well as outdoor gatherings of more than 250. And businesses will be required to have their employees work remotely to the extent possible.

There are no changes to gyms and fitness facilities, but they are “directed to prioritize outdoor physical fitness activities.” All activities must follow the mask mandate and social distancing.

“This is the virus speaking,” he says. “The virus is making the rules here, we’re just trying to anticipate what those rules are and doing what we can to reduce the risk that virus is going to do a lot of damage to Pennsylvania.”

[..]

The Pennsylvania Licensed Beverage and Tavern Association released a statement in response to the order:

"Today Pennsylvania pumped the breaks on reopening of taverns and restaurants. The revised statewide mitigation order in part now limits the industry to 25% indoor occupancy, and requires all patrons seated indoors to be at a booth or table, and ordering food.

"At a time when the industry is already struggling, this makes matters worse.

"The Pennsylvania Licensed Beverage and Tavern Association calls upon the state to develop a bailout package, specific for the industry.

"Our Members are paying their yearly licensing fees to the state, but not being allowed to operate fully. In addition, business loans, rent, utilities, and industry vendors still must be paid out of reduced revenue.

"For starters, Pennsylvania should immediately eliminate all state fees associated with running a tavern or restaurant. In addition, higher discounts should be provided to licensed establishments purchasing liquor from the state. Furthermore, additional financial assistance should be included.

"In today's news conference, Governor Wolf said that the state is at a tipping point which forced it to act to prevent COVID-19 spread. Let's not forget that the tavern and restaurant industry also is at a tipping point. Without help, we will see more small business restaurants and taverns not survive."

[..]

- https://pittsburgh.cbslocal.com/2020/07/15/gov-tom-wolf-coronavirus-mitigation-efforts/

****

July 15, 2020, 11:29PM (Amir-ul Kafirs to group):

Re: 'The Virus Is Making The Rules': Gov. Tom Wolf Imposes Statewide Restrictions On Bars, Restaurants And Larger Indoor Gatherings – CBS Pittsburgh

Our governor has clearly lost his mind:

"This is the virus speaking," he says. "The virus is making the rules here..."

Hhmm.. well I guess that's grounds for impeachment! After all, I don't think the virus was elected!

""During the past week, we have seen an unsettling climb in new COVID-19 cases," Gov. Wolf says.

""When we hit our peak on April 9, we had nearly two thousand new cases that day with other days' cases hovering around 1,000. Medical experts looking at the trajectory we are on now are projecting that this new surge could soon eclipse the April peak. With our rapid case increases we need to act again now.""

Almost as an afterthought this is eventually followed by:

"The health department reported 994 new positive virus cases Wednesday, bringing the statewide total to more than 97,000. The health department reported the results of nearly 29,000 virus tests, the highest one-day total since the beginning of the pandemic.

"Health officials also reported 26 new deaths."

That's 994 new positive cases out of 29,000 people tested. That's roughly 3%. Then the 26 deaths are roughly 3% of that. Note that the 26 new deaths aren't explained. I think we can be pretty sure they aren't among young people who've been out partying at bars. Representatives of the tavern industry have this to say:

"Our Members are paying their yearly licensing fees to the state, but not being allowed to operate fully. In addition, business loans, rent, utilities, and industry vendors still must be paid out of reduced revenue."

Can you imagine? I'd be ppppiiiiissssssssseeeeddddd if I were them!!

I found it amusing that there was an ad for this product on the same page:

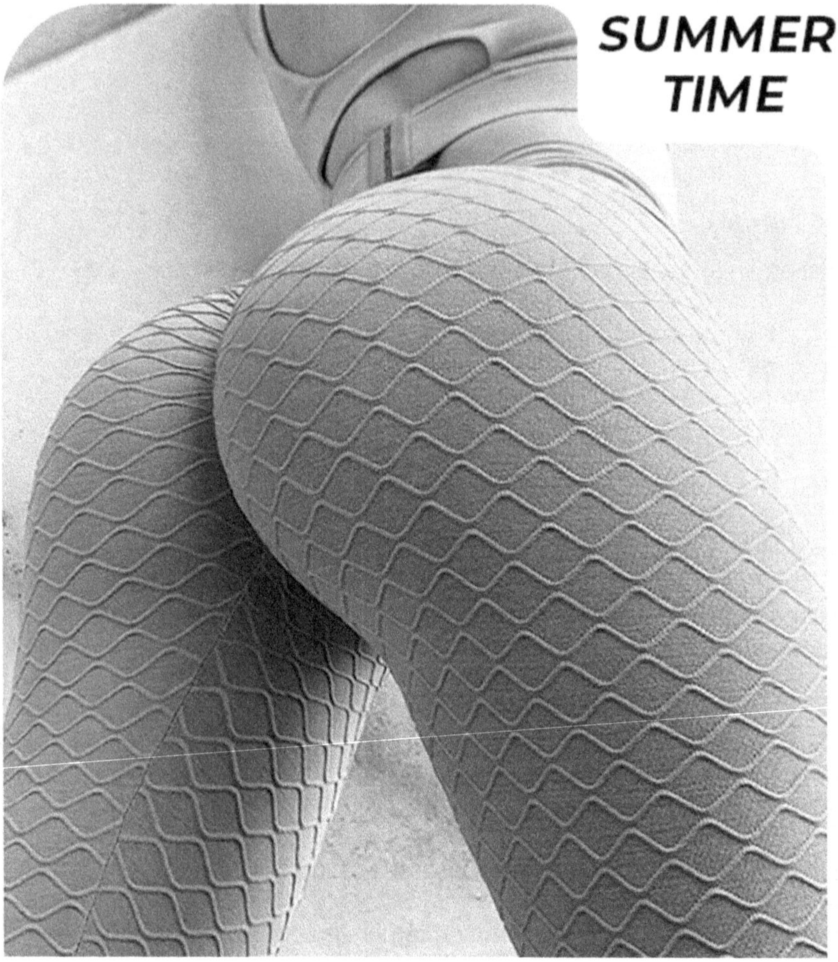

****

July 16, 2020, 12:02AM (Amir-ul Kafirs to group):

HERETICS: Children

Another mild-mannered one:

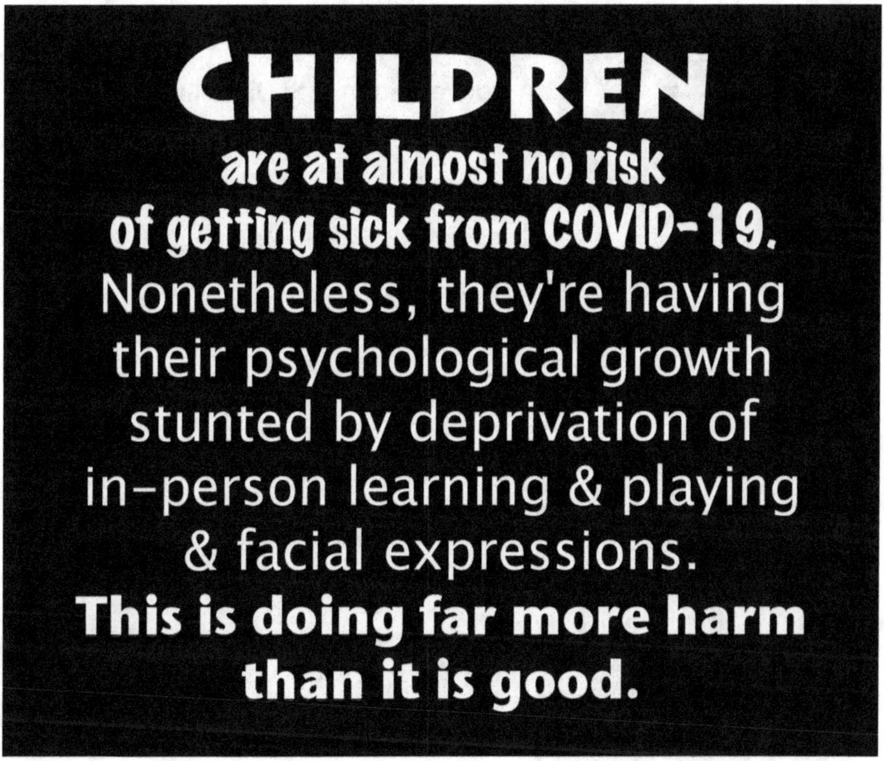
CHILDREN
are at almost no risk
of getting sick from COVID-19.
Nonetheless, they're having
their psychological growth
stunted by deprivation of
in-person learning & playing
& facial expressions.
This is doing far more harm
than it is good.

****

8 Comments 2 Shares

Like Comment Share

001a Would you go volunteer to be in a classroom right about now?

Like · Reply · 1d

002a 001 of course! If u consider any news beyond the mass media, u will know the risk is miniscule to none. Check out this short video for starters: https://m.youtube.com/watch?feature=share&v=A2rbIDYczvY

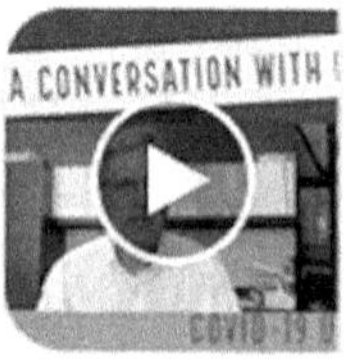

YOUTUBE.COM

A Conversation with Dr. Kelly Victory

Love · Reply · 1d 2

002b 001 also consider what Senator Jensen has to say: https://www.facebook.com/1492673654369368/posts/2357005124602879/

Love · Reply · 1d 2

002c 001 & here is an excellent artucle on the entire virus situation: https://off-guardian.org/.../07/second-wave-not-even-close/

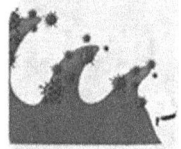

OFF-GUARDIAN.ORG

Second wave? Not even close.

Love · Reply · 1d 2

001b 002 My main sources are DemocracyNow, MedPageToday and afriend who is an immunology researcher. I consider these to be reliable journalism, not " mass media" and real science. As far as I'm concerned everything you cite is BS. And BTW, yes, get off your cushion and go volunteer! I dare you. How about on the Navajo Reservation for instance or in a poor neighborhood in Miami. Find out there if this is real. Go poll musicians in NOLA. You're apparently in an an alternate reality.

Like · Reply · 1d

[Editor's interpolation: At this point, I wasn't reading the comments anymore because I was traveling & because the comments had so consistently become abusive. As such, I didn't know about 001's attacks until Inquiring Librarian called the HERETICS' attention to them in the email that follows this. When I read them I was truly appalled. 001 *assumes*, incorrectly, that Inquiring Librarian doesn't work with children when, in fact, it's a major part of their profession to do so & a part of their everyday life. 001 further tells Inquiring Librarian to "Go poll musicians" which is *another incorrect assumption* insofar as both Inquiring Librarian & their partner *are musicians.* 001's instant dismissal of Dr. Kelly Victory, Doctor/ Senator Jensen, & JB Handley's excellent article without, obviously, having

***any clue* about who they were or what they said or what their qualifications are shows that 001 is a classic *Bourgeois Quasi-Intellectual of the New Dark Ages.* I immediately unfriended & blocked 001, *may they rot in a dungeon of their own choosing.*]**

003a 001
Can you explain why you dismiss the things that 002 posts as "BS"? Why do you think these doctors would lie?

I work in a school and can't wait to get back into the classroom. I have two children and they desperately need to interact with their peers.
The quarantine focuses solely on the virus, while there are many other aspects of life that are being negatively effected.
I believe, as many doctors do, that we can focus on protecting the vulnerable without shutting down all of society.
(Democracy Now, as much as I enjoy it, does have a political bias.)

2
Love · Reply · 1d

002d 001 i am a public librarian. I interact with all walks of life ever day in an inner city library, and I also live in a very poor section of my city. In fact, i work at a child centered library (that also serves many of the elderly in the neighborhood) and many of my patrons are dying to get their kids back to school, without masks. I agree with Breen Casey, Democracy Now is very politicized, and i would add, misguided, it is npr but just a bit deeper and more thoughtful. It is clear we do not agree and i can't imagine you took the time to read or listen to anything i shared with you. The best way to even attempt to hash this out reasonably without mudslinging will be to chat again in a few years and look back on these events. In my opinion, based on simply what i observe around me and the many highly credentialed scientists, lawyers, and medical professionals i follow, the big pharmaceutical companies have basically hijacked our medical system... Throw the corrupted WHO and GAVI into the mix with their faulty vaccine profiteering, and the whole western world has been sucked in, with 3rd world countries tossed in as unethical and highly protested testing grounds (something i find to be absolutely reprehensible, heartbreaking, and shockingly criminal beyond words).

3
Love · Reply · 1d · Edited

Write a reply...

004b There's also this happy yet underreported news from Childrens Hosptial of Pittsburgh:
"....the experience to date is reassuring that many, if not most, children with chronic illnesses will recover without needing to be admitted to the hospital."

https://www.chp.edu/our.../infectious-diseases/covid-19

I don't know why I bother. Most of you don't like to see any facts that aren't morbid doom and gloom.

CHP.EDU

www.chp.edu

Love · Reply · 18h 1

Write a comment...

****

July 16, 2020, 2:27PM (Inquiring Librarian to group):

RE: HERETICS: Children

By now, some of you may have seen the vitriolic comments on this one on social media. I got attacked by one of Amir-ul Kafirs's social media friends... crazy stuff! As I was sending them links in my comment, I was wondering what kind of, if any, response they would give me. And I wondered if they were a rabid covid fear supporter, how would they attack me, and how quickly would they attack me? I mean, they could have waited a few hours to at least lead me to believe they MAY have looked at and listened to the information I quoted for them. But no, they wrote back swinging within a few minutes. Thankfully, Naia Nisnam graciously came to the rescue to ease me of my cyber bullying slap in the face. Even though the person attacking my comment was clearly misguided, they were VICIOUS!! I of course, had to respond to their comment on my comment. I am wondering if they could possibly save face and come back swinging with more hate and venom. What is funny and typical, is they could not possibly have had the time to listen to the 2 videos I quoted for them, or read the JB Handley article that I also linked them to. It's amazing how sure of themselves these ill-informed believers are.

****

July 16, 2020, 6:49AM (Dick to group):

RE: HERETICS: Children

Hi tENT

I had an idea that I'd like to propose to you:

Why don't you do a News Program? "The Heretic News"... It could present, with your brand of humor, the immense amount of facts you glean from all the articles you read... It could be weekly, or bi-weekly...or just a one shot deal... you could have guests...it could be like perfomance art meets reality.... it could have a theme at the opening...a logo... whatever you felt like doing really... anyway it's an idea

I could help with certain aspects of it...I'd love to write a theme, maybe design the logo... or anything else... I could be the Paris Correspondant....Inquiring Librarian could cover Louisiana.... we could shoot it on our phones...

****

July 16, 2020, 2:42PM (Inquiring Librarian to group):

Here is a whole bunch of information on the corruption within the CDC: https://childrenshealthdefense.org/advocacy-policy/cdc-corruption-deceit-and-cover-up/

& this dramatic rant from Jon Rappoport also addresses some of this, more succinctly:
https://blog.nomorefakenews.com/2020/07/16/mr-trump-deliver-knockout-blow-to-traitorous-cdc/

It seems that they are big vaccine supporters, in part due to their public/private partnerships with big pharma. & they are great at skewing and sometimes removing their collected data as best serves their interests.

****

CDC: Corruption, Deceit and Cover-Up

With the global vaccine market now at tens of billions of dollars, vaccine safety should be of utmost concern to the Centers for Disease Control (CDC). But instead, rather than testing and monitoring the health effects of vaccines and patient injuries truthfully to the American public and making critical and necessary corrections in the program, the CDC has become a mouthpiece for industry and has protected the 'all vaccines for all children' policy despite peer-reviewed science to the contrary.

According to a UPI Investigative article written in the early 2000s, the CDC owned at least 28 vaccine patents. They are also in charge of vaccine promotion (getting the public to take vaccines) and vaccine safety. The CDC, like other large bureaucratic agencies, also has a revolving door to industry that comes with inherent conflicts of interests. Common sense should have told us that this system was doomed to fail.

The documents below, some of which **[were]** obtained by the Freedom of Information Act (FOIA) show a pattern of deceit perpetrated by the CDC on the American public and world stage for over 25 years. The Children's Health Defense believes that the vaccine safety should be taken from the CDC.

- https://childrenshealthdefense.org/advocacy-policy/cdc-corruption-deceit-and-cover-up/

****

Dispatches from the War: Mr. Trump, deliver a knockout blow to the traitorous CDC

by Jon Rappoport
July 16, 2020

"...against all enemies, foreign and domestic..."

Let's get domestic.

I promise you, Mr. President, if you send a hundred FBI agents into the CDC and remove millions of their files as evidence, you'll discover this federal agency is entirely corrupt, and has been for decades.

While the Department of Justice prepares indictments, make a public declaration that your administration will ignore all their COVID case numbers and recommendations. They're criminal liars. That's their whole game.

Let me help you out with four examples. Face it, you're not good with details, so you may want a team to summarize the following revelations for you.

ONE: The Atlantic, May 21, 2020, has a story, headlined, "How could the CDC make that mistake?"

I'll give you the key quotes, and then comment on the stark inference The Atlantic somehow failed to grasp.

"We've learned that the CDC is making, at best, a debilitating mistake: combining test results that diagnose current coronavirus infections with test results that measure whether someone has ever had the virus...The agency confirmed to The Atlantic on Wednesday that it is mixing the results of viral [PCR] and antibody tests, even though the two tests reveal different information and are used for different reasons."

"Several states—including Pennsylvania, the site of one of the country's largest outbreaks, as well as Texas, Georgia, and Vermont—are blending the data in the same way. Virginia likewise mixed viral and antibody test results until last week, but it reversed course and the governor apologized for the practice after it was covered by the Richmond Times-Dispatch and The Atlantic. Maine similarly separated its data on Wednesday; Vermont authorities claimed they didn't even know they were doing this."

"'You've got to be kidding me,' Ashish Jha, the K. T. Li Professor of Global Health at Harvard and the director of the Harvard Global Health Institute, told us when we described what the CDC was doing. 'How could the CDC make that mistake? This is a mess'."

"The CDC stopped publishing anything resembling a complete database of daily [COVID] test results on February 29. When it resumed publishing test data last week [the middle of May]..."

First of all, notice the CDC stopped reporting complete case numbers on a daily basis, for two and a half months. Remember that. I'll cover a more egregious CDC stoppage in a minute.

But here is the main event: The Atlantic fails to mention the true outcome of this "test-combining mistake" at the CDC—which, in fact, is a purposeful maneuver. Only the PCR should be used for case-counting (according to the conventional experts).

You take those two types of tests, the antibody and the PCR...put them together, add up those results which suggest COVID in any relevant or irrelevant way, and voila, you have inflated case numbers. Which is exactly what the CDC wants. They're in the business of raising false alarms and promoting epidemics. That's called a crime.

TWO: In August of 2014, a long-time researcher at the CDC, William Thompson, publicly admitted that he and his co-authors intentionally lied in their study of the MMR vaccine.

They concluded the vaccine did not raise the risk of autism. But they knew this was a fabrication. Their data (which they threw out in the trash) pointed to an increased risk of autism in very young African American children.

Thompson refused to speak with the press, after he published his confession on his attorney Rick Morgan's website. Thompson said he would testify at a Congressional hearing. Despite efforts, a hearing never materialized. Thompson remained silent, and the CDC reassigned him to another unit.

No one at the CDC has been prosecuted for this crime.

THREE: In the fall of 2009, during the so-called Swine Flu epidemic, CBS investigative reporter, Sharyl Attkisson, discovered the CDC had secretly stopped counting cases in the US.

Yet, the agency was claiming tens of thousands of Americans had the epidemic disease.

She found out why the CDC had gone dark. Here is an excerpt from an interview I did with Attkisson:

Rappoport: "In 2009, you spearheaded coverage of the so-called Swine Flu pandemic. You discovered that, in the summer of 2009, the Centers for Disease Control, ignoring their federal mandate, [secretly] stopped counting Swine Flu cases in America. Yet they continued to stir up fear about the 'pandemic,' without having any real measure of its impact. Wasn't that another investigation of yours that was shut down? Wasn't there more to find out?"

Attkisson: "The implications of the story were even worse than that. We discovered through our FOI efforts that before the CDC mysteriously stopped counting Swine Flu cases, they had learned that almost none of the cases they had counted as Swine Flu was, in fact, Swine Flu or any sort of flu at all! The interest in the story from one [CBS] executive was very enthusiastic. He said it was 'the most original story' he'd seen on the whole Swine Flu epidemic. But others pushed to stop it [after it was published on the CBS News website] and, in the end, no [CBS television news] broadcast wanted to touch it. We aired numerous stories pumping up the idea of an epidemic, but not the one that would shed original, new light on all the hype. It was fair, accurate, legally approved and a heck of a story. With the CDC keeping the true Swine Flu stats secret, it meant that many in the public took and gave their children an experimental vaccine that may not have been necessary."

Total CDC fakery. Turning a Nothing into a "pandemic" and selling it. Needless to say, that is a crime.

But it isn't end of the story.

[..]

- https://blog.nomorefakenews.com/2020/07/16/mr-trump-deliver-knockout-blow-to-traitorous-cdc/

****

July 17, 2020, 6:49PM (Amir-ul Kafirs to group):

Here is a whole bunch of information on the corruption within the CDC:

I looked at this but I'm not going to read every article linked to at the moment, if ever.

& this dramatic rant from Jon Rappoport also addresses some of this, more succinctly

Alright, this guy. I don't really have any trouble believing his claims that the CDC manufactures pandemics & then supports profiting off of them. After all, that's what we seem to be in the midst of now. HOWEVER, it's this sort of thing that I find hard to take:

"I assure you, Mr. Trump, the four examples I've cited are only a particle of a sliver of a tip of the scandal. The CDC has been operating as a criminal agency inside the United States for a very long time.

"Sending in the FBI to seize records, indicting and prosecuting hundreds, at the very least, of their employees and top executives, and cutting the agency off from any input whatsoever concerning COVID, would mark a tremendous service to the nation."

Is this guy's every solution to *send in the troops?!* & does he actually believe that Rump would do anything that's good for anybody other than himself?!

It seems that they are big vaccine supporters,

Are there any government health agencies that're taking a more cautious line regarding vaccines? It seems unlikely. Everyone's afraid of being tarred the way that annoying Science reporter tarred Kennedy: "are you trying to put us back in the dark ages?" (or whatever it was she said) — just like everyone's afraid of being called a "Conspiracy Theorist". Nobody seems to be afraid of milking the Big Pharma cash cow. Money talks & health care walks.

****

July 16, 2020, 8:40PM (Amir-ul Kafirs to group):

I'm sitting in a Day's Inn in MI near a nice lake after having driven 7.5 hrs to buy a used vibraphone. I'm watching a scifi movie called R.I.P.D.. I haven't looked at my social media today. Judging by what Linda says I have a new enemy I'll be blocking soon. It's 'funny', I literally have spent too much of my life being hated simply bc I clear-headly express thoughtful but unpopular opinions. Oh, well.

****

July 16, 2020, 9:01PM (Inquiring Librarian to group):

RE: HERETICS: Children

If i posted what i thought, like u do, i am positive most of my friends would attack me also and i would unfriend them all. Lately i have posted a few vague things that have gotten little to no comment from my sheep friends, and a couple got the message wrong assuming i was too ignorant to understand the obvious that i was in actuality tearing apart and using to allude to today's 'situation'.

****

July 17, 2020, 3:08AM (Dick to group):

TR: Free virtual summer camps

I'm transfering a mail from microsoft, I assume many of you received it, but just in case, here it is
it's about virtual summer camps
what a hellish idea
instead of sending kids to real lakes, camp sites, the beach, or whatever, they use the computer and build digital skills
i think this confirms the ideas about the desocializing of kids
it's like in the future they will have no lives outside of the computer

De : Microsoft Store
Envoyé : vendredi 17 juillet 2020 05:39
À :
Objet : Free virtual summer camps

Spark curiosity with free virtual summer camps

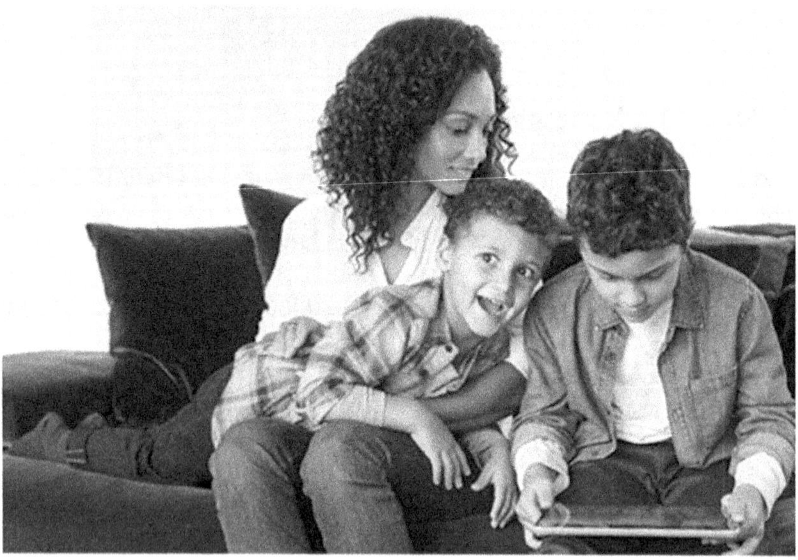

Make good use of free time with the Summer Passport for Digital Fun: a series of interactive workshops for kids. They'll be so busy having fun, they'll forget they're building valuable digital skills.

****

July 17, 2020, 6:57PM (Amir-ul Kafirs to group):

Re: TR: Free virtual summer camps

what a hellish idea

Absolutely hellish & against everything that makes summer camps valuable & important. HOWEVER, it does serve Bill Gates's apparent interests perfectly: reroute everyone's socialization away from actual human contact to mediated contact & turn them into zombies for big business: the perfect Asperger's Syndrome Manchurian Candidiates!

Naia Nisnam was offered to run such a camp & declined.

****

July 17, 2020, 3:13AM (Dick to group):

a guy I follow who does film analysis posted this

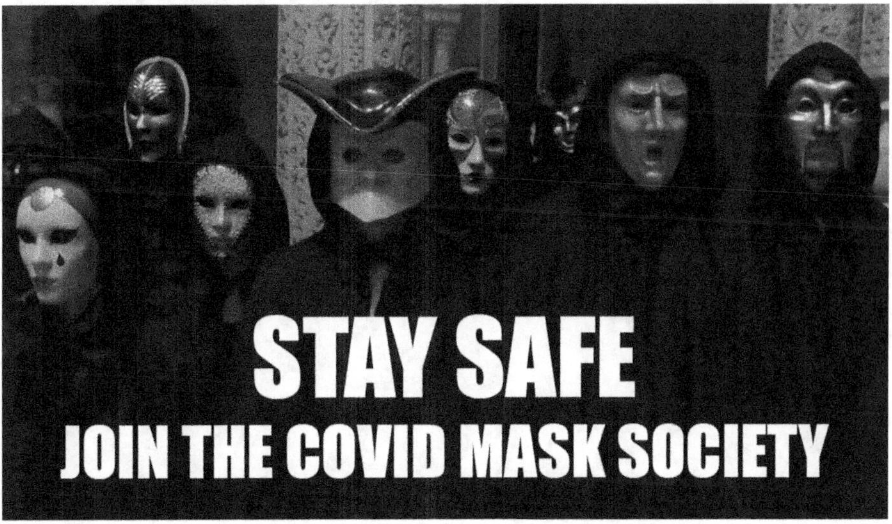

****

July 17, 2020, 5:41PM (Amir-ul Kafirs to group):

Why don't you do a News Program? "The Heretic News"...

Dick, ***I'd love to do it*** & it might be fun for everyone but I'm so overextended right now it's insane. I have more projects that're laying barely touched than I can even stand to think about. I've been totally neglecting my feature about _____. I have a new short I should be working on. I have 3 book reviews to write. I have 2 new notation apps to install & learn. I have 2 pieces of (M)Usic to (d) compose. I have something like 20 new instruments in my house to place, tune, & play. They're taking up so much space right now I can barely walk around. Basically, I spend so much of every day just replying to emails here that I have very little time for anything else. I haven't even worked on the HERETICS book except to accumulate the HERETICS emails into monthly files. In addition to all that, I'm *trying to have some fun*. Naia Nisnam & I are both close to losing our minds here surrounded by so many zombies & we try to at least go to a drive-in movie once a week. Even that takes planning & time. I feel like my life is falling apart around me. I hardly slept at all last night & that coupled with all the driving is making me feel like I might collpase at any moment. &, yet, I'm still going to work on emails here until I can't stand it anymore (which might be soon).

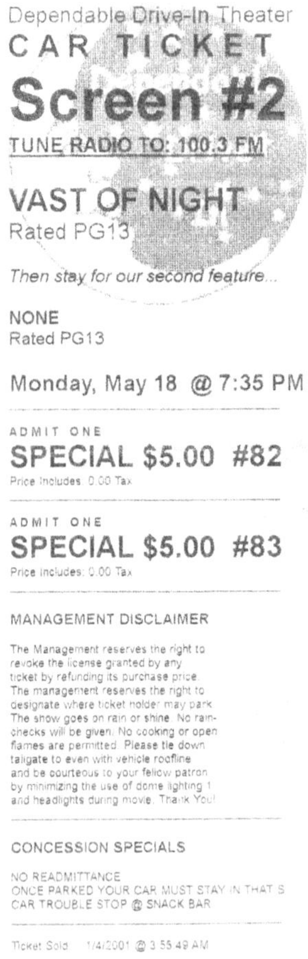

Dependable Drive-In Theater
CAR TICKET
Screen #2
TUNE RADIO TO: 100.3 FM

VAST OF NIGHT
Rated PG13

Then stay for our second feature...

NONE
Rated PG13

Monday, May 18 @ 7:35 PM

ADMIT ONE
SPECIAL $5.00 #82
Price Includes: 0.00 Tax

ADMIT ONE
SPECIAL $5.00 #83
Price Includes: 0.00 Tax

MANAGEMENT DISCLAIMER

The Management reserves the right to revoke the license granted by any ticket by refunding its purchase price. The management reserves the right to designate where ticket holder may park. The show goes on rain or shine. No rain-checks will be given. No cooking or open flames are permitted. Please tie down taligate to even with vehicle roofline and be courteous to your fellow patron by minimizing the use of dome lighting 1 and headlights during movie. Thank You!

CONCESSION SPECIALS

NO READMITTANCE
ONCE PARKED YOUR CAR MUST STAY IN THAT S
CAR TROUBLE STOP @ SNACK BAR

Ticket Sold 1/4/2001 @ 3:55:49 AM

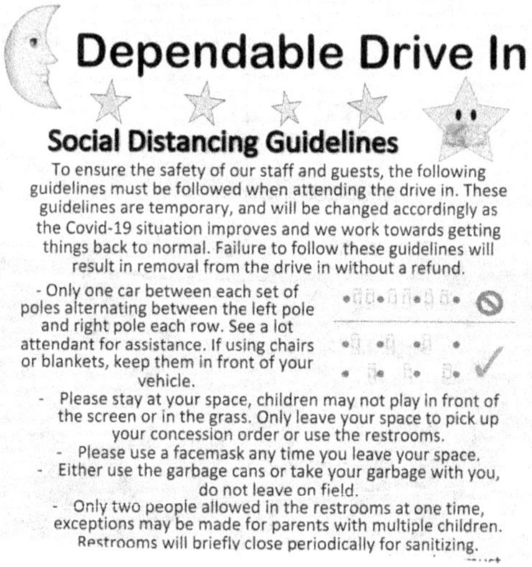

Dependable Drive In

Social Distancing Guidelines

To ensure the safety of our staff and guests, the following guidelines must be followed when attending the drive in. These guidelines are temporary, and will be changed accordingly as the Covid-19 situation improves and we work towards getting things back to normal. Failure to follow these guidelines will result in removal from the drive in without a refund.

- Only one car between each set of poles alternating between the left pole and right pole each row. See a lot attendant for assistance. If using chairs or blankets, keep them in front of your vehicle.
- Please stay at your space, children may not play in front of the screen or in the grass. Only leave your space to pick up your concession order or use the restrooms.
- Please use a facemask any time you leave your space.
- Either use the garbage cans or take your garbage with you, do not leave on field.
- Only two people allowed in the restrooms at one time, exceptions may be made for parents with multiple children. Restrooms will briefly close periodically for sanitizing.

****

July 17, 2020, 5:56PM (Dick to group):

I understand, I know how busy you are, good luck with it
Let's just keep the idea in our heads and maybe one day the moment will arrive when it could be useful
I am dealing , too, with a lot of stuff - my son and my brother are both having

problems (of different types but problems anyway)
and other stuff too is making like hard, essentially I feel drugged half the time and can hardly stand it anymore
Anyway, hang in there and keep trying to have fun, I think that's important at a time like this !

****

July 17, 2020, 6:04PM (Amir-ul Kafirs to group):

RE: HERETICS: Children

Even though the person attacking my comment was clearly misguided, she was VICIOUS!!

As far as I'm concerned, she looked like a total fool to anyone paying attention who isn't similarly afflicted with ZOMBIEISM. I mean she lectured you to get off your ivory tower (not the expression she used but something similar) & get out & work with real kids when, HEY!, that's already your profession! Then she wrote off your links as "BS" without, obviously, having the slightest clue about what they are. Then she listed NPR & a few other things as her sources as if they're obviously perfect. At this point the Democrats have become so desperate to get rid of Rump that NPR has probably become the liberal equivalent to Fox 'News'.

ANYWAY, that despicable commenter: We lived in a 2 floor deluxe apartment in BalTimOre originally leased to rich young'un _____ in 1988. Commenter & I lived there until 1989 when they bought a house & their partner, _____, & another person named _____ & I moved in with her. Strangely, I remember what everyone EXCEPT commenter did for a living. I was closer to everyone else BUT commenter but we were friends. Commenter & _____ broke up in 1991ish & _____ & I moved into a warehouse in downtown BalTimOre. I don't remember _____ being an artist or a political activist or even a particularly politically concerned person or a scholar or, really, much of anything else. They must've had money or they wouldn't have been able to buy the house we lived in. I imagine they were a bit of a yuppie.

The point is that their incredible pomposity against what I wrote & against Inquiring Librarian & Naia Nisnam defending it isn't in any way that I know of justified by their being some sort of long-term 'Social Justice Warrior'. They're like someone who meets a black person & then explains civil rights to a political activist with her new expertise or meets a Jew & explains the holocaust to an anti-nazi. I keep having this kind of experience over & over again: people who know next to nothing lecturing me on things I'm an expert on. Imagine my having read roughly 5,000 books & having written about 1,500 of them & being published as a writer in about 2,000 instances. Now imagine someone who's just learned that the word "in" is a preposition. Now imagine this "in" person skims about one book a year & lectures me on English, saying something like: *You should really read Hemingway* — when, of course, I would've read Hemingway when I was a teenager. SO, Good Riddance to despicable commenter.

Dick might appreciate this: I used to joke that BalTimOre was so right wing that even the left wing was right wing. That's an exaggeration, of course, but most of these people that I'm unfriending & blocking on social media are old BalTimOre 'friends': people that I know as very conservative who're posing as liberals. _____, e.g., sold a commissioned miniature diorama on the theme of the Star-Spangled Banner to President Bush Sr. Can you imagine me doing something like that?!

don't fuck 'em!

****

July 17, 2020, 6:12PM (Amir-ul Kafirs to group):

RE: HERETICS: Children P.s.

P.s. One of the sickest things about despicable commenter's attack was their implication that I'd be afraid to work with kids right now!! That boggled my mind given that it had never occurred to me to be afraid of being around kids & given that I'm around Naia Nisnam's kids just about every week, with none of us wearing a mask. Commenter's a very ordinary person who's quite probably never taken a risk in her life while I've been taking major risks since I was about 14 if not younger. At that age I had a guy hold a switchblade to my throat & tell me he was going to cut my throat. I told him to go ahead. He didn't. I don't think commenter's ever had the chutzpah to rock the boat at all. & this is the type of person who attacks me?! What an asshole.

****

July 17, 2020, 6:15PM (Amir-ul Kafirs to group):

[COVID MASK SOCIETY]

I deduce that's from "Eyes Wide Shut".

****

July 17, 2020, 6:19PM (Dick to group):

yeah, it is
the guy is interesting, his name is Rob Ager
he makes film analysis videos, some are better than others but when he does Kubrick he seems to be at his best
he is also interested in conspiracy theories as a phenomenon
i wrote him to ask what he thought about the covid-19 business, maybe he'll do something, if he did, it could be interesting

****

July 17, 2020, 5:01PM (Amir-ul Kafirs to group):

RE: HERETICS: Children (Thought Police)

1st, I'm truly sorry that Inquiring Librarian & Naia Nisnam were lambasted by that idiot commenter. HOWEVER, I'm deeply touched that you 2 came to my defense & that you did it so eloquently without having to resort to anything as nasty as what commenter was saying. I'll write about that in more detail later. Starting yesterday morning around 8:30 I drove 15.5 hours out of the next 27.5 hours to go to Michigan to get a vibraphone I bought. Given that I HATE driving long-distance that was quite a feat for me. I'm still burnt-out from it & slowly recovering. I have managed to eek out the following text panel as a spoof on commenter & her ilk so I hope that Inquiring Librarian & Naia Nisnam get a good laugh out of it. I don't specifically mention commenter, of course, but I think the spirit of what it's aimed at is pretty clear. I've already unfriended & blocked them so they won't see it.

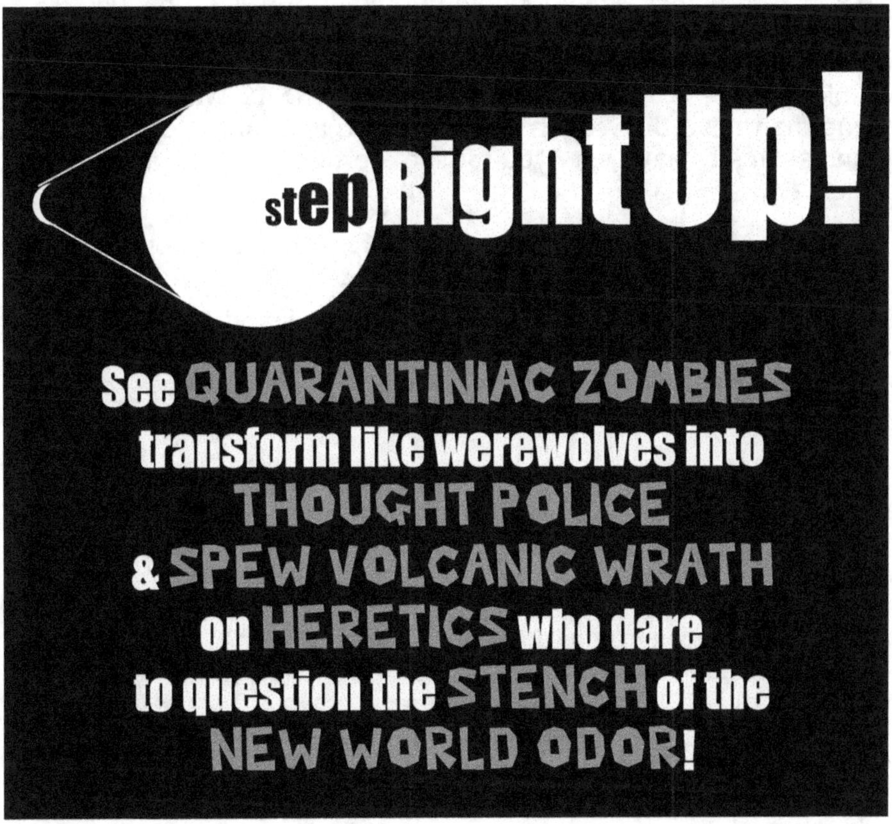

****

July 17, 2020, 6:30PM (Naia Nisnam to group):

Another doctor who seems to make logical sense

The False-Positive Panic Over COVID-19 - LewRockwell

https://www.lewrockwell.com/2020/07/no_author/the-false-positive-panic-over-covid-19/

****

The False-Positive Panic over COVID-19

By Neil A. Kurtzman, MD
Mises.org
July 17, 2020

Imagine an articulate chief lemming bragging that not only had his followers jumped off a cliff, but that they had done so in far greater numbers than any other slice of the rodents. This is the position occupied by the US regarding testing for COVID-19.We've done more testing than any other country and bragged a lot about doing so; but no one seems to have survived to give a proper interpretation of the results.

To begin with, the tests currently in use do not test for the entire virus, rather they just test for various fragments of it. Many of the results are thus false, sometimes false positives and sometimes false negatives. This means one has to interpret their results with caution. Our medical authorities, to say nothing of our political ones, don't seem to be able to do this.

All medical students are taught the basics of screening in their introductory statistics course. The problem is that most of them either didn't go or slept through the course. The rest immediately forgot what they had learned.

When testing for anything, a medical professional needs to know the positive predicative value (PPV) of the test as well as the negative predictive value. I'll focus on the former.

In order to know the PPV—i.e., the percent likelihood that a positive test is a true positive—the sensitivity of the test must be known as well as prevalence of the disease, at least to an approximate degree. According to a recent article in the *New England Journal of*

Medicine, the sensitivity of the tests for COVID-19 is about 70 percent. The prevalence in any of the tested populations is not yet known, so we cannot calculate the PPV, although we can calculate what it would be at any prevalence level we want to assume. I'll get back to this below.

A test for COVID-19 that is 70 percent sensitive will only catch 70 percent of the tested subjects with the disease. Therefore, 30 percent will falsely test negative. Additionally, Bayes's theorem, the mere mention of which defeats the numeracy of all but the most resolute of physicians, says that a 70 percent sensitive test will be positive in 30 percent of the tested population that doesn't have the disease. (I am assuming a specificity that is also 70 percent. The specificity of the various tests used has not been given.) Consider testing for COVID-19 in 1 million subjects, none of whom harbors the virus. Three hundred thousand will test positive.

[..]

The Johns Hopkins COVID-19 tracker that is widely used and quoted considers a confirmed test to be equal to a positive test. This is an error of epic dimensions for the reasons just stated.

[..]

How does one estimate the PPV of a COVID-19 test? At 70 percent sensitive there's no need to. Such a test is so contaminated with both false positives and negatives that its use is virtually without utility. Suppose we had a test that was 95 percent sensitive and specific. The PPV is the number of true positives divided by the sum of true and false positives. To make this calculation we must assume a prevalence of the virus in the sampled group. Let's start with a prevalence of 1 percent. If we test 10,000 subjects, 100 will carry the virus. Of these, 95 will test positive. Bayes's theorem says 495 (5 percent of the 9,900 patients) without the virus will also have a positive result. That's 495 false positive tests. The PPV in this hypothetical sample is 95/95+495, or about 16 percent.

Now assume our population (again 10,000 subjects) has 50 percent true positives. Here our PPV is 95 percent (4700/ 4700+250). The relationship of PPV to prevalence is given in the figure below. Note that even with a 95 percent sensitive test we'll be overwhelmed with false positive results if our tested population has a low prevalence for the virus. The more we test, the more false positives we're likely to get if our testing is not focused.

Effects of Prevalence Sensitivity=95% Specificity=95%

Population's Prevalence	Predictive Value of a Positive Test
0.1%	1.9%
1.0%	16.1%
2.0%	27.9%
5.0%	50%
50%	95%

It should be obvious from the data above that all the testing we have done and continue to do has likely confused more than enlightened. The virus is real and in the wild. How should we effectively deal with it? The best indicator of our status is how many people are in the hospital because of a *clinical* diagnosis of viral pneumonia. More specifically, how many are in the ICU. Note that testing here is unnecessary, as the assumption today is that any case of viral pneumonia is caused by the coronavirus.

[..]

Neil A Kurtzman, MD, is Grover E. Murray Professor Emeritus and University Distinguished Professor Emeritus at Texas Tech University Health Sciences Center.

- https://www.lewrockwell.com/2020/07/no_author/the-false-positive-panic-over-covid-19/

****

July 17, 2020, 7:59PM (Amir-ul Kafirs to group):

Re: Another doctor who seems to make logical sense

Ok, I read it. It seems reasonable to me but then I'm not in any way even remotely an expert on such things so a contrary argument might also seem reasonable.

****

July 18, 2020, 8:54AM (Dick to group):

here is a video by that film analysis guy, it's a sort of predictive video, he made it on 20 march
It's a bit chatty but I find he has some interesting ideas here and there
some of his predictions seem to have come true
I also find interesting the optimism which shows itself from time to time about a possible change for the better...i felt that too for a short time at the beginning of the lock-down but it quickly dissappeared

https://www.youtube.com/watch?v=ZtLUZ3W_G8Q&fbclid

Thoughts on Covid 19: social and psychological effects of the pandemic? - YouTube
Most discussion of the Coronavirus topic is about the short term effects of the pandemic. Here's my thoughts on the potential long term effects. WEBSITE: htt...

****

July 18, 2020, 12:30PM (Amir-ul Kafirs to group):

I only got 1:29 into this before it froze on my computer. I liked it so far. I'll probably add it to my PANDEMIC PANIC playlist because he talks about people's desire for the apocalypse which I don't think any of the other videos that I've linked to do. That's important stuff & it helps explain much of the fervent believer attitudes of people: it's like the end times have come for them & they're ready to sacrifice all sanity to it (as long as its 'safe', of course).

****

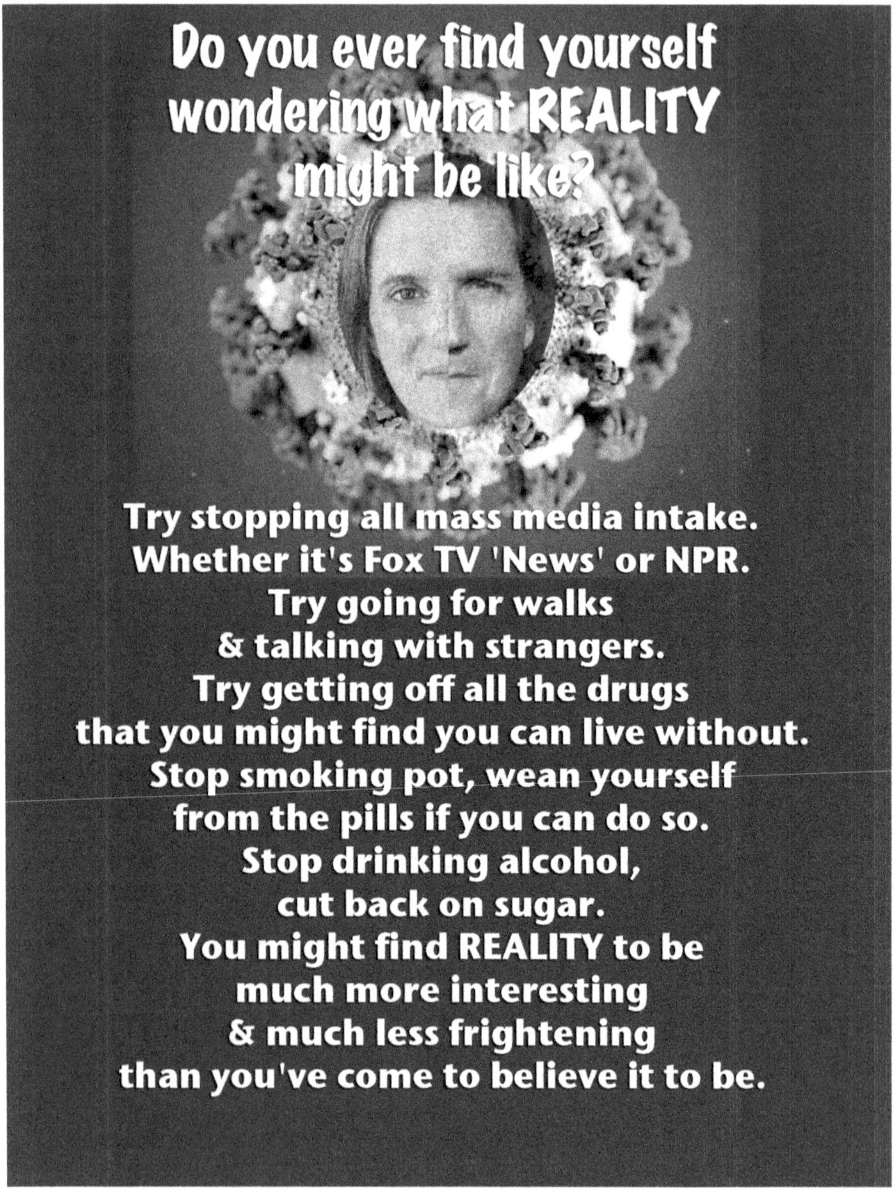

****

July 18, 2020, 12:33PM (Amir-ul Kafirs to group):

Re: HERETICS: Reality

In case you didn't figure it out that's Amy Goodman of NPR on the left & Tucker Carlson of Fox TV 'News' on the right.

****

July 18, 2020, 12:37PM (Dick to group):

Re: HERETICS: Reality

I like it a lot glad you kept coffee off the list

****

July 18, 2020, 12:58PM (Dick to group):

what you wrote is interesting, i recall when trump was elected many people said that to a great degree it was they wanted change -any change at all just to escape what could be called " the loop of the known" in politics
if that mood prevails, people will probably line up to have bio-metric chips, vaccines... boredom is what leads people to self-mutilation and all sorts of other undesirable activities

****

July 18, 2020, 2:07PM (Amir-ul Kafirs to group):

I was actually fairly moderate in my list of proposed abstentions. Withdrawal from the mass media is the most important part. I hope people realize that I'm implying that NPR & Fox TV 'News' *are the coronoavirus.*

****

July 18, 2020, 8:08PM (Amir-ul Kafirs to group):

Re: Free virtual summer camps pt 2 Rob Ager vid

I'm a little over halfway thru this one now. I find it a bit boring to watch because not much changes about it visually, it's just him talking. STILL, I think he nails it pretty good & covers multiple facets. The one thing he seems to get 'wrong' is that it can't become a right-left issue. Whew! Did he miss that one! I've been cutting back & forth between this & "Nazis at the Center of the Earth" (https://youtu.be/vxBs7WgqOCk) which has the nazi torture doctor, Joseph Mengele, as a survivor of WWII who continues his 'research' underground under Antarctica. It seems like a good mix for creating the special 'mood'.

****

July 18, 2020, 8:40PM (Amir-ul Kafirs to group):

Re: Free virtual summer camps pt 3 Rob Ager vid

One of the things that he discusses that interests me is the closing of borders. It's funny how liberals seem to think they're defying Rump by being pro-quarantyranny but it's always seemed to me that Rump's biggest issue has been closing borders & now he's getting that at a far more profound level than he could've achieved any other way.

ALSO, Ager's "optimism"? I think that's where he's the most foolish. He thinks people will become more competitive & that that's a good thing. Competitiveness in its typical capitalist manifestation usually just means more dirty tricks. He thinks people will get a 'reality check' & start to reconsider what's most important in their life. I don't see that happening at all. He thinks people will become more health-conscious. I don't see that as very likely either. It seems more likely that too many people will put their health-care in the hands of doctors who're little more than pushers for big pharma & that they'll get even less exercise than they did previously.

****

July 19, 2020, 9:05AM (Amir-ul Kafirs to group):

HERETICS: Nazi Killer Nurses

Well, lest I get less cynical & pessimistic about the medical profession I just had to find this:

"CARING CORRUPTED - The Killing Nurses of The Third Reich"

https://youtu.be/Rz8ge4aw8Ws

Cizik School of Nursing has created a REMI Platinum Award-winning documentary film that tells the grim cautionary tale of nurses who participated in the Holocaust and abandoned their professional ethics during the Nazi era. The 56-minute film, Caring Corrupted: the Killing Nurses of the Third Reich, casts a harsh light on nurses who used their professional skills to murder the handicapped, mentally ill and infirm at the behest of the Third Reich and directly participated in genocide.

****

July 19, 2020, 9:46AM (Amir-ul Kafirs to group):

HERETICS: Scenarios for the Future of Technology and International Development

In case Event 201's suspicious prescience wasn't enough for you, here's the Rockefeller Foundation & GBN (Global Business Network)'s "Scenarios for the Future of Technology and International Development" from 2010 attached as a PDF. I quote from page 19. This was called to my attention by a friend in

Canada.

"During the pandemic, national leaders around the world flexed their authority and imposed airtight rules and restrictions, from the mandatory wearing of face masks to body-temperature checks at the entries to communal spaces like train stations and supermarkets. Even after the pandemic faded, this more authoritarian control and oversight of citizens and their activities stuck and even intensified." - p 19

In general, this particular "Scenario" that I quoted from is not particularly accurate in its prediction but it's close enough to be an uncomfortable fit. Keep in mind that the Anonymous movement's release on COVID-19 ("Anonymous Message To Bill Gates (proof and evidence from other sources in description)": https://youtu.be/iUNoiHrplcw) explained Bill Gates's 'philanthropy' as a PR move similar to that of Rockefeller in the earlier 20th century. SO, it's interesting to see the Rockefeller Foundation ahead of Gates again in pandemic predicting.

****

July 20, 2020, 9:07AM (Dick to group):

New habits...

Seen today at the post office... It says together we are learning new habits to simplify daily life.... masks are obligatory as of today and at the bottom it says 'even under the mask let's share a smile'!!

****

July 20, 2020, 9:47AM (Amir-ul Kafirs to group):

Re: New habits...

It says together we are learning new habits to simplify daily life....

"simplify daily life"?! How about 'minimize our enjoyment of life' instead?

it says 'even under the mask let's share a smile'!!

Alotof good that'll do. How about a demonic grimace instead? It's not like anyone will notice the difference.

****

July 20, 2020, 10:11AM (Amir-ul Kafirs to group):

HERETICS: It's just fucking endless..

Here's another one I came across thanks to Twitter:

https://labourbehindthelabel.org/covid-19-support-workers/

It's a call for help from a garment-industry labor-supporting organization. Here's a sample:

4. Prioritise worker safety: Brands and suppliers that continue production must comply with World Health Organisation guidance on social distancing and PPE to prevent spread of COVID-19. This includes all retail workers, factory workers, logistics workers, warehouse and delivery workers.
5. Respect the right to refuse work: Workers who stop working due to COVID-19 risks must not be penalized. Brands should ensure that all workers in their supply chains can self-isolate or stay at home if they have COVID-19 symptoms, without risking their employment.

That's an excerpt from this:

Dear Marks & Spencer, Primark, Next, Asda, Arcadia, ASOS & Boohoo,
COVID-19 has exposed deep inequalities embedded into global supply chains. It is vital that brands ensure that workers in their supply chains do not pay the greatest price for the pandemic. Please will you protect the workers who make your clothes by committing to:
1. Honour contracts: Brands should publicly confirm that they will not cancel orders and that they will pay originally agreed amounts on schedule. Brands should agree to requests from suppliers to extend deadlines and should not apply delay sanctions.
2. Pay wages and protect jobs: All employees and supply chain workers, who were working at the onset of the crisis, regardless of employment status should be paid their legally mandated wages and benefits, including severance payments and arrears.
3. Bailout the workers: Brands should support the capacity of employers to maintain workers' employment and wages (including, rehiring previously dismissed workers). Brands must act ethically and work to ensure that government bailouts in producing and consumer countries financially support employees and workers in their supply chains.
4. Prioritise worker safety: Brands and suppliers that continue production must comply with World Health Organisation guidance on social distancing and PPE to prevent spread of COVID-19. This includes all retail workers, factory workers, logistics workers, warehouse and delivery workers.
5. Respect the right to refuse work: Workers who stop working due to COVID-19 risks must not be penalized. Brands should ensure that all workers in their supply chains can self-isolate or stay at home if they have COVID-19 symptoms, without risking their employment.
6. Put people before profits: Shareholders should not be getting dividends and CEOs should not be getting bonuses whilst staff and supply chain workers are going unpaid.
7. Rebuild a more equitable industry: In the aftermath of the pandemic, brands

must commit to proper human rights due diligence to create more sustainable and resilient supply chains. Now is the time for brands to ensure that in the future all workers are paid a living wage, have safe and secure working conditions and access to social protection benefits.
Do let me know what you plan to do.
Yours truly,
Your Signature

Ordinarily, I might support something like this except for my disagreement with the basic premise which is that there's an extraordinary health crisis. In other words, there's no call for brands to recognize how ridiculous this all is there's just a call for them to impose better medical police state conditions. SO, instead of maybe acknowledging the worker's right to reject WHO guidelines as deranged, at best, & insidious, at worst, they're expected, once again, to comply 'for their own good'.

****

July 20, 2020, 10:45AM (Amir-ul Kafirs to group):

HERETICS: 2 things meant to convince me

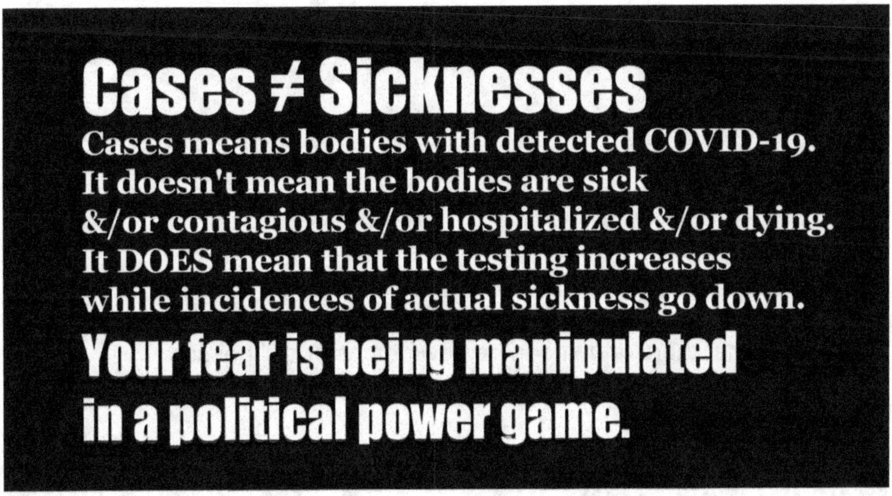

Cases ≠ Sicknesses
Cases means bodies with detected COVID-19.
It doesn't mean the bodies are sick
&/or contagious &/or hospitalized &/or dying.
It DOES mean that the testing increases
while incidences of actual sickness go down.
Your fear is being manipulated
in a political power game.

Remember when I posted that to social media a few days ago?

I thought what I was saying was obvious & clear.

A friend named ______ posted 2 links to 2 Johns Hopkins webpages that he thought might convince me that what I was saying isn't true. Not wanting to be like the people who refuse to look at what we link to but post violent opposition to it without having any idea of what it is I went to look at both webpages. The 1st one presents:

Rate of Positive Tests in the US and States Over Time

- https://coronavirus.jhu.edu/testing/individual-states/usa?fbclid=IwAR0b35Kw7UHKg8SFqPAdSiWCD-hfJFSN2sJB3zPn9oDwBG-cQN872shrdxU

& has this chart:

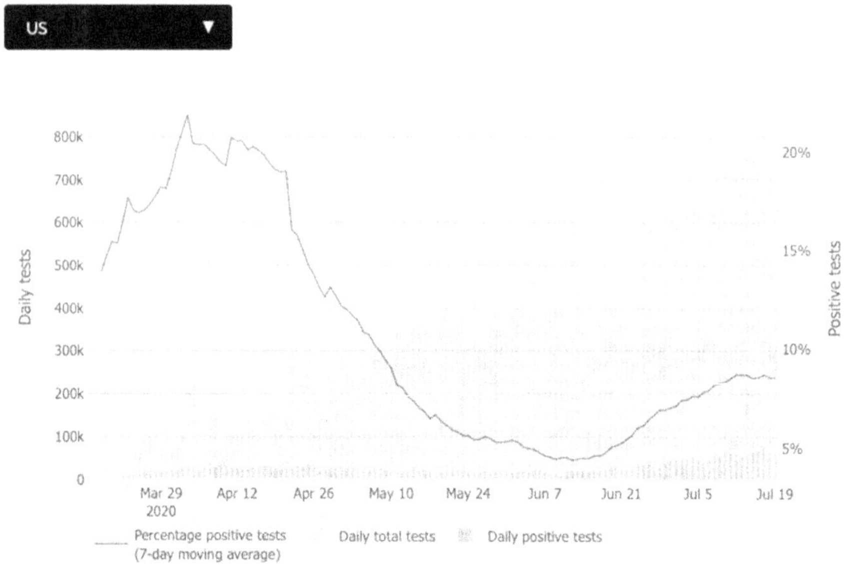

As far as I can tell, it says nothing other than what I'm trying to point out the emptiness of: viz: that if you test more people you'll find more cases but that that doesn't mean that there're going to be new deaths or sicknesses.

The 2nd one is called:

Timeline of COVID-19 policies, cases, and deaths in your state

A look at how social distancing measures may have influenced trends in COVID-19 cases and deaths

- https://coronavirus.jhu.edu/data/state-timeline/new-deaths/pennsylvania

& has this chart:

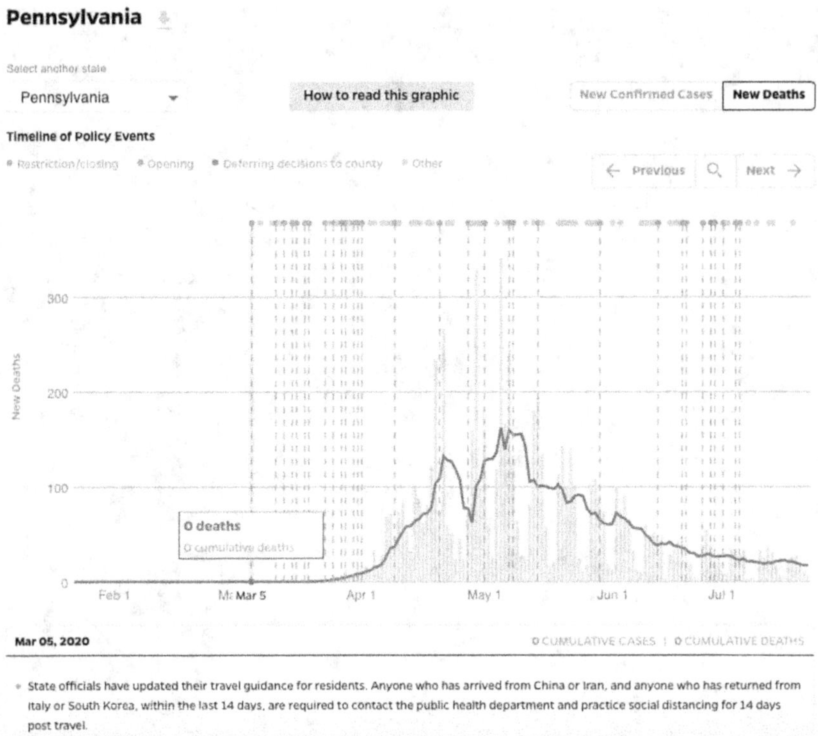

As far as I can tell, it says nothing other than what I'm trying to point out: that deaths are going down (except, apparently, in FLA, a retirement state with, therefore, a high percentage of older people that we can expect a higher likelihood of dying from) independent of the cases tested positive for. I also don't see how this tells us what the effects of social distancing have been on these statistics. if I understand the color coding correctly, the death stats rise & fall independent of the measures taken to hypothetically prevent new deaths.

SO, apparently what I thought was a clear statement didn't reach _____ at all. In other words, the usual signs of BRAIN-BLOCK are at work.

****

July 20, 2020, 11:39AM (tENT to group):

HERETICS: BRAIN-BLOCK

Are you exhibiting signs of
BRAIN-BLOCK?
When someone suggests that you read an article or look at statistics that you fear may go contrary to entrenched positions that have come to dominate your life do you automatically insult the person without really having any idea of what the articles say or the statistics show?
Then you may have BRAIN-BLOCK, a serious mental health condition that's destroying your ability to THINK FREELY.
This is not incurable & probably won't result in your death.
It's simply a symptom of your fear of being rejected by your preferred subculture.
TRY CLEAR-THINKING TODAY!
You'll make enemies but they weren't worth being friends with in the 1st place.

****

July 20, 2020, 2:59PM (Dick to group):

Re: HERETICS: BRAIN-BLOCK

This is a little bit cheesy but to a certain degree it reminds me of the current world situation:
https://www.youtube.com/watch?v=30JSXzfwSLs

****

July 20, 2020, 5:41PM (Amir-ul Kafirs to group):

Re: HERETICS: BRAIN-BLOCK

This is a little bit cheesy but to a certain degree it reminds me of the current world situation:
https://www.youtube.com/watch?v=30JSXzfwSLs

Do you know Anne McGuire's work? (http://www.vdb.org/artists/anne-mcguire) She made a movie called "Strain Andromeda The" & another called "Adventure Poseiden The". Both take the original movies & reorder the shots in reverse order — something that completely fucks with the dramatic tension of them.

****

July 20, 2020, 5:44PM (Inquiring Librarian to group):

Re: HERETICS: 2 things meant to convince me

Yes. I get this same brick wall brainedness every time I try to approach someone with the thought of considering the logic of all of this. I too have provided graphs, articles, prominent well credentialed scientists' and medical professional's views. All to no avail. I just get shot down, criticized, told it's all bs, and sometimes they even try, like Amir-ul Kafirs's friend, to brainlessly 'school' me in the 'science'.
I have given up on trying to open new people's minds. I'm instead concentrating on trying to fish for new people in hiding who realize the pandemic is really a scamdemic. I have found several over the past few weeks. We are all freaked out. It just plain sucks. I'm at my wits end with this nonsense. I'm considering now just how I can survive in a new way of life when I flee the obvious forcible injection that we will all be faced with within a year's time. I have had to unfollow most of my social media friends because I cannot deal with their idiotic pleading for more lockdowns, screaming for a 'vaccine' cureall, and ratting on their friends. It disgusts me. It is looking more and more to me like society as a whole will be split in the not too distant future. If the biomedical technocrats do not basically kill us, then those of us who chose not to be forced into their lifestyle will create an alternate society where we can live more naturally, we will have our own neighborhoods and businesses and schools and stores and farms, etc... This is in my ideal world because I feel like the old world is not coming back.

I found this James Corbett podcast interesting:
https://www.corbettreport.com/mybody/

& here is another great new C.J. Hopkins article:
https://consentfactory.org/2020/07/20/globocap-uber-alles/?fbclid=IwAR0u3em5bnSpHVlgytDUVQpzZysVl7bKn9BPWX7bQxIFnnY2WCq4oIi0qi4

& here is an exciting debate this coming Thursday that will be very interesting to watch. RFK Jr. rarely has a chance to debate over vaccines with anyone of significance, because most people know he will crush them with his knowledge. This could help our situation:
https://childrenshealthdefense.org/news/vaccine-debate-is-on-robert-f-kennedy-jr-vs-alan-dershowitz/

****

July 20, 2020, 6:25PM (Amir-ul Kafirs to group):

Re: HERETICS: 2 things meant to convince me

I was just about to get off the internet when I saw this message so this reply will be a short one.

Yes. I get this same brick wall brainedness every time I try to approach someone with the thought of considering the logic of all of this.

I don't think the situation's hopeless. Even the most brainwashed person has some entry point.

This could help our situation:
https://childrenshealthdefense.org/news/vaccine-debate-is-on-robert-f-kennedy-jr-vs-alan-dershowitz/

I'm not going to check this out right now but I'm definitely interested. Do any of you know who Alan Dershowitz is? I have a vague memory of him starting out as some sort of 'leftist' lawyer & then almost immediately becoming the guy-who-gets-rich-criminals-off. Here's a sample paragraph from his Wikipedia description:

"Dershowitz has been involved in several high-profile legal cases, including as a member of the defense team for the impeachment trial of Donald Trump. As a criminal appellate lawyer, he won 13 of the 15 murder and attempted murder cases which he had handled, and has represented a series of celebrity clients, including Mike Tyson, Patty Hearst, and Jim Bakker. His most notable cases included the successful appeal of Claus von Bülow's 1982 conviction for the attempted murder of his wife, Sunny, and the 1995 O. J. Simpson murder trial, in which he served on the legal "Dream Team", alongside Johnnie Cochran and F. Lee Bailey, as an appellate adviser. Dershowitz was also a member of the legal defense teams for the prominent sex offenders Harvey Weinstein and Jeffrey

Epstein, his personal friend. In 2006 he helped to negotiate a non-prosecution agreement on Epstein's behalf." - https://en.wikipedia.org/wiki/Alan_Dershowitz

I think you'll agree that's quite a selection of clients. It's strange that he couldn't get Jim Bakker off. It's hard for me to not think of him as the scum-of-the-earth so him debating Kennedy must really be something.

****

July 20, 2020, 7:23PM (BP to group):

Re: HERETICS: 2 things meant to convince me

Infuriating, ain't it?! Remember: In the beginning it was all about flattening the curve, don't overwhelm the hospital system. OKAY. I can understand that. But we knew it was gonna make it's way. And the hospital system, from what I can see, is NOT overwhelmed. Scary? Yea, sure. But no one ever said no one is ever going to die again. Be it lockdowns, masks, whatever, this thing creeps and crawls. Countless articles -- a major one recently that the "smart" people tout -- saying NYC combatted it best. Uhhhhh: No! And another big Times article taking down Sweden for their silly ways. But of course getting it all wrong! It was never about herd immunity there. It was about a BALANCE. A balance that we all need! Sooooo, a bit that drives me crazy is that the stereotypical liberal (or whatever it is they are labeled) always cites how the USA is a bunch of primitives compared to our enlightened friends over yonder in the Euro World. And there is truth to that! I don't always agree, but I definitely want to follow their lead and open up the garsh dang schools. It's a black out in the States pertaining to that info. Apparently the NFL (football league for you weirdo art people) just announced that there will be NO fan attendance this year. Stadiums that sit 80,000 plus people are now incapable of social distancing. REEEE DICK U LESS

****

July 20, 2020, 10:22PM (Inquiring Librarian to group):

HERETICS: Dr. Andrew Kaufman, July 17th Interview

I really 'enjoyed' this interview by Del Bigtree of Dr. Andrew Kaufman.
https://www.bitchute.com/video/w7TZzZFXX1ar/
I've listened to several interviews of Dr. Andrew Kaufman over the past few months concerning the 'pandemic'. This guy is great, and credentialed up the wazoo. Here, he discusses the idea of viruses, like bacteria, actually occurring naturally in the body, and coming out and causing harm when the body is under stress, and also coming out to repair and rework parts of your body internally when other parts go awry. That is really just a small shred of what Kaufman says in this. It is interesting, in the end, I shuddered a bit to consider, that he considered also, if this 'virus' really isn't a 'virus' per se in the sense that we consider a virus coming at us from the 'outside', what the hell are they planning

on injecting into our bodies?? I've been wondering this WAY TOO MUCH lately. It was 'nice' to hear a 'real' scientist actually mention this creepy unknown. Also, in a more hopeful direction, he ended with mentioning that many, many, many more real scientists are coming forward to dispute the absurdly, obviously, flawed narrative of this plandemic.

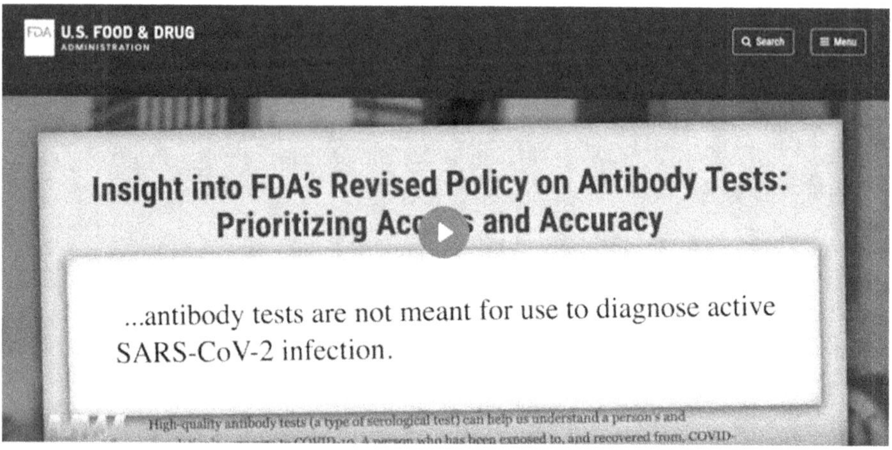

DEL BIGTREE INTERVIEWS DR ANDREW KAUFMAN - 17TH JULY 2020 | TH

WATCH

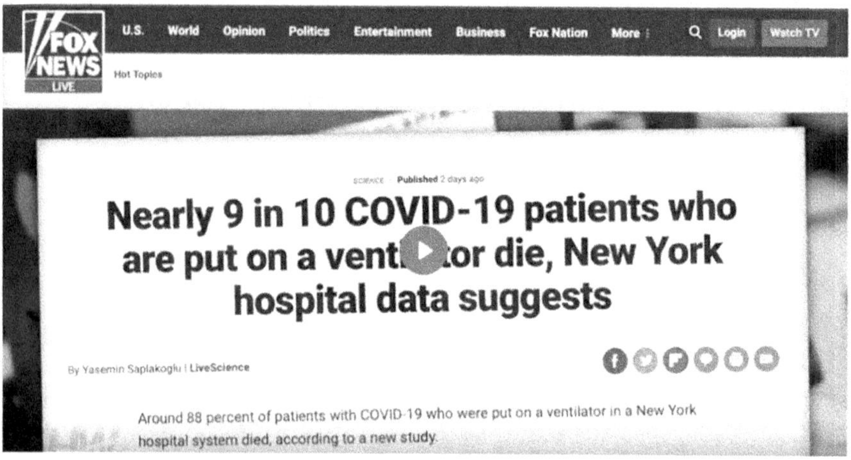

Well, here you go, it's a great interview, if you have the time to sit through it. I do my morning exercises and all of my cooking, many of my rides to the store and work, to this stuff. I've listened to hours and hours and hours and hours of interviews and talk shows on covid 19 over the past few months. My mind is really reeling with all of the information it is absorbing. It makes going to work daily and needing to live the lie such an out of mind and body experience. It's so hard to relate to or even acknowledge the fears and 'intellectual' banter pervading my staff who FULLY believe all of the nonsense. Obviously, I am grateful to be getting a paycheck.

Be well all. I'm losing my mind here in Louisiana. Does anyone want to move out to Montana or hide in the deep woods of New Hampshire with me? I feel like the time to hide is coming. I hope I am just being paranoid. I am honestly quite scared. But I am trying to keep from letting this get the best of me. I tend to get going when the going gets tough, but I dread these dark clouds forming.

****

July 20, 2020, 10:26PM (Inquiring Librarian to group):

Re: HERETICS: It's just fucking endless..

Something similar came to me in my email this weekend, from my local/national union. It was so obnoxious, citing the CDC and WHO and masks, etc... that I immediately felt nauseous from it and then promptly deleted it. I was tempted to write the sender back to give him/her a piece of my mind. But I restrained myself by taking a deep breath and clicking the delete button.

Well, that is that on that. I got my new ancient piano tuned this past weekend. I'm heading off to plunk out my struggling monkey tunes on it and feel grateful I still have another night in good health with a lovely roof over my head that will hopefully not be taken from me in the name of this insidious 'reset'.

****

July 20, 2020, 10:32PM (Inquiring Librarian to group):

Re: HERETICS: Reality

I think Amir-ul Kafirs's last statement, " I hope people realize that I'm implying that NPR & Fox TV 'News' *are the coronavirus."* is what John Waters was getting at in his graduation speech that I shared a couple of weeks ago. The students are the "vaccine", thus he would have been underhandedly implying the media is the 'virus'. Anways, I love this meme or whatever you call it, that Amir-ul Kafirs made.

****

July 21, 2020, 8:06AM (Amir-ul Kafirs to group):

HERETICS: Predictions

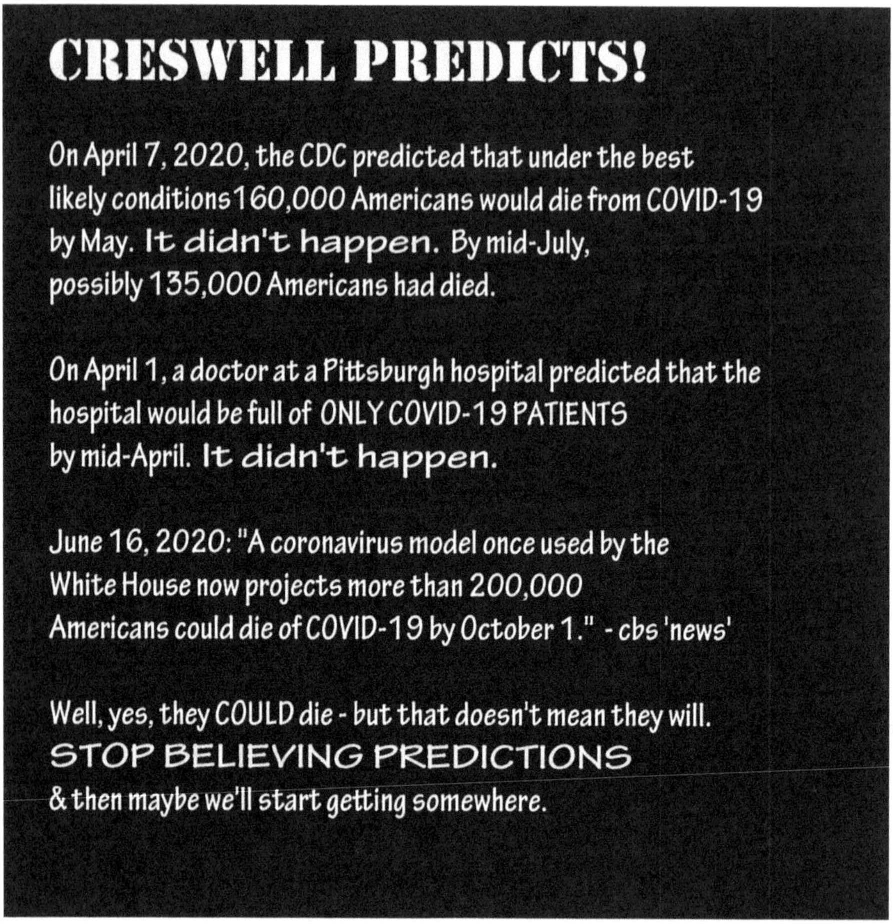

CRESWELL PREDICTS!
On April 7, 2020, the CDC predicted that under the best likely conditions 160,000 Americans would die from COVID-19 by May. It didn't happen. By mid-July, possibly 135,000 Americans had died.
On April 1, a doctor at a Pittsburgh hospital predicted that the hospital would be full of ONLY COVID-19 PATIENTS by mid-April. It didn't happen.
June 16, 2020: "A coronavirus model once used by the White House now projects more than 200,000 Americans could die of COVID-19 by October 1." - cbs 'news'
Well, yes, they COULD die - but that doesn't mean they will.
STOP BELIEVING PREDICTIONS
& then maybe we'll start getting somewhere.

****

July 21, 2020, 8:44AM (Amir-ul Kafirs to group):

HERETICS: "Wearing Masks Saves Lives" censored on YouTube

Well, "Wearing Masks Saves Lives" lasted online for about 9 days before someone flagged it. It's so easy for anyone to censor anything these days if it's online. Fortunately, it's still on the Internet Archive but even there there never seem to be ANY views so I have to wonder what's happening with that. Here's the message from YouTube followed by my appeal:

YouTube

Hi onesownthoughts,

As you may know, our Community Guidelines describe which content we allow – and don't allow – on YouTube. Your video Wearing Masks Saves Lives was flagged to us for review. Upon review, we've determined that it may not be suitable for all viewers and it has been placed behind an age restriction.

Video content restrictions

If a video contains violent or graphic content that appears to be posted in a shocking, sensational, or disrespectful manner, it's less likely to be allowed on YouTube. We also don't allow content that's intended to incite violence or encourage dangerous activities. We review content on a case by case basis and will only make limited exceptions for appropriate educational, documentary, artistic, and scientific contexts, where the purpose of posting is clear.

In light of this, we ask that uploaders post as much information as possible in the title and description of their video to help us and viewers understand the primary purpose of the video. Please note, even with this additional context, it's still not acceptable to post violent or gory content that's primarily intended to be shocking, sensational, or disrespectful and this type of content is prohibited on YouTube. Learn more here.

How you can respond

If you believe this was a mistake, we'd like to hear from you. To appeal this age restriction, please submit this form. Our team will thoroughly review your appeal and will contact you again very soon.

For more information on YouTube's Community Guidelines, please visit our Help Center.

Sincerely,
- The YouTube Team

Reduced to their 800 word limit:

Whoever flagged my video entitled "Wearing Masks Saves Lives" did not do so to call attention to its purported "violence" they did so to censor its anti-propaganda message. There're many valid opinions from doctors that wearing masks not only don't save anyone's life but actually are bad for both physical and mental health. People such as yourselves who yield to such censorship efforts would do well to remember Pastor Niemöller's famous poem about the German Nazi Era, an abridged version of which follows:

Then they came for the Jews, and I did not speak out—

Because I was not a Jew.
Then they came for me—and there was no one left to speak for me.

The more you give in to the type of person who flagged this video, the more you allow Free Speech to be destroyed.

****

Fulll version:

Whoever flagged my video entitled "Wearing Masks Saves Lives" did not do so to call attention to its purported "violence" they did so to censor its anti-propaganda message. There're many valid opinions from doctors that wearing masks not only don't save anyone's life but actually are bad for both physical and mental health. People such as yourselves who yield to such censorship efforts would do well to remember Pastor Niemöller's famous poem about the German Nazi Era, an abridged version of which follows:

First they came for the socialists, and I did not speak out—
Because I was not a socialist.
Then they came for the trade unionists, and I did not speak out—
Because I was not a trade unionist.
Then they came for the Jews, and I did not speak out—
Because I was not a Jew.
Then they came for me—and there was no one left to speak for me.

The "violence" in my movie in which a stopped car is bumped up against by a walking person who pretends to fling off of it is far from gory. Obviously, more violent images abound EVERYWHERE in our society, including on YouTube, where they constitute a central aspect of entertainment and so-called 'news'. The more you give in to the type of person who flagged this video, the more you allow Free Speech and other Civil Liberties to be destroyed. This is far from a joke, it's a very serious erosion of society.

****

July 21, 2020, 10:20PM (Inquiring Librarian to group):

Re: "Wearing Masks Saves Lives" censored on YouTube

Yes! Amazing letter Amir-ul Kafirs!!! I'm sure they will ignore it . But if it's not robots 'reading' it, it might make them think a little.

And boy that sucks someone ratted on it and it was taken down. The nerve!!! So many things are being taken off of Youtube and so many people are being thrown in to fb jail. It's ridiculous. Welcome to "Pravda!". I have mostly moved to Bitchute to listen to the videos and podcasts I'd like to hear. Sadly the audiences on this platform are much sparcer than on Youtube. But the audiences seem to grow by day. I see big promise in these other platforms. But to be honest, Bitchute is the only one I've checked out so far. It's wonderful so far for me at least though. Can you, Amir-ul Kafirs, make a Bitchute channel?? I will subscribe right away!! =] I love that you throw creativity and humor into your work. Most of my Bitchute channels are so serious. I was seriously considering how much better off my friends that died too young/too soon were than all of us after a weekend of Bitchute centered covid related listening. I mean, seriously I was feeling like a glass of cyanide wouldn't be so bad right now. The humor is needed. I stand firm on not becoming a victim, to fight the good fight until the end catches me, not me catching the end.

****

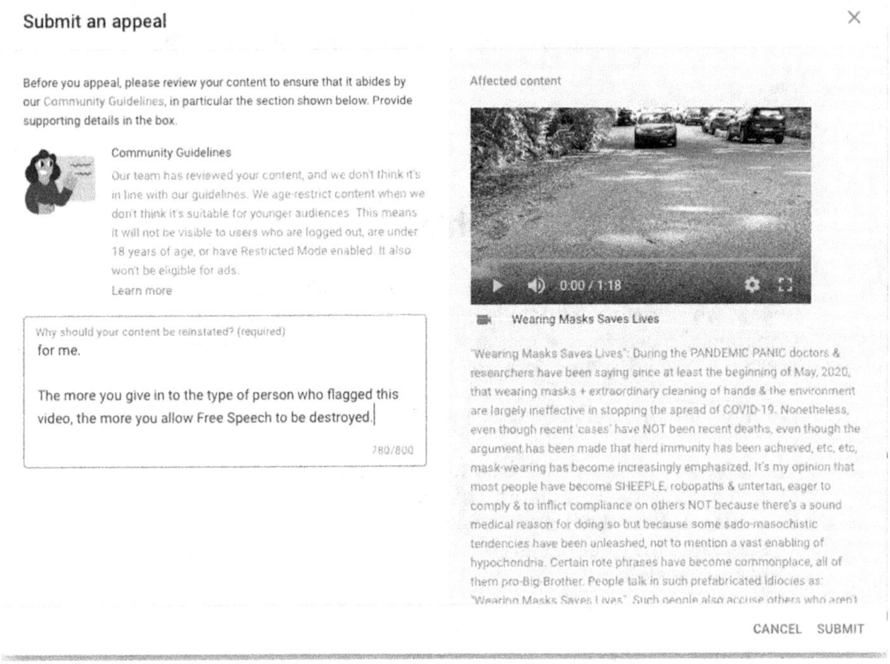

****

July 21, 2020, 8:47AM (Dick to group):

RE: HERETICS: "Wearing Masks Saves Lives" censored on YouTube

wow, sorry to hear this
amazing people flag videos
whatever happened to freedom of speech

****

July 21, 2020, 10:21AM (Amir-ul Kafirs to group):

Re: HERETICS: "Wearing Masks Saves Lives" censored on YouTube

amazing people flag videos

I've made a new text panel addressing CENSORSHIP that refers to FLAGGING. That, hopefully, will go up in 2 days.

whatever happened to freedom of speech

It actually doesn't bother me much that it's been age restricted. It was never intended for children anyway & I always state as much about all my videos on YouTube. What bothers me is that any repressive &/or stupid &/or neurotic QUARANTINIAC can flag something of mine & cause something restrictive to happen to it. Here's the reply that I got from my YouTube appeal:

YouTube

Dear onesownthoughts,

Thank you for submitting your video appeal to YouTube. After further review, we've determined that while your video does not violate our Community Guidelines, it may not be appropriate for a general audience. We have therefore age-restricted your video.

For more information please visit the YouTube Help Center.

We apologize for the delay. Due to the recent global health crisis related to COVID-19, a number of our normal review processes have been disrupted and are experiencing delays. To stay up to date on any changes in our services—and our broader response to COVID-19—please check the Help Center.

Sincerely,
- The YouTube Team

While they "apologize for the delay" in their response because of some "global health crisis", they actually replied almost immediately — making it seem likely to me that anything mask &/or COVID-19 related is high priority.

****

July 24, 2020, 10:01PM (Amir-ul Kafirs to group):

Re: "Wearing Masks Saves Lives" censored on YouTube

Amazing letter Amir-ul Kafirs!!! I'm sure they will ignore it . But if it's not robots 'reading' it, it might make them think a little.

I have some hope that they read both my notes to the movie & my appeal letter & that that's why they only age-restricted & aren't even claiming that it violates their Community Guidelines. Maybe it's overly optimistic of me but knowing that their censorship policies are somewhat guided by ADL (Anti-Defamation League) people I think there's a chance that the quote from Pastor Niemöller might hit home. I mean, I seriously think that what's essentially happening is akin to a neo-nazi coup d'etat with a thousand year reich agenda so I can honestly appeal to the dangers along those lines.

so many people are being thrown in to fb jail.

I'm actually amazed I've only been censored on Facebook a couple of times. I think a part of it is that they mainly censor & fact-choke people with huge followings, which excludes me. PLUS, there's a tiny chance that I get a little respect from SOMEBODY as a 'famous artist' & that that earns me a little leeway.

Can you, Amir-ul Kafirs, make a Bitchute channel??

I think I already am a member because I subscribed to Spiro Skouras's channel or some such. So far, though, I've never been censored on the Internet Archive so I prefer that philosophically. Their mission statement appeals to me the most. They seem to have a Free Speech philosophy & an availability of information philosophy that's relatively unmarred by other political agendas. I'll use BitChute if I get forced out of everything else. I don't know what their upper file size limit is or if one has to pay to post. I have looked at a few of these alternate channels but I wasn't that impressed by any of them. YouTube sucks in some ways but it definitely reaches the most people. PLUS I can link to it on Goodreads which I can't do with the Internet Archive or Vimeo. Vimeo was fine until they started getting desperate for money.

I love that you throw creativity and humor into your work. Most of my Bitchute channels are so serious.

I get the impression they're mostly humorless & uncreative - kindof like the horrible movies that've been made in attempts to refute Michael Moore's work.

I stand firm on not becoming a victim, to fight the good fight until the end catches me, not me catching the end.

Even though we're a really small part of the resistance to this that doesn't mean we're absolutely useless. Every oppositional voice helps crack the PR of the dominant narrative a bit more.

****

July 24, 2020, 10:08PM (Amir-ul Kafirs to group):

Re: "Wearing Masks Saves Lives" censored on YouTube

And boy that sucks someone ratted on it and it was taken down.

I should clarify: IT WASN'T TAKEN DOWN, it was just age-restricted, which is fine with me because it's not really intended for kids. I went to it on a different computer than the one I usually use & it opened up fine without even any sort of disclaimer.

****

July 21, 2020, 1:25PM (Amir-ul Kafirs to group):

Re: HERETICS: 2 things meant to convince me

It was the younger people that were scared/freaked out.

Let's hope that they don't age into adults who continue to believe all this PANDEMIC PANIC nonsense.

Remember: In the beginning it was all about flattening the curve, don't overwhelm the hospital system. OKAY. I can understand that. But we knew it was gonna make it's way. And the hospital system, from what I can see, is NOT overwhelmed.

Right. Even those investigative reporter nurses countered the claim that the NYC hospitals were overcrowded. Now, NYC is being shuffled down the memory tube & Florida's the new poster child. Fear must march on.

Scary? Yea, sure. But no one ever said no one is ever going to die again.

It's funny isn't it that older people such as myself (66, had pneumonia twice, been diagnosed as diabetic) are often NOT afraid. I know I'm going to die eventually but it's not feeling like it's going to be anytime soon & I'm not particularly worried about it. The medical industry doesn't give us immortality, it gives us constant fear of death. I tried to explain to the last dr I went to that I'm not afraid of dying, I'm afraid of having my quality of life decline. If I had listened to her my quality of life would've declined considerably & my fear of death would've been constant. She literally tried to terrorize me into thinking/feeling like I was going to die any minute. Instead, I'm still in good health 10 months later.

Be it lockdowns, masks, whatever, this thing creeps and crawls. Countless articles -- a major one recently that the "smart" people tout -- saying NYC combatted it best. Uhhhhh: No!

Believe that one & they'll tell you another!! All those deaths didn't happen without hospital intervention. Anyone who had the misfortune to live in NYC at the time deserves pity. I was much more fortunate to live in Pittsburgh.

I definitely want to follow their lead and open up the garsh dang schools.

Yeah, the schools should reopen. Of course, I think EVERYTHING should reopen.

Stadiums that sit 80,000 plus people are now incapable of social distancing. REEEE DICK U LESS

Right, like they couldn't just seat 20,000 people in there instead if they must follow their stupid social distancing rules. Then again, the team owners & football players are all millionaires, they're not going to be hurting no matter what. In the meantime, the taxpayer pays for the stadiums so one crowd makes money while the other has it vacuumed away.

****

July 21, 2020, 4:05PM (Amir-ul Kafirs to group):

Re: HERETICS: Dr. Andrew Kaufman, July 17th Interview

I really 'enjoyed' this interview by Del Bigtree of Dr. Andrew Kaufman.
https://www.bitchute.com/video/w7TZzZFXX1ar/

I'm trying to get through this one now. I'm finding it very interesting. 1st Kaufman's claim that there were basically 4 papers that established the virus & the disease associated with it as real, 2nd his statement that the actual virus was never isolated enough to prove that it is what the claims made for it were. That, in itself, is fantastic. I may have to interupt my paying attention to it because Naia Nisnam & I are going out to the woods to make a movie of us painting (I've got a silly idea to establish a "School of Negativity"). I'll make a movie of that. I'm expecting her arrival in the next half-hour or so. ANYWAY, thanks for this link, it's great stuff. I'm thinking of compiling a list of doctors that're questioning the MONOLITHIC NARRATIVE & he'll be on there. Being reminded of the others would be helpful.

Kaufman says that no tests were ever conducted to prove that the pathogen even causes an illness.

Here's what the notes on BitChute state:

AN INCONVENIENT COVID TRUTH
MIT, Duke, and Medical University of South Carolina graduate Dr. Andrew Kaufman, MD, joins Del for a mind-blowing discussion detailing what we

actually know about the #COVID19 virus itself, and the very inconvenient truth every American needs to know.
#WhatIsCovid #InconvenientTruth #Covid #Coronavirus #TheHighWire #DelBigtree #AndrewKaufman

Kaufman speculates that what they're testing for may even be a sample of our own RNA that comes to the fore under a variety of circumstances & doesn't even necessarily indicate the presence of a virus. Bigtree asks Kaufman to try to convince him that the body produces such things from the inside. I find this possibility very exciting. It seems that this is called "Terrain Theory" (although I may've misunderstood) & this is associated with Natural Healing. I need to research this more. He also mentioned "Dark Field Microscopy" which is a way of observing live cells rather than dead ones — something, again, of particular interest to me.

One thing that's a bit strange to me is how similar Andrew Kaufman & James Corbett look to one another:

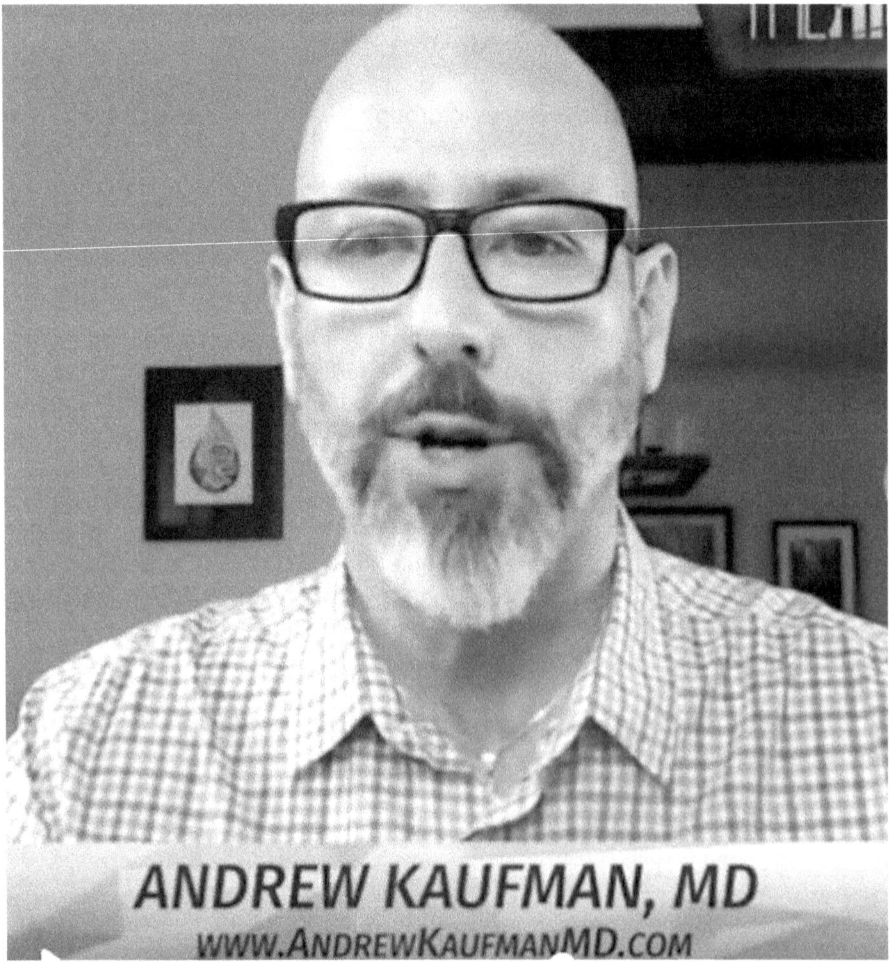

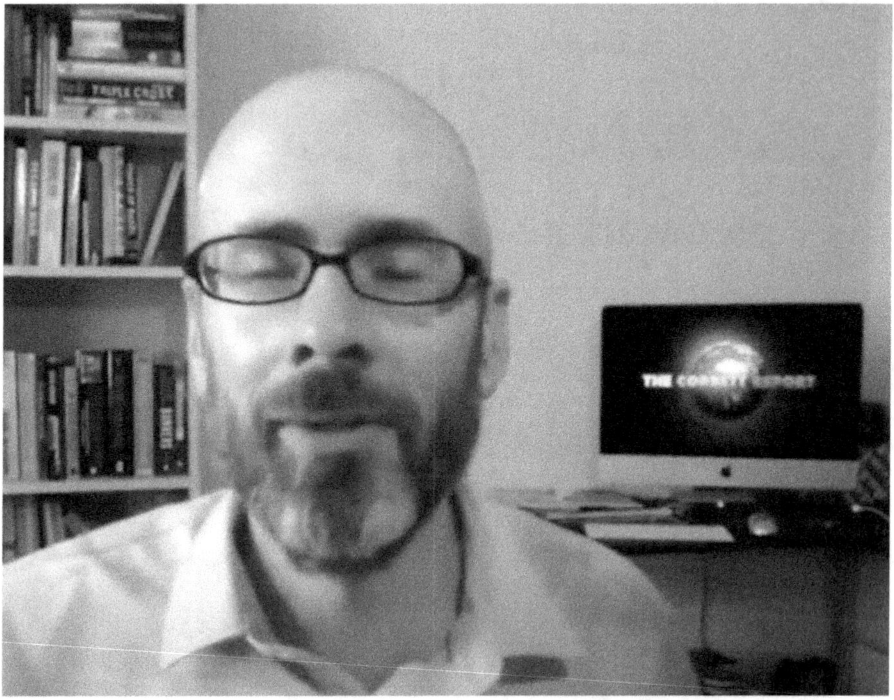

This is a somewhat common gay man look. **[The assumption here being that they're both gay which may not be the case]** I have at least one gay artist friend who looks pretty similar. I'd hate to find out that these guys are actually the same person or twins or some such. Fortunately their voices are too different for me to go down that route!

Another good concept: pleomorphism.

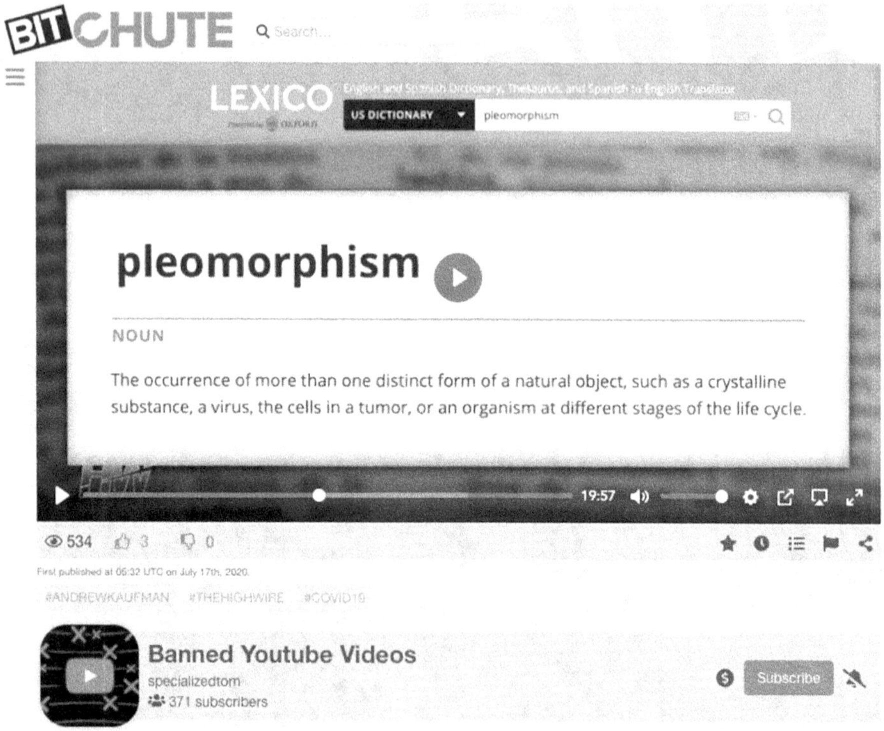

Research Karl Friston's saying that up to 80% of the population might not even be able to get the virus.

It's also great to see that there's a Democrat who's questioning the validity of the tests:

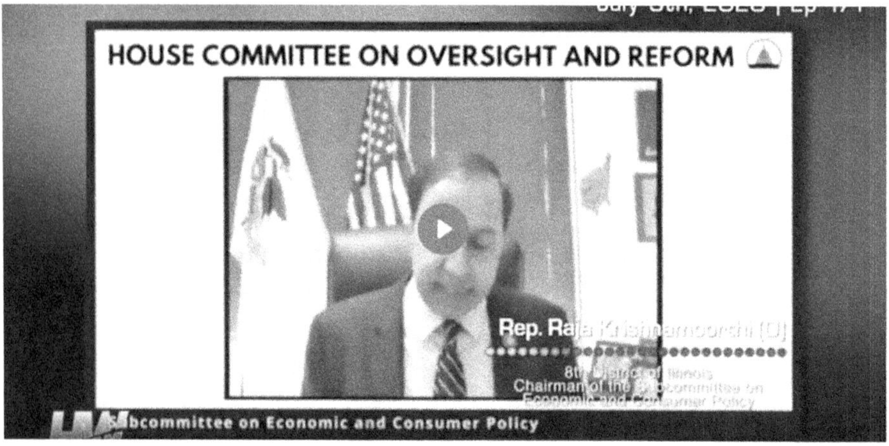

Research Dr. Cameron Kyle-Sidell, MD:

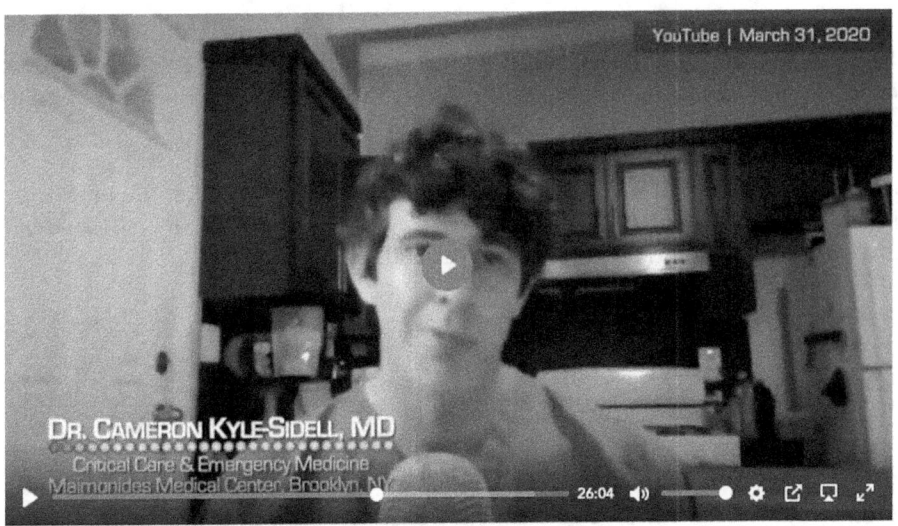

This doctor says the COVID-19 patients he's treated don't have symptoms similar to pneumonia but instead look like people suffering from high altitude oxygen deprivation. This means that giving people oxygen instead of putting them on ventilators is what helps them. I thought ventilators meant that people were being given oxygen so I guess I need to understand that more.

Kaufman says that doctors are being prevented from sending corpses for autopsies & that's preventing actual knowledge of cause of death. Kaufman also speculates that Kyle-Sidell's symptom description also sound like cyanide poisoning. Very interesting. Kaufman says that Kyle-Sidell was silenced after this & taken off ICU duty.

I've made some feeble attempts to find reliable PANDEMIC PANIC suicide data & Kaufman refers to suicide & an image of a New York Times article is shown:

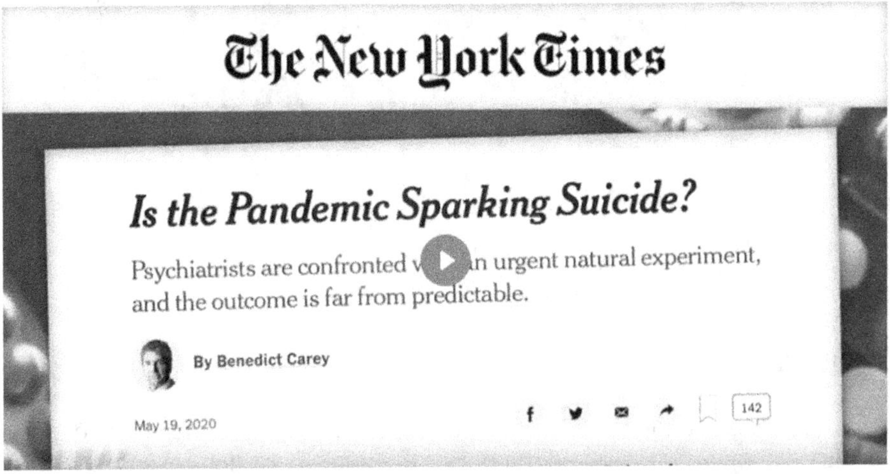

[Editor's interpolation: Note that the headline says: "*Is the Pandemic Sparking Suicide?*". It seems to be that it would be more accurate to ask: "*Is the Quarantine Sparking Suicide?*" but the New York Times isn't likely to go there.]

Given the NYT's poor record of reliability recently I'll have to look at that article directly to decide what I think about it. In my feeble research there's been the inevitable fact-choker dominance of increased suicide claims.

Kaufman says that street drugs have remained available & that people having more 'free time' coupled with their 'stimulus checks' has enabled deeper addiction problems. This is part of his claim, which I tend to agree with, that the lockdown is causing many of the deaths rather than preventing them.

Around 36:30 Del Bigtree asks the big question of "Who's behind this?". Kaufman says that of the big pandemic predictive things produced by the Rockefeller Foundation, Event 201, & the World Economic Forum that the latter's is the most "impressive". I've heard from Naia Nisnam that they've looked at their website & found it particularly disturbing so I'm sure I need to look at that:

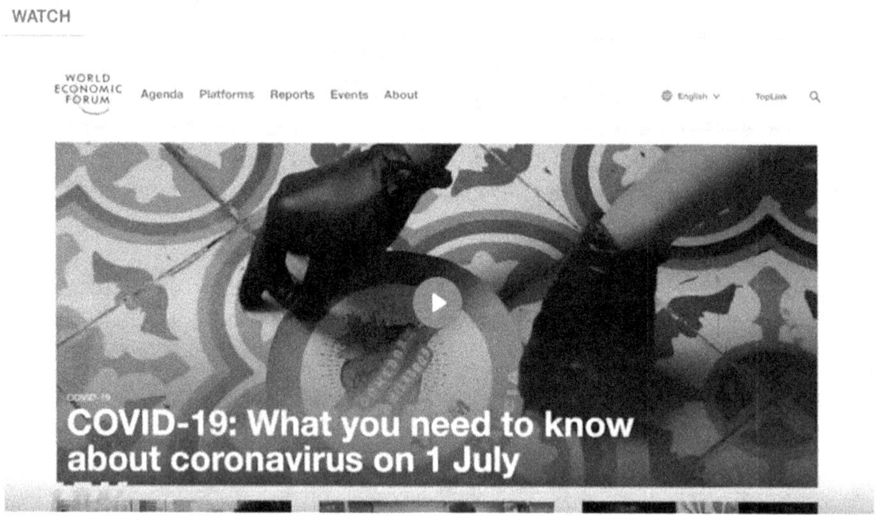

This was truly great. I'm very glad i made it through the entire thing. I linked to it on social media.

****

July 21, 2020 (______'s comments on the above on social media):

______: Very interesting! It would have been great to see this scientist in dialogue with his colleagues who uphold the opposite (official) position/research perspective. It's such dialogues that are becoming less and less possible in the current climate, and this is, to me, the greatest problem and danger of the current info climate.

_____: Ok, although I totally agree on the extreme dubiousness of the global shutdown policies (and lack of transparency thereof), I wasn't quite convinced by his virology argument and, as I was way too curious to wait for an actual experts debate to ever happen (which would probably be never) so, I went and did a short research myself. I read the first (available online, I guess) case of novel coronavirus detection from 2012 and they used antigen detection and then genetic sequencing to detect the virus. Then, I researched (again as I had already looked into the matter in the beginning of the pandemic but was fuzzy on the respective details) methods of isolating viruses, as I remember there were more than one, unlike what he is saying in this interview, and sure, the protocol of genetic sequencing is one of the main virus detection protocols. There is little, if anything, strange or unus**[u]**al in the methods used to isolate the novel coronavirus, as far as my verification went. You can check it out yourself: https://academic.oup.com/cid/article/31/3/739/297506

_____: Just saying, it seems that, if there is anything dubious about the isolation of the virus, it goes deeper than the argument presented in this interview. However, this interview gave me a better orientation/understanding as to why some people seem to believe there is no virus at all. Until now, I thought it was merely a combination of strange/suspicious policy behaviours coupled with the fact that many people lived in places or moved in circles where they hadn't had first hand experience or contact with infected people, e.g.

Amir-ul Kafirs's reply:

Amir-ul Kafirs: I'm in no position to argue one way or the other about this. I liked what Kaufman had to say in general & couldn't pick any of it apart with my nonexistent expertise. I'll leave it to people more qualified than myself to duke it out (which doesn't include Fact Chokers) but for the meantime Kaufman still appeals to me more than most. Still, I appreciate your input. I don't mean to naysay it, I'm admittedly liking him on the basis of what's understandable to me.

****

July 21, 2020, 5:14PM (Dick to group):

Here's an interesting video
I have to say however the choice it seems to present between politicians and the technocrats doesn't make me optimistic...meaning since all the politicians seem to have sold out, it doesn't seem like a real choice
people have to start doing things themselves as far as I can tell...but I wouldn't know how to structurally put that in place

https://www.youtube.com/watch?v=HKdsL57SUZo&feature=share

The Global Elite & The Coronavirus Coup D'état With Patrick Wood - YouTube
In this interview, Spiro is joined by Patrick Wood who is a leading and critical expert on Sustainable Development, Green Economy, Agenda 21, 2030 Agenda and...

****

July 24, 2020, 9:46PM (Amir-ul Kafirs to group):

Here's an interesting video

FUCK. Yet-another video I don't feel I have time to watch just now, if ever. I do intend to compile a timeline of these things & then I hope that either Naia Nisnam or I will go through them ALL & make representative screenshots & summaries of important points. Dick, if you ever have time to do something like this it would be much appreciated but if people don't want to do such things I certainly understand & I don't want you to feel inhibited about sharing links.

****

July 21, 2020, 5:59PM (Naia Nisnam to group):

COVID-19 Mortality Is Going Down in ICUs — What This Means

https://www.healthline.com/health-news/covid-19-mortality-is-going-down-in-icus-what-this-means-for-the-pandemic

****

Fact Checked

COVID-19 Mortality Is Going Down in ICUs — What This Means for the Pandemic

- Deaths from COVID-19 in ICUs have dropped by about a third since the start of the outbreak.
- Though the decline is substantial, health experts say the mortality rate for ICU patients with COVID-19 is higher than what's observed with other viral pneumonias.
- Health experts think better treatment and more resources may explain the mortality drop.

New research from the United Kingdom suggests the overall mortality rate for patients with COVID-19 in the intensive care unit (ICU) has dropped by about a third since the beginning of the pandemic.

The study, published in the journal Anaesthesia, tracked mortality in COVID-19

ICUs and recorded a decline from above 50 percent in March to 42 percent in May.

The findings are consistent across the globe — from Europe to Asia and North America.

Health experts suspect the drop is due to a few factors: Criteria for ICU admission has evolved, doctors have a better understanding of how to treat COVID-19 symptoms and complications, and healthcare facilities have more resources, compared with the start of the pandemic when the world was underprepared.

Though the decline is substantial, health experts say the mortality rate for ICU patients with COVID-19 is higher than what's observed with other viral pneumonias.

"While we are certainly glad the mortality rate has declined and not as high as some of the earlier reports, this still represents a dangerous disease with regards to risk of death as well more long-term risks of disability," said Dr. Jonathan Siner, a Yale Medicine pulmonologist, critical care physician, and medical director of the medical ICU.

More patients in the ICU are surviving

To better understand how the mortality rate amongst patients with COVID-19 in the ICU has changed, the researchers conducted a systematic review and meta-analysis looking at 24 observational studies.

They examined the health outcomes of 10,150 patients and identified a massive drop in the mortality rate recorded in ICUs across the globe.
The rate fell from above 50 percent at the end of March to 42 percent at the end of May.

According to the researchers, the findings are consistent around the world, despite continental differences in treatments being administered and ICU admission criteria.

The mortality rate is dropping, but it's still high

Doctors are optimistic that the mortality rate is dropping, but say the current mortality rate of 42 percent is still high.

For comparison, the mortality rate for other viral pneumonias treated in the ICU is about 22 percent, the study states.

"It's definitely still high, twice the usual mortality in ICU for viral pneumonia," said Dr. Eric Cioe-Pena, the director of global health at Northwell Health in New Hyde Park, New York.

Additionally, acute respiratory distress symptom (ARDS) — a severe lung complication some patients with COVID-19 experience — is known to have a mortality rate of 40 Trusted Source to 60 percent, according to Siner.

Siner says the mortality rate for patients severely ill with COVID-19 — and ARDS — is influenced by how severe the lung damage is, if other organs like the kidneys and brain are injured or inflamed, and whether the patient has other health problems.

Why the mortality rate dropped

Doctors now have a better grasp on how to treat COVID-19 and the complications it causes, compared with the start of the pandemic.
Back in February and March, COVID-19 was a new disease and doctors were in the early stages of experimenting with different treatment options.

Months later, doctors have identified a few drugs, like remdesivir and corticosteroids, that improve the course of the disease.

Doctors also have a better idea of who should be admitted to the ICU and how to best manage their symptoms with oxygen support and ventilators.

[..]

Written by Julia Ries on July 17, 2020 — Fact checked by Jennifer Chesak

- https://www.healthline.com/health-news/covid-19-mortality-is-going-down-in-icus-what-this-means-for-the-pandemic

****

July 22, 2020, 3:31AM (Amir-ul Kafirs to group):

Re: COVID-19 Mortality is Going Down in ICUs — What This Means

I read this one. As per the section of the Andrew Kaufman interview that I analyzed somewhat yesterday in which Dr. Cameron Kyle-Sidell, MD, stated that the COVID-19 patients he'd been dealing with appeared to have symptoms more in keeping with high-altitude sickness, an explanation of the following:

"Though the decline is substantial, health experts say the mortality rate for ICU patients with COVID-19 is higher than what's observed with other viral pneumonias."

would be that this is because it's NOT a viral pneumonia but is, instead, oxygen-deprivation. As such, the higher mortality rate would be because COVID-19 is being treated for being something that it's NOT & this treatment would be causing further damage rather than solving the problem.

****

July 22, 2020, 3:31AM (Amir-ul Kafirs to group):

HERETICS: Anti-Immigration

Liberals believe that by embracing Draconian measures as part of the PANDEMIC PANIC they're countering the Right-Wing. However, such measures as border closures & generally restricted travel serve Right-Wing Anti-Immigration purposes more than Rump's ridiculous border wall ever could. Think again, Liberals, you're destroying Civil Liberties.

****

July 22, 2020, 11:58AM (Inquiring Librarian to group):

HERETICS: "1986"

I listened to another great Del Bigtree interview this morning.
https://www.bitchute.com/video/nxyF0ayZO7ku/
This one here is with Andrew Wakefield, the media and industry shamed doctor who has been relentlessly persecuted for years for his studies into the link between autism and childhood vaccinations. He also made the movie "Vaxxed" addressing the issues of children damaged by vaccinations and interviews with the affected families. I have not seen this yet, but hope to.

His latest movie has just been released. It is called "1986". It is about the 1986 Childhood injury act that gave indemnity/no liability for vaccine manufacturers who injure children.

Consider also, mentioned in this interview, that there is a new act, the "Public Readiness and Emergency Preparedness Act", acronym, "PREP, that gives full indemnity to all involved in the current vaccine manufacture and distribution for covid 19.
https://www.phe.gov/Preparedness/legal/prepact/Pages/prepqa.aspx

"The Public Readiness and Emergency Preparedness Act (PREP Act) authorizes the Secretary of the Department of Health and Human Services (Secretary) to issue a declaration (PREP Act declaration) that provides immunity from liability (except for willful misconduct) for claims of loss caused, arising out of, relating to, or resulting from administration or use of countermeasures to diseases, threats and conditions determined by the Secretary to constitute a present, or credible risk of a future public health emergency to entities and individuals involved in the development, manufacture, testing, distribution, administration, and use of such countermeasures. A PREP Act declaration is specifically for the purpose of providing immunity from liability, and is different from, and not dependent on, other emergency declarations."

& check out the 1st 2 FAQ's answered (all FAQ's can be found on the above linked website, but these 1st 2 are so nefarious they'll knock your socks off right off the bat!).

"**1. What is Immunity from Liability?**

Immunity means that courts must dismiss claims brought against any entity or individual covered by the PREP Act. Claims that courts must dismiss include claims for any loss that is related to any stage of design, development, testing, manufacture, labeling, distribution, formulation, labeling, packaging, marketing, promotion, sale, purchase, donation, dispensing, prescribing, administration, licensing or use of a countermeasure recommended in a Declaration. This includes, but is not limited to, claims for:

death;
physical, mental, or emotional injury, illness, disability, or condition or fear of any such injury, illness, disability, or condition;
any need for medical monitoring; or
property damage or loss, including business interruption loss.

The only exception is for claims of willful misconduct. (See Question 3: Are There Any Limitations on Immunity From Liability?).

2. Who May be Afforded Immunity from Liability Under a PREP Act Declaration?

A Declaration may provide liability immunity for covered persons. Covered persons may include, at the Secretary's discretion:

Manufacturers of countermeasures;
Distributors of countermeasures;
Program planners, i.e., individuals and entities involved in planning, administering, or supervising programs for distribution of a countermeasure, e.g., State or local governments, Indian tribes, or private sector employers or community groups that establish requirements or provide guidance, technical or scientific advice or assistance, or provide a facility;
Qualified persons, i.e., persons who prescribe, administer, or dispense countermeasures such as healthcare and other providers or other categories of persons named in a Declaration, e.g., volunteers;
Officials, agents, and employees of any of these entities or persons; and

The United States."

Holy Moly!! Run for the hills and absolutely AVOID this 'vaccine'!!

****

July 21, 2020, 4:37PM (Naia Nisnam to group):

https://www.weforum.org/great-reset/

There is a video on here that is a little over an hour long. I haven't made through the whole thing yet. I highly suspect that this is the real reason behind the pandemic but I'd like to hear what all of you think.

The timing is strange- in 3-6 months they came up w this whole plan? I can find mention of the wef wanting a global economic reset as far back as 2017 and I barely looked. I imagine they've been working on this plan for a long time.
The release date of this information, this video, to the public coincides w the George Floyd murder. Potential anti-globalization activists were completely distracted.

Their plan sounds like a splendid new utopia...
Tell me what you guys think.

****

July 21, 2020, 10:14PM (Inquiring Librarian to group):

Re: HERETICS: Dr. Andrew Kaufman, July 17th Interview

First off, thank you Amir-ul Kafirs for putting so much into listening to and sharing the Dr. Andrew Kaufman podcast. I am glad you loved it too and so glad that you share it on social media.

Naia Nisnam, I actually did listen to the whole drole World Economic Forum. It certainly does sound splendid. But coming from the voices and corporations represented, it could likely have a terrifying dark side. I would imagine that anyone else on this email group could dissect this better than me. All things economic are honestly over my head. I did not inherit any intelligence at all in that part of my brain. But, here is a short article on a negative spin of the World Economic Forum gathering:
https://off-guardian.org/2020/07/20/the-great-reset-fraud/?fbclid=IwAR3NmvQKNjnIVIFgg6w44xJxZZu3bkJ6utVx85eHA45RwM79NYNpKkesniA

"The Great Reset Fraud

Like everyone, I would love to live in a pollution-free world. I would love to see human civilization strike a balance with nature and at the risk of sounding like a naïve idealist, I sincerely do believe that this is ultimately our destiny as a species."... "

False Remedies to the Oncoming Meltdown

Many false solutions will be presented as society wakes up to the burning building it is trapped in, and unless our minds have become aware of those false solutions, (not to mention those arsonists managing this fire from the top), then many well-intentioned souls from all walks of life may sign onto their own death warrants and accidentally usher in a solution far worse than the disease they sought to remedy."...
If you want to go full paranoid, I listened to this talk this morning with "Patrick Wood who is a leading and critical expert on Sustainable Development, Green Economy, Agenda 21, 2030 Agenda and historic Technocracy." https://www.bitchute.com/video/Hp1nrC5CAswn/?fbclid=IwAR3cNnWcwFtfWminexSM3tSdxt1zhHEkLDn56GKwi0ucvMFVmpQHX5PZKK4

It is a Spiro interview of Patrick Wood.

I know some of you aren't fond of Spiro. But Spiro barely talks in this. And what Patrick Wood discusses in this talk directly addresses what the World Economic Forum discusses, but the dark side and the long standing history since the 1930's of this type of reset, including the eugenics movement and how it affected his mother who was sterilized at a young age (Patrick Wood was adopted).

Ok, I'll leave the rest of this up to you all to figure out. My specialty is viruses and vaccines and the biomedical policing of the braindead.

****

July 22, 2020, 8:20PM (Naia Nisnam to group):

I finally listened to the full Kaufman interview. It is hard for me to follow the science as Ive never studied anything beyond biology 101.

But-
A week or 2 before Plandemic came out, a friend sent me an interview w Dr Judy and she said similar things about the RNA code existing naturally in our bodies. She theorized that it had become activated in many many people as a response to last years flu vaccine. It would be interesting to know what percentage of people testing positive for Covid had taken last years flu vaccine. (Gates himself admits that that particular year's flu vaccine was only 45 percent effective...)

****

July 22, 2020, 9:37PM (Naia Nisnam to group):

I just watched the Patrick Wood video. He makes complete sense to me. The

one thing I can't agree w him on is his sense of hope.
If he's banking on enough of the American people to educate themselves and declare that they will not comply to actually make a difference- I don't believe that at all. Americans love their tech, they don't care that they're under constant surveillance, they love staying home, ordering everything online, binge watching whatever and interacting w others only via social media. Americans love their stupid masks and the power it gives them- the power to feel self righteous, to feel like they're doing something great for the world wo doing anything at all. Americans will love being told that the new world economy is all about environmentalism and equality.
I'm feeling like we're all screwed, there's nothing to be done about it, and I'd be better off if I didn't know anything and could go about my life being comfortably dumb.
Sorry if that's depressing but... that's where I am.

****

July 22, 2020, 6:33PM (Naia Nisnam to group):

Forced County COVID-19 Lockdown of Ventura Apt Building at 137 S. Palm St. | Citizens Journal

https://www.citizensjournal.us/forced-county-covid-19-lockdown-of-ventura-apt-building-137-s-palm-st/

****

Forced County COVID-19 Lockdown of Ventura Apt Building at 137 S. Palm St.

Added by **Citizen Reporter** *on July 20, 2020.*

By Kevin Daly & George Miller

Lockdown was lifted today after results came in and only one positive test occurred.

On July 17, Ventura County forcibly locked down a seven story public housing (Ventura Housing Authority) apartment building at 137 S. Palm St in Ventura. You can view the lockdown order (unsigned) and a letter from the building manager below. The order claims its authority emanates from California Code 12030 and 120175.
It says **"This order shall remain in force until rescinded by the Health Officer in writing. Violation or failure to comply with this Order may result in "civil detention" and is a misdemeanor punishable by imprisonment, fine or both."**
We were told and the letter from the apartment manager states that the building is locked down, quarantine is mandatory until test results are received, no one is allowed in or out of the building except "essential workers" and that COVID-19 testing in the building is mandatory.

[..]

After the tests results came in today, 7-20-20, only one more positive . The lockdown was rescinded, but residents were asked to avoid interaction, going out and to wear masks and socially distance. Dr. Levin is recommending retesting in a week or two.
Levin said this was a unique set of circumstances and was done out of an abundance of caution due to the very vulnerable population of residents. The county wanted to avoid situations like have occurred in nursing homes we've all read about.
We'll let you know if we hear more.

[..]

- https://www.citizensjournal.us/forced-county-covid-19-lockdown-of-ventura-apt-building-137-s-palm-st/

****

July 22, 2020, 9:34PM (Amir-ul Kafirs to group):

HERETICS: "Pandemic" (2008 movie) pt 1

I ordered 2 movies called "Pandemic" online within the past few weeks & I'm watching one of them now to compare it to what's been happening in 'real life'. This 1st one is:

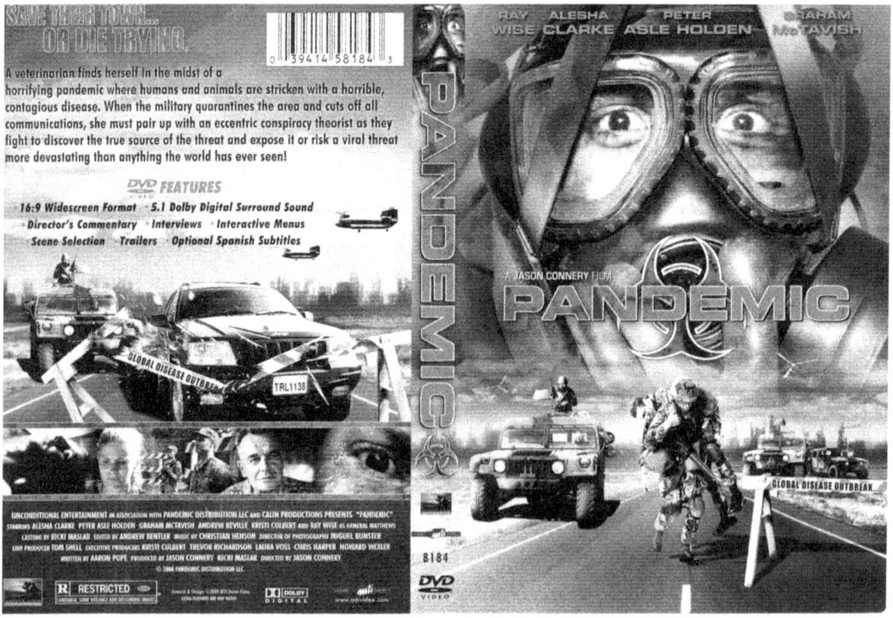

Pandemic

R 2008 · Thriller/Disaster · 2h 18m

The Army places a town under quarantine, and a veterinarian (Alesha Clarke) joins forces with a conspiracy theorist (Peter Asle Holden) when a contagious illness strikes humans and livestock.

Initial release: 2008
Director: Jason Connery

I'm going to watch a bit & then write some notes & post them here.

The movie starts with a long shot showing a man on horseback in sillhouette riding on a ridge. Shots gradually show him closer. He's a modern-day rancher in his early 40s in apparent good health. He gets back to his ranch & puts the horse in a stall. His heart then starts to beat violently, he falls over & tries to make it out of the barn but his blood vessels in his face start to rupture & his orifices start to bleed & he appears to die. This happens within seconds.

In a new scene we see a veternarian drive her pick-up truck home. She has an urgent message from a client who demands that she go to his ranch immediately. She gets there & a horse is lying on the ground, it's face covered in blood. The vet very quickly decides that it '*must be a virus*'. It seems to me that she has basically nothing to go on to make that diagnosis. The rancher says that '*they must've put it in the water*'. He appears to be a "Conspiracy Theorist'. He's somewhat hysterical, he gets a shotgun to shoot the horse because he '*can't stand to see her suffer*'. The vet tries to talk him out of it without success. She gets another call from another ranch with a similar case. The rancher tells the horse that he '*loves her*' & then shoots her in the head with the shotgun. It seems to me that the rancher is being pretty hasty to kill a creature he '*loves*' just because it's been sick for an hour or so.

The vet is at home trying to research the symptoms. She can't find anything online on the health database she's accessing. The TV's on in the background. There's a news report about finding the dead rancher & the vet realizes that the symptoms seem the same. The coroner's name is mentioned. The vet goes to the coroner's office where she barges in past the receptionist & asks to see the dead rancher. She tells the coroner about the horses. They decide to call the CDC. The coroner calls them & tells them that they've got a '*viral outbreak*'.

Some military vehicles arrive, presumably the same night, with a general who orders the town of "Diablo" locked down discretely so the town doesn't panic. All this on the basis of a rather hasty conclusion phone call from the coroner. They use a general for this? The Conspiracy Theorist rancher is shown hiding behind a wagon wheel looking paranoid.

STAY TUNED FOR MORE PARANOID PREPARATION OF THE MASSES!!

****

July 22, 2020, 9:40PM (Naia Nisnam to group):

HERETICS: "Pandemic" (2008 movie) pt 1

I don't even have the words to comment but here's this:

https://www.google.com/amp/s/www.latimes.com/entertainment-arts/tv/story/2020-04-01/pandemic-netflix-documentary-coronavirus%3f_amp=true

****

A Netflix series predicted a global pandemic. It was dismissed as 'a show about the flu'

By MEREDITH BLAKE STAFF WRITER
APRIL 1, 20206:56 PM

Not if but when.

It's the rallying cry uttered over and over again by the doctors, scientists, humanitarian workers and public health officials profiled in "Pandemic: How to Prevent an Outbreak." Structured like a globe-trotting thriller, the Netflix documentary series follows dedicated men and women on the front lines of the battle against the next devastating disease to ravage the human population — an event they are all certain is just around the corner.

Turns out they were right.

In a freakish coincidence of timing, "Pandemic" premiered on Netflix in late January, just as the novel coronavirus was beginning its rampage. Over six episodes, the series issues uncomfortably prescient warnings about the risk of a new respiratory virus that could, within a matter of months, overwhelm the planet. It brings epidemiological science to life in unexpected ways — not with dry data but through compelling characters located in far-flung, seemingly unconnected places, from a crowded animal market in Vietnam to an under-resourced hospital in rural Oklahoma.

"There were already a lot of scary science documentaries where you had people sitting in a room talking about the potential for a new virus to spread around the world," says executive producer Sheri Fink, a reporter for the New York Times with experience in infectious disease. (She covered the H1N1 flu pandemic in 2009 and the Ebola outbreak in West Africa in 2014.) "We thought we would try to go around the world and give a sense of the lives of these people who felt passionate [about] and devoted their lives to trying to detect pandemics."

These subjects include Susan Flis, a retired nurse who volunteers to give out flu shots at the U.S.-Mexico border in Arizona; Jacob Glanville, an entrepreneur trying to develop a universal flu vaccine; Michel Yao, a doctor with the World

Health Organization attempting to contain an Ebola outbreak in the Democratic Republic of the Congo; and Dr. Syra Madad, the infectious disease specialist preparing New York's municipal hospitals for the next pandemic.

Scientists and healthcare workers are the story's heroes but there are also antagonists: One story line follows Caylan Wagar, a home-schooling mother of five and anti-vaccine activist in Oregon who, in the midst of a historic measles outbreak, fights against stricter immunization laws. The documentary shows how a constellation of distinct forces including a growing distrust of scientific authority, global instability and a lack of funding for public health infrastructure makes us more vulnerable to a deadly new disease.

Filmed over the course of the 2018-2019 flu season, "Pandemic" is full of what-if scenarios — many involving Madad's work in New York City — that have now come to fruition. Minutes into the first episode, a team of medical workers covered head to toe in protective gear run through a simulation to test their readiness for a major flu outbreak in the city. Madad, who is overseeing the drill, warns them: "If you're not protected, if you can't protect yourself, then how are you going to protect others?" Later, she lays out a hypothetical scenario in which a single traveler arriving by plane in New York City could trigger an overwhelming outbreak that would, within weeks, incapacitate the city. She's also seen pleading with politicians about resources for pandemic preparedness.

It's very strange [to] look back and see that we sort of took this trip through exactly what is happening right now.

"PANDEMIC" CO-DIRECTOR DOUG SHULTZ

Sound familiar?

"The work of prevention and preparedness — it's challenging to make that real to people before the bad thing happens and makes people care about it," says Fink.

Isabel Castro, one of the series' directors, recalls the apathetic response she got from friends and family when she told them about the project she was working on. "Everyone would be like, 'Oh you're making a show about the flu?' They would talk about it dismissively and I would be like, 'No, this is a big deal.' So it's very surreal for these same people now to be watching the show and to be like, 'Oh my God. I can't believe it happened in our lifetime.'"

Production wrapped a few months before the coronavirus outbreak began in China. Ironically, it was a relatively mild flu season in the United States, but even a mild flu season is enough to overwhelm Holly Goracke, the only doctor at a hospital in Jefferson County, Okla.

[..]

'Pandemic: How to Prevent an Outbreak'

Where: Netflix
When: Any time

Rating: TV-14 (may be unsuitable for children under the age of 14)

****

July 22, 2020, 9:54PM (Amir-ul Kafirs to group):

HERETICS: "Pandemic" (2008 movie) pt 2

The military quickly block the roads with large red-striped barriers & razor-wire. Beefy soldiers in camou fatigues holding automatic weapons man the blockades. 6 or so troop carriers arrive at the coroner's office where the clerk, the coroner, & the vet still are. The clerk summons the 2 doctors who're astonished by this large military presence so soon after they called the CDC. It's explained to them by a very authoritarian captain that he'll need their cooperation because '*surely they understand the need to contain the virus*'. They somewhat reluctantly agree.

It's daytime & the locals are gathered in a diner looking a bit disgruntled. A rancher is talking to the vet at the diner counter. A voice over an announcement sound-system is telling everyone that they'll be under quarantine until it's deemed no longer necessary, which is possibly implied to be soon. The rancher talking with the vet is being informed by her that the government's going to take care of it. He says; '*Like they did in New Orleans? Like they did at 3 Mile Island? Like they did with AIDS?*'. He's obviously skeptical but he likes the vet so he's somewhat mollified. The vet leaves.

I'D THOUGHT I COULD GET THROUGH THE WHOLE MOVIE TONIGHT BUT I'M ALREADY SICK OF IT SO I MIGHT NOT CONTINUE UNTIL TOMORROW. **Think of it as a HERETICS serial!**

****

July 23, 2020, 5:17AM (Amir-ul Kafirs to group):

HERETICS: "Pandemic" (2008 movie) pt 3

The veterinarian returns home where she tries to get on the internet but gets an error message. She tries to use her landline, that doesn't work either. She tries to use her cell-phone, that doesn't work. Exasperated, she gets in her truck to drive back into town but her way is blocked. She insists that one of the soldiers use his communication device to arrange a meeting between her, the captain, & the general. That works & they allow her through the blockade.

The disgruntled rancher who was questioning the government's ability to handle the situation is shown training a horse. He suddenly collapses & bleeds profusely from his skin & dies within seconds.

The vet is allowed into the military encampment where the captain shows her into a tented office complex where she meets the general. The environment of this command center is bustling but the general tells everyone but the captain & the vet to leave. The general is affable & tries to charm the vet into being less aggressive. She demands to know why communications are shut down & the general informs her that the townspeople must not be allowed to communicate with the outside world or they'll cause panic. The veterinarian asks whether the general thinks that people should be allowed the right to communicate & he tells her that rights aren't his concern. She says "This is bullshit." She leaves.

She goes to the coroner's office. The coroner & the clerk appear to not be there. The vet notices that there's a new body bag in the morgue so she puts on a mask & gloves & goes in & unzips the bag & sees the bloodied face of the disgruntled rancher. She's upset. She notices another body bag & looks at the name-tag on it. It may've had the name of the coroner on it but the shot seems to've been left ambiguous. She hears people & hides out of sight & notices that soliders are bringing in another body. After they're gone, she slips off her gloves & leaves, face-mask still on. So far, none of the soldiers have been wearing masks or gloves.

****

A sidenote here is that ever since this QUARANTYRANNY began I've been having trouble with my internet. Avoiding paranoia, I've attributed the trouble to a heavier demand on the service. It's common for me to get this message:

Safari Can't Find the Server

Safari can't open the page
"https://www.youtube.com/watch?v=DEnv8pb7yIA"
because Safari can't find the server "www.youtube.com".

It's also common for me to not be able to send emails. Usually if I close the Mail app & reopen it it works. It took most of the day to download notation software that I paid for, something that should've only taken a short while. We should take into consideration the possibility that we might not be able to communicate with each other eventually.

****

July 23, 2020, 9:08PM (Amir-ul Kafirs to group):

HERETICS: "Pandemic" (2008 movie) pt 4

The veterinarian drives around town on her way home from the coroner's office having a soul-searching moment while she looks at the townspeople who wave hi & at the soldiers performing various functions. The editing is a tad more free here & there's a woman singing as the soundtrack. She gets home & thinks there's an intruder so she gets out her cattle-prod & walks around her house eventually going in the front door which has wafted open. Eventually she finds a man hunched over in her kitchen & she cattle-prods the back of his neck. He turns around in pain & it's the conspiracy theory rancher, named Spencer, who shot his horse near the beginning. He begs her to put down the prod &, after some hesitation, she does.

He's excited & somewhat incoherent but he tells her that 'they're after him'. He's seen the soldiers & thinks they're there to get him. His story comes out jumbled but apparently both his grandfather & his father were involved in some sort of secret military stuff which he saw & has been informing the public about. He'd moved to Diablo County to hide out thinking THEY wouldn't be able to find him there.

He explains a little more coherently to the questioning vet that the military has picked Diablo County for a preparedness exercise because it's the most sparsely populated county in the US & it'll be easy to cover up the deaths. He claims that they introduced the virus, despite basically zero evidence so far it's now being taken for granted that it's a virus, into the water from just over the county line. He asks her how long it took for them to respond when she & the coroner contacted the CDC & she said "About a half hour." He explains that it was so fast because they were waiting for the call.

The vet wants to know what his 'facts' are. He says he can't tell her why he knows this. She tells him he has to leave, he says that if he does they'll kill him, that they're searching his house now, that he came there on foot through the woods, that they don't know he's there.

Cut to soldiers guarding the gate to the military camp. 2 carloads of civilians show up demanding to see the general & saying that if there's a vaccine they want it. The spokesperson soldier says that he has orders to not admit anyone. The spokesperson civilian is being aggressively insistent. The soldier keeps telling him to "Stand down." Eventually, the soldier fires a shot into the air & aims the gun at the civilian & they all leave with the civilian saying "This is bullshit!"

In the meantime, the coroner's clerk, Brian, has taken advantage of the distraction & snuck in. He gets caught but successfully gets in to see the Captain who's looking at Top Secret info on his computer. Brian tells him he's feeling sick, that there's a rumor around town that the military has a vaccine & he volunteers to be a test subject. The Captain appears to like him & agrees to give it to him as long as he doesn't tell anyone. Brian's given a shot.

Cut to the vet & the theorist driving. The theorist is hiding on the floor of the passenger side of the pick-up. The vet wants him to sit on the seat but he insists it's necessary. She notices that they're being followed. The theorist proposes an escape plan but the vet stops the truck & gets out to go talk to the follower(s). As she approaches their car they back up quickly & the car stops, possibly stalling. She shouts out at them asking if this is a game. The theorist grabs her & pushes her in the passenger seat of her truck & takes off as the driver. They proceed to try to shake pursuit.

They pull off into the scrub, the Captain & another soldier get out of the car that was following & with pistols held at arm's length tell them to exit their vehicle. When they get close they realize that they've made their escape on foot. Spencer says they have to cross over the county line. The Captain gets more soldiers & they set off in pursuit with raised rifles with lights on the ends. The Captain says he wants them alive. Spencer stops & writes something on a piece of paper & stuffs it in the vet's clothes & tells her to keep it for when they need it. She wants to know what it is. He says it's a map. The soldiers start firing at them & they start running some more.

Spencer pulls out a handgun to the vet's surprise. He tells her to run, she does, a solider raises a rifle to shoot at her & Spencer shoots the solider, apparently killing him. The vet gets captured by a solider, the Captain?, & Spencer tries to get in a shot. Someone gets shot in the leg. They both get captured & the General is there & he says "Thank God we found you." The vet wants to know what's going to happen to Spencer & the General says "He'll be taken care of." They're both taken away.

STAY TUNED FOR THE THRILLING CLIMAX!

****

July 24, 2020, 11:58AM (Amir-ul Kafirs to group):

HERETICS: "Pandemic" (2008 movie) pt 5 (END)

[I forgot to mention in my last report that Spencer has a revelation that this ISN'T a preparatory exercise but an aggressive test of a bio-weapon on US citizens in preparation for its use elsewhere.]

Cut to Brian getting something out of the fridge. He looks at his hand & smells it.

Cut to the vet with the General. She's asking about Spencer. The General says he's being looked after. The General says that the virus has quadrupled in strength, that it's mutating. He needs her to keep the townspeople calm as the voice of reason. He says that otherwise people will become volatile. She says 'Like Spencer?' Yes, like Spencer. She says that he shot in self-defence. The General says that he'll tell that to the solider he shot, he was a good soldier. He asks her how well does she know Spencer, she counters with "How well do you know him?" The General reveals that Spencer served under him in airborne Special Forces. The General says Spencer was a "rising star" but that one day "he went away" & that they tracked him at 1st but then they lost him.

He says he worked for the Cubans 1st, for the Shining Path, etc — anyone who opposed US foreign policy. The vet says: "He was a terrorist?" The General replies: "Or a Freedom Fighter, depending on your point-of-view." The General says that Spencer has been developing the skills he'd been taught in the military & that he's been honing them & developing new weapons. The implication might be that Spencer has actually precipitated this situation by putting a bioweapon in the water. The General then reveals that Spencer is his son.

The scenes cut back & forth between Spencer in a dark room arguing with the Captain & the General cunningly fishing for information from the vet. Spencer inquires about the vet & is informed that she's being "debriefed" by the General. This upsets Spencer since he knows how tricky his father is. The General talks in his usual disarming affable way but a bit of his true nature peeps through when he asks the vet to imagine how "embarrassed" he is that his only son is a threat to the US. The vet subtly seems to catch on to the General's true uncaring & career-advancing nature but doesn't let on (other than in slight acting). Spencer is told he'll never see the light of day again.

The Captain tells Spencer he's going to have to do what he has to do to protect the country & he gets out a needle kit. Spencer says "You're going to put me down!" The Captain says it's just a vaccine. They get into a fight & Spencer gets shot & killed.

The General & the vet are driving in a military vehicle & the vet is looking at papers & photos that the General has given her to look at. One of them is of Brian, the coroner's clerk, as a corpse with the usual bloody face. The General explains that he volunteered for the vaccine & that it didn't work. He says that's the Captain's department. If Spencer had been given the 'vaccine' he could've been listed as a virus casualty. The vet comments that Brian looks worse than the others. She speculates that it could be a genetic mutation OR that the vaccine could be mixing with the virus, accelerating it & making it worse. The General says "Hhmm" & reaches for something out of shot.

He was reaching to open his door. Apparently, the vehicle was stopped at the vet's house, presumably her truck's been taken away or left at the spot where she & Spencer left it. She says "What are you doing?" The General says: "I was going to walk you to your door." She says something about being beyond chivalry now & he acquiesces. The vet gets in her house & lays on her couch flashing back to scenes with Spencer. She keeps peeping out the window. It's ambiguous but it seems that the military vehicle is still there. She gathers up bottles of water & puts them in a backpack.

The next scene shows her running through the woods with the backpack on. She stops & looks at the map Spencer gave her. She leaves all but one bottle of water behind & continues running. The vet reaches her destination, the next county over that's not under quarantine & it's daytime & we see that she's dying. She flashes back to the General giving her a glass of water. She realizes that he gave her the bioweapon.

The 'news' on a TV being watched by the Captain 'reports' that the vet has died in a car crash when her truck drifted off the road. Next, the TV reports that a virus is effecting livestock in Afghanistan & that there're some reports that humans are exhibiting similar symptoms. A leader of an Al Queda splinter group has been one of the casualties.

A puppy is shown running along the side of the road. It may be the same road next to which the vet died. A boy in a passing car sees the dog & begs his dad to pull over so they can pick it up. They do. We see the dog's face poking out the open window & see that it's showing signs of the disease. We hear the boy ask his dad if they can keep the dog when they get back to LA. The implication is obvious: the pandemic is out.

****

Ok, this wasn't a great movie — but I'm trying to get a handle on what kind of pandemic stories there are out there in pop culture. I think this one was a made-for-TV movie, I assume it was seen by millions. It definitely puts an anti-government / pro-Conspiracy-Theorist spin on things & promotes "freedom fighter" sympathies. Obviously, it also ends 'hopelessly'.

****

July 24, 2020, 10:34PM (Amir-ul Kafirs to group):

Re: HERETICS: "Pandemic" (2008 movie) pt 1

I don't even have the words to comment but here's this:

https://www.google.com/amp/s/www.latimes.com/entertainment-arts/tv/story/2020-04-01/pandemic-netflix-documentary-coronavirus%3f_amp=true

Yeah, OK, this article &, apparently, the doc series that it's about, is a crock of shit. I didn't really mind it that much, though, until it got to this part:

"Scientists and healthcare workers are the story's heroes but there are also antagonists: One story line follows Caylan Wagar, a home-schooling mother of five and anti-vaccine activist in Oregon who, in the midst of a historic measles outbreak, fights against stricter immunization laws. The documentary shows how a constellation of distinct forces including a growing distrust of scientific authority, global instability and a lack of funding for public health infrastructure makes us more vulnerable to a deadly new disease."

Needless to say, I'm immediately sympathetic to the "antagonist", regardless of what I might think about her otherwise, because her position is being completely disrespected.

****

THE CONTEXT

The Covid-19 crisis, and the political, economic and social disruptions it has caused, is fundamentally changing the traditional context for decision-making. The inconsistencies, inadequacies and contradictions of multiple systems –from health and financial to energy and education – are more exposed than ever amidst a global context of concern for lives, livelihoods and the planet. Leaders find themselves at a historic crossroads, managing short-term pressures against medium- and long-term uncertainties.

THE OPPORTUNITY

As we enter a unique window of opportunity to shape the recovery, this initiative will offer insights to help inform all those determining the future state of global relations, the direction of national economies, the priorities of societies, the nature of business models and the management of a global commons. Drawing from the vision and vast expertise of the leaders engaged across the Forum's communities, the Great Reset initiative has a set of dimensions to build a new social contract that honours the dignity of every human being.

Find out more about the Great Reset

Read more

OUR CONTRIBUTION

The World Economic Forum has developed a reputation as a trusted platform for informed collaboration and cooperation between all stakeholders – reinforced by a track record of success over five decades. The Forum now offers its experience in building purpose-driven communities in service of the extraordinary challenge and opportunity the world faces for a "Great Reset". The Forum provides an unparalleled platform for creating, shaping and delivering collaborative solutions for the future through its:

THE GREAT RESET

Can the tools of finance build back better?

The solutions to the COVID crisis have to work for all and the planet. If businesses do not solve this, the liabilities will be beyond measure and assets will have no value.

Michael Izza 22 Jul 2020

THE GREAT RESET

We need multilateral cooperation and a reset to recover better

With a desire for global cooperation, we can work out – together – what the Great Reset will look like and how we can make it a reality.

Feike Sijbesma 21 Jul 2020

THE GREAT RESET

3 ways digital businesses can enable the Great Reset

Updating business models for a digital-first world, led by purpose, is now an imperative for almost every company.

Manju George and Nokuthula Lukhele 17 Jul 2020

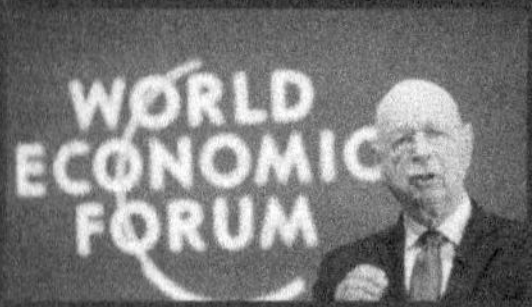

THE GREAT RESET

Klaus Schwab's vision of a post-COVID world, and how the economy can work with nature - this week's Great Reset podcast

World Economic Forum Founder Klaus Schwab's book on the Great Reset; and a report that shows how working with nature can deliver millions of jobs.

Robin Pomeroy 17 Jul 2020

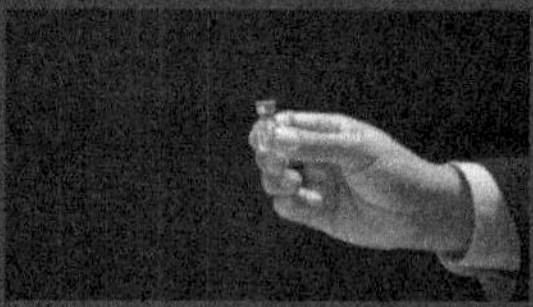

COVID-19

How the massive plan to deliver the COVID-19 vaccine could make history – and leverage blockchain like never before

Eradicating COVID-19 could mean distributing up to 19 billion vaccine doses. Leveraging blockchain can make that distribution equitable.

Punit Shukla, Amey Rajput, and Sid Chakravarthy 17 Jul 2020

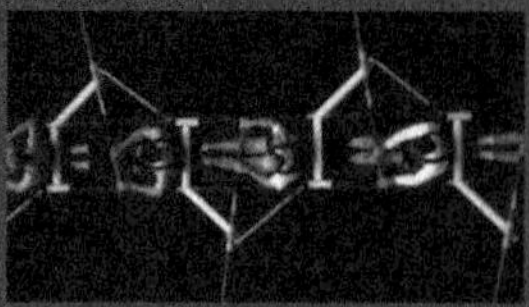

THE GREAT RESET

To reinvent the future, we must all work together

COVID-19 has exposed our flaws - and given us a chance to fix them once and for all. Here is a five point plan of action to get us on the right track.

Robert E. Moritz 17 Jul 2020

ISRAEL

Hugging a tree in Israel to beat the coronavirus blues

Israel's Nature and Parks Authority is encouraging people to hug a tree to help overcome the sense of detachment that coronavirus social-distancing rules can bring.

Jeffrey Heller · Reuters 17 Jul 2020

THE GREAT RESET

COVID-19 has created a unified ethos of urgent action in Africa. This model can achieve lasting change

COVID-19 has shifted the cultural context: suddenly previous obstacles to change are surmountable as bigger ones are overcome, and an ethos of urgent action takes hold.

Elsie S. Kanza 17 Jul 2020

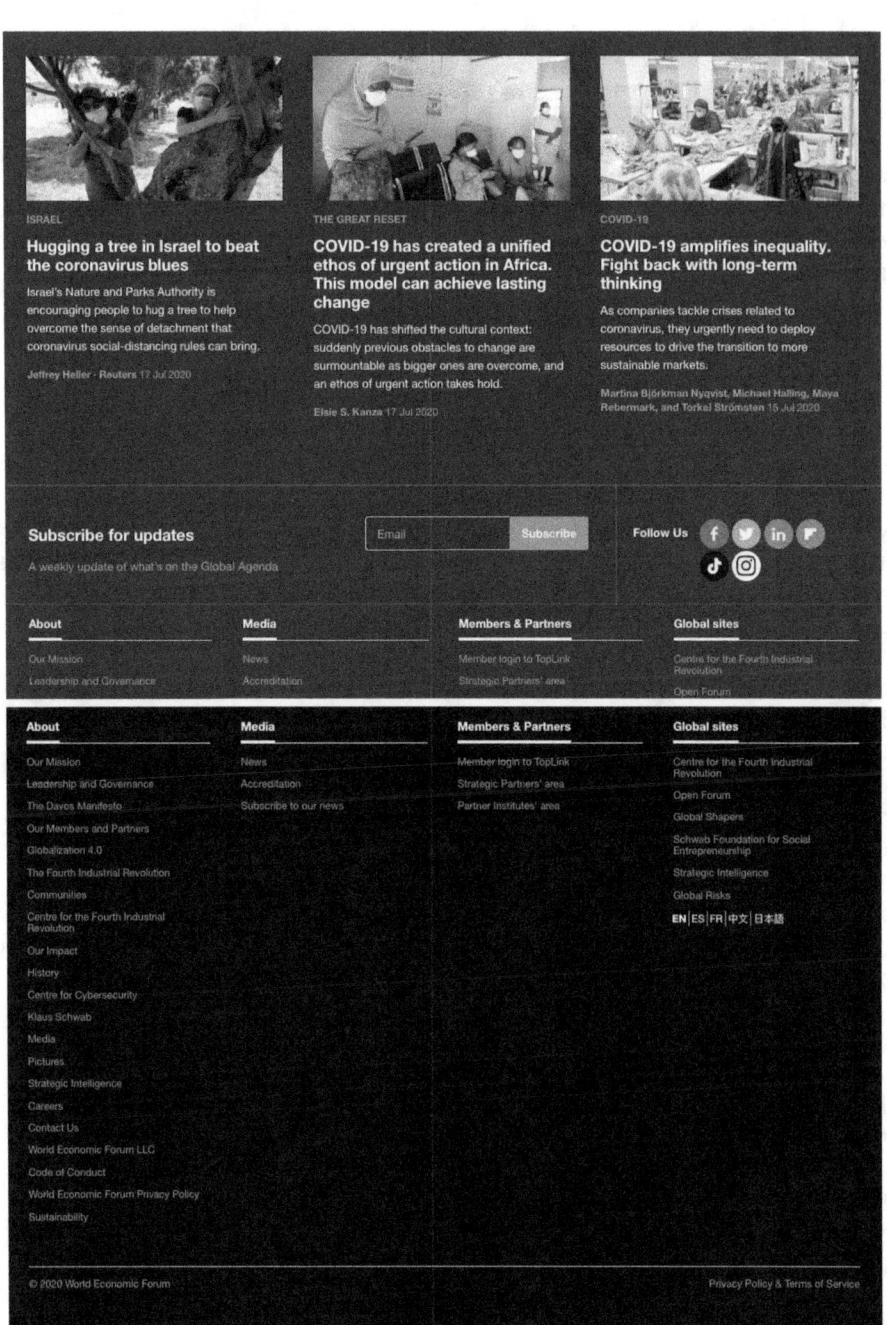

COVID-19

COVID-19 amplifies inequality. Fight back with long-term thinking

As companies tackle crises related to coronavirus, they urgently need to deploy resources to drive the transition to more sustainable markets.

Martina Björkman Nyqvist, Michael Halling, Maya Rebermark, and Torkel Strömsten 15 Jul 2020

Subscribe for updates

A weekly update of what's on the Global Agenda

Email Subscribe

Follow Us

About

Our Mission
Leadership and Governance

Media

News
Accreditation

Members & Partners

Member login to TopLink
Strategic Partners' area

Global sites

Centre for the Fourth Industrial Revolution
Open Forum

About

Our Mission
Leadership and Governance
The Davos Manifesto
Our Members and Partners
Globalization 4.0
The Fourth Industrial Revolution
Communities
Centre for the Fourth Industrial Revolution
Our Impact
History
Centre for Cybersecurity
Klaus Schwab
Media
Pictures
Strategic Intelligence
Careers
Contact Us
World Economic Forum LLC
Code of Conduct
World Economic Forum Privacy Policy
Sustainability

Media

News
Accreditation
Subscribe to our news

Members & Partners

Member login to TopLink
Strategic Partners' area
Partner Institutes' area

Global sites

Centre for the Fourth Industrial Revolution
Open Forum
Global Shapers
Schwab Foundation for Social Entrepreneurship
Strategic Intelligence
Global Risks

EN | ES | FR | 中文 | 日本語

Privacy Policy & Terms of Service

****

July 22, 2020, 10:12PM (Amir-ul Kafirs to group):

[The World Economic Forum's "Great Reset"]

I highly suspect that this is the real reason behind the pandemic

I've only watched the 1st few minutes. I'll watch it all eventually but I have to take it in small doses. One of the things that struck me is that it states something like "We all have a role to play." Unfortunately, what seems to be taken for granted is that these "roles" are predetermined for us, there's no room for individualism here! Somehow, we're supposed to 'feel good' that there's a script for all of us to unquestioningly follow. **I don't feel good about that at all!!!!!**

****

July 23, 2020, 5:52AM (Amir-ul Kafirs to group):

I can literally only take about a minute of this one at a time so my comments on it will be very stretched out over multiple emails. One of the participants is from the IMF, the International Monetary Fund. Anti-Globalization activists will remember that the IMF & the World Bank have both long since been exposed as userers, as organizations posing as for the general good of 'developing economies' whose real purpose is to control the politics in those countries & to, essentially, extract all natural resources & otherwise bankrupt them — making them feeble dependent states. The introductory montage to all this is somewhat in the style of "Koyaanisqatsi", a film that I imagine most or all of you have seen that was pioneering in its use of sophisticated camerawork to present "Life Out of Balance" (the Hopi meaning of the title). Interestingly, when I was verifying the spelling online this was listed NOT as a Hopi word but as English. "Koyaanisqatsi" had no narration & had a compelling soundtrack by Philip Glass. It seems to me that this introductory montage is meant to communicate a similar feel: a variety of things are shown, including George Floyd protestors & astronauts in free-fall. The 'message' seems to be that these are the extremes of our world today & the background for the WEF's planning.

Wikipedia has a long entry on the WEF that begins with this:

The **World Economic Forum** (**WEF**), based in Cologny-Geneva, Switzerland, is an NGO, founded in 1971. The WEF's mission is cited as "committed to improving the state of the world by engaging business, political, academic, and other leaders of society to shape global, regional, and industry agendas". It is a membership-based organization, and membership is made up of the world's largest corporations.

The WEF hosts an annual meeting at the end of January in Davos, a mountain resort in Graubünden, in the eastern Alps region of Switzerland. The meeting brings together some 3,000 business leaders, international political leaders, economists, celebrities and journalists for up to five days to discuss global issues, across 500 public and private sessions.

The organization also convenes some six to eight regional meetings each year in locations across Africa, East Asia, Latin America, and India and holds two further annual meetings in China and the United Arab Emirates. Beside meetings, the organization provides a platform for leaders from all stakeholder groups from around the world – business, government and civil society – to collaborate on multiple projects and initiatives. It also produces a series of reports and engages its members in sector-specific initiatives.

Due to its prominence as an international community of leaders from business, politics, arts and media, the World Economic Forum and particularly its annual meeting in Davos are among others criticised regarding the public cost of security, the formation of a wealthy global elite without attachment points to the broader societies, undemocratic decision processes, gender issues and a lack of financial transparency.

- https://en.wikipedia.org/wiki/World_Economic_Forum

It was founded by Klaus Schwab 49 years ago & his introductory speech is up next so I'll try to endure that.

He says that we're in the midst of the most severe crisis since WWII or some such. Since this meeting is centered around COVID-19(84) I assume that this is the 'crisis' he refers to. Since I find the supposed basis for this 'crisis' to be largely imaginary I'm immediately put off by this. The 'crisis', for me, is the way the whole social fabric is being changed using COVID-19(84) as an excuse. Therefore, the only thing that the WEF is likely to do is to further exploit this farce to the advantage of the big corporations & politicians that they gather together. Schwab makes the astounding claim that 75 years ago people came together to bring us decades of increased peace & global cooperation. Really?! That's funny, what I've personally noticed is continual war. I wonder whether the people of Korea, Vietnam, Laos, Cambodia, Iraq, Iran, Syria, Libya, Guatemala, Nicaraugua, El Salvador, Afghanistan, etc, etc, feel that there's been 'increased peace & global cooperation'?! Schwab also mentions that "prosperity has been brought to hundreds of millions of people around the world". Is that like the 'prosperity' that was brought to Bhopal??? Where Union Carbide had a horrible chemical accident that killed many with little or no recompanse or responsibility taken?!

SO, I just went back to the video but it's no longer playing for me & I wanted to confirm details regarding Bhopal but that search won't work either. It's 5:47AM, is the internet really so busy around here?! Presumably I won't be able to send this email either so we'll see what I have to do about that.

ANYWAY, I really don't mean to be so negative — it's just that I feel that it's important to cry "Bullshit!" when I see it & I am sure am seeing alotof it!!

****

July 23, 2020, 10:53AM (Amir-ul Kafirs to group):

The **Bhopal disaster**, also referred to as the **Bhopal gas tragedy**, was a gas leak incident on the night of 2–3 December 1984 at the Union Carbide India Limited (UCIL) pesticide plant in Bhopal, Madhya Pradesh, India. It is considered among the world's worst industrial disasters. Over 500,000 people were exposed to methyl isocyanate (MIC) gas. The highly toxic substance made its way into and around the small towns located near the plant.

Estimates vary on the death toll. The official immediate death toll was 2,259. In 2008, the Government of Madhya Pradesh had paid compensation to the family members of 3,787 victims killed in the gas release, and to 574,366 injured victims. A government affidavit in 2006 stated that the leak caused 558,125 injuries, including 38,478 temporary partial injuries and approximately 3,900 severely and permanently disabling injuries. Others estimate that 8,000 died within two weeks, and another 8,000 or more have since died from gas-related diseases. The cause of the disaster remains under debate. The Indian government and local activists argue that slack management and deferred maintenance created a situation where routine pipe maintenance caused a backflow of water into a MIC tank, triggering the disaster. Union Carbide Corporation (UCC) argues water entered the tank through an act of sabotage. The owner of the factory, UCIL, was majority owned by UCC, with Indian Government-controlled banks and the Indian public holding a 49.1 percent stake. In 1989, UCC paid $470 million (equivalent to $845 million in 2018) to settle litigation stemming from the disaster. In 1994, UCC sold its stake in UCIL to Eveready Industries India Limited (EIIL), which subsequently merged with McLeod Russel (India) Ltd. Eveready ended clean-up on the site in 1998, when it terminated its 99-year lease and turned over control of the site to the state government of Madhya Pradesh. Dow Chemical Company purchased UCC in 2001, seventeen years after the disaster.

Civil and criminal cases filed in the United States against UCC and Warren Anderson, UCC CEO at the time of the disaster, were dismissed and redirected to Indian courts on multiple occasions between 1986 and 2012, as the US courts focused on UCIL being a standalone entity of India. Civil and criminal cases were also filed in the District Court of Bhopal, India, involving UCC, UCIL and UCC CEO Anderson. In June 2010, seven Indian nationals who were UCIL employees in 1984, including the former UCIL chairman, were convicted in Bhopal of causing death by negligence and sentenced to two years imprisonment and a fine of about $2,000 each, the maximum punishment allowed by Indian law. All were released on bail shortly after the verdict. An eighth former employee was also convicted, but died before the judgement was passed.

- https://en.wikipedia.org/wiki/Bhopal_disaster

****

July 23, 2020, 11:41AM (Amir-ul Kafirs to group):

Schwab also mentions that "prosperity has been brought to hundreds of millions of people around the world".

I've seen this announcement of prosperity before in at least 3 other contexts. They were all situations where rich white guys were obviously obvlivious to the economic realities of many or most people. President McKinley announced widely that there was prosperity in the United States. He was assassinated by the anarchist Leon Czolgosz. Czolgosz was one of the many children of the era who had had to work in a factory by something like age 10. The life he saw around him wasn't prosperous except for the rich factory owners who were exploiting the child labor. McKinley was such a "Fat Cat" that when an attempt was made in autopsy to find the bullet that killed him they were unable to do so (or so the story's told). Another example is that when the cameraman who'd been on "Independence Day" (a film I hated) gave a presentation at the Andy Warhol Museum of a "Koyaanisqatsi"-styled film-in-progress (without any of the social observation saving graces) he was making he explained that "Everyone can afford to buy a cool car now". What world he lived in was pretty obvious from the stupidity of his film & he was very out-of-touch with reality. Some similar statement was made by an audience member at a Berrigan brother talk at CMU. These people actually seem to believe that everyone is as rich as they are. How anyone could be that out of touch with reality is beyond me.

"The COVID-19 crisis has shown us that our old systems are not fit anymore for the 21st century."

The underlying assumption of all this is that there're people **qualified & entitled** to control how things are done in the world. I am basically opposed to that. That's the same type of arrogant privilege that those articles in *The Atlantic* also tout. The lawyers will censor the internet for us, they know what's best for us. NOT. Yep, the privileged elites have the wisdom to understand the poor feeble-minded children under their self-appointed care. Klaus Schwab is making the claim that equality is going to be created under the WEF's vision. REALLY? Does that mean everyone in the world will have the privileges that he & his cronies were probably mostly *born with?!* I think not — because it's the very inequalities that create & maintain this privilege.

Schwab talks about the "post-corona era". Again, I think this is a completely artificial construct. Imagine if he were saying the "post 2019 flu era": people would be saying *What the fuck is this guy talking about?!* — but because COVID-19(84) has been exaggerated into a disaster of WWII proportions (it's not even close) he can act like we really 'need' the WEF's planning to save us from the brink of total annhilation. The thing is, this brink of annhilation has been brought on by the very people who are now going to 'save us from it'. Unfuckingbelievable.

He speaks out against "nationalism" in the same breath as "racism". So whose internationalism / post-nationalism will 'we' be practicing? Somehow I don't think it'll be the internationalism of Belarus, e.g.. I mean it's not going to be internationalism, it's going to be *doing things in the way that the dominating imperialist countries want it done*. It's just the new colonialism. One of the things that's interested me about this COVID-19(84) is seeing how the few countries that've had the strength to resist being sucked up into the global plan have each refuted the PANDEMIC PANIC narrative in their own ways. Swedish spokespeople said they believed in the intelligence of their people as they see fit, no lockdown. Lukashenko in Belarus has referred to "coronapsychosis" & has said that it's better to die standing than on your knees. He claims, if I understand correctly, that NO-ONE in Belarus has died from COVID-19. Whether that's true or not I have no way of knowing but my friend in Belarus hasn't reported any extraordinary deaths that he's noticed. In short, it seems to me that maintaining nationalism under these conditions has turned out to be a good thing.

Schwab claims that "we have a choice to remain passive which would lead to an amplification of many of the problems that we see today." The thing is, he's not proposing that the masses not remain passive, he wants them to be SHEEPLE, even though that's not explicitly stated. He wants the **leaders** to not be passive. Fine, Lukashenko's not being passive, how does he like that?! Oh, that's right, not only do the leaders have to be not passive they all have to be on the same page. Yep, the answer is to "build a new social contract". The thing is that a contract is signed by 2 agreeing parties, what's being forced upon us here is much more akin to the treaties that Native Americans were forced to sign with the European invaders — anything good in it for them was definitely NOT something that was going to be honored by the people drawing up the contracts.

NOW, I'M ONLY 3:30 INTO THIS PIECE OF SHIT & I'M ALREADY SO WORKED UP IT'S ALMOST UNBEARABLE.

****

July 23, 2020, 1:34PM (Amir-ul Kafirs to group):

One thing that's funny about this is how Schwab talks somewhat like Dr Strangelove. None of my English-speaking German friends say "ze" instead of "the" but Schwab does. Schwab promotes a vision of living more harmoniously with nature. Of course, technology is presented as a big part of this. Now, truthfully, I like technology, I'm typing this on a computer, I'm sending the message to you folks via the internet; I make movies, I make electronic (M)Usic, etc, etc. I am definitely a product of this 'civilization' AND I consider humans to be animals & what we do to be 'natural' no matter how extremely out-of-kilter it is with the rest of nature. BUT, when I think of "living harmoniously with nature" I think of deer wandering through the woods & eating all day. I don't think that's what the WEF has in mind. Humans are always going to be the extreme to which tool-making can go. That's always going to make us causing destruction to the mostly non-tool based rest of nature. I'll be happy to see humans pollute less & leave less of a footprint but there's no way that's ever going to be 'harmonious' with the rest of nature unless we become total anarcho-primitivists — which I'm not going to do. & if I'M NOT GOING TO DO IT I think we can be sure that the forces that the WEF represents are going to do it even less.

"We have to mobilize all consituents of our global society to work together": I'd call that **forced labor** because there's no way ALL of us want the same thing. I'm 100% sure that I don't want the same thing that Schwab & co want & I'm 100% sure that he could care less what I want & that he'll try to impose it upon me 'for my own good'.

Schwab lists the various professions represented but emphasizes "above all, the younger generation". Who, exactly, is representing the "younger generation"? Is it Skinny Woman (my new archetype of a person who I think has gone dreadfully wrong)? Next up is some guy from the UN. I'm 4:45 in.

****

July 23, 2020, 4:43PM (Amir-ul Kafirs to group):

The United Nations Secretary General António Guterres says: "The microscopic virus has closed down entire countries & economies." Nope, it's this type of false logic that keeps people in La-La Land. The people who're manipulating the narrative of the virus are the ones shutting down the countries & the economies, they're the ones that should be blamed. A virus has no power to do such a thing. He also refers to "the lawlessness of cyberspace" as one of the "warning signs that we must heed". Yep, there you have it: in order to bring the world back to a place where it won't be so endangered by a virus we must also suppress the "lawlessness of cyberspace" which, as far as I can tell, means **suppress any narrative contrary to the WEF's about what's actually happening here.** It's incredible, really, how transparent these people are. &, yet, how many idiots will fall for this shit?!

He further recommends "strong unity & solidarity — particularly for developing countries". In other words, it's the same old same old propaganda that's been used to cover up crimes by Globalization for a very long time. I'm up to 6:19. This is truly some of the most insidious euphemistic language I've ever witnessed.

****

July 23, 2020, 6:25PM (Amir-ul Kafirs to group):

On to Caroline Ansti of PACT. There's a continued verbal bowing down to His Royal Highness, the Prince of Wales, who's in attendance. This ROYAL FAMILY SHIT really does have staying power, doesn't it?! People just eat it up, it's old school celebrity culture. She intros him & he begins to speak by clarifying that it's been 38 years now that he's been trying to put people & the planet central. He just reiterates the same tired myths about the world coming to a standstill because of the virus & because we didn't have the mechanisms to deal with it. I tend to think that if COVID-19 had been left to its own devices some of the old & sick would've died, probably considerably less than those that the hospitals 'helped' along their way. I think hardly anyone would've noticed anything, it would've just been the usual: "Oh, did you hear? 92 year old Joe passed away." & that would've been that.

Then he moves on to Climate Change & its being a "devastating reality for many people". This is a more complicated subject for me. I've read 2 novels about climate change: Michael Crichton's "State of Fear", which refutes climate change & which I think is horrible (I've written a scathing review of it if anyone's interested), & Kim Stanley Robinson's "Green Earth", which presents climate change as a reality & which I thought was excellent (I also wrote a long review of that). I'm still not convinced one way or another. I can say that in my personal experience that the winters have gotten progressively warmer & less snowy in the last 55 years. That, however, is close to meaningless.

HRH goes on to list the other pandemics we've gone through including bird flu, swine flu, ebola, SARS, etc. The problem here is that all of those were exaggerated, but not near the degree that COVID-19 has been, & that NONE of them turned out anywhere close to what they were predicted to be. If anything, they could be used as examples of how ridiculous the induced fears are. No such luck here. In fact, this is where he starts to get particularly scary because he starts talking about how these diseases originate from animals & about how we need to change the relationship between domestic & wild animals, blah, blah, blah. I'm rooting for the animals being left far more alone than they are now. He's proposing taking action to restore a balance with nature but I suspect that the subtext means more like control-freaking on everything even more than we do now. What he says after that I find basically unobjectionable: giving back to nature as much as we take from 'her', pro-biodiversity, etc.

HRH repeats the myth about the 75 years after WWII seeing unprecedented growth, blah, blah. The basic underlying attitude here is that powerful humans must take control of EVERYTHING & HRH & his cronies are the ones to do it. It seems to me that nature would do just fine if humans intervened ***less***. I've been saying for probably the last 50 years or so that *there's no system that's suitable for all situations.* Hence, the fewer systems or the more flexible ones the better.

One aspect of my orchestra's, HiTEC's, structure was precisely that it was highly systematic at the same time it basically allowed anyone to do *whatever* as long as they were *thinking.* I'm not sure anyone in the group ever understood that.

I'm not opposed to the more ecological statements he makes until he gets to the part of how to restore the economy. That's where it starts to get too Big Brother for me. Basically he's not talking about letting people go back to their original jobs he's talking about creating new jobs that're more "sustainable" & better for the ecology, etc. ***But it's not like people are being given a fucking choice, are they?!*** Just like they weren't given a choice when the Industrial Age started that has been the ongoing main contributor to the destruction of the environment in the 1st place! After this, at about 13:00, the image freezes & the video continues but there's no sound.

SO, end of pt 6. HRH was the most tolerable one of the lot so far.

****

July 24, 2020, 6:26PM (Amir-ul Kafirs to group):

16:10: HRH shuts up. Back to Caroline Ansti of PACT. She intros Kristalina Ivanova Georgieva-Kinova (a Bulgarian economist serving as Chairwoman and Managing Director of the International Monetary Fund since 2019). GROAN. I'm not sure I can stand this. "Now is the time to think what history would say about this crisis & now is the time for all of us to define our own role." Somehow, I don't think that by "all of us" she means the 7.5 billion people who're going to be effected by the decisions of the 119 member IMF. By "all of us" I think she means the same thing that everyone else seems to mean: all participants in the WEF's meeting. The rest of us don't get a vote, we're just to do what we're told &/or manipulated into. "Worrisome signs: 170 countries are going to finish this year with a smaller economy than with which they started." Gee, I wonder why? Could it be because they were scared into ruining their own economies so that the global robber barons could impose their own self-benefitting structure on them? The IMF specializies in stepping into countries in a bad economic way & finishing them off while pretending to help, laughing all the way to the (World) bank — kindof like the doctors at Elmhurst Hospital, eh?! "unless we act", "great opportunity for reset": it was their 'acting' that caused the problem in the 1st place & their "reset" will be the final nail in the coffin — all 'for our own good', of course.

The IMF forsees a "massive injection of fiscal stimulus": this means loan-sharking. They're not GIVING AWAY THE MONEY. Of course, the IMF is talking about stimulating more "green" & "fairness". Why don't I believe her? They'll do that as long as there's massive profit for them involved. That's why the word "opportunities" keeps coming up in everyone's speeches. "Reforestation": in the past "reforestation" has meant planting product trees in areas where there was once biodiversity. Imagine devastating an environment for resource extraction & then planting only pine trees to replace it. Presto chango! That's "reforestation": even though all the endangered species that aren't of any use for capitalism are destroyed there's a new crop of trees available for turning into lumber.

"We know that the digital economy is the big winner of this crisis." Wow, I'm sure she didn't think that was in any way self-damning but I think that sortof says it all: there's a "winner" to the 'crisis': those are the businesses that've benefited from having their smaller competitors forced into destruction by the QUANRANTYRANNY. Here's an image that I found on Naia Nisnam's social media timeline:

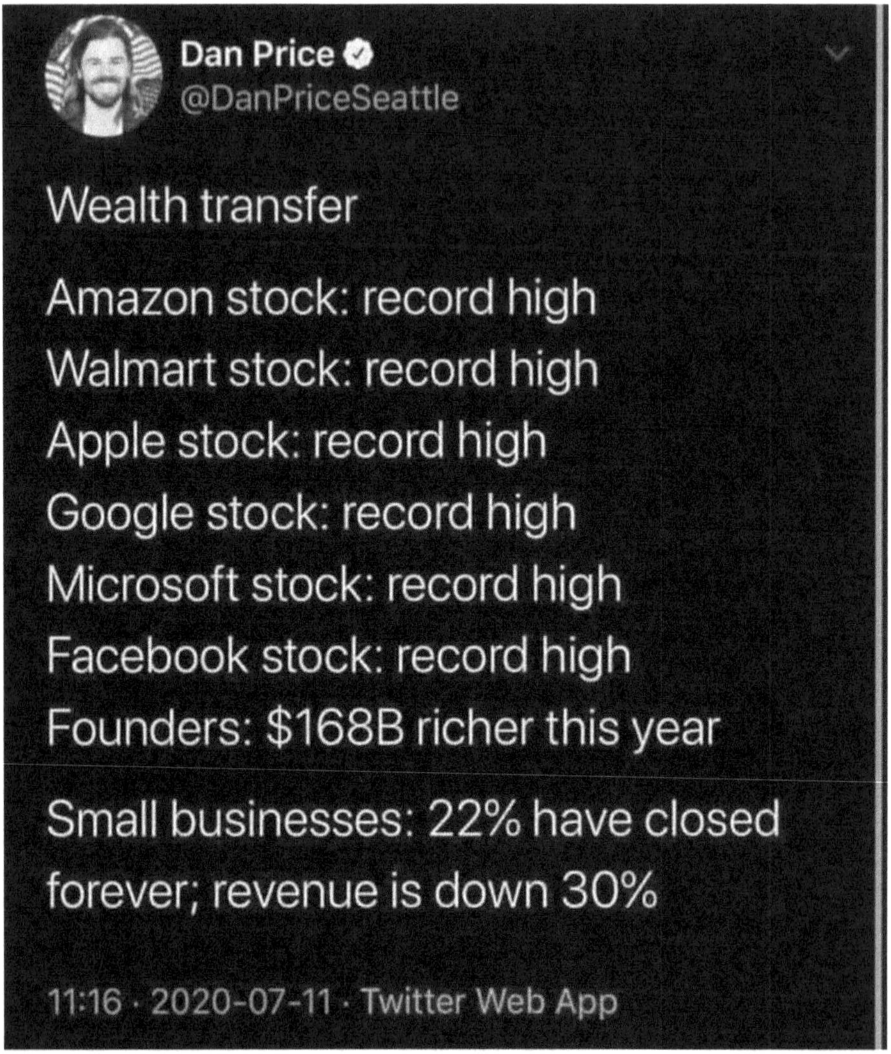

SO, there we have SOME of the "winners". I'm sure there're even BIGGER ones that aren't so obvious.

Then she promotes the IMF & the World Bank's goals to "shrink the digital divide".

"We know that this pandemic, if left on its own, is going to deepen inequality." Really? By what? Mainly killing off poor people in NYC? The deepened inequality is 100% the result of economic manipulation by these global corporate players. "We take care of the most vulnerable peoples, then we can have a better world for all." Nothing has changed about this really. It's just the Catholic Church all over again. The stroke of genius is in convincing people that COVID-19 is a much bigger health threat than it actually is & using it accordingly. That's working big time. Everything else is the same old same old Globalization false promise.

She mentions the IMF's "one trillion dollars" & "tremendous engagement on the policy side": Money talks & you'd better walk the way the say.

24:23: It goes back to Klaus Schwab. He emphasizes a "long-term perspective" which I don't think is bad in & of itself but is still evocative for me of a 'thousand year reich'. He wants companies to report not only on their finances but also on how they're serving the environment AND "SOCIAL COHESION". What, exactly, is "SOCIAL COHESION"? Cohesion implies to me an absence of difference, an absence of dissent.

Okay, 25:50: it froze again & the sound stopped again so I'll stop here for the moment.

****

July 24, 2020, 6:33PM (Amir-ul Kafirs to group):

Re: HERETICS: Dr. Andrew Kaufman, July 17th Interview

A week or 2 before Plandemic came out, a friend sent me an interview w Dr Judy and she said similar things about the RNA code existing naturally in our bodies. She theorized that it had become activated in many many people as a response to last years flu vaccine. It would be interesting to know what percentage of people testing positive for Covid had taken last years flu vaccine.

It's interesting that in the 2008 "PANDEMIC" movie I just watched & gave you the long description of that the hero, the veternarian, speculates that the vaccine might *accelerate* the action of the virus. As I understand it, & Inquiring Librarian's more the expert here, that's something similar to what Kennedy says about a possible thing with the COVID-19 vaccine. **[Pathogenic Priming]**

****

July 24, 2020, 9:14PM (Amir-ul Kafirs to group):

Re: HERETICS: "1986"

I listened to another great Del Bigtree interview this morning.

Oh, well, in the interest of even looking at & copying & pasting all the HERETICS emails of the past few days I'm going to have to pass on checking out this interview for right now at least but I'm hoping that in the interest of the HERETICS book that someone will have the time to get through the whole thing, take some screen shots, & write a summary that covers its main points. Inquiring Librarian, I know you're already overworking yourself but if you ever have the time to write a summary of any of these things you post links to while you're in the midst of watching/listening-to them & the time to take a few representative screen shots (preferably in full screen mode to try to get the best resolution) that would be very helpful & would reduce what is at the moment an impossible workload for me.

"The Public Readiness and Emergency Preparedness Act (PREP Act) authorizes the Secretary of the Department of Health and Human Services (Secretary) to issue a declaration (PREP Act declaration) that provides immunity from liability (except for willful misconduct) for claims of loss["]

WELL! That sure is convenient isn't it? Just not for the patient who's really taking a big risk to get involved with such folks.

****

July 24, 2020, 9:25PM (Amir-ul Kafirs to group):

Forced County COVID-19 Lockdown of Ventura Apt Building at 137 S. Palm St. | Citizens Journal

https://www.citizensjournal.us/forced-county-covid-19-lockdown-of-ventura-apt-building-137-s-palm-st/

I read this article. The whole incident seems like it wouldn't have happened without the current climate of fear & people trying 'to do the right thing' which generally seems to mean acting like Big Brother. Here's an explanatory excerpt:

****

The building is run by the Ventura Housing Authority and has elderly and behavior health cases living there - 74 units in total, mostly singles. Some residents are mobile, some not.

A resident fell, was hospitalized and tested positive for COVID-19. The building management went on full alert. Common areas had already been shut down, but they also disabled the keys and residents couldn't get back in if they left and returned. Some called the police, who told the management they couldn't do that. So, the County Health Dept was involved and quarantined the place at management's request, Levin told me.

Two more residents became ill, tested positive. The laundry area was closed.

After the tests results came in today, 7-20-20, only one more positive . The lockdown was rescinded, but residents were asked to avoid interaction, going out and to wear masks and socially distance. Dr. Levin is recommending retesting in a week or two.

Levin said this was a unique set of circumstances and was done out of an abundance of caution due to the very vulnerable population of residents. The county wanted to avoid situations like have occurred in nursing homes we've all read about.

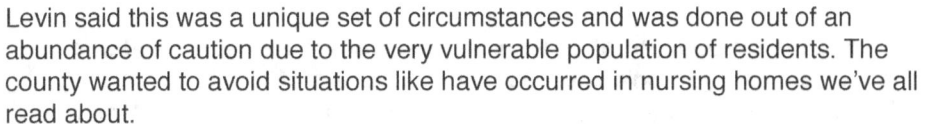

****

Maybe the worst part about it for me is that the residents' keys were made to not work. I can imagine that going horribly awry.

****

July 22, 2020, 5:48PM (Inquiring Librarian to group):

HERETICS: Dershowitz/RFK Jr. Mandatory Vaccinations Debate Tomorrow

Robert F. Kennedy Jr. will be debating the topic of mandatory vaccinations tomorrow morning, 8:45am EST. Alan Dershowitz said this recently: "Let me put it very clearly: you have no constitutional right to endanger the public and spread the disease, even if you disagree. You have no right not to be vaccinated...And if you refuse to be vaccinated, the state has the power to literally take you to a doctor's office and plunge a needle into your arm."

Here is the link to the debate, which I am sure will be recorded: https://childrenshealthdefense.org/news/vaccine-debate-is-on-robert-f-kennedy-jr-vs-alan-dershowitz/

****

July 22, 2020, 8:40PM (Naia Nisnam to group):

Re: HERETICS: Dershowitz/RFK Jr. Mandatory Vaccinations Debate Tomorrow

Thanks for the link. It's hard to believe people still listen to anything Dershowitz has to say. He defends the shittiest of shit bags, he helped Epstein get his 13-month vacation at rich-person jail in 2005, and I'm hoping he goes down hard when Ghislaine Maxwell (who he continues to defend in the media) goes to trial...
I'm currently feeling disgusted with the whole world.

****

July 24, 2020, 9:32PM (Amir-ul Kafirs to group):

Re: HERETICS: Dershowitz/RFK Jr. Mandatory Vaccinations Debate Tomorrow

Robert F. Kennedy Jr. will be debating the topic of mandatory vaccinations tomorrow morning, 8:45am EST.

Well, I missed this but **I certainly want to check out the video of it at some point. Linda, can you post the relevant link as part of this thread?** If you don't do so I can probably find it in the messages that you sent me but, as I've expressed before, making it a part of these emails makes it easier for me to document it all. THANKS!

Alan Dershowitz said this recently: "Let me put it very clearly: you have no constitutional right

Wow! That's such an obnoxiously hateful statement that I find it hard to accept it as anything other than what DERSHOWITZ IS BEING PAID TO SAY BY BIG MONEY INTERESTS.

****

July 24, 2020, 10:16PM (Amir-ul Kafirs to group):

I just watched the Patrick Wood video. He makes complete sense to me. The one thing I can't agree w him on is his sense of hope.

I realize it's hard to not give up hope but I also think it's a bit too simple to give in to hopelessness. Here's a quote from a message that Inquiring Librarian sent me about the Kennedy / Dersshowitz debate:

Kennedy killed it! Over 45k views in 4hrs, 6.3k likes, 75 dislikes.

45,000 likes!! That's incredibly impressive & VERY HOPEFUL. You & I have the misfortune to be mainly connected to liberal culture, which was fine UNTIL they caved in to the big COVID-19 myth. Now, it's like they're all zombies. Under such social conditions, where we're both unfriending people at an unprecedented rate, it's hard to not feel down. Add to that the utter prevalence of mask-wearing around here & it's almost too much to bear.

Americans will love being told that the new world economy is all about environmentalism and equality.

You probably haven't had a chance to read my ongoing commentary about The Great Reset but, yeah, this environmentalism & equality business is one of the biggest hoaxes I've ever witnessed &, yeah, I'll bet people will fall for it rather than remembering who's saying it & what their previous record has been.

I'm feeling like we're all screwed, there's nothing to be done about it,

Oh, well, at the risk of being a cliché version of myself: RESISTANCE IS FERTILE.

and I'd be better off if I didn't know anything and could go about my life being comfortably dumb.

You could never be comfortable with being dumb.

Sorry if that's depressing but... that's where I am.

Ever thought about becoming an extreme boxer?

****

July 23, 3:56AM (Amir-ul Kafirs to group);

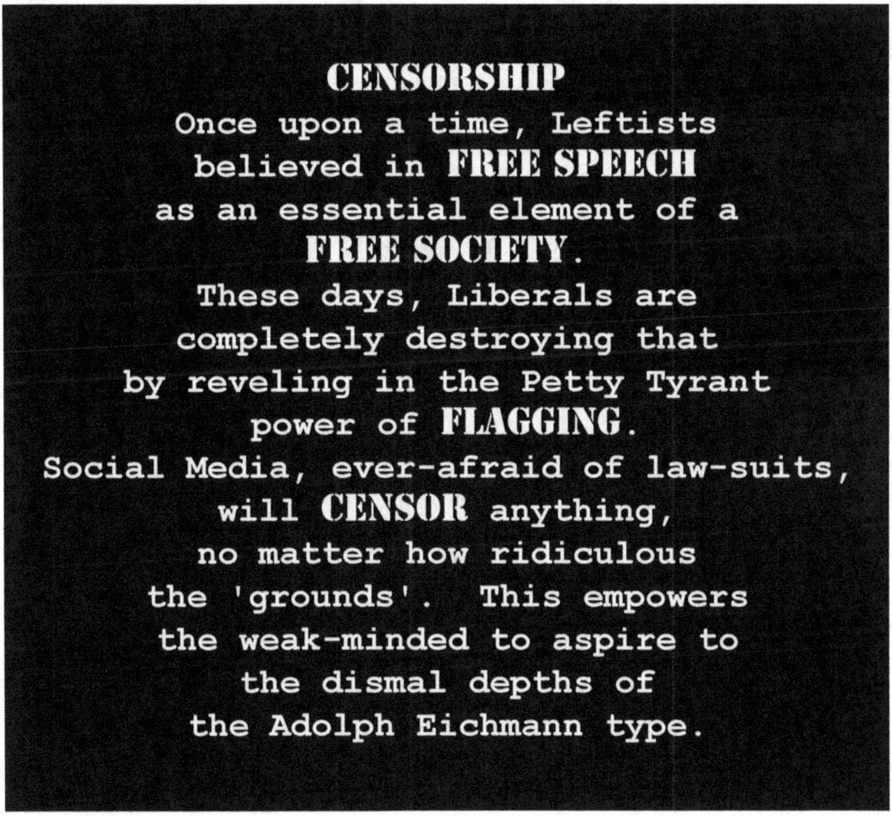

CENSORSHIP
Once upon a time, Leftists
believed in FREE SPEECH
as an essential element of a
FREE SOCIETY.
These days, Liberals are
completely destroying that
by reveling in the Petty Tyrant
power of FLAGGING.
Social Media, ever-afraid of law-suits,
will CENSOR anything,
no matter how ridiculous
the 'grounds'. This empowers
the weak-minded to aspire to
the dismal depths of
the Adolph Eichmann type.

****

July 23, 2:00PM (Amir-ul Kafirs to group):

HERETICS: Illiberalism

Here's an article by somebody who also writes for *The Atlantic*, which I've come to hate, that I think is pretty good. It's doesn't directly address COVID-19(84) but it's obviously about these times.

- tENT

A Taxonomy of Fear

There is a pattern in the way speech is silenced. Understanding it can help us stand up to the illiberalism of this moment.

Emily Yoffe
Jul 21

We live in a time of personal timorousness and collective mercilessness. There might seem to be a contradiction between being fearful and fearless, between weighing every word you say and attacking others with abandon. But as more and more topics become too risky to discuss outside of the prevailing orthodoxies, it makes sense to constantly self-censor, feeling unbound only when part of a denunciatory pack.

Institutions that are supposed to be guardians of free expression—academia and journalism in particular—are becoming enforcers of conformity. Campuses have bureaucracies that routinely undermine free speech and due process. Now, these practices are breaching the ivy wall. They are coming to a high school or corporate HR office near you.

The cultural rules around hot button issues are ever-expanding. It's as if a daily script went out describing what's acceptable, and those who flub a line—or don't even know a script exists—are rarely given the benefit of the doubt, no matter how benign their intent. Naturally, people are deciding the best course is to shut up. It makes sense to be part of the silenced majority when the price you pay for an errant tweet or remark can be the end of your livelihood.

Do these problems really matter so long as we have a president who daily tramples on rights, civil discourse, and the rule of law? They do. Of course, we must keep our focus on the danger this administration presents. But it is also our moral and strategic obligation to vigorously defend the principles of a free society. Upholding these values will help us defeat Trumpism.

The process by which sinners are punished and apostates expelled can seem random. But there are rules and patterns to the ways in which speech is being silenced. Analyzing and understanding these can help us stand up to the illiberalism of this moment, whether it comes from the left or the right.
To that end, here is my taxonomy of fear.

The Perils of Safety

James Bennet's resignation from his position as the editorial page editor of the *New York Times* quickly became the genesis story of today's debate about "cancel culture." Bennet was pressured to depart after he ran an op-ed by Tom Cotton, a Republican Senator from Arkansas, whose argument that the military should be used to respond to riots caused an uproar among the paper's staff.

At first, A. G. Sulzberger, the paper's publisher, publicly expressed his support for the decision to run the op-ed. But that quickly changed after Black employees asserted not just that Cotton's argument was morally repugnant, or that he failed to make it in a way that met the *Times*' standards, but that the piece threatened their lives. "Running this puts Black @nytimes staff in danger," many of them tweeted.

The language used by the *Times* staffers is indicative of a wider trend. In *The Coddling of the American Mind*, Greg Lukianoff and Jonathan Haidt describe the recent emergence and rapid spread on college campuses of what they call "safetyism," a view that "equates emotional discomfort with physical danger." Safetyism, they write, teaches students "to see words as violence and interpret ideas and speakers as safe versus dangerous."

Confronted with words, ideas, or decisions they dislike, a growing number of people are asserting that they are in danger of suffering psychological or even bodily harm. But when one party asserts that a debate threatens their very well-being, it is hard to deliberate on policy—or topics such as race and gender. The result is a narrowing of the space for public discussion and an inability to teach ever more ideas and books.

As Harvard Law professor Jeannie Suk Gersen has chronicled in the *New Yorker*, for example, law professors find it increasingly difficult to teach rape law because some students consider the subject too disturbing. "Student organizations representing women's interests now routinely advise students that they should not feel pressured to attend or participate in class sessions that focus on the law of sexual violence, and which might therefore be traumatic," she writes. "Some students have even suggested that rape law should not be taught because of its potential to cause distress."

But, as Suk Gersen has pointed out, it was feminists who fought for the overhaul of deeply sexist rape laws, and it is sexual assault victims who will be hurt if lawyers do not learn about the subject. In practice, safetyism will make some of the most vulnerable people in our society less safe.

Contamination by Association

[..]

Emily Yoffe is a contributing writer at *The Atlantic* and a member of *Persuasion*'s Board of Advisors.

- https://www.persuasion.community/p/a-taxonomy-of-fear?utm_campaign=post&utm_medium=web&utm_source=copy

****

July 23, 4:25PM (Amir-ul Kafirs to group):

HERETICS: Elizabeth Warren: Extend & Expand the Eviction Moratorium

Recorded Live
U.S. Senator Elizabeth Warren

- https://www.facebook.com/watch/live/?v=213362043306941&notif_id=1595531373395388&notif_t=live_video

I'm watching this now. Of course I support the concern over impending evictions essentially caused by the quarantyranny so this is interesting to check out since it's argumentation in favor of bills that their proponents are expecting Rump & others to block. Almost everyone is wearing a mask but Warren isn't. Unfortunately, she's also taking the Democratic party line about the nature of the pandemic. Too bad, she's a bit of a disappointment.

****

July 24, 2020, 11:59AM (Amir-ul Kafirs to group):

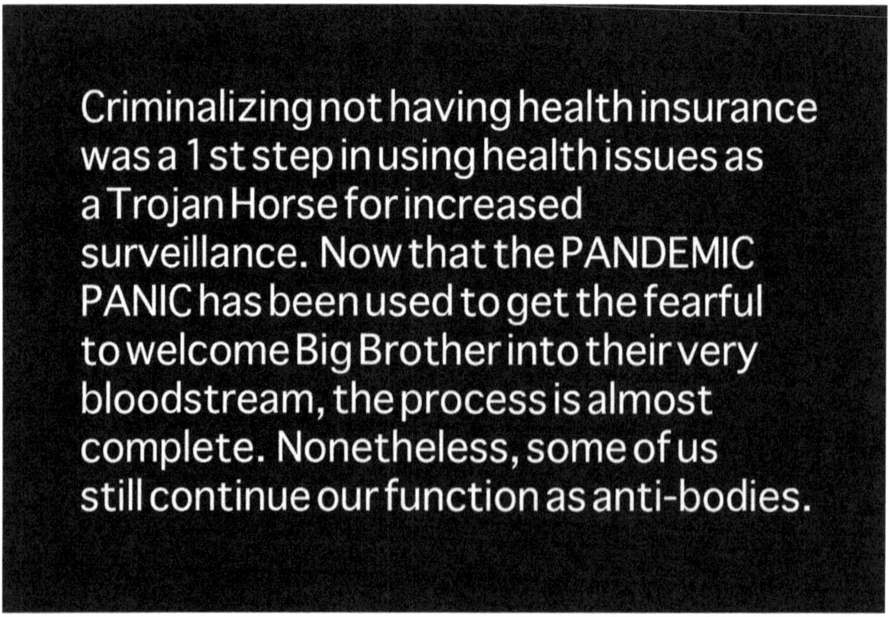

Criminalizing not having health insurance was a 1st step in using health issues as a Trojan Horse for increased surveillance. Now that the PANDEMIC PANIC has been used to get the fearful to welcome Big Brother into their very bloodstream, the process is almost complete. Nonetheless, some of us still continue our function as anti-bodies.

****

July 24, 2020, 5:29PM (Inquiring Librarian to group):

HERETICS: Hope from a Coon Ass State, and Stately Canada

Hola All,

This is a sign of hope from Canada:

Lawsuit against Trudeau Government: Constitutional Lawyer Rocco Galati and the Lies and Crimes of the COVID Operation

https://www.globalresearch.ca/rocco-galati-lies-crimes-covid-operation/5719222

& Hope from my dear state of Louisiana, it's at times like this that I LOVE my coon ass redneck liberty loving state-mates. They are thinking, and they are investigating and they are going public with their findings:

Louisiana's Parish And Local Officials Continue Questioning COVID Numbers

https://thehayride.com/2020/07/louisianas-parish-and-local-officials-continue-questioning-covid-numbers/?fbclid=IwAR357IXgk8p9PzMV1nMNav1sm_Br98e94Fcdt-ErRpSVjAvBlg-x0WlpHnc

My favorite quote from the article is this one, "Terrebonne's total death count from all causes is right on target for an average year."

& exposure of corruption galore in Louisiana in this article:

What We Know About Federal Funding, Louisiana Politics And COVID-19

July 24th, 2020

https://thehayride.com/2020/07/what-we-know-about-federal-funding-louisiana-politics-and-covid-19/?fbclid=IwAR367GZcM91qBLUwK3aSJI1DgqGksJEoqlOqKdSacLhgRpNvfSPkJXGvi6I

****

Lawsuit against Trudeau Government: Constitutional Lawyer Rocco Galati and the Lies and Crimes of the COVID

Operation

By Rocco Galati and Mark Taliano
Global Research, July 23, 2020

Celebrated Canadian Constitutional lawyer ***Rocco Galati*** *characterizes the COVID Operation as "the biggest example of misinformation and lies on a global scale that we've seen."*

The Constitutional challenge that he is filing with the Ontario Superior Court seeks to pull back the shroud of secrecy imposed by the Trudeau and Ford governments which, he says, are currently and have been "ruling by decree" beneath the pretexts of "COVID Measures" and "Emergency Measures".

Specifically, he is seeking "declatory and injunctive" relief against COVID measures. The Canadian Broadcasting Corporation (CBC) is also named as a defendant since it is publicly funded with a public mandate under the Broadcast Act and has a "duty of care."

Both Prime Minister Trudeau and Premier Ford refuse to divulge the substance and source of their "medical advice", and the media, including the CBC, are guilty of extraordinary censorship.

Whereas mayors in North America have proudly met with Bill Gates for advice, he has obvious conflicts of interest, and he is neither a doctor nor an expert.

Ontario's world-renowned Sick Kid's Hospital, on the other hand, is well qualified to weigh in on these matters. In a recent peer-reviewed study conducted by two expert virologists, aided by twenty experts, **the hospital has advised against social distancing and masking**, (1) **saying that social distancing and masking import drastic psychological harm on children.**

Galati reminds us of the impacts of societies' fascistic reactions to COVID.

- State diktats have assisted in premature deaths of people in Long Term Care Facilities.
- 170,000 scheduled surgeries (including heart and cancer surgeries) in Canada were postponed,
- suicides have spiked,

The Guardian reported that in the month of April 2020 alone, there were 10,000 extra dementia patient deaths in England and Wales. (2) The World Food Bank notes that 130 million additional people will be on the brink of starvation due to COVID measures (already one child starves to death every 29 seconds on planet earth).

Galati explains how all of **the COVID statistics have been manipulated,** saying, for example, that if the primary cause of death is cancer, but COVID is evident or presumed, then the Cause of Death is listed (falsely) as COVID.

The government's reactions to COVID amount to "state crimes". Galati's lawsuit should be a strong step in freeing ourselves from these destructive globalist tentacles.

Amanda Forbes interviews **Rocco Galati**

***Rocco Galati** is Toronto based Constitutional Lawyer*
***Mark Taliano** is a Research Associate of the Centre for Research on Globalization (CRG) and the author of **Voices from Syria**, Global Research Publishers, 2017. Visit the author's website at https://www.marktaliano.net where this article was originally published.*

Notes

(1) John C.A. Manley, "Toronto Children's Hospital Recommends Back to School without Masks or Social Distancing. Detailed Report." Global Research, 21 July, 2020.
(https://www.globalresearch.ca/back-school-without-masks-social-distancing-advises-sickkids-hospital/5719018) Accessed 22 July, 2020.
(2) The Guardian, "Extra 10,000 dementia deaths in England and Wales in April." 5 June, 2020.
(https://www.theguardian.com/world/2020/jun/05/covid-19-causing-10000-dementia-deaths-beyond-infections-research-says) Accessed 22 July, 2020.

- https://www.globalresearch.ca/rocco-galati-lies-crimes-covid-operation/5719222

****

Louisiana's Parish And Local Officials Continue Questioning COVID Numbers

July 24th, 2020 MacAoidh

Over the last couple of weeks we've picked up a lot of traffic here at The Hayride passing along a pair of reports from two parish governments – Red River and DeSoto – who have pushed back against the escalated numbers of COVID-19 cases coming out of Gov. John Bel Edwards' press conferences and news releases. Both noticed evidence that the case counts have been inflated by counting people who tested positive more than once as separate cases, something the Louisiana Department of Health has vehemently denied they're doing.

Red River and DeSoto Parish are not the only ones finding disparities, however. Sheriff Scott Franklin in LaSalle Parish has similarly uncovered some fluff in the numbers, and his brother penned an op-ed in the Jena Times (reprinted on the paper's Facebook page) which challenges Edwards' record-keeping.

Caldwell Parish has also reported irregularities, as noted in the link above.

And then there's this e-mail we received from President-elect Archie Chaisson in Lafourche Parish…

I've read the last two articles about the COVID numbers from Red River and DeSoto. I wanted to let you know that I've tried to tell everyone since the second or third week of this that the data is wrong, including the Governor's Counsel and Dr. Billioux with DHH to no avail. We know that we have people on our list that are not even Lafourche residents in addition to daily "unknown" residents because the spreadsheet we get doesn't even have an address on it. So if it doesn't have an address then now do they even know it's in Lafourche??

We take the daily list we get from DHH and between our Sheriff's Office and 911 System we run the names and addresses to confirm their location. We remove the inconsistencies and come up with a true number for Lafourche. For example, July 19 the stat showed 86 new cases for Lafourche but our count was 81 based on the list provided by DHH. We operate a day behind so I don't have the July 20 numbers yet from 911. It's only five people but you take five cases every day then it adds up quickly. Another large example is July 14-15, the state showed a two day total of 109 but after our work its was only 72 cases. That is a starker example of how bad it is.

Just wanted to pass that along to let people know it's a wide spread issue. If you have any questions please reach out to my office.

Next door to Lafourche Parish is Terrebonne, where we're told there have also been questions about the numbers though the parish hasn't gone public with any inconsistencies. But a local official did send us this…

Terrebonne's total death count from all causes is right on target for an average year.

100% of COVID related deaths tested positive, although COVID was not always the cause of death. (I need to follow up on the causes of death listed on death certificates.)

100% of COVID related deaths had co-morbidities. Nearly all had multiple. The most common one was hypertension. (It's not the high blood pressure itself but the medication for high blood pressure that makes a person vulnerable because it changes the way the virus affects the body.)

Average age of COVID related deaths is 75.

64% of COVID related deaths were nursing home residents. (45 out of 70)

Death count of senior citizens from all causes is also right on target for an average year. (Average 200 per year. 2020 so far: 104)

Terrebonne has 2 hospitals. All in-hospital COVID related deaths are from one of them. The other had zero.

That hospital difference – both are admitting COVID patients. It could be VERY significant to look at because the one with zero deaths is the "charity" hospital – Chabert Hospital. Think about that!

These stories from parish government people around the state aren't hard to find, though Louisiana's legacy media isn't working very hard to find them. They cast a long shadow of doubt over whether we're getting a straight story from Edwards and the Louisiana Department of Health.

[..]

- https://thehayride.com/2020/07/louisianas-parish-and-local-officials-continue-questioning-covid-numbers/?fbclid=IwAR357IXgk8p9PzMV1nMNav1sm_Br98e94Fcdt-ErRpSVjAvBlg-x0WlpHnc

****

What We Know About Federal Funding, Louisiana Politics And COVID-19

July 24th, 2020 MacAoidh

From a source very familiar with the legislative appropriations process, some perspective on exactly how federal funding colors Gov. John Bel Edwards' response to COVID-19 and his recent obsession with case counts.

If you paid attention to Edwards' most recent press conference on the virus, which took place yesterday, you probably noticed as we did that he's very long on scolding the public about mask-wearing, but a bit short of emphasis on actually treating people who have COVID-19. Many have explained this by concluding Edwards really only cares about drawing down as much federal money as possible in order to replace state and local revenue lost to his shutdowns. Whether that's partially or completely true, we can't say.

What we can say, per our source, is the following…

- Louisiana has received approximately $3 billion in direct federal aid so far. That doesn't include money which has gone to private citizens – PPP, the boosted unemployment payments which are set to run out in a week, and stimulus checks. It also doesn't include FEMA dollars which are still flowing in.
- Of that $3 billion, $1.8 billion of it is CARES Act money. The state has

also received funding from a number of other federal sources. Some $150 million came in from the feds that went directly to public and private universities in the state, most of which was "off the books." Plus the $1.8 billion wasn't the only CARES Act money which came in; there was some $280 million to K-12 schools, there were smaller grants like a $14 million chunk to the Louisiana Department of Agriculture and Forestry for emergency food bank assistance, some $15 million that went to the state's Councils on Aging to help with Meals on Wheels programs, $24 million for a rental assistance program, $20 million for the state's unemployment insurance pool, cash to support libraries and museums, and on and on.

- Some $524 million of that $1.8 billion in core CARES Act funding was aimed at local governments. This is where things start to become interesting.
- The local money isn't supposed to be used to replace lost tax revenue, for obvious reasons – you don't want perverse incentives leading to local governments gratuitously locking down their own economies. But with so much of the virus response handled at the state level, the lost tax revenue really is the prime fiscal effect of COVID-19.
- So how to allocate that $524 million? Well, a formula was set up which allocated 30 percent of it to the 64 parishes based on their populations, and 70 percent of it would be allocated based on case count as of the day the funding bill was passed – which was June 1.
- But the Legislature didn't include the allocation table as part of the funding bill, and that gave some wiggle room to Commissioner of Administration Jay Dardenne to make changes to the case-count allocation.
- As a result, Dardenne has turned that 70 percent pool of money into a moving target, changing total allocations as case counts change. It's beginning to look like an arbitrary, Byzantine process by which the locals are now incentivized to find more cases of COVID-19 and spend more federal money in something like a bizarre pageant with Jay Dardenne as the judge. The money is being doled out in phases, so the competition for federal dollars is ongoing.
- The federal government put strings on the cash, so the locals have to qualify their expenditures in order to receive that funding. As we understand it, testing is one of those qualified expenditures. So there have been nearly 1.2 million COVID-19 tests done in Louisiana, a number equal to a quarter of the state's population.
- The Legislative Auditor has been tasked with verifying those local government expenditures. At some point we'll see a report on how that money is being spent. We probably won't think very fondly of the results of that report.
- It's a common opinion at the Capitol that the 1.2 million COVID-19 tests have come not out of any scientific basis but purely to run up a maximum case count. Particularly since there's a Phase 4 stimulus plan being negotiated in Congress which started in the Senate at a trillion dollars, and Edwards is busy wrangling Louisiana's congressional delegation to

seek as much of that $1 trillion in federal relief money as possible.

Nowhere in any of this is a consideration for Louisiana businesses or the state's private sector. It took a strident, unified effort by the legislature to carve out a couple hundred million in federal CARES Act money for grants to business, which Edwards reluctantly signed after complaining that the money was coming out of the local governments' mouths. There are now 345,000 Louisianans who have filed active unemployment claims, which means the state has a double-figure unemployment rate even after what's being described as a mass exodus to other states the size of which we won't be able to ascertain for months to come.

In the meantime, legislators this week were broadsided with a poll asserting that Louisiana residents were wholly behind Edwards' handling of the virus and staunchly opposed to the petition circulating in the House with about two-thirds of the Republican delegation having signed it which would cancel Edwards' emergency declaration and force him to allow the state to go back to normal. The poll was commissioned by Leading Louisiana, a 501(c)4 organization formed by House Speaker Clay Schexnayder and Senate President Paige Cortez, and that's a point of contention with several legislators we talked to this week.

Why? Because those legislators think it was a push-poll aimed at discrediting the legislators who have signed the petition. They point to the third question asked in the survey, which they thought was particularly loaded...

There are a number of moving parts here, but among them a few things rankle. First, the poll leaked to Sam Karlin at the Baton Rouge Advocate almost immediately after it was released to legislators. While it's possible that Karlin got it from one of the legislators, the ones we talked to think the leak was more direct. An Advocate article essentially marginalizing those House members who have signed the petition followed shortly thereafter.

But the poll's second question was also a sore spot. It asked respondents whether they had approved of the performance of the state's hospitals vis-a-vis COVID-19, which seemed a little peculiar.

The pieces come together when, as a number of legislators we talked to told us, one considers that the political consultant who is the executive director for Leading Louisiana and works with Schexnayder as his consultant also has a six-figure contract to do communications work for Franciscan Missionaries, the organization which runs Our Lady of the Lake, Our Lady of Lourdes and St. Elizabeth's hospitals in Baton Rouge, Lafayette and Gonzales, respectively. Over the weekend there was an Advocate article quoting OLOL's head as saying the petition would be disastrous to the state's COVID-19 response, and that was seen as connected to the release of the poll.

[..]

- https://thehayride.com/2020/07/what-we-know-about-federal-funding-louisiana-

politics-and-covid-19/?
fbclid=IwAR367GZcM91qBLUwK3aSJl1DgqGksJEoqlOqKdSacLhgRpNvfSPkJXGvi6I

****

July 24, 2020, 5:52PM (Inquiring Librarian to group):

HERETICS: RFK Jr. Debate w/ Dershowitz & Kennedy Attacker from the Inside

Admittedly, I am behind on the last 2 days of everyone's posts. But the weekend is here, and I've not stopped my obsessive research on this whole debacle.

If you have not yet seen it, check out RFK Jr.'s debate with Alan Dershowitz. I think it was fabulous. Kennedy killed it. Barely after 24 hours of it's posting it has 225,757 Views, 13,000 Likes, & just 178 Dislikes
https://www.youtube.com/watch?v=IfnJi7yLKgE&feature=share&fbclid=IwAR01MMgxqUqABkbhFaGCf449cC4ecawGjr35lNeDVRs9hZANZ41eqVvurxQ

Then I noticed this guy, Dr. Shiva, who is bashing Kennedy, to be expected I suppose. There could be some truth to what he says, I don't know, but Dr. Shiva seems like an angry guy looking to divide and he also has pretty bad video making skills for a guy that is supposed to have so many degees in so many technical fields, he seems unreal to me, but I could be totally wrong, this is my gut feeling... The Kennedys have always been mesmerizing and RFK Jr. is no exception. Note that Dr. Shiva threw Kennedy under the bus FIRST in a somewhat subpar videorecording explaining the pandemic scam in simple talk to the layfolks. Note also, that RFK Jr's Nephew is running against this Dr. Shiva for Senate in Massachusetts. Crazy twisted ties here.
Ok, here is Dr. Shiva's freak out on and retaliation on RFK Jr.
https://shiva4senate.com/kennedy-lawsuit/?fbclid=IwAR2XbhttjZuqvknFpyWyFp4-twXhGxh1gvFSvJ-D-IBDfqW8VwRDS7b0Exw
& his original video that bashed Kennedy (and all of the Kennedys) about half way through:
https://www.youtube.com/watch?v=wxv8LBfRCEo&feature=youtu.be&fbclid=IwAR0un-GAqoB-BuLMnRvV7AFfBznx6w-y7S6m9VbLlqUBxc9y9wSWpTGmVSM

& here is Kennedy's rebuttal to Dr. Shiva's original video bashing of him and his family. This rebuttal is what sparked Dr. Shiva to decide to try to sue Kennedy:
https://childrenshealthdefense.org/news/critical-questions-for-dr-shiva-about-his-attempts-to-splinter-the-health-freedom-movement/?fbclid=IwAR03Iwq9ClDqHL-iQ8tzP9WqmGxIfAlrhql-t-bJNh6KEOqz8xdOLWM-47A

****

July 24, 2020, 11:11PM (Amir-ul Kafirs to group):

Re: HERETICS: Hope from a Coon Ass State, and Stately Canada

This is a sign of hope from Canada:

Lawsuit against Trudeau Government: Constitutional Lawyer Rocco Galati and the Lies and Crimes of the COVID Operation

What can I say?! I wish this lawyer the best of luck. The bulk of the article appeared earlier in this. Note the lawyer's 1st quote: "***Rocco Galati*** *characterizes the COVID Operation as "the biggest example of misinformation and lies on a global scale that we've seen."*" I'd go along with that! ALSO, Naia Nisnam, you might want to research this more: "Ontario's world-renowned Sick Kid's Hospital, on the other hand, is well qualified to weigh in on these matters. In a recent peer-reviewed study conducted by two expert virologists, aided by twenty experts, **the hospital has advised against social distancing and masking**, (1) **saying that social distancing and masking import drastic psychological harm on children.**" in case you ever try to make a case at the school where you work.

& Hope from my dear state of Louisiana

Louisiana's Parish And Local Officials Continue Questioning COVID Numbers

Another very useful article about the inflating of statstics that we've all come to know well right now but that I think Dr. Kelly Victory talks about most clearly in one of her videos on YouTube. Anyway, this article nails it too:

"We take the daily list we get from DHH and between our Sheriff's Office and 911 System we run the names and addresses to confirm their location. We remove the inconsistencies and come up with a true number for Lafourche. For example, July 19 the stat showed 86 new cases for Lafourche but our count was 81 based on the list provided by DHH. We operate a day behind so I don't have the July 20 numbers yet from 911. It's only five people but you take five cases every day then it adds up quickly. Another large example is July 14-15, the state showed a two day total of 109 but after our work its was only 72 cases. That is a starker example of how bad it is."

& exposure of corruption galore in Louisiana in this article:

What We Know About Federal Funding, Louisiana Politics And COVID-19

Sheesh. Just a taste:

- So how to allocate that $524 million? Well, a formula was set up which allocated 30 percent of it to the 64 parishes based on their populations, and 70 percent of it would be allocated based on case count as of the day the funding bill was passed – which was June 1.
- But the Legislature didn't include the allocation table as part of the funding bill, and that gave some wiggle room to Commissioner of Administration Jay Dardenne to make changes to the case-count allocation.
- As a result, Dardenne has turned that 70 percent pool of money into a moving target, changing total allocations as case counts change. It's beginning to look like an arbitrary, Byzantine process by which the locals are now incentivized to find more cases of COVID-19 and spend more federal money in something like a bizarre pageant with Jay Dardenne as the judge. The money is being doled out in phases, so the competition for federal dollars is ongoing.

Thanks, as usual, for the helpful info!

****

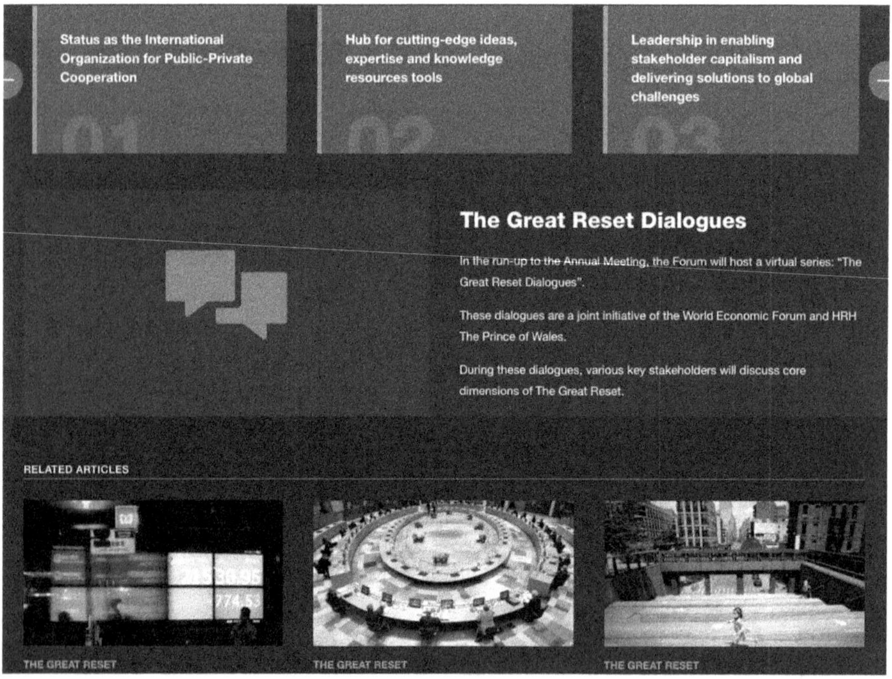

****

July 24, 2020, 11:32PM (Amir-ul Kafirs to group):

Re: HERETICS: RFK Jr. Debate w/ Dershowitz & Kennedy Attacker from the Inside

Crazy twisted ties here.

Sheesh, what a twisted web. Once again, I'm not going to take the time to watch all this stuff right now. In 30 minutes it'll be midnight & I'll upload a new text panel (I don't call them "memes" because I think that's an incorrect use of the word - it might be more accurate to say "Thought for the Day". After I get that online it's time to get off the computer. As usual, I've spent an insane amount of time just reading emails & articles & trying to archive them & reply. I did design some new protest signs today that I got a little work done on making. Now all I need is a situation in which to use them.

****

July 25, 2020, 12:04AM (Amir-ul Kafirs to group):

HERETICS: World Economic Forum

Inspired by suffering through the beginning of "The Great Reset":

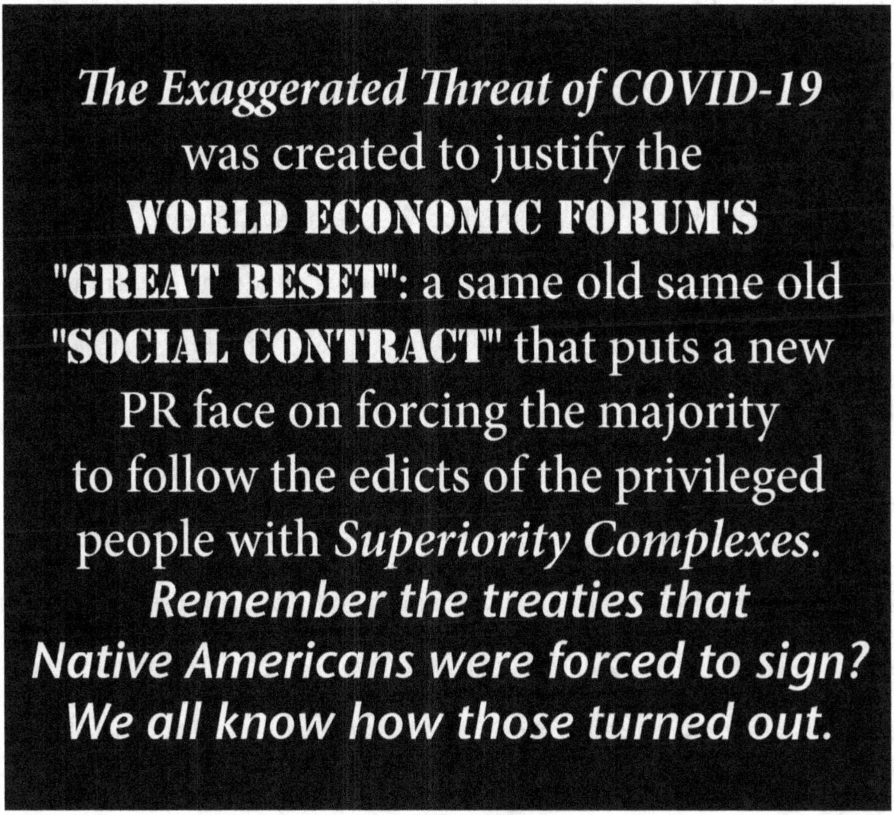
The Exaggerated Threat of COVID-19
was created to justify the
WORLD ECONOMIC FORUM'S
"GREAT RESET": a same old same old
"SOCIAL CONTRACT" that puts a new
PR face on forcing the majority
to follow the edicts of the privileged
people with *Superiority Complexes.*
Remember the treaties that
Native Americans were forced to sign?
We all know how those turned out.

****

July 25, 2020, 8:57PM (Inquiring Librarian to group):

HERETICS: Are we taking new HERETICS?

I have a new HERETIC friend who lives in California. I haven't mentioned it to him yet, but I thought I'd ask you first, in case he would be interested. He's feeling really stifled by the restrictions in California/Oakland right now. He's really bright and insightful and has been sharing a lot of interesting information with me on the pandemic debacle via social media. He is an old friend of friends from way back in my undergraduate years. He is a musician and an artist and has a real gift to see through bullshit and writes well. I think he could be a great addition and would add a U.S. state. Although, honestly, I'm not sure he'd even want to join us. But I thought I'd ask you all first. =] He is a Kennedy, actually related to the famous Kennedy's.

****

July 26, 2020, 12:24AM (Amir-ul Kafirs to group):

Re: HERETICS: Are we taking new HERETICS?

I've been thinking about this lately. As you probably remember, at 1st I tried including anyone that I thought might add something substantially skeptical & heretical to the mix so I tried my friend _____, who asked to be removed (I think it was 'too much' for him) & _____, who's probably too busy doing other things that're more important to him (& who's not really political). Phill added _____, who only piped in a tiny bit & who eventually faded away. Recently, I've thought of asking 2 friends in Canada if they'd like to join. They'd have plenty to add, they're both very smart & critical. BUT, I seem to've decided to NOT invite them. WHY? It seems to me that even with this small group of 6 of us we're all completely overwhelmed & can't keep up with the amount of posts with links. It's all I can do to read everyone's emails &, recently, I haven't had time to watch any of the linked-to movies. I try to at least read all the articles but I've probably missed a few. Because I'm trying to take all the input & somehow turn it into a book, these emails are an insane amount of work for me &, truthfully, my life is somewhat slipping away from me. I'm being crushed by the heat, I'm barely making it through the days, & even though I get SOMETHING done every day I'm working at an unprecedentedly slow pace. SO, for me, even adding *one more person* would be like the straw that broke the camel's back. As such, I hope we stay with just the 6 of us. On the other hand, I think it's up to the individual to decide whether they really want more people involved here. The problem, again for me, is that I have a sense of purpose that goes beyond just a casual sharing of whatever relevant things we come across. My purpose is to organize it all into something coherent that can be presented to a larger public. Since that's essentially *my purpose alone*, I need to keep it within limits. Anything that pushes it beyond those limits will be even more unmanageable than what I'm trying to do now & may even turn the proposed book into something undoable (if it's not already).

****

July 26, 2020. 12:10AM (Amir-ul Kafirs to group):

HERETICS: Viral Economy

Another one inspired by the WEF's "Great Reset":

In a speech to the World Economic Forum, the United Nations Secretary General António Guterres says: "The microscopic virus has closed down entire countries & economies." Nope, it's this type of false logic that keeps people in La-La Land.
The people who're manipulating the narrative of the virus are the ones shutting down the countries & the economies, they're the ones that should be blamed. A virus has no power to do such a thing.
He also refers to "the lawlessness of cyberspace" as one of the "warning signs that we must heed". Yep, there you have it: in order to bring the world back to a place where it won't be so endangered by a virus we must also suppress the "lawlessness of cyberspace" which, as far as I can tell, means suppress any narrative contrary to the WEF's about what's actually happening here. It's incredible, really, how transparently dishonest these people are.

****

Like Comment Share

001a Virus makes people uneasy with patronizing establishments.
Rational precaution begets lockdowns.
How is this conflated into some grand conspiracy?

Reply · 7h 1

Amir-ul Kafirs Have you seen the World Economic Forum's "The Great Reset"? I doubt that you'll change your mind about what you're saying from watching it but you might at least get some context. Even watching the 1st 10 to 20 minutes might help with that.

Like · 7h 1

001b A flood has no power to erect barriers preventing driving over washed out roads
Except for the way that the existence of flooding necessitates such measures.
But yeah, the people who put up the barriers put them up. Not the floods.
+1 for factuality.
-3 for pretending that the dots don't connect.

Reply · 7h

Amir-ul Kafirs It helps to've been an anti-Globalization activist, as I was, in order to have this perspective.

Like · Reply · 7h 1

Amir-ul Kafirs The pompousness of 'grading me' is, unfortunately, typical. You, obviously, have no idea what I'm talking about.

Like · Reply · 7h 1

Write a reply...

002a another perspective -
https://www.northjersey.com/.../americans.../5194987002/

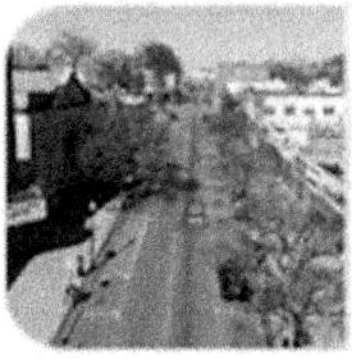

NORTHJERSEY.COM

Americans stopped the economy, not politicians. And we will restart it

Like · Reply · 7h 1

003a Difficult times or not ?

Like · Reply · 6h

Amir-ul Kafirs Yes, difficult times. I'm simply trying to maintain my own perspective here. I call things as I see them. As an Anti-Globalization activist I've seen the IMF, e.g., destabilize economies so they could move in as global loan sharks, control the politics,, extract the resources, & create dependent states. I see the same thing at play here. The PANDEMIC has become such a sacred thing that calling attention to the economic opportunism that surrounds it is absolutely taboo for some people. That, of course, limits intelligent discourse & further enables the destruction of the economy. It's no joke that as many people have been deprived of their living as have been. This knee-jerk reaction to describe any observations that go contrary to the Party Line as "Conspiracy Theory" & to then dismiss them, no matter how much evidence there is to back them up, is pernicious & reinforces Censorship Culture.

****

July 26, 2020, 1:06PM (Amir-ul Kafirs to group):

HERETICS: Who stopped the economy?

Commenter 002, who I unfriended (but never blocked) long ago on social media because of what I considered to be abusive comments, posted a link to this article as a comment on my "Viral Economy" text panel (uploaded July 26, 2020). Not wanting to completely ignore things that people post going contrary to my own opinions, I occassionaly look at what's linked to, which is probably more than they ever would do in response to me. Interspersed throughout the article in **bold [brackets]** is my commentary. I've posted a select part of this as my reply to commenter 002. I'll probably block them after I give them time to read it.

Americans stopped the economy, not

politicians. And we will restart it

Steve Horwitz Special to the USA TODAY NETWORK
Published 4:33 a.m. ET May 17, 2020 Updated 10:51 a.m. ET May 17, 2020

[OK, I immediately take exception to the title: It's outright claiming that all small business people closed their businesses as a grassroots democratic gesture in solidarity with government-expressed health concerns. That's the same kind of specious fake logic that claiming that 'the virus shut down the economy' is. I'll address this more below.]

As the various states and localities continue to develop plans for opening up their economies from the COVID-19 lockdowns, we need to think carefully about what it means to "restart" an economy, and, more fundamentally, what exactly constitutes "the economy."

The rhetoric from Washington, D.C. and the state capitals is that the president and the various governors have it within their power to restart their economies. And in some cases, we see even more local levels of government asserting that such a restart is within their purview. In one sense, they are all correct: lifting the legal constraints they have all put in place is a necessary condition for the resumption of economic activity.

But doing is not sufficient to ensure the restart they desire. The only people who can really restart the economy are us. Only when we — All Americans — decide that we are comfortable with resuming various kinds of economic activity because we believe it to be safe will that activity happen. You can open the cage door, but that does not mean the animal will come out.

[Right, because some people only feel safe in their cage. There will never come a time when "All Americans" "decide that we are comfortable with resuming various kinds of economic activity" precisely because many Americans live in a state of almost constant paranoia now. The main thing that will help destroy this paranoia will be a new propaganda campaign that tells the BELIEVERS that it's now safe. Until then, the weak-minded will live in a constant state of hypochondriac fear.]

Politicans and the media (not to mention economists) too often treat the economy as if it were some giant machine with various dials and buttons that can be pushed to produce particular results. So if we just push the "restart" button, the machine will come to life.

Economies, however, are not machines. They are much more like human ecosystems with all of the connections, complications, and unpredictability such systems contain.

Understanding how economies operate has to begin with understanding human choices and the constraints under which we choose.

In the case of the lockdowns, it is important to realize that people were out in front of closing down the economy. The evidence is pretty clear that we began withdrawing well before governments at all levels turned practice into legal decrees. Schools, restaurants, gyms, and houses of worship began to close or move to virtual before they were mandated to do so. Cell phone data indicate that people began to practice social distancing and forms of quarantine before governments acted.

[I think this is a total lie. Business owners closed their businesses out of fear of being fined or otherwise penalized. Even when they did that they thought that it was very temporary & not something that had the possibility of ruining their business for good. Certainly there were at least a few people who shut down their businesses in advance cooperation with what they'd been told was coming but mainly out of fear — fear of penalty AND fear of disease, a fear that had been inculcated in them by propaganda.]

We stopped the economy, not the politicians. And we will restart it.

[Again, bullshit, without the top-down imposition of law there would NOT have been a shutdown. That's like a policeman saying that someone that they killed commited suicide by stepping in front of their gun while they were firing it. Such a tactic was actually tried when the state murdered the MOVE people in 1982 in Philadelphia.]

That restart will happen when people believe that engaging in various forms of economic activity is sufficiently safe. Those beliefs will be a combination of their assessment of the virus and their confidence in what firms are doing to make going to stores, restaurants, and the like hospitable and safe.

[Really? What about all those BIG BUSINESS CHAINS that stayed open the whole time? Home Depot, Target, Dunkin' Donuts, etc..]

Two considerations are important here.

First, we need make sure that the public has a reasonably accurate assessment of the risks associated with various activities. For example, we are pretty sure COVID-19 does not transmit through food, and we know that hand-washing is about the most effective preventative step we can take. We also know that some demographic groups are more vulnerable than others. With surveys showing significant majorities opposing opening up various activities, it would be good to make sure those perceptions are based on fact more than fear. It is those perceptions that will drive the behavior that determines how and when the economy restarts.

Second, sellers will have a big role in the timing and shape of any restart. Governments at all levels have already shown that they will want to regulate the way that sellers and service providers structure their businesses as they reopen. There are always dangers in one-size-fits-all approaches, but the problem here is that these can prevent market competition from discovering new practices that both meet safety standards and satisfy customers.

[My point above is that the economy only shut down for small businesses.

Mega-businesses, the same businesses that've been forcing Mom & Pop businesses into bankruptcy all along, continued operating & CONTINUED FORCING MOM & POP BUSINESSES INTO BANKRUPTCY. This shut-down hasn't been for 'safety', that's just a euphemism to keep the weak-minded in La-La Land, it's been to further enable big businesses to monopolize. Home Depot put every smaller hardware store out of business in my area. One by one, the 3 hardware stores I gave my business to went under. This was BEFORE the quarantine. The quarantine accelerated this process even further.]

The main benefit of giving firms as much leeway as possible in figuring out how to persuade potential customers that their business is safe is that it is only through the diversity of approaches that this competition produces that we discover what works best.

Neither governments nor private firms know ahead of time which will work. Allowing for competition in how firms structure their safety protocols will produce better results than the heavy-handed approach of politicians.

The economy is not a machine with a restart button. It's a complex set of human relationships that rests on individual perceptions and choices. Rebuilding those relationships and generating economic activity will take time and will be driven by the people's perceptions of what is safe and what is not, not the dictates of politicians.

The economy is us.

Steven Horwitz is the Distinguished Professor of Free Enterprise at Ball State University in Muncie, Indiana. He is also Dana Professor of Economics Emeritus at St. Lawrence University in Canton, New York.

- https://www.northjersey.com/story/opinion/2020/05/17/americans-stopped-economy-not-politicians-and-we-restart/5194987002/?fbclid=IwAR2YdbpVpKFYZeDjZNQ5qAokSuMr-cog05Apg8so7UJAYI4FQEeM8lpxxSI

****

July 25, 2020, 9:11PM (Inquiring Librarian to group):

HERETICS: The Resistance is Growing

As you all know by now, I am obsessed with this pandemic being centered around the awful vaccine being developed. I wanted to share this absurd article that I found on Google last night. I was trying to find a link between the different vaccine skeptic groups. Of course, all I found was pro-vaccine propaganda. At this point the internet is so censored against vaccine skeptics, that the only way you can find vaccine skeptical information is by knowing the exact site/source you are looking for and going right to it.

Ok, so here is the absurd article. I read it and did discover that all of my vaccine skeptic sources are linked and seem to work symbiotically together. The brilliant thing about this article (for vaccine skeptics), is that it proves without a doubt that big pharma is squirming and is losing the battle to promote 'safe' vaccines. The antivaxx movement appears to be winning more and more people once the facts are revealed. What is nuts is this article is calling the antivaxxers liars with no science, but in reality it is the vaccine propaganda pushers who are lying and have no science to prove vaccines are safe. And the public is learning this and learning it rapidly.
https://www.mediamatters.org/coronavirus-covid-19/most-notorious-anti-vax-groups-use-facebook-lay-groundwork-against-novel?fbclid=IwAR1tvyDXA9HH2AWdcYiYXzBSh2agGT9BhMIXwimiYAPIO_w5cUDtfbKIJUc

The most notorious anti-vax groups use Facebook to lay the groundwork against the novel coronavirus vaccine

I found 2 priceless quotes in this article:
1. "After Buzzfeed News identified anti-vaccine ads in January, a Facebook spokesperson paradoxically responded, “Facebook does not have a policy that bans advertising on the basis that it expresses opposition to vaccines. Our policy is to ban ads containing vaccine misinformation."
2. "There's evidence that even brief exposure to anti-vaccination information changes attitudes. According to a 2010 study published in *Health Psychology*, “Accessing vaccine-critical websites for five to 10 minutes increases the perception of risk of vaccinating and decreases the perception of risk of omitting vaccinations as well as the intentions to vaccinate.” The phenomenon does not appear to work in reverse: A study that attempted to change attitudes with “direct pro-vaccination messages” found that those messages actually reinforced misguided beliefs. In fact, common ways that anti-vaccine information is countered are typically ineffective."

Lastly, 2 days ago I was invited to join a group called "Health Freedom Louisiana". https://www.healthfreedomla.org/
I am still waiting on my acceptance, But I wrote to them on their social media page last night with a few questions. I found out from the representative that was responding to me on social media, the following in regard to my not yet hearing back from them on my acceptance: "We are a tad overwhelmed with membership requests at the moment - over 90 - and we try to vet new members as well as possible on social media, so don't give up on us if it takes a while to get to your request.

Once we get you in, we have regional groups that we can add you to, we have smaller local groups too.:))"

This gives me a lot of hope!

****

The most notorious anti-vax groups use Facebook to lay the groundwork against the novel coronavirus vaccine

Health experts say vaccine rejection could imperil efforts to get the novel coronavirus outbreak under control in the US

WRITTEN BY TIMOTHY JOHNSON
PUBLISHED 07/09/20 10:01 AM EDT

Key takeaways:

- The three most prominent U.S. anti-vaccination organizations -- National Vaccine Information Center, Children's Health Defense, and Informed Consent Action Network -- are using Facebook and other major social media platforms to lay the groundwork for widespread coronavirus vaccine rejection.
- Facebook allows these groups to identify their organizations with descriptors like "Educational Research Center" and "Medical & Health" organization.
- Facebook's current policies surrounding vaccine misinformation include de-ranking accounts and posting "educational units" to some anti-vaccine misinformation. But the Facebook pages for NVIC, CHD, and ICAN and those groups' leaders do not contain any warnings from Facebook about the organization's purposes.
- The groups' pages are rife with vaccine conspiracy theories and other coronavirus misinformation. For example, NVIC has promoted conspiracy theories about Bill Gates and vaccine development, CHD has promoted the falsehood that wearing masks does not reduce the likelihood of coronavirus spread, and ICAN's leader has claimed even the "biggest vaccine advocates in the country" are "sounding the alarm" on coronavirus vaccine development.
- Facebook pages for NVIC, CHD, ICAN and their associated leaders and media projects have a combined more than 950,000 followers. This represents the tip of the iceberg; according to a recent report, anti-vaxxers have a combined Facebook following of 58 million people.
- Academic research on approaches similar to Facebook's to counter anti-vaccine misinformation suggests Facebook's current policies will not be effective in countering coronavirus vaccine misinformation.
- A growing share of Americans say they will refuse to receive a coronavirus vaccine, which could greatly harm efforts to get the disease under control in the U.S.

As novel coronavirus cases spike in the U.S. and numerous efforts are underway to develop a vaccine, the most prominent U.S. anti-vaccination organizations are using Facebook and other social media platforms to poison the well against a potential vaccine -- even though the consequence of widespread vaccination rejection in the U.S. would be an additional public health disaster.

In March 2019, Facebook said it "implemented new policies to de-rank accounts spreading vaccine misinformation in their search results," according to ABC News. Later that year, Facebook and Instagram (which Facebook owns) announced they had partnered with the WHO and Centers for Disease Control and Prevention to "start posting educational units about vaccines on 'vaccine-related searches on Facebook, Facebook Groups and Pages that discuss vaccines, and Invitations to join Facebook Groups that discuss vaccines.'" In theory, Facebook bans ads that include vaccine misinformation, but enforcement has been spotty. Anti-vaccine content on Facebook may be fact-checked by Facebook's third-party fact-checking program. Additionally, Facebook has a policy to take action against coronavirus misinformation, though the methods Facebook uses have been criticized as ineffective and scattershot in their application. After Buzzfeed News identified anti-vaccine ads in January, a Facebook spokesperson paradoxically responded, "Facebook does not have a policy that bans advertising on the basis that it expresses opposition to vaccines. Our policy is to ban ads containing vaccine misinformation."

There's evidence that even brief exposure to anti-vaccination information changes attitudes. According to a 2010 study published in *Health Psychology*, "Accessing vaccine-critical websites for five to 10 minutes increases the perception of risk of vaccinating and decreases the perception of risk of omitting vaccinations as well as the intentions to vaccinate." The phenomenon does not appear to work in reverse: A study that attempted to change attitudes with "direct pro-vaccination messages" found that those messages actually reinforced misguided beliefs. In fact, common ways that anti-vaccine information is countered are typically ineffective. A 2014 study published in *Pediatrics* tested the following four messaging strategies "designed to reduce vaccine misperceptions and increase vaccination rates for measles-mumps-rubella (MMR)":

(1) information explaining the lack of evidence that MMR causes autism from the Centers for Disease Control and Prevention; (2) textual information about the dangers of the diseases prevented by MMR from the Vaccine Information Statement; (3) images of children who have diseases prevented by the MMR vaccine; (4) a dramatic narrative about an infant who almost died of measles from a Centers for Disease Control and Prevention fact sheet; or to a control group.

None of the four approaches "increased parental intent to vaccinate a future child" and the study warned that attempts to "correct false claims about vaccines may be especially likely to be counterproductive." Based on these findings, it seems unlikely the "educational units" Facebook affixes to some vaccine misinformation would be sufficient in stopping the spread. Another negative factor in play at Facebook and other social media outlets is that research suggests that anti-vaccination content tends to be more popular than pro-vaccine content and anti-vaccine messages -- aided by the fact that their arguments need not be premised on scientific research -- tend to use stronger rhetorical devices compared to pro-vaccination efforts.

Given the fraught conditions surrounding the effects of anti- and pro-vaccine messaging, one solution, of course, would be for social media platforms to root out and remove anti-vaccine misinformation rather than include a disclaimer or appeal to an authority that may actually reinforce anti-vaccine attitudes.

There are growing concerns that vaccine rejection will prevent the United States from overcoming the novel coronavirus pandemic

Support in the U.S. for vaccination generally has been on a downward trend for the past two decades. A January 2020 poll released by Gallup found that 84% of Americans believe it is "important" to vaccinate children, down from 94% in 2001. The poll found that support for vaccination has declined "among almost all subgroups of the U.S. public." Gallup attributed the decline in support for vaccination to the spread of false information about vaccines, in particular the debunked link between vaccines and autism, writing of false vaccination claims, "While they are not as pervasive and are being exposed as untrue, these counterarguments are still getting through, perhaps explaining why public support for vaccines remains lower than at the start of this century."

[..]

- https://www.mediamatters.org/coronavirus-covid-19/most-notorious-anti-vax-groups-use-facebook-lay-groundwork-against-novel?fbclid=IwAR1tvyDXA9HH2AWdcYiYXzBSh2agGT9BhMIXwimiYAPIO_w5cUDtfbKIJUc

****

July 26, 2020, 7:49AM (Amir-ul Kafirs to group):

Re: HERETICS: The Resistance is Growing

It's interesting: I, personally, don't get vaccinated because I've had the ongoing philosophy referred to in my emails before that I think my body's immune system is far more profoundly functional & 'wiser' than anything doctors & pharma is going to do & because I think that mild exposure to anything not completely toxic functions as a natural immunization. Furthermore, I continue to assert that big business & capitalism in general wants people to buy EVERYTHING from them — convinced that what we have naturally & for free couldn't possibly be worthy.

Ok, so here is the absurd article.

As usual, there's no room given for the possibility that there might be any validity to anti-vaccine positions. Everyone's a "quack" or 'discredited' or whatever. The very complete demonizing, the position that any anti-vaccination opinion is inherently invalid is probably a factor in people's not trusting articles such as this one. Maybe there are just too many people who've been alive long enough to've gone without vaccinations & been just fine.

The most notorious anti-vax groups

"most notorious", of course, just means most widely belonged-to & most successful.

"Facebook does not have a policy that bans advertising on the basis that it expresses opposition to vaccines. Our policy is to ban ads containing vaccine misinformation."

Ha ha! Finally Facebook does something that doesn't completely embrace censorship-culture! I reckon that's at least partially because there's money in it for them.

There's evidence that even brief exposure to anti-vaccination information changes attitudes.

That's wonderful. I'd like to think that all this Fact-Choking & Censorship Culture will fail because there're some shreds of common sense & skepticism in a larger quantity of people than seems to be the case. Remember the old question: *What if there were a war & nobody came?* Well, what if nobody got vaccinated (obviously that won't happen) & COVID-19 doesn't produce a wave of deaths? I think there'll be over-reporting of deaths, I think people will die IN the health care system as a result of said system's malpractices. How many more Elmhursts will there be?

we try to vet new members as well as possible on social media

Cool. I imagine they're vetting them for Trojan Horse people whose soul purpose in trying to join is to attack from within.

****

July 25, 2020, 9:20PM (Inquiring Librarian to group):

HERETICS: Quantum Dot Tags

Here is a fun video by James Corbett.
https://lbry.tv/@DrewMedia:5/Democracy_Down_Raw_Files_James_Corbett:5

He begins with information on the new delivery method for our upcoming experimental coronavirus vaccines. This new delivery method uses "Quantum Dot Tags" that are "something like a barcode tattoo", injected into the skin using a "micro-needle array patch".

****

July 26, 2020, 8:28PM (Dick to group):

I had a thought, perhaps it's too borderline to be taken seriously but here it is.

If you use the basic code of a=1, b=2, etc. then Covid 19 equals Covid AI.

AI of course means ARTIFICIAL INTELLIGENCE.

Now, if you take the World Economic Forum great reset theory seriously with its talk of the 4th Industrial Revolution, the universal application of AI is the stated objective of all that is happening.

Finally viruses and the concept of 'the viral' are synonymous with AI so it all makes for a possible rather cynical in-joke on the part of the covid masterminds.

****

July 26, 2020, 8:51PM (Amir-ul Kafirs to group):

Re: HERETICS: Who stopped the economy?

1st, my thanks to Dick & Inquiring Librarian for commenting on the Viral Economy thread. It continues to amaze me that things that people post to 'refute' me & the dismal level of pseudo-intelligence that they represent. That article that commenter 002 posted is so moronic & flagrantly false that commenter 002's thinking it's somehow 'smart' would boggle my mind if I didn't already know what an idiot they are. I blocked them now too.

If you use the basic code of a=1, b=2, etc. then Covid 19 equals Covid AI.

AI of course means ARTIFICIAL INTELLIGENCE..

I think it's a wonderful idea. It appeals to my simple encoding mind enormously.

****

July 26, 2020, 8:59PM (Amir-ul Kafirs to group):

HERETICS: Co-opting Anonymous

Let the co-optation begin!:

Sponsored Create Ad

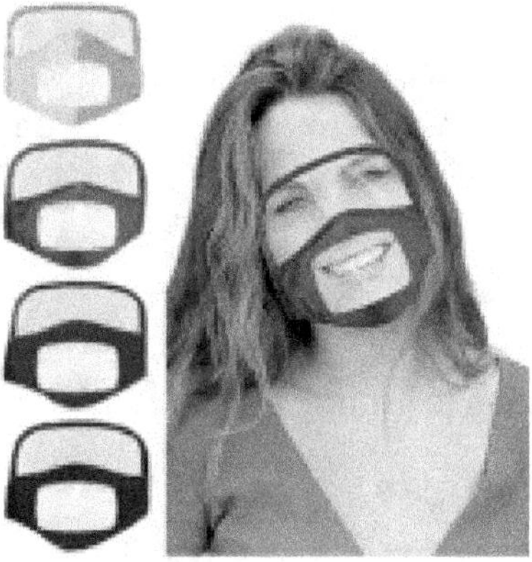

10% off sitewide
ivrose.co.uk
🔥🔥 Buy 3 get 15% off, Buy 4 get 20% off
🔥🔥 Up to 75% off! 🎉🎉 Free shipping order over...

😸 Safe delivery 😸 buy 1 get 2nd 20% off 🛒
https://chicmetoday.com/products/nd6073-c...
😸 Only $5.99 🔥
fashionable,breathable,washable and reusable
😸 A must for fashion people~

****

July 26, 2020, 10:46PM (BP to group):

Re: HERETICS: Who stopped the economy?

Jaw dropping. Totally clueless. I can't comment further, you did that well enough Amir-ul Kafirs. Shit like this is just too much for me to handle. USA Today via NorthJersey.com, no less. Yea, every shopkeeper was slamming their doors shut. Disgusting.

****

July 26, 2020, 10:18PM (Inquiring Librarian to group):

Re: HERETICS: Are we taking new HERETICS?

Yes. This makes total sense. I was hoping you/someone would say this. I think we are already so overwhelmed. And my friend is trying to move now from Oakland to Joshua Tree because he is so freaked out by how brainwashed everyone is in Oakland and he's lost his record shop due to the shutdowns. He says that people in Joshua Tree are way less brainwashed. aka: he has a lot on his plate right now.

****

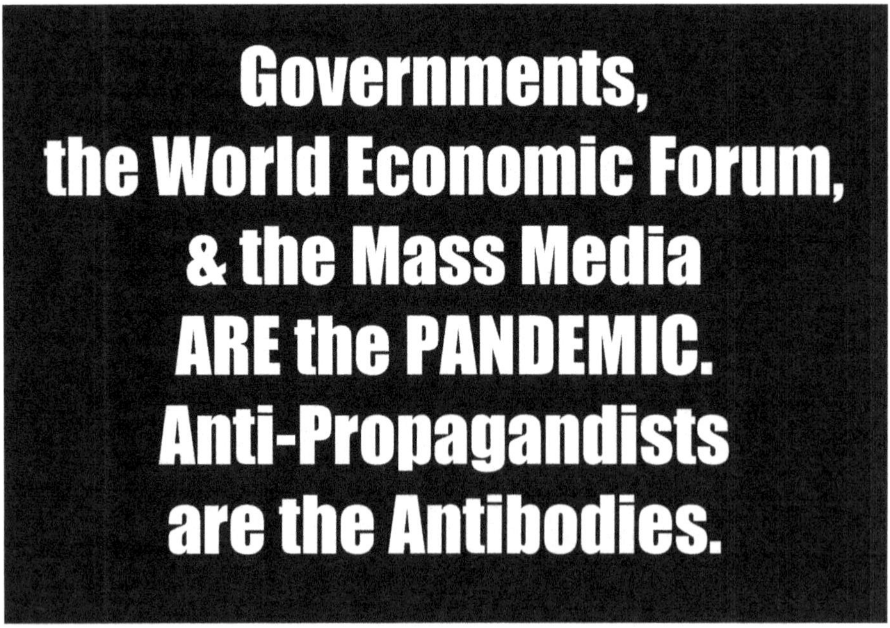
Governments,
the World Economic Forum,
& the Mass Media
ARE the PANDEMIC.
Anti-Propagandists
are the Antibodies.

****

July 28, 2020 (photos at rest stop from Amir-ul Kafirs):

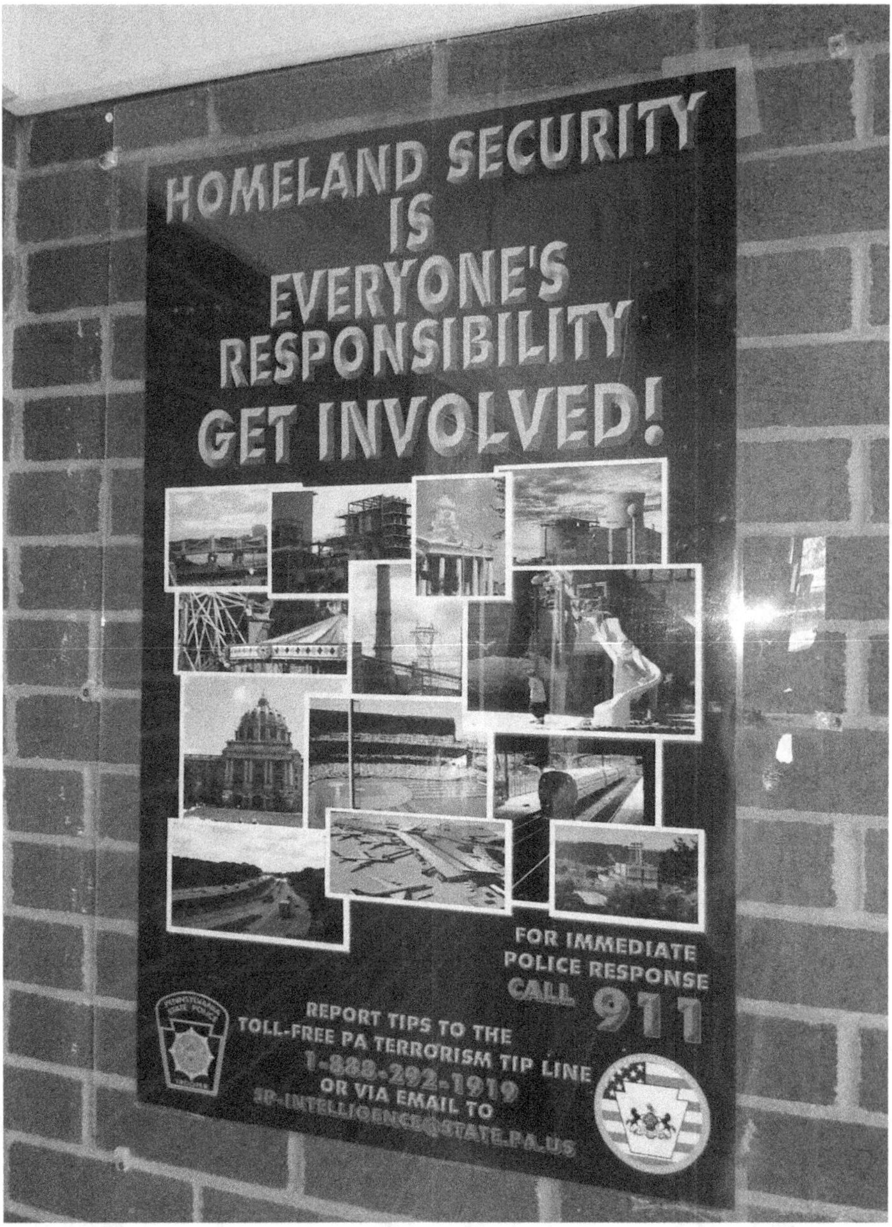

****

July 27, 2020, 5:13AM (Dick to group):

RE: HERETICS: Anti-Propagandists

very good!

*
unbelievably, just after writing about Tom Hanks in my essay for the proposed book, a friend posted this
https://www.youtube.com/watch?v=EmWDUmFV6yY&fbclid
so my suspicions weren't groundless at all
he makes his appearance at about 1:50 secs

WHO Cares What Celebrities Think - #PropagandaWatch - YouTube
SHOW NOTES: https://www.corbettreport.com/?p=37227 WHO cares what celebrities think? WHO cares, that's who! Or, more to the point, WHO wants you to care what...

****

July 27, 2020, 10:45AM (Inquiring Librarian to group):

Re: HERETICS: Anti-Propagandists

Yes, this one is excellent! I've gotten really obsessed with each of Corbett's reports throughout each week. This one is short, and very informative. I believe that in this, it was indicated that the same pr firm that was hired to promote good feelings about the Gulf war is being used to push this current celebrity feel good about destroying the economy over a fake pandemic. Everything these days is becoming so unreal. I just started delving into David Icke. As nutty as this guy has been pegged as for years, I have to say, he seems right on point on what is going on now. At least David Icke ends this show that I'll link below positively. According to David Icke, we the people have the power to not be scared and we the people can fight back against that 1%. We are many more than the 1%. Coming to work every Monday, I am usually so depressed to walk in the door to work with people who believe everything like worker drone bees. I guess time will tell what will happen to these people and to people like us. I plan to fight back with the Louisiana Health Freedom group for starters, but they have to let me into their group first. I will give them another week and then I will check in with them again. Given my job that I am still desperately trying to hold onto, I cannot go at combating this alone, but in an established group, I will have more power to fight back.

Here is the David Icke thing I listened to, it's a good 2.5 hours long. It's a great cooking, showering, and exercising one.
https://www.bitchute.com/video/H4W7FwBy0Ukh/?fbclid=IwAR0icfqjjJbNO7huEiaTXvHiXsuRyTs8gphuPGDc2ocWEJR8Hgt9nDmUOWs

****

July 28, 2020 (photos at rest stop from Amir-ul Kafirs):

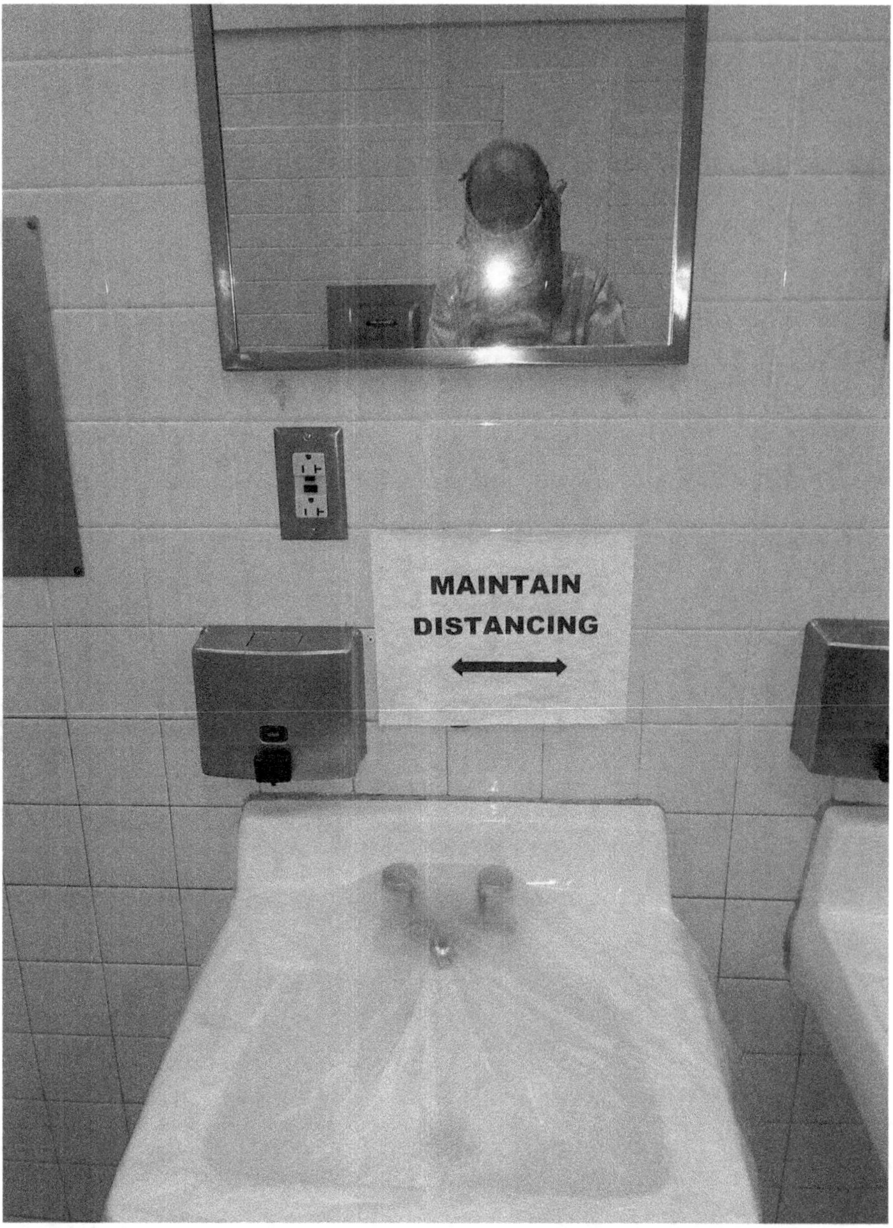

****

July 28, 2020, 8:51PM (Amir-ul Kafirs to group):

HERETICS: Masks vs Non-Masks

It appears that I've decided to just not worry about how many enemies I make with these things, the sheer JOY of saying such direct things is worth it.

Amir-ul Kafirs
3d ·

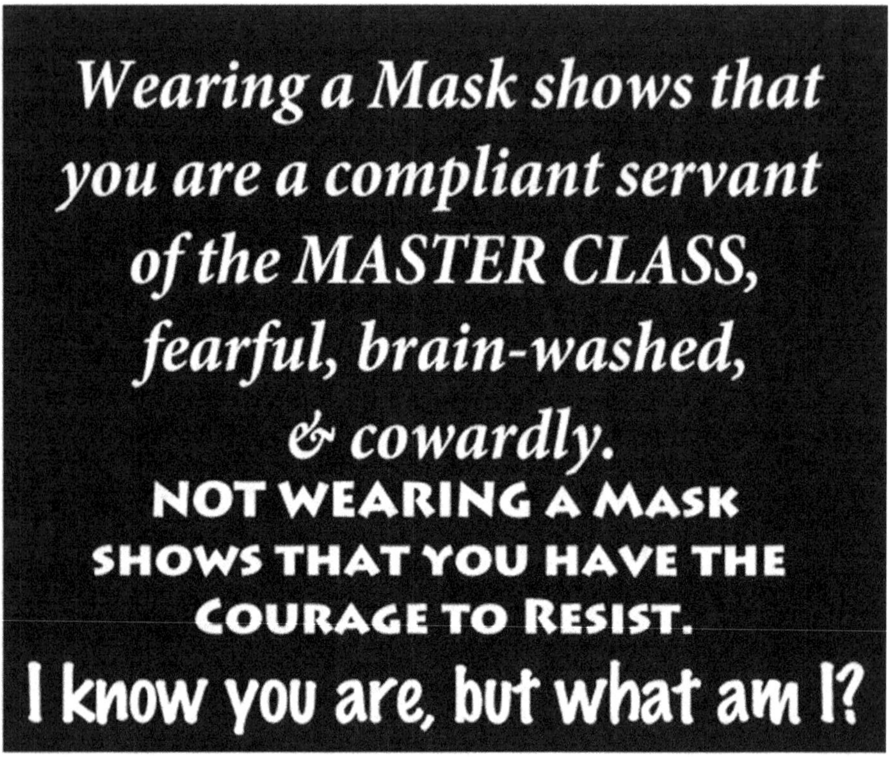

Wearing a Mask shows that
you are a compliant servant
of the MASTER CLASS,
fearful, brain-washed,
& cowardly.
NOT WEARING A MASK
SHOWS THAT YOU HAVE THE
COURAGE TO RESIST.
I know you are, but what am I?

Monty Cantsign and 4 others 22 Comments

Like Comment Share

001a You're joking, tENT, right? Please tell me you're joking.
Like · Reply · 3d 6

002a alive
Like · Reply · 3d 1

003a a compliant servant of common sense
2
Like · Reply · 3d

004a Oh is this why you blocked Andrew? Cuz you're actually an anti mask person? Jeebus. Tent, what the hell?
1
Like · Reply · 3d

Amir-ul Kafirs Actually, I blocked him because he insulted me.
Like · Reply · 1m

Write a reply...

004b You're an avid fan of over utilizing fonts and apparently not a fan of protecting your neighbors and friends from a deadly disease?
2
Like · Reply · 3d

005a Oh no
Like · Reply · 3d

006a Brainwashed by the PHS and NDMS in the '90s with training for dealing with airborne pathogens.
1
Like · Reply · 3d

007a Not. C'mon, Tent. Did you know the Czech Republic got its numbers down to near-zero through mask-wearing exclusively.
1
Like · Reply · 3d

008a wow, tEnt, you have really lost it. this is sad and pathetic. i once had a lot of respect for you. sorry to see you go.
2
Like · Reply · 3d

009a Wtf. This is not about courage. It is about public health.

Like · Reply · 3d 3

010a Too much urethane in your life?

Like · Reply · 3d

011a Tent, I really hope that you do not believe this. There is plenty of easily available, researched, documented, scientific evidence proving that mask wearing prevents the spread of Covid-19. Are you into Trump and Breitbart and Infowars now? Where is th... See More

Like · Reply · 2d 3

012a DERP

Like · Reply · 2d

013a Have you crossed to the dark side living up there?

Like · Reply · 2d 1

014a Either you're currently engaged in the single-least-interesting conceptual art piece in the history of an often uninteresting genre or you're dumb as a box of rocks. I suspect that a lot of people are going to drop you if you don't drop this.

Like · Reply · 2d

014b You're playing on my last nerve.

Like · Reply · 2d

015a If I don't wear a mask I cannot go in the liquor store or the supermarket. So I wear a mask because I like to eat drink and be merry

Like · Reply · 2d 1

001b Though I do like the idea of generating a huge Facebook thread with one comment as an art project.

Like · Reply · 2d

016a I'm sensible.

Like · Reply · 3h

017a

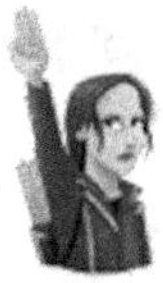

Like · Reply · 52m

Amir-ul Kafirs 014c : As the guy who told me that you wanted to rape me when you had AIDs I've always valued your health advice & am glad to have you set me straight. Thank you for pointing out the error of my ways.

Like · Reply · 4m

Write a comment...

[Commenter 001 at least manages to maintain a little distance & humor, commenter 009 at least attempts to address the surface content of the text, commenter 015 is pragmatic in a somewhat self-mocking way, & commenter 017 recognizes the Fascism of the GROUPTHINK]

There's so much that I can say about the string of responses to my obvious provocation: One is that people easily have their chains jerked. In fact, their chains are *so easily jerked* that doing so is like flipping a post-hypnotic suggestion switch on Pavlovian Zombies. Most of these people are Manchurian Candidates programmed by mediated non-experience into being suppressors of Free Thinkers. This, unfortunately, is what I've been commenting about all along: viz. that people are being manipulated by mass media signals into having completely predictable responses.

Would it have been really *so difficult to have engaged me in some way that didn't involve insulting me?* After all, I was speaking in *generalities*, not attacking specific people in personal ways. What makes the defensive reactions even more telling is that *not one single person got far enough into the 3 sentence text to TAKE INTO CONSIDERATION the last sentence.* The last sentence being "I know you are but what am I?"

I imagine that most native English speakers will recognize this as a

common children's fighting sentence. One child insults another & they retort in a way meant to reflect the insult back. The idea here being that exchanging insults is completely childish. So what do the commenters do? Insult me.

I'm not a Scientologist & I'm not in favor of Scientology but reading William S. Burroughs did get me interested in their "E-Meter" which they use to monitor emotional response to trigger words. The idea being, as I understand it, that if a person has a strong emotional response to a trigger word, such as something taken to be insulting, they need to work on neutralizing their reaction so that they can be more 'objective'.

Fortunately, I had another relevant text panel ready to go for the next day. It was my hope that people who would get angry about this 1st text would then be able to distance themselves more after reading the 2nd one.

****

July 29, 2020, 12:28PM (Amir-ul Kafirs to group):

HERETICS: Divide & Conquer

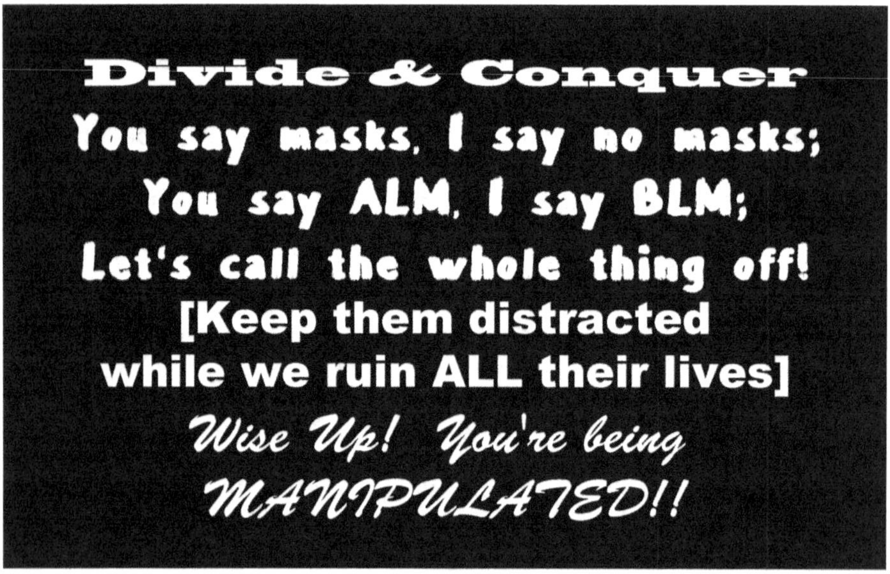

Divide & Conquer
You say masks, I say no masks;
You say ALM, I say BLM;
Let's call the whole thing off!
[Keep them distracted
while we ruin ALL their lives]
Wise Up! You're being
MANIPULATED!!

****

July 28, 2020 (photos at rest stop from Amir-ul Kafirs):

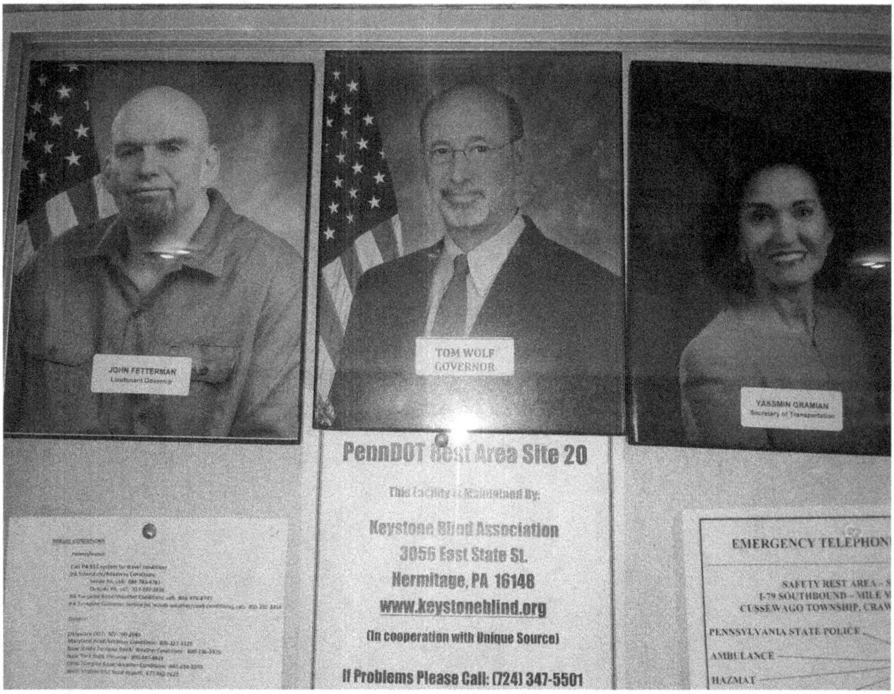

****

July 30, 2020, 3:47AM (Dick to group):

Re: HERETICS: Anti-Propagandists

I saw this posted on social media (see below) by the only multi-millionaire I know, none other than _____ (for those of you who don't know him, he's the son of an extremely successful real estate developer)
I can't get over it
I saw a similar thing (a video in French) from a guy here who said that normal people have no right to decide for themselves on health issues because they are untrained (ie not doctors, biologists, etc)
It seems like the idea of people making up their own minds, even at the risk of being wrong, is no longer acceptable
In a sense, if this is extended, why should people even be allowed to vote? that should be reserved for only those with degrees in political science
Or since very few people are nutritionists, they shouldn't be allowed to buy their own food
Or in fact, let's face it, they shouldn't be allowed to think because very few have studied logic, philosophy or... you get the point
This mask business is truly a stroke of genius... the fact that not wearing a mask means you are a socially irresponsible, selfish egoist putting **other's lives** at risk is the trump card in every argument that disallows whatever reasoning a non-mask wearer may have
non-mask wearers are (according to the various articles) alternatively irresponsible, less eductated, morally deficient (I wonder what the whole list

would consist of?) - it's kind of incredible
Since when has America been the land of the socially responsible? It's like a joke. The whole place is built on the idea to get rich (like ______) and sharing isn't exactly a virtue as I recall it from my time there, at least not among the so-called 'haves'...

https://www.nytimes.com/2020/07/27/opinion/us-republicans-coronavirus.html

****

Opinion

The Cult of Selfishness Is Killing America

The right has made irresponsible behavior a key principle.

By Paul Krugman
Opinion Columnist
July 27, 2020

America's response to the coronavirus has been a lose-lose proposition.

The Trump administration and governors like Florida's Ron DeSantis insisted that there was no trade-off between economic growth and controlling the disease, and they were right — but not in the way they expected.

Premature reopening led to a surge in infections: Adjusted for population, Americans are currently dying from Covid-19 at around 15 times the rate in the European Union or Canada. Yet the "rocket ship" recovery Donald Trump promised has crashed and burned: Job growth appears to have stalled or reversed, especially in states that were most aggressive about lifting social distancing mandates, and early indications are that the U.S. economy is lagging behind the economies of major European nations.

So we're failing dismally on both the epidemiological and the economic fronts. But why?

[..]

You see, the modern U.S. right is committed to the proposition that greed is good, that we're all better off when individuals engage in the untrammeled pursuit of self-interest. In their vision, unrestricted profit maximization by businesses and unregulated consumer choice is the recipe for a good society.

Support for this proposition is, if anything, more emotional than intellectual. I've long been struck by the intensity of right-wing anger against relatively trivial regulations, like bans on phosphates in detergent and efficiency standards for light bulbs. It's the principle of the thing: Many on the right are enraged at any suggestion that their actions should take other people's welfare into account.

This rage is sometimes portrayed as love of freedom. But people who insist on the right to pollute are notably unbothered by, say, federal agents tear-gassing peaceful protesters. What they call "freedom" is actually absence of responsibility.

[..]

- https://www.nytimes.com/2020/07/27/opinion/us-republicans-coronavirus.html

****

July 30, 2020, 5:50AM (Amir-ul Kafirs to group):

Re: HERETICS: Anti-Propagandists

(for those of you who don't know him, he's he son of an extremely successful real estate developer)

His father also wrote a book on the shopping mall as the new religious center.

It seems like the idea of people making up their own minds, even at the risk of being wrong, is no longer acceptable

Alas, you're exactly right. I read the opinion piece & I found it utterly despicable. Who would've ever thought that I'd find myself in the position of defending the so-called 'right'?! But, then, the question is: Are we even talking about the 'right' anymore?! I quote from the opinion piece:

"This rage is sometimes portrayed as love of freedom. But people who insist on the right to pollute are notably unbothered by, say, federal agents tear-gassing peaceful protesters. What they call "freedom" is actually absence of responsibility."

There's the usual conflating at work. The "people who insist on the right to pollute" are presented as the same people who're unbothered by "federal agents tear-gassing peaceful protestors" are presented as the 'right'. But can such a generalization be accurately made? It seems to me that one primary characteristic of the 'right' is an objection to "federal agents" asserting their power over people in general. PLUS, whoa, what an oversimplification, ultimately the key approach of this piece, to say that "What they call "freedom" is actually absence of responsibility." I think that what people call freedom is more accurately depicted as the ability to live one's life without having the details of it dictated by federal 'authority'.

Or in fact, let's face it, they shouldn't be allowed to think because very few have studied logic, philosophy or... you get the point

&, indeed, I think your point is exactly correct. This is what society is being remade into at a level I've never seen before, the level where free-thinking individualists are simply 'irresponsible': relinguish your self-determination ENTIRELY & you'll be an exemplary good citizen — & there are plenty of SHEEPLE baaing to do this.

non-mask wearers are (according to the various articles) alternatively irresponsable, less eductated,

Of course, less-educated means not falling in line with propaganda professors like this guy.

Since when has America been the land of the socially responsable? It's like a joke. The whole place is built of the idea to get rich (like ______)

& _____'s wealth is based on inherited money. Would they have been able to start their bar/restaurant without it? The place where I couldn't even get hired as a dishwasher? Sometime in the last few years _____ friend-requested me on social media, as did the conservative founder of a weekly paper. I ignored them both.

****

July 27, 2020, 11:00AM (Inquiring Librarian to group):

Re: Fw: MAYOR CANTRELL ANNOUNCES NEW RESTRICTIONS TO HELP REDUCE COMMUNITY SPREAD OF COVID-19

I woke in disbelief and anger to an official message. How absurd?! My mayor is destroying my city. This is unbelievable, and I am guessing she will not stop here.

The article ends with this humdinger:

Dr. Avegno also announced that the federal government has agreed to send surge testing resources to New Orleans. These resources — similar to what is being offered in Baton Rouge — will allow the City to significantly increase the number of tests offered to residents in the region daily. The program will be supported by the Louisiana National Guard and will begin next Tuesday (July 28) at the UNO Lakefront Arena as a drive-thru testing site with the hours of 8 a.m. to 6 p.m. Rotations will be made in the weeks to come at the sites of university partners around the city.

More information will be available on ready.nola.gov/testing."

When this mass testing was done in Baton Rouge, the LA state capital, the government was actually offering free McDonalds meal tickets to anyone who tested, whether they were sick or not..., go get tested, everyone... free junkfood

for you! I mean, REALLY??!!
http://ldh.la.gov/index.cfm/newsroom/detail/5682

****

July 28, 2020 (photos at rest stop from Amir-ul Kafirs):

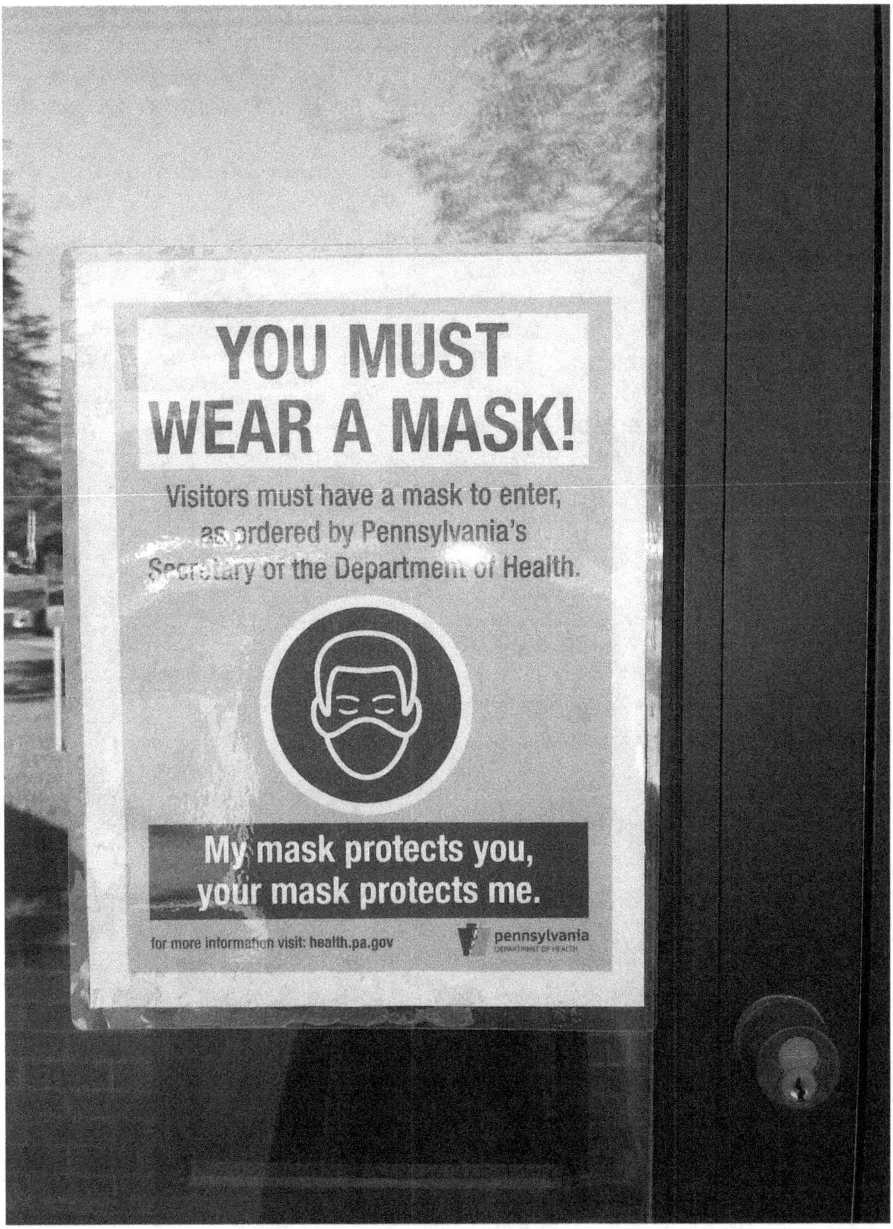

****

Local McDonald's giving free Value Meal vouchers to first 500 people to get tested for COVID-19 Tuesday at Alex Box Stadium

July 13, 2020
The first 500 people who show up for testing Tuesday, July 14 at LSU's Alex Box Stadium's Geaux Get Tested site will receive a coupon for a McDonald's Value Meal. Valluzzo Companies, owner of more than 40 McDonald's locations in Baton Rouge, is offering the meal deal to help encourage people to get tested for COVID-19.
The LSU test site, as well as other sites in Baton Rouge, Gonzales and Zachary, are part of the federal government's effort to support communities that have been identified as COVID-19 hotspots, or communities where there has been a recent and intense level of new cases and hospitalizations related to the ongoing outbreak.
"Valluzzo Companies has generously provided Value Meal coupons to encourage people to get a free COVID-19 test," said Kim Hood, test site director for the Louisiana Department of Health. "This free testing is only available to the community through the end of the week. Anyone who is experiencing symptoms or who is concerned they may have been exposed to someone with the virus is encouraged to get tested. The test sites are quick and efficient, and wait times are short.""

****

July 30, 2020, 6:09AM (Amir-ul Kafirs to group):

Re: MAYOR CANTRELL ANNOUNCES NEW RESTRICTIONS TO HELP REDUCE COMMUNITY SPREAD OF COVID-19

Dr. Avegno also announced that the federal government has agreed to send surge testing resources to New Orleans.

The more testing, the more 'cases', presumably the more federal aid money for politicians to skim off of.

the government was actually offering free McDonalds meal tickets to anyone who tested,

That's truly 'funny'. Talk about sick humor! How about a free 32 ounce soda?

****

July 27, 2020, 3:08PM (BP to group):

As I've said a hundred times already, I am seriously burnt. Maybe that's not it really. Let's say I'm depressed. And reading the news and the hysteria pushes me further in that direction. A week until the kids and I get in the car. Looks like we are going to make it. Headed to Massachussetts and NJ is not banned....yet! But I feel better now that I'm close. Was really worried Mass would find an excuse to keep us out (or quarantine for 14 days upon arrival....which really doesn't work for a ten day holiday, does it?)

Spotted this bit on Alex Brenson's twitter: a woman who says she and partner have not left their one bedroom apartment in Brooklyn for 134 days. Okay. Let us see how she makes a living: National Correspondent, Time Mag. And her book:

The Ones We've Been Waiting For: How a New Generation of Leaders Will Transform America Hardcover – February 18, 2020

https://www.amazon.com/Ones-Weve-Been-Waiting-Generation/dp/0525561501

We're fucked!

****

July 30, 2020, 6:19AM (Amir-ul Kafirs to group):

a woman who says she and partner have not left their one bedroom apartment in Brooklyn for 134 days.

Ok, once upon a time such a person would've been unequivocably considered a paranoid agoraphobic.

****

July 30, 2020, 5:10AM (Amir-ul Kafirs to group):

HERETICS: Unfriend & Block

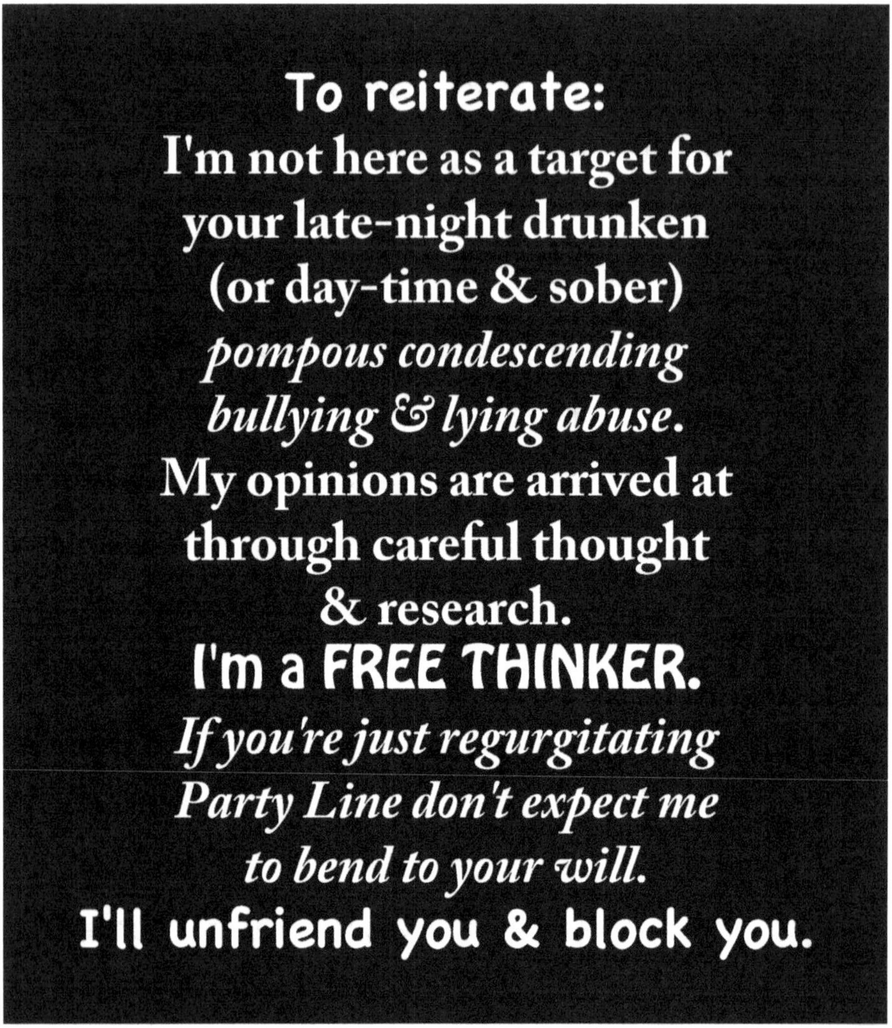
To reiterate:
I'm not here as a target for
your late-night drunken
(or day-time & sober)
pompous condescending
bullying & lying abuse.
My opinions are arrived at
through careful thought
& research.
I'm a FREE THINKER.
If you're just regurgitating
Party Line don't expect me
to bend to your will.
I'll unfriend you & block you.

****

July 27, 2020, 4:20PM (BP to group):

Stumbled upon this one today which made me think of your AI Sauce bit.

Rep. Paul Gosar spells out 'Epstein Didn't Kill Himself' in tweets

https://nypost.com/2019/11/13/rep-paul-gosar-spells-out-epstein-didnt-kill-himself-in-tweets/

And a bit of UFO stuff, too!

****

July 27, 2020, 3:31PM (BP to group):

Please Lord, can the Universities terminate these people?

SHUT IT DOWN, START OVER, DO IT RIGHT

An open letter to America's decision makers, on behalf of health professionals across the country.
https://uspirg.org/resources/usp/shut-it-down-start-over-do-it-right

****

Dear decision makers,

Hit the reset button.

Of all the nations in the world, we've had the most deaths from COVID-19. At the same time, we're in the midst of "reopening our economy," exposing more and more people to coronavirus and watching numbers of cases -- and deaths -- skyrocket.

In March, people went home and stayed there for weeks, to keep themselves and their neighbors safe. You didn't use the time to set us up to defeat the virus. And then you started to reopen anyway, and too quickly.

Right now we are on a path to lose more than 200,000 American lives by November 1st. Yet, in many states people can drink in bars, get a haircut, eat inside a restaurant, get a tattoo, get a massage, and do myriad other normal, pleasant, but non-essential activities.

Get our priorities straight.

More than 117,000 Americans had died of COVID-19 by mid-June. If our response had been as effective as Germany's, estimates show that we would have had only 36,000 COVID-19 deaths in that period in the United States. If our response had been as effective as South Korea, Australia, or Singapore's, fewer than 2,000 Americans would have died. We could have prevented 99% of those COVID-19 deaths. But we didn't.

The best thing for the nation is not to reopen as quickly as possible, it's to save as many lives as possible. And reopening before suppressing the virus isn't going to help the economy. Economists have gone on record saying that the only way to "restore the economy is to address the pandemic itself," pointing out that until we find a way to boost testing and develop and distribute a vaccine, open or not, people will not be in the mood to participate.

[..]

Matthew Wellington
Public Health Campaigns Director, U.S. PIRG

[..]

- https://uspirg.org/resources/usp/shut-it-down-start-over-do-it-right

****

July 30, 2020, 10:39AM (Amir-ul Kafirs to group):

Re: Please Lord, can the Universities terminate these people?

Here's the recurring justification for just about anything:

"Right now we are on a path to lose more than 200,000 American lives by November 1st. Yet, in many states people can drink in bars, get a haircut, eat inside a restaurant, get a tattoo, get a massage, and do myriad other normal, pleasant, but non-essential activities."

It's a PREDICTION. Because, according to this PREDICTION, 200,000 Americans may die by November 1st Draconian measures must be taken. Maybe that many people will be dead by then, maybe the statistics will be manipulated to make that seem to be the case. I don't know & neither do these 'experts' — but they claim to, I don't claim to, & they don't convince me.

****

July 30, 2020, 10:47AM (Amir-ul Kafirs to group):

Re: Please Lord, can the Universities terminate these people?

On Jul 27, 2020, at 3:54 PM, Inquiring Librarian wrote:

Lets rush them in now for a gene altering covid vaccine. I mean NOW! They see the urgency, shoot them up.

Right. The obvious thing being that we're not telling them what to do but they're trying to tell us what to do. The openly stated basis for this is that any reason we might have for feeling differently about any of these matters is discounted regardless of whether they know what it is. They're the 'experts', we're to be their test subjects. No basis we could possibly have for saying NO could ever be valid, according to them. As far as I'm concerned, even an *intuitive* rejection of the imposed health plans are valid. I don't buy the we're-responsible-for-other-people's-health argument at all.

****

July 27, 2020, 10:02PM (Inquiring Librarian to group):

HERETICS: Public Health Quarantine Doctors Ad & Frontline Doctors Speak Out

Hi All, I found a great one today from my friend in California. One of his friends is a doctor. She was looking for jobs this past fall, 2019. And she took a screen shot of a job she had considered applying for. You can see the job description here:

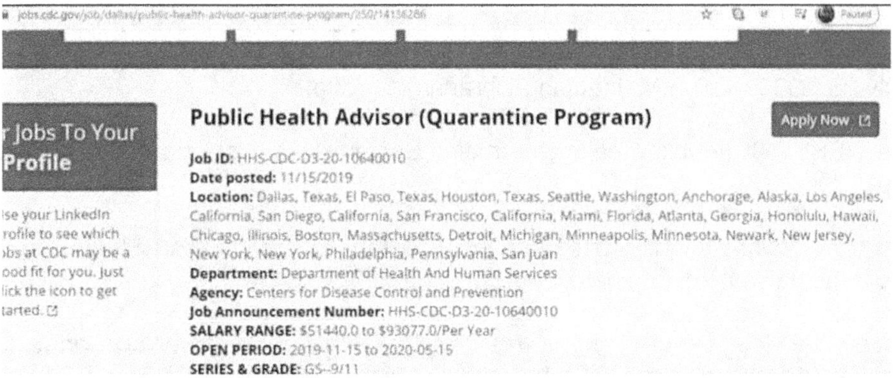

Next, take a listen to, or read the transcript of, this here group of frontline doctors from across the country doing a press conference in front of the U.S. Supreme Court today. It was up on Facebook and I tried to share it with a few people. Within an hour of my sharing it, it was taken down.

For now at least, it is here on Youtube:
https://www.youtube.com/watch?v=n9yKtoYxd5Q

I found this link here to the transcript of the press conference:
https://www.rev.com/blog/transcripts/americas-frontline-doctors-scotus-press-conference-transcript

****

Jul 27, 2020

America's Frontline Doctors SCOTUS Press Conference Transcript

A group of American doctors calling themselves "America's Frontline Doctors" held a press conference on COVID-19, hydroxychloroquine, and more outside the Supreme Court of the United States. Read the transcript of their press conference here.

Warning: This press conference has been flagged & taken down by multiple social media platforms for containing "misleading" or "false" information. Rev does not condone the use of any COVID-19 treatments outlined in this press conference.

[..]

- https://www.rev.com/blog/transcripts/americas-frontline-doctors-scotus-press-conference-transcript

****

July 28, 2020, 12:04PM (Inquiring Librarian to group):

Re: HERETICS: Public Health Quarantine Doctors Ad & Frontline Doctors Speak Out

We have advancement of this issue that I posted yesterday. I consider this to be monumental in the fight against the covid nazis.

1st off, the video I shared above was taken off of facebook. It won't be long before it disappears from Youtube. You can watch all 3 hours of it here on Bitchute:
https://www.bitchute.com/video/YfQuHY1qQVqY/?fbclid=IwAR3Xnq8mJNKOPPYNKCS5auXrohTHq0Z1fmi18IED09VgWN2RX5PPtPhwWls

& here is a quick commentary on the removal. I know you all might think Breitbart is evil. But to be honest, this is on my side now. I support supporting these doctors.
https://www.breitbart.com/tech/2020/07/27/facebook-censors-viral-video-of-doctors-capitol-hill-coronavirus-press-conference/amp/?fbclid=IwAR1rlNPhkcjzUtWTXMu6kIoJythfwaMcApZB3mDOnrXuTCwU3fwtP5dPdh8

"Facebook has removed a video posted by Breitbart News earlier today, which was the top-performing Facebook post in the world Monday afternoon, of a press conference in D.C. held by the group America's Frontline Doctors and organized and sponsored by the Tea Party Patriots. The press conference featured Rep. Ralph Norman (R-SC) and frontline doctors sharing their views and opinions on coronavirus and the medical response to the pandemic. YouTube (which is owned by Google) and Twitter subsequently removed footage of the press conference as well."

From my local Health Freedom Louisiana organization.... Please note "SIXTEEN MILLION VIEWS"!!!! This is phenomenal!!

****

July 29, 2020, 12:56AM (Inquiring Librarian to group):

Re: HERETICS: Public Health Quarantine Doctors Ad & Frontline Doctors Speak Out

& the drama carries on... I posted this on Facebook in response to a fellow Heretic's post about the press conference:

Can you even believe how horribly the mainstream media are trying to bash and discredit these doctors?? It was so awful reading the slander and twisting of words and thoughts in today's 'news'. I actually tried to get a 'friend' to listen to the doctors, before he publicly lambasted them on facebook with a CBS "News" slander of the press conference. His level of denial and inability to listen actually drove me to tears and unfriending this 'friend', who has a PhD in Cognitive Science, nonetheless??!! The doctors came back to say a word against the slander today, (of course this was removed from mainstream social media within hours of being posted). Thank goodness Bitchute continues to save the day: https://www.bitchute.com/video/pwK1uoxaWWDk/

****

July 29, 2020, 2:23PM (Inquiring Librarian to group):

Re: HERETICS: Public Health Quarantine Doctors Ad & Frontline Doctors Speak Out

I realize the videos I shared are really looooonnng. Maybe it will be best to start backwards. Yesterday, after the mass media completely slandered all of these doctors who spoke outside the Supreme Court in D.C., the doctors came back and defended themselves. I feel like these doctors are the key to our medical freedom right now, possibly the key to the end of this tyranny we are all facing right now. I am serious about this. It is the first ammendment and free speech that is being taken away to silence our most important people who are fighting back. This is MASSIVELY IMPORTANT right now. The fact that the press has taken down every recording of these physicians talking over the past 3 days means that what they have to say is what the media/big pharma/big tech (GATES and his cronies of the vaccine and Global Reset world that is being based around biomedical tyranny) DO NOT want you or anyone to hear. And they will take great lengths to brainwash you into thinking these legitimate doctors are quacks and viciously discredit them. And they will do their best to make sure the public simply cannot hear the voices of these doctors.

Here is the video clip, this one is less than 1 hour long. It's really important to hear and share. You can try to throw it up on fb, but it will be taken down pretty rapidly. & if you are upset about the Tea Party Patriots or the Breitbart thing,

please just get over that. This is beyond political. These doctors just needed someone to give them a voice and those groups gave it to them.
https://www.bitchute.com/video/pwK1uoxaWWDk/

You can carry on after watching this to see how the mainstream media is 'lambasting' (thank you Amir-ul Kafirs for the new and exciting word that fits so much these days, sadly) these doctors and in particular Dr. Immanuel. Dr. Immanuel is from Cameroon, in Africa, where she got her initial medical training. She is very religious, and she does wax on the poetic and preacher-like rant here and there. But to be honest, all that she said in this press conference struck me as so true and so heartfelt. BLM should be here defending her, instead, the hypocrisy is rife with people attacking and falsely discrediting her honesty and passion.

Check out this article in the Washington Post. I am not going to copy and paste it. Just click on the link and read it so that you can also see the pretty young and very serious 'fact checker' 'debunking' what the professional real doctors have said.

Trump retweeted a video with false covid-19 claims. One doctor in it has said demons cause illnesses.

https://www.washingtonpost.com/technology/2020/07/28/stella-immanuel-hydroxychloroquine-video-trump-americas-frontline-doctors/

Ok, here are a few highlights, but I urge you to read the whole bit of nonsense:

The video showed a group that has dubbed itself America's Frontline Doctors, standing on the steps of the Supreme Court and claiming that neither masks *[YAY!! I support this!! Thank you!!]* nor shutdowns *[Yay no. 2!! I even more support these physicians!! Tell me more!!]* are necessary to fight the pandemic, despite a plethora of expertise to the contrary. It was live-streamed by the conservative media outlet Breitbart and viewed more than 14 million times *[Holy Moley, that's a lot of views before big tech got their greedy hands on it to take it down, Big Tech, I'll say you failed here!! Power to the nonbrainwashed people! These physicians need to be heard and shared!!]* — fueled by a tweet by Donald Trump Jr. and multiple retweets by President Trump, which have since been deleted.

"The doctors who appear in the viral video include James Todaro *[I have been following him for several months, he is awesome and has seen through the bs for some time]*, an ophthalmologist and bitcoin investor who was one of the earliest proponents of hydroxychloroquine, and Simone Gold, a Los Angeles-based doctor and lawyer who has long claimed that lockdowns will kill more people than the coronavirus *[Yes!!!! I believe she is right. Thank you Simone Gold for being honest and intelligent and I would love for you to be my doctor some day. You are one of my new heros. I love you.. Truly, I love you and your fellow frontline physicians. Please keep up the amazing work].* But Immanuel stands out for beliefs that are particularly out of step with scientific consensus."

"As the Daily Beast's Will Sommer first noted, Immanuel has asserted that many gynecological issues are the result of having sex with witches and demons ("succubi" and "incubi") in dreams, a myth that dates back at least to the "Epic of Gilgamesh," a Sumerian poem written more than 4,000 years ago. She falsely claims that issues such as endometriosis, infertility, miscarriages and STIs are "evil deposits from the spirit husband." *[???????!!! The Daily Beast?? I mean COME ON!! ?? Can I just swear here... WHAT THE F*=%# PEOPLE??!!! Ultimately, I do not care if she believes in demons or the antichrist or aliens. To me this is part of her culture, like many in S. America, Magical Realism is cultural, a way of storytelling, a way of working with intuition and with nature and the mind body experience. I believe what she, and all of the fazilion other doctors speaking in the press conference say. She is right, they are right. Why is the mass media picking on only 3 of the at least 15 doctors speaking at the press conference? Enough said. I still sleep with a stuffed yellow mouse and honestly Qanon is looking more and more true and appealing to me daily, does that make me a bad cat mom or an incompetent librarian? No. I do not think so.]*

"Hello Facebook put back my profile page and videos up or your computers will start crashing till you do," she tweeted. "You are not bigger that God. I promise you. If my page is not back up face book will be down in Jesus name." *[Yes! Dr. Immanuel gets emotional and throws Jesus, and possibly a bit of sorcery, in here and there, but heck, I'm all for it. Thank you Dr. Immanuel for your passion and your culture from Cameroon honestly fascinates me. Keep up the good work! I love you and your penchant for magical realism while you do honest work to save us all, which is what, I believe, you are doing. Thank you so much. I am humbled by your strength and intelligence, Love, Librarian and free thinker in cowardly hiding.]*

& let's support HCQ here...
https://childrenshealthdefense.org/news/fauci-steering-the-pandemic-narrative-toward-vaccine-solutions-is-nothing-new/
& pull out of this, the Lancet and New England Journal of Medicine's retraction of their falsified HCQ discrediting studies (which are also explained in detail by several of these now censored "Frontline Physicians".
https://www.thelancet.com/journals/lancet/article/PIIS0140-6736(20)31324-6/fulltext

Note, nowhere in the press conference did Dr. Immanuel say anything about demons. And if she's said it in the past, it's important to respect her Cameroonian heritage where her descendents were likely infiltrated by rabid western white evangelists that would have converted her descendents at some point. The point is, Dr. Immanuel was very professional in her speeches at the conference. You will note in the Bitchute rebuttal of the doctors above, that at the end of the recording, a white black lives matter lunatic guy was telling Immanuel that HE was more black than her. & there was another woman in a face shield yelling at the doctors the whole time. Dr. Immanuel is also a religious preacher, what she says on her own time as a preacher is her business. Let's talk to her congregation and her in particular if you want to know what she thinks about religion, etc...

& lets be honest here, the article above uses TRUMP in the headlines to grab readers, to bias them right away. This should not be politicized, this is life saving medicine which knows no party lines. And to tell you the truth, I think Trump is right on this. He is pushing therapeutics over vaccines, I have listened to a few of his recent press conferences lately. I have heard it from the horse's mouth. I know he is head of Operation Warp Speed, but I actually wonder about this now. He supports HCQ, and he is right to do so, HCQ & Zinc. My mom is a retired nurse, decades as an ICU and CCU (Cardiac Care Unit) nurse. She knows HCQ is safe. The Lancet journal about HCQ was false propaganda. They overdosed already half dead people with deathly amounts of HCQ, more than you would ever give anyone without expecting death. The Lancet journal article had to be retracted, too many doctors came out and reported it as false. Dr. Zelenko in NY has interview after interview supporting HCQ.

Anyways, this all is absolutely worth your checking out. I see it as a turning point. The media and censors are locking down. But the word is out, en masse.

****

Internet Culture

Trump retweeted a video with false covid-19 claims. One doctor in it has said demons cause illnesses.

By
Travis M. Andrews and
Danielle Paquette
July 29, 2020 at 10:17 a.m. EDT

[..]

In the viral video, Immanuel made the unsubstantiated claim that hydroxychloroquine is a "cure for covid," the disease caused by the coronavirus. As a previous Post story put it: "There is no known cure for the novel coronavirus or the disease it causes, according to the Centers for Disease Control and Prevention and the World Health Organization. Multiple studies have disputed claims that antimalarial and antiviral drugs such as hydroxychloroquine, azithromycin and chloroquine can help treat or even prevent the coronavirus. Last month, the FDA revoked an emergency approval that allowed doctors to prescribe hydroxychloroquine to covid-19 patients even though the treatment was untested."

Hydroxychloroquine's false hope: How an obscure drug became a coronavirus 'cure' I The Fact Checker

Claims about hydroxychloroquine to treat covid-19 have gained traction despite a lack of scientific evidence. How did this happen? (Elyse Samuels, Meg Kelly, Sarah Cahlan/The Washington Post)

[..]

- https://www.washingtonpost.com/technology/2020/07/28/stella-immanuel-hydroxychloroquine-video-trump-americas-frontline-doctors/

****

JUNE 11, 2020

Fauci: Steering the Pandemic Narrative Toward Vaccine "Solutions" Is Nothing New

By the Children's Health Defense Team

Since the emergence of HIV in the early 1980s, Dr. Anthony Fauci has acquired decades of experience being the front man for a network of powerful Big Pharma and Big Medicine interests. This network (one of the most conspicuous members of which is Fauci's friend and patron Bill Gates) profits handsomely from regularly declared epidemics and pandemics via the unending flow of cash that such events inevitably direct to pharmaceutical interventions—and especially vaccination.

Fauci's father was a pharmacist, and Fauci himself has specialized in the pharmacological "regulation" of the human immune system. He hitched his professional wagon to vaccines early on, and his agency's single-minded focus on vaccine "solutions"—and simultaneous denial of serious vaccine-created problems such as vaccine failure and pathogenic priming—has long threatened to suffocate other avenues of exploration, whether for prevention or treatment.

Although Fauci has never been able to deliver on the promise of an HIV vaccine made when he took the helm of NIAID (the National Institute of Allergy and Infectious Diseases) in 1984, he has been highly successful—for decades—in attracting billions for HIV vaccine research. And as new threats like Ebola and Zika have emerged, the groundwork laid during the HIV era has allowed vaccines to continue to monopolize both attention and funding.

Fauci is not only a productive agency fundraiser but also a prolific publisher. The National Library of Medicine search engine (PubMed) pulls up nearly 300 publications that he has authored or co-authored over the last two decades. And many of these—like Fauci's 2017 remarks at Georgetown University that the Trump administration should expect a "surprise outbreak" within "the next few years"—not only foreshadow future events but also provide major hints of his network's vaccine bias.

In 2003, for example, Fauci and coauthors (including then-CDC-director Julie Gerberding) spelled out a vision in Science for a "global vaccine enterprise." Although their focus back then was on HIV, the proposed measures sound eerily similar to what many of these same players have called for in conjunction with COVID-19 vaccines—including "quickly measuring the effectiveness of vaccine protection as prototype vaccine candidates are identified," expanding manufacturing resources "to speed [vaccine candidates'] use in human trials" and "systematically explor[ing] . . . delivery systems for vaccines." It should probably come as no surprise, then, to discover similar fortune-telling tendencies in some of Fauci's other publications.

In other words, the high mortality was the result of poorly understood viral-bacterial interactions rather than of a virus on its own.

The 1918-1919 pandemic

A century before COVID-19, the Spanish flu was one of the most famous—and society-scarring— pandemic episodes in global history. In a 2007 analysis in The Journal of Infectious Diseases, Fauci and NIAID co-author David Morens examined some of the "unusual epidemiologic features" and patterns associated with the deadly pandemic. The 1918-1919 pandemic differed from current events in terms of the age groups affected, with the Spanish flu responsible for "extraordinary" excess mortality in healthy adults in their twenties and thirties, while COVID-19 has targeted older adults and individuals with underlying chronic conditions. Nonetheless, several of the NIAID authors' observations are intriguing in light of the phenomena being observed today. For example:

- The 1918-19 influenza pandemic presented a number of "seemingly new and severe clinical forms of disease" that frequently proved fatal, including an "acute aggressive" type of pneumonia and an "acute respiratory distress-like syndrome" (ARDS) involving cyanosis (lack of oxygen in the blood). Individuals with COVID-19, too, have displayed numerous symptoms considered "unusual" for classic respiratory viruses, including the "emergency warning signs" of cyanosis and ARDS-like breathing difficulties.
- In 1918-1919, cytokine storms ("a deleterious overexuberant release of proinflammatory cytokines") may have contributed to the mortality seen in young and otherwise healthy adults. Cytokines are cell signaling

proteins that play an important role in the immune response but which, in some circumstances, can apparently "go rogue." Researchers writing in March in The Lancet argued that patients with severe COVID-19 illness, too, are showing signs of "virally driven hyperinflammation" or what they call "cytokine storm syndrome." In their 2007 publication, Fauci and Morens offered little explanation for cytokine storms other than to suggest that they might be triggered by "unappreciated host or environmental variables."

- Based on the events of 1918-1919, Fauci and Morens speculated in 2007 that an individual's response to a new virus might "depend on the history of previous exposures." Although the two authors did not consider vaccine exposure as a form of "previous exposure," a January 2020 Pentagon study indicates that they should have. The study found that members of the military who received an influenza vaccine had a 36% increased odds of going on to develop a coronavirus infection. Other studies have likewise pointed to increased risks of viral respiratory infections—both influenza and non-influenza—from flu shots. Shouldn't researchers be taking vaccination history into account when examining the "staggering" number of COVID-19 deaths that have occurred in nursing home residents subjected to annual influenza and pneumococcal vaccine requirements?

[..]

- https://childrenshealthdefense.org/news/fauci-steering-the-pandemic-narrative-toward-vaccine-solutions-is-nothing-new/

****

Retraction—Hydroxychloroquine or chloroquine with or without a macrolide for treatment of COVID-19: a multinational registry analysis

Mandeep R Mehra

Frank Ruschitzka
Amit N Patel
Published:June 05, 2020DOI: https://doi.org/10.1016/S0140-6736(20)31324-6

After publication of our *Lancet* Article,1 several concerns were raised with respect to the veracity of the data and analyses conducted by Surgisphere Corporation and its founder and our co-author, Sapan Desai, in our publication. We launched an independent third-party peer review of Surgisphere with the consent of Sapan Desai to evaluate the origination of the database elements, to confirm the completeness of the database, and to replicate the analyses presented in the paper.

Our independent peer reviewers informed us that Surgisphere would not transfer the full dataset, client contracts, and the full ISO audit report to their servers for analysis as such transfer would violate client agreements and confidentiality requirements. As such, our reviewers were not able to conduct an independent and private peer review and therefore notified us of their withdrawal from the peer-review process.

We always aspire to perform our research in accordance with the highest ethical and professional guidelines. We can never forget the responsibility we have as researchers to scrupulously ensure that we rely on data sources that adhere to our high standards. Based on this development, we can no longer vouch for the veracity of the primary data sources. Due to this unfortunate development, the authors request that the paper be retracted.

We all entered this collaboration to contribute in good faith and at a time of great need during the COVID-19 pandemic. We deeply apologise to you, the editors, and the journal readership for any embarrassment or inconvenience that this may have caused.

[..]

****

July 30, 2020, 2:43PM (Amir-ul Kafirs to group):

Re: HERETICS: Public Health Quarantine Doctors Ad & Frontline Doctors Speak Out

She was looking for jobs this past fall, 2019. And she took a screen shot of a job she had considered applying for. You can see the job description here:

OK, that is truly amazing & vvvveeeerrrrrryyyyy useful in solidying the position that advance planning went into this current situation.

I found this link here to the transcript of the press conference:

I didn't watch the video but I did read the transcript. I found it interesting. 'Coincidentally', *the next day after you posted this*, I got an email from a friend linking to an article making fun of the doctor from Cameroon. Here's the email that I wrote to him today:

On Jul 28, 2020, [name removed to keep their identity secret] wrote:

Trumps New COVID Doctor Claims Demon Sperm Is Responsible For Disease https://www.patheos.com/blogs/progressivesecularhumanist/2020/07/trumps-new-covid-doctor-claims-demon-sperm-is-responsible-for-disease/?fbclid=IwAR2VYKtakFIEzZtTMSI8SIDcEVF92UrYYVWVcGbCtqR9D54oLJiKKm3gU_o

Now, I admit, that ordinarily, as a person who detests religion, I would just appreciate this for its camp value.

ALAS, in these times, where the vicious propaganda is flying fast & furious, a headline such as the above seems pretty transparent as something meant to bias people against the doctor, to dismiss them as a total idiot, which they very well may be. SO, I read a transcript of what this doctor said at a recent press conference & I paste it below. I should explain that I have no opinion about hydroxychloroquine. I hope to avoid ALL treatments for COVID-19 &, fortunately, I haven't gotten sick yet so, so far, so good. From the beginning ventilators have struck me as a bad idea & I haven't come across any believable info contradicting this. SO, my purpose in sharing this is to give you a chance to read the doctor's actual words. You might find them, as I do, adequately reasonable & not full of "demon sperm" talk. That doesn't mean she hasn't said things about "demon sperm" elsewhere, maybe she has — but I think the reason for character-assassinating her probably has more to do with the things she says below because her narrative goes so much against the mainstream one.

Dr. Stella Immanuel: (05:27)
Hello, I'm Dr. Stella Immanuel. I'm a primary care physician in Houston, Texas. I actually went to medical school in West Africa, Nigeria, where I took care of malaria patients, treated them with hydroxychloroquine and stuff like that. So I'm actually used to these medications. I'm here because I have personally treated over 350 patients with COVID. Patients that have diabetes, patients that have high blood pressure, patients that have asthma, old people … I think my oldest patient is 92 … 87 year olds. And the result has been the same. I put them on hydroxychloroquine, I put them on zinc, I put them on Zithromax, and they're all well.
Dr. Stella Immanuel: (06:12)
For the past few months, after taking care of over 350 patients, we've not lost one. Not a diabetic, not a somebody with high blood pressure, not somebody who asthma, not an old person. We've not lost one patient. And on top of that, I've put myself, my staff, and many doctors that I know on hydroxychloroquine for prevention, because by the very mechanism of action, it works early and as a prophylaxis. We see patients, 10 to 15 COVID patients, everyday. We give them breathing treatments. We only wear surgical mask. None of us has gotten sick. It works.
Dr. Stella Immanuel: (06:46)
So right now, I came here to Washington DC to say, America, nobody needs to die. The study that made me start using hydroxychloroquine was a study that they did under the NIH in 2005 that say it works. Recently, I was doing some research about a patient that had hiccups and I found out that they even did a recent study in the NIH, which is our National Institute … that is the National …

NIH, what? National Institute of Health. They actually had a study and go look it up. Type hiccups and COVID, you will see it. They treated a patient that had hiccups with hydroxychloroquine and it proved that hiccups is a symptom of COVID. So if the NIH knows that treating the patient would hydroxychloroquine proves that hiccup is a symptom of COVID, then they definitely know the hydroxychloroquine works.

Dr. Stella Immanuel: (07:42)

I'm upset. Why I'm upset is that I see people that cannot breathe. I see parents walk in, I see diabetic sit in my office knowing that this is a death sentence and they can't breathe. And I hug them and I tell them, "It's going to be okay. You're going to live." And we treat them and they leave. None has died. So if some fake science, some person sponsored by all these fake pharma companies comes out say, "We've done studies and they found out that it doesn't work." I can tell you categorically it's fixed science. I want to know who is sponsoring that study. I want to know who is behind it because there is no way I can treat 350 patients and counting and nobody is dead and they all did better.

Dr. Stella Immanuel: (08:21)

I know you're going to tell me that you treated 20 people, 40 people, and it didn't work. I'm a true testimony. So I came here to Washington DC to tell America nobody needs to get sick. This virus has a cure. It is called hydroxychloroquine, zinc, and Zithromax. I know you people want to talk about a mask. Hello? You don't need mask. There is a cure. I know they don't want to open schools. No, you don't need people to be locked down. There is prevention and there is a cure.

Dr. Stella Immanuel: (08:48)

And let me tell you something, all you fake doctors out there that tell me, "Yeah. I want a double blinded study." I just tell you, quit sounding like a computer, double blinded, double blinded. I don't know whether your chips are malfunctioning, but I'm a real doctor. I have radiologists, we have plastic surgeons, we have neurosurgeons, like Sanjay Gupta saying, "Yeah, it doesn't work and it causes heart disease." Let me ask you Dr. Sanjay Gupta. Hear me. Have you ever seen a COVID patient? Have you ever treated anybody with hydroxychloroquine and they died from heart disease? When you do, come and talk to me because I sit down in my clinic every day and I see these patients walk in everyday scared to death. I see people driving two, three hours to my clinic because some ER doctor is scared of the Texas board or they're scared of something, and they will not prescribe medication to these people.

Dr. Stella Immanuel: (09:35)

I tell all of you doctors that are sitting down and watching Americans die. You're like the good Nazi … the good one, the good Germans that watched Jews get killed and you did not speak up. If they come after me, they threaten me. They've threatened to … I mean, I've gotten all kinds of threats. Or they're going to report me to the bots. I say, you know what? I don't care. I'm not going to let Americans die. And if this is the hill where I get nailed on, I will get nailed on it. I don't care. You can report me to the bots, you can kill me, you can do whatever, but I'm not going to let Americans die.

Dr. Stella Immanuel: (10:09)

And today I'm here to say it, that America, there is a cure for COVID. All this foolishness does not need to happen. There is a cure for COVID. There is a cure for COVID is called hydroxychloroquine. It's called zinc. It's called Zithromax. And it is time for the grassroots to wake up and say, "No, we're not going to take this any longer. We're not going to die." Because let me tell you something, when somebody is dead, they are dead. They're not coming back tomorrow to have an argument. They are not come back tomorrow to discuss the double blinded study and the data. All of you doctors that are waiting for data, if six months down the line you actually found out that this data shows that this medication works, how about your patients that have died? You want a double blinded study where people are dying? It's unethical. So guys, we don't need to die. There is a cure for COVID.

****

July 30, 2020, 2:53PM (Amir-ul Kafirs to group):

Re: HERETICS: Public Health Quarantine Doctors Ad & Frontline Doctors Speak Out

It won't be long before it disappears from Youtube.

Speaking of which, I got yet-another notice that my "Wearing Masks Saves Lives" movie has been age-restricted. It was as if they didn't know that this already happened. SO, I assume that means that another flagging has occurred. I have to wonder how long it'll be before they ban it altogether.

I support supporting these doctors.

The important point is to support supporting the doctors. If the 'left' won't do so then *shame on the left*. Even if the doctors are wrong I think it's important to have their opinions out there. They, obviously, don't think they're wrong or they wouldn't be sticking their professional necks out.

Please note "SIXTEEN MILLION VIEWS"!!!!

Of course, "16,000,000 views" might only mean a few seconds each time. That's still mind-boggling & it shows that people are looking for alternative views on the subject — even if it's just because what members of their political party endorse it's better than only paying attention to the dominant narrative.

****

July 30, 2020, 3:10PM (Amir-ul Kafirs to group):

His level of denial and inability to listen actually drove me to tears and unfriending this 'friend', who has a PhD in Cognitive Science, nonetheless??!!

This is a recurring problem for me. Basically, I realize that I have almost complete contempt for most other people but that I still accept people as friends & curb my contempt in favor of liking them for whatever qualities I can find. Unfortunately, when I find them doing what I call "regurgitating the party line" my reasons for liking them tend to disappear & all the reasons I've had for being contemptuous of them come to the fore. I'm actually not happy about this but I can still understand why it's the way it is.

Bitchute continues to save the day

Bitchute's apparent lack of censorship is going a long way to endear it to me. I wonder, though, if they censor things that might seem to be extremely 'leftist'. All of the things we watch there are probably acceptable to 'right wingers'. The point is, I don't know how 'free speech' supporting Bitchute actually is. I don't know how 'free speech' supporting I WOULD BE if I were running such a platform. I wouldn't want to support a KKK ad, e.g., so I'm not sure how I'd deal with such things.

****

July 30, 2020, 5:55PM (Inquiring Librarian to group):

I have to interject here. I think it is important not to judge what is going on now along 'party' lines as in liberals vs. conservatives. When we do this, we are dividing sides that would normally be united. Those doctors speaking were speaking under the Tea Party/Breitbart platform. But that was the platform that gave them a platform on which to speak, basically they provided the stage that gave them their voice to the world. It says nothing about the political bent of any of those doctors. No where in the approximately 5 hours of listening to these doctors did anyone divulge anything political. It was pretty amazing in fact. To be honest, I start to cringe when I am listening to something about the current situation and someone starts throwing politics into it.

That being said, Bitchute...
It is believed that Bitchute is nonpartisan. Yes, it has some extreme conservative stuff on it. But it also has just as much liberal stuff on it, from what I can tell. And let's be honest here, with what is going on, party lines seem to be pretty blurred, to me at least. I mean, we are talking about health care, life and death situations in the medical world. This was also the point of these 'Frontline Doctors', that politics should have nothing to do with medicine right now. As RFK Jr. states, children are not democrats or republicans, they are just kids, this isn't about what political party you adhere to. Also, said by RFK Jr. when asked if he's lost faith in the Democratic party by Del Bigtree (Note: Kennedy says he is a lifelong democrat and still sticks by his party, Del, also a lifelong democrat is waivering because his very right to free speech is being taken away by the neoliberal takeover of the democratic party), that if the democrats actually knew (meaning the little people like us, not the 'leaders'), what vaccines and the medical industry/ big pharma are/have been doing, if what they have been doing was not censored, then they would certainly agree with the vaccine skeptics, realize they

are being lied to about the lockdown, masks, and the pandemic, etc...

On Bitchute, Derick Broze - "The Unconscious Resistance" - has his channel, James Corbett of the "Corbett Report", The Last American Vagabond has their channel (they are on the stance that the 2 party system is a lie designed to divide and conquer), etc. Bitchute is just a fledgling platform that the many that are currently being censored off of the major media platforms can use to get their message out. If you had not noticed, in the past 2 weeks, this week in particular, Facebook and Youtube have been purging their platforms of SO MANY antivaxx and anti plandemic sites. It's been a phenomenal week of Censorship.

Just because you've already been given way too many videos from me. Here is a 2 hour rant, complete with all sources from Del Bigtree about being censored, the Frontline Doctors, the plandemic, etc. Del is a lifelong democrat, but like many of us, we are starting to doubt our own party. I admire Kennedy for still having hope in the party, as he warns much harm has and will continue to be done by the republican party. At this point, how do we save the first amendment to free speech?

This was yesterday's intro to today's 2 hour talk. Short and funny. I believe Phil already posted it on his social media page.
https://www.facebook.com/watch/?v=284963176119841
Fake hashtags,
"#Cats #FluffyPuppies #EpicFails #TedTalk #ShoeTying #Shoes #CatsofInstagram #CatsofFacebook #Puppies"
The real content is on large flash cards... Brilliant! 100% Facebook approved content.

Ok, I can't share today's Highwire show with you because it was already taken down by facebook, just a couple hours after it aired. When it comes back up, I will share it on the new platform, which may very well be Bitchute and I guarantee it is not conservative, unless you consider free speech and the 1st amendment and the right to live without forced toxic medical intervention to be 'conservative'.

****

July 30, 2020, 6:08PM (Amir-ul Kafirs to group):

I realize the videos I shared are really looooonnng.

For me, yes, too long. I, of course, have my own movies in progress, which I'm grossly neglecting. I'm still glad you provide the links so that I can at least enter them into the general HERETICS record but I don't have time to look at them. Even having gone away to Erie on a trip that was a mere 37 hours has set me back on email communication by days. One thing is that I try to read everyone's emails here & give at least a cursory reply to show you all that I, at least, am paying attention.

The fact that the press has taken down every recording of these physicians talking over the past 3 days means that what they have to say is what the media/ big pharma/big tech (GATES and his cronies of the vaccine and Global Reset world that is being based around biomedical tyranny) DO NOT want you anyone to hear.

I agree, so I'm glad to've been able to have the time to read the transcript of what they said.

And they will do their best to make sure the public simply cannot hear the voices of these doctors.

Indeed — & that's one of the worst signs of what's happening these days.

This is beyond political.

I agree. I just wish they'd had the opportunity to be presented more neutrally. Unfortunately, the wonderful net neutrality is being eroded away rapidly with public health as the pretext.

But to be honest, all that she said in this press conference struck me as so true and so heartfelt.

I agree.

fueled by a tweet by Donald Trump Jr. and multiple retweets by President Trump, which have since been deleted.

It's nice to know that even Rump can be censored because I get his damn tweets without ever choosing to 'follow' him & I can't figure out a way to stop them, to 'unfollow' him.

"The video showed a group that has dubbed itself America's Frontline Doctors, standing on the steps of the Supreme Court and claiming that neither masks *[YAY!! I support this!! Thank you!!]* nor shutdowns *[Yay no. 2!! I even more support these physicians!! Tell me more!!]* are necessary to fight the pandemic, despite a plethora of expertise to the contrary.

"despite a plethors of expertise to the contrary": a more honest article might bring up that there's also expertise that supports what they're saying: the 14 studies reported on in the CDC's own journal, Dr. Yealey in Pittsburgh, & Dr. Victory. But, of course, the article's intention isn't to be fair, it's to make them look like an isolated group of lunatics. They aren't.

It was live-streamed by the conservative media outlet Breitbart and viewed more than 14 million times *[Holy Moley, that's a lot of views before big tech got their greedy hands on it to take it down, Big Tech, I'll say you failed here!! Power to the nonbrainwashed people!*

I wish I could say that those 14,000,000 are "nonbrainwashed" but their watching the video doesn't necessarily indicate that. It might just mean that they're brainwashed by the lesser of the mainstream narratives.

Ultimately, I do not care if she believes in demons or the antichrist or aliens. To me this is part of her culture,

She's from Africa. I don't find it too hard to believe that belief in demons & suchlike is so central to the African culture that speaking in those terms is a way of making her patients relate to her. It's not far from, say, "virus" to "demon". In English we have the expression "to demonize"; Immanuel is *being demonized here.*

I still sleep with a stuffed yellow mouse

I hope you're using birth control.

I love you and your penchant for magical realism

I'm not sure I'd agree with calling this "magical realism". When I think of "magic realism" I think of a specific tendency of Latin American story-telling. Even in that context the term is overused to refer to *all* Latin American story-telling, no matter how inappropriate. Anyway, it might not be that important but you might want to be more careful using the term.

I am humbled by your strength and intelligence

Yeah, it's great that they're taking the risk to speak publicly — it took courage. I hope it doesn't ruin their careers.

Here's an amusing quote from the article:

"Others, though, found it demonstrably less amusing. Physician and scientist Eugene Gu tweeted, “Just because someone is a doctor it doesn’t mean that person is smart. ... Think for yourself.”"

That's exactly what we're trying to do here, eh?! That's the 1st admission I've seen by a physician that doctors aren't necessarily smart. Ha ha!

& let's support HCQ here...

Here's an interesting quote from the above, which I'm still in the midst of reading:

"

- Based on the events of 1918-1919, Fauci and Morens speculated in 2007 that an individual’s response to a new virus might “depend on the

> history of previous exposures." Although the two authors did not consider vaccine exposure as a form of "previous exposure," a January 2020 Pentagon study indicates that they should have. The study found that members of the military who received an influenza vaccine had a 36% increased odds of going on to develop a coronavirus infection. Other studies have likewise pointed to increased risks of viral respiratory infections—both influenza and non-influenza—from flu shots. Shouldn't researchers be taking vaccination history into account when examining the "staggering" number of COVID-19 deaths that have occurred in nursing home residents subjected to annual influenza and pneumococcal vaccine requirements?

"

The very next paragraph has also grabbed my attention:

"In 2008, Fauci, Morens and another NIAID author published an even more exhaustive analysis of the 1918-1919 pandemic, reviewing still-available postmortem samples as well as information from published autopsy series. Although their analysis excluded nonpulmonary causes of death, the three authors concluded that it was influenza virus infection "in conjunction with bacterial infection" that led to most of the 1918-1919 deaths. In other words, the high mortality was the result of "poorly understood" viral-bacterial interactions rather than of a virus on its own. "Without this secondary bacterial pneumonia," the three wrote, "most patients would have recovered.""

I hope I can keep that in mind if & when I ever get into yet-another-stupid-conversation-comparing-the-Spanish-Flu-to-COVID-19.

ANYWAY, I read the whole article, I found it excellent.

& pull out of this, the Lancet and New England Journal of Medicine's retraction of their falsified HCQ discrediting studies

OK! Here's a relevant paragraph of their retraction:

"Our independent peer reviewers informed us that Surgisphere would not transfer the full dataset, client contracts, and the full ISO audit report to their servers for analysis as such transfer would violate client agreements and confidentiality requirements. As such, our reviewers were not able to conduct an independent and private peer review and therefore notified us of their withdrawal from the peer-review process."

That puts *Lancet* on my list-of-sources-to-be-trusted (actually, I don't have such a list unless it's a 'mental note' one). It's good to know that they had the courage to retract something they published.

Note, nowhere in the press conference did Dr. Immanual say anything about demons.

I agree. I think the biggest fear of her detractors is *not* any beliefs she may have in demons & Jesus & such-like ***but in how reasonable & common-sensical she is in the press conference.***

And to tell you the truth, I think Trump is right on this.

Well, I keep saying this: Rump *is a politician* — he puts on an act for his perceived demographic. I'm not going to EVER trust anything he says.

****

July 30, 2020, 6:31PM (Amir-ul Kafirs to group):

1st, I have to say, I'm not sure who you're addressing this to, it seems to be me since, as far as I can tell, I'm the only one commenting here on what you've been posting. Anyway, it seems that you're being defensive without actually reading what I write so I'll explain that I basically agree with you about the uselessness of the politics, etc. But I think you'd have to be in denial if you think that people's party affiliations aren't influencing what they'll pay attention to & what they'll agree with.

I think it is important not to judge what is going on now along 'party' lines as in liberals vs. conservatives.

Having said that many times myself already in many instances here & elsewhere I have to ask: who is your interjection aimed at?

I start to cringe when I am listening to something about the current situation and someone starts throwing politics into it.

I'm thankful that they didn't mention politics. Dr. Victory also mentioned that this is not about politics, I agree with her. Nonetheless, if the doctors were speaking on a stage with swastikas on it it would amount to more than just a platform being provided for them. The Tea Party knows that *they* can use the doctors for *their* political purposes — even if the doctors don't share them. I'm grateful that the doctors have an uncensored platform to get their ideas out there & I'm glad to be able to read their opinions in the transcript.

It is believed that Bitchute is nonpartisan. Yes, it has some extreme conservative stuff on it. But it also has just as much liberal stuff on it, from what I can tell. And let's be honest here, with what is going on, party lines seem to be pretty blurred, to me at least.

Again, Linda, you're being too defensive. I'm not a democrat or a republican. I find them both contemptible. I'm a free thinker, I can agree with anyone that I find inspired &/or reasonable, etc. I didn't diss Bitchute, I expressed gratitiude for its being uncensored. I just don't know it well enough to know exactly HOW uncensored it is. I'm a member, but I've never posted anything there. As I've stated before, I prefer the Internet Archive because their mission statement is about freedom of speech & information. Maybe Bitchute's is too, I don't know.

****

July 30, 2020, 12:23PM (Inquiring Librarian to group):

The HighWire/Del Bigtree - Deplatformed by YouTube

So, you may have heard about the "Highwire", Del Bigtree's independent news media site:
https://thehighwire.com/

Yesterday, Youtube removed all of his videos from his website. There was no warning, he never got flagged or reprimands. But, he discusses vaccine safety and he is completely on the nonsense lies that we are being manipulated with right now. He is intelligent, honest, and shares some of the best satire and real news with excellent sources of what insanity is going on right now. He sticks to the facts and the facts right now are weapons against the establishment.

Here is my favorite so far of his. It is priceless, and less than 3 minutes long. Here he is making fun of Bill Nye, the Science Guy's trying to sell the idea that vaccines are safe:
https://www.facebook.com/HighWireTalk/videos/422232484819416/?d=null&vh=e

Here is Del reacting, late last night, to having his website deplatformed by Youtube, less than 6 minutes long, showing that we are Winning! (i like his positive attitude):
https://www.youtube.com/watch?feature=youtu.be&t=17&v=jXgxYhZp_-o&app=desktop

& this one is awesome! Here he is, in 30 minutes, explaining the facts and math behind why it is so unlikely for you to die from covid 19, including t-cell immunity vs. antibody immunity, real math crunching the numbers, and the superior effectiveness of natural immunity over vaccine-induced immunity.
https://www.facebook.com/HighWireTalk/videos/1022854141465102/?d=null&vh=e

Honestly, all of Del's stuff is great. It has a sense of humor, it is confident, and it is reaching for the positive aspects in moving forward with what we are dealing with right now (the opposite of Spiro). He also interviews a lot of great scientists, local leaders, and doctors. His team is working on finding newer and safer platforms... stay tuned for the new and improved website and secure videos!

****

July 30, 2020, 11:52PM (Inquiring Librarian to group):

Re: The HighWire/Del Bigtree - Deplatformed by YouTube

Hi Everyone,

Here is the Del Bigtree Highwire video from today's talk show that was taken down about 1 hour after the live feed ended. I think that the show here is brilliant. It goes pretty in depth about the Front Line Doctors,with a lot of clips from their summit and into HCQ. Again, I think this is a pretty big step into outing the pharmaceutical industry's nonsense. But I am perhaps just naive, which I fully accept is very possible.
https://lbry.tv/@nobody:d/the-cyber-attack-on-truth:3?fbclid=IwAR0jrWgM8f0_c7M8Eae-bMYHhl2mbxHvBG0zTv2a0HN3j2e8smfzFO-348o

****

July 30, 2020, 11:57PM (Inquiring Librarian to group):

Ok, so the Front Line Doctors Website is back up. Along with all of their videos, their website had also been taken down by big tech. How disgusting.

Here it is:
https://americasfrontlinedoctorsummit.com/?fbclid=IwAR2t-MCY98oMyUanj3QkEkx2gFoFZXHZcvcUzoTuas_Qytxd0laSRq5cHYw
from the front page:

"American life has fallen casualty to a massive disinformation campaign. We can speculate on how this has happened, and why it has continued, but the purpose of the inaugural White Coat Summit is to empower Americans to stop living in fear.

If Americans continue to let so-called experts and media personalities make their decisions, the great American experiment of a Constitutional Republic with Representative Democracy, will cease."

****

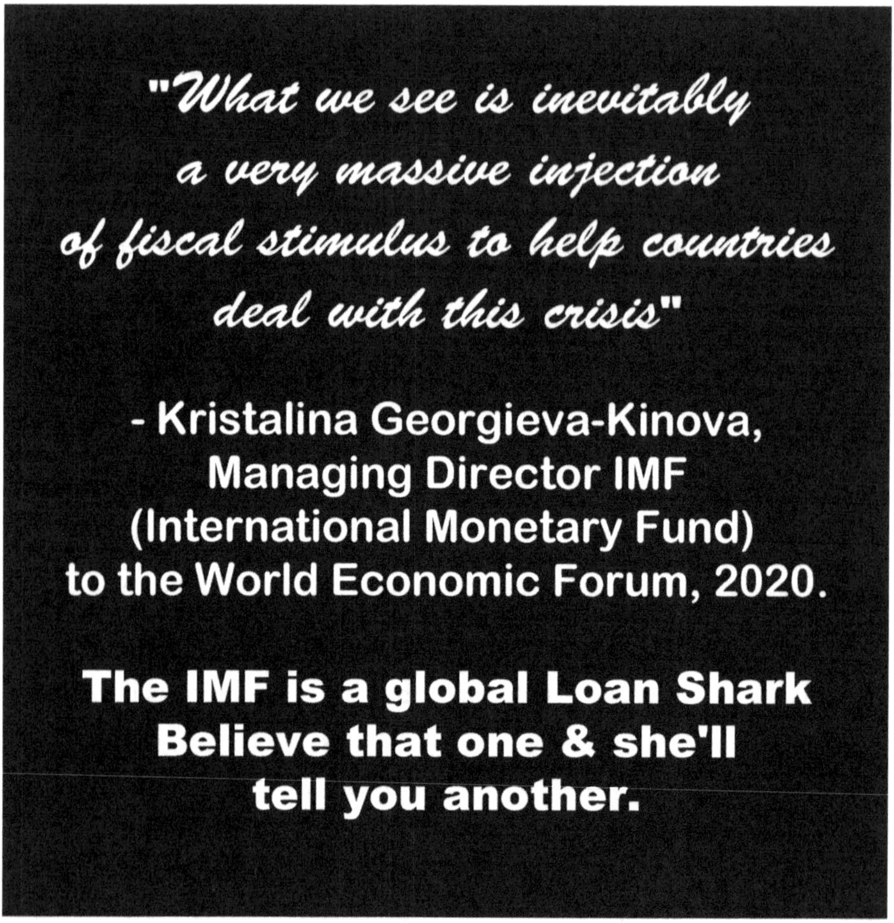
"What we see is inevitably
a very massive injection
of fiscal stimulus to help countries
deal with this crisis"
- Kristalina Georgieva-Kinova,
Managing Director IMF
(International Monetary Fund)
to the World Economic Forum, 2020.
The IMF is a global Loan Shark
Believe that one & she'll
tell you another.

****

July 31, 2020, 2:50AM (Amir-ul Kafirs to group):

HERETICS: Tooth Fairy

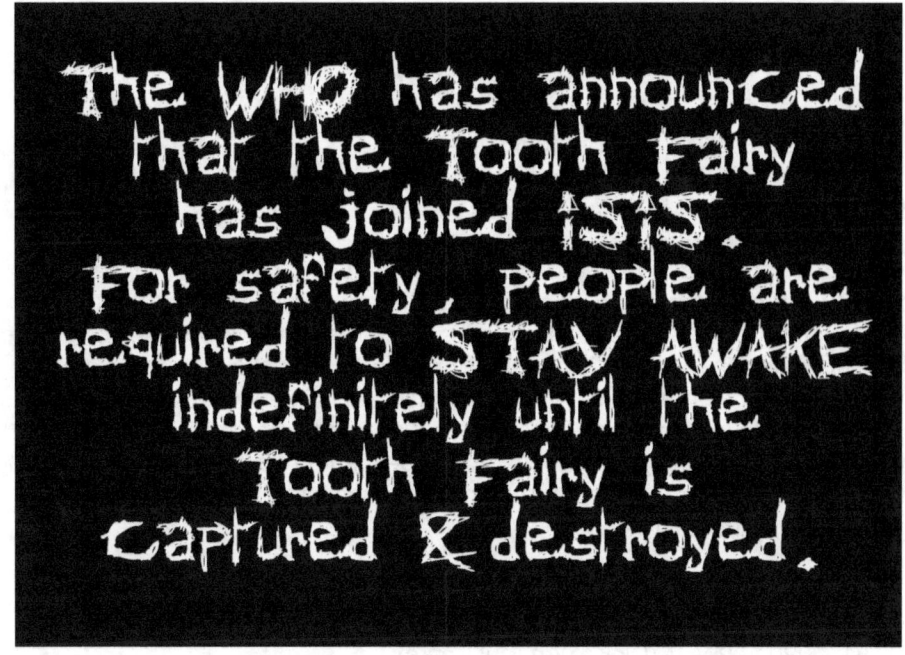

****

July 31, 2020, 6:37AM (Dick to Amir-ul Kafirs):

On July 4, Dick wrote to Amir-ul Kafirs about a classical radio station announcer & a pandemic related post he made on his blog. The following is another such post:

"20 weeks in isolation and I have not relied on a single delivery service. I walk to the stores about once or twice a week. Drive my car about once a month. Three months ago I had some Chinese food delivered. The only time."

****

July 31, 2020, 8:12AM (Amir-ul Kafirs to Dick):

a strange and I feel sad bravado

"20 weeks in isolation"

It's hard for me to see that as anything other than masochism.

****

July 31, 2020, 8:15AM (Dick to Amir-ul Kafirs):

yeah i agree

masochism is kind of what I meant by a sad bravado

****

July 31, 2020, 8:26AM (Amir-ul Kafirs to Dick):

masochism is kind of what I meant by a sad bravado

Yeah, it's a sort of passive aggressive challenge: *Look, I can deny myself more than you* ***& it's for the good of others.*** But it's not for the good of others, it's out of total hatred for himself AND others. It's a sickness that wishes itself on others. It's what I called in my mom "sympathetic magic" & "Munchausen Syndrome by Proxy". In other words, the self-righteousness of it is intended to set an example but the example is akin to self-flaggelation, it seems to me that the desire is for *other people to self-flaggelate so that they'll get caught up in the frenzy of hurting themselves like he is.* Maybe I'm reading too much into it with my amateur psychoanalysis but that's my intuitive take.

****

July 31, 2020, 8:29AM (Dick to Amir-ul Kafirs):

I think you hit the nail right on the head !
It's that!
And there were 'like's and 'loves' comments!
It's madness! That means he's been in the house 5 months
It's sick

****

July 31, 2020, 8:29AM (Amir-ul Kafirs to group):

"School of Negativity" notes - 1080p - 6:29

https://youtu.be/XZcHF6FWKf0

"School of Negativity": I was getting some supplies from a store when I noticed that they had black canvases for sale. This inspired me to imagine painting in negative. I've generally found the QUARANTYRANNY oppressive & the emphasis on masks suffocating so it occurred to me that this might be a good time to create a "School of Negativity". Always trying to think of new activities to keep my friend Naia Nisnam & myself entertained & sane during these times I further imagined going into a natural environment & painting a negative landscape with 2 black canvases screwed together somewhat askew to disrupt the usual rectangularity. One thing led to another & to a trip to Lake Erie, the world's 11th largest lake that also happens to be conveniently close to where we live AND someplace that neither of us had been to before. The painting is completely amateurish but I think we both enjoyed the attempt to paint in negative while simultaneously struggling against the wind & getting baked by the sun.

****

July 30, 2020, 6:01AM (Dick to group):

HERETICS: another questionnaire

I'm curious, what names do you all recall given to non-mask wearers?

I recall :

Psychopaths
Less educated
Selfish

Also, can anyone think of an argument to counter the claim that not wearing a mask endangers other's lives?

****

July 31, 2020, 3:11AM (Amir-ul Kafirs to group):

Re: HERETICS: another questionanaire

Also, can anyone think of an argument to counter the claim that not wearing a mask endangers other's lives?

Unfortunately, the basis for any argument that I might have would be doing what's natural because I think that nature functions well, just like the human body's immune system, when allowed to work with minimal interference. What that means in this instance is that the body breathes in in order to bring fresh air in & breathes out to expel no-longer fresh air. To me, anything that inhibits this process is unhealthy. As I've mentioned before in relation to my own life I feel like mild exposure to one's environment, which includes the inhalation of a small quantity of someone else's exhalation, is an immunization. I started with the word "Unfortunately" because I think such an argument is only accepted by fellow naturists & is rejected by anyone who believes 1st & foremost in human intervention into EVERYTHING, hence believing in medicine more than in nature &/or one's own immune system. My personal opinion about this belief in human intervention is that it causes the most severe problems. Nature doesn't produce nuclear weapons & chemical warfare, at least not in any way except through human 'ingenuity'. & things like the bombing of Hiroshima & Nagasaki, the Bhopal Union Carbide disaster, the Chernobyl nuclear accident, mustard gas in the trenches of WWI are the things that defeat the human immune system. A virus, however, unless COVID-19 (if it even exists as we're told it does) is manufactured in a lab, is a product of nature & is less severe than an explosion or radioactivity.

****

July 31, 2020, 6:22AM (Dick to group):

Thanks!
Your position seems reasonable to me
Today, by the way, there is a heat wave here in Paris... wearing a mask is going to be like a torture

****

July 31, 2020, 8:20AM (Amir-ul Kafirs to group):

I was thinking about it more. When I wear a mask I feel suffocated, both physically & psychologically. Not only do I feel that it's inhibiting my breathing, I feel like it's inhibiting a more psychological flow. Obviously, wearing a mask is blocking one's primary means of self-expression, speaking (& singing, etc), but also one's sense of taste & smell. All of these things combine to produce what I call "**Unconscious Suffocation**". Not only do ***I*** feel suffocated but I feel an empathetic suffocation when I see other people with masks on — it's akin to seeing a child pull a plastic bag over their head, there's an instinctual urge to rush to remove the bag/mask.

****

July 31, 2020, 12:56PM (Inquiring Librarian to group):

HERETICS: Censorship & the FCC

I am not sure if you are aware of this. But in the U.S., this week, the U.S. Government has done the following:

Commerce Department Files Petition to Clarify Liability Protections for Online Platforms and Protect Against Censorship

Here is the official government declaration of the Petition:
https://www.commerce.gov/index.php/news/press-releases/2020/07/commerce-department-files-petition-clarify-liability-protections-online?fbclid=IwAR1x4CFmmlp5JYbAIQOVGo0uzJ7vLEIinDay4YRPDbeBecF76lieWxhoqxI

Sounds like what we want, right? It appears to be cracking down on the censors, not those platforms being censored. Or am I being delusional?
Here is all 57 pages of the petition if you care to dive deeply into it.
https://www.ntia.gov/files/ntia/publications/ntia_petition_for_rulemaking_7.27.20.pdf

Then check out this crazy CNN article which to me states that the U.S. government is trying to crack down on the censors so that big tech platforms stop taking down legitimate information.

Trump is moving forward with his plan to regulate social media

https://www.cnn.com/2020/07/27/tech/fcc-social-media-petition/index.html
CNN seems to be unsuccessfully attempting to warp this petition into something nefarious, but I cannot see that outside of the title of the article (which I find to be misleading if you actual read the article which makes the point that the government is trying to 'regulate' social media by getting them to stop censoring so much information). They keep mentioning Trump and 'mail in voting', which to me, seem like lures/triggers to get people riled up against stopping censorship. Aka: Trump is stupid and wrong and how silly that he thinks his posting [mis]information about mail in voting is so stupid that OF COURSE, it must be censored, aka: Censorship is GOOD! We need Censorship. Do you follow the 'logic'? Trump is being used as a pawn to get you to think censorship is needed and ok?

It appears that CNN is claiming that the federal government should not interfere with big tech's internet and social media censorship. Their argument makes no sense to me. CNN is actually defending the censors/censorship. Am I reading this wrong?

Remember, this week, the Frontline Doctors were Censored on Monday. This petition was filed on Monday. Also, this week, Del Bigtree's Highwire was deplatformed by Youtube. And Del's video from yesterday was taken down by Facebook 1 hour after its live feed. All of these here who were censored this week were speaking out, with facts and real medical knowledge, about the hazards of vaccines and pointing out that the vaccines are not necessary. Now they are censored. Perhaps the above Petition is what we want. Without censorship of those who speak out about vaccines and those that offer viable alternative treatments for Covid, we would have more power to fight the elites who wish to enslave us, specifically they wish to enslave us through Covid. Am I crazy?

****

Commerce Department Files Petition to

Clarify Liability Protections for Online Platforms and Protect Against Censorship

FOR IMMEDIATE RELEASE

Monday, July 27, 2020

Office of Public Affairs
(202) 482-4883
publicaffairs@doc.gov(link sends email)

Today, the National Telecommunications and Information Administration (NTIA) filed a petition for rulemaking with the Federal Communications Commission (FCC) on behalf of U.S. Secretary of Commerce Wilbur Ross seeking to clarify regulations related to section 230 of the Communications Decency Act.

The petition was filed in response to the May 2020 Executive Order on Preventing Online Censorship. It calls on the FCC to make clear when online platforms can claim section 230 protections if they restrict access to content in a manner not specifically outlined under the Act.

"Many Americans rely on online platforms to stay informed and connected, sharing their thoughts and ideas on issues important to them, which can oftentimes lead to free and open debate around public policies and upcoming elections," **said Secretary of Commerce Wilbur Ross**. "It has long been the policy of the United States to foster a robust marketplace of ideas on the Internet and the free flow of information around the world. President Trump is committed to protecting the rights of all Americans to express their views and not face unjustified restrictions or selective censorship from a handful of powerful companies."

The petition also seeks further clarity from the FCC:

- Whether, and to what degree, Section 230 of the Communications Decency Act provides protection for social media's content moderation decisions
- The conditions under which content moderation and editorial decisions by social media companies shape content to such a degree that section 230 no longer protects them
- Social media's disclosure obligations with respect to their content moderation practices

A link to the petition can be found here.

BUREAUS AND OFFICES

National Telecommunications and Information Administration

- https://www.commerce.gov/index.php/news/press-releases/2020/07/commerce-department-files-petition-clarify-liability-protections-online?fbclid=IwAR1x4CFmmlp5JYbAIQOVGo0uzJ7vLEIinDay4YRPDbeBecF76lieWxhoqxI

****

In the Matter of)
Section 230 of the
Communications Act of 1934)
To: The Commission

Before the

FEDERAL COMMUNICATIONS COMMISSION Washington, DC 20554

)
File No. RM-_____

PETITION FOR RULEMAKING OF THE
NATIONAL TELECOMMUNICATIONS AND INFORMATION ADMINISTRATION

July 27, 2020

National Telecommunications and Information Administration
U.S. Department of Commerce 1401 Constitution Avenue, NW Washington, DC 20230
(202) 482-1816

I.
II.
III.
IV.
V. 230
A. Act
B.
C.
D.
E.

1. 2. 3. 4.

TABLE OF CONTENTS

In the Matter of)
Section 230 of the
Communications Act of 1934)
To: The Commission
Before the
FEDERAL COMMUNICATIONS COMMISSION Washington, D.C. 20554
)
File No. RM-_____
PETITION FOR RULEMAKING OF THE
NATIONAL TELECOMMUNICATIONS AND INFORMATION ADMINISTRATION

[..]

- https://www.ntia.gov/files/ntia/publications/ntia_petition_for_rulemaking_7.27.20.pdf

****

Trump is moving forward with his plan to regulate social media

By Brian Fung, CNN Business

Updated 7:41 AM ET, Tue July 28, 2020

(CNN Business) The Trump administration took a key step on Monday toward fulfilling the president's executive order on social media, formally asking the FCC to develop regulations that could apply to Facebook, Twitter and other tech platforms.

The petition for rulemaking puts the ball in the FCC's court. The agency must now decide whether to agree to President Donald Trump's call for FCC oversight of internet platforms. Trump and other Republicans have long criticized companies, including Facebook (FB) and Twitter (TWTR), for allegedly censoring conservatives; the companies have denied the claims.

"President Trump is committed to protecting the rights of all Americans to express their views and not face unjustified restrictions or selective censorship from a handful of powerful companies," said Commerce Secretary Wilbur Ross in a statement.

FCC spokesman Brian Hart said the agency will carefully review the petition.

Under Trump's May executive order, a branch of the Commerce Department known as the National Telecommunications and Information Administration was expected to call on the FCC to "clarify" Section 230 of the Communications Decency Act, the law that has shielded tech companies from much litigation over internet content since its passage in 1996.

Trump's social media order was introduced and signed days after Twitter applied a warning label to his tweets that said they were "potentially misleading." Twitter highlighted two of Trump's tweets that claimed, without evidence, that mail-in voting would lead to widespread voter fraud. Trump later threatened to "strongly regulate" or shut down social media platforms. Since then, Trump has continued his attacks against Twitter.

Donald J. Trump

So disgusting to watch Twitter's so-called "Trending", where sooo many trends are about me, and never a good one. They look for anything they can find, make it as bad as possible, and blow it up, trying to make it trend. Really ridiculous, illegal, and, of course, very unfair!
6:41 PM · Jul 27, 2020

Legal experts say the executive order is on shaky ground, as the FCC has traditionally avoided regulating internet companies. The order is already facing at least one legal challenge that claims it is unconstitutional.

Jessica Rosenworcel, a Democratic FCC commissioner, said the agency should steer clear of the request.

"The FCC shouldn't take this bait," Rosenworcel said in a statement. "While social media can be frustrating, turning this agency into the President's speech police is not the answer. If we honor the Constitution, we will reject this petition immediately."

- https://www.cnn.com/2020/07/27/tech/fcc-social-media-petition/index.html

****

July 31, 2020, 7:04PM (Amir-ul Kafirs to group):

Re: HERETICS: Censorship & the FCC

Aka: Trump is stupid and wrong and how silly that he thinks his posting [mis]information about mail in voting

The entire voting system can be rigged, I think, mainly by just having the Electoral College overide the popular vote. I do believe that the Florida vote that resulted in Bush Jr getting elected was rigged. I do believe that mail-in voting can be rigged & that the fear of going to the polls is just ridiculous. One of the people I unfriended & blocked on Facebook thinks that the fear of going to the polls is ***absolutely real*** — I think he's absolutely insane. I have no problem believing that both Republicans & Democrats will rig elections & that this time it's the Democrats who will be the most likely suspects in the rigging of this upcoming election. Since they're also the ones pushing for mail-in voting it seems reasonable to me that they must have a technique figured out for rigging that.

Trump is being used as a pawn to get you to think censorship is needed and ok?

Yeah, I can see that. He doesn't help things by constantly making pronouncements that're truly imbecelic, by wanting to build the border wall, by calling COVID-19 the "Chinese Virus", etc.

we would have more power to fight the elites who wish to enslave us, specifically they wish to enslave us through Covid. Am I crazy?

I'm 100% against internet censorship & I do think that such censorship will benefit the COVID-19(84) Global Dictatorship that has descended upon us.

****

July 31, 2020, 9:05PM (Amir-ul Kafirs to group):

It appears to be cracking down on the censors, not those platforms being censored. Or am I being delusional?

I read that one. It's just a short thing. Yeah, it seems like what we want. I can't really evaluate it though without understanding what "section 230 of the Communications Decency Act." is all about, which I don't.

It appears that CNN is claiming that the federal government should not interfere with big tech's internet and social media censorship. Their argument makes no sense to me. CNN is actually defending the censors/censorship. Am I reading this wrong?

I read this. I don't see it the way you do but, again, without understanding current internet law it's impossible for me to understand what this actually means. The article claims that Rump wants the FCC to oversee social media platforms to make sure they're not censoring conservative content, which Rump claims they are. If the FCC doesn't oversee internet providers then I think that's a good thing, I think it's more likely to result in more freedom of speech than less. I've been censored by YouTube & Facebook & Wikipedia. I'm not a conservative, so that's one example of censorship of a non-conservative. Legally, this must be an insanely complicated issue. Facebook & YouTube must have whole legal teams working on the issue of how to control content. The question is: If the FCC steps in does that improve matters or make it worse? I don't think it necessarily makes it better. The move by microbroadcasters ('pirate' radio people) has been toward more freedom from the FCC. Since that's more my neck of the woods I'm more inclined in that direction. One of the primary things the FCC did early on was stop radio stations from having enormous broadcast power that would blow other smaller wattage stations away. I'm fine with that. What hasn't happened is the prevention of mass media from gradually being monopolized by a smaller & smaller group of mega-rich people. I'm not happy about that. These people know that the more they control the media the more they control popular opinion. It's more than a little ironic that Rump complains about censorship of conservatives because newspapers & TV are almost exclusively owned by conservative interests & they routinely censor any content that goes against those interests. As such, social media, if it's censoring conservatives, is one of the only places left where conservatives can't run the show.

Alas, though, as we've discussed before, what's happening now goes above & beyond 'conservatives vs liberals'. No matter what face is put on things what we've got here is an oligarchy of people who believe they are destined to rule vs a many-headed hydra who refuses to cooperate with the new slavery. The FCC, being a government agency, would be better than a privatized oversight organization but that doesn't mean it would be any good. I see more hope in resistance to censorship in the myriad ways it's already happening — in websites that're elusively out-of-control. Essentially, in what I call "Guerrilla Playfare". But that's all very fragile.

Now they are censored.

But they still managed to reach millions of people.

they wish to enslave us through Covid. Am I crazy?

I think we have to keep in mind that COVID-19(84) is being used as a pretext to censor — but, ultimately, the censorship will go wwwaaaayyyy beyond just preventing health information from being heard, *everything* contrary to the MONOLITHIC NARRATIVE will be censored. I don't believe that *any person in a major position of power* wants their enemy's positions to be uncensored & freely available. Rump's been at the forefront of claiming that there's "fake news" & all the rest. It's my opinion that **he** just wants to be the one who says what's fake & what's real. I don't trust that.

****

July 31, 2020, 1:23PM (Inquiring Librarian to group):

HERETICS: Library Positive 'cases'

Libraries are closing. Albeit this is temporary, but it's ridiculous and does not bode well for our future

Meanwhile, I learned today that the 5G towers are being constructed in the French Quarter as I type this. How awful. According to 'conspiracy theorists', these are all about mass surveillance and also the wireless technology at this depth is extremely polluting and cancerous.
https://childrenshealthdefense.org/news/5g-and-wireless-technology-health-effects/
"***clear evidence that this radiation [5G/microwave radiation] causes cancer and breaks DNA.***"

****

OCTOBER 15, 2019

5G and Wireless Technology Health Effects

By Dafna Tachover, Contributing Writer

I was invited to give a short presentation on 5G & Wireless Technology health effects to the Beverly Hill's City Council. Seventy years of science, including thousands of studies showing clear evidence of harm, the human evidence and the evidence of fraud, cannot be conveyed in 15 minutes. As an experienced telecommunication and computers' officer who understands the technology, as an attorney trained to evaluate evidence, and has actually litigated this issue in the Israeli Supreme Court, and as an advocate who is working daily with adults and many children who have become sick, there is no doubt – the evidence of adverse health effects from wireless technology, including from cell phones, Wi-Fi, wireless "smart" utility meters and cell towers is conclusive.

... clear evidence that this radiation [5G/microwave radiation] causes cancer and breaks DNA.

Adverse changes have been ignored

Nothing has changed in our way of life in the past 35 years as drastically as the adoption of wireless technology. Adverse changes in human, animal, and plant health have been occurring dramatically over the same time frame, but the obvious correlation and the evidence have been ignored.

The public is being misled to believe that wireless technology, which emits microwave radiation, is safe and that there is "no evidence" it is harmful. According to the "safety" guidelines adopted by the Federal Communication Commission (FCC) in 1996, Radio and Microwave frequencies used for wireless technology, are harmful only if they create a temperature change in tissue. This is known as the thermal effect. These guidelines were already obsolete when adopted. The non-thermal harm is scientifically proven including by studies of our own government.

Most recently, on November 1, 2018, the final report of the Federal Government National Toxicology Program (NTP), the government expert agency on toxins, was published. The $30 million 19-year study found CLEAR EVIDENCE that this radiation causes cancer and breaks DNA. This study confirmed what other studies already showed decades ago including reports and studies by the Navy, Air-Force, NASA, and the EPA which recognized and documented the profound bio-effects of wireless technology.

Federal laws and FCC regulations enabled this forced deployment by removing any barriers, preempting municipal authority, and giving the wireless industry almost unlimited access to our public rights of ways.

Forced deployment

The NTP study should have been a game changer and put a halt to further deployment of wireless technology. The NTP scientists said that the public should be informed. Instead, The FCC has been fast-tracking the deployment of 5G. 5G is the infrastructure for the internet of things and is intended to wirelessly connect 20 billion more devices and for that purpose, deploy 800,000 more cell towers and launch 20,000 satellites which will exponentially increase our exposure to this harmful radiation.

The deployment of the 800,000 5G "small" cell antennas on poles near every few homes has begun and is progressing quickly. Most of these antennas are 4G and some will utilize millimeter wave frequencies. Studies show profound bio-effects from millimeter waves as well. Federal laws and FCC regulations enabled this forced deployment by removing any barriers, preempting municipal authority, and giving the wireless industry almost unlimited access to our public rights of ways.

These antennas are being forced on residents within a few feet of their homes without their informed consent, and they are being prevented from effectively objecting from their installation on any grounds, including health. These antennas may be smaller but because of their proximity, they increase the levels of radiation on our streets by thousands of times. Families who have had these "small" antennas installed near their homes are becoming sick, sometimes within days after they are installed. There is a reason why insurance companies refuse to insure the wireless industry for health effects.

If you don't want to wake up in the morning and have a 5G cell tower a few feet from your children's bedroom window, it is time to become informed and help efforts to get US cities and states to "Just Say No" to the FCC & 5G.

- https://childrenshealthdefense.org/news/5g-and-wireless-technology-health-effects/

****

July 31, 2020, 9:21PM (Amir-ul Kafirs to group):

Re: HERETICS: Nola Library Positive 'cases'

Libraries are closing. Albeit this is temporary, but it's ridiculous and does not bode well for our future

Basically, it's just overkill. A 'case', as we discussed many times, doesn't mean much of anything. Even if we were to take all this pseudo-concern over public health seriously, which I don't at all, there's no way that "deep cleaning" the library is going to help & there's no way that deaths are going to be stopped. We're not immortal, live with it.

"***clear evidence that this radiation [5G/microwave radiation] causes cancer and breaks DNA.***"

I don't have any trouble believing that microwave radiation causes cancer & I don't have any trouble believing that more microwave 'towers' are going to cause more of it. Alas, I'm equally certain that young people, especially, will be creaming their jeans over having quicker access to the banal.

****

July 31, 2020, 9:44PM (Amir-ul Kafirs to group):

July 31, 2020, 8:48PM (Naia Nisnam to group):

Her beliefs about demons fucking women are beyond absurd and have no place in science or medicine.
Why did the other doctors include her in the platform? Didn't they realize that crap would make it easy to discredit them all?

That's part of the way propaganda works — everyone is discredited by association with one person. IMO it shouldn't be that way: fine, discredit that doctor as, essentially, a 'witch doctor' — but don't throw out everyone else.

My guess is that no one knew how insane she was until the press dug up that

2013 video.

Keep in mind that at one time, probably even NOW, most doctors identified as being associated with a religion, in this country usually Christianity. Christians believe that God impregnanted a virgin woman who gave birth to God's son. God's son was killed & buried in a cave. He then was reborn & got out of the cave. Christianity is as full of bizarre shit as any religion — but you won't find the news 'exposing' an ordinary Christian doctor as a nut-case.

Personal Thoughts on the Covid-19 Pandemic
Part Two
- Dick Turner, Artist/Composer, Paris

My first observations on the Covid-19 situation were written from the perspective of someone who experienced an event and tried to make sense of it in terms of what he'd seen and heard as it unfolded. That is, there I was, information began to present itself to me in various ways, I tried to understand it.

In this short paper I'd like to discuss what I believe are the philosophical – historical underpinnings of the Covid-19 "pandemic" and why I think so many people are in line with the current mindset.

*

I will begin way out in left field.

In his "Treatise on Orchestration" Nicolai Rimsky-Korsakov presents a very interesting idea, an idea which, for all purposes is *inconceivable in today's world*. He says that when thinking about orchestral sound and the use of instruments *there are some things that should not be done*.

This idea of having the possibility for a novel effect but purposely not taking advantage of it is unthinkable in the modern world. I would say that almost all the "more advanced" music written since he penned that idea has been to some degree a refutation of his idea, beginning in fact with his famous student Igor Stravinsky. (I have long felt that in Le sacre de printemps Stravinsky, in youthful rebellion set out to do the exact opposite of many of his teacher's precepts. I think that the short section of "The Sage" is a satirical musical portrait of his teacher in fact.)

I believe that this idea of *purposefully not doing something* is alien to us because we are no longer religious; that is, religion no longer plays an active role in our lives. We may have ideas about God, or consider ourselves to have a spiritual bent but these ideas, too, only prove the difference between today and the world in which Rimsky wrote his book, a world that was already changing.

Only the religiously orthodox can understand that rule. Only those who have some form of inner moral law can understand that rule.

They have no choice because *they have the law*.

The non-orthodox, as I will show later, if an opportunity presents itself, must take advantage of it. It is a necessity to them; it is the essence of their being.

They have no choice because *they do not have the law*.

I believe this is the predicament of this current moment in history for certain new ideas have arrived, certain new possibilities, and I believe that mankind will be powerless to not put them in place.

*

I will not try to hide that the following ideas are written from a so-called "conspiratorial perspective". Specifically I believe the Covid-19 "pandemic" is a tool being used to put in place the so-called Agenda 2050 of the World Economic Forum, which I believe to be the mouthpiece of the so-called "1%". But even if I am mistaken, and I sincerely hope that I am, I want to discuss a larger issue that I feel has been brought into the public eye by this event – the eventual ubiquitous use of AI and bio-technology.

*

I have long felt that the 21rst century hasn't yet begun. Each century seems to have its own identity, at least that's how it seems to have gone since the end of the Middle Ages.

Here's my historical breakdown of the last 600 years and my

apologies to official historians one of which I am not.
Everyone knows that the Middle Ages came to an end with the Renaissance. This is the "Official End" because as Huizinga (A great Dutch historian, I am referring to his book *The Waning of the Middle Ages*) points out there's always some overlap between identified historical periods when new ideas start to take force over older ones. The Renaissance was Reason and Science based as opposed to Faith based. Think of Leonardo's drawings and compare them to illustrated manuscripts and nothing else needs to be said.

> By the way, I think that in fact there is no real end to anything and that even today certain "mediaeval mindsets" still exist (as for example the End of the World panic when we moved into the year 2000AD). I think that probably, even among the most modern populace that probably stone-age behaviors still exist… who knows maybe eating meat is one of them? My point is simply *mindsets change in response to new information*.

Next, conveniently for my purposes, about 100 years later, in 1492 America was "discovered" by the West. What does this mean or rather, imply? It means and implies that ship building, compasses, navigational theory; in short, it means that technology had developed so highly that long sea voyages were possible.
This gave rise to a merchant class that rivalled the Royalty in power and a growing tradesman class, the development of cities, specialized business activities, etc. A lot of infra-structure was put into place, to put it another way.
Again, almost like clockwork, 100 years later, around 1600 saw Colonialism take force as the reigning mode of Western thought-in-action.

> Small aside: let us not be hypocritical about the past.

> First, why trade when you can steal and get away with it? And secondly, why pay people if you can enslave them? Please don't think I am personally in favor of these systems but please try to admit their reality within a radically different social context.

In short this was a time of the continued expansion of Western power, living high on the hog so to speak.

1700 is marked by a new kind of event: Europe was the only thing happening on a global scale. And when that kind of self-assurance takes place *it allows people to relax*. It was the first time in modern history where people felt comfortable enough to just sit on their asses and think. Think about it: Encyclopedias and Philosophical treatises seem to show up every other week.

Please consider that what happens when people think is that they reconsider what they already know and hold it up to question. They become interested in reform, justice, equality, etc. They also become interested in tearing down what exists and making it better… Or at least, that's the intention.

Well, they were successful and in 1789 came the French Revolution, which was the beginning of the 19th century, again, about 100 years since the last major change. It inspired people and to a large degree *invented a new idea of what it meant to be a human being*. Or maybe it's better to say, it consolidated ideas that had been developing over time.

Three of these ideas that would take on tremendous significance later are: evolution, the non-existence of the soul and ideas about the unconscious mind.

It also was the kicking into high gear of the Industrial Revolution which, again conveniently for my 100 year historical plan progressed and in 1914, again about 100 years later, allowed the World to go crazy.

Here the important word is the WORLD: For WWI was, along with WWII a few years later, for better or (to be honest) worse, a global war, a global event. Maybe the first one.

NOTE: I have long felt that war serves two purposes

- To speed up historical events (it takes hundreds of years to build a city, it takes a few days or even hours to destroy one)
- To allow people to get to know each other in the only way they trust, i.e. through fighting

These wars established the USA as the one world power. They also brought the final end of colonialism and began the process of bringing, maybe forcing is a better word, the once colonized or subjugated nations onto the world economic stage – notably for our purposes, China.

And voilà, *that's my personal take* on the historical setting for what I now propose to expand upon.

*

So here we are.

It's already 2020! It's time to get the show on the road. Something's got to change, the question is, what? We need some changes to stay on track historically.

First, a small aside:

The problem with modern reality is war is no longer possible even though *it's what we* want and probably need for psychological reasons*.

*I use the word "we" to suggest a sort of collective unconscious. I do not mean to imply that all people feel this way down to the last man. My point is rather that though the 1% may always start the wars, that it takes two to tango and without the compliance of the so-called "masses" there would be no wars.

The unavailability of world war is due, as I'm sure you guessed, to the existence of the Hydrogen bomb.

Since we cannot kill each other on a controlled global

scale we are left to stagnate. But, unlike the 18th century when the stagnation was due to a lopsided prosperity and reflection, we now stagnate like trapped monkeys in a cage. We sit in our cage and try to contemplate the past and desire to correct it, we look at the future through the bars of our cage and all we want is change, it makes no difference what change, anything will do if just to distract us from the condition of being ourselves.

Pertinent Childhood Memory: I once saw a gorilla in a cage in the Baltimore Zoo. It sat there under a garish yellow light looking as miserable as miserable can be. I noticed that he was vomiting, eating his vomit and then re-vomiting just to entertain himself in his endless hellish limbo-like boredom.

Anything to escape! A war would seem like a blessing in fact. For a war is something like getting drunk, you drink yourself senseless so you then can wake up and feel repentant for a while before you go out *to tie another one on*.

Meanwhile, in the background something had been happening, four things in fact:

First, the resources of the world became concentrated in the hands of a very small group of people

Second Auschwitz, which made humanity no longer trust itself

Third, as mentioned previously, non-Western nations have entered into the Global economic arena. This has had the effect of introducing cultural relativism.

Fourth, there have been huge advances in artificial intelligence and bio-tech research. **But so far, few of these have been put into active use.**

An Observation:

Any child knows the agony of the night before Christmas. The child knows that there are toys waiting for him beneath the tree but that he must wait to open them! If he could he'd just get it over with, but no, convention dictates he must wait.
I think that these developments in AI and bio-tech research are like the toys beneath the Christmas tree and the small group of people who somehow own everything (perhaps only because *we allow them to own it*) are the children. They are sick of waiting and want to open up the toys! After all, the toys are all there waiting to be played with.
Besides, they have another motivation – they know that *they are the only ones with toys* and that the situation is essentially if not *totally unfair*. And so they feel double urge to make sure they can get those toys open and in active use so that they can hold on to what they have for as long as possible, **forever if possible**.
Now, they can't **JUST DO IT** as the popular mind numbing slogan goes. No, they can't just impose this on the world. Why? Because of the 17th century and all its philosophy about equality, human rights, etc.
So they have to impose it upon us with our agreement! And though this is a challenge, they are up for it! Remember, they know that the caged gorilla wants change, it's sick of eating its puke, "Just get me out of this cage and I'll be happy" I can imagine him pleading to himself. He wants to go to the bar and get drunk – but he can't because he knows *this time it will kill him*.

> NOTE: When in France where I live, the so-called yellow vests were protesting, one of the arguments aimed against them was that they were out of step with the times, unable to adapt to the modern world, hopelessly

> anachronistic in their thinking. Well, that's how I see anyone who is against this AI-Bio-tech world being presented. You can't fight progress I hear booming from every quarter.
>
> I believe what is needed to install the new AI, bio-technocracy is to show that freedom and the human are ideas attached to previous times and are now outmoded and impediments to progress.

No the 21rst century hasn't yet begun – it's waiting but it needs an event.

Someone might say: Well what about 911? That was a major event and the world did seem to change afterwards.

911 was a preliminary event to the degree that it consolidated the new era of surveillance so it was a really good start towards the New World Order. But there was a problem: how could it be used to implement bio tech and ubiquitous AI? That was a real challenge!

As I showed at the start of this paper century defining events are linked to technology. Thus, it would seem logical that the new technology would usher in a new century. And here we have them! AI and Bio-tech…

But there is, as I see it, a problem.

In the past the West **turned outward** in reaction to its technological advances. This is no longer an option, because there is no West anymore. It's gone, it's a memory, nostalgia, Europe is now a theme park.

> NOTE: It is a belief of mine *that anything once identified no longer exists* as an active force. Thus, what, for example, we call racism today did not exist in the early days of slavery. To confuse the modern idea of racism and the historical idea of racism is a major error. It is for this reason that I believe racism no longer exists as a

> reality in the West but only as an *identity tool*. Real racism is an unspoken thing and there are no words for it, it is a position. Racism is an idea that developed in exact relation to the development of people's consciousness of their changing perspective on slavery. As an example of this I recommend "The Mutiny on the Elsinore" by Jack London, a fascinating book on this subject.

We cannot turn outwards because there is a problem – the cage! **Our cage.** *The cage will not change* so we must change what's in the cage, that is, *ourselves*. We cannot turn outward, so now we must direct the changes against ourselves. However this is self-destructive.

We want to fight but we can only beat ourselves.

And what use is thinking *if it can lead to Auschwitz*?

Consider in this context if you will something mentioned earlier in passing: the death of the idea of the human soul and the gradual sidelining of religion. The importance of this cannot be overestimated. The death of the soul means one thing and one thing only: that we are material like any other material. The sidelining of religion means another thing: the end of an external moral law. Moral law was the bulwark against the chaos of outer reality. Right or wrong it provided a framework for choice. The world as it is presents endless possibilities and moral law allows us to choose according to a relationship with an eternal God. In the absence of moral law people are doomed to go through all the variations, doomed to try everything because there is no ultimate authority.

It is not difficult to see how Auschwitz developed out of such a predicament. For in the absence of God all thoughts, all actions are equal. Again, JUST DO IT, a slogan which I feel could have easily replaced ARBEIT MACH FREI.

One of the main "conspiratorial" lines of argumentation in the

Covid-19 business is that it is being used to implement the putting in place of the so-called fourth industrial revolution, namely, AI and Bio-tech.
The question is can a small group of people actually usher in a century changing event or must this happen in an organic way?
The danger, as I see it, is that this new century *could be the last* due to the desire for change at any price, the abandoning of choice, the inability to leave the cage and the desire for self-directed abuse in combination with bio-tech and AI realities.
For the goal is to surrender being human and start acting like machines.
The goal is the eradication of what has become our random savage consciousness. (Savage because according to psychoanalytic theory that while we may have no inner moral law we certainly have an inner law of monumental inescapable monstrous selfishness: it is called the Id.)

> Small quasi-metaphysical note: As I write this I am struck by the horror of our situation and where perhaps the people who want to install a technocracy probably feel they are doing humanity a favor. Look at what used to be called the gentiles! A group of lost soulless, lawless ambient-meat-beings, doomed to go through every possible choice variation until the end of time.
> Of course Nietzsche suggested that the Will and Work should replace God and the Soul but so far, very few people have taken up his suggestion…

So, to escape the horns of this dilemma, we need to eradicate consciousness.
And the eradication of consciousness is easily enacted by allowing others to dictate what you think and do.
When this happens, a sort of magic takes place where your cage is no longer a cage because you have voluntarily decided to stay

in it, you stay in the cage and maybe you even cover your mouth to be extra safe, meaning extra distant from your own capacity or need to think.

Wasn't the confinement this exact situation in a miniature way?

It may seem impossible that a small group of people impose their will upon the entire human race but recall Justinian who commanded that all his subjects become Christian: "Through This Thall Shalt Conquer!" he saw written in the sky. The difference is, at least theoretically, that today we are individuals capable of self-directed thought and choice.

So it is interesting that the Covid-19 business is acting to limit our self-directed thought and choice to impose a global reality upon us.

I have no conclusions to draw and I cannot read the future. The question however presents itself to me: will people find the strength and courage to be human or will they surrender to imagined historical forces forced upon them to escape the burden of thought?

But if I had to make a guess, here's what I have to offer if this new agenda is put into place. The Middle Ages are known as a time when things "froze" in place. There was an official dogma which no one questioned either because it never occurred to them to question it or because they were afraid to be labelled a heretic and be subsequently burned alive, tortured to death, etc.

Well, if the small group of people who want to install this new technocracy on a global scale succeed I think we will enter into a new Middle Ages of sorts, call it perhaps the Middle Ages of Progress; it would be just as mind numbing as we suppose the last one was (though probably much worse) and, if by chance we actually survived it, it will be looked back upon, in 600 years or so, as a sort of period where what was the Clergy had been transformed into the Technocrats to dictate to everyone the party line which, if swayed from would not call forth death, but some form of electrode induced mind change.

It would be a time of ***endless meaningless progress***; progress with no aim, progress not towards something but just endless movement into empty space.

Progress has been traditionally always progress in terms of the development of the human spirit and of human knowledge. That is, it served the idea that human beings could be perfected, intellectually, socially, morally. But as I have shown, the idea of the human along with that of the spirit have been attacked to the point of non-existence.

This has caused a radical change in the definition of progress.

The progress we see today turns that idea on its head and people (or the ambient-meat-machines we have been defined into) become the raw material for the technology meant to serve them. We will serve it, it will not serve us.

Transhumanism is not about perfecting the human but humanizing the machine or inversely, machining humans to serve tasks. This would be the last step in the abdication of the Will, the soul, and of any vestige of inner moral law.

Perhaps that's what the "collective consciousness" desires, only time will tell. The danger as I see it is that, if made, this choice removes choice from future generations who perhaps could feel differently if asked to make a choice in the matter.

I'd mentioned earlier that one of the results of the global wars in the 20th century was the emergence onto the world stage of what had been previously colonies or countries that had been dominated by the West. At the present moment the most successful of these is China. And China is in the forefront of installing AI and bio-tech into every aspect of the lives of its citizens. They are incredibly practical using the organs of condemned men for transplants is the best example. Why throw them in the garbage? Meat is meat.

This is not racist culturally bigoted China bashing by the way for *Western eyes look hungrily at China* and only wish they could install these same practices into the lives of their own countries. But for the moment we have in place all those philosophical writings from the 18th century… that's a problem. But it's being worked on and soon I suspect we will be free to move forward.

Well, that's enough of a pep talk.

I'm personally in favor of radically increased Freedom; Freedom *despite the dangers of endless variation*; Freedom everywhere and in all things, **particularly my own mind**.

Freedom is the opposite of control and sadly, control is the direction I see things moving in. And if it is true that we can no longer turn outward and wage a drunken war, well so much the better! Let us then turn inward to change ourselves, revolutionize ourselves but ***consciously*** each according to his or her desire with respect towards others. This could be the new goal and I think it is limitless.

Who knows? Maybe we'll finally get it right.

Dick Turner

1 August 2020

The author wishes to warmly thank tENTATIVELY a cONVENIENCE for his valuable suggestions and close reading of this article.

HERETICS emails - August, 2020

August 1, 2020, 4:12AM (Dick to group):

RE: "School of Negativity" movie online

Great, I will be a Card carrying Member of The School of Negativity
Yes, I have a printer

I was thinking - an example of the positive aspect of negativity is being against forced mask wearing
it is a "negative" position (being against legislated mask wearing), but in fact the desired outcome is "positive" (human freedom)

****

August 1, 2020, 9:54AM (Amir-ul Kafirs to group):

On Jul 31, 2020, at 10:17 PM, Inquiring Librarian wrote:

On the demons thing. It honestly does not bother me.

It doesn't necessarily bother me, either — but as someone who's been a HERETIC my whole adult life I might be what you could call 'hypersensitive' to belief systems that can turn murderous fast. What if a believer in demons were to decide that I'm possessed by one because I deny that Jesus is an historic personage? Exorcising the 'demon' from me through torture & murder is the way the Catholic Church went for OVER FOUR HUNDRED YEARS & that sort of stuff isn't just about 'cultural difference' it's about getting the masses whipped up into enough of a frenzy to commit any atrocity in 'the name of the public good' — just like the pandemic is being used now.

Anyways, here is an RFK Jr. quote article on Freedom of Speech.

He is good at expressing things quickly in a way that many people can probably understand & relate to.

****

August 1, 2020, 5:09AM (Dick to Amir-ul Kafirs):

I don't want to dwell on it but you'd written you felt depressed and I'm sorry to hear it
I hope it passes soon
I am also dealing with the feelings you described - being tired, feeling depressed,

etc. it's been going on for a while
I was concerned about it so I saw my doctor and had a blood test, happily there were no negative indications
Thus in my case I think it's tied to my being alone
I think it's also tied to this covid business
I find that the onslaught of every aspect of life by politicians, various doctors, and "the man on the street" complying blindly with whatever rule is sent their way is making me feel like many values I felt were, well for lack of a better phrase, eternal or at least unquestioned (personal freedom) are for many people just empty words (to quote J Cage...) and they really want to be controlled and told what to do
(And it's true, the more I think about ______'s post, the more I feel he is a sort of monster...can you imagine what he'd accept handed down from above, he wouldn't care if we were all locked up for years)
Maybe this acceptance of authority is a way to escape a feeling of personal responsibility, maybe freedom is too much for a lot of people, after all, very few actually make use of it
It reminds me of being given permission to kill, as in a war, it takes away the personal element of choice (or at least perhaps it does, I never was in a war)
finally I feel that my vision of art is being affected because it seems to me that art & culture are under the most ferocious assault that I've ever seen
I feel surrounded by idiots
In fact, I feel very marginalised, which is normal really, but these days the feeling has grown exponentially that the thing I've dedicated my life to has no meaning for most people on the planet and if it was just flushed down the toilet they wouldn't even care
these thoughts, though a bit dark are meant to be helpful to the degree that you aren't alone
anyway, hang in there

****

August 1, 2020, 10:26AM (Amir-ul Kafirs to Dick):

I hope it passes soon

Well, it's been a central facet of my life since I was, what?, 14? Obviously tying in to the onslaught of adolescence. The 1st time I slit my wrists I was 18 — but one friend of mine did something like that when she was EIGHT.

I think it's also tied to this covid business

Yes, of course! I mean this is quite possibly the lowest point I've seen society sink to. I've been thinking of making a text panel that says: "I feel like Wittgenstein at the border of Spain" — but only people like yourself would understand it & it would make us all more depressed so I won't do it.

they really want to be controlled and told what to do

I really hope it's not that bad but it sure seems to be. For me, this is pretty much the way I've felt about most people for most of my life but I've been able to live with it because it hasn't been so overtly manifested. Now we have THE MASKS as the 'badge of honor' to show us all the people who're willing to give up their freedom, who don't feel suffocated, whatever. I was serious when I said that even seeing other people wear masks makes me feel suffocated. I HATE seeing burkas.

(And it's true, the more I think about ______'s post, the more I feel he is a sort of monster...can you imagine what he'd accept handed down from above, he wouldn't care if we were all locked up for years)

He's almost like a poster boy for this era. When I read that blog-post of his about confining himself for 120 days ("The 120 Days of Sodom") I felt a revulsion for him — like I said it feels like being in the same room with someone else's vomit.

It reminds me of being given permission to kill, as in a war, it takes away the personal element of choice (or at least perhaps it does, I never was in a war)

Yeah, I've thought about that alot. Lewis Yablonsky's "Robopaths" has about the best breakdown of that sort of thing that I've ever read.

I feel very marginalised, which is normal really,

Yep. Not only do most people HATE what I do, they don't even have the slightest idea of what it is! Not even Naia Nisnam has the slightest interest. When we went to Lake Erie they were talking about how different we are, about how they have NO interest in painting, in art, in music. I offered to give them one of my 'business cards': they're hand-cut-out, unusual. They had NO interest in even looking at it to see what it was. I gave it to them anyway.

but these days the feeling has grown exponentially that the thing I've dedicated my life to has no meaning for most people on the planet and if it was just flushed down the toilet they wouldn't even care

Sad but true. The people who get the most pleasure out of the things that you & I care about are usually the people who are also makers. Since we were painting Lake Erie I tried to explain how remarkable Turner's paintings of water & sky are. Naia Nisnam'd never heard of him & had no interest.

these thoughts, though a bit dark are meant to be helpful to the degree that you aren't alone

Oh, I know that you & I are roughly in a similar state of mind for similar reasons.

anyway, hang in there

I just keep doing what I've always done — which is thinking about what's happening around me & putting out what I make for the world to mostly not care about &/or be hostile toward. But, really, I think most people would rather that I just SHUT THE FUCK UP so they can peacefully repeat their puppet-speak without having me question it.

ANYWAY, best wishes to both of us!! Just keep making your work, it's the best we can do.

Cheerio,

yr pal,

Amir-ul Kafirs

****

August 1, 2020, 10:40AM (Inquiring Librarian to group):

I suppose the point also is that there were about 12, I believe, of these doctors speaking. The covid positive media realize the summit was long, many ppl won't actually listen to it. They will focus on that 1 doctor the media slandered and call it a day. We are focusing here on 1/12 of the speakers and nothing to do with what she said at the summit, but what she has said in ministry. This is all good and well, but it gets us nowhere on the point of the summit and the aftershock that it sent across the nation, and arguably across the world.

2 days after the summit, hydroxycholoroquine was outlawed from being used for covid in Ohio. The Governor there actually stepped in and stopped this because it is/was criminal to cut ppl off from a proven legitimate treatment.

Ohio pharmacy board reverses ban on hydroxychloroquine as coronavirus treatment after DeWine's request

By Max Filby
The Columbus Dispatch
Posted Jul 29, 2020 at 5:47 PM Updated Jul 30, 2020 at 7:21 AM

https://www.dispatch.com/news/20200729/ohio-pharmacy-board-reverses-ban-on-hydroxychloroquine-as-coronavirus-treatment-after-dewinersquos-request

It is also important that this summit is important to many conservatives (and many liberals like myself and my friend in California). My sister, a nurse, and my mom, a nurse, were both very receptive to the summit. My sister invited me to a closed 'conservative' social media group that focuses on all topics covid. I joined! I am finally able to share my research and voice on the absurdities of covid with this massive group of individuals. I am able to share all of my links and articles and videos with these people. Many of them have a baseline idea of what is going on. I am able to share the in-depth background and sources to their ideas. I feel like I am doing something to educate people who are willing to hear something beyond mass media propaganda related to covid, without hating my guts. They know something is wrong, I lead them to what exactly is wrong, from my research. Ok, that is a tangent. You see, this is so much bigger than HCQ and Dr. Immanuel. I would say 99% of my 'liberal' friends HATE ME right now and think I am CRAZY. They will listen to NOTHING I say. My sister gets it. My mom gets it. My dad gets it. These people that are a part of this closed conservative group get it. I mean, at this point if anyone will listen to me/us, I am game. To me this is about life and death. Enslavement vs. freedom and free speech.

The summit also covered masks, the psychology of the lockdowns, child psychology as pertains to the lockdowns with actual anecdotes of real working class families struggling through this, the safety of schools reopening, the corruption in the school board in ca and the teacher's union, etc.

From their website, https://americasfrontlinedoctorsummit.com/ , which is now back up, Here is the Agenda that they followed:

1st Day Agenda

8:30 am: Coffee, Opening Remarks
9:00 am: Panel #1 Schools
10:00 am: Topic #2 The Virus/Disease Facts
10:20 am: Topic #2 Hoaxes Identified
10:40 am: Panel #2 Hoaxes Demonstrated
11:10 am: Panel #2 Medical Cancel Culture
11:30 am: Topic #3 Fear
11:45 am: Topic #4 Public Policy
12:00 pm: Lunch
1:00 pm: Capitol Hill Photo Op
2:00 pm: Capitol Hill Press Conference
4:00 pm: Panel 2: HCQ
5:00 pm: Topic #4: Follow the Money
5:30 pm: Panel #3: Lockdowns
4:00-8:00 pm: Individual Physician Interviews

**Tentative Congressional Meetings: 4-6 pm

Physicians & Congresspersons can discuss any healthcare related topic.

& then there was this:

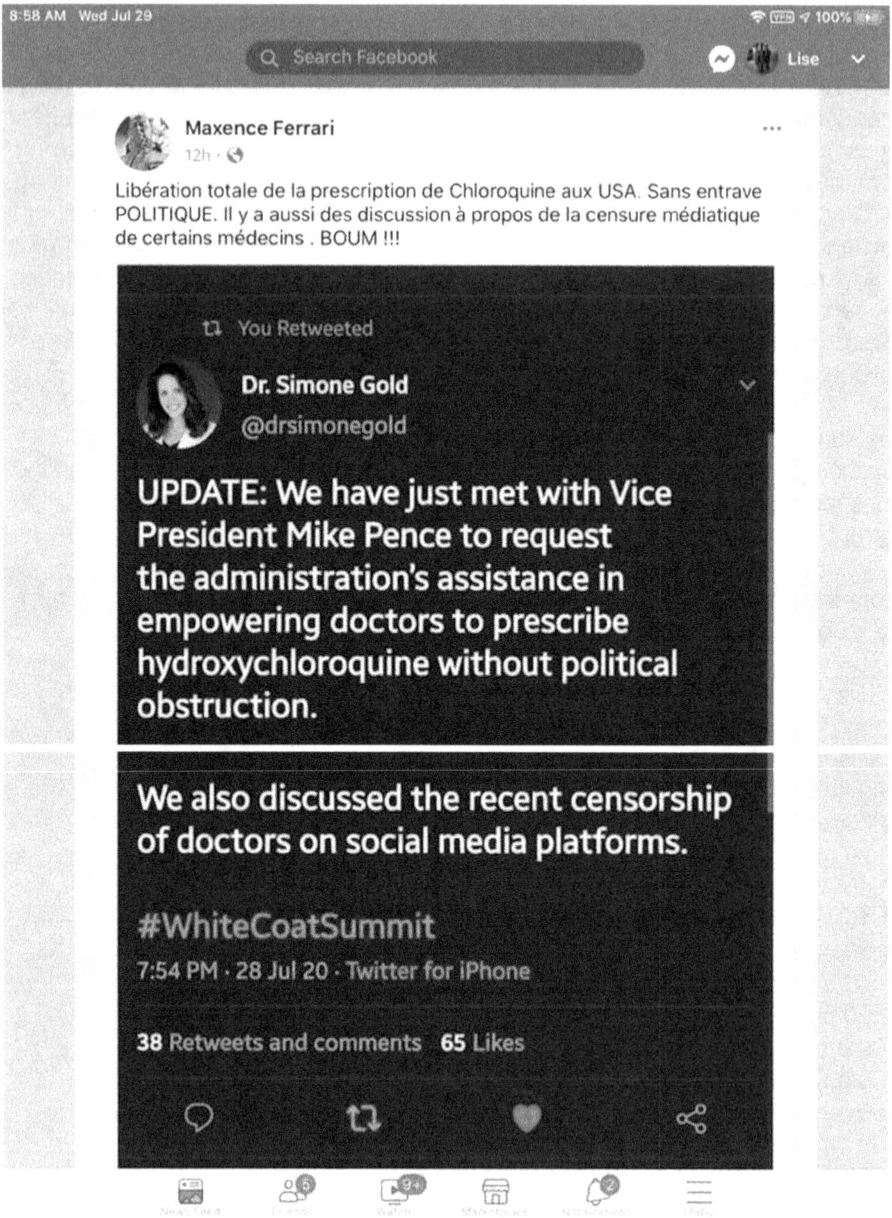

****

Ohio pharmacy board reverses ban on hydroxychloroquine as coronavirus treatment after DeWine's request

[redacted]

President Donald Trump and his administration kept up their out-sized promotion Monday of an anti-malaria drug not yet officially approved for fighting the new coronavirus, even though scientists say more testing is needed before it's proven safe and effective against COVID-19. Trump trade adviser Peter Navarro championed hydroxychloroquine in television interviews a day after the president publicly put his faith in the medication to lessen the toll of the coronavirus pandemic. **By** Max Filby

The Columbus Dispatch

Posted Jul 29, 2020 at 5:47 PM
Updated Jul 30, 2020 at 7:21 AM

Hydroxychloroquine has been touted by President Donald Trump as a way to treat and prevent the coronavirus. The Ohio pharmacy board planned to ban the drug as a COVID-19 treatment until Gov. Mike DeWine spoke up about it.

The State of Ohio Board of Pharmacy has changed course on its ban of hydroxychloroquine and chloroquine as coronavirus treatments following the governor's urging to do so.

Beginning Thursday, pharmacies, clinics and other medical institutions were to be prohibited from dispensing or selling the drugs to treat COVID-19, according to regulations issued by the State of Ohio Board of Pharmacy. They could still be used in clinical trials, said Cameron McNamee, director of policy and communications for the board.

That regulation change has since been pulled back by the board though. Instead, the board now plans to reexamine the issue with the assistance of the State Medical Board of Ohio, clinical experts and other stakeholders to determine its next steps, according to an announcement.

The board's shift came after Gov. Mike DeWine asked the state pharmacy board on Thursday morning to rescind its plan to ban hydroxychloroquine and chloroquine as treatments for the virus.

July 29, 2020

DeWine said the decision of how to treat COVID-19 should instead be between patients and their doctors. The Ohio State Medical, the oldest and largest physician-led organization in Ohio, also said it supported a reversal of the ban.

“The Board of Pharmacy and the State Medical Board of Ohio should revisit the issue, listen to the best medical science and open the process up for comment and testimony from experts,” DeWine said in a prepared statement.

[..]

Dispatch reporters Rick Rouan and Lucas Sullivan contributed to this story.

- https://www.dispatch.com/news/20200729/ohio-pharmacy-board-reverses-ban-on-hydroxychloroquine-as-coronavirus-treatment-after-dewinersquos-request

****

Press Conference of America's Frontline Doctors

American life has fallen casualty to a massive disinformation campaign. We can speculate on how this has happened, and why it has continued, but the purpose of the inaugural White Coat Summit is to empower Americans to stop living in fear.

If Americans continue to let so-called experts and media personalities make their decisions, the great American experiment of a Constitutional Republic with Representative Democracy, will cease.

- https://americasfrontlinedoctorsummit.com

****

August 1, 2020, 11:12AM (Amir-ul Kafirs to group):

HERETICS: BLM in Nursing Homes

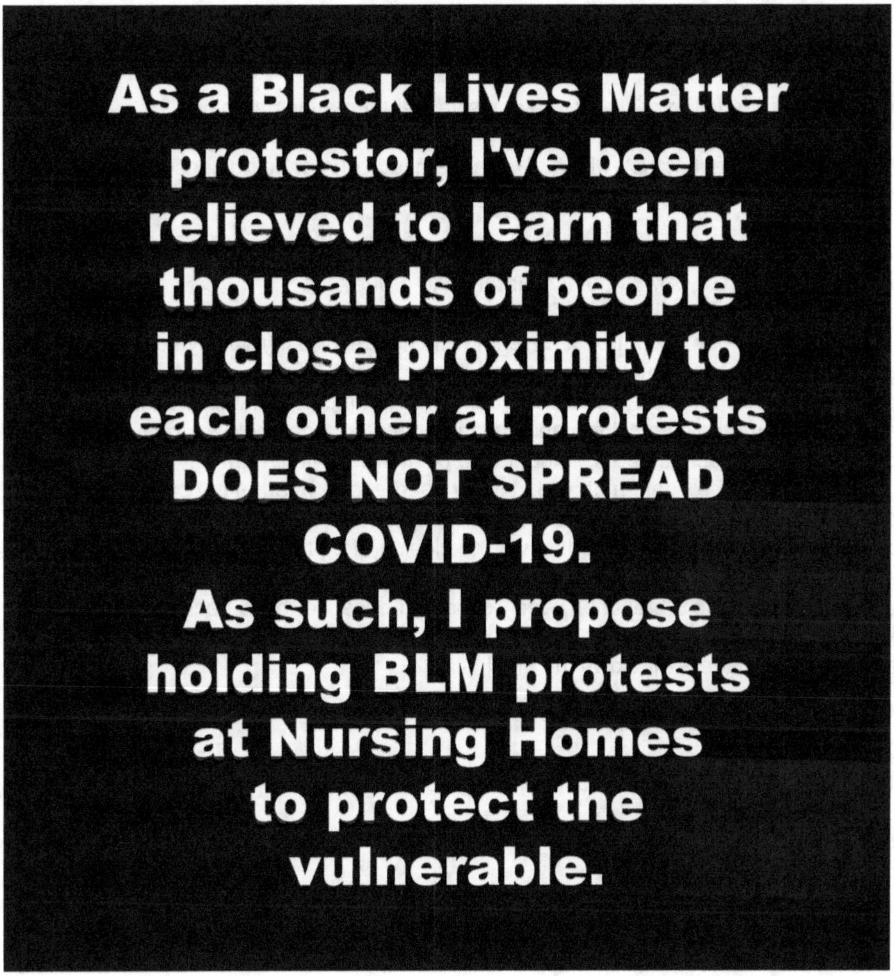
As a Black Lives Matter protestor, I've been relieved to learn that thousands of people in close proximity to each other at protests DOES NOT SPREAD COVID-19.
As such, I propose holding BLM protests at Nursing Homes to protect the vulnerable.

****

August 1, 2020, 2:35PM (Amir-ul Kafirs to group):

The Governor there actually stepped in and stopped this because it is/was criminal to cut ppl off from a proven legitimate treatment.

I'm all in favor of its being available. As the article states, it's now an issue between doctor & patient, as it should be. Otherwise, I have no position on the effectiveness or non-effectiveness of hydroxycholoroquine. Some people say one thing, others say another. Personally, I'd rather avoid ANYTHING that doctors prescribe these days so I hope I don't find myself in a position of being forced into one or another. I'm more afraid of ventilators & hospitals than I am of anything else.

It is also important that this summit is important to many conservatives (and many liberals like myself and my friend in California).

It's important to me that any medical opinion that goes contrary to the dominant (& VERY

DOMINEERING) narrative is out there in force. I like the "Frontline Doctors" mission statement:

American life has fallen casualty to a massive disinformation campaign.

& wish them the best of luck with it. I wish them luck on not being censored too.

****

August 1, 2020, 10:24AM (Inquiring Librarian to group):

I'm just feeling a loss of control. I have a lovely house, and my back yard garden is my get-a-way. During the day I have scented flowers and butterflies everywhere, and birds on my birdfeeder. At night I have a night blooming nightshade family tree that smells heavenly with moths everywhere and cats at my feet. If I can hold on to this, I have nothing to be depressed about. What is the point in worrying, right? I don't want to fight with friends because I get emotional. I likely need a form of art of my own outside of gardens collecting old lamps. My entire library system was thrown under the bus yesterday morning on social media over the closing of 3 branches due to 1 "Case". How can this be? And how can it be that we were thrown under the bus not for being so ridiculous as to close 3 branches over 1 case, but because these hecklers on social media think that the libraries should be closed down permanently because they are dangerous covid super spreaders. It blows my mind.

****

August 2, 2020, 1:43PM (Amir-ul Kafirs to group):

Look, I need to take a step back here.

I'm sure we're all on edge. I know I am. Fortunately, in my neighborhood, almost no-one wears a mask. That helps. They're just people going about their lives as they ordinarily would. But on social media it's easy for me to imagine a crowd forming, a mob coming to my house & setting it on fire. That's how paranoid I am. I had my place in Baltimore set fire to in 1985, it could happen again.

I need to stop sending you all so many links and news items and jokes and this and that,

I'm glad to get this info from you & I'm glad to be able to set it into the HERETICS record but, as I've explained, I don't have time to check out all the videos because, unlike you, I don't just listen to them. Instead I try to watch them & do something more proactive with them — like take screenshots or write a synopsis, to put them on my YouTube PANDEMIC PANIC playlist. I notice that one's been censored off already but I'm not sure which one. As such, it takes *time* that I just don't have. I'm trying to do so many other things & I'm STILL neglecting most of my life. AND I'm exhausted. AND unbearably lonely.

I wake him with my typing on my computer and that upsets him.

Can't you move your computer to somewhere where he can't hear the typing? Can't he sleep somewhere else?

There are no jobs to be had in this city right now.

You should have a contingency plan. The house across the street from me sold for $318,000.00 or something like that. I don't know what it's like in Louisiana but it's supposedly a Seller's Market around here. Maybe you can sell your house & live off of that money somewhere else that's less crazy than Louisiana.

I hate myself for being lazy and becoming a librarian. I should have gone at least into nursing.

Being a librarian is a good thing. Think of how depressed you'd be if you were a nurse right now.

I am confident if this vaccine is mandatory and I am forced into it, I will die.

Remember, you're making a prediction. Predictions are only valid once they become true. I find life almost unbelievably hellish right now but in the back of my mind there's always the old saying "*This, too, shall pass.*"

Good luck to all of us,

I'll try to be less touchy in the future,

****

August 2, 2020, 1:50PM (Amir-ul Kafirs to group):

these hecklers on social media think that the libraries should be closed down permanently because they are dangerous covid super spreaders. It blows my mind.

Yes, it's heinous to an extreme — but the people who worked out the psychology of this &, yes, unfortunately, I DO think most of this bad behavior was preplanned & forseen by the people who imagined shutting down the economy at the same time as requiring people to wear muzzles, knew that they'd be training Pavlovian Attack Dogs, dogs that would accept the muzzle but go berserk when unfettered. What I, personally, *wouldn't have expected* is how many of those people are 'friends of mine': supposedly caring, liberal people — even people supposedly with 'talent' (even If I, personally, have always found them mediocre). Alas, this lesson learned is a lesson never to be forgotten.

****

August 2, 2020, 10:37AM (Inquiring Librarian to group):

HERETICS: The War on Everything

I want to know what you think of these ideas, of Denis Rancourt, and then of C.J. Hopkins. They are thinking in the same train of thought. I feel they may be correct. It is a scary thing to consider.

1. Denis Rancourt:

Denis Rancourt

Admin · 4d

IMO. This is not just Pharma wanting to sell vaccines.

This is geopolitical on the largest scale. It is driven by the loss of USA-based hegemony to a growing and powerful China, which is organizing around the USA monetary and trade dominance. China's presence in the world threatens the USA-power-based global elite everywhere. Their answer is to demonize China, to isolate from China, to exclude China from Africa, Latin America, much of Asia, the Middle East... This military and economic occupation of its traditional occupied territories, while not trading with China will destroy the USA and Western middle-working classes... so these classes are a threat (Brexit, Yellow Vests, Trump land, etc.) and must be neutered and prevented from everything. COVID-19, the medical totalitarianism achieves that and destroys society, while the professional and managerial classes sleep through the most destructive erosion of everything, thinking they will be safe, but many will not be safe. Only police numbers will grow. Put another way: this is to destroy Trump and his plan for a strong domestic middle and working class. The Elite need global exploitation, not domestic distributed growth.

2. C.J. Hopkins (in relation to the recent protests against lockdowns in Germany... Go Germany!!! =]):

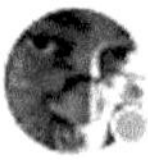

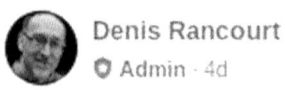

CJ Hopkins

3h ·

Here's The New York Times, calling the people who protested the corona-totalitarianism in Berlin yesterday "neo-Nazis," and here are a few photos of those people. Maybe some of my old (and former) friends in New York could explain to me again how The New York Times is a "serious," "respectable" newspaper that I should trust, and not just a neo-Goebbelsian GloboCap propaganda organ.

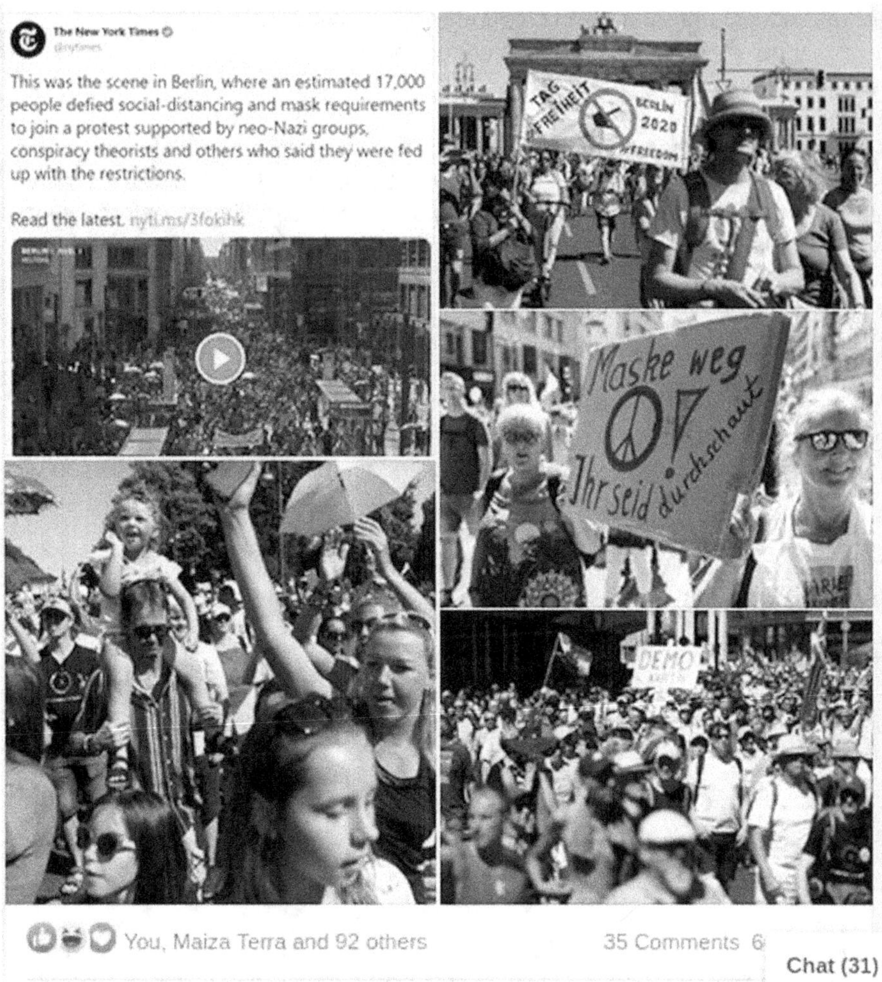

https://www.nytimes.com/aponline/2020/08/01/world/europe/ap-virus-outbreak-germany.html

Thousands Protest in Berlin Against Coronavirus Restrictions

By The Associated Press

BERLIN — Thousands protested Germany's coronavirus restrictions Saturday in a Berlin demonstration marking what organizers called “the end of the pandemic” — a declaration that comes just as authorities are voicing increasing concerns about an uptick in new infections.

With few masks in sight, a dense crowd marched through downtown Berlin from the Brandenburg Gate.

Protesters who came from across the country held up homemade signs with slogans like “Corona, false alarm,” “We are being forced to wear a muzzle,”

"Natural defense instead of vaccination" and "We are the second wave." They chanted, "We're here and we're loud, because we are being robbed of our freedom!"

Police used bullhorns to chide participants to adhere to social distancing rules and to wear masks, apparently with little success. They tweeted that they drew up a criminal complaint against the rally's organizer for failing to enforce hygiene rules, then said shortly afterward that the organizer had ended the march.

Police estimated about 17,000 people turned out. The demonstrators were kept apart from counterprotesters, some of whom chanted "Nazis out!"

Protesters continued to a subsequent rally on a boulevard running through the city's Tiergarten park, which police estimated drew 20,000 people. Police declared that event over as organizers again failed to get demonstrators to wear masks or keep their distance.

Protests against anti-virus restrictions in Germany have drawn a variety of attendees, including conspiracy theorists and right-wing populists.""

****

August 2, 2020, 12:26PM (Amir-ul Kafirs to group):

Re: HERETICS: The War on Everything

I want to know what you think of these ideas, of Denis Rancourt, and then of C.J. Hopkins.

I respect Rancourt's acknowledgement of & observation of this mess as a global phenomena. Naturally, I think he's correct about that. I can't honestly say that I understand the US/China competition enough to say that China is really a threat to US economic hegemony. Maybe it is, maybe it isn't. I also find it hard to believe that Rump is really working toward making a strong middle & working class. I DO think that this medical tyranny is eroding the middle & working class lifestyles & that that's for the benefit of an oligarchy. Rancourt ends with: "The Elite need global exploitation, not domestic distributed growth." I can go along with that. I'm less sure of what he postulates leading up to this conclusion.

2. C.J. Hopkins (in relation to the recent protests against lockdowns in Germany... Go Germany!!! =]):

It's great to see the pictures of people. Unfortunately, the constant demonization of anti-maskers as right-wing nuts makes it so that the NY Times calling these folks "neo-nazis" is immediately suspect. A big problem with that is that for people with limited political understanding they're going to make being a "neo-nazi" *look like a good thing* ***because they're resisting the muzzle.*** In other words, such demonizing is going to start back-firing.

Protesters who came from across the country held up homemade signs with slogans like “Corona, false alarm,” “We are being forced to wear a muzzle,” “Natural defense instead of vaccination” and “We are the second wave.”

They chanted, “We’re here and we’re loud, because we are being robbed of our freedom!”

Naturally, I can relate to the slogans & I don't see anything in the least "neo-nazi" in them. I've made some new protest signs that I'm sure most people will find completely incomprehesnible &, therefore, 'insane'. Anything that normal people don't understand = insanity. This despite the fact that normal people don't understand much of anything.

****

August 2, 2020, 5:13PM (Amir-ul Kafirs to group):

On Aug 2, 2020, at 2:44 PM, dick turner wrote:

do you know about the Japanese doctors who experimented on un anesthetized chinese during WW2?

I met a Chinese woman when I was working at the Smithsonian long ago who was still outraged about "The Rape of Nanking" where the Chinese commited most of their atrocities. I have the book of that name but I haven't read it. I've seen Frank Capra's footage from there in "Why We Fight" too. At any rate, I'm somewhat aware of their atrocities & perhaps I should've made reference to them as well as those of the nazis but I didn't want to go too deeply into that sort of thing because I was staying fairly close to the personal backstory. Maybe in the body of the book but I doubt that I'll have time or energy — the book is already too complex as it is, I don't know how I can possibly ever get it done.

****

August 2, 2020, 5:45PM (Amir-ul Kafirs to Dick):

I think that in the long run they'll both be happy if they discipline themselves to write something but that 1st step is pretty hard. It comes naturally for you & me but even I have to push myself pretty hard sometimes when I'm depressed & these are extraordinarily bad circumstances even though in relation to the horrors of generations before us it's not bad at all!! Imagine if we'd had to live through WWII!! Humans create such nightmares for ourselves.

****

August 2, 2020, 3:02PM (Amir-ul Kafirs to group):

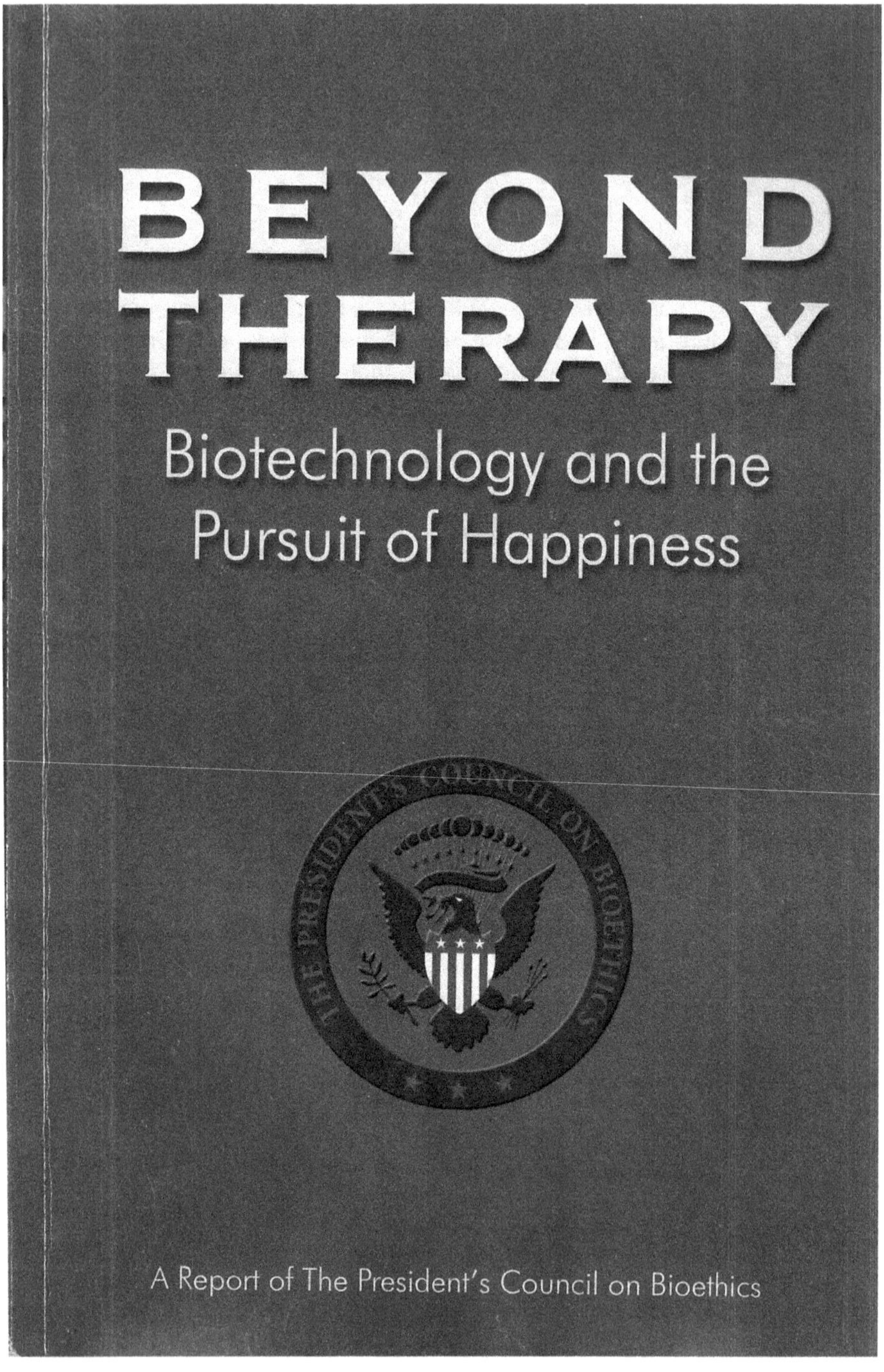

HERETICS: "Beyond Therapy"

This is a book I picked up in Erie. It was published in October, 2003, by "The President's Council on Bioethics" & seems to be basically about new techniques for altering mental life & for doing things like bioengineering 'better children'. If I had the time &/or energy I'd read & review this for the HERETICS book. As usual, it seems that the implication is that nature just isn't good enough & that those clever scientists & doctors are really going to improve on it. Naturally, I doubt that.

****

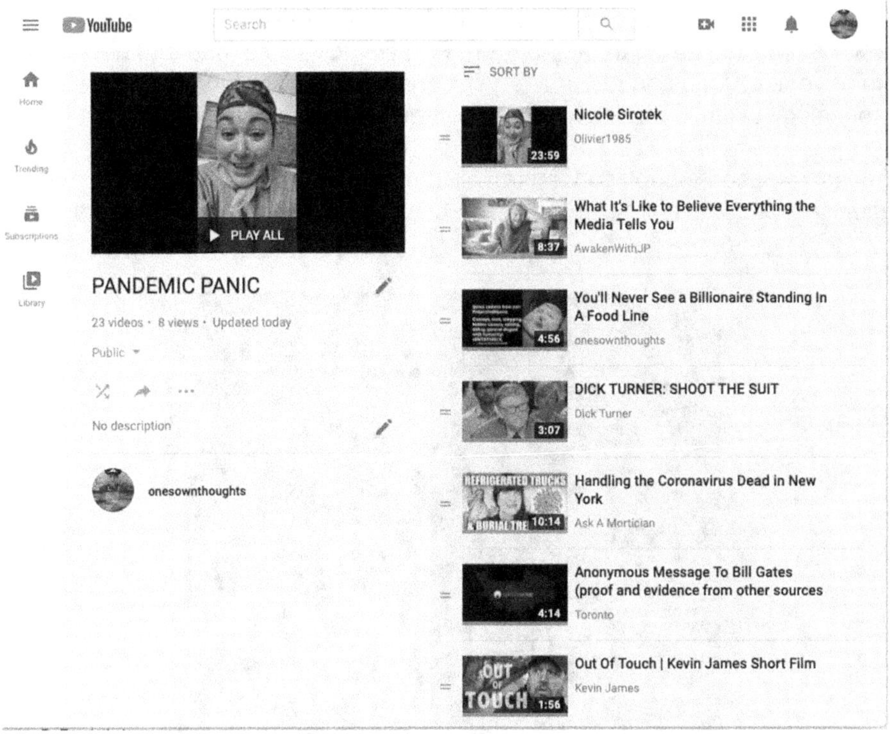

****

August 2, 2020, 6:28PM (Inquiring Librarian to group):

Re: HERETICS: "Beyond Therapy"

I am sure the book will be fascinatingly terrifying. And absolutely, the natural body's immune system will always be superior to the human artificially manufactured one. For years, I've felt full faith in my own immune system. I instinctively knew that I absolutely should never get a flu shot. From my studies on vaccines, I am confident I will never get another vaccination.

& here I will segue into another video! YAY!!! This one is amazing (they all are!). This here dives into fauci's level of corruption and what happens to doctors who call him out and don't follow his corrupt orders:
https://m.youtube.com/watch?v=6YqkRpvn6jY

Mikovits worked as a molecular biologist in vaccines at the ft. Detrick molecular bioweapons lab. She discovered animal derived illness jumping from animal cell linings to humans through vaccines. Something called xmrv's. Something to do with causes behind aids, chronic fatigue syndrome, covid 19, etc.
Dr Fauci tried to get her to retract her study findings, because they hurt the vaccine industry severely by exposing that they were causing immediate animal to human diseases that would in nature take centuries to happen. Aka: the vaccine industry caused many deaths and illnesses. Mikovits refused to retract the study, despite threats from the nih/fauci, so fauci set her up, discredited her work, bankrupted her, banned her from Fort Detrick's labs, and had her arrested with never a charge and never a day in court. She is back working now as an immunologist with plant derived immunotherapy, which I support.

She just released a book concerning all of these NIH based corruptions and their casualties, patients and scientists. The book is called "Plague of Corruption: https://www.skyhorsepublishing.com/9781510752245/plague-of-corruption/

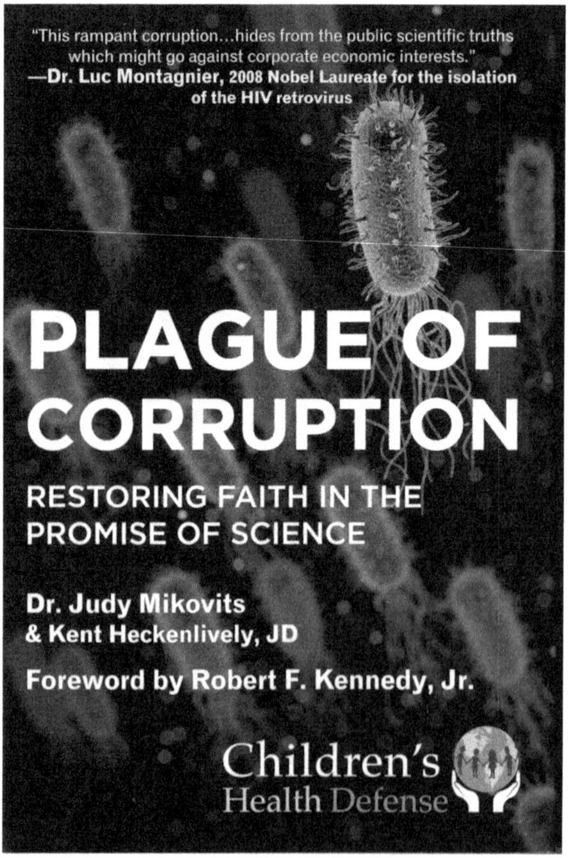

& realize too, Fort Detrick and Wuhan contain bioweapons labs from which the latest coronavirus escaped from.

****

August 3, 2020, 7:02PM (Amir-ul Kafirs to group):

dives into fauci's level of corruption and what happens to doctors who call him out and don't follow his corrupt orders:

I watch the 1st 10:42 of this. I liked it enough to add it to my PANDEMIC PANIC YouTube playlist.

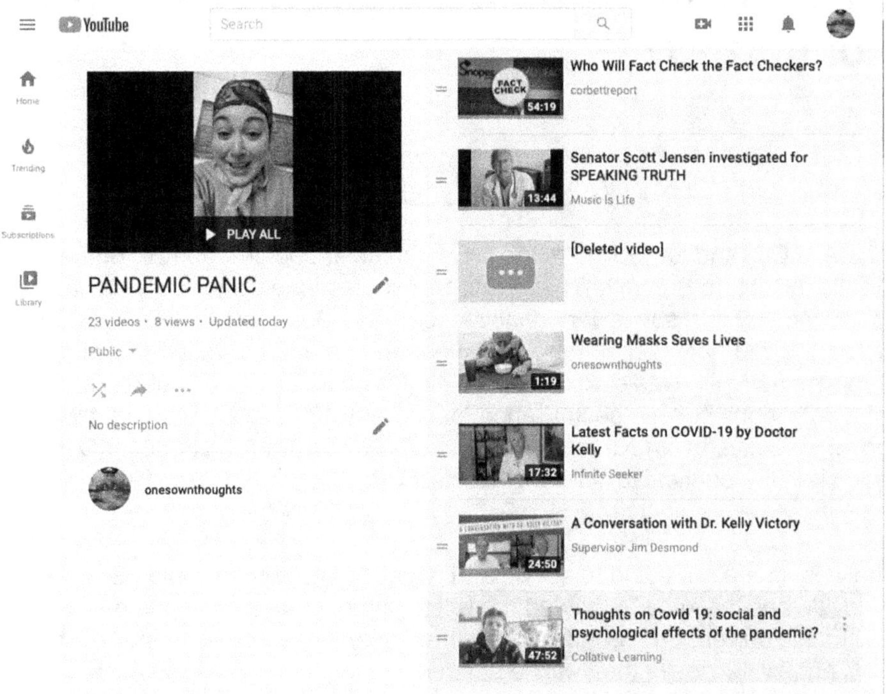

Fort Detrick and Wuhan contain bioweapons labs from which the our latest coronavirus escaped from.

I have no particular problem believing this & I find Mikovits's argument that the ability of the virus to jump from animals to humans could've only happened with lab assistance compelling but I also still keep an open mind that the latest coronovirus doesn't originate this way.

****

August 2, 2020, 11:55PM (Inquiring Librarian to group):

More on HCQ (Hydroxychloroqine)

Hola everyone,

Here is some fun information on the Hydroxychloroqine insanity:

This is about the nonsensical censorship of the drug and some of the corruption leading to its censorship.

July 30, 2020

Two-Tiered Medicine: Why Is Hydroxychloroquine Being Censored and Politicized?

https://childrenshealthdefense.org/news/two-tiered-medicine-why-is-hydroxychloroquine-being-censored-and-politicized/?itm_term=home&fbclid=IwAR0Ve1wEls-qLU7T312qWgK35pJgJrZA2KTOFGleVmUEyTuDTzyfrskPA6w

& here is Dr. (and Lawyer) Simone Gold, the chief doctor organizer of the Frontline Doctors Summit. This is just 11 minutes long. She really has a lot to share and say and she is very qualified to do so. One thing that really struck me in this, is HCQ has been in use for 70 years (my mother, a retired icu and ccu nurse verifies this) was starting to be pulled from an over the counter drug to a list 2 poisonous substance in France on January 13th, 2020. The drug was proven effective by an NIH study in "Virology" under Fauci in 2005 for Sars Cov 1 which is 78% identical to Sars Cov 2 (otherwise known as Covid 19). https://www.facebook.com/740512463/videos/10158373798967464/

The wolves are out trying to eat up and discredit Dr. Simone Gold. She, like Mikovits, has the knowledge and the will to speak to take down the biomedical part of this current new world order. If they take these people in the NIH and CDC and WHO down, they will be outed as guilty of murder through their disinformation campaign.

****

JULY 30, 2020

Two-Tiered Medicine: Why Is Hydroxychloroquine Being Censored and Politicized?

[..]

both have the reputation of being safe if dosed properly. The most problematic sequelae have been the emergence of drug-resistant malaria and, with long-term use and higher-than-recommended doses, retinopathy.

On March 13, 2020, Dr. Todaro and a coauthor published an online white paper that pointed to the CDC's 2005 chloroquine research and outlined the early and successful use of CQ in Covid-19 patients in South Korea and China. Noting these promising results and the fact that China had zeroed in on CQ "after several screening rounds of thousands of existing drugs," the two physicians urged the U.S. to give America's medical profession an immediate green light to prescribe CQ and HCQ for Covid-19 patients. Instead, the doctors were met with Google's removal of their white paper.

Around the same time, France reported positive results for HCQ use in combination with the antibiotic azithromycin. The French doctor achieving these results, Dr. Didier Raoult, has been writing for years about the potential to "recycle" CQ and HCQ for 21st century viral and other infections. More recently, a Michigan study of patients hospitalized with a Covid-19-related admission and treated early confirmed that both HCQ alone and HCQ plus azithromycin can significantly reduce Covid-19-linked mortality. Other studies have highlighted the success of a triple combination of HCQ, azithromycin and zinc, a known antiviral. CQ/HCQ rapidly increase intracellular zinc levels—important given that the individuals most likely to be Covid-19 patients (the elderly and those with comorbid chronic conditions) tend to be zinc-deficient.

As of late July, a tally of 65 studies around the world indicated that 100% of the studies that assessed HCQ for Covid-19 pre-exposure prophylaxis (PrEP), post-exposure prophylaxis (PEP) or early use showed "high effectiveness," as did 61% of the studies examining HCQ use in later stages of illness. Describing a "natural experiment" in Switzerland, Yale's Dr. Risch has noted:

On May 27, the Swiss national government banned outpatient use of hydroxychloroquine for COVID-19. Around June 10, COVID-19 deaths increased four-fold and remained elevated. On June 11, the Swiss government revoked the ban, and on June 23 the death rate reverted to what it had been beforehand.

Even with the mixed results for late use, some clinicians have described "clear-cut and dramatically positive clinical responses" in individuals treated "when breathing was already very difficult and continuing to worsen." In six patients:

...[S]ignificant improvement in breathing was seen within about four hours after the first dose, with a complete clinical recovery seen after about an average of three days. [...] The rapidity with which the shortness of breath evolved in all these individuals strongly suggested that respiratory failure secondary to COVID-19-induced acute respiratory distress syndrome was imminent.

... [clinical trials] that were supposed to lay questions about HCQ safety and effectiveness to rest administered non-therapeutic, toxic and potentially lethal doses of HCQ (four times higher than standard doses) to thousands of study participants.

A nefarious agenda

The media's flagrant misrepresentation of the HCQ science is bad enough, but the willingness of top-tier journals to finagle the science in an anti-HCQ direction is even more shocking. In early June, scrutiny from dozens of independent scientists forced The Lancet to retract a study it had published just 13 days previously—a "study out of thin air" that used apparently fabricated data to undermine CQ/HCQ therapy. The debacle has since become known as #LancetGate. (The same day as the Lancet retraction, the New England Journal of Medicine retracted a separate Covid-19-related study that relied on unverifiable data sourced from the same company that supplied the data for the Lancet study.) The French health minister used the Lancet study results as justification to ban HCQ's use despite widespread public interest in and support for the drug.

[..]

- https://childrenshealthdefense.org/news/two-tiered-medicine-why-is-hydroxychloroquine-being-censored-and-politicized/?itm_term=home&fbclid=IwAR0Ve1wEls-qLU7T312qWgK35pJgJrZA2KTOFGIeVmUEyTuDTzyfrskPA6w

****

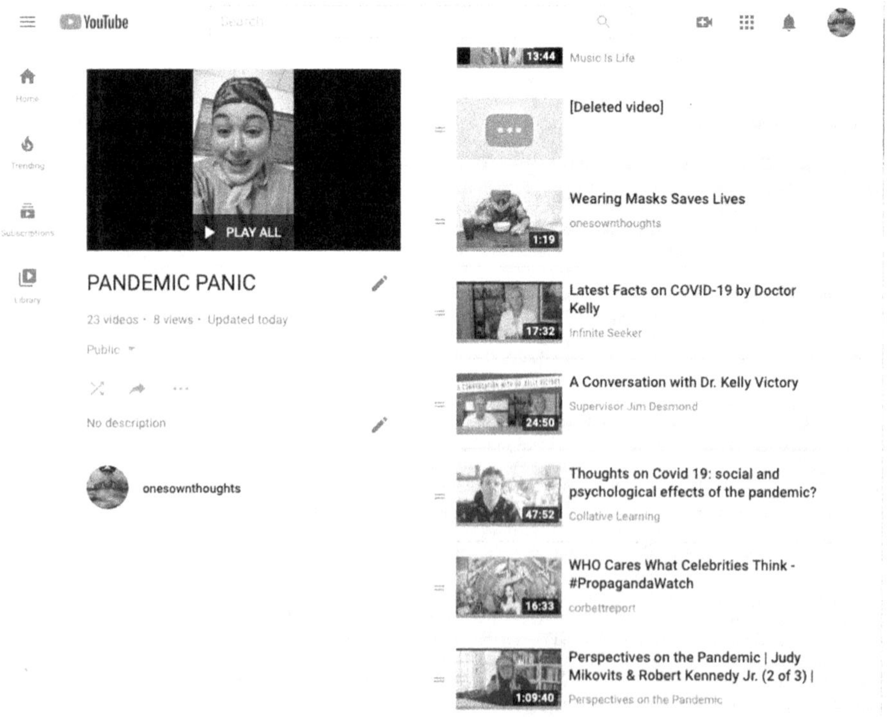

****

August 3, 2020, 8:49PM (Amir-ul Kafirs to group):

Re: More on HCQ (Hydroxychloroqine)

Two-Tiered Medicine: Why Is Hydroxychloroquine Being Censored and Politicized?

Another good article, I appreciate your directing me to it. I quote:

"tens of thousands of Covid-19 patients "are dying unnecessarily" for "reasons having nothing to do with a correct understanding of the science." The expert making that dire assessment—Yale epidemiology professor Harvey Risch, MD, PhD—believes that in the future, "this misbegotten episode regarding hydroxychloroquine will be studied by sociologists of medicine as a classic example of how extra-scientific factors overrode clear-cut medical evidence.""

The gist of the article is that HCQ has been demonstrated to work many times but that it's not profitable or 'sexy' to use it so it's defamed instead.

& here is Dr. (and Lawyer) Simone Gold, the chief doctor organizer of the Frontline Doctors Summit. This is just 11 minutes long.

Yeah, that's great. I shared it on Facebook with this as a preface:

To all the people who will say IN ADVANCE that what this doctor has to say is invalid (without having any significant idea of why that's supposedly the case) I simply ask you to listen to her talk for the length of this short interview.

If they take these people in the NIH and CDC and WHO down, they will be outed as guilty of murder through their disinformation campaign.

I'd love to see that happen but the mere possibility of it is something that's going to keep a very tight lid on everything.

****

August 3, 2020, 9:01PM (Amir-ul Kafirs to group):

HERETICS: Question for Dick & Phil

My friend Tom DiVenti (who published Dick's book) & I have had a short message exchange where I wrote:

"I don't believe that the quarantine is a necessary health measure, I believe that it's being used as a way to destroy mom & pop level business in order to create a dependency state"

& Tom countered with:

"The mom and pop theory is valid maybe here but not around the world."

I'm curious about what you, Dick, are seeing in Paris, & you, Phil, are seeing in Amsterdam. Here, small businesses almost across the board are being bankrupted by the lockdown while the giant corporate chains are open & making more money than ever. Is it the same there?

****

August 3, 2020, 9:25AM (Amir-ul Kafirs to group):

HERETICS: Scapegoating

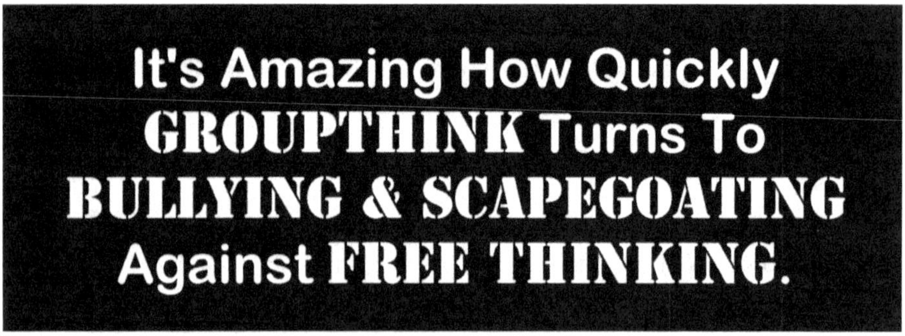
It's Amazing How Quickly
GROUPTHINK Turns To
BULLYING & SCAPEGOATING
Against FREE THINKING.

****

August 3, 2020, 10:13PM (Inquiring Librarian to group):

I've been listening to the most recent David Icke London Real episode, no. 5. Icke brings up the idea that there actually is not a virus or real illness floating around out there. He is leaning strongly on the side that there is no virus, just as Dr. Andrew Kaufman said. Icke says that the whole illness thing is a big fake. The 1% in charge of this whole debacle would not actually unleash a real virus or illness, because they could too easily lose control of it. And control is what those in charge want. And as such, they would have ultimate control to psychologically operate the 'pandemic' in any way they like, the symptoms, the causes, the modes of transmission, to best suit the 1%'s needs. I am honestly really suffering through this episode. It is dreadfully creepy and depressing and lacks most of the usual positivity of the other episode I saw of his. He has a great point though, the 1% is a few. We are many. What we need to do is organize and resist. Of course, keeping us separated will make this harder. But I do see it happening. Sadly, our own liberal party seems to be most prey to the manipulation. And then he goes on to discuss, if there is no virus, what is in this vaccine?? He deduces it will be dna editing technology and nanotechnology, both of which are things I have heard. A friend of mine in Illinois and I both agree that we think that such technology already has existed and has been injected into our younger generations in the form of vaccinations, and the older populations who would get a flu shot. That is all crazy talk, but is it... So, Icke explains that these technologies being injected into us would slowly transform the human race, something brave new world-esqe, into the human being a transhuman connected/networked computer-like to a hive mind. The human would no longer think independently. The human ability to breed outside of a test tube would become obsolete. You will notice, Icke points out, that the vaccine is going to supposedly require multiple injections and new injections each year, as the fictitious virus mutates. So as such, the transhuman mind will become more complete with each vaccination. And then there is 5G.. another conspiracy theory nightmare all tied in to this.

For the 1st time since I can remember, the conservatives feel warm and fuzzy to me. Most of the sites that I spy on of theirs, are absolutely opposed to vaccinations and especially this covid one. Just don't hate me for saying that. If I have to hear David Icke say one more time, we are heading for the new Hunger Games, I might have to grab all of my cats, and hop in the car to take refuge at the beach for a day alone to hash this all out, then pack my things and hide away in a cabin deep in the sheltering woods of a remote New Hampshire mountain. Amir-ul Kafirs got me started on the idea of moving. I like this idea. But my dream is a crazy place like a little town in Iowa or S. Dakota (or NH), where there supposedly are no lockdowns or mask mandates. But I did notice that most of their libraries are closed.

Ok, if anyone wants to watch this grueling 3.5 hour video (I am about 2.75 hours in and ready to jump off the nearest cliff... or the less cowardly coping mechanism would be to finally confront Health Freedom Louisiana and find out if they have rejected me from joining their group or if they are still 'vetting' me. =/). To bring this full circle, even Icke says it will be difficult for us to resist alone. But to join a group of resistance is what we need... enter for me locally Health Freedom Louisiana!

http://login.londonreal.tv/index.php?action=social&chash=1c9ac0159c94d8d0cbedc973445af2da.166&s=4782a770acb2d164130a6271ffdd389a

****

August 3, 2020, 10:13PM (Amir-ul Kafirs to group):

So as such, the transhuman mind will become more complete with each vaccination. And then there is 5G.. another conspiracy theory nightmare all tied in to this.

I've been reading SF since the 1960s so my mind is open to a much broader variety of possibilities than most people. Right now I'm reading a SF book called "Kaleidoscope Century" (1995) by a guy named John Barnes. In it, thre's a war called "The War of the Memes". Memes, contrary to the overused incorrect association of boxes with image & text that're shared on social media, are self-replicating AIs. Basically what happens in the story is that competing memes start fighting over control of all human beings. A human can surrender to a meme & give up free will altogther in exchange for becoming a part of the meme's superorganism. It seems incredibly relevant to now. I'll be using a brief excerpt from it as one of my text panels. Here's the beginning of the text. I'll share the full excerpt when I show you the finished text panel. I'm sure it'll resonate with many or all of us here. Basically, the scene is that 2 mercenaries in the pay of one of the memes have been sent to assassinate 2 people who're part of a resistance movement against meme control. They've broken into their house & the old man they're about to kill is talking to them.

"The old guy went on. "Well, I can understand why a lot of people choose to run a meme, to invite it into their existence. Really, I do; there are plenty of people out there whose own personalities will never allow them any happiness, who tie themselves in one knot after another, people for whom the biggest curse in the world is freedom of choice because they're programmed to keep choosing wrong and blaming themselves for it.["]"

- John Barnes, ***Kaleidoscope Century*** (1995)

http://login.londonreal.tv/index

Thanks for the link. I'm definitely not going to watch this one anytime soon if ever but I'm glad to add it to the database. It's fascinating to just see all the places where such videos can appear that're independent of YouTube.

****

August 4, 2020, 7:25AM (Dick to group):

Re: HERETICS: Question for Dick & Phil

I have noticed a number of places that have closed but nothing on a massive scale
When you say mom and pop businesses what do you mean exactly?
Here for example there are small resturants in about 8 out of 10 cafés
The situation if very different than in the other place I lived, Baltimore
People here live in their "quarter" and go to local businesses a lot...it's strange,

many people are still living in the quarter where they were born
I take walks pretty regularly and I have seen "going out of business permanently" signs whether this is due to the lock-down or the normal ups & down of business, I can't say

****

August 4, 2020, 9:37PM (Amir-ul Kafirs to group):

Re: HERETICS: Question for Dick & Phil

The question is: Have they closed because of the damage done to the business by the lockdown?

When you say mom and pop businesses what do you mean exactly?

I mean businesses that have individual owners that aren't part of a big franchise or big corporation. SO, local restaurants, bookstores, flower shops, hardware stores, etc..

Here there were once hardware stoes in almost every neighborhood. Then Home Depot came in & they all went out of business. That was before the quarantine. Now, because of the quarantine the same process has dramatically accelerated. Almost all, if not all, corporate chain stores have miraculously stayed open as "essential", even Dunkin' Donuts which is about as non-essential as it gets. As Naia Nisnam has pointed out, a locally owned bakery called Patty Cake (or some such) has had to close during the lockdown. I don't know whether it's gone out of business but a few months of no income couldn't have helped.

****

August 4, 2020, 10:16PM (Amir-ul Kafirs to group):

HERETICS: PANDEMIC 2016 movie

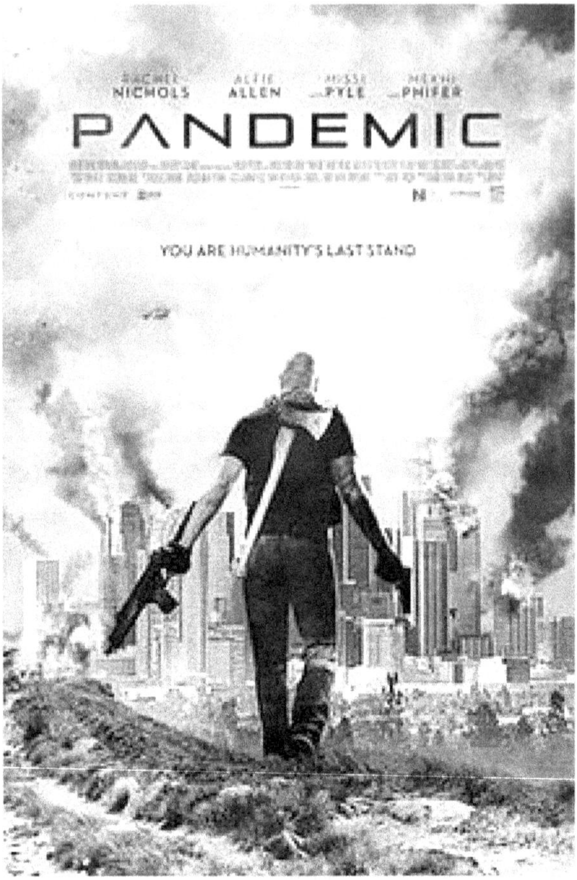

Theatrical release poster

Directed by	John Suits

Produced by	Gabriel Cowan John Suits
Written by	Dustin T. Benson
Starring	Rachel Nichols Alfie Allen Paul Guilfoyle Pat Healy Danielle Rose Russell Missi Pyle Mekhi Phifer
Music by	Alec Puro
Cinematography	Mark Putnam
Edited by	Nicholas Larrabure
Production company	New Artists Alliance
Distributed by	XLrator Media
Release date	February 26, 2016 (FrightFest Glasgow) April 1, 2016 (United States)
Running time	91 minutes

OK, I've started watching the 2nd of the "Pandemic" movies in my collection. This one's from 2016. It starts off with home movies of a couple with a teenaged daughter. The movies & stills are from significant moments in the daughter's life such as her birthday party & her singing a song on stage at what appears to be some sort of school event. This cuts to the woman of the couple in a somewhat grim basement looking at her cellphone. That's where she was just looking at the images we 1st saw. She looks at something that we don't see that apparently has a camera in it & repeats over & over again what seems to be a mission statement.

Cut to her in what seems like a military environment being briefed about the gear she's about to put on & the mission she's about to undertake. It turns out that she's a doctor working with a military team whose job it is to find survivors of a pandemic & bring them back to the compound she's in. The head doctor who's briefing her takes her on a tour of the cells in which the 5 types of pandemic casualties are located. Type 1 is possibly curable, type 2 is hemmorhaging, type 3 has suffered massive brain damage from the hemmorhaging, type 4 is "hibernating". The doctor explains that at 1st it was thought that they were dead because they have no detectable vital signs but it turns out that they revive & that whoever revives 1st will immediately kill whoever is around them without knowing why. Type 5 are permanently extremely violent & homicidal.

The head doctor takes the woman doctor outside where she sees that some casualties are being shot & put in mass graves. The head doctor says that he's not proud of that but that that's what has to be done. The woman doctor, henceforth 'our hero', is hooked up with a team about to go on a mission. The head doctor pulls her aside & tells her to turn off her helmet radio & then explains to her that if she's infected she shouldn't tell anyone but that she should come back & get treated immediately. Anyone else who's infected has to be left behind. It might be her helmet that she's talking to near the beginning. It protects her head from the outside air, has a camera that's always on, night-vision, a headlight, & a radio.

****

A thought comes to me: who funded these Pandemic movies? If I'm going to wax conspiratorial it would be interesting to find if any funding for this came from any group that's connected to the PANDEMIC PANIC now.

****

August 5, 2020, 6:22AM (Amir-ul Kafirs to group):

Re: HERETICS: PANDEMIC 2016 movie pt 2

Each team has a driver, driving a school bus with wire mesh over the windows (akin to prisoner transport buses), a navigator, a gunner, & a doctor. The driver is immediately hostile. The doctor is hypothetically in charge of the team but there's resistance to that. The gunner gives the doctor a bat & tells her to pretend that it's like the "Whack-A-Mole" game: if someone starts to get into the bus hit them over the head & knock them out (kill them). They go into a tunnel that ends with a heavily guarded large door. As soon as the door opens a mob of infected people start trying to pour in & get gunned down. They try to get into the bus & one thing leads to another & they start to get in. There's total mayhem with hemmorhaging infected people acting like zombies & getting killed. That finally ends with no-one on the crew hurt. The doctor has chosen a route of the 3 routes given to the team but the driver picks a different way to go because the route the doctor has picked is through the suburbs where everybody's type 5.

The gunner explains that in downtown it's all gangs of armed types 2 & 3.

Their destination is a hospital where a previous team that didn't return found a large number of survivors. The gunner on this team was married to the gunner on our hero's team. He had asked for permission to hunt for the missing team from the head doctor who denied it. Nonetheless, it seems that his plan is to look for the missing team anyway. The doctor is being ignored as the leader of the group because she's too "fresh".

The team on the bus tell their stories, the doctor's from LA, where they are now, but she'd been moved to NYC to work on a vaccine, which hasn't been developed yet but looks promising. The navigator had had a lover (child?) whose picture she still carries who died of leukemia before the pandemic started. The driver is a felon on work release. The gunner had been a traffic cop.

There's a woman in the middle of the road who's yelling for them to stop begging to be got out of there. They stop, there's a wall to the side that has what look like Missing Persons notices covering it. The doctor clumsily tests the woman, finds out she isn't infected & they try to get her out of there but she's chained to a manhole cover & it turns out that she's bait in a trap & infected people rise up out of hiding & start attacking. The gunner kills many people but gets injured & barely makes it back onto the bus. He's angry at the doctor because she's not violent enough & the gunner thinks she's going to get them all killed by being so unable to kill the infected quickly enough.

****

August 5, 2020, 3:44PM (Amir-ul Kafirs to group):

Re: HERETICS: PANDEMIC 2016 movie pt 3

The doctor is clumsily dressing an arm wound of the gunner. He asks her whether she's been trained for the field. He asks where she praticed as a doctor. She said she did lab research. Disgusted, the gunner finishes wrapping his arm himself.

The bus is moving through downtown LA, there're people milling about on the sidewalks, these people are ignoring the bus. The team is talking about what to do. They're not stopping to test the apparently non-violent people outside, they have one destination. The driver says that what they're really doing is getting guinea pigs to take back to the compound to test the vaccine on. He tells the doctor to ask what "Quarantine A" is when they get back. I reckon that's where the guinea pigs go. It further comes out that the team, other than the doctor, have to 'earn their keep', they're not fed otherwise.

They see another schoolbus, the gunner threatens to kill the driver if he doesn't stop. They do, the gunner gets off & gets into the other bus. Everyone on it seems dead, he finds his gunner wife, also dead. Back at the team's bus, the doctor is standing in the open back doorway waiting for the gunner to return when hands grab her ankles & pull her out onto the street. Two deranged & angry looking men are attacking her, maybe to kill her, maybe to rape her. The navigator shoots the 2 men with a flare gun & the doctor grabs the axe that one of them was carrying & slashes one of their chests with it. The gunner gets off the other bus & shoots the other man & helps the doctor up.

They keep going. Their destination is a school, not what I 1st thought. The gunner asks the doctor if she's ever seen the infected becoming cannibals. She says no. Apparently his wife's body had been cannibalized. They get to the school & all 4 go in. The school seems deserted but it's very dark inside so they're relying on their helmet lights. The driver finds food & take his helmet off to start eating. The gunner stays with him. The 2 women, the navigator & the doctor, continue their search for surviviors. As usual, the audience is being set up for something bad to happen to the separated team. The driver asks the gunner what he thinks of the doc. The gunner just shakes his head.

****

August 5, 2020, 6:48PM (Amir-ul Kafirs to group):

Re: HERETICS: PANDEMIC 2016 movie pt 4

The doctor suggests that the 2 women separate. She has the ulterior motive of trying to find a working cell phone that she can use to try calling her daughter & husband. She finds one in a bag on the floor but it's broken. She goes into a bathroom where the sinks are covered in plastic. There's blood covered plastic around the handicapped stall. She opens it & there's a man there who appears to be dead (he may be a 'hibernator', phase 4). She touches him, he falls back, she gets his cell-phone & tries the call again. Her daughter answers. The doctor asks her why she hasn't answered before & the daughter answers that her dad had told her to only turn the phone on once a day. The doctor asks whether her husband is there & the daughter says he's gone out for help. The daughter's scared. The mom says she'll be there for her very soon. The navigator appears at the bathroom door & the gunner's voice is heard over the radio saying "You called for us?" The navigator says "I found something."

The team goes to a room that's barricaded from the inside. They try to get the doors open, initially failing. The doctor wanders off into a different room following the sound of a woman singing "Hush, Little Baby". The doctor sees her back & approaches her telling her that she won't hurt her. The woman turns around, she appears to've hemorrhaged, she appears to be cradling a baby. She begs the doctor to take the baby saying it's not infected. The doctor says that she'll have to test its blood 1st. The rest of the team has entered the room. The woman puts the baby down. It's unclear to me whether it's an actual human baby or a doll. If it's a human, it's dead & partially decayed or eaten. The doctor says that they can't take the baby. The woman's upset. Eventually, the driver stabs her in the throat & kills her.

The team's planning to leave but the navigator insists that they get into the barricaded room. The gunner shoots the door & they go in & it's a gym with a large quantity of people laying on the floor on mats &/or in sleeping bags. It appears that the team is too late. The team decides to leave but mayhem breaks lose again as a mob of infecteds comes after them. The usual mass murder & chaos ensues, the team has to jump out a 2nd floor window, the gunner stays behind & kills quite a few, including in hand-to-hand combat, before his helmet is crushed & he's killed. The driver runs off to the bus ahead of the women but when he appears to reach there a mob of infecteds appears to get him. The women try to get in touch with the compound but they appear to be out of radio range so they decide that they have to find somewhere to hide before night comes because it's far worse at night.

They're out on the streets, it's night, there're sounds of nearby violence, they hide in a van & the doctor grabs a screwdriver for protection. A man opens the back door of the van & she stabs him in the throat. It takes a while for him to die. The 2 women open a store roll-up door & go inside what seems to be a lamp shop. The navigator pulls out the picture that she carries that I thought was of her fiancée but it's actually her young son. She talks about wishing she had him back. The navigator says that a team will be sent out for them because she's a doctor but that they don't care about the navigator so she has to stay with the doctor if she wants to be saved. The 'doctor' reveals that she's not a doctor, that she found the doctor's ID in NYC where she was on a business trip, that she impersonated the doctor because it was the only way she could get back to LA & to her family. The navigator's pissed, blaming the doctor for gunner's death. The doctor-impersonator says that once the compound people realize that she's an imposter they won't send a team out for them.

****

August 5, 2020, 8:54PM (Amir-ul Kafirs to group):

Re: HERETICS: PANDEMIC 2016 movie pt 5

They search the store for water & weapons. A stage 5 infected breaks in. They turn off their head-lamps & switch to night-vision. The infected finds them, knocks the navigator aside & down, probably briefly unconscious, & hits the doctor-imposter's helmet hard enough to disable the night-vision. A struggle ensues with a ball-peen hammer, the women are losing but the driver, who I'd thought was dead, appears & stabs the infected through the neck.

The driver informs them that there's another doctor at a nearby hospital holing up with some survivors. They communicate by radio & arrange for what's left of the team to meet them there, to hot-wire an ambulance, & to take everyone away. It turns out that the driver's got a bad chest wound & is, therefore, in stage 1 infection. The doctor-imposter had been told to not bring anyone like that back but she says that if the driver helps her retrieve her family from the suburbs that she'll get him back into the compound for treatment. The driver goes out without his helmet to see whether the coast is clear.

The driver is walking ahead in his civvies when a car pulls up & the people in it interrogate him, wanting whatever he has. He has nothing but says that he saw a bus a few blocks away so they just hit him & let him go to go after the fictional bus. The 3 of them get to a fence, the driver jumps over, the navigator stops, panicked because she can't find the picture of her dead son. She finds it in the street but a car comes along & hits her & the occupants take her away. The doctor-impresonator follows them on foot & gets to them as they're ripping out the navigator's innards & eating them.

The doctor-impersonator uses her last 2 bullets to kill 2 of them, some run away, the remaining one begs for mercy but she beats his head in. The driver comes up & hugs her. They get to the hospital but the doctor won't let them in because he says the driver's infected. They meet in the garage where after the driver hot-wires the ambulance the doctor won't let them come along because he'd worked with the doctor that the impersonator was pretending to be so the doctor knew she was fake.

The driver hot-wires another ambulance & they barely get out of the garage because of the usual horde of infecteds. They drive at night over deserted highways & the driver tells the doctor-impersonator that he was on to her fairly early on but he congratulates her on being a good con artist. They get to the psuedo-doctor's house, she goes inside & finds her daughter hiding. The driver waits outside in the ambulance with the moror running. The 'doctor' tests her daughter & finds that she's infected but lies to her about that. The fake doctor takes entirely too long & follows a trail of blood to the garage where she finds her dead husband in the trunk of the car where he'd closed himself in to protect his daughter. There's a video camcorder with a note on it telling whoever finds him to look at the tape. The tape briefly tells his story.

The driver & the ambulance are surrounded by stage 5 infecteds & he starts honking the horn. The woman gets her daughter to wear the suit, the driver comes to the door pursued by infecteds & the woman stabs as many as she can while they get to the upstairs. They all jump out the window but not before the driver's too injured to go on anymore. The mother & daughter make it to the ambulance & drive to the compound. They're attacked by infecteds outside the compound but the soldiers open up & start shooting. Since the 'doctor''s no longer wearing a suit they wound her & contact the head doctor to tell them that someone from the missing unit is back. The head doctor assumes it's the 'doctor' & tells the soldier to take her to Quarantine A. The soldier says that he's been ordered to not let anyone in who appears infected but the head doctor insists.

****

August 6, 2020, 1:35AM (Amir-ul Kafirs to group):

Re: HERETICS: PANDEMIC 2016 movie pt 6 (end)

The last shot is as if from the helmet cam of the daughter. The solider follows the head doctor's order & carries the suited figure inside the compound & the wire mesh gate is closed. The mother is seen lying on her side watching the daughter get taken away while mobs are running past her back & forth. Unrealistically, none of them are trampling her. The daughter is to be taken to Quarantine A which the driver had previously announced was where people are taken as guinea pigs for vaccine testing.

All in all, this one was much worse than the 2008 PANDEMIC movie that I described previously. Even though it had higher production values it was just basically yet-another zombie movie. There wasn't even any greater context, it was just fear-triggering mayhem.

****

August 4, 2020, 4:02PM (Inquiring Librarian to group):

HERETICS: New JB Handly Article, Incl. the enforced mental disorders. BONUS->Australian Tyrrany

J.B. Handly has written another amazing article on "Lockdown Lunacy". Here he argues, with plenty of facts & figures, that in the U.S., we have reached herd immunity... aka "It's Over".
https://childrenshealthdefense.org/news/lockdown-lunacy-3-0-its-over/
A quick quote from the beginning:

Have we lost our collective minds? Yes.

You may not be one of them. In fact, I'm guessing the people who actually take the time to read my blog posts are the few remaining who haven't been subsumed by the panic, but can we agree that most have?

[..]

& you really should read the whole linked article, "When Will The Madness End?" https://www.aier.org/article/when-will-the-madness-end/

By the same author, Jeffrey A. Tucker, in the same magazine as the above "When Will The Madness End" article, The American Institute for Economic

Research, is a shocking article on the fascist leadership's crackdown in the Australian state of Victoria.

https://www.aier.org/article/madness-in-melbourne/

Here are a list of restrictions from the article in Melbourne, take a deep breath... It's a dystopian nightmare:"

Police may now enter anyone's home **without a warrant.**

Curfew 8:00pm.

$1,652 fine if outside without "a valid reason" – an amount being raised by the day

Can't visit any family or friends.

$200 fine for no mask (mandatory masks at all times).

Can only exercise once per day, for up to 1 hour.

Only one person per household, per day can leave the house (including for groceries).

Can't go more than 3 miles from your home.

Weddings are illegal.

No gatherings of any size.

Army is on the streets fining/arresting people.

"Since March 21, a total of 193,740 spot checks have been conducted by police across Victoria."

Protests/activism is illegal; people have already been arrested for peaceful gatherings.

Media is EXTREMELY biased, calls protesters "right wing conspiracy nutjobs" and won't allow discussion of whether these lockdowns are right or not.

Several thousand people were placed under house arrest and unable to leave for ANY reason, with food rations delivered by the army, leading to appalling levels of personal trauma.

Australia won't release how many fines they've given out, but an ABC news report says it's over $5.2 million so far.

Streets of Melbourne are empty, even in a city of 5 million+ people. People are HATEFUL to each other, everyone is cannibalising their neighbours (calling police to report any little infraction of the rules and turning on each other like some socialist hellhole).

Billboards outside on the street that say in capital letters: "WHAT ARE YOU DOING? STAY HOME." They feel extremely oppressive, like we're being yelled at by a very oppressive government.

The Victorian Premier Daniel Andrews shows complete and utter disdain for us, constantly blaming us. He's blamed children (yes, really) for not taking this seriously enough. Every chance he gets, he tells us it's OUR fault the virus is spreading (even though that's what viruses do – they spread).

It's not just the Victorian Premier – the Australian Prime Minister Scott Morrison is just as terrible. He's encouraged all of this, and he was responsible for the first lockdown.

1984 dystopian language: billboards everywhere saying "Staying apart keeps us together." Have they gone mad?

There's probably more but at this point I honestly lost track of all the insanity that's happened.

All because 147 people died in the state of Victoria (total population is 6.359 million), almost all of the deaths are over 70 with comorbidities, same as everywhere else in the world."

****

JULY 30, 2020

LOCKDOWN LUNACY 3.0—It's over.

By J.B. Handley, CHD Contributing Writer

If you're hoping the COVID-19 pandemic will go on forever, this post may disappoint you. And, I get it. We have gone frothing-at-the-mouth nuts over a slightly above-normal virulence virus, with a unique and obvious age-distribution pattern that should have made containment easy and panic completely unnecessary. And, if you're living in the United States, like I am, you probably think my declaration that this pandemic is "over" to be somewhere between wishful thinking and incredibly premature, and I hear you, too, although forgive me if I'm not sure you're the one thinking clearly, given some of the things I've recently read. I promise to support my assertion with data, and the wisdom of people far more expert than me who are having a harder time being heard in the present climate of…bats#@t crazy.

Have we lost our collective minds? Yes.

[..]

Jeffrey A. Tucker of the American Institute for Economic Research put it best in his excellent essay on July 10 titled, When will the Madness End?:

[..]

****

When Will the Madness End?

I was sitting in the green room in a Manhattan television studio on the day that the storm seemed to hit. It was Thursday, March 12, 2020, and I was waiting anxiously for a TV appearance, hoping that the trains wouldn't shut down before I could leave the city. The trains never did shut but half of everything else did. On this day, everyone knew what was coming. There was disease panic in the air, fomented mostly by the media and political figures. A month earlier, the idea of lockdown was unthinkable, but now it seemed like it could happen, at any moment.

A thin, wise-looking bearded man with Freud-style glasses sat down across from me, having just left the studio. He was there to catch his breath following his interview but he looked deeply troubled.

"There is fear in the air," I said, breaking the silence.

"Madness is all around us. The public is adopting a personality disorder I've been treating my whole career."

"What is it that you do?" I asked.

"I'm a practicing psychiatrist who specializes in anxiety disorders, paranoid delusions, and irrational fear. I've been treating this in individuals as a specialist. It's hard enough to contain these problems in normal times. What's happening now is a spread of this serious medical condition to the whole population. It can happen with anything but here we see a primal fear of disease turning into mass panic. It seems almost deliberate. It is tragic. Once this starts, it could take years to repair the psychological damage."

I sat there a bit stunned, partially because speaking in such apocalyptic terms was new in those days, and because of the certitude of his opinion. Underlying his brief comments were a presumption that there was nothing particularly unusual about this virus. We've evolved with them, and learned to treat them with calm and professionalism. What distinguished the current moment, he was suggesting, was not the virus but the unleashing of a kind of public madness.
I was an early skeptic of the we-are-all-going-to-die narrative. But even I was unsure if he was correct that the real problem was not physical but mental. In those days, even I was cautious about shaking hands and carrying around sanitizer. I learned later, of course, that plenty of medical professionals had been trying to calm people down for weeks, urging the normal functioning of society rather than panic. It took weeks however even for me to realize that he was right: the main threat society faced was a psychological condition.

I should have immediately turned to a book that captivated me in high school. It is Extraordinary Popular Delusions and the Madness of Crowds by Charles Mackay (1841). I liked reading it because, while it highlighted human folly, it also seemed to indicate that we as a civilization are over that period in history. It allowed me to laugh at how ridiculous people were in the past, with sudden panics over long hair and beards, jewelry, witches, the devil, prophecies and sorcery, disease and cures, land speculation, tulips, just about anything. In a surprising number of cases he details, disease plays a role, usually as evidence of a malicious force operating in the world. Once fear reaches a certain threshold, normalcy, rationality, morality, and decency fade and are replaced by shocking stupidity and cruelty.

He writes:

In reading the history of nations, we find that, like individuals, they have their whims and their peculiarities; their seasons of excitement and recklessness, when they care not what they do. We find that whole communities suddenly fix their minds upon one object, and go mad in its pursuit; that millions of people become simultaneously impressed with one delusion, and run after it, till their attention is caught by some new folly more captivating than the first. We see one nation suddenly seized, from its highest to its lowest members, with a fierce desire of military glory; another as suddenly becoming crazed upon a religious scruple; and neither of them recovering its senses until it has shed rivers of blood and sowed a harvest of groans and tears, to be reaped by its posterity.... Men, it has been well said, think in herds; it will be seen that they go mad in herds, while they only recover their senses slowly, and one by one.

[..]

by Jeffrey A. Tucker

- https://www.aier.org/article/when-will-the-madness-end/

****

Madness in Melbourne

Melbourne, that glorious city in the state of Victoria in Australia, granted me some of the best travel days of my life during two separate trips each lasting a full week.

A happy, civilized, highly educated people are here living amidst modern architecture, inspiring bridges, and natural beauty, a place where even the police are kind, and when you ask them for directions they reply with a smile, and when you say thank you, they say "No worries."

Now there are big worries in Melbourne.

The Premier has imposed a vicious police state without precedent in this country's history. His name is Dan Andrews (a sweet-sounding name that masks the tyrant he has become), and he tweets out pictures of empty streets to brag about what he has achieved in the name of suppressing a virus.

Tacitus's line about the Roman empire comes to mind: "Where they make a desert, they call it peace."

Australia is the only country in the world that has a law that people can't be mean to each other. Now it is host to one of the world's meanest governments. The catastrophe began with a spring lockdown before there were any cases of C-19 much less deaths. The ethos in Australia was one of extreme exclusion and suppression of the virus, not as bad as New Zealand but pretty bad. The rest of the world can catch this disease, but Australia would use its geographical isolation and political intelligence to ban the virus. The virus will be in awe and know to stay away forever.

It's not a good theory because that's not how viruses work.

Still, it seemed to work, at first. That's because the virus had yet to arrive.

When the virus did arrive, the futility of the suppression strategy was revealed. Melbourne had set up quarantine hotels for people arriving from abroad or returning from cruises. They would spend 14 days in isolation to purge themselves of possible infection. Then all would be okay. There was a problem: the wiley virus escaped.

[..]

This is lockdown ideology at work. It is tyranny without limit, at the expense of all human dignity, decency, and rights. The politicians make a desert and call it health.
Like everywhere else on the planet, Melbourne will have to reach herd immunity from C-19 at some point. Those who deny that are risking not only liberty and health but civilization itself.

[..]

Jeffrey A. Tucker is Editorial Director for the American Institute for Economic Research. He is the author of many thousands of articles in the scholarly and popular press and eight books in 5 languages, most recently The Market Loves You. He is also the editor of The Best of Mises. He speaks widely on topics of economics, technology, social philosophy, and culture. Jeffrey is available for speaking and interviews via his email. Tw | FB | LinkedIn

- https://www.aier.org/article/madness-in-melbourne/

****

August 4, 2020, 4:08PM (Amir-ul Kafirs to group):

Re: HERETICS: New JB Handly Article, Incl, the enforced mental disorders. BONUS->Australian Tyrrany

OK! I've read & copied all 3 articles. They're all very useful.

Have we lost our collective minds? Yes.

"I'm a practicing psychiatrist who specializes in anxiety disorders, paranoid delusions, and irrational fear.

I loved this one BUT it's unfortunate that the practicing psychiatrist isn't identified. Of course, that's an ongoing problem isn't it? People are afraid to identify anyone because they're afraid of the harm that may be inflicted on them.

Here are a list of restrictions from the article in Melbourne

Having spent a considerable amount of time in Melbourne (maybe 6 weeks) I can safely say that it's one of my favorite cities in the world. I mention that because the violations of its civil liberties are so insane that it's like reading about a friend being beaten to death or something else similarly horrible.

****

August 4, 2020, 9:27PM (Inquiring Librarian to group):

Re: HERETICS: "Beyond Therapy"

David Icke just wrote a new book, "The Answer", centering around his theories of life and on the plandemic and his suggestion of solutions. I would like to get it. https://shop.davidicke.com/us/product/the-answer-by-david-icke/

My list of impt books to purchase is growing... Given free libraries may soon become a thing of the past, i feel i have an excuse to buy books again... And tell myself it was ok to buy that new large bookshelf!

****

August 5, 2020, 5:28PM (Amir-ul Kafirs to Dick):

Re: HERETICS: Question for Dick & Phil

On Aug 4, 2020, at 10:11 PM, dick turner wrote:

No I can't say if I've seen more out of business signs lately
I'll try to see if there are government statistics

Thanks. That would be helpful. I'm beginning to suspect that the deliberate destruction of small businesses is more a phenomena in places where there's American big business hegemony. In other words, if France doesn't have huge American chain stores like Target, Home Depot, CVS, etc, then there's probably no destruction of small competing businesses.

What do you think?

****

August 4, 2020, 12:42PM (Amir-ul Kafirs to group):

HERETICS: My New FB Postings

I've gotten a little behind in keeping you updated on my social media posts so here're the latest 4. One of them just has "tyrrany" corrected to "tyranny", another is a sharing of something that Inquiring Librarian shared with me (bless 'em!).

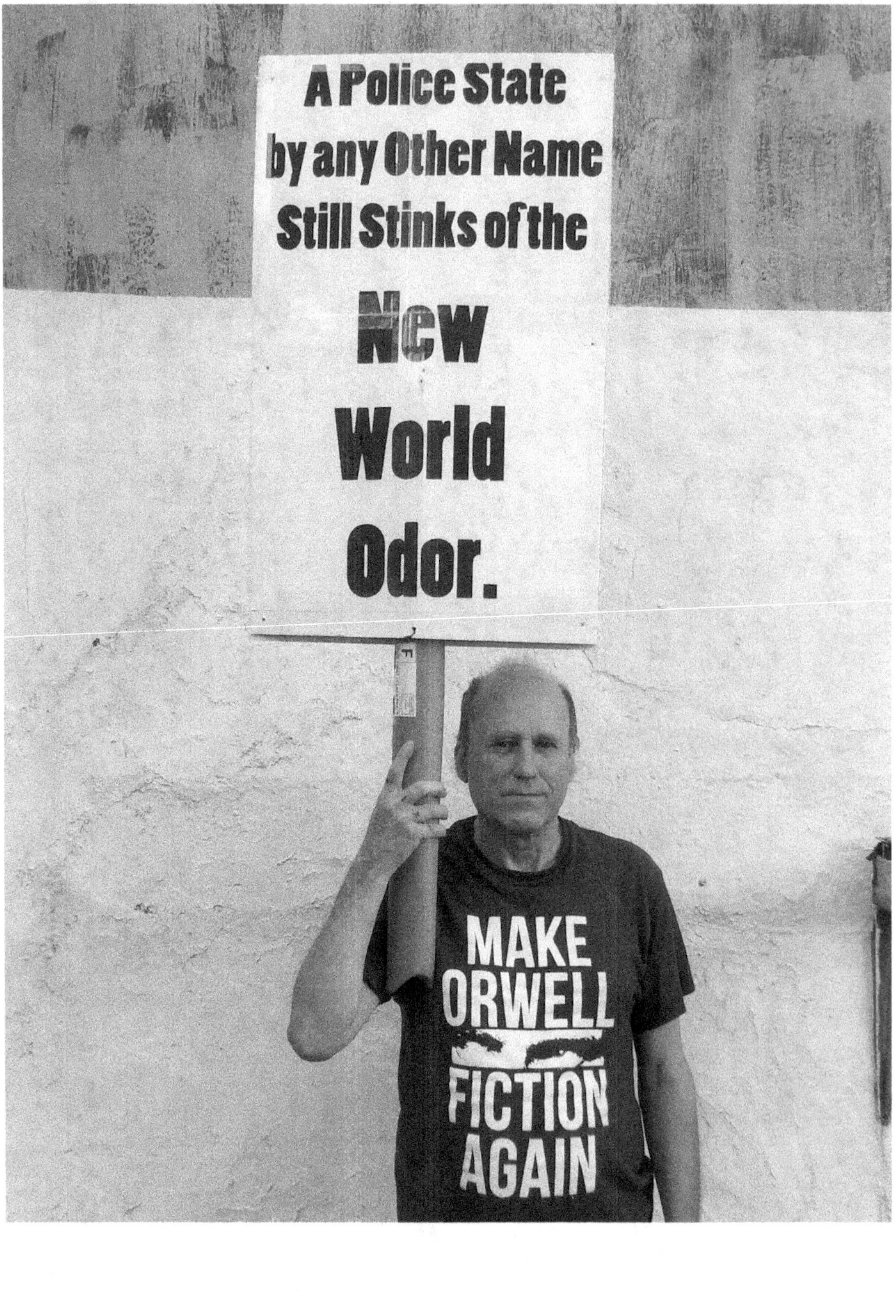

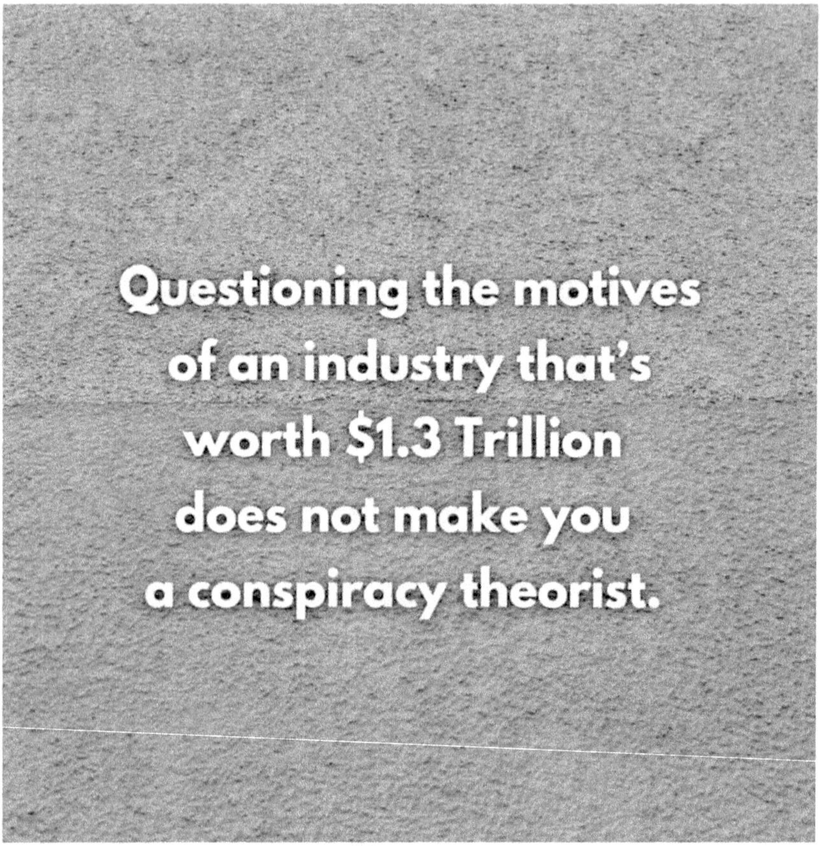
Questioning the motives
of an industry that's
worth $1.3 Trillion
does not make you
a conspiracy theorist.

Dunkin' Donuts
= ESSENTIAL;
Public Libraries
= NONESSENTIAL.
Crime Scene:
"Nuthin' to look at here,
just keep movin'."

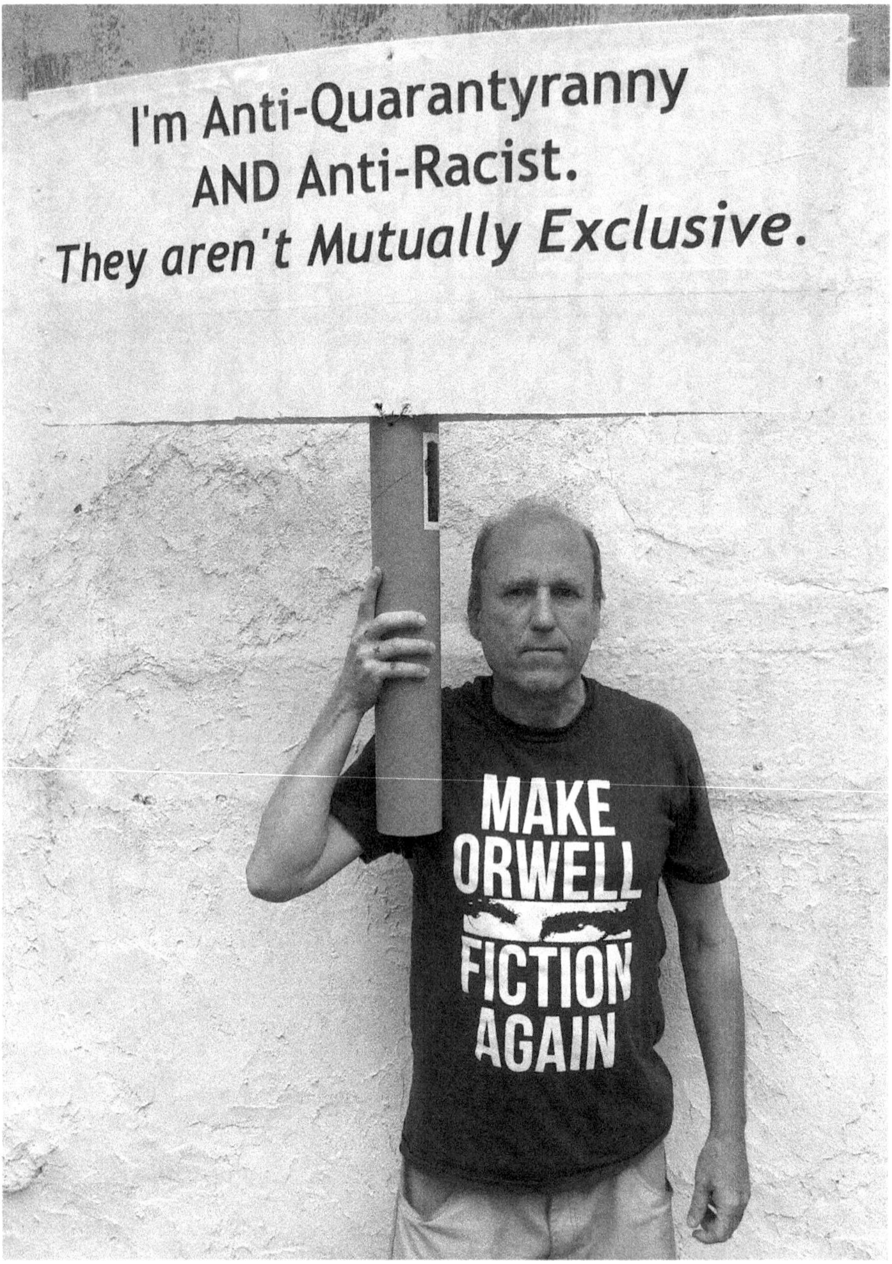

****

August 5, 2020, 5:38AM (Amir-ul Kafirs to group):

HERETICS: the Kaleidoscope Century text panel

"The old guy went on. "Well, I can understand why a lot of people choose to run a meme, to invite it into their existence. Really, I do; there are plenty of people out there whose own personalities will never allow them any happiness, who tie themselves in one knot after another, people for whom the biggest curse in the world is freedom of choice because they're programmed to keep choosing wrong and blaming themselves for it. There's no meme out there that's as cruel to the people running it as their own personalities would be. They should have the choice to pick up one, even though that's the last choice they can ever make.

""But you and I—or you and this Yuri, if that's really his name, and Monica, and me, probably your Murphy, if he's still alive, all of us—for some reason we're fussy. We want to make those choices. The thought of not making them makes us even more unhappy than our own failures. We can't help it, we only want happiness we can get for ourselves, as ourselves, by our own efforts and choices.["]"

- John Barnes, ***Kaleidoscope Century*** (1995)

****

August 5, 2020, 6:451AM (Dick to group):

local (bad) news

The mayor of Paris wants to impose masks
where there are large groups of people
i.e. where people meet & socialize !!!
French article below

here's the traduction (translation)

By Christine Henry and Quentin Laurent (with Marie Boyer)
August 4, 2020 at 5:18 p.m., modified August 5, 2020 at 6:01 a.m.
After Lille, Bayonne, Biarritz, Le Touquet, Troyes or in Ile-de-France, Enghien-les-Bains or Alfortville, Anne Hidalgo, the town hall (PS) of Paris in turn asks for the wearing of the compulsory mask outdoors in some areas of the capital.

“The goal is to slow the resumption of the Covid-19 epidemic. The incidence rate (Editor's note: number of cases per 100,000 inhabitants) fell from 24 at the end of last week to 27. The movement has been slow but steady for a month. We are waiting for a second wave. It is urgent to strengthen barrier gestures if we do not want to achieve a new confinement,” explains Anne Souyris, EELV deputy to the mayor of Paris in charge of health.

Anne Hidalgo wants to impose the mask outdoors on Parisians
“Discussions between the services of the police prefecture (PP) and those of the town hall of Paris took place to study the measures to be put in place in view of the evolution of epidemiological data, in particular that of wearing a mask in exterior ”, we confirm to the PP without giving further details.

Quays of the Seine, Canal Saint-Martin and target markets
There is no question for the mayor of the capital to generalize the wearing of the mask in the streets. Only areas frequented by a large number of people are targeted, in particular the banks of the Seine or the Canal Saint-Martin, crowded with people at aperitif time, but also open markets, certain parks and gardens, shopping streets or near stations where many travelers without a mask meet.

For the time being, the list of sites has not yet been finalized. “We will rely on feedback from the borough mayors to define the zones as precisely as possible. Wearing a mask is painful, especially in hot weather. If the areas are chosen intelligently, the Parisians will wear it, ”assures the deputy who hopes that the prefectural decree will be taken quickly. “We have to act on a case-by-case basis, as in Germany. The French government has understood this and is moving in this direction, ”continues the elected Parisian.

VIDEO. Covid-19: Castex calls for "vigilance" to avoid "widespread reconfinement"

"It's not too soon ! Frankly, if it can avoid a second confinement, I am for making this effort. Moreover, I find this decision a little late," asserts Marine Loiseau, 28, designate cross textile this Tuesday early evening on the Parisian quays. An opinion that does not seem to be shared by a shopkeeper who manages a refreshment bar near the Louis-Philippe bridge a little further: “I'm afraid that might discourage people from coming. "

In Nice, Christian Estrosi (LR) had not waited for the green light from the government: “My decision to make the wearing of a mask compulsory outside has been constant since the start of confinement. But neither the government nor the administrative courts had considered that this provision could be applicable,” he said Monday on RTL. He had created controversy in early May, by issuing an order requiring the wearing of a mask in the public space of his city.

Well respected in Lille city center
In the North, the prefect has imposed the wearing of masks in certain public areas of the Lille metropolitan area, while information suggested an increase in cases. Martine Aubry "understands the relevance of the measure", we commented to the office of the mayor (PS) of Lille, where we also observe that the obligation seems "particularly well respected in the city center" .

"The State must listen to the mayors, they are the ones who know their city, where are the concentrations of population", comments for his part Philippe Laurent, mayor (UDI) of Sceaux and secretary general of the association of mayors of France. He had taken a decree requiring the wearing of a mask in early April, before being challenged by the Council of State. "The government has changed its discourse on the subject, but it is because now we have masks ...", observes the elected representative of Hauts-de-Seine.

https://www.leparisien.fr/paris-75/le-port-du-masque-bientot-obligatoire-a-paris-04-08-2020-8363397.php#xtor=EREC-1481423604-[NL75]---${_id_connect_hash}@1

****

August 5, 2020, 2:44PM (Amir-ul Kafirs to Dick):

Re: May I use "Dark Ages of Progress"?

On Aug 5, 2020, at 2:25 PM, dick turner wrote:

sure, be my guest

it's a compliment !

you could thank me in a comment in the post if you want , not in the text

Here's what I made:

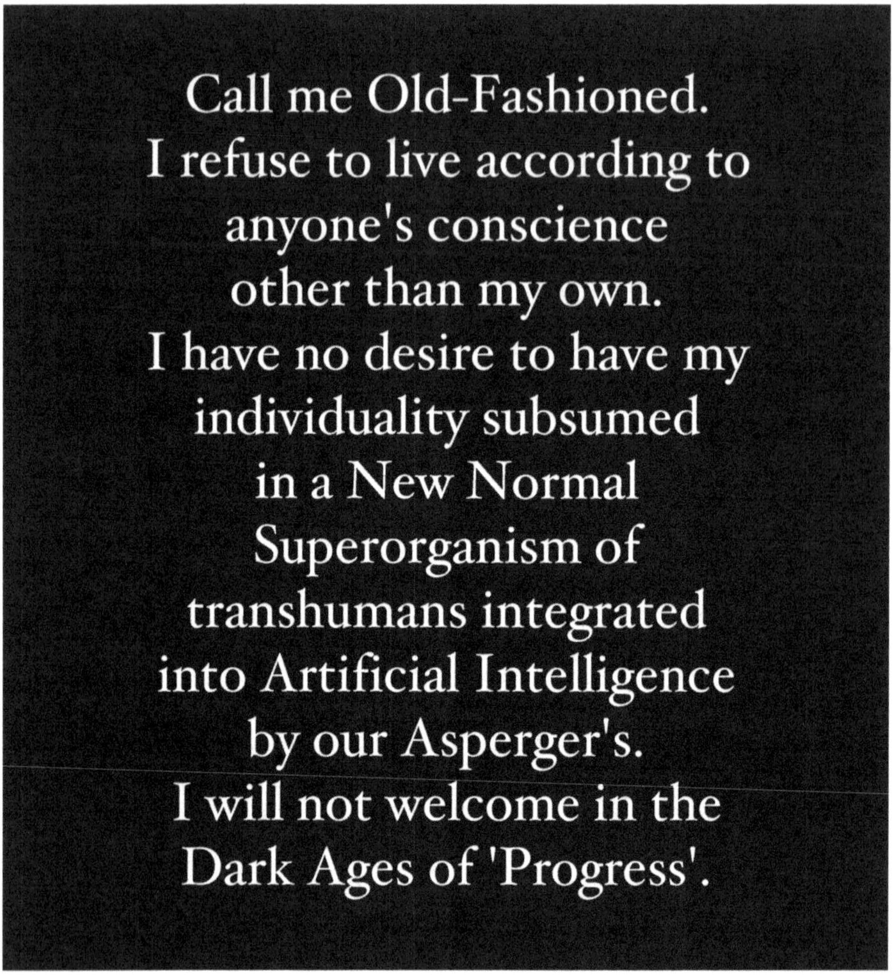

Call me Old-Fashioned.
I refuse to live according to anyone's conscience other than my own.
I have no desire to have my individuality subsumed in a New Normal Superorganism of transhumans integrated into Artificial Intelligence by our Asperger's.
I will not welcome in the Dark Ages of 'Progress'.

****

August 5, 2020, 4:27PM (Amir-ul Kafirs to group):

I need some help here

Back in the beginning of April the CDC's Journal published an article that was a summary of 14 studies that each concluded that masks & sterilizing, etc, was not effective. I can't find the article right now. I know Naia Nisnam alluded to it at least once in one of their posts & I probably heard of it because of someone else's post. I'd like to access that article again. Can anyone help?

****

August 5, 2020, 4:43PM (Inquiring Librarian to group):

Re: I need some help here

Here it is:
https://wwwnc.cdc.gov/eid/article/26/5/19-0994_article

****

August 5, 2020, 4:44PM (Amir-ul Kafirs to group):

Bless you Inquiring Librarian!

You have just been granted eternal happiness!

****

August 5, 2020, 4:50PM (Inquiring Librarian to group):

Yay!!! OCD Librarian to the Rescue!!

****

August 5, 2020, 5:33PM (Inquiring Librarian to group):

Re: HERETICS: "Beyond Therapy"

I'm going to order it out of my next paycheck. I'm trying to space things out. I feel like books like this are ready to be the 1st banned when censorship takes a stronger stranglehold. I have a list now of 5 books to order that I can keep to fight off this war on the natural body.

-Plague of Corruption, by: Judy Mikovitz
-The Virus & the Vaccine, by: Debbie Bookchin
-The Answer, by: David Icke
-Why You Can't Trust the Pharmaceutical Companies, by: Marcia Angell
-Virus Mania, by: Torsten Engelbrecht and Claus Köhnlein, M.D., most updated copy here:
https://www.bookdepository.com/Virus-Mania-Torsten-Engelbrecht/9783751942539?utm_medium=api&utm_campaign=Bookfindercom&a_aid=Bookfinder&utm_term=9783751942539&utm_content=Virus-Mania&utm_source=book_link&selectCurrency=USD

****

August 5, 2020, 5:41PM (Inquiring Librarian to group):

Re: HERETICS: New JB Handly Article, Incl. the enforced mental disorders.

BONUS!!->Australian Tyrrany

I can visualize the friends being beaten to pulps in Melbourne... It sounds like a true dystopian nightmare. Did you know that Australia's government is completely wrapped up in big pharma and the vaccine industry?
Polly Tommey, the mother of an autusic child that was injured by the MMR vaccine, was banned for 3 years from Australia because she brought the movie, "Vaxxed", that she co-produced to Australia for public screenings. I believe she was thrown out of and banned from all of Australia for something like "bioterrorism". I heard her say it in an interview, but I cannot find the exact damning term on the web right now.

From the article below on the "Vaxxed" movie website, you can dig further into the issue here:
"The Australian Prime Minister, Malcolm Turnbull, recently passed a stringent new mandatory vaccination law that requires all children to be fully vaccinated to receive government child-care benefits and rebates. His wife, Lucy Turnbull, is also Chair of Australian pharma corporation, Prima BioMed, which has worked in collaboration with the pharmaceutical companies Novartis and GlaxoSmithKline. It appears that the Australian government has deep ties to the pharmaceutical industry and that it has decided that it's in its best interest to ban an individual who it perceives as threatening to these financial interests."
https://vaxxedthemovie.com/vaxxed-producer-banned-from-australia-censorship/

I believe that Scott Morrison is now the Prime Minister there, as of 2019. I would imagine he also has his hands in the vaccine pot of gold. Regardless, Lucy Turnbull is likely still in.

Now, let's take a moment of silence to weep for those in Melbourne, and also to thank our lucky stars it's not that bad here.. yet.

****

Vaxxed Producer Polly Tommey Banned From Australia For Three Years In An Unprecedented Attempt To Censor The Film By The Australian Government

FOR IMMEDIATE RELEASE
Los Angeles, August 10, 2017– In an unprecedented censorship attempt by the Australian Government, Polly Tommey, one of the producers of *Vaxxed: From Cover-Up to Catastrophe,* was banned from re-entering Australia for three years following the recent Australian tour of the film. The Australian government gave this reason for the ban, "…if the wider Australian community had been made

aware of Ms. Tommey's presence in Australia promoting an anti-vaccination film and conducting anti-vaccination seminars, there is a risk that the Australian community would react adversely and thereby would be a risk to the good order of the Australian community."

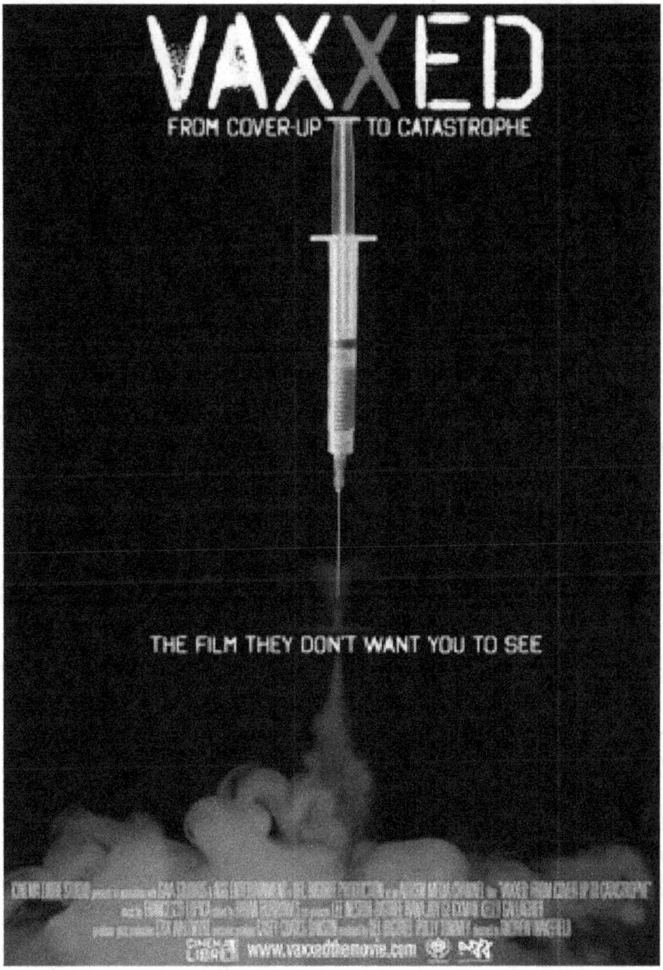

Vaxxed, at its core, is about a whistleblower from the U.S. Centers for Disease Control, who revealed that the CDC concealed and destroyed data on their 2004 study that showed a causal association between the MMR (measles, mumps and rubella) vaccine and autism. The film is not, and has never been, an anti-vaccination film. The ban demonstrates that the Australian government is attempting to shut down all debate on the topic of vaccine safety, and prevent their citizens from having access to a robust, honest discourse about the possible risks of vaccination.

The Australian press was equally at fault for propagating a misinformation campaign about the film while it was touring Australia, printing several slanderous and totally false articles about *Vaxxed*. The result of that targeted campaign was that the film was given a new-found visibility in Australia, and subsequently all the remaining screenings of *Vaxxed* sold out with long waiting lists. Despite their government and media's attempt at censoring the film and attempting to prevent their citizens from seeing it, thousands of Australians came out to view the film during the two-week tour, making it one of the most successful *Vaxxed* tours to date.

The Australian Prime Minister, Malcolm Turnbull, recently passed a stringent new mandatory vaccination law that requires all children to be fully vaccinated to receive government child-care benefits and rebates. His wife, Lucy Turnbull, is also Chair of Australian pharma corporation, Prima BioMed, which has worked in collaboration with the pharmaceutical companies Novartis and GlaxoSmithKline. It appears that the Australian government has deep ties to the pharmaceutical industry and that it has decided that it's in its best interest to ban an individual who it perceives as threatening to these financial interests.
"The decision of the Australian government to ban one of the producers of *Vaxxed* for three years is totally shocking and unacceptable. Polly Tommey is the mother of an autistic child who was vaccine injured from the MMR vaccine, and was touring Australia to give a voice to other families of vaccine injured children. This is an extreme freedom of speech infringement and should not be tolerated. We strongly condemn such action, which didn't happen in any other part of the world where the film was played. We will not, and have never in the past, allowed censorship to block the public from learning about the crucial message in our film. The actions of the Australian government, and others who attempt to censor this film, will only help delay real scientific advancements in vaccine safety that are desperately needed," says Philippe Diaz, Chairman of Cinema Libre Studio.

FILM LINKS:

www.vaxxedthemovie.com I @vaxxedthemovie I facebook.com/vaxxedthemovie

# # #

For interviews:
Jamie Coker Robertson,
jamievaxxed@gmail.com

- https://vaxxedthemovie.com/vaxxed-producer-banned-from-australia-censorship/

****

August 5, 2020, 9:57PM (Inquiring Librarian to group):

HERETICS: Humor for Today

My sister sent me this humor today. She knows I'm losing it. She's on our side with this pandemic. She is a nurse.

Here is the Song, it's a "Monster Mash" Covid spoof:

https://www.youtube.com/watch?v=_gdYtMGvedw

Here is the series of jokes:

I don't know who to give credit to, but this is hilarious.

So we're into our 5th month of defeating COVID-19. These words made me laugh. But there's a lot of truth mixed in to consider. . .

1. So let me get this straight, there's no cure for a virus that can be killed by sanitizer and hand soap?

2. Is it too early to put up the Christmas tree yet? I have run out of things to do.

3. When this virus thing is over, I still want some of you to stay away from me.

4. If these last months have taught us anything, it's that stupidity travels faster than any virus on the planet.

5. Just wait a second – so what you're telling me is that my chance of surviving all this is directly linked to the common sense of others? You're kidding, right?

6. If you believe all this will end and we will get back to normal just because we reopen everything, raise your hand. Now slap yourself with it.

7. Another Saturday night in the house and I just realized the trash goes out more than me.

8. Whoever decided a liquor store is more essential than a hair salon is obviously a bald-headed alcoholic.

9. Remember when you were little and all your underwear had the days of the week on them. Those would be helpful right now.

10. The spread of Covid-19 is based on two factors: 1. How dense the population is and 2. How dense the population is.

11. Remember all those times when you wished the weekend would last forever? Well, wish granted. Happy now?

12. It may take a village to raise a child, but I swear it's going to take a whole vineyard to home school one.

13. Did a big load of pyjamas so I would have enough clean work clothes for this week.

****

August 5, 2020, 10:05PM (Inquiring Librarian to group):

HERETICS: Front Line Doctor's Summit, Pt. 2

I know you are all excited for another video... a 3 hour one! You can tell I have a stunning social life, right? I think it consists solely of my creepy tall neighbor staring at me on occasion over the 6 foot fence separating our yards.

Anyways, this here is pt. 2 of the Frontline Doctor's Summit from 2 weeks ago. I managed to miss this one. I remember it was said to be 6 hours long. I watched 3 hours inside, and then the 2 hours outside. But man... THIS video says it ALL. In this video, 2 doctors really stand out, Dr. Scott Barbour, MD from Georgia, and Dr. James Todaro, MD. Both doctors completely call out the pandemic as full of lies and manipulation from the pharmaceutical companies which control the scientific journals and treatments, etc... I'm too tired to explain this well or clearly. If you have 3 hours to spare, this is totally worth it. I can see why the media would want to silence and toss this one under the rug. & it does address hcq, in the beginning, a scientist goes in depth how hcq works on covid 19. But for me, the meat of this is in the early to middle... the calling out of the big players in this scamdemic.

https://www.bitchute.com/video/E7f4nTAR0gMF/

****

August 6, 2020, 2:02AM (Amir-ul Kafirs to group):

Re: HERETICS: Front Line Doctor's Summit, Pt. 2

I know you are all excited for another video... a 3 hour one!

I continue to be thankful to just enter another link in my burgeoning database.

You can tell I have a stunning social life, right?

Isn't that a part of how this whole thing works? To alienate people to the point of insanity? I'm proud of all of us for staying on point to the extent that we have.

****

August 6, 2020, 2:20AM (Amir-ul Kafirs to group):

HERETICS: Posting on social media

I'd previously been posting a new Thought for the Day text panel after midnight because I was eager to get them out there. Now I have the opinion that many of the people who attack me are alcoholics who're drunk then so I've decided it's better to hold off on posting them until early morning when I wake up & most of the drunks are probably still sleeping it off.

Thanks to Naia Nisnam for apparently leaving a comment to direct a mutual friend to something I posted. I couldn't bear to even look at it right now but I think that's what Naia Nisnam did. One of the ongoing things that I find irritating is this high & mighty tone that people take that I know are literally at an intellectual level lower than where I was as a 9 year old — even though they're adults. SO, one friend of mine asks for "scientific evidence" as if he'd be able to understand scientific evidence as differentiated from a hole-in-the-ground. He wouldn't. SOO, I've decided to stop looking at my social media timeline comments at all. It's too frustrating & I let it get to me too much. I made that decision before, probably back in March or April, but I've been slipping. I'll still continue to post things everyday (or thereabouts) but I'll ignore it otherwise so I don't waste any time or emotions on it.

Here's the next text panel I'll upload:

If you're so concerned
about HEALTH
why don't you
LOSE SOME WEIGHT,
STOP BEING AN
ALCOHOLIC,
& EAT LESS SUGAR.
You're much less likely
to die with the assistance
of COVID-19 that way.

****

August 6, 2020, 3:39PM (Inquiring Librarian to group):

Heretics: Hydroxychloroquine In Depth & Stanford Resistance to the Mainstream Media Narrative

I found more fun stuff on Hydroxychloroquine. 1st, is an article about the Louisiana Attorney General's support of the use of Hydroxychloroquine, and a Newsweek article which criticizes his response to Facebook when he defends the Front Line Doctors and even states that he is taking HCQ. I have separated each article/study by asterisks [*****************].

****

The Jeff Landry-Facebook-HCQ Kerfuffle
"...Let's remember that it was in Murdock's own publication that the head of epidemiology at Yale, Dr. Harvey Risch, posted a full-throated defense of hydroxychloroquine and called it a cure for COVID-19...We're pushing remdesivir, which is a new drug whose side effects aren't fully known. And we're rushing vaccines to market which may or may not be effective or even safe. But HCQ is "potentially dangerous?"
And Landry is a kook for calling out Facebook over their refusal to allow people to even post information about HCQ from America's Frontline Doctors or others who have had positive experiences with HCQ? It's like we're in the Twilight Zone. *Newsweek* runs a piece from the head of epidemiology at Yale Medical School that supports everything America's Frontline Doctors had to offer, and then *Newsweek* sends one of its reporters out to trash the entire argument as "false and potentially dangerous" and Landry for noting the whiff of fascism and censorship coming off Big Tech as they squelch the debate.
What in the hell is going on here?"
https://thehayride.com/2020/08/the-jeff-landry-facebook-hcq-kerfuffle/

****

MEDICINE
(UN) CENSORED

A Study Out of Thin Air

by James M Todaro, MD (Columbia MD, @JamesTodaroMD)

May 29, 2020

Misinformation is bad. Misinformation in medicine is worse. Misinformation from a prestigious medical journal is the worst. Herein is a detailed look at the controversial Lancet study that resulted in the World Health Organization ending worldwide clinical trials on hydroxychloroquine in order to focus on patented therapeutics.

https://www.medicineuncensored.com/a-study-out-of-thin-air

Then, check out Dr. Todano's "Medicine Uncensored" website. He created this so that voices could be heard about effective medications for covid, and other illnesses, without censor, and with well documented evidence of efficacy. You can see at the start here he goes into detail on the Lancet Journal's retracted fake 'study' that steered the world away from HCQ when it was first released, before it was justifiably retracted as 'fake'.

****

Here is a Washington Times article discussing Dr. Todaro's new website, "Medicine Uncensored". This is the whole article, I loved it all. It is spot on with everything I heard and also a good summary of parts of James Todano's excellent talk at the Front Line Doctor's summit, part 2 of the inside summit:

Doctor goes on offensive after coordinated attacks on hydroxychloroquine

Dr. James Todaro stood on the steps of the Supreme Court last week to join fellow doctors in touting hydroxychloroquine as a viable early-stage treatment for those who contract the coronavirus — and says he was stunned by the backlash.

Video of the doctors triggered the internet, with Twitter pulling down tweets that showed clips of the event, even suspending the account of presidential son Donald Trump Jr., insisting that the doctors and anyone on social media who backed them were spreading bad medicine amid the pandemic.

"I've never seen so many different institutional levels attack," said Dr. Todaro, a former physician turned investment manager with Blocktown Capital. "It seems like a coordinated effort to discredit hydroxychloroquine."

The treatment, a favorite topic of President Trump especially early in the pandemic, has become a dividing line in America. Many scientists and doctors dismiss it out of hand. Some states have banned its use as a COVID-19 treatment. The Food and Drug Administration has issued strict cautions about its use — though the agency says decisions about it should be left to doctors and patients.

It's one of many fractures surrounding the coronavirus, pulling back the curtain on the kind of fierce medical debates that usually play out in academic journals and conferences, not on cable news shows.

Dr. Todaro is not the most famous member of the hydroxychloroquine club. Dr. Vladimir "Zev" Zelenko in New York did the "clinical legwork" in support of the Zelenko protocol, the controversial early treatment regimen that uses a three-drug cocktail of hydroxychloroquine, azithromycin and zinc.

But Dr. Todaro has been one of the most effective combatants in the public debate, instrumental in getting retractions from the world's most prestigious medical journals and a growing social media audience.

He's even the unexpected possessor of a Twitter "blue check" signifying verified status — "I was kind of surprised I got that," he told The Washington Times.

He zealously guards his privacy. When asked where he lives and his age, he said, "In the Midwest" and "mid-30s."

He trained as an ophthalmologist at Columbia University medical school, graduating in 2014, but has since allowed his license to lapse. In addition to the investments, he runs a website, Medicine Uncensored, and says he neither holds drug company stocks nor has placed bets on them, short or long.

Dr. Todaro says he launched Medicine Uncensored because he was startled by the offensive against medicines that he considers safe, effective and affordable. The push against non-patented hydroxychloroquine has come on two fronts, he said, one medical; the other political.

"If it seems like the medical system (e.g., NIH, WHO, medical journals, institutional experts) is rigged against hydroxychloroquine," he tweeted recently, "it's because it is." The political side of the anti-hydroxychloroquine push he chalks up to hatred for Mr. Trump, but Dr. Todaro insists that alone cannot account for the fury and the breadth of anti-hydroxychloroquine sentiment.

"Many attribute this negative publicity to anti-Trump sentiment from mainstream media outlets including CNN, MSNBC, Washington Post, New York Times and Huffington Post. This thesis does not entirely hold up to scrutiny though," he wrote in a July essay at Omni.

In fact, as Dr. Todaro points out, at a March 19 press conference in which Mr. Trump heralded hydroxychloroquine, he also mentioned another drug that has been widely embraced by the medical community and media since — remdesivir.

"The media attacked hydroxychloroquine but gave remdesivir a pass when at that time there was no clinical evidence of remdesivir's effectiveness," Dr. Todaro said.
Studies have shown remdesivir slices coronavirus' mortality rate and helps about one-third of coronavirus patients get better quicker. But it also represents a more expensive option, with analysts putting the profits for Gilead Pharmaceutical, its maker, north of $1 billion.

Nevertheless, within 48 hours of Mr. Trump's press conference, Gilead's share price plunged 20%.

"You might also call it a competition killer, hydroxychloroquine," Dr. Todaro said. "It's very hard to make money off it, even if there is grassroots support for it it's really hard to have a financial interest in it."

Hydroxychloroquine's critics argue its benefits appear to be limited to the early stages of the virus and that in sicker patients it can bring on potentially dangerous cardiovascular complications, especially if paired with azithromycin.

One study published in the prestigious medical journal The Lancet in May said hydroxychloroquine's use to treat COVID-19 led to "an increased risk of in-hospital mortality."

"We were unable to confirm a benefit of hydroxychloroquine or chloroquine, when used alone or with a macrolide, on in-hospital outcomes for COVID-19. Each of these drug regimens was associated with decreased in-hospital survival and an increased frequency of ventricular arrhythmias when used for the treatment of COVID-19," the study reported.

That study now has a "RETRACTED" in large red letters on the Lancet website — thanks in large part to Dr. Todaro, after it was shown that the study's data wasn't put together by doctors but by a shadowy online group known as Surgisphere that refused to make the data available for an audit.

"I was flabbergasted by that," Dr. Todaro said. "They say, 'oh, the peer-review process is so rigorous and it's very much intact,' but this phony study wasn't caught by any of their authors or Lancet editors? That's never happened before."

Lost in the controversy surrounding some of Dr. Todaro's thesis is the fact he thinks remdesivir works, too. He wants to expand the weapons in medicine's anti-coronavirus arsenal, not undermine other treatments, he said.

In the process, however, he has found himself an outsider, an Ivy League-educated doctor now branded an iconoclast at best, a villain at worst.

"You have to be terrified of it," he said of the "coordinated effort" to make his position suspect. "I think what I'm offering should be seen as a hub of information."

https://m.washingtontimes.com/news/2020/aug/2/dr-james-todaro-launches-medicine-uncensored-after/

****

& here you can see Dr. James Todano's study on the positive use of HCQ on patients from March 13th, 2020. This was removed/censored from the internet at some point in the 'pandemic'. But he has gotten it back up here.

An Effective Treatment for Coronavirus (COVID-19)

Presented by: James M. Todaro, MD (Columbia MD, jtodaro2@gmail.com) and Gregory J. Rigano, Esq. (grigano1@jhu.edu)

In consultation with Stanford University School of Medicine, UAB School of Medicine and National Academy of Sciences researchers.

March 13, 2020

https://docs.google.com/document/d/e/2PACX-1vTi-g18ftNZUMRAj2SwRPodtscFio7bJ7GdNgbJAGbdfF67WuRJB3ZsidgpidB2eocFHAVjIL-7deJ7/pub

****

Ok, so James Todano went to Stanford. Stanford seems to have at least 2 awesome covid containment skeptics who have been vocal expressing their resistance to the government pandemic response!! Yay!! After James Todaro, there are 2 actual professors there who are doing major studies and getting their names out there against what is going on. They are Professor Michael Levitt, and Professor John Ionnidis.

- **Michael Levitt** - Levitt is a nobel prize-winning structural biology professor at Stanford who has been tracking the coronavirus consistantly for the past 6 plus months. He is one of several scientists who have been advocating against the lockdown and backing alternative theories on the future of the Covid-19 pandemic. Levitt is not an epidemiologist, but has been studying the disease, using methods and data different from what most epidemiologists have been using. He has been making predictive models that go against those designed by Gates https://www.stanforddaily.com/2020/08/02/qa-michael-levitt-on-why-there-shouldnt-be-a-lockdown-how-hes-been-tracking-coronavirus/ & here is his team helping me compile his awesome data: https://med.stanford.edu/levitt.html
- **John P.A. Ionnidis** is a professor of medicine and professor of epidemiology and population health, as well as a professor by courtesy of biomedical data science at Stanford University School of Humaniteis and Sciences, and co-director of the Meta-Research Innovation Center at Stanford (METRICS) at Stanford University. https://www.statnews.com/2020/03/17/a-fiasco-in-the-making-as-the-coronavirus-pandemic-takes-hold-we-are-making-decisions-without-reliable-data/

****

The Jeff Landry-Facebook-HCQ Kerfuffle

August 5th, 2020 MacAoidh

Check out this Newsweek piece about Louisiana Attorney General Jeff Landry's letter to Facebook, and see if you can spot the horrendous journalism in it…

The Louisiana attorney general has complained to Facebook about its removal of a viral video filled with lies about COVID-19 treatments.

In a letter to CEO Mark Zuckerberg dated August 3, Republican AG Jeff Landry accused the social media platform of "showing political bias" by deleting a clip that spread last month after being hosted by the far-right website Breitbart News.

"It seems you and your team at Facebook choose to censor or misuse your algorithms to downplay voices on one side of issues while failing to do so on the other. This now appears to be true when it comes to treatments for COVID-19," he wrote.

"I am asking that you respect the agency and intelligence of the American people to make their own decisions, free from your Orwellian benevolence," he added.

The footage—which was taken during an event organized by an unknown group dubbed "America's Frontline Doctors"—contained false and potentially dangerous claims about the viral disease that has killed more than 155,000 people in America.

The group, claiming to consist of physicians who had treated COVID-19 patients, met at the steps of the U.S. Supreme Court in Washington, D.C. on July 27.

Did you catch it?

"False and potentially dangerous claims."

Says who?

Jason Murdock is the author of this piece…

Jason Murdock is a staff reporter for Newsweek.

Based in London, Murdock previously covered cybersecurity for the International Business Times UK and B2B tech for V3.co.uk. Winner of The Drum's 'Digital Writer of the Year' award in 2017. Contact: j.murdock@newsweek.com
If Jason Murdock was a medical doctor, you'd expect that would be in his bio. And no, covering cybersecurity might give you some expertise on computer viruses but not the organic kind. Sorry.

Who is this guy to say that the things the America's Frontline Doctors folks said were "false and potentially dangerous?"

Let's remember that it was in Murdock's own publication that the head of epidemiology at Yale, Dr. Harvey Risch, posted a full-throated defense of hydroxychloroquine and called it a cure for COVID-19.

Why would Newsweek run Risch's op-ed if it was "false and potentially dangerous?"

We've been struggling to understand this complete collapse of any semblance of objectivity in major news organs over the past couple of years, brought out in stark relief by the COVID-19 panic and the legacy media's coverage of it. We're not going to declare that Risch is correct and that hydroxychloroquine, along with zinc and azithromycin, is a cure for COVID. We've seen a whole lot of anecdotal evidence to that effect, and then we've seen public health bureaucrats and hospital administrators come running out with their hair on fire to declare that it doesn't work at all.

We already know there's a financial piece to this, with respect to remdesivir and the amount of money that can be made if it becomes the universal treatment for COVID. At something like $3,000 per course of medication, compared to maybe $50 for the HCQ protocol, you're looking at the ability to make a serious markup off dosing COVID patients with it.

And if remdesivir works better than HCQ, great. It's worth $2,950 a head to keep people from dying of COVID.

But it's worth pointing out that over four million Americans have had HCQ prescribed to them for lupus and rheumatoid arthritis over the years, and it's pretty well tested despite the sudden claims it's "potentially dangerous." HCQ has been the go-to medication for malaria for better than half a century, and somehow it's "potentially dangerous." This is a drug that's available over the counter in most of the world, for crying out loud.

To call it unpersuasive to say HCQ is some hidden killer in the medicine cabinet is to be charitable. "Clear bullshit" is a more apt description.

It's worthwhile to note at this point that Landry isn't just some blowhard politician where this question is concerned. He tested positive for COVID-19 a few weeks back. When that happened, Landry's doctor prescribed HCQ, and whether it worked or not on him, Landry was asymptomatic the entire time until he tested negative for the virus later. He takes prescription meds for allergies, and it's possible those might have had an effect on keeping the virus from doing anything to him, but it's a fact that Landry took HCQ when he had the virus, didn't get sick and then tested negative.

[..]

- https://thehayride.com/2020/08/the-jeff-landry-facebook-hcq-kerfuffle/

****

A Study Out of Thin Air

by James M Todaro, MD (Columbia MD, @JamesTodaroMD)

May 29, 2020

Misinformation is bad. Misinformation in medicine is worse. Misinformation from a prestigious medical journal is the worst. Herein is a detailed look at the controversial Lancet study that resulted in the World Health Organization ending worldwide clinical trials on hydroxychloroquine in order to focus on patented therapeutics.

Study Overview

In brief, the Lancet study is a multinational registry analysis assessing the effectiveness of hydroxychloroquine or chloroquine with or without macrolide therapy (e.g. azithromycin) in treatment of COVID-19 in hospitalized patients. The study was very large (perhaps impossibly so, but we will address that later) and included 96,032 patients, of which 14,888 were in treatment groups. The study found that hydroxychloroquine and chloroquine with or without macrolide therapy resulted in significantly increased risk of both in-hospital mortality and de-novo ventricular arrhythmia during hospitalization. **In summary, the authors concluded that hydroxychloroquine and chloroquine are actually harmful and increase risk of death when used for in-hospital treatment of COVID-19.**

The Lancet study was released on Friday, May 22. After deliberating over a weekend, on Monday, May 25, the World Health Organization hastily announced the cessation of all COVID-19 clinical trials on hydroxychloroquine in 17 different countries. **Instead of performing its own due diligence, the WHO immediately relied on an observational study cloaked in the reputation of the nearly 200-year old medical journal *The Lancet*.**

After its publication, a grass-roots investigation by hundreds of physicians and researchers worldwide revealed irreconcilable inconsistencies in the data that *The Lancet's* peer-review process overlooked. The study is now found to have inconsistencies with data from national registries of hospitalized COVID-19 patients. The authors continue to hide data sources in a black box controlled by an unknown corporation called Surgisphere.

Surgisphere

Only one peer-reviewed publication prior to the Lancet study.

Surgisphere appears to be the sole provider of the data for the Lancet study, and boasts itself to be a real-time global research network that "performs cloud-based healthcare data analytics" using machine learning and artificial intelligence.

Based on the Lancet study, it must be a very large, sophisticated network indeed to have partnered with hundreds of hospitals worldwide with the capability of retrieving detailed patient data in real-time.

One would expect a multinational database such as this to be a treasure trove coveted by researchers. Strangely, this is not so. Surgisphere has a razor thin folder of contributions to past publications. Besides the Lancet publication, Surgisphere's only other peer-reviewed publication is one entitled Cardiovascular, Drug Therapy, and Mortality in Covid-19 that was published on May 1, 2020 in The New England Journal of Medicine.

The Research section of Surgisphere's website features twenty-three "Case Studies from Around the World" as evidence of their prior work and product features. The vast majority of these "case studies" lack scientific substance and actually consist of short letters, press releases or potential use-cases for its database.

In place of actual research, the website appears primarily promotional and gives the impression of an immature tech company with lofty goals as opposed to a global database with real-time data on millions of patients.

A company with only five employees, most of which joined only two months ago.

According to LinkedIn, Surgisphere has five employees, only one of which has a medical degree—the founder Dr. Sapan Desai. The remaining four employees appear to have little to no science or medical background, but with a plethora of experience in business development and sales & marketing. The team's personnel consist of a VP of Business Development and Strategy, VP of Sales and Marketing and two freelance writers creating content for Surgisphere.

With the exception of the founder, the entire Surgisphere team joined the corporation only 2-3 months ago. Actually, according to LinkedIn, the VP of Sales & Marketing is still employed by another tech company, W.L. Gore & Associates. Prior to February 2020, Surgisphere appears to have had a single employee, the founder.

A shrouded internet history.

The internet trail behind Surgisphere is peculiar to say the least. Mostly because it isn't there. The Internet Archive (Wayback Machine) has records on more than 439 billion web pages and has long served as a tool to view webpages as they existed in the past. I've used the tool hundreds of times and am frequently surprised by the breadth of its database. Even some of the most obscure webpages have historical snapshots available. In the rare circumstances where a historical snapshot is not available, the Wayback Machine's response is "Wayback Machine doesn't have that page archived." A far less common response—one I've never seen before—is "Sorry. This URL has been excluded from the Wayback Machine."

It's this last response that is delivered when searching https://surgisphere.com/ in the Wayback Machine.

There are primarily two ways for companies to hide internet histories. First, they can insert special codes into their websites to hide from the Wayback Machine's automated crawlers. Secondly, companies can request the removal of their historical snapshots, but there's no guarantee the Internet Archive will honor these requests. Both of these practices are highly unusual and almost exclusively used for obscuring nefarious activities.

A list of subsidiary companies without substance.

A deeper dive into Surgisphere reveals three subsidiary companies: Surgical Outcomes Collaborative, Vascular Outcomes and Quartz Clinical. On each of the homepages of these three websites, the Surgisphere copyright is publicly visible near the bottom of the page.

[..]

Data inconsistencies were found nonetheless.

Strike #1. Australia is unique because it is both a country and continent, which makes data obfuscation more challenging. Thus, it is no surprise that false data was first discovered in Australia. The Guardian reported yesterday that the number of COVID-19 deaths included in the Lancet study for Australia exceeded the total nationally recorded number of COVID-19 deaths. The Lancet study reported 73 deaths from the continent of Australia, but records show that Australia had only a total of 67 COVID-19 deaths by April 21. When confronted with this inconsistency, the lead author of the study, Dr. Mandeep Mehra, admitted the error but dismissed it as simply a single hospital that was accidentally designated to the wrong continent.

Strike #2. North American data from the study is highly suspicious. The study reports that 63,315 hospitalized patients with COVID-19 met inclusion criteria prior to April 14, 2020. A review of the well-curated data from the COVID Tracking Project by *The Atlantic* shows that there were only 63,276 patients hospitalized with COVID-19 by April 14. It is theoretically possible that Surgisphere also collected patient data from Canada and Mexico. However, both of these countries had a tiny number of COVID-19 hospitalizations in comparison to the USA. On April 16, Canada reported 2,019 COVID-19 hospitalizations. Although data is not readily available on COVID-19 hospitalizations in Mexico, the country had only 5,014 positive cases and 332 deaths by April 14. Based on common rates of case-to-hospitalization ratios, it is likely that Mexico had fewer than 1,000 COVID-19 hospitalizations. Thus, the total number of COVID-19 hospitalizations in North America (USA, Canada and Mexico) by April 14 is about 66,000.

Are we to believe that Surgisphere truly had relationships and data exchange agreements with 559 hospitals in the USA, Canada and Mexico that captured detailed patient records for 63,315 COVID-19 patients out of a total of 66,000 patients? These figures do not even include the 2,230 patients with COVID-19 who did not meet the inclusion criteria, meaning that Surgisphere is claiming they have patient data on even a greater number than 63,315 patients.

Strike #3. The study reports patient data from Africa that requires sophisticated patient monitoring technology and electronic medical record systems. An open letter to The Lancet signed by 146 physicians and medical researchers believes this to be unlikely. For the data to be valid, nearly 25% of all COVID-19 cases and 40% of all deaths in the continent would have occurred in Surgisphere-affiliated hospitals with sophisticated electronic patient data recording and monitoring capable of detecting and recording "nonsustained [at least 6 sec] or sustained ventricular tachycardia or ventricular fibrillation." In the setting of a highly contagious virus, continuous cardiac monitoring is not always utilized as it increases high-risk patient contact for healthcare workers. **A combination of cardiac monitoring practices during COVID-19 and the sophisticated equipment necessary to do so make it highly unlikely that cardiac arrhythmia data is available for such a large percentage of patients in Africa.**

[..]

Surgisphere Responds

Surgisphere responded to inquiries by refusing to provide any additional details on the data sources and instead asking physicians and researchers to trust them.

Does a corporation that appeared out of thin air two months ago deserve this trust?

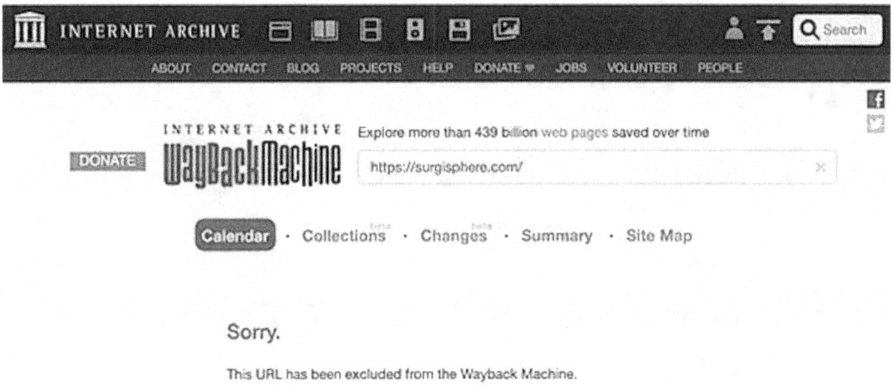

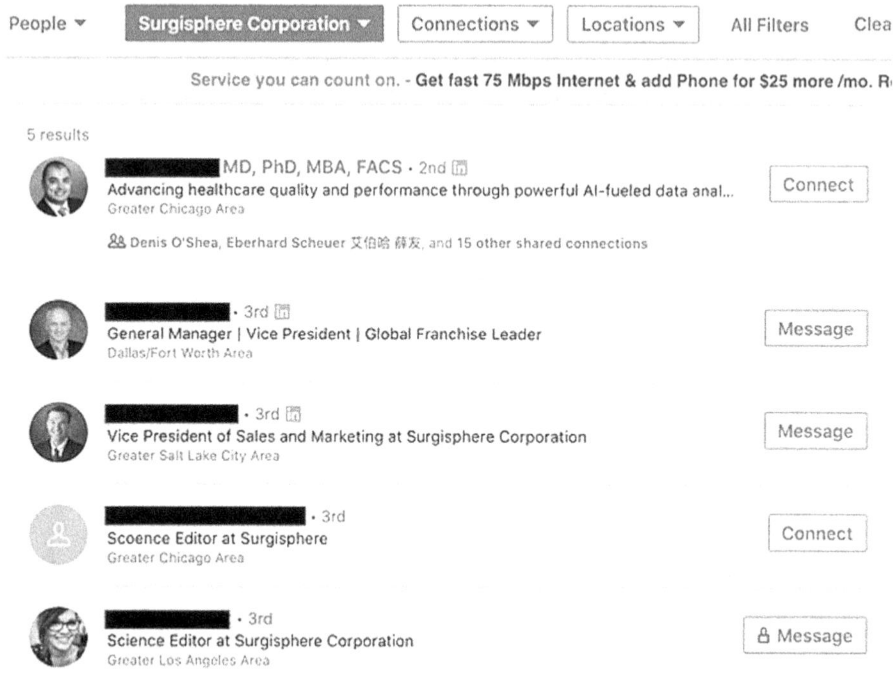

People ▾ | Surgisphere Corporation ▾ | Connections ▾ | Locations ▾ | All Filters | Clea

Service you can count on. - Get fast 75 Mbps Internet & add Phone for $25 more /mo. R

5 results

[redacted] MD, PhD, MBA, FACS · 2nd
Advancing healthcare quality and performance through powerful AI-fueled data anal...
Greater Chicago Area
Denis O'Shea, Eberhard Scheuer 艾伯哈 薛友, and 15 other shared connections
Connect

[redacted] · 3rd
General Manager | Vice President | Global Franchise Leader
Dallas/Fort Worth Area
Message

[redacted] · 3rd
Vice President of Sales and Marketing at Surgisphere Corporation
Greater Salt Lake City Area
Message

[redacted] · 3rd
Scoence Editor at Surgisphere
Greater Chicago Area
Connect

[redacted] · 3rd
Science Editor at Surgisphere Corporation
Greater Los Angeles Area
Message

- https://www.medicineuncensored.com/a-study-out-of-thin-air

****

An Effective Treatment for Coronavirus (COVID-19)_

Updated automatically every 5 minutes

An Effective Treatment for Coronavirus (COVID-19)

Presented by: James M. Todaro, MD (Columbia MD, jtodaro2@gmail.com) and Gregory J. Rigano, Esq. (grigano1@jhu.edu)

In consultation with Stanford University School of Medicine, UAB School of Medicine and National Academy of Sciences researchers.

March 13, 2020

SPANISH: https://docs.google.com/document/d/e/2PACX-1vR1adodKPhWalV9djnerI2x_v1LGgGyhZZxpl0O5r-

ZNyDdagqFq1rTCxXBqaeicfxgvypDOqKCZVyV/pub
Translation by: Celia Martínez-Aceves (**Yale** B.S. Candidate 2021; celia.martinez-aceves@yale.edu), Martín Martínez (**MIT** B.S. 2017 ; martin.martinez.mit@gmail.com)

ITALIAN: https://docs.google.com/document/d/e/2PACX-1vSjPNh_WX6FXUIE3OaA3ScsW7yIH3-SpZyYzElNQUNuJvDmD9eFzM29mVXeaYRY-rjGv52wkrZNa7tb/pub
Translation by: Google Translate and edited by Ross Shulman, **Cornell University** MS '20 ross.shulman@gmail.com

Summary

Recent guidelines from South Korea and China report that chloroquine is an effective antiviral therapeutic treatment against Coronavirus Disease 2019. Use of chloroquine (tablets) is showing favorable outcomes in humans infected with Coronavirus including faster time to recovery and shorter hospital stay. US CDC research shows that chloroquine also has strong potential as a prophylactic (preventative) measure against coronavirus in the lab, while we wait for a vaccine to be developed. Chloroquine is an inexpensive, globally available drug that has been in widespread human use since 1945 against malaria, autoimmune and various other conditions.

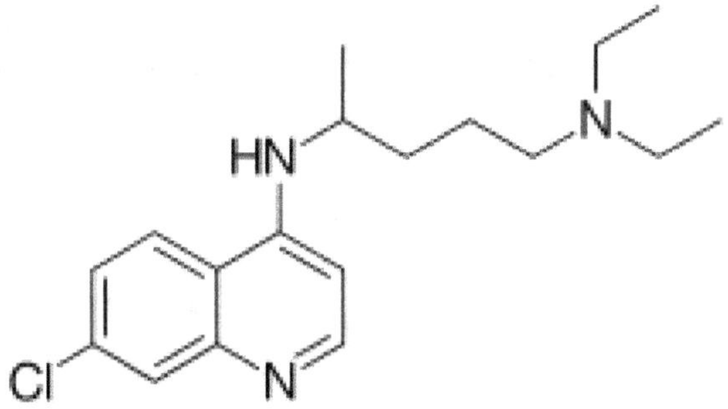

Chloroquine: $C_{18}H_{26}ClN_3$

Background

The U.S. CDC and World Health Organization have not published treatment measures against Coronavirus disease 2019 ("COVID-19"). Medical centers are starting to have issues with traditional protocols. Treatments, and ideally a preventative measure, are needed. South Korea and China have had significantly more exposure and time to analyze diagnostic, treatment and preventative options. The U.S., Europe and the rest of the world can learn from their experience. According to former FDA commissioner, board member of Pfizer and Illumina, Scott Gotlieb MD, the world can learn the most about COVID-19 by paying closest attention to the response of countries that have had significant exposure to COVID-19 before the U.S. and Europe.

As per the U.S. CDC, "Chloroquine (also known as chloroquine phosphate) is an antimalarial medicine… Chloroquine is available in the United States by prescription only… Chloroquine can be prescribed for either **prevention or treatment** of malaria. Chloroquine can be prescribed to adults and children of all ages. It can also be safely taken by pregnant women and nursing mothers."

CDC research also shows that "chloroquine can affect virus infection in many ways, and the antiviral effect depends in part on the extent to which the virus utilizes endosomes for entry. Chloroquine has been widely used to treat human diseases, such as malaria, amoebiosis, HIV, and autoimmune diseases, without significant detrimental side effects."

The treatment guidelines of both South Korea and China against COVID-19 are generally consistent, outlining chloroquine as an effective treatment.

[..]

Treatment Guidelines from South Korea

According to the Korea Biomedical Review, the South Korean COVID-19 Central Clinical Task Force guidelines are as follows:

1. If patients are young, healthy, and have mild symptoms without underlying conditions, doctors can observe them without antiviral treatment;

2. If more than 10 days have passed since the onset of the illness and the symptoms are mild, physicians do not have to start an antiviral medication;

3. However, if patients are old or have underlying conditions with serious symptoms, physicians should consider an antiviral treatment. If they decide to use the antiviral therapy, they should start the administration as soon as possible:

… chloroquine 500mg orally per day.

4. As chloroquine is not available in Korea,

doctors could consider hydroxychloroquine 400mg orally per day (Hydroxychloroquine is an analog of chloroquine used against malaria, autoimmune disorders, etc. It is widely available as well).

5. The treatment is suitable for 7 - 10 days, which can be shortened or extended depending on clinical progress.

Notably, the guidelines mention other antivirals as further lines of defense, including anti-HIV drugs.

Treatment Guidelines from China

According to China's Novel Coronavirus Pneumonia Diagnosis and Treatment Plan, 7th Edition, the treatment guidelines are as follows:

1. Treatment for mild cases includes bed rest, supportive treatments, and maintenance of caloric intake. Pay attention to fluid and electrolyte balance and maintain homeostasis. Closely monitor the patient's vitals and oxygen saturation.

2. As indicated by clinical presentations, monitor the hematology panel, routine urinalysis, CRP, biochemistry (liver enzymes, cardiac enzymes, kidney function), coagulation, arterial blood gas analysis, chest radiography, and so on. Cytokines can be tested, if possible.

3. Administer effective oxygenation measures promptly, including nasal catheter, oxygen mask, and high flow nasal cannula. If conditions allow, a hydrogen-oxygen gas mix (H_2/O_2: 66.6%/33.3%) may be used for breathing.

4. Antiviral therapies:

... chloroquine phosphate (adult 18-65 years old weighing more than 50kg: 500mg twice daily for 7 days; bodyweight less than 50kg: 500mg twice daily for day 1 and 2, 500mg once daily for day 3 through 7) …

Additionally, the Guangdong Provincial Department of Science and Technology and the Guangdong Provincial Health and Health Commission issued a report stating "Expert consensus on chloroquine phosphate for new coronavirus pneumonia: … clinical research results show that chloroquine improves the success rate of treatment and shortens the length of patient's hospital stay."[9] The report further goes on to cite research from the US CDC from 2005 as well as research from the University of Leuven University in Belgium regarding chloroquine's effectiveness against SARS coronavirus at the cellular level.[10]

Like the South Korean guidelines, notably, other antivirals (e.g. anti-HIV drugs) are listed as further lines of defense. The most research thus far has been around chloroquine.

Chloroquine as a prophylactic (preventative) measure against COVID-19

According to research by the US CDC, chloroquine has strong antiviral effects on SARS coronavirus, both prophylactically and therapeutically. SARS coronavirus has significant similarities to COVID-19. Specifically, the CDC research was completed in primate cells using chloroquine's well known function of elevating endosomal pH. The results show that "We have identified chloroquine as an effective antiviral agent for SARS-CoV in cell culture conditions, as evidenced by its inhibitory effect when the drug was added prior to infection or after the initiation and establishment of infection. The fact that chloroquine exerts an antiviral effect during pre- and post-infection conditions suggest that it is likely to have both prophylactic and therapeutic advantages."

The study shows that chloroquine is effective in preventing SARS-CoV infection in cell culture if the drug is added to the cells 24 h prior to infection.

[..]

- https://docs.google.com/document/d/e/2PACX-1vTi-g18ftNZUMRAj2SwRPodtscFio7bJ7GdNgbJAGbdfF67WuRJB3ZsidgpidB2eocFHAVjIL-7deJ7/pub

****

Q&A: Michael Levitt on why there shouldn't be a lockdown, how he's been tracking coronavirus

By Zenobia Lloyd on August 2, 2020

Michael Levitt is a Nobel Prize-winning structural biology professor at Stanford who has been tracking the coronavirus consistently for the past six months. He is one of several scientists who have been advocating against the lockdown and backing alternative theories on the future of the COVID-19 pandemic. Levitt is not an epidemiologist, but has been studying the disease, using methods and data different from what most epidemiologists have been using.

The Stanford Daily (TSD): How did you generate your first few predictions on the coronavirus?

Michael Levitt (ML): I started to look at the numbers when there was no one looking at the numbers — on Jan. 27 and Jan. 28. There were only a few cases in two places after six days. The first thing I was really concerned about was the death rate in the province of Hubei, where the outbreak started, and then the rest of China.

What I noticed right from the very beginning is that the case fatality ratio was more than 10 times higher inside Hubei than outside Hubei.

Many people generally look at the number of cases, the number of deaths, the death rate, but there was something that I did then, which was probably out of ignorance, that ended up being very useful: Looking at the number of deaths today divided by the number of deaths yesterday, and calculating the ratio and the percent increase.

When I looked at the percent increase, it went from a 100 to 120 to 144 percent increase and so on. And that becomes a very big number, very quickly. When I did this on Feb. 1, I noticed that the numbers for the ratio of deaths today over deaths yesterday had gone from a 30% increase on the 28th of February down to an 18% increase. After four days it had gone down steadily from a 30% increase per day to an 18% percent increase.

I didn't publish it anywhere. I made a two-page PDF and sent it out to people through WhatsApp and then actually got on a flight. It ended up getting like 2 million [views] pretty quickly and suddenly I actually had skin in the game. So I started to study the numbers every single day. I wrote 24 reports in February, each day, just doing a bit more analysis, and trying to predict when the pandemic would end.

TSD: For your earlier predictions, were there any mistakes that you made or anything that you didn't account for when making them?

ML: There were a lot of things. It's very hard to know what the ending total number of deaths will be, but there are ways to try and calculate it. You can look at the number of cases per day over the number of new deaths per day.

This is now done very commonly. And then when the number of cases gets to a peak, you can predict that the number of deaths are around a third of the way through. It's a rough estimate, but if you know exactly where the peak is, then it *usually* does work.

Going off of the only numbers that I already had, it basically quite clearly said that inside Hubei, there would be a few thousand deaths, and outside of Hubei in China there would only be a few hundred deaths. And that was enough to give people more confidence in understanding the virus, though I don't think it really prepared the rest of the world for what was going to end up happening.

TSD: How has your outlook changed over the course of the past four months as COVID-19 spreads and new research comes out?

ML: I don't think it really has changed. I have overall been pretty consistent in my opinion. One thing that did change for me was that I used to never use Twitter at all. I thought Twitter was stupid. And then I first used it for COVID-19 towards the end of March when I had just started studying cases in New York City.

A lot of people would see my tweets and actually sent me helpful information, and I was really impressed. It's a great way to get information.

TSD: What do you wish that people had understood at the start of the coronavirus pandemic?

ML: Firstly, one thing that was not publicized in the very beginning, that was actually known, was the age distribution of the deaths.

People who were older had a much higher chance of dying, but the trouble was that, comparatively, there aren't that many old people in China. It's a relatively young country, with a small proportion of the population over the age of 85, whereas in places like Italy, half of the deaths were over 85.

But when this paper came out in the middle of February, no newspapers picked it up and they really should have. They should have said, "Look, this really is a disease that's going to affect old people."

TSD: Is there any policy that you think should have been implemented initially around the world or in the U.S. specifically?

ML: I know one policy that I would have implemented, but it's something no one will talk about.

People live and they die, and it's very sad because we all have people that we've loved who have died and it's terrible, but we know that that's the way the world works.

And it seems to me that dying at 70 isn't the same as dying at the age of 17, no matter how great you think you are and how important you are. The fact is that a 17 year old has, let's say, 60 years of life in front of him, and a 73 year old has maybe five years of life ahead of him.

I saw lots of reports on the amount of deaths from COVID-19 compared to the deaths from the Vietnamese war. Well, maybe the numbers were the same, but the deaths from the Vietnamese war were people in their twenties being sent to defend their country. And it isn't the same thing.

One thing that also I found disturbing was The New York Times ran a front page where they listed the names of the first hundred thousand COVID-19 fatalities. How many of those people died from lots of other reasons? 90% of the people who died from COVID-19 have heart problems, lung problems and other conditions.

During the time that a hundred thousand people died from COVID, another 500,000 people died due to other problems. They shouldn't be any more celebrated than the 500,000 people. This ended up making people incredibly scared because they were publicizing this instead of telling people that all the deaths of COVID-19 in the whole world are three or four days worth of natural deaths, which is the truth.

But no one was brave enough to discuss it. People didn't want to say that if you were 95, you had heart problems and died of COVID, but it wasn't just a terrible tragedy. It isn't a tragedy.

You have something like 8,000 people who die every day in the U.S. and you don't hear about them. And so this is something which I thought was a mistake. It wasn't making it easy for the policymakers to make decisions based on this information because they would be called the "granny killer." The trouble is that the drop in the economy is going to kill many people as well.

Because when you have poverty, life expectancy goes down. If you're going to take a very moral stand, you can't say these deaths matter; those deaths just don't matter.

[..]

- https://www.stanforddaily.com/2020/08/02/qa-michael-levitt-on-why-there-shouldnt-be-a-lockdown-how-hes-been-tracking-coronavirus/

****

Welcome to the Levitt Lab!

Since 28 January 2020, Levitt, his Stanford group and an international team of volunteers have worked tirelessly on data analysis of COVID-19. While widely distributed, our work has been hidden from search engines due to failure of our 25-year old lab website at www.csb.stanford. Follow us on Twitter. Relevant links follow:

2 Feb to 2 Mar. All 22 almost-daily Analyses of COVID-19 in China released by email, WhatsApp, Twitter and WeChat. The shows the best and the worst of real-time science, typos and all.
14 Mar. Analysis of China and Rest of the World. This is a key analysis full of Tables and Figures that is not easy to comprehend; it is the basis of all my subsequent work.
20 Mar. Calcalist Interview with Ari Libsker (Hebrew):
"Israeli Nobel Laureate: Coronavirus spread is slowing" (In English in Jerusalem Post)
22 Mar. LA Times Interview with Joe Mozingo
Why this Nobel laureate predicts a quicker coronavirus recovery: 'We're going to be fine'
22 Mar. The Medium, a first post on the *Excess Burden of Death associated with coronavirus*. This is for saturation of infection, like that on the Diamond Princess which may lead to herd immunity.
25 Mar. *How Accurate are the Number of UK and US Deaths Predicted by Ferguson et al. (2020)?*
16 Apr. Particularly clear Radio New Zealand interview with Dave Campbell: 'No evidence that Covid-19 is causing huge loss of life' (listen)
2 May. Lockdown TV in London, James Billot & Freddie Sayer. *Nobel prize-winning scientist: the Covid-19 epidemic was never exponential*
15 May. Two YouTube podcasts
Exponential_Growth_is_Scarry_Michael_Levitt_14May20 and
Curve_Fitting_for_Understanding_Michael_Levitt_14May2020

[..]

- https://med.stanford.edu/levitt.html

****

A fiasco in the making? As the coronavirus pandemic takes hold, we are making decisions without reliable data

By JOHN P.A. IOANNIDIS MARCH 17, 2020

The current coronavirus disease, Covid-19, has been called a once-in-a-century pandemic. But it may also be a once-in-a-century evidence fiasco.
At a time when everyone needs better information, from disease modelers and governments to people quarantined or just social distancing, we lack reliable evidence on how many people have been infected with SARS-CoV-2 or who continue to become infected. Better information is needed to guide decisions and actions of monumental significance and to monitor their impact.

Draconian countermeasures have been adopted in many countries. If the pandemic dissipates — either on its own or because of these measures — short-term extreme social distancing and lockdowns may be bearable. How long, though, should measures like these be continued if the pandemic churns across the globe unabated? How can policymakers tell if they are doing more good than harm?

Vaccines or affordable treatments take many months (or even years) to develop and test properly. Given such timelines, the consequences of long-term lockdowns are entirely unknown.

The data collected so far on how many people are infected and how the epidemic is evolving are utterly unreliable. Given the limited testing to date, some deaths and probably the vast majority of infections due to SARS-CoV-2 are being missed. We don't know if we are failing to capture infections by a factor of three or 300. Three months after the outbreak emerged, most countries, including the U.S., lack the ability to test a large number of people and no countries have reliable data on the prevalence of the virus in a representative random sample of the general population.

This evidence fiasco creates tremendous uncertainty about the risk of dying from Covid-19. Reported case fatality rates, like the official 3.4% rate from the World Health Organization, cause horror — and are meaningless. Patients who have been tested for SARS-CoV-2 are disproportionately those with severe symptoms and bad outcomes. As most health systems have limited testing capacity, selection bias may even worsen in the near future.

The one situation where an entire, closed population was tested was the Diamond Princess cruise ship and its quarantine passengers. The case fatality rate there was 1.0%, but this was a largely elderly population, in which the death rate from Covid-19 is much higher.

Projecting the Diamond Princess mortality rate onto the age structure of the U.S. population, the death rate among people infected with Covid-19 would be 0.125%. But since this estimate is based on extremely thin data — there were just seven deaths among the 700 infected passengers and crew — the real death rate could stretch from five times lower (0.025%) to five times higher (0.625%). It is also possible that some of the passengers who were infected might die later, and that tourists may have different frequencies of chronic diseases — a risk factor for worse outcomes with SARS-CoV-2 infection — than the general population. Adding these extra sources of uncertainty, reasonable estimates for the case fatality ratio in the general U.S. population vary from 0.05% to 1%.

That huge range markedly affects how severe the pandemic is and what should be done. A population-wide case fatality rate of 0.05% is lower than seasonal influenza. If that is the true rate, locking down the world with potentially tremendous social and financial consequences may be totally irrational. It's like an elephant being attacked by a house cat. Frustrated and trying to avoid the cat, the elephant accidentally jumps off a cliff and dies.

Could the Covid-19 case fatality rate be that low? No, some say, pointing to the high rate in elderly people. However, even some so-called mild or common-cold-type coronaviruses that have been known for decades can have case fatality rates as high as 8% when they infect elderly people in nursing homes. In fact, such "mild" coronaviruses infect tens of millions of people every year, and account for 3% to 11% of those hospitalized in the U.S. with lower respiratory infections each winter.

These "mild" coronaviruses may be implicated in several thousands of deaths every year worldwide, though the vast majority of them are not documented with precise testing. Instead, they are lost as noise among 60 million deaths from various causes every year.

[..]

- https://www.statnews.com/2020/03/17/a-fiasco-in-the-making-as-the-coronavirus-pandemic-takes-hold-we-are-making-decisions-without-reliable-data/

****

August 7, 2020, 5:50AM (Amir-ul Kafirs to group):

Ok, no videos. But a fazillion

One of my favorite numbers!!

Lancet Journal's retracted fake 'study' that steered the world away from HCQ when it was first released, before it was justifiably retracted as 'fake':

Wow, "Surgisphere" is right up there with Eric W. Dolan & *Psy Post*. Remember my July 12, 2020, 7:14PM (tENT to group): HERETICS: Psy Post & Eric W. Dolan?

- **Michael Levitt**

This guy says things that I think are very important that should be obvious but seem to be generally overlooked:

"And it seems to me that dying at 70 isn't the same as dying at the age of 17, no matter how great you think you are and how important you are. The fact is that a 17 year old has, let's say, 60 years of life in front of him, and a 73 year old has maybe five years of life ahead of him.

"I saw lots of reports on the amount of deaths from COVID-19 compared to the deaths from the Vietnamese war. Well, maybe the numbers were the same, but the deaths from the Vietnamese war were people in their twenties being sent to defend their country. And it isn't the same thing. "

****

August 7, 2020, 6:17AM (Amir-ul Kafirs to group):

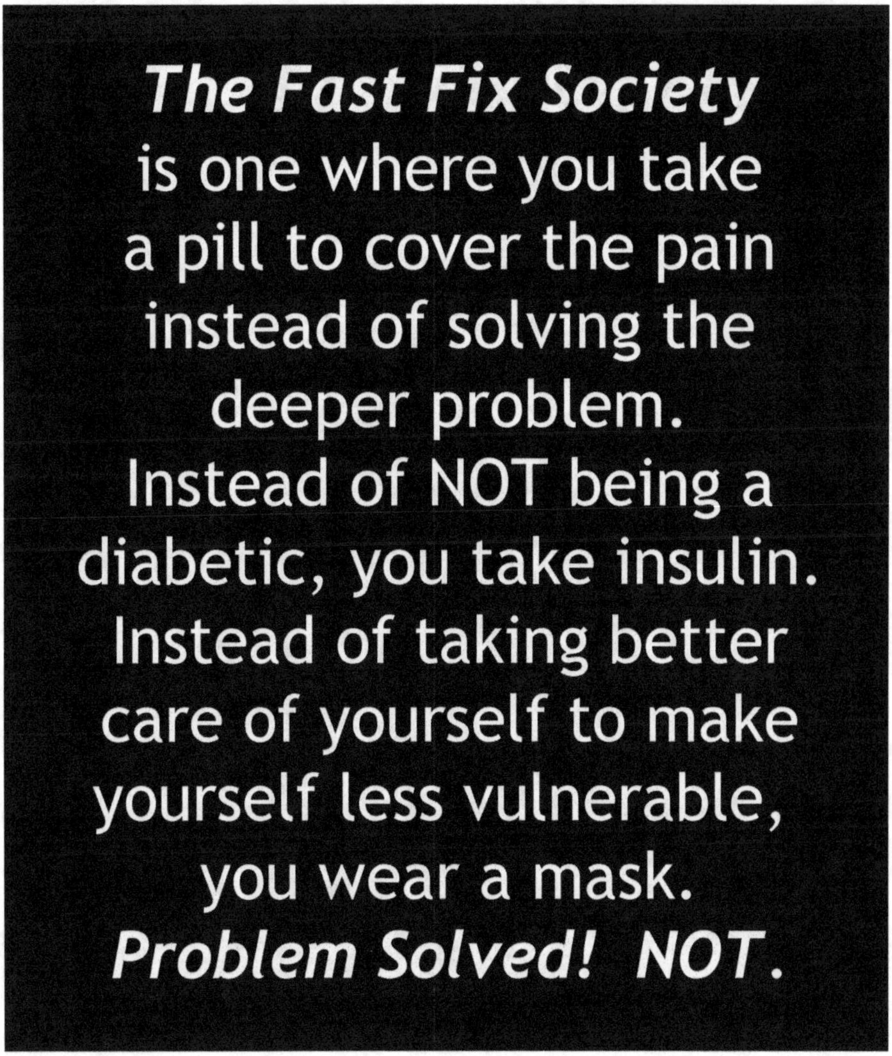

The Fast Fix Society
is one where you take
a pill to cover the pain
instead of solving the
deeper problem.
Instead of NOT being a
diabetic, you take insulin.
Instead of taking better
care of yourself to make
yourself less vulnerable,
you wear a mask.
Problem Solved! NOT.

****

August 7, 2020, 6:22AM (Amir-ul Kafirs to group):

HERETICS: Antibody 1

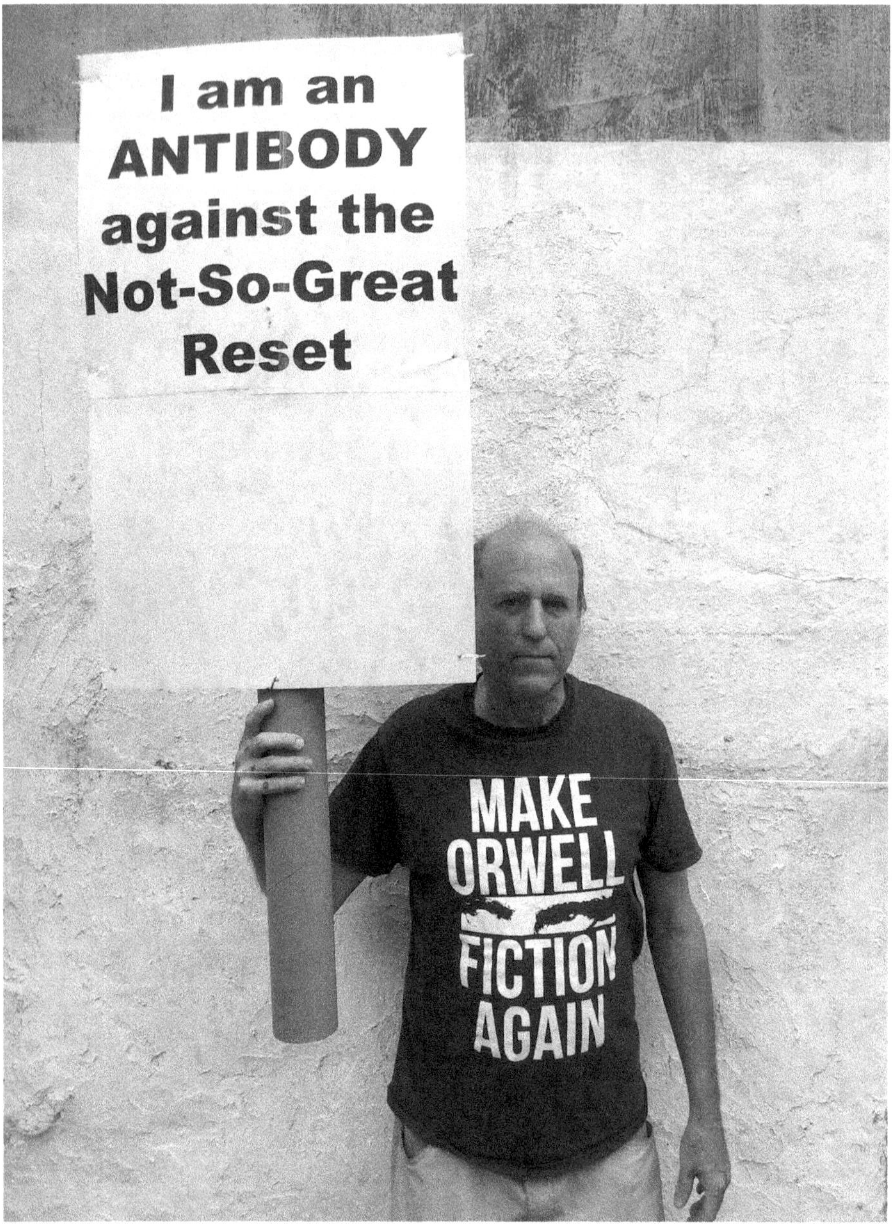

****

August 7, 2020, 12:42PM (Inquiring Librarian to group):

HERETICS: Performance Appraisal Portal

This image pisses me off every time I log into my staff Performance Appraisal portal site. How stupid, to put a mask on Benjamin Franklin. He is likely rolling over in his grave. When the RNA vaccine induced Zombie apocalypse hits, I hope Ben comes back and eats the hell out of the 'brains' of Fauci and all the other head honchos. They even made his eyes look stressed out. Yes, of course he'd be stressed out. These assholes in charge are destroying our country. But I can bet he would not stoop to wear a mask and he'd fight back hard.

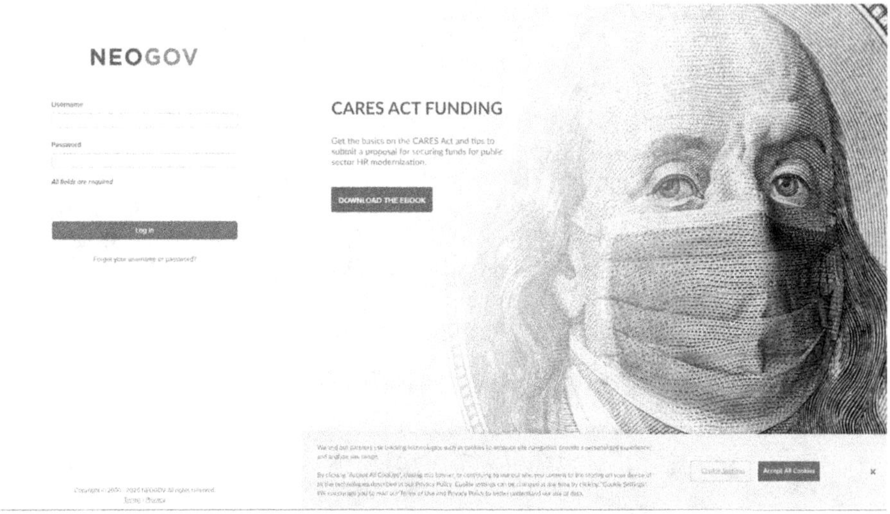

****

August 7, 2020, 1:01PM (Amir-ul Kafirs to group):

Re: HERETICS: Performance Appraisal Portal

This image pisses me off every time I log into my staff Performance Appraisal portal site. How stupid, to put a mask on Benjamin Franklin.

Ha ha! It'll be a nice image to subvert though!

****

August 7, 2020, 1:50PM (Inquiring Librarian to group):

HERETICS: Disgusting Article & Hopeful Talk Show

Let's start with the disgusting first. I like to save the good things for the last.

Defeat COVID-19 by requiring vaccination for all. It's not un-American, it's patriotic.

Make vaccines free, don't allow religious or personal objections, and punish those who won't be vaccinated. They are threatening the lives of others.

"To win the war against the novel coronavirus that has now killed over 158,000 people in this country, the only answer is compulsory vaccination — for all of us. And while the measures that will be necessary to defeat the coronavirus will seem draconian, even anti-American to some, we believe that there is no alternative. Simply put, getting vaccinated is going to be our patriotic duty."
https://www.usatoday.com/story/opinion/2020/08/06/stop-coronavirus-compulsory-universal-vaccination-column/3289948001/?fbclid=IwAR1HQGkg_nzQh64MFwCpRZvTLUe84EpwGMHmoRLoZ-IAIM9MNrjMwX5-6hA
1 word from me - DISGUSTING!!
****

But here is another great one from Del Bigtree's Highwire. Sounds like the people may be winning, major protests in England and in Germany this past week, Moderna board members selling their stocks down to zero, censorship is opening the eyes of the people, Trust in the vaccine is down now to 40% of those polled who would actually take the damn thing. It was taken off of Facebook within an hour or so of it being live streamed:

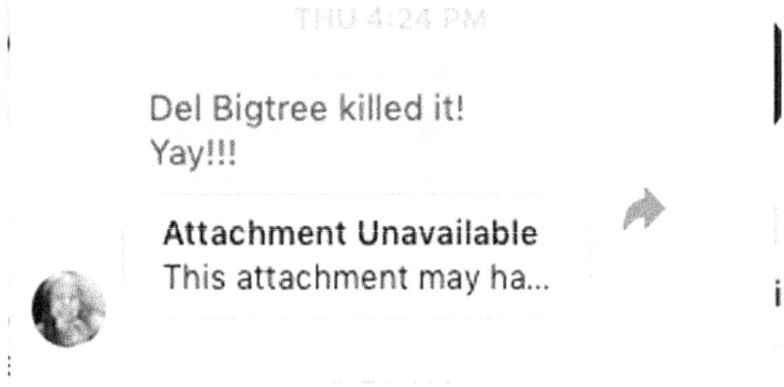

THE HIGHWIRE: THE FRONTLINE PUSHBACK! (BANNED ON FB AND YOUTUBE)

https://www.bitchute.com/video/GysupvP1dHOU/

****

Defeat COVID-19 by requiring vaccination for all. It's not un-American, it's patriotic.

Make vaccines free, don't allow religious or personal objections, and punish those who won't be vaccinated. They are threatening the lives of others.

Dr. Michael Lederman, Maxwell J. Mehlman and Dr. Stuart Youngner
Opinion contributors

[..]

Severe penalties for non-compliance

Nor is there an alternative to vaccine-induced herd immunity in a pandemic. Relying on enough people becoming infected and then immune is dangerous, as exemplified by the Swedish experience where the COVID-19 mortality rate exceeds that of its more cautious neighbors. Broad induction of immunity in the population by immunization will be necessary to end this pandemic. In simple terms, a refusal to be vaccinated threatens the lives of others.
So here's what America must do when a vaccine is ready:

▶ Make vaccinations free and easily accessible.

▶ Exempt only those with medical contraindications to immunization. It is likely that more than one vaccine platform will prove effective (as was the case for polio vaccines) and, as a result, medical conditions that prohibit all COVID-19 vaccines will be rare.

▶ Do not honor religious objections. The major religions do not officially oppose vaccinations.

▶ Do not allow objections for personal preference, which violate the social contract.

[..]

- https://www.usatoday.com/story/opinion/2020/08/06/stop-coronavirus-compulsory-universal-vaccination-column/3289948001/?fbclid=IwAR1HQGkg_nzQh64MFwCpRZvTLUe84EpwGMHmoRLoZ-IAIM9MNrjMwX5-6hA

****

August 7, 2020, 6:14PM (Amir-ul Kafirs to group):

Re: HERETICS: Disgusting Article & Hopeful Talk Show

Defeat COVID-19 by requiring vaccination for all. It's not un-American, it's patriotic.

USA Today is an 'interesting' publication for an academic to publish in, isn't it? Something aimed at, what? A 6th grade reading level? Anyway, this appeal to "patriotism" is just an attempt to corral in the conservatives to 'do their duty'. Yes, DISGUSTING.

****

August 7, 2020, 2:33PM (Inquiring Librarian to group):

Stop Bit Burning . Com

I saw this great interview of Zack Vorhes today. He is organizing a class action lawsuit against google supported platforms. The concept is a modern take on fighting book burning.
https://www.stopbitburning.com/
He is a former Google employee who became a whistleblower against Google, sending a 950 page document with evidence on Google's dirty business on censorship and swaying elections to the DOJ (Dept. of Justice) in D.C, before Google got a hold of him.

Here is Zack's website: "Google Leaks: Censorship Exposed"
https://www.zachvorhies.com/

If you want to see the interview with Zack, it's here. I found it fascinating: https://www.bitchute.com/video/loJJXTILtMUb/

****

August 7, 2020, 6:28PM (Amir-ul Kafirs to group):

Re: Stop Bit Burning . Com

He is organizing a class action lawsuit against google supported platforms.

It's interesting that your email coincides with a related one that I also got today. The following is the beginning of it:

Notice of Class Action Settlement re Google Plus – Your Rights May Be Affected
You are not being sued. This notice affects your rights. Please read it carefully. On June 10, 2020, the Honorable Edward J. Davila of the U.S. District Court for the Northern District of California, granted preliminary approval of this class action Settlement and directed the litigants to provide this notice about the Settlement. You have received this notice because Google's records indicate that you may be a Settlement Class Member, and you may be eligible to receive a payment from the Settlement. Please visit www.GooglePlusDataLitigation.com for more information. The Final Approval Hearing on the adequacy, reasonableness, and fairness of the Settlement will be held at 9:00 am on November 19, 2020 in San Jose Courthouse, Courtroom 4, 5th Floor located at 280 South 1st Street, San Jose, CA 95113. You are not required to attend the Final Approval Hearing, but you are welcome to do so at your own expense.

Summary of Litigation

Google operated the Google+ social media platform for consumers from June 2011 to April 2019. In 2018, Google announced that the Google+ platform had experienced software bugs between 2015 and 2018, which allowed app developers to access certain Google+ profile field information in an unintended manner. Plaintiffs Matthew Matic, Zak Harris, Charles Olson, and Eileen M. Pinkowski thereafter filed this lawsuit asserting various legal claims on behalf of a putative class of Google+ users who were allegedly harmed by the software bugs

("Class"). Google denies Plaintiffs' allegations, denies any wrongdoing and any liability whatsoever, and believes that no Class Members, including the Plaintiffs, have sustained any damages or injuries due to the software bugs.

****

August 7, 2020, 6:05PM (Phil to group):

Re: HERETICS: Book in Progress: PLEASE ANSWER!!

Sorry all for going off the radar a from this group for a while. Things have gotten a bit busy here and I have less time and as a result I have fallen some pages behind in keeping up with the emails. I will hopefully do a bit more of an update on whats going on here early next week but at the moment I have to go to bed and sleep. I have been up since 5 and gotta go to work tomorrow and the next day.

As far as the moms and pops businesses questions I don't have the details and would have to look into it more. Certainly The Netherlands has been hit hard economically like everywhere. A lot of people have lost jobs...I'll try and look up the details later. I think quite a lot of restaurants have closed down. I know it has also hit architectural businesses hard.

Sorry I did not get a text done.
I feel fine about using the name Phil Bradley for the book. As for as 'activist' I am not 100 percent sure about but also have no problems with it so if I come with another suggestion use it. There is nothing in these emails. that I have a problem with as far as being published. Sorry I missed your personal backstory...the link is expired now.

****

August 7, 2020, 6:18PM (Phil to group):

Re: HERETICS: "Beyond Therapy"

Looks like a scary book. The antidote book is 'Against Therapy' by Jeffery Mason. I read it a long time back....

****

August 7, 2020, 9:41PM (Dick to Amir-ul Kafirs):

The photo I mentioned

https://images.app.goo.gl/NdLaWQA2KMyoeFHG9

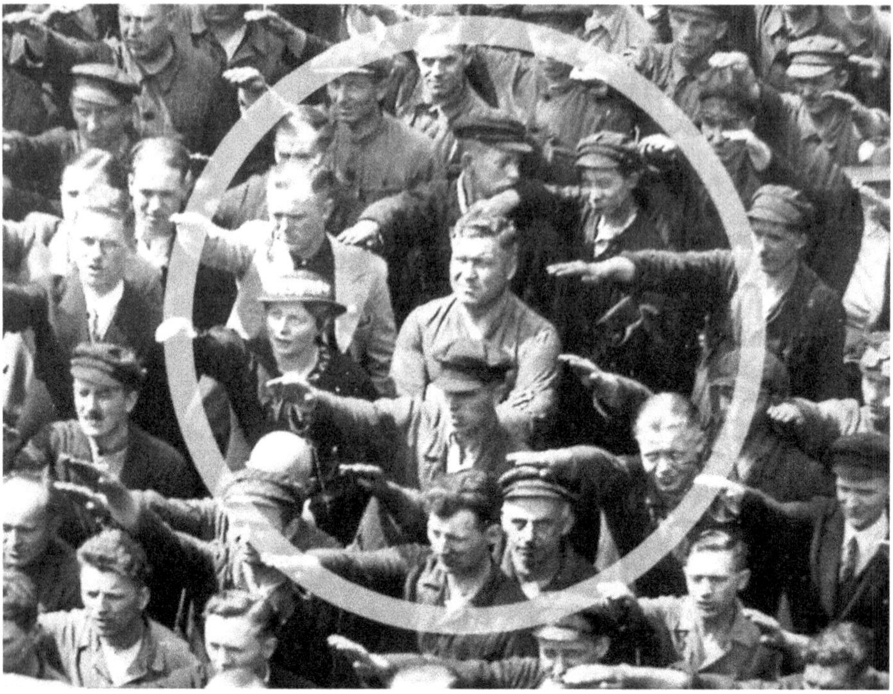

****

August 8, 2020, 9:03AM (Amir-ul Kafirs to Dick):

RE: The photo I mentioned

On Aug 8, 2020, at 9:01 AM, dick turner wrote:

I thought of a caption for it
something like

"people reaching for free masks and look at the loser who doesn't want one!"

Ha ha! This was the caption I put:

When I was a child, I refused to recite the Pledge of Allegiance in Elementary School. I was the only one in my class to do so. That wasn't something taught to me by any adults, such as my parents, that was my own decision. As an adult I went to an open-to-the public rehearsal of the Pittsburgh Opera where everyone but me stood & put their hand over their heart during the Star Spangled Banner. On another occasion I wasn't alone for a change when a small group of us didn't stand & put our hands over our hearts for the National Anthem before a Roller Derby game. One member of that small group of contestaires is still friendly to me here. Recently, I think I was alone again in not participating in such a process at a drive-in movie theater. BEWARE OF

GROUPTHINK.

****

August 9, 2020, 11:23AM (Inquiring Librarian to group):

HERETICS: Science & Health Feedback "Fact-Checked"

I know some time back, we were all wondering who on earth the science and health feedback people were, who funds them, and how accurate are they? Well, this article is a hilarious fish slap in the face to the fact checkers that attacked the original article.

Ok, start with the Fact Check Feedback from the authors of the original article:

Fact-Checking a "Fact-Checker": A Response to HealthFeedback.org

Rosemary Frei

On July 12 an organization called Health Feedback posted a review of my and Patrick Corbett's July 2 OffGuardian article on the bombshell revelations of Bulgarian Pathology Association President Dr. Stoian Alexov. They stamped it "inaccurate."

This article is a refutation of Health Feedback's so-called fact-checking. I show why Dr. Alexov's statements, in fact, fit the evidence, and punch plenty of other holes in Health Feedback's claim that our article is "clearly wrong" and has "very little credibility."

Health Feedback's review is fatally faulty right off the top, when the review's unnamed author **mistakes my co-author Patrick Corbett for James Corbett of The Corbett Report**: the screencap at the top of the review is from James Corbett's June 16 interview with me.

The review also takes a swipe at outlets that reposted our article: it notes Media Bias/Fact Check dubbs GlobalResearch.ca and Australian National Review "conspiracy websites..."

https://off-guardian.org/2020/08/06/fact-checking-a-fact-checker-a-response-to-healthfeedback-org/?fbclid=IwAR0hQgH9xtcouq1UX_--jdKvKhvGvAEhlv_-eKlifAxRzy424mmtajq2bFs

The article is really long and really complicated. But, you get the gist from diving into the article.

****

In case you want to read the original article, it is linked in the above article, but here it is anyways:

"No one has died from the coronavirus" Important revelations shared by Dr Stoian Alexov, President of the Bulgarian Pathology Association

Rosemary Frei and Patrick Corbett

https://off-guardian.org/2020/07/02/no-one-has-died-from-the-coronavirus-president-of-the-bulgarian-pathology-association/

****

& here is the Health Feedback crappy 'Fact Check' of the original article:

People have died from the coronavirus, contrary to article claiming to report pathologist's "revelations" on COVID-19

https://healthfeedback.org/claimreview/people-have-died-from-the-coronavirus-contrary-to-article-claiming-to-report-pathologists-revelations-on-covid-19/

(Note: It looks like the already took the James Corbett photo off of the top of the article, Ha HA!!!!!)

****

People have died from the coronavirus, contrary to article claiming to report pathologist's "revelations" on COVID-19

CLAIM

"no one has died from the coronavirus"

VERDICT

INACCURATE

SOURCE: Patrick Corbett, Rosemary Frei, OffGuardian, 2 Jul. 2020

DETAILS

Inaccurate: Contrary to the article's claims, people have died from COVID-19. This is evident from the excess mortality seen in 2020, in which a higher number of deaths are occurring relative to previous years before the pandemic. As reported by several published studies, antibodies specific for SARS-CoV-2 have also been discovered and the novel coronavirus has been shown to cause COVID-19.

KEY TAKE AWAY

People have died from COVID-19. This is evident from the excess mortality observed in 2020 compared to previous years before the pandemic occurred. Monoclonal antibodies that bind to SARS-CoV-2 have also been discovered and reported in published studies, and pathologists have been using such antibodies, as well as other techniques like in situ hybridization which do not require antibodies, to detect SARS-CoV-2 infection in human tissue.

FULL CLAIM: "no one has died from the coronavirus"; "no novel-coronavirus-specific antibodies have been found"; "the novel coronavirus has not fulfilled Koch's postulates"; "the inability to identify monoclonal antibodies for the virus suggests there is no basis for the vaccines"; "the WHO is creating [worldwide] chaos is by prohibiting almost all autopsies of people deemed to have died from COVID-19"

Originally published by OffGuardian, this article makes numerous claims about the COVID-19 pandemic that have been republished in other outlets such as GlobalResearch.ca and Australian National Review, both of which have been described as conspiracy websites by Media Bias/Fact Check. The article purportedly discloses "important revelations" by Stoian Alexov, a Bulgarian pathologist and president of the Bulgarian Pathology Association, which he allegedly made during a webinar organized by the European Society of Pathology (ESP). The article has received more than 60,000 interactions on social media including Facebook and Twitter.
Health Feedback reached out to several scientists regarding the veracity of Alexov's claims, including members of the ESP leadership, who responded with a joint clarification on behalf of the Society. You can read the ESP's official clarification in full here.

REVIEW

Claim 1:

The article states that Alexov claims that "No one has died from the coronavirus" and that no antibodies specific to SARS-CoV-2 have been identified. It goes on to say that "Dr. Alexov made his jaw-dropping observations in a video interview summarizing the consensus of participants in a May 8, 2020, European Society of Pathology (ESP) webinar on COVID-19."

The webinar referenced in the article, titled "COVID-19: Unprecedented Daily Challenges in Pathology Laboratories across Europe" was indeed organized by the ESP. However, although Alexov is a member, he is not listed among the presenters. Therefore, the claim that Alexov made his remarks at a "consensus of participants" during the ESP webinar—with the implication that his comments were accepted as part of the scientific or medical consensus—is false. The complete proceedings were recorded and are publicly available on the ESP's YouTube channel.

Claim 2:

"no novel-coronavirus-specific antibodies have been found"

This is false. Several published studies report the discovery of antibodies that bind specifically to SARS-CoV-2, the causative agent of COVID-19, as well as antibodies against SARS-CoV-2 in people who had been previously infected[1-4].

[..]

Claim 5:

"the novel coronavirus has not fulfilled Koch's postulates"

Koch's postulates are a set of criteria used to determine whether a certain microorganism is the cause of a disease. They were originally developed by Robert Koch, a German physician who won the Nobel Prize for Physiology or Medicine in 1905 for his work on tuberculosis. The original postulates are as follows:

1. The microorganism must be found in abundance in all organisms suffering from the disease, but should not be found in healthy organisms.
2. The organism must be isolated from a host containing the disease and grown in pure culture.
3. Samples of the organism taken from pure culture must cause the same disease when inoculated into a healthy, susceptible animal in the laboratory.
4. The organism must be isolated from the inoculated animal and must be identified as the same original organism first isolated from the originally diseased host.

While these postulates remain an important foundation for establishing the cause of an infectious disease even today, scientists have also recognized that there are limitations to these criteria. Vincent Racaniello, a virologist and professor at Columbia University's College of Physicians & Surgeons, wrote in his blog post that "Despite the importance of Koch's postulates in the development of microbiology, they have severe limitations, which even Koch realized." For example, Vibrio cholerae, the causative agent of cholera, could be isolated from both sick and healthy people, invalidating postulate #1.

Other notable exceptions to the original postulates that Racaniello pointed out are viruses, such as poliovirus, which causes illness of varying severity and does

not manifest in the same way for all infected individuals. For example, fewer than 1% of individuals infected by polio are affected by paralysis. Additionally, "Postulates #2 and #3 cannot be fulfilled for viruses that do not replicate in cell culture, or for which a suitable animal model has not been identified." Consequently, over the past decades, scientists have found it necessary to modify Koch's postulates to adapt the criteria for the study of viral diseases[11-13].
Ian Lipkin, professor of epidemiology and director at the Center for Infection and Immunity of Columbia University's Mailman School of Public Health, told Health Feedback that many published studies have already demonstrated that SARS-CoV-2 fulfills Koch's postulates[14-16]. Specifically, researchers isolated SARS-CoV-2 from COVID-19 patient samples, propagated the virus in cell cultures in the laboratory, and infected non-human primates with the cultured virus. The infected primates displayed the same signs of COVID-19 as humans, including lung damage and pneumonia. Finally, the researchers were able to detect the virus in the infected animals. With these findings, all four of Koch's postulates are met, demonstrating that SARS-CoV-2 is the cause of COVID-19.

[..]

- https://healthfeedback.org/claimreview/people-have-died-from-the-coronavirus-contrary-to-article-claiming-to-report-pathologists-revelations-on-covid-19/

****

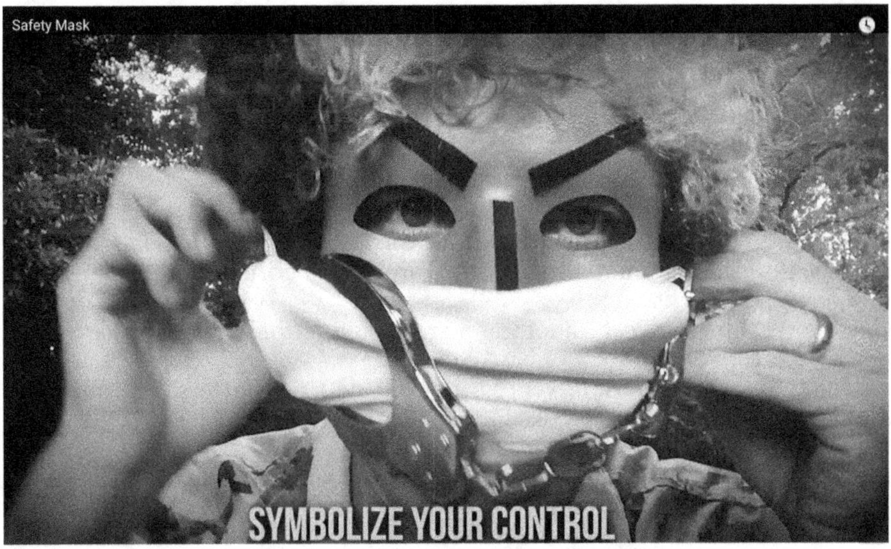

(still from an online video called "Safety Mask")

****

August 9, 2020, 4:00PM (Amir-ul Kafirs to group):

HERETICS: Thought for the Day (One 'Truth')

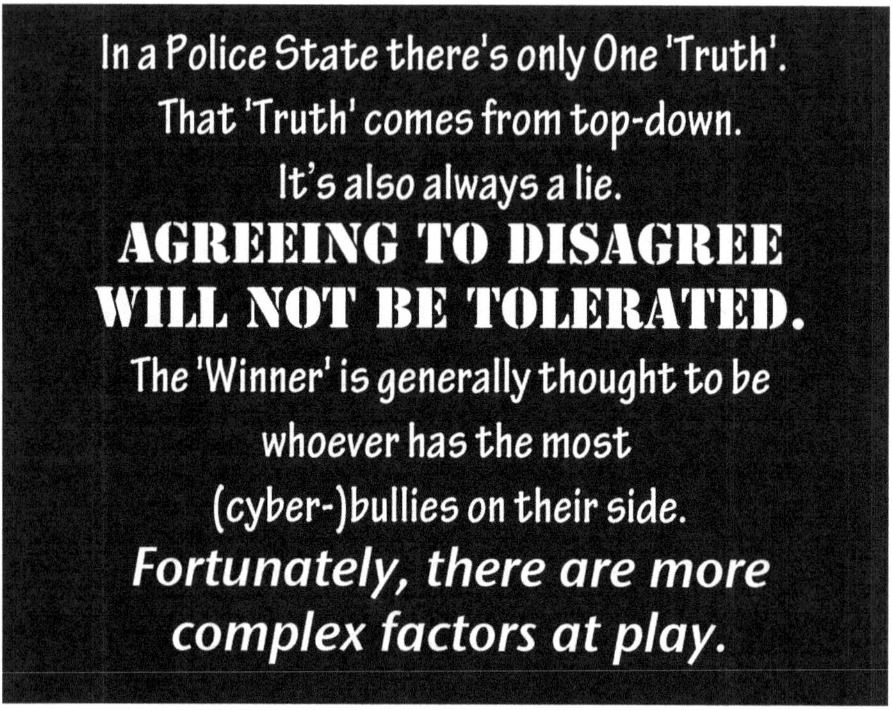

In a Police State there's only One 'Truth'.
That 'Truth' comes from top-down.
It's also always a lie.
AGREEING TO DISAGREE
WILL NOT BE TOLERATED.
The 'Winner' is generally thought to be
whoever has the most
(cyber-)bullies on their side.
Fortunately, there are more
complex factors at play.

****

August 10, 2020, 9:38AM (Dick to group):

HERETICS: Social Studies

I don't know if anybody has been following the Lebanon situation, but Macron, the French president went there uninvited and began criticising the government

today the Washington Post said it was a great example of "leadership" !

(Macron is among the most fervent European Union Supporters, his approval ratings are terrible here so it looks like a polishing up of his image)

going there univited, as another French politician said would be like if there was a disaster in Marseille and Trump or Putin went there uninvited to "help out" and give their advice on the Government here

It can't help but make me think that this is part of the"one world government" idea, Macron was groomed by his experiences in the Rothschild banks and they are supporters of the WEF

There were rumors, quickly quelled, that the Mossad had actually bombed the port, there is a film showing a bombing in fact

https://www.weforum.org/organizations/edmond-de-rothschild-sa

Groupe Edmond de Rothschild | World Economic Forum
The World Economic Forum is an independent international organization committed to improving the state of the world by engaging business, political, academic and other leaders of society to shape global, regional and industry agendas. Incorporated as a not-for-profit foundation in 1971, and headquartered in Geneva, Switzerland, the Forum is tied to no political, partisan or national interests.

****

August 10, 2020, 9:49PM (Amir-ul Kafirs to group):

Re: HERETICS: Social Studies

I don't know if anybody has been following the Lebanon situation,

I wasn't even aware of any of this because I'm so completely wrapped up in trying to get work done on this book. I finally organized all the May emails & articles together. Next I only have to do June & then I can move on to a larger overview.

as another French politician said would be like if there was a disaster in Marseille and Trump or Putin went there uninvited to "help out" and give their advice on the Government here

Seems pretty incredibly pompous & arrogant.

****

Groupe Edmond de Rothschild

The Edmond de Rothschild Group was founded in 1953 by Baron Edmond de Rothschild and has been presided over since 1997 by Baron Benjamin de Rothschild. The Group is active in asset management, private banking, corporate finance, private equity and fund administration. As of 31 December 2014, the Group had CHF 163 billion of assets under management and 2,700 employees spread across 31 offices, branches and subsidiaries. Since February 2015, Baroness Ariane de Rothschild is

Chair of the Executive Committee.

- https://www.weforum.org/organizations/edmond-de-rothschild-sa

****

August 10, 2020, 10:30AM (Amir-ul Kafirs to group):

HERETICS: Muzzle Training

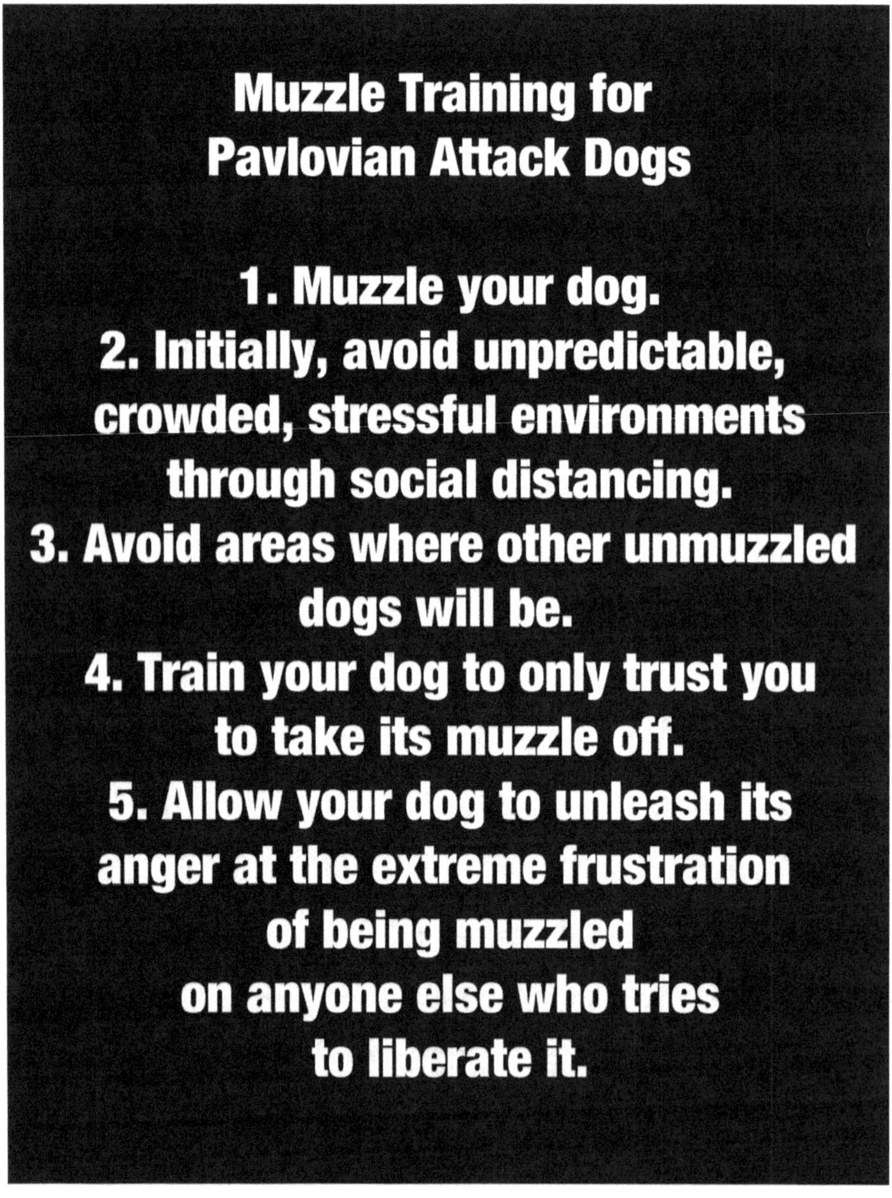

Muzzle Training for
Pavlovian Attack Dogs
1. Muzzle your dog.
2. Initially, avoid unpredictable, crowded, stressful environments through social distancing.
3. Avoid areas where other unmuzzled dogs will be.
4. Train your dog to only trust you to take its muzzle off.
5. Allow your dog to unleash its anger at the extreme frustration of being muzzled on anyone else who tries to liberate it.

****

August 10, 2020, 9:57PM (Amir-ul Kafirs to group):

Re: HERETICS: Muzzle Training

On Aug 10, 2020, at 10:40 AM, Inquiring Librarian wrote:

Bravo! I am sure this will piss many off, because the truth hurts.

I only have 3 more of these text panels made & I'll continue to post one one-a-day on social media until they're gone & then I might put my social media acct in some sort of suspended animation or get rid of it altogether. I barely even look at it anymore because I'm so tired of how many stupid hostile posts there are. I'm beginning to think of it as the "Amir-ul Kafirs" project whose day is done. A part of the problem is that I have new ideas every day for new text panels. I made one new one today on CHILD ABUSE that I felt was too important to not make. I hope I don't feel so compelled in the future because I feel that it's important to spend my time working on the book & on getting it done & then *moving on to other things in my life.*

****

August 10, 2020, 5:21PM (Inquiring Librarian to group):

HERETICS: Humor from the Deep South, Louisiana Cajun-Style

I joined a social media group called, "Recall John Bel Edwards". Edwards is my crappy dictatorial Governor. I believe he rivals Pennsylvania's Wolf for being a total Hitler Asshole.

One of the group's posts yesterday was this. Apparently the Governor is aware of our page and he's pissed and is now threatening us. I got carried away because here you've got most of it cut and pasted for time immemorial. One of my favorite insults was, "Then he needs to quit being a dick-tater" (tater tots are huge here in Louisiana).:

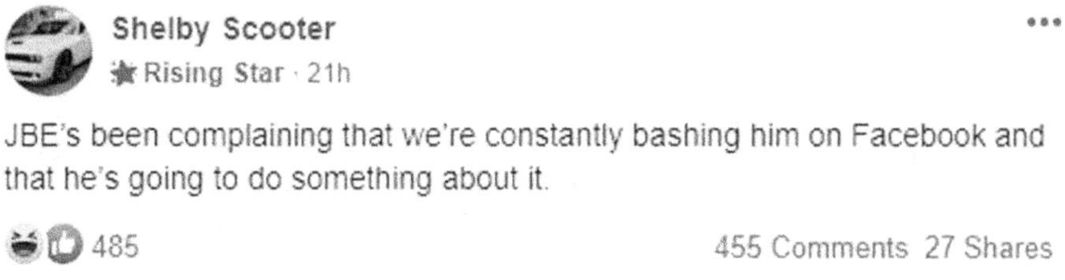

Shelby Scooter

Rising Star · 21h

JBE's been complaining that we're constantly bashing him on Facebook and that he's going to do something about it.

485 455 Comments 27 Shares

Jennifer Hyatt-Barnes He's a little pansy bitch!!

Like · Reply · 21h 12

Marsha Pivert Dale Who let him into our group?

Like · Reply · 21h 8

Jo Ann Rhodus Marsha Pivert Dale its his watch dogs

Like · Reply · 21h 1

Jennifer Hyatt-Barnes Jo Ann Rhodus his watch dog can kiss all of our asses

Like · Reply · 21h 5

View 1 more reply

Alex Prompradit Poor thing..here ya go

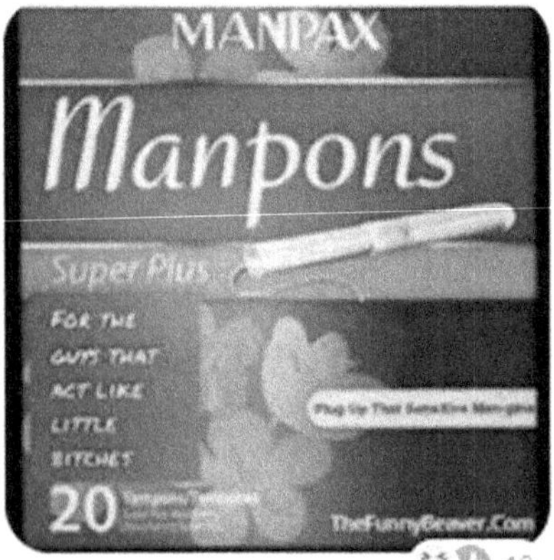

Like · Reply · 21h 16

Sheila Gunn Oneil Alex Prompradit , glad to see you got the correct size Alex!

Like · Reply · 21h 2

Andre Maria Daigle Awe! Someone get him a pacifier! He's such an asshole!

5

Like · Reply · 21h

Derrick Doumit Fuck jbe do something I dare him

3

Like · Reply · 21h

Jennifer Hyatt-Barnes Derrick Doumit looks like he might have to Handel up on the whole state we all sick of him

3

Like · Reply · 21h · Edited

Jed Simon

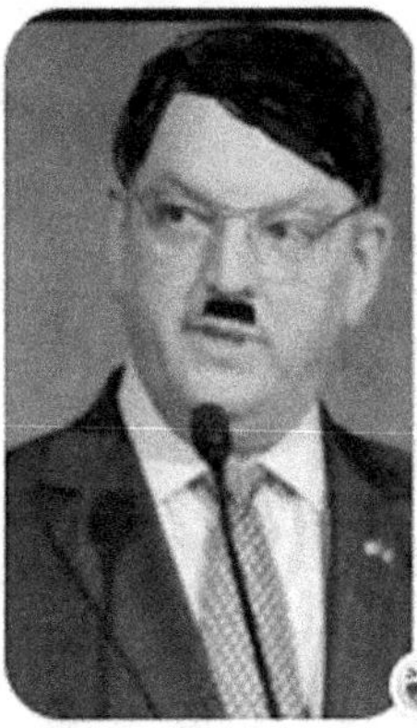

13

Like · Reply · 21h

David Allen Jed Simon
There is a sign between Hammond and Baton Rouge that this would look nice on.

Like · Reply · 21h

Eddy White Jed Simon yes indeed !! Love it

Like · Reply · 4h

Dale Dupree Tell him to meet us face to face.

Like · Reply · 21h 7

Therese Lefebvre Atwell Why are corrupt lying commie tyrants always so thin skinned?
Do they really think we are stupid enough to believe in and approve of their BS?

Like · Reply · 21h 5

Matt Elliott Is he upset nobody tagged him?

Like · Reply · 21h 2

Vivian Rouly To hell with him. Candyass, snowflake

Like · Reply · 21h 3

Mike Scherer Ol' turtle lookin motherfucker

9

Like · Reply · 21h

Judy Guyre Aymond

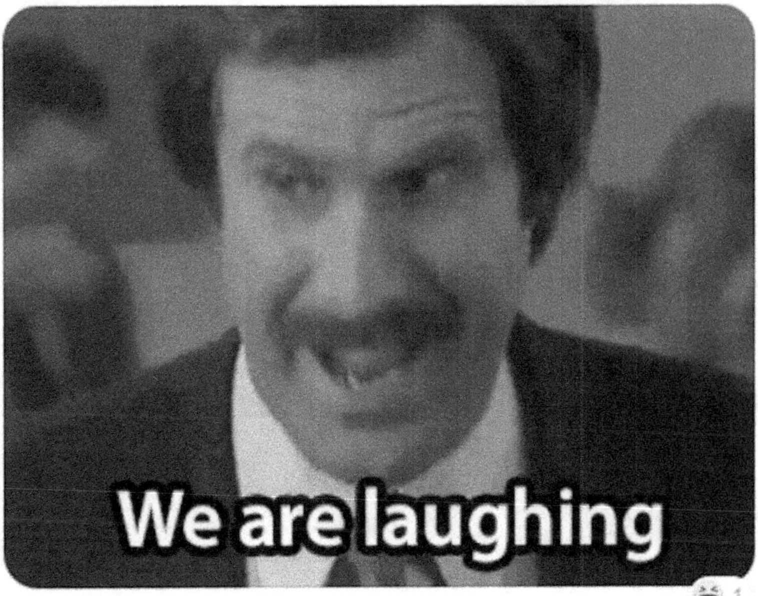

1

Like · Reply · 21h

Hank Broodkoorn

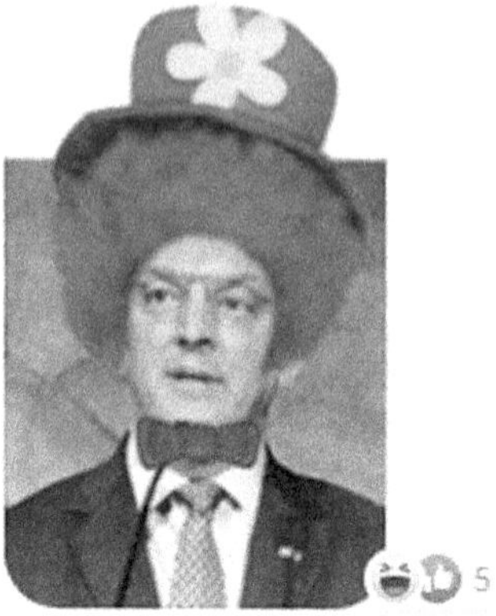

Like · Reply · 21h

Lane Braud Sr Lmfao he not going to do shit

Like · Reply · 21h 2

Samuel Lato He'll close the bars, oh wait, ge already did that

Like · Reply · 21h 3

[Editor's interpolation: The quantity of anti-Governor-Edwards posts provided by Inquiring Librarian was considerably more numerous than what I've included above. One of the things that interests me about these is that he's derided both as being like Hitler *and* as a "corrupt lying commie tyrant" — making the comments appealing to &/or originating from both the 'left' & the 'right']

****

August 10, 2020, 10:04PM (Amir-ul Kafirs to group):

Re: HERETICS: Humor from the Deep South, Louisiana Cajun-Style

"Recall John Bel Edwards".

Amazing. So much insulting going around! I wonder if there's one like this for every governor or at least for Governor Wolf?

****

August 10, 2020, 10:50PM (Naia Nisnam to group):

State-by-state breakdown of federal aid per COVID-19 case

These numbers are more complicated than I thought. It seems they reflect only the first round of money given out to states but is not reflective of what will happen with the second round of grant money?

I have a headache from trying to understand the plan for my teenager's online learning. I can't make sense of this article right now but I had mentioned it to Amir-ul Kafirs yesterday and want to at least send the link:

https://www.beckershospitalreview.com/finance/state-by-state-breakdown-of-federal-aid-per-covid-19-case.html?fbclid=IwAR0S_uxPi4XuN5ci8_O8iS-xF5ZLYBfukDDe0bipfQJJmYXk2f6tVy0N9-Y

****

State-by-state breakdown of federal aid per COVID-19 case

Ayla Ellison (Twitter) - Tuesday, April 14th, 2020

HHS recently began distributing the first $30 billion of emergency funding designated for hospitals in the Coronavirus Aid, Relief, and Economic Security Act. Some of the states hit hardest by the COVID-19 pandemic will receive less funding than states touched relatively lightly, according to an analysis by *Kaiser Health News*.
The first round of grants will be distributed based on historical share Medicare revenue, not based on COVID-19 burden. Therefore, hard-hit states like New York will receive far less per COVID-19 case than most other states.
HHS said it doled out the first slice of funding based on Medicare revenue to get support to hospitals as quickly as possible. The agency said the next round of grants "will focus on providers in areas particularly impacted by the COVID-19 outbreak," rural hospitals and other healthcare providers that receive much of their revenues from Medicaid.
Below is a breakdown of how much funding per COVID-19 case each state will receive from the first $30 billion in aid. *Kaiser Health News* used a state breakdown provided to the House Ways and Means Committee by HHS along with COVID-19 cases tabulated by *The New York Times* for its analysis.

Alabama
$158,000 per COVID-19 case
Alaska
$306,000
Arizona
$23,000
Arkansas
$285,000
California

$145,000
Colorado
$58,000
Connecticut
$38,000
Delaware
$127,000
District of Columbia
$56,000
Florida
$132,000
Georgia
$73,000
Hawaii
$301,000
Idaho
$100,000
Illinois
$73,000
Indiana
$105,000
Iowa
$235,000
Kansas
$291,000
Kentucky
$297,000
Louisiana
$26,000
Maine
$260,000
Maryland
$120,000
Massachusetts
$44,000
Michigan
$44,000
Minnesota
$380,000
Mississippi
$166,000
Missouri
$175,000
Montana
$315,000
Nebraska
$379,000
Nevada

$98,000
New Hampshire
$201,000
New Jersey
$18,000
New Mexico
$171,000
New York
$12,000
North Carolina
$252,000
North Dakota
$339,000
Ohio
$180,000
Oklahoma
$291,000
Oregon
$220,000
Pennsylvania
$68,000
Rhode Island
$52,000
South Carolina
$186,000
South Dakota
$241,000
Tennessee
$166,000
Texas
$184,000
Utah
$94,000
Vermont
$87,000
Virginia
$201,000
Washington
$58,000
West Virginia
$471,000
Wisconsin
$163,000
Wyoming
$278,000

- https://www.beckershospitalreview.com/finance/state-by-state-breakdown-of-federal-aid-per-covid-19-case.html?fbclid=IwAR0S_uxPi4XuN5ci8_O8iSxF5ZLYBfukDDe0bipfQJJmYXk2f6tVy0N9-Y

****

August 11, 2020, 6:50AM (Amir-ul Kafirs to group):

Re: State-by-state breakdown of federal aid per COVID-19 case

If I understand this correctly, & it's hard to believe, here's the highest example of what one state got **PER COVID-19 PATIENT!**:

West Virginia
$471,000

Per ***patient?!*** That's out of $30,000,000,000.00 of funding. The state to get the smallest amount per patient was:

New York
$12,000

New York, according to the current CDC data, has had 426,000 confirmed cases & 32,361 deaths.

West Virginia, according to the same CDC data, has had 7,754 confirmed cases & 141 deaths.

Since the money is "the first $30 billion of emergency funding designated for hospitals in the Coronavirus Aid, Relief, and Economic Security Act" & since, I assume?, the "confirmed cases" aren't all hospital connected I don't know how to calculate how much money was actually gotten. Even an estimate would inevitably be wildly off.

Thanks for sending this. It's far more extreme than I'd imagined.

****

August 10, 2020, 11:22PM (Naia Nisnam to group):

US COVID death rate by age range

The color coded graph is at the bottom:

https://www.cdc.gov/nchs/nvss/vsrr/covid_weekly/index.htm

****

Weekly Updates by Select Demographic and

Geographic Characteristics

Provisional Death Counts for Coronavirus Disease 2019 (COVID-19)

Updated: August 5, 2020

Note: Provisional death counts are based on death certificate data received and coded by the National Center for Health Statistics as of August 5, 2020. Death counts are delayed and may differ from other published sources (see Technical Notes). Counts will be updated every Wednesday by 5pm. Additional information will be added to this site as available.

List of Topics

1. Age and sex
2. Race and Hispanic origin by jurisdiction and by age
3. Place of death
4. Comorbidities
5. Excess deaths
6. State and county data files

Age and sex

Table 1 has counts of death involving COVID-19 and select causes of death by sex and age group for the United States.

Table 1. Deaths involving coronavirus disease 2019 (COVID-19), pneumonia, and influenza reported to NCHS by sex and age group. United States. Week ending 2/1/2020 to 8/1/2020

Select Measure

COVID-19 Deaths

Reporting Period

Week ending 2/1/2020 through 8/1/2020Week ending 2/1/2020 through 8/1/2020

NOTE: Provisional death counts are based on death certificate data received and coded by the National Center for Health Statistics as of the date of analysis and do not represent all deaths that occurred in that period.
SOURCE: NCHS, National Vital Statistics System. Estimates are based on provisional data.

- https://www.cdc.gov/nchs/nvss/vsrr/covid_weekly/index.htm

****

August 11, 2020, 8:04AM (Amir-ul Kafirs to group):

Re: US COVID death rate by age range

The color coded graph is at the bottom:

A convenient feature of the chart, which I can't capture with a screen-shot, is that you can move the cursor along the timeline to get specific death counts.

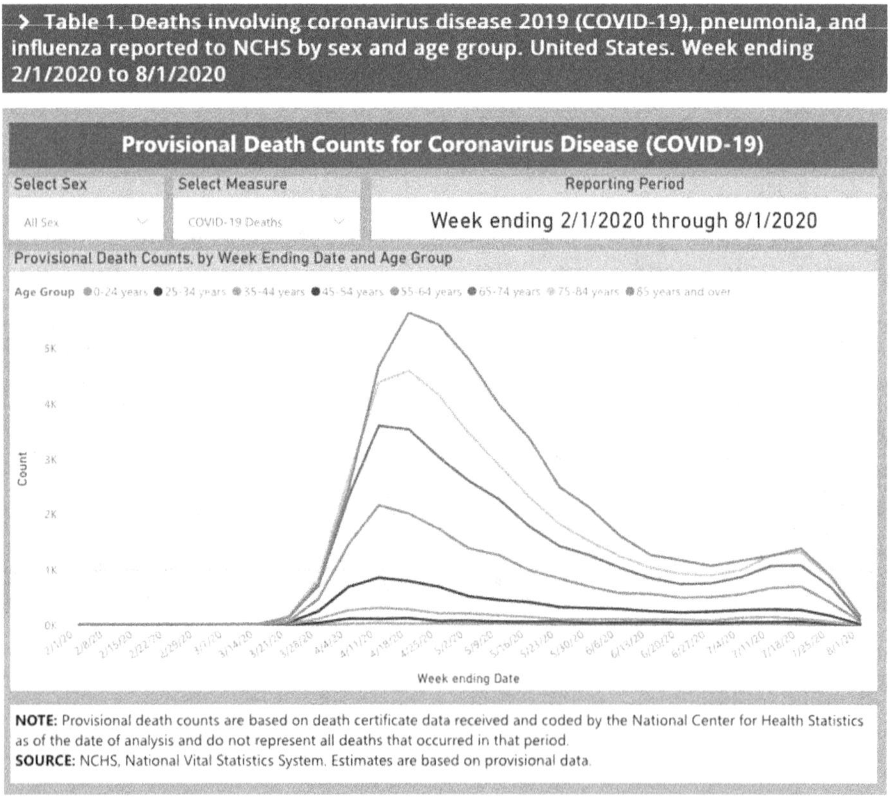

Hence, the peak shows 17 deaths IN ONE WEEK in the 0-24 range & 5,642 in the 85 or older range. 5,642 divided by 17 = 331.882 (etc) so a person in the 0-24 age range had 1/3rd of 1% of a chance of dying as someone 85 or older. That was at the peak of April 14, 2020. As of August 1, 2020, IN ONE WEEK there was **ONE** death in the 0-24 range & **157** in the 85 & older range. That's in the entire US. Note that the chart isn't just for COVID-19 but also includes pneumonia & the flu. I mean obviously I'm biased here but I'm trying to read this data straight & I just can't get any reasonable health justification for a continued quarantine in August (or earlier for that matter). It's interesting that the rapid rise of deaths happened in the 1st 4 weeks of the quarantine & that the downward slope has occurred during the continued quarantine. It seems to me that supporters of the lockdown would have a hard time using these statistics to say that the quarantine was effective. It also seems to me that the progress of deaths followed a typical peak & fall that a non-quarantined situation might have. SO, I'll test that.

I do a search for CDC data for "Provisional Death Counts for pneumonia & influenza Disease 2018". Now, admittedly, it's 7:30AM, I'm too half-awake to be doing this right now but I've gotten 'sucked in'. I suspect that the above chart is an improvement on previous CDC data presentation brought about by the emphasis on providing COVID-19 data. Anyway, here goes:

Table 1: Estimated influenza disease burden, by age group — United States, 2017-2018 influenza season

	Symptomatic Illnesses		Medical Visits		Hospitalizations		Deaths	
Age group	Estimate	95% Cr UI	Estimate	95% Cr UI	Estimate	95% Cr UI	Estimate	95% Cr UI
0-4 yrs	3,678,342	(2,563,438 -7,272,693)	2,464,489	(1,695,054 - 4,904,296)	25,644	(17,871 - 50,702)	115	(0 - 367)
5-17 yrs	7,512,601	(5,899,989 - 10,199,144)	3,906,553	(3,002,375 - 5,356,724)	20,599	(16,177 - 27,965)	528	(205 - 1,392)
18-49 yrs	14,428,065	(12,258,820 - 19,396,710)	5,338,384	(4,262,260 -7,333,716)	80,985	(68,809 - 108,874)	2,803	(1,610 - 6,936)
50-64 yrs	13,237,932	(9,400,614 -23,062,957)	5,692,311	(3,895,925 - 10,028,080)	140,385	(99,691 - 244,576)	6,751	(4,244 - 15,863)
65+ yrs	5,945,690	(3,907,025 - 11,786,777)	3,329,586	(2,139,716- 6,623,717)	540,517	(355,184 -1,071,525)	50,903	(35,989 - 83,230)
All ages	44,802,629	(39,322,959 - 57,928,172)	20,731,323	(17,978,392 - 27,248,302)	808,129	(620,768 -1,357,043)	61,099	(46,404 - 94,987)

* Uncertainty interval

Table 2: Estimated rates of influenza-associated disease outcomes, per 100,000, by age group — United States, 2017-2018 influenza season

	Illness rate		Medical visit rate		Hospitalization rate		Mortality rate	
Age group	Estimate	95% Cr UI	Estimate	95% Cr UI	Estimate	95% Cr UI	Estimate	95% Cr UI
0-4 yrs	18,448.1	(12,856.5 - 36,475.0)	12,360.2	(8,501.3 -24,596.7)	128.6	(89.6 - 254.3)	0.6	(0.0, 1.8)
5-17 yrs	13,985.6	(10,983.6 - 18,987.0)	7,272.5	(5,589.3 -9,972.2)	38.3	(30.1 - 52.1)	1.0	(0.4, 2.6)
18-49 yrs	10,469.7	(8,895.6 - 14,075.1)	3,873.8	(3,092.9 - 5,321.7)	58.8	(49.9 - 79.0)	2.0	(1.2, 5.0)
50-64 yrs	20,881.1	(14,828.2 - 36,378.8)	8,978.9	(6,145.3 -15,818.0)	221.4	(157.2 - 385.8)	10.6	(6.7, 25.0)
65+ yrs	11,690.6	(7,682.1 -23,175.5)	6,546.7	(4,207.2 -13,023.8)	1,062.8	(698.4 - 2,106.9)	100.1	(70.8, 163.7)

* Uncertainty interval

Note that these are JUST for the flu, no pneumonia, & have a different age range specification. The all-ages deaths from flu in the 2017-2018 season in the US was 94,987. Now according to online CDC data (https://www.cdc.gov/coronavirus/2019-ncov/cases-updates/us-cases-deaths.html) there have been 161,842 deaths from COVID-19 in the US so far. I searched for recent data on pneumonia/flu deaths in the US & only got data as recent as 2018, not 2020 (https://www.cdc.gov/nchs/pressroom/sosmap/flu_pneumonia_mortality/flu_pneumonia.htm). Another search yielded "49,157" deaths for pneumonia in 2018 in the US. (https://www.cdc.gov/nchs/fastats/pneumonia.htm) Now, I really should get back to bed so I'm going to be totally cavalier here:

I'm going to treat the 161,842 COVID-19 deaths as if they might possibly be really flu & pneumonia deaths as well & I'm going to subtract a previous recent year's stats for those 2:

161,842 minus 94,987 (flu) & 49,157 (pneumonia) = 17,698 COVID-19 deaths.

You get the idea. I'm just experimenting here so this is not to be taken as some chiseled-in-stone conclusion but if one were to be skeptical about COVID-19 statistics this would be one way to greatly reduce them. I didn't find flu & pneumonia statistics for the same time as COVID-19 except where they're lumped together in the original chart that inspired this mini-tirade so I've used earlier (but still fairly recent) data.

****

Understanding the Numbers: Provisional Death Counts and COVID-19

Provisional death counts deliver the most comprehensive picture of lives lost to COVID-19. These estimates are based on incoming death certificates, which are the most reliable source of death data and contain information not available anywhere else, including information about the place of death, other causes that contributed to the death, and race and ethnicity.

How it works

The National Center for Health Statistics (NCHS) uses data from death certificates, which are sent to NCHS daily, to produce provisional COVID-19 death counts. These include deaths occurring within the 50 states, the District of Columbia, and Puerto Rico.

NCHS also provides summaries that examine deaths in specific categories and in greater geographic detail, such as deaths by county or by race and Hispanic origin.

COVID-19 deaths are identified using a new ICD–10 code. When COVID-19 is reported as a cause of death – or when it is listed as a "probable" or "presumed" cause – anywhere on the death certificate, the death is coded as **U07.1.** This can include cases with or without laboratory confirmation.

Why these numbers are different than counts from other sources

Provisional death counts may not match counts from other sources, such as media reports or numbers from county health departments. Our counts often track 1-2 weeks behind other data because:

- **Death certificates take time to be completed.** There are many steps to filling out and submitting a death certificate. Waiting for test results can create additional delays.
- **States report at different rates.** Currently, 63% of all U.S. deaths are reported to NCHS within 10 days of the date of death, but there is significant variation between states.
- **It takes extra time to code COVID-19 deaths.** While 80% of death records are processed and coded electronically at NCHS within minutes, most deaths from COVID-19 cannot be coded electronically and must be coded by a person, which takes an average of 7 days.
- **Other reporting systems use different definitions or methods for counting deaths.**

Things to know about the data

Provisional counts are not final and are subject to change. Counts from previous weeks are continually revised as more records are received and processed.

Provisional data are not yet complete. Counts will not include all deaths that occurred during a given time period, especially for more recent periods. However, the completeness of the data can be estimated by examining the average number of deaths reported in previous years.

Death counts should not be compared across states. Some states report deaths to NCHS on a daily basis, while other states report deaths weekly or monthly. State vital record reporting may also be affected or delayed by COVID-19 response activities.

To view the provisional death counts or for more detailed technical information, visit our Provisional Death Counts for Coronavirus Disease (COVID-19) page.

Centers for Disease Control
and Prevention
National Center for Health Statistics

****

August 11, 2020, 7:06PM (Dick to group):

Though I haven't found any hard statistics, I was speaking with a very knowledgeable friend who told me that the covid-19 'pandemic' has forced 70% of the nightclubs in Paris to close as well as many small businesses but that the real disaster has been felt in 'les provinces' that is, smaller towns where many small businesses have gone under.

I can verify that in the quarter where I usually hang out more than half the places are shut, this could be because of August, but it's really strange to see

He also told me that Macron may use Article 93 (I think that was the number) which would give him absolute control if a planned anti covid measures demonstration takes place on 12 September...

Also, as of yesterday, a city map has been issued that shows where masks are obligatory in Paris, basically wherever people habitually meet

In short, it is a nightmare

****

August 12, 2020, 9:49AM (Amir-ul Kafirs to group):

But are there any big corporate chains in France? That're still thriving? Or is that mainly an American thing?

Also, as of yesterday, a city map has been issued that shows where masks are obligatory in Paris, basically wherever people habitually meet

In the biggest of the 2 parks I go to regularly here, Frick Park, mask use is on the decline. In the slightly smaller park, Schenley Park, it seems on the uprise. Yesterday when I went for a walk there most people had on masks or put them on as soon as they saw me. If they didn't have masks they clutched their shirts to their mouths. Even though I don't think it's their intention, this creates a situation where they're reacting to me, personally, rather than following a general health procedure. Psychologically, it's insidious.

In short, it is a nightmare

Indeed. One that we can't wake up from.

****

August 12, 2020, 7:40AM (Dick to group):

a cartoon...

This says "Coronavirus with the homeless"

"Why aren't we contaminated?"

"Because we don't have a television"

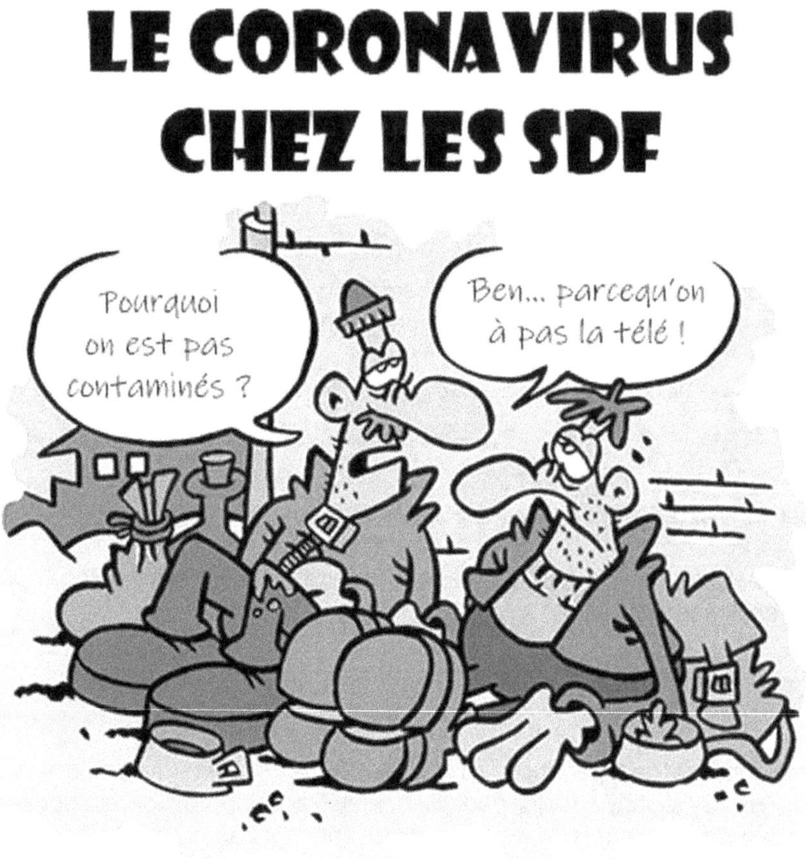

****

August 12, 2020, 9:56AM (Amir-ul Kafirs to group):

Re: a cartoon...

That's great! Where did that appear publicly? I can't imagine such a cartoon appearing in any of the mainstream newspapers here in the US! Not in the New York Times, not in USA Today — not in the Pittsburgh Post Gazette, not in ANY Pittsburgh 'news'paper 'left' OR 'right'!!

****

August 12, 2020, 9:56AM (Amir-ul Kafirs to group):

HERETICS: Thought for the Day (Problem Solving)

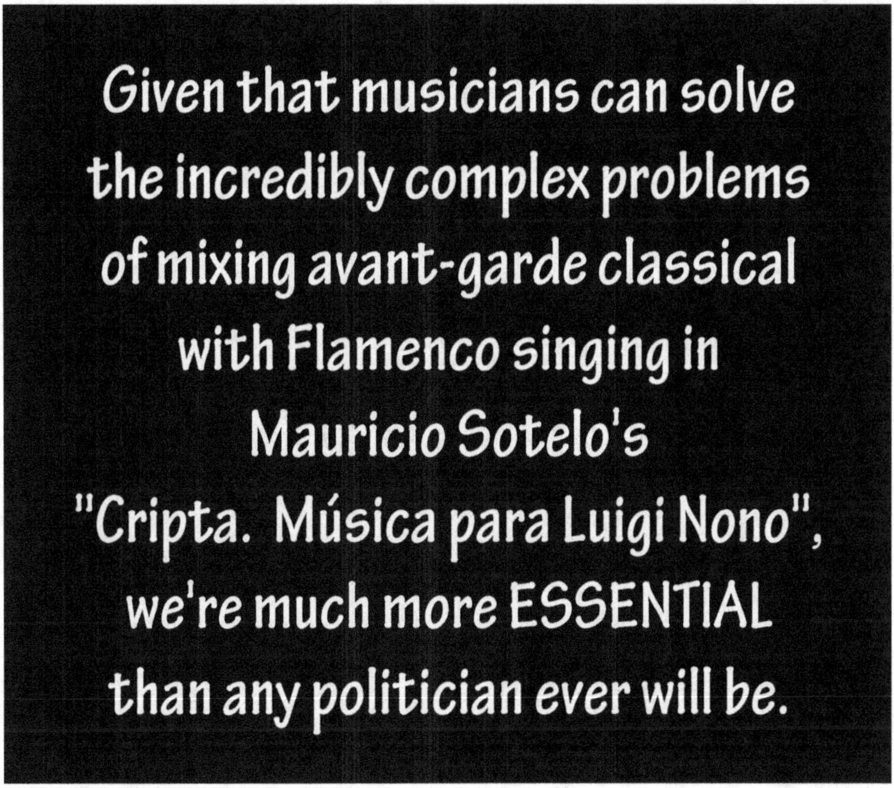
Given that musicians can solve
the incredibly complex problems
of mixing avant-garde classical
with Flamenco singing in
Mauricio Sotelo's
"Cripta. Música para Luigi Nono",
we're much more ESSENTIAL
than any politician ever will be.

****

August 12, 2020, 9:54AM (Dick to group):

yes, there are big chains here
they are particularly present in the provinces kind of like walmart

I few i recall are

LeClerc - like walmart
Leroy Merlin - like home depot
Castorama - like home depot too
Casino - food
Decathalon -sporting goods
FranPrix - food

****

August 12, 2020, 10:00AM (Amir-ul Kafirs to group):

yes, there are big chains here

But what I'm getting at is: Are they all thriving? While the small businesses go under?

****

August 12, 2020, 10:00AM (Dick to group):

RE: HERETICS: Thought for the Day (Problem Solving)

I like this one, too
Nice attack from an abstract angle !

****

August 12, 2020, 10:05AM (Amir-ul Kafirs to group):

RE: HERETICS: Thought for the Day (Problem Solving)

I'm trying to provide a variety of approaches.

Do you like Flamenco music? I love it. The singer on the piece referred to is called Arcangel. I generally appreciate the guitar playing the most but the singing & dancing are phenomenal too.

****

August 12, 2020, 10:03AM (Dick to group):

yes, they are doing very well, that was my point

it's like in the states, the billionaires all are making out like bandits

the biggest one, Arnault (I think that's his name) owns a large nimber of the media sources to boot

the same friend told me that during the lockdown, macdonalds drive-thrus were allowed to stay open in the provinces and the wait was sometimes more than 3 hours

****

August 12, 2020, 10:13AM (Amir-ul Kafirs to group):

it's like in the states, the billionaires all are making out like bandits

Right, exactly, under the guise of a PANDEMIC the big corporate chains shut down the small business competition that many of us prefer & then their business gets even BIGGER. Now those small business owners, if they want to survive, will just have to become managers for the chain stores.

****

August 12, 2020, 11:45AM (Amir-ul Kafirs to group):

On Aug 12, 2020, at 10:19 AM, dick turner wrote:

when I go out and see people wearing these masks in 110° heat I feel like I am living in a sort of proto Zombie Third reich

That's essentially what it is. Except, I suppose that it's the FOURTH REICH, the Zombie Fourth Reich. I wonder if there's a new safety symbol that's the equivalent of the swastika.

****

August 12, 2020, 11:11AM (Amir-ul Kafirs to group):

HERETICS: Toll Booths

Naia Nisnam & I were talking the other day about how during the PANDEMIC toll booths have become transitioned to all-electronic. They told me that Pennsylvania's toll booth workers are permanently out of work because the system won't be going back to human labor if & when the PANDEMIC PANIC is over. I told them that the toll booth workers are still on the job in other states that I've recently driven through such as Ohio.

SO, I got to thinking about it & started wondering how many states are permanently switching to electronic tolling. I found this article:

https://www.governing.com/topics/mgmt/no-more-toll-booth-collectors.html

which as of July 27 only lists 6 such states & doesn't include Pennsylvania:

"A growing number of states are eliminating toll plazas entirely in some areas and moving to all-electronic systems. At least six — California, Colorado, Florida, Georgia, Massachusetts and Texas — have swapped traditional toll booths for cashless systems on some roads or bridges,"

It IS actually more efficient, I'll give it that, but there's an aspect to it that doesn't seem to be questioned much, viz: **IT'S DRAMATICALLY INCREASED SURVEILLANCE.** Before, when you paid a toll-booth person in cash, who you were & where you were going wasn't any of their business. NOW, IT IS THEIR BUSINESS. The government knows when & where you've driven.

It's a continuation of what happened with the parking meters in Pittsburgh. Until very recently one just put coins in the meter, that was it. NOW, we put in our license plate number. That creates a record of where the car has been parked.

When I remarked about this to the Reverend Ivan Stang of the Church of the SubGenius 7 years ago & expressed my surprise that no-one that I knew was complaining about this as Big Brother he said something like "That's because everybody *wants to be under survelllance now.*" It's as if people feel like being under surveillance makes them the star of their very own 'reality' TV show.

****

August 12, 2020, 11:57AM (Amir-ul Kafirs to group):

Re: HERETICS: Toll Booths

there's an aspect to it that doesn't seem to be questioned much, viz: **IT'S DRAMATICALLY INCREASED SURVEILLANCE.**

Ok, I take that back. There ARE people questioning it. Here's an excerpt from the article I linked to:

"Cashless Tolling Concerns

"Unions aren't the only critics. Some motorists say the transponder and camera-based system invades their privacy and they worry that a data trail on their travel is being created.

""We would like drivers to have the choice of being able to pay in cash or electronically," said John Bowman, vice president of the National Motorists Association, a driver's rights group. "There are people who don't want a transponder on their vehicle for privacy reasons. They don't want to be tracked where they go.""

****

August 12, 2020, 11:56AM (Inquiring Librarian to group):

Re: a cartoon...

Nice cartoon Dick! And yes, I see this daily in Louisiana. I have a gaggle of drunk old dudes that congregate daily on the corner of the block where I live. Not a single one of them has been picked off by the 'virus'. One even has a trach in his neck. He drinks himself to a slouch in his chair, or against another drunk old guy next to him each day. You gotta be kitten me if this virus is that deadly but hasn't so much as nicked these dirty, unhealthy elderly folks who are way off the wagon.

****

August 12, 2020, 11:51AM (Dick to group):

When you talk about a swastika I think of this poster one sees everywhere

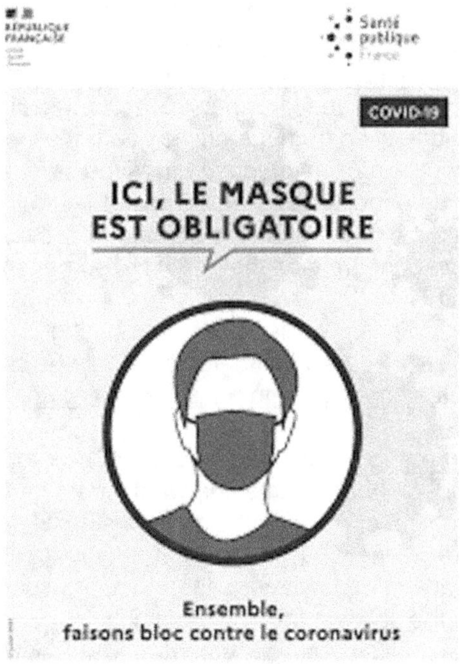

****

August 12, 2020, 12:04PM (Inquiring Librarian to group):

Here let me try to make everyone feel even worse. Check out this bioethics professor's article on "Morality Pills". By the end he suggests that we need to sneak this into the water supply to 'fix' those noncompliant little imps (like us).

https://theconversation.com/amp/morality-pills-may-be-the-uss-best-shot-at-ending-the-coronavirus-pandemic-according-to-one-ethicist-142601?fbclid=IwAR0RCxMruaA2J-4WAzTu2iAt93Z-2vFTpB6roifGXXWUU2U9DtROKmlRB1k

****

'Morality pills' may be the US's best shot at ending the coronavirus pandemic, according to one ethicist

Parker Crutchfield, Western Michigan University
August 10, 2020 8.07am EDT

COVID-19 is a collective risk. It threatens everyone, and we all must cooperate to lower the chance that the coronavirus harms any one individual. Among other things, that means keeping safe social distances and wearing masks. But many people choose not to do these things, making spread of infection more likely. When someone chooses not to follow public health guidelines around the coronavirus, they're defecting from the public good. It's the moral equivalent of the tragedy of the commons: If everyone shares the same pasture for their individual flocks, some people are going to graze their animals longer, or let them eat more than their fair share, ruining the commons in the process. Selfish and self-defeating behavior undermines the pursuit of something from which everyone can benefit.

Democratically enacted enforceable rules – mandating things like mask wearing and social distancing – might work, if defectors could be coerced into adhering to them. But not all states have opted to pass them or to enforce the rules that are in place.

My research in bioethics focuses on questions like how to induce those who are noncooperative to get on board with doing what's best for the public good. To me, it seems the problem of coronavirus defectors could be solved by moral enhancement: like receiving a vaccine to beef up your immune system, people could take a substance to boost their cooperative, pro-social behavior. Could a psychoactive pill be the solution to the pandemic?

It's a far-out proposal that's bound to be controversial, but one I believe is worth at least considering, given the importance of social cooperation in the struggle to get COVID-19 under control.

[..]

Promoting cooperation with moral enhancement

It seems that the U.S. is not currently equipped to cooperatively lower the risk confronting us. Many are instead pinning their hopes on the rapid development and distribution of an enhancement to the immune system – a vaccine.

But I believe society may be better off, both in the short term as well as the long, by boosting not the body's ability to fight off disease but the brain's ability to cooperate with others. What if researchers developed and delivered a moral enhancer rather than an immunity enhancer?

Moral enhancement is the use of substances to make you more moral. The psychoactive substances act on your ability to reason about what the right thing to do is, or your ability to be empathetic or altruistic or cooperative.

[..]

****

August 12, 2020, 12:13PM (Inquiring Librarian to group):

Re: HERETICS: Toll Booths

There are very few tolls in Louisiana, that I know of. I grew up in Pennsylvania, outside of Philly, near King of Prussia. I went to college at the U. of Delaware. It was insane how many toll roads there are in PA and DE. I HATED them!!! And they were getting increasingly more expensive as time passed. I also remember the toll for the tunnel just outside of Baltimore. I went through one time with zero cash on me. They let me through anyways but said they'd take a photo of my license plate and send me the $1 or $2 toll bill. They never did.

In Louisiana, we had one toll going from the east to west bank of Nola. That toll was completely removed about 2 years ago. There is another one over Lake Pontchartrain. But I haven't been over it since the pandemic started. Louisiana as whole is pretty resentful of these mandates and changes, and quite hostile towards them I would say. I find it a relief to get out of the city where people who value and fight for civil liberties live. I've never felt so proud of my backwoods neighbors in this state.

And great news! I've finally been granted entry into the Health Freedom Louisiana group!! I can't wait to find like minded folks. I'm still eyeing Iowa for escape.

****

August 12, 2020, 12:30PM (Naia Nisnam to group):

Re: HERETICS: Toll Booths

I've heard that here in PA they plan to have only the busiest of the toll booths (at state border crossings and major interchanges) open. This is info from a friend of my moms who worked at a small toll interchange.

Amir-ul Kafirs, I lost the chain where we laughed at the comments about the Louisiana governor and you wondered if our governor wolf was facing similar hilarious derision.
24 members of our state legislature did try to have him impeached back in June. Unfortunately, most of the jokes are aimed at our state secretary of health, Rachel Levine, bc shes transgendered. That is increasing hostility from leftists towards the anti-lockdown movement in PA.
I had wondered at how PA, w so many conservatives, ended up with a transgendered secretary of health. Turns out it's because most people didn't know. Now everyone's watching her. I wish they'd focus only on the messed up things that she's done instead of gender issues. But I also hate it when the msm makes fun of Trump's bad hair and orange skin instead of focusing only on the messed up things that he says and does.

This is a link to a Forbes article about PA's governor wolf and how he's managed to continue with his illegal orders:

https://www.forbes.com/sites/markchenoweth/2020/07/02/when-the-wolf-at-the-door-is-your-governor/?fbclid=IwAR2pOwpISMY85uY0ujmWHTK4AU8RscTzSepy4B4xEkPPCp8gGeUG3jQZWxU#53bfc74a5927

****

When The Wolf At The Door Is Your Governor

Mark Chenoweth Contributor
Policy
I cover U.S. legal issues, especially the Administrative State.

The novel coronavirus pandemic has many Americans struggling to keep the wolf from the door of their homes and businesses. For Pennsylvanians, the threat has become all the more menacing, because the wolf at their doors is the governor—and the state supreme court just invited him in.
Like many of his counterparts across the country, Gov. Tom Wolf unilaterally declared a state of emergency in response to the pandemic. In a Proclamation of Disaster Emergency issued on March 6, he put himself in charge of the state's response to Covid-19 to the exclusion of the elected legislature. Since that date he has issued multiple executive orders with binding legal effect—that is, new rules or suspensions of laws (with at least temporary effect)—never approved by the legislature.
As in many states, the State of Disaster Emergency gives the governor ostensibly temporary powers to bind the citizenry without legislative participation. While efficient in cases of true cataclysm—particularly when a legislature is unable to convene—such executive edicts do not benefit from the careful deliberation and democratic input and legitimacy of a full legislative process. Nor do the governor's rules keep the law-passing separate from the law-executing—as the state constitution requires. Rather, he has now consolidated both powers in a way that enables him to target favored or disfavored businesses or industries (or, say, favor gatherings for social protest purposes, but disfavor gatherings for religious worship purposes).

One question worth asking is whether the emergency declaration was even necessary to fight the coronavirus effectively. Might compliance with new safety policies be higher—and thus enhance everyone's safety—if those rules were adopted by a bipartisan legislature rather than dictated by one man? Other questions include whether the declared emergency is lawful and when will it end? On April 13, in the *Friends of Danny DeVito v. Wolf* case, the Pennsylvania Supreme Court turned away an earlier challenge to the governor's assumption of emergency powers, implying that a vote of the legislature could end it: "As a counterbalance to the exercise of the broad powers granted to the governor," it wrote then, "the Emergency Code provides that the General Assembly by concurrent resolution may terminate a state of disaster emergency at any time." Shortly after the governor renewed the state of disaster emergency on June 6 (which had expired after 90 days), the General Assembly exercised the counterbalancing power noted by the Supreme Court and passed a concurrent resolution on June 9 to terminate the governor's emergency powers immediately. After hearing daily from constituents that the governor's lockdown orders are killing businesses they had built over decades and are destroying their livelihoods, legislators from both parties evidently decided they had waited long enough. The bipartisan vote in the state house was 121-81, including all Republicans and 12 Democrats in favor, and the vote in the state senate was 31-19, with all Republicans and 2 Democrats in favor. Together more than 60% of the legislature voted to end the governor's unilateral rule.

[..]

****

August 12, 2020, 5:33PM (Amir-ul Kafirs to group):

24 members of our state legislature did try to have him impeached back in June.

It seems that impeachment is impossible. It would be really interesting if it worked at least some of the time. Rump would be gone, Wolf would be gone. Both would be a huge improvement.

I wish they'd focus only on the messed up things that she's done instead of gender issues.

Agreed. That'll change eventually because there'll be transgendered conservatives eventually, if not already.

makes fun of Trump's bad hair and orange skin instead of focusing only on the messed up things that he says and does.

More ad hominem arguments.

This is a link to a Forbes article about PA's governor wolf

Excellent article. Consider this excerpt:

"Shortly after the governor renewed the state of disaster emergency on June 6 (which had expired after 90 days), the General Assembly exercised the counterbalancing power noted by the Supreme Court and passed a concurrent resolution on June 9 to terminate the governor's emergency powers immediately. After hearing daily from constituents that the governor's lockdown orders are killing businesses they had built over decades and are destroying their livelihoods, legislators from both parties evidently decided they had waited long enough. The bipartisan vote in the state house was 121-81, including all Republicans and 12 Democrats in favor, and the vote in the state senate was 31-19, with all Republicans and 2 Democrats in favor. Together more than 60% of the legislature voted to end the governor's unilateral rule.

"

Rather than accept that bipartisan action by the democratically-elected legislature, taken under the same statute that authorized him to declare an emergency in the first place, Governor Wolf refused to relinquish his special powers. When state legislators sued seeking to force an end to the state of emergency, he asked the Pennsylvania Supreme Court to exercise its aptly named king's bench jurisdiction to decide the case.
"On July 1, the state supreme court in *Wolf v. Scarnati et al.*, held 4-1-2 that a vote by both houses of the legislature counts for nothing. All four justices backing Governor Wolf's position (JJ. Wecht, Baer, Donohue and Todd) were elected to the state supreme court as Democrats. This slim court majority abandoned the logic of "counterbalance" that had supported its April decision in the *Friends of Danny DeVito* case. As a result, Gov. Wolf now wields single-handed executive power greater than any seen in Pennsylvania since the American Revolution got rid of King George III."

In other words, Governor Wolf is literally now the dictator of Pennsylvania. To me, that makes him worse than Rump.

****

August 12, 2020, 12:14PM (Naia Nisnam to group):

I'd be offended by the "morality pill" concept if it wasn't so funny... Maybe if we give everyone a dose of "magic mushrooms" the sociopaths that are running the world and ruining our lives would become empathetic and end the pandemic by admitting that it's a farce.

****

August 12, 2020, 12:32PM (Amir-ul Kafirs to group):

I read somewhere or saw in a documentary that Hitler is reputed to've designed the swastika / hackencross images that becme the symbol for nazism (of course it was taken from 'Aryan' culture). I've always figured that that was where his artistic training paid off because the image was very catchy. This image of the suffocated person isn't nearly as catchy.

****

August 12, 2020, 3:10PM (Amir-ul Kafirs to group):

"The scenario in which the government forces an immunity booster upon everyone is plausible. And the military has been forcing enhancements like vaccines or "uppers" upon soldiers for a long time. The scenario in which the government forces a morality booster upon everyone is far-fetched. But a strategy like this one could be a way out of this pandemic, a future outbreak or the suffering associated with climate change. That's why we should be thinking of it now."

Right, governments have been forcing drugs on soldiers for a long time. Is that supposed to be a good thing? Didn't Hitler use methadone addiction as a way to control soldiers? The US military got author Alice Sheldon (James Tiptree, Jr) addicted to speed during WWII so that she could work long hours. Parker Crutchfield has as much of a sense of ethics as a dog turd.

****

August 12, 2020, 3:15PM (Amir-ul Kafirs to group):

On Aug 12, 2020, at 12:33 PM, dick turner wrote:

no, it isn't
but it is everywhere

&, unfortunately, "everywhere" is where it needs to be to work the way it does.

Have you seen any graffiting over them? I've seen little or no graffiting against the lockdown anywhere I've been. That's almost incredible to me. That's almost more of a sign of complacency than anything else.

****

August 12, 2020, 3:18PM (Amir-ul Kafirs to group):

I'd be offended by the "morality pill" concept if it wasn't so funny...

I've mentioned a documentary called "Demon Rum" about the prohibitionist/pro-nazi-car-manufacturer Henry Ford & his "Morality Squads" that visited worker homes & prevented them from getting promotions if their homes seemed 'immoral', ie: if there was any drunkeness going on. SO, there is a precedent for this sort of thing.

Maybe if we give everyone a dose of "magic mushrooms"

Ha ha! Do you remember when the Yippies said they were planning to put LSD in the water? I'm sure they never had the slightest intention of doing that but it scared the straight world big time.

****

August 12, 2020, 12:40PM (Naia Nisnam to group):

Re: a cartoon...

I love this cartoon, it's super funny and so on point.
A few months ago I talked with a homeless guy who told me he thinks it's all

bullshit because he knows people in a few different camps around the city and no one has gotten sick. I know from experience that those guys don't socially distance- they share smokes and pass around bottles of booze. My guess is that most of the homeless have been exposed to the virus but haven't gotten sick enough to go to the ER. As long as they can avoid shelters, they aren't going to be tested.... Maybe the next time the government needs a surge in cases, they'll go out and test the homeless.

****

August 12, 2020, 4:21PM (Dick to group):

interesting, no I haven't seen grafitti over them !

****

August 12, 2020, 4:23PM (Inquiring Librarian to group):

Then, in the dark recesses of the night, we all need to get to work!!

****

[Dick shared multiple images of detourned mask enforcement posters that he'd designed]

August 12, 2020, 4:23PM (Dick to group):

I am going to print a number of these on adhesive paper, i'll keep them on me and put them up when I can and am not being watched

if anybody has ideas to add to it, let me know

****

August 12, 2020, 5:43PM (Amir-ul Kafirs to group):

Thanks for that. I never liked Shepard Fairey's work that much but this is a perfect repurposing of it considering that he was the one who brought us that Obama HOPE poster.

****

August 12, 2020, 5:48PM (Dick to group):

i'm glad you suggested the idea because it's something i can do to feel constructive

****

August 12, 2020, 5:53PM (Amir-ul Kafirs to group):

No point in just sitting around & twiddling our thumbs.

Speaking of which, I was planning on retiring from social media after posting the last of my text panels tomorrow but, for better or worse, I was inspired to make 3 more today so I'm not sure what's going to happen.

****

August 12, 2020, 5:55PM (Dick to group):

here's my first batch !

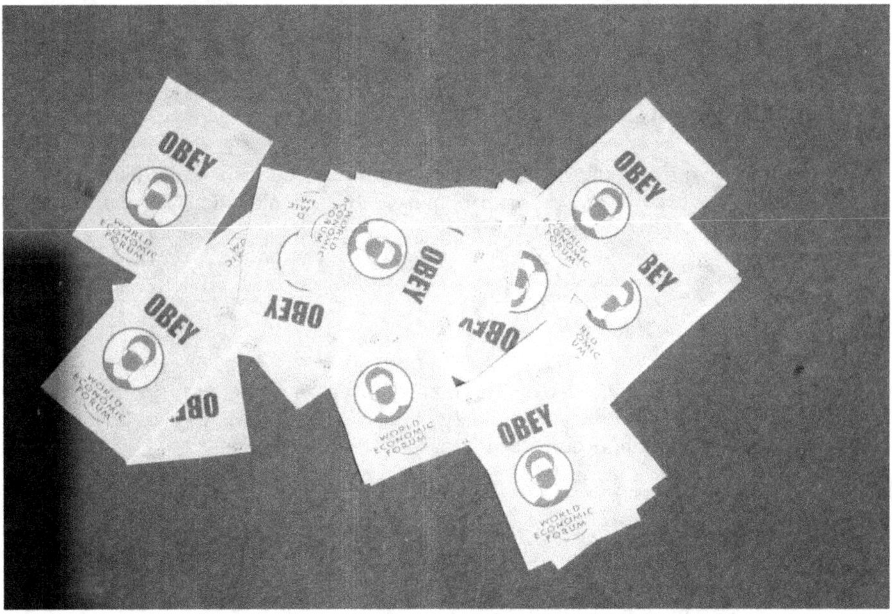

****

August 12, 2020, 5:58PM (Amir-ul Kafirs to group):

HERETICS: WikiLeaks

I follow WikiLeaks on Twitter & here's something that I found interesting today:

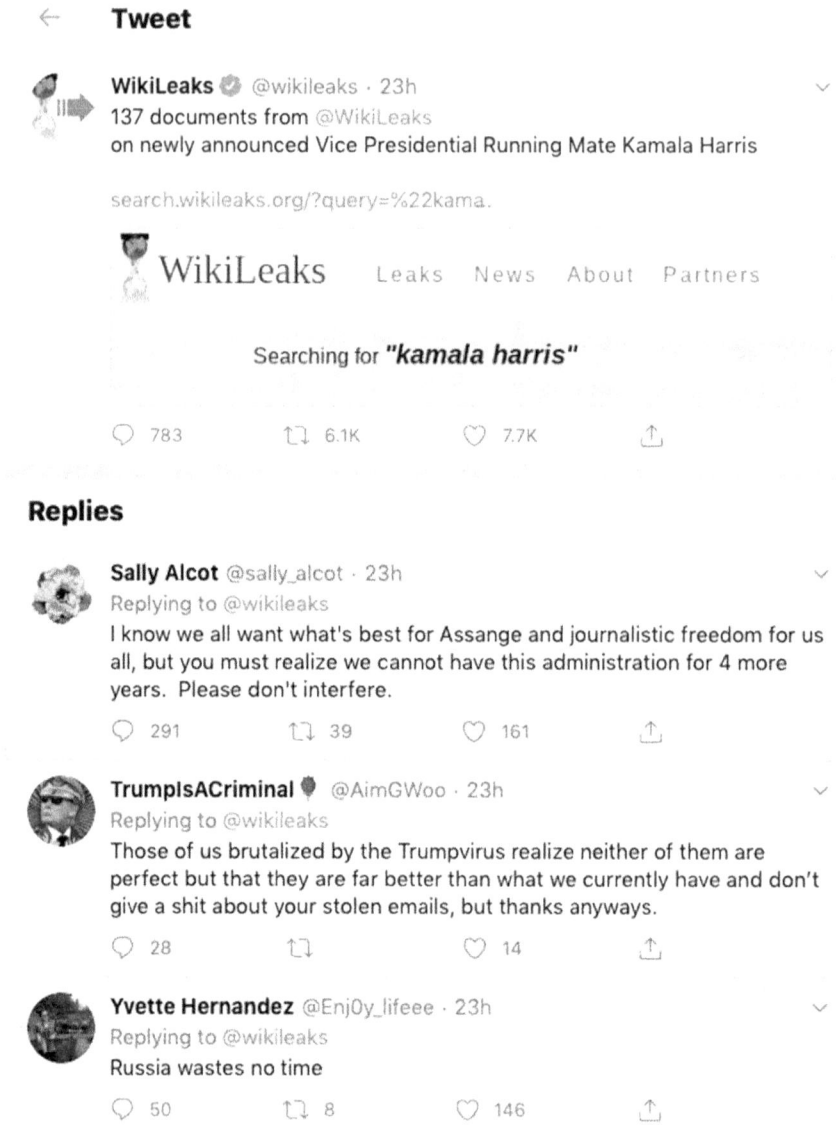

Tweet

WikiLeaks @wikileaks · 23h
137 documents from @WikiLeaks
on newly announced Vice Presidential Running Mate Kamala Harris

search.wikileaks.org/?query=%22kama.

WikiLeaks Leaks News About Partners

Searching for ***"kamala harris"***

783 6.1K 7.7K

Replies

Sally Alcot @sally_alcot · 23h
Replying to @wikileaks
I know we all want what's best for Assange and journalistic freedom for us all, but you must realize we cannot have this administration for 4 more years. Please don't interfere.

291 39 161

TrumpIsACriminal @AimGWoo · 23h
Replying to @wikileaks
Those of us brutalized by the Trumpvirus realize neither of them are perfect but that they are far better than what we currently have and don't give a shit about your stolen emails, but thanks anyways.

28 14

Yvette Hernandez @Enj0y_lifeee · 23h
Replying to @wikileaks
Russia wastes no time

50 8 146

Kamala Harris is the Vice Presidential nominee to accompany Biden. I don't know when that was announced but it must have been recently, like today? ANYWAY, there're already WikiLeaks about her. I looked at a few of them, I didn't notice anything substantially incriminating so the content may not be a big deal but I DO think it's interesting that these 'leaks' are appearing so soon. Note the responses that I included in my screenshot.

****

August 12, 2020, 6:09PM (Dick to group):

HERETICS: WikiLeaks

A social media friend wrote this:

In 2015-16, I lost a lot of friends by trying to speak up against a corrupted Democratic Primary process, and media, trying to warn my friends that it was going to mean Trump, if they didn't stand up to stop what was happening. I was called every condescending name in the book for it, as if I were some crazy Alex Jones type for saying so. All while the media claimed Clinton had a 98.1% chance of winning. It was the very definition of gaslighting. And after they lost our country to Trump, instead of waking up and demanding that all that corruption be addressed, so many friends here went the other direction: no time for any criticism of corporate media, or the Democratic Party.
So then came 3 1/2 years of watching friends obsess on neo-con conspiracy theories about Russia - thinking themselves liberal for it - and refusing to look at the history of those (Republicans) they began putting up as heroes, and casually throwing around McCarthy'ism as a way to silence progressives, who demanded we speak about issues, instead. And nothing but excuses for Democratic leadership as they caved to the right wing on issue after issue, with hollow theatrical speeches getting all the attention, instead of how Democratic leadership was actually voting. Endless escalations of pentagon/ DHS funding, a historic number of Trump judges fast-tracked, funding his wall, all of it. Until finally this year, another round of obviously corrupted primaries and media, and acceptance of vote tallies in which the math simply made no sense. Then COVID...so no more time for discussion.
Now with Biden / Harris, they are announcing that our primary process is officially meaningless - as 2 of the LEAST popular candidates throughout the primaries are suddenly described as having 'won'. No time to talk about that, either. Because then you'll be accused of 'supporting Trump'. It's so obvious from the outside, and yet I see so many friends here, terrified into accepting it.
Both Joe Biden and Kamala Harris (as well as everyone else planned for their administration) are absolutely Republican in terms of their policies. Looking past Joe Bidens' embarrassing dementia, terrible history, and credible rape accusations, if you don't know what Kamala Harris has done in her past as a prosecutor, you need to - as her being black, and a woman have been meaningless in terms of her refusal to prosecute corporate criminals, promotion of the neo-con war machine, support for a surveillance state, and criminally brutal treatment of non-violent offenders in California.
This is a woman who willfully refused to release non-violent prisoners after a court order to do so, with the (literal) excuse that they were needed for low-cost prison labor. Think about what that means. She wouldn't prosecute Steve Mnuchin, for what her own dept. described as over a thousand criminal violations, after he donated to her campaign. So many other examples of corruption in Harris' history. How she laughed about smoking weed ("I am Jamaican!") while locking up thousands of people for the same thing. And during the primaries she was so unpopular for these reasons, she had to drop out before anyone even voted. Yet now, corporate America is telling you that she's your next president - and HOW did that happen, exactly? Even if you choose to

accept Joe Biden's overnight rise from tanking all year to sudden domination - as the DNC did nothing while people in poor communities were forced to wait in 7 hour lines when attempting to vote - if it were by the number of votes that were counted, they'd still be talking about VP Bernie Sanders. How did that become Kamala Harris instead? How do some 80% of Dems support Medicare 4 All, while the DNC refuse to even allow the term into their (meaningless) platform draft? We have been SHIT on by these people, and Kamala Harris being black and a woman mean nothing.
If we accept this level of corruption again, even tacitly or with criticism attached, we won't be allowed to criticize her actions in the future - as she will obviously take over for Biden immediately - without our being willfully mis-labeled as 'Trump supporters' - or even dumber, 'Russian puppets'. So with Kamala Harris, we can literally say at this point, that the Democratic Party have anointed a candidate for president that NO ONE has voted for - not even a pretense of democracy anymore.
So while I do hate and fear Donald Trump, I cannot support the Democratic Party with my vote. Electing Biden/Harris will do NOTHING to stop the economic collapse, nothing to stop the evictions, nothing to stop police misconduct, nothing to end the wars, nothing to provide Americans healthcare, nothing re: climate change, nothing to raise wages, nothing. And I will be openly critical towards anyone here who tries to pretend otherwise. I won't be intimidated with name calling, or people unfriending me, or trying to blame me for Trump - as if my vote or lack thereof would even matter. These aren't liberals, nor are they centrists, they won't be 'moved to the left' on anything, and it's a monumental mistake to allow them to blackmail your support.

****

August 12, 2020, 8:52PM (Amir-ul Kafirs to group):

Re: HERETICS: WikiLeaks

Well, I don't know jackshit about Kamala Harris but I'm long-since past any hope that someone is going to do something for the people based on their being black or a woman. At any rate, your friend's tirade makes perfect sense to me as a critique of the Democratic Party at this point in time. As one former friend of mine recently told me: "All's fair in love & war." He's a staunch democrat. The thing is, *All is NOT fair in love & war* because there is NO LOVE, it's *all war & it's all* ***unfair*** & it's these very self-justifying morons who make it that way.

****

August 13, 2020, 12:00AM (Inquiring Librarian to group):

Re: HERETICS: WikiLeaks

Yes, your friend's tirade also makes perfect sense to me. Thank you for sharing. I'd love to pick your friend's brain a bit to see more of how he/she is feeling beyond that rant. I know several staunch democrats who are jumping ship in the election because it is becoming all too clear which demon is more insidious. It's a very sad time for the United States. On a brighter note, at least more Americans, myself included, are waking up to a lot of the corruption. I think there may be hope for the future of the democratic party to regroup and recover at some point in the future, enough of us are seeing with clearer eyes. RFK Jr. hasn't given up on the party. He said that most Democratic voters have good hearts and mean well, but they have been misled and if we could just get through to them, change would happen. I believe this also. It is too late for this election, but in 4 years, as long as we're not murdered or transhuman slave dumbots, I see a sea change in the Democratic party.

****

August 13, 2020, 10:39AM (Phil to group):

Re: HERETICS: Book in Progress: PLEASE ANSWER!!

I have fallen way behind in this list at the moment. I will try and catch up and also try and read soon peoples contributions to the book. Here is a generally up date with some not so directly relevant personal situation info.

work situation
I can't remember exactly what I wrote about my work situation last time. It came down to the franchisees (our bosses) wanting us to sign an agreement that had three parts to it. First they wanted to take away five days of holidays the amount of holidays that we would be allocated for the time we were in quarantyranny. I did not have a big problem with this. The second part they wanted to divide our holiday allowance (for me just over 1,000 euro) into two payments Half in July (when it would normally all be paid) and half in December (I guess to give them some breathing room for other depts). The final part was basically a bit complicated to explain but translates to a donation to the company (in my case around 400 euros) which would be taken out of my second holiday allowance. So my company has became a charity now. In the end I compromised on two parts of the agreement but not on the donation to the company. A couple of weeks later after I had signed my agreement I actually needed my full vacation allowance. I had to write to my bosses to ask them if it would be possible to pay all my allowance in July. Luckily that gave me my full holiday allowance on the same day. Some staff agreed to everything and others to none of it and some just to some of it.

World Economic Forum
I protested the Wold Economic Forum meeting that was held in Melbourne on September 11, 2000 held in the Crown Casino. It was a national blockade. The protest successfully disrupted the meeting. Many sessions had to be cancelled and delegates had to be flown in by helicopter onto a pad on top of the building. I went to the protest in Melbourne with a group of anarchists from Adelaide. The following year we had a get together at my house (where Amir-ul Kafirs once stayed). The son of one of those present rang his father with the news. We all

ended up spending the rest of the evening watching 9/11 news live. that was useful for me because I remember seeing a lot of stuff that was swept under the carpet later that aroused my curiosity.
Last year I remember seeing a lot of short WEF videos shared on social media. I remember it was good propaganda because there were some videos that I agreed with content wise and almost considered sharing.

Phil Bradley Project
I had thought of collaborating with other Phil Bradleys on a project. I think it would be a fun idea. There is one on social media that interacts with me from time to time. https://www.facebook.com/phil.bradley.927543 I found it amusing that there were Phil Bradleys that share interests or previous interests of mine such as a drummer (i was a drummer in some bands for a little while), wing chun (I practiced wing chun for about three years once) and an Australian green party politician (I was involved with setting up the south Australian branch of the Australian Greens)

****

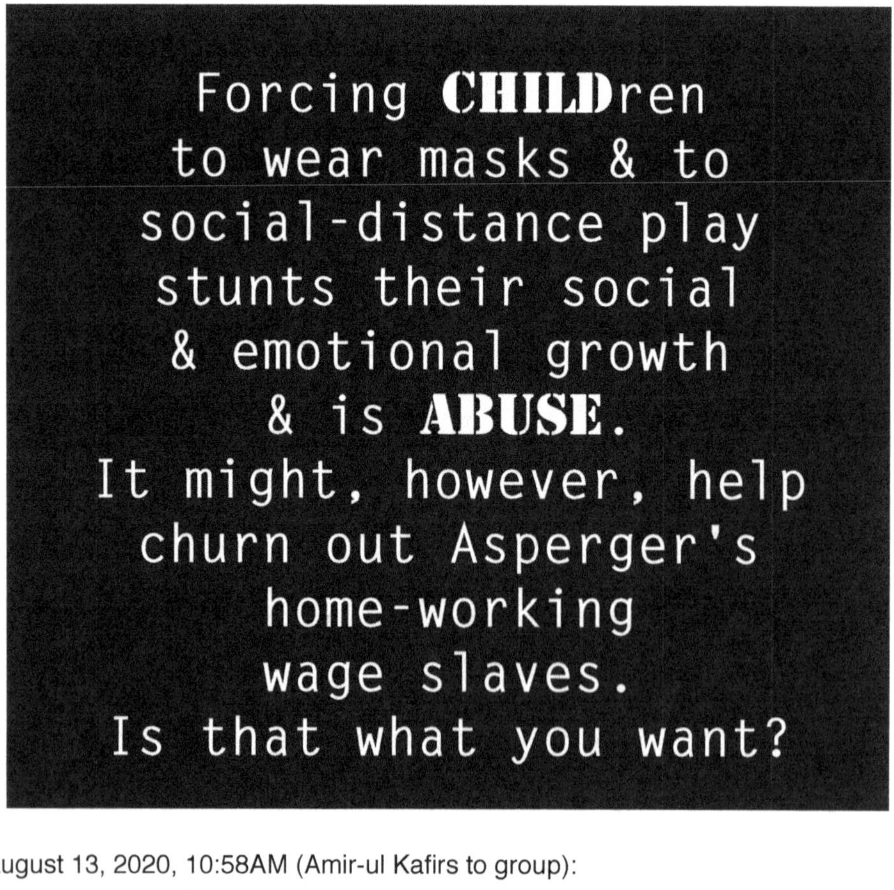
Forcing CHILDren
to wear masks & to
social-distance play
stunts their social
& emotional growth
& is ABUSE.
It might, however, help
churn out Asperger's
home-working
wage slaves.
Is that what you want?

August 13, 2020, 10:58AM (Amir-ul Kafirs to group):

HERETICS: CHILD ABUSE

This was to be my LAST social media post but, oh well, there are 3 more ready & waiting.

****

August 13, 2020, 11:05AM (Inquiring Librarian to group):

HERETICS: CHILD ABUSE

This one is GREAT! I manage a kid-centered library. It breaks my heart daily to see kids with masks (& sometimes face shields). We accidentally left green frostinged cupcakes on a library table about a month ago. A nice family with masked kids came in. Within 5 minutes, the kids were maskless, flying around the library, chasing each other and screaming, with green frosting on their faces. The masks did not come back on. The parents did not care. It was bliss.

****

August 13, 2020, 11:05AM (Amir-ul Kafirs to group):

Re: HERETICS: CHILD ABUSE

This one is GREAT!

I'm glad you like it. It's nice to know that the 3 people I know who work with kids the most, you, Naia Nisnam, & a woman in Pittsburgh who runs her own pre-school all are on the same page with I consider to be *common sense observations:* viz that masking up in childcare situations is just about as emotionally & socially bad as it gets.

****

August 13, 2020, 8:15PM (Inquiring Librarian to group):

HERETICS: Dr. Scott Atlas - Just Added to the U.S. Corona Virus Task Force

GREAT NEWS!!! Dr. Scott Atlas has been added to the U.S. Coronavirus Task Force!! Why is this good news?? It is because I have been following him for some time. He is VERY well credentialed, **Atlas** received a Bachelor of Science degree in biology from the University of Illinois in Urbana-Champaign and his MD from the Pritzker School of Medicine of the University of Chicago. He currently serves as the Robert Wesson Senior Fellow at Stanford University's Hoover Institution. Notice again, he is from Stanford. A lot of good ppl are coming from Stanford in this pandemic!!

He wants to end the lockdowns, based on hard science (on which he is a true expert). He wants kids to go back to school. He states unabashedly, with

scientific backing from this and other countries, that kids are not carriers of the virus and they do not die from it. He believes in natural herd immunity and thinks we are over testing and politicizing the virus in ways that are killing Americans. Read more here:
HowToRe-OpenSocietyUsingEvidence,MedicalScience,andLogic
https://www.hsgac.senate.gov/imo/media/doc/Testimony-Atlas-2020-05-06.pdf

And see how much the neoliberal fascists squirm, trying to lambast and shame Atlas. Their derision of Atlas in this 'news' cast is to me, insulting, shameless and pure lies and propaganda...they are squirming because Atlas can take Fauci, the vaccine Czar, out:
Keilar: Dr. Atlas wouldn't know science if it kicked him in the Atlas

https://www.cnn.com/videos/politics/2020/08/13/brianna-keilar-fact-check-trump-new-coronavirus-adviser-scott-atlas-crn-vpx.cnn?fbclid=IwAR2RGzKxoRdvTwODqzciZDJVcjQ2Gb5jmxWccsrOn7fELeaov6TiUl15VtQ

I do not know his stance on vaccinations. But I know he is NOT Fauci, who is basically the Vaccine Czar/Drug Lord of the NIH who profits wildly off of mass vaccinations since that is the industry he works and has gotten filthy rich in (not plandemic conflict of interest there, right??).

****

How To Re-Open Society Using Evidence, Medical Science, and Logic

Scott W. Atlas, MD, is the David and Joan Traitel Senior Fellow at Stanford University's Hoover Institution and the former Chief of Neuroradiology at Stanford University Medical Center.

The consequences of the COVID-19 pandemic have been enormous. As of the first week of May, more than 70,000 Americans have died. If it were compared as a separate country, the New York area would rank, by far, as number one for deaths per capita. Given that three to four weeks typically elapses before death, thousands more already infected will also succumb to the virus. That said, the direct daily toll from the infection has markedly declined throughout the United States, including the epicenter of New York. The curves have been flattened – the stated goal of the isolation has been accomplished – for both hospitalizations per day and deaths per day.

We now have an even greater urgency, due to the severe and single-minded policies already implemented. Treating Covid-19 "at all costs" is severely restricting other medical care and instilling fear in the public, creating a massive health disaster, in addition to severe economic harms that could generate a world poverty crisis with almost incalculable consequences. Half of neurosurgery patients still refuse to come in for treatment of diseases that if left untreated risk brain hemorrhage, paralysis, and death, even when their doctors directly reassure them. Transplants from living donors are down 85 percent from the same period last year. Missed biopsies of now undiscovered cancers number thousands per week. That doesn't include the latest reports of skipping two-thirds to three-fourths of cancer screenings, most childhood vaccinations, and treatment for new strokes and known cancer.

We also know that total isolation *prevents* **broad population immunity and** *prolongs* **the problem.**

We know from decades of medical science that infection causes individuals to generate an immune response – antibodies – and the population later develops immunity. Indeed, that is the *main purpose* of widespread immunization in other viral diseases – to assist with "herd immunity". In the Covid-19 epicenter New York City, higher immunity is likely, although undoubtedly muted by the extreme isolation policies, as more than 20 percent of those tested had antibodies. A similar finding was reported in Boston. That fact has been *incorrectly* portrayed as an urgent problem requiring mass isolation. On the contrary, infected people are the immediately available vehicle for establishing widespread immunity. By transmitting the virus to others in lower-risk groups who then generate antibodies, pathways toward the most vulnerable people are blocked, ultimately eradicating the threat. While we do not know with certainty that antibodies from Covid-19 stop infection, it is expected, based on decades of virology science, including other coronavirus respiratory viruses, where immunity post-infection is thought to last for a year or more. That's why scientists are hopeful about using Covid-19 antibodies to treat the sickest patients; that's the basis for the drive to generate a vaccine.

There are two critical aspects of this urgently needed, targeted re-entry plan. First, policymakers must apply logic and critical thinking to the data we have acquired, instead of continuing to prioritize hypothetical projections – projections that need to be readjusted every few days, highlighting their inaccuracy - and then combine that evidence with decades of established medical science. Second, we must demonstrate and fully convey the logic underlying the plan to reassure a public that has become almost paralyzed with panic and fear.

Reassuring the public about re-entry requires repeating the facts – what we know - about the threat and who it targets. By now, multiple studies from Europe, Japan, and the US all suggest that the overall fatality rate is far lower than early estimates, perhaps below 0.1 to 0.4%, i.e., ten to forty times lower than estimates that motivated extreme isolation. And we also now know who to protect, because this disease - by the evidence - is not equally dangerous across the population. In Detroit's Oakland County, 75 percent of deaths were in those over 70; 91 percent were in people over 60, similar to what was noted in New York. And younger, healthier people have virtually zero risk of death and little risk of serious disease – as I have noted before, under one percent of New York City's hospitalizations have been patients under 18 years of age, and less than one percent of deaths at any age are in the absence of underlying conditions.

Here are specific, science-based, logical steps to strategically end the lockdown and safely restore the pathway to normal life:

First, let's finally focus on protecting the most vulnerable – that means nursing home patients. Given that older people with underlying conditions are obvious set-ups for serious complications from respiratory infections, it is difficult to excuse policies that allowed 20,000 nursing care residents to die - 30 percent of all deaths in the US, more than half of the total in some states, particularly when they already live under controlled access. Urgently needed, targeted protection would include strictly regulating all who enter and care for nursing home members by requiring testing and protective masks for all who interact with these highly vulnerable people. Moreover, nursing home workers should be tested for Covid-19 antibodies, and if negative, for virus to exclude infection, to ensure safety of senior residents. No Covid-19-positive patient can resume residence until definitively cleared by testing.

We must continue to educate and inform the public about what they have already successfully learned regarding the at-risk group. That means issuing rational guidelines advising the highest standards of hygiene and appropriate social distancing while interacting with elderly friends and family members at risk, including those with diabetes, obesity, and other chronic conditions.

Second, those with mild symptoms of the illness should strictly self-isolate for two weeks. It's not urgent to test them – simply assume they have the infection. That includes confinement at home, having the highest concern for sanitization, and wearing protective masks when others in their homes enter the same room.

Third, open all K-12 schools. If under 18 and in good health, you have nearly no risk of serious illness from Covid-19. Exceptions exist, as they do with virtually every other clinically encountered infection, but that should not outweigh the overwhelming evidence to the contrary. Again, standards for consciously protecting elderly and other at-risk family members or friends, including teachers in higher-risk groups, should still be employed.

Fourth, open most businesses, including restaurants and offices, but require new standards for hygiene, disinfection, and sanitization via enforceable, more stringent regulations than in the past. It is reasonable to post warnings for customers who are older or in other ways vulnerable. Avoid unnecessary requirements for spacing of customers, though – it is not logical that otherwise healthy adults, especially younger age groups, should be isolated or maintain a six-foot spacing from each other. If infection is still prevalent, socializing among these low-risk groups represents the opportunity for developing widespread immunity and eradicating the threat.

[..]

- https://www.hsgac.senate.gov/imo/media/doc/Testimony-Atlas-2020-05-06.pdf

****

Keilar: Dr. Atlas wouldn't know science if it kicked him in the Atlas

CNN Right Now

Months into the coronavirus pandemic, President Donald Trump announced Dr. Scott Atlas as a medical adviser for the White House coronavirus task force. CNN's Brianna Keilar breaks down Dr. Atlas's controversial stance on Covid-19.

****

August 13, 2020, 8:22PM (Inquiring Librarian to group):

Re: HERETICS: Dr. Scott Atlas - Just Added to the U.S. Corona Virus Task Force

Here is another excellent interview of Dr. Atlas, you can click on the bottom for the transcript:
https://podcasts.la.utexas.edu/cepa/podcast/scott-atlas-covid-19-interview/

****

Scott W. Atlas, M.D.is the Robert Wesson Senior Fellow at the Hoover Institution of Stanford University and a Member of Hoover Institution's Working Group on Health Care Policy.

Dr. Atlas investigates the impact of government and the private sector on access, quality, pricing, and innovation in health care and is a frequent policy advisor to government and industry leaders in these areas. During the 2008, 2012, and 2016 presidential campaigns, he was a Senior Advisor for Health Care to a number of candidates for President of the United States. He has also advised several members of the United States Senate and House of Representatives and testified to Congress on health care reform. His most recent book is entitled Restoring Quality Health Care: A Six-Point Plan for Comprehensive Reform at Lower Cost (Hoover Press, 2016). Some of Dr. Atlas's previous health policy books include In Excellent Health: Setting the Record Straight on America's Health Care System (Hoover Press, 2011), Reforming America's Health Care System (Hoover Press, 2010), and Power to the Patient: Selected Health Care Issues and Policy Solutions (Hoover Press, 2005). Dr. Atlas had a Fulbright award to collaborate with academic leaders in China on structuring health care solutions for China, and also participated with leaders from government and academia on the World Bank's Commission on Growth and Development. He has also advised leaders on health care and medical technology in several countries outside the US, including Latin America, Southeast Asia, and Europe. Dr. Atlas has published and been interviewed in a variety of media, including the Wall Street Journal, Forbes Magazine, CNN, USA Today, Fox News, London's Financial Times, BBC Radio, The PBS News Hour, Bloomberg Radio, Brazil's Correio Braziliense and Isto E, Italy's Corriere della Sera, Argentina's Diario La Nacion, and India's The Hindu.

Dr. Atlas is also the editor of the leading textbook in the field, the best-selling Magnetic Resonance Imaging of the Brain and Spine, now in its 5th edition and officially translated from English into Mandarin, Spanish, and Portuguese. He has been editor, associate editor, and a member of the boards of numerous scientific journals and national and international scientific societies over the past three decades. His medical research centered on advanced applications of new MRI technologies in neurologic diseases. While Professor of Radiology and Chief of Neuroradiology at Stanford University Medical Center from 1998 until 2012 and during his previous faculty positions, Dr. Atlas trained over 100 neuroradiology fellows, many of whom are now leaders in the field throughout the world.
He lectures on a variety of topics, most notably the role of government and the

private sector in health care quality and access, global trends in health care innovation, and the key economic issues related to the future of technology-based medical advances. In the private sector, Dr. Atlas is a frequent advisor to start-up entrepreneurs and companies in the life sciences and medical technology.

Dr. Atlas has received numerous awards and honors in recognition of his leadership in the field. He is recognized internationally as a leader in both education and clinical research and had been on the Nominating Committee for the Nobel Prize in Medicine and Physiology for several years. He has been named by his peers in The Best Doctors in America every year since its initial publication, as well as in regional listings, such as The Best Doctors in New York, Silicon Valley's Best Doctors, and other similar publications. He was honored to receive the 2011 Alumni Achievement Award, the highest career achievement honor for a distinguished alumnus from the University of Illinois in Urbana-Champaign, his alma mater.

Dr. Atlas received a BS degree in biology from the University of Illinois in Urbana-Champaign and an MD degree from the University of Chicago School of Medicine.

Guests

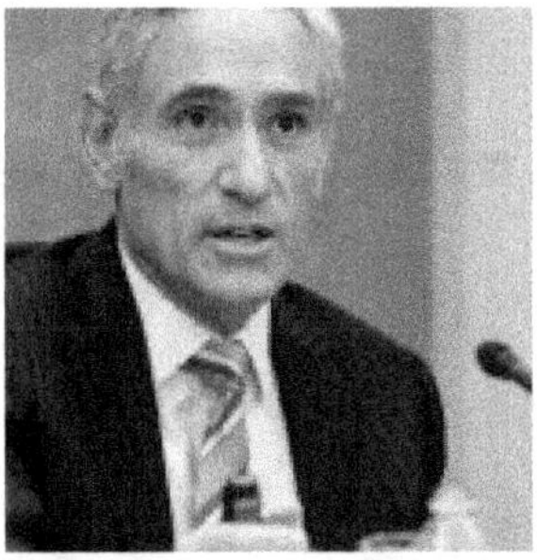

Scott Atlas
Robert Wesson Senior Fellow at Stanford University

Welcome to Policy McCombs. A data focused conversation on tradeoffs.

I'm Carlos Kavala from the Saban Center for Policy at the University of Texas at Austin. A pleasure to have Dr. Scott Atlus from the Hoover Institution, where he's a senior fellow and also a former professor and chief neuro radiologist at the Stanford Medical School Center Medical School. Scott, thanks for joining us here. Thanks for having me. So we're here in June 2nd, 2020, and I want to have a conversation about our policies and the decisions made leading up to this day associated with the pandemic of October 19. So let's go back to March or even before that went. When were you started to get nervous or concerned about what was coming our way and what data and information where you're looking at?

Then let's say, you know, late February, March, you're a well, you know, I'm like a every human being I have. My first reaction was I was afraid, you know, because that's just the normal inclination of something is as bad as what was said originally about the fatality rate. And, you know, sort of the assumption that this was we were what's called medically naive to this infection, meaning it was brand new and a, nobody would have any immunity, et cetera, as the first reports were sort of really sensationalizing things so early. I would say in in February, things started to come out about who was really being impacted.

And yet there was this public discourse. And then eventually in March, I started writing about this. I think I may have written in February. I don't remember that. But the reality was that the data coming out was suddenly in the public sphere discussion where people I don't know why. Maybe because we live in an era of hyperbole and we live where if you do a Google search, you're an expert and our society confers expertise to people who have none, but they happen to be successful in some other walk of life or their ranch or whatever the rationale for it is. And so there was a public discussion, incredibly naive to what medical science says and really took off to be a very fearful discussion. And a lot of it was because of these hypothetical projections that were from, you know, early on statistical models. But by virtue of being very early are very problematic by definition because there's very little actual data entering and it's just about a hypothetical. And somehow this became the discussion. The narrative was really based on worst case scenario hypothetical. People were afraid it was a bad mix.

[..]

- https://podcasts.la.utexas.edu/cepa/podcast/scott-atlas-covid-19-interview/

****

August 14, 2020, 4:58AM (Amir-ul Kafirs to group):

HERETICS: Legless

I prefaced this one on social media with:

Today's approach is in the style of an SF dystopic flash fiction:

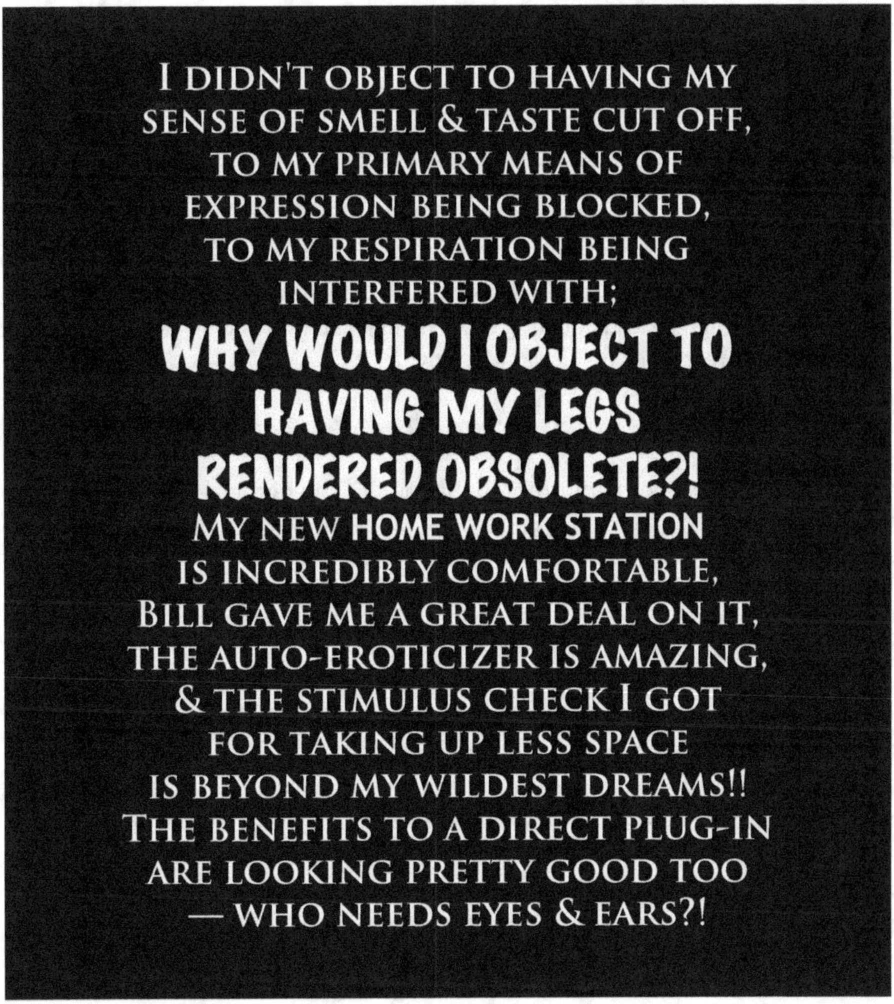
I DIDN'T OBJECT TO HAVING MY
SENSE OF SMELL & TASTE CUT OFF,
TO MY PRIMARY MEANS OF
EXPRESSION BEING BLOCKED,
TO MY RESPIRATION BEING
INTERFERED WITH;
WHY WOULD I OBJECT TO
HAVING MY LEGS
RENDERED OBSOLETE?!
MY NEW HOME WORK STATION
IS INCREDIBLY COMFORTABLE,
BILL GAVE ME A GREAT DEAL ON IT,
THE AUTO-EROTICIZER IS AMAZING,
& THE STIMULUS CHECK I GOT
FOR TAKING UP LESS SPACE
IS BEYOND MY WILDEST DREAMS!!
THE BENEFITS TO A DIRECT PLUG-IN
ARE LOOKING PRETTY GOOD TOO
— WHO NEEDS EYES & EARS?!

Perhaps that will help my largely 'undercultured' social media readership have a little understanding that I'm experimenting with different ways of presenting commentary within a deliberately limited format.

****

August 14, 2020, 5:32AM (Amir-ul Kafirs to group):

Re: HERETICS: Dr. Scott Atlas - Just Added to the U.S. Corona Virus Task Force

That does seem to be good news although I still find him to be more pandemic-happy than I'd prefer. E.G.:

"**Second**, those with mild symptoms of the illness should strictly self-isolate for two weeks. It's not urgent to test them – simply assume they have the infection. That includes confinement at home, having the highest concern for sanitization, and wearing protective masks when others in their homes enter the same room."

Still, his concluding last few sentences are promising:

"Smart, safe re-entry cannot be delayed by fear or hypothetical projections, because we have direct data on risk and experience with managing it. The goal of the strict isolation has been accomplished. Let's stop underemphasizing empirical evidence and established medical science while instead doubling down on hypothetical models. Science and logic must prevail over fear and worst-case scenarios."

Keilar: Dr. Atlas wouldn't know science if it kicked him in the Atlas

I didn't watch this. I take it for granted that any Rump nominee will be opposed as if he's an idiot. While such an approach probably still works with most of the people I'm 'friends' with on social media it's long since worn thin for me. It's 'funny', though, that he'd be found so objectionable, even though I know it's not ultimately about what he says as what he represents politically, because what he says strikes me as common-sensical. Take this, e.g.:

"**Fourth**, open most businesses, including restaurants and offices, but require new standards for hygiene, disinfection, and sanitization via enforceable, more stringent regulations than in the past. It is reasonable to post warnings for customers who are older or in other ways vulnerable. Avoid unnecessary requirements for spacing of customers, though – it is not logical that otherwise healthy adults, especially younger age groups, should be isolated or maintain a six-foot spacing from each other. If infection is still prevalent, socializing among these low-risk groups represents the opportunity for developing widespread immunity and eradicating the threat."

Of course, I find that common-sensical whereas the knee-jerk opponents are bound to depict it as utter madness. Oh, well.

I do not know his stance on vaccinations.

In the statement you link to he says this:

"While we do not know with certainty that antibodies from Covid-19 stop infection, it is expected, based on decades of virology science, including other coronavirus respiratory viruses, where immunity post-infection is thought to last for a year or more. That's why scientists are hopeful about using Covid-19 antibodies to treat the sickest patients; that's the basis for the drive to generate a vaccine."

So, I reckon the implication is that a vaccine is a good thing. He might just be being circumspect.

****

August 14, 2020, 5:53AM (Inquiring Librarian to group):

Re: HERETICS: Dr. Scott Atlas - Just Added to the U.S. Corona Virus Task Force

I agree on the heavy handed lockdown part. But i then noticed that article was from April. I think the other articles posted were more recent. :)

This 1 is August 13th.
https://www.google.com/amp/s/wjla.com/amp/news/nation-world/one-on-one-with-dr-scott-atlas

This 1 here is from late June:
https://podcasts.la.utexas.edu/cepa/podcast/scott-atlas-covid-19-interview/

It is possible Atlas is not referring to vaccines in the article, but to herd immunity and also "passive immunity approaches', as described here:
https://www.bmj.com/content/370/bmj.m2722
"The devastating pandemic caused by the SARS-CoV-2 coronavirus appears to be a prime candidate for traditional prevention (vaccines) and passive immunity approaches. Passive immunity, using convalescent plasma from recovered patients or monoclonal antibodies with high levels of neutralising antiviral activity, have potential for both therapy and prevention".

****

One on one with Dr. Scott Atlas

by SCOTT THUMAN, Sinclair Broadcast Group Chief Political Correspondent Thursday, August 13th 2020

WASHINGTON (SBG) - During the coronavirus crisis, many people have been getting their guidance from Dr. Anthony Fauci, Dr. Deborah Birx, and other members of the White House task force.
But there's a new doctor who also has the president's ear — and he's making a concerted push to get schools up and running.
Sinclair's Chief Political Correspondent Scott Thuman was at the White House today to question Dr. Scott Atlas. Here is part of their exchange.

Dr. Scott Atlas: “It's very, very, low, extremely low risk to children. There's not zero risk to anything, in fact, in life, but to be very precise, the risk to children is extremely low.”
Scott Thuman: “You've been a strong advocate of getting kids back to school. What about the fear of transmission, because we see, for example, the schools in Georgia, the photo goes viral? Several dozen tested positive. Does that cause

us to say we need to hit the brakes at all?"
Dr. Scott Atlas: "It shouldn't. And I'll explain why. There is no data that shows that the disease is transmitted in a significant amount from children to adults. There is no, there are several types of studies to look at that for. One is contract tracing. There is one as recently as August 2 from Switzerland, shows that there is no significant transmission."
Scott Thuman: "We were in this building we interviewed Dr. Birx and asked about transmission rate from children under the age of 10 and she said 'I know children under 10 can get infected. What I don't know is how many transmit the virus'. So who's right?"
Dr. Scott Atlas: "It's not a matter of being right or wrong. It's a matter of looking at the data. It's easy to say we don't know everything — that's true. I'm not going to dispute that, but there's no disease in the world that we know everything about. There's a preponderance of evidence here that children are not a significant source of the infection. One of the world's best pediatric hospitals, their recommendation is no mask no spacing."
Scott Thuman: "Do you agree with that?"
Dr. Scott Atlas: "Well, I think I do and here's the logic: if there's no risk to children, no significant risk I should say, then what are you protecting them from? If kids get the infection in this school that's still okay. The goal of public policy is not to prevent healthy people from getting the infection. The goal of public policy, public policy is to prevent high-risk individuals from getting the infection. But that has nothing to do with locking down schools to stop people who have no problem with the disease from getting an infection."

[..]

- https://wjla.com/news/nation-world/one-on-one-with-dr-scott-atlas

****

Editorials
Vaccines, convalescent plasma, and monoclonal antibodies for covid-19
BMJ 2020; 370 doi: https://doi.org/10.1136/bmj.m2722 (Published 09 July 2020)

Worldwide, many covid-19 vaccines are at various phases of development.Trials are also investigating convalescent plasma as a containment option or supportive therapy for patients with covid-19. Understandably, there is great public expectation that these efforts will be successful, but caution is necessary with respect to both vaccines and passive immunity.

Vaccines

Many candidate vaccines target the virus spike protein, a molecule essential for the virus to bind to the angiotensin converting enzyme 2 receptor complexes in the cell membrane as a first step for infection. Studies of SARS-CoV-2 genomic sequences indicate that regions encoding the receptor binding domain of the spike protein are highly conserved, providing hope for a successful vaccine directed at a stable target. However, substantial mutations (albeit rare) in the spike protein close to the receptor binding domain are described along with other drift variants. The effect of these mutations on protein expression and the antigenicity required to provoke an antibody response (or to interact with passive antibody) is unclear.

There are further reasons for caution over covid-19 vaccines. Over a decade, attempts to develop vaccines against SARS and MERS, caused by related coronaviruses, have been unsuccessful. Attempts to produce vaccines against other RNA viruses, such as dengue, resulted in candidates that were not protective, and some exacerbated disease through antibody dependent enhancement. Although there is no evidence that the SARS-CoV-2 vaccine candidates produce antibody dependent enhancement, it remains a possibility. Furthermore, covid-19 disproportionately affects older age groups, where immune senescence leads to poorer quality immune responses. Vaccines may be less effective in those with greatest need. Additionally, infections with other coronaviruses and challenges with experimental vaccines have resulted in short term (1-2 years) protective immunity. Vaccine effectiveness and duration may therefore require repeated vaccinations and the use of adjuvants to improve responses.

[..]

- https://www.bmj.com/content/370/bmj.m2722

****

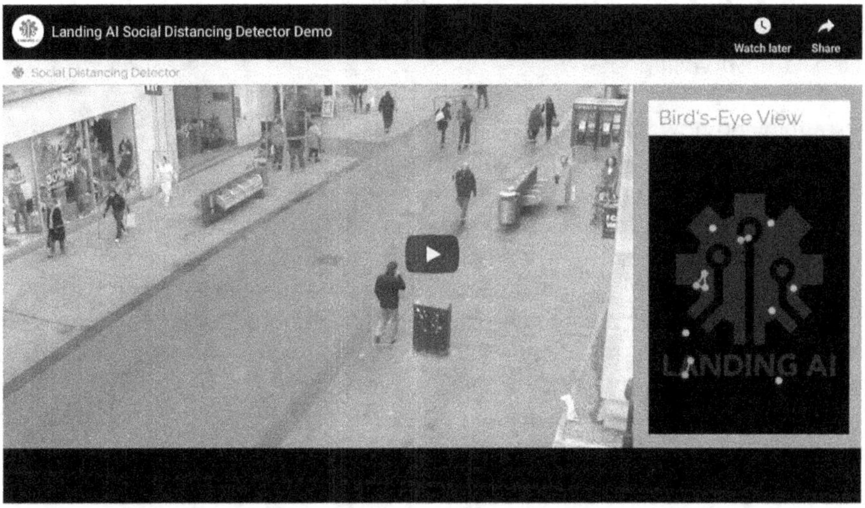

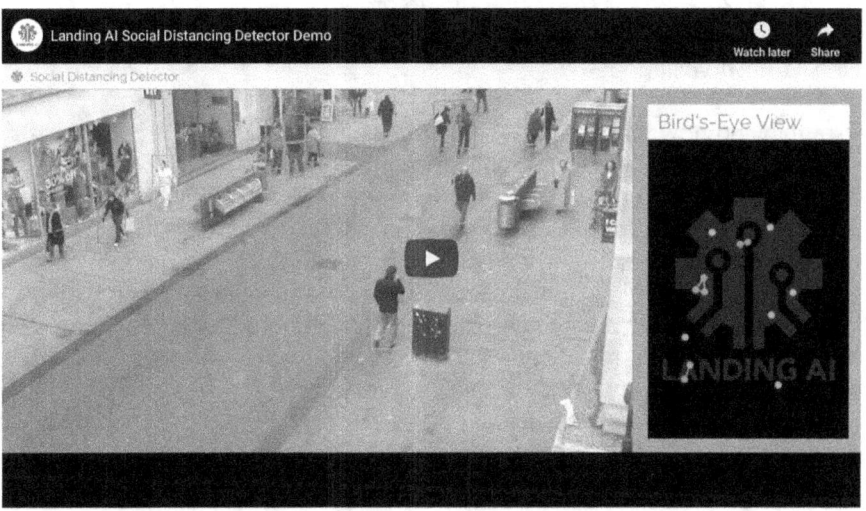

This demo video is performed on the public "OXFORD TOWN CENTRE" dataset

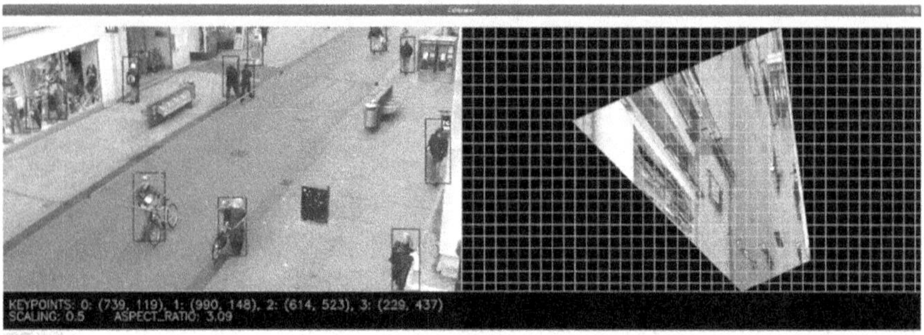

On the left is the original perspective view overlaid with a calibration grid. On the right is the resulting bird's eye view Note that the sides of the street lie completely parallel to the green grid.

****

August 14, 2020, 11:11AM (Naia Nisnam to group):

European doctors speak out against CoronaScam

I've only skimmed these and won't have time to read through it all today but thought I'd share...
The more doctors I see speaking out, the more hope I have:

https://acu2020.org/english-versions/

****

August 15, 2020, 8:34AM (Amir-ul Kafirs to group):

HERETICS: Surveillance

SO, I'm thinking now that I have to have a cut-off point of when I make & take new things for the (still very hypothetical but getting there) BOOK & **TOMORROW** will be 5 months since I made my 1st PANDEMIC PANIC post on social media so I think that tomorrow is when I'll make my last post there & tomorrow will be the last day when I cull from these emails for the book. I'm not sure what I'm going to do with my social media page, I've been looking at the settings to see if there's a way I can temporarily suspend it or if I can stop all comments. I think Phil has his page set up that way so I'll see if I can figure out how to do that. That way people (mainly myself) can still access it as an historical database but it can't just be used as a place for people to dump on me. SO, here's the 2nd-to-the-last of the text panels:

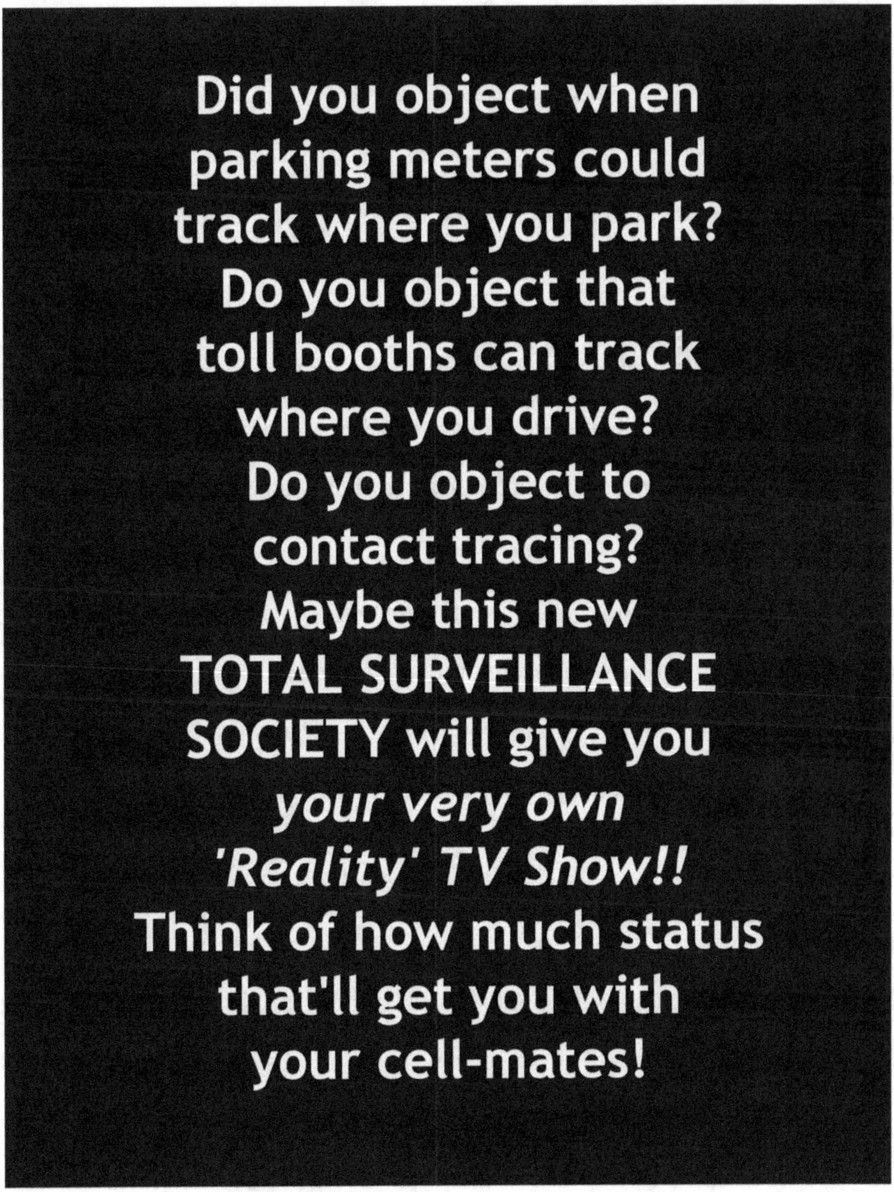

Did you object when
parking meters could
track where you park?
Do you object that
toll booths can track
where you drive?
Do you object to
contact tracing?
Maybe this new
TOTAL SURVEILLANCE
SOCIETY will give you
your very own
'Reality' TV Show!!
Think of how much status
that'll get you with
your cell-mates!

****

August 15, 2020, 7:13PM (Amir-ul Kafirs to group):

HERETICS: Kamala Harris

Inquiring Librarian sent me a link to an article about Kamala Harris on Consortiumnews:

https://consortiumnews.com/2020/08/13/kamala-harriss-distinguished-career-of-serving-injustice/?fbclid=IwAR3w2WhM5bGinzK_r7H3Jbls8CbQupXbBd4QVxokHK48INUNB5hcJc5j85k

They depict her as what I'd consider to be a typical rising star DA —> Attorney General: somone willing to sell out justice for power, business as usual. Here're some excerpts:

"Harris, who served as San Francisco district attorney from 2004 to 2011 and California attorney general from 2011 to 2017, describes herself as a "progressive prosecutor." Harris's prosecutorial record, however, is far from progressive. Through her apologia for egregious prosecutorial misconduct, her refusal to allow DNA testing for a probably innocent death row inmate, her opposition to legislation requiring the attorney general's office to independently investigate police shootings and more, she has made a significant contribution to the sordid history of injustice she decries."

"Harris refused DNA testing that could exonerate Kevin Cooper, a likely innocent man on death row, and she opposed statewide body-worn police cameras. Harris favored criminalizing truancy, raising cash bail fees and keeping prisoners locked up for cheap labor. She also supported reporting arrested undocumented juveniles to Immigration and Customs Enforcement, covering for corrupt police lab technicians and blocking gender confirmation surgery for a transgender prisoner. A U.S. District Court judge concluded that withholding the surgery constituted cruel and unusual punishment in violation of the Eighth Amendment."

"Although many of Harris's prosecutorial actions harmed people of color, a notable one helped the white "foreclosure king" — Steve Mnuchin, now Trump's Treasury secretary.

Mnuchin was CEO of OneWest Bank from 2009-2015. A 2013 memo obtained by *The Intercept* alleges that "OneWest rushed delinquent homeowners out of their homes by violating notice and waiting period statutes, illegally backdated key documents, and effectively gamed foreclosure auctions."
After a yearlong investigation, the California attorney general's Consumer Law Section "uncovered evidence suggestive of widespread misconduct." In 2013, they recommended that Harris prosecute a civil enforcement lawsuit against the bank.

"Without any explanation," Harris's office declined to initiate litigation in the case. Mnuchin donated $2,000 to Harris's Senate campaign in February 2016. It was his only donation to a Democratic candidate.

In January 2017, the Campaign for Accountability claimed that Mnuchin and OneWest Bank used "potentially illegal tactics to foreclose on as many as 80,000 California homes," and called for a federal investigation."

SO, since I've never heard of Consortiumnews & since they give a pretty negative view of Harris I was curious about what type of Fact Choker spin there might be on them so I checked a Wikipedia entry about the now deceased founder, Robert Parry, 1st:

"**Robert Parry** (June 24, 1949 – January 27, 2018) was an American investigative journalist. He was best known for his role in covering the Iran-Contra affair for the Associated Press (AP) and *Newsweek*, including breaking the Psychological Operations in Guerrilla Warfare (CIA manual provided to the Nicaraguan contras) and the CIA involvement in Contra cocaine trafficking in the U.S. scandal in 1985.
He was awarded the George Polk Award for National Reporting in 1984 and the I.F. Stone Medal for Journalistic Independence by Harvard's Nieman Foundation in 2015.
Parry was the editor of ConsortiumNews.com from 1995 until his death in 2018."

- https://en.wikipedia.org/wiki/Robert_Parry_(journalist)

He seems to be depicted with surprising appreciation there.

Then I checked a media bias site:

"Factual Reporting: **MOSTLY FACTUAL**
Country: **USA**
World Press Freedom Rank: **USA 48/180**
History
Consortium News is an alternative independent news source established in 1995 by Robert Parry, who passed away in 2018. It is considered the first alternative investigative journalism internet news source. Consortium News covers stories deeply and has been responsible for uncovering scandals and important information that was not found/covered by the mainstream media. The website does not disclose current ownership.
Read our profile on United States government and media.
Funded by / Ownership
The website lacks transparency and does not disclose ownership. Funding appears to be derived from donations.
Analysis / Bias
Consortium News has articles that many on the right may consider left biased: https://consortiumnews.com/2014/04/30/the-fat-cats-of-fast-food/
While also having articles the left won't like: https://consortiumnews.com/2017/05/19/do-high-level-leaks-suggest-a-conspiracy/
The reporting from consortium news cites itself as trying to find the truth. However, I would say that they do often report on things with a left leaning focus. With articles like the above pro-minimum wage or anything regarding the environment. I can see how some on the left would feel that articles like the above or another titled "Europe May Finally Rethink NATO Costs" can come off as right leaning. The reality is that truth has no side. Sometimes somebody on the right is correct and somebody on the left is wrong. The bigger issue is that the political environment of America has been moving the goal posts, of left and right, to the right for the last 30+ years. Meaning that somebody who is "left"

today may in fact have been right 20 years ago. Consortium News has experts from various backgrounds and not just pure journalist which also helps with its reporting to keep it as centered as one can get these days. They have articles about Hillary, Obama, Bush, and Trump all of which have negative things to say about them. They cite factual data with real sources and with minimum usage of loaded wording that you often find in other online only magazines. I would put this news source in your feed to get a more grounded perspective on many of the issues that are shaping up today.
The best way to describe Consortium News, is Wikileaks, without the leaks. They reject imperialism no matter what side is controlling it. They also often do not have a favorable view of President Trump: VIPS Memo to the President: Is Pompeo's Iran Agenda the Same As Yours?
A factual search reveals they have not failed a fact check.
Overall, we rate Consortium News Left-Center Biased based on story selection and advocacy that mildly favors the left. We also rate them Mostly Factual in reporting due to a lack of transparency despite a clean fact check record. (D. Van Zandt 11/3/2016) (M. Allen 6/3/17) Updated (7/27/2019)"

- https://mediabiasfactcheck.com/consortium-news/

SO, it's interesting to me that the media bias people credit them with being "Left-Center Biased" & mainly give them a slightly low rating because their ownership is not transparent.

IN OTHER WORDS, Consortium News ISN'T lambasted as 'right wing' or 'extremist'. I wonder if that'll change as Harris's political career advances.

The relevance, of course, to HERETICS is the apparent emphasis of the Democrats on upping the Medical Police State to its maximum if & when elected.

****

August 16, 2020, 7:56AM (Amir-ul Kafirs to group):

HERETICS: Billionaire Surveillance + shutting off

At the bottom is my last text panel regarding the PANDEMIC PANIC to be posted to social media. I need to move onto different things in my life. ALSO, I reposted a black & white version of my 1st social media post regarding the PANDEMIC PANIC made 5 months ago on March 16, 2020. I don't announce this on social media but I've changed all my Timeline & Tagging settings from being very open to basically being closed. People can't comment on my timeline or tag me anymore. I won't be checking my social media timeline anymore. While some social media friends have impressed me with their intelligence & wit I've been generally dismayed by the comments. There's been almost no willingness whatsoever to be open to the idea that there's a mind control operation in progress. I've spent 5 months trying to address this in various ways but I've come up against a wall of propaganda-speak. Enough is enough. If you want to communicate with me PLEASE do so using email instead of social media. SO, here're the 2 posts:

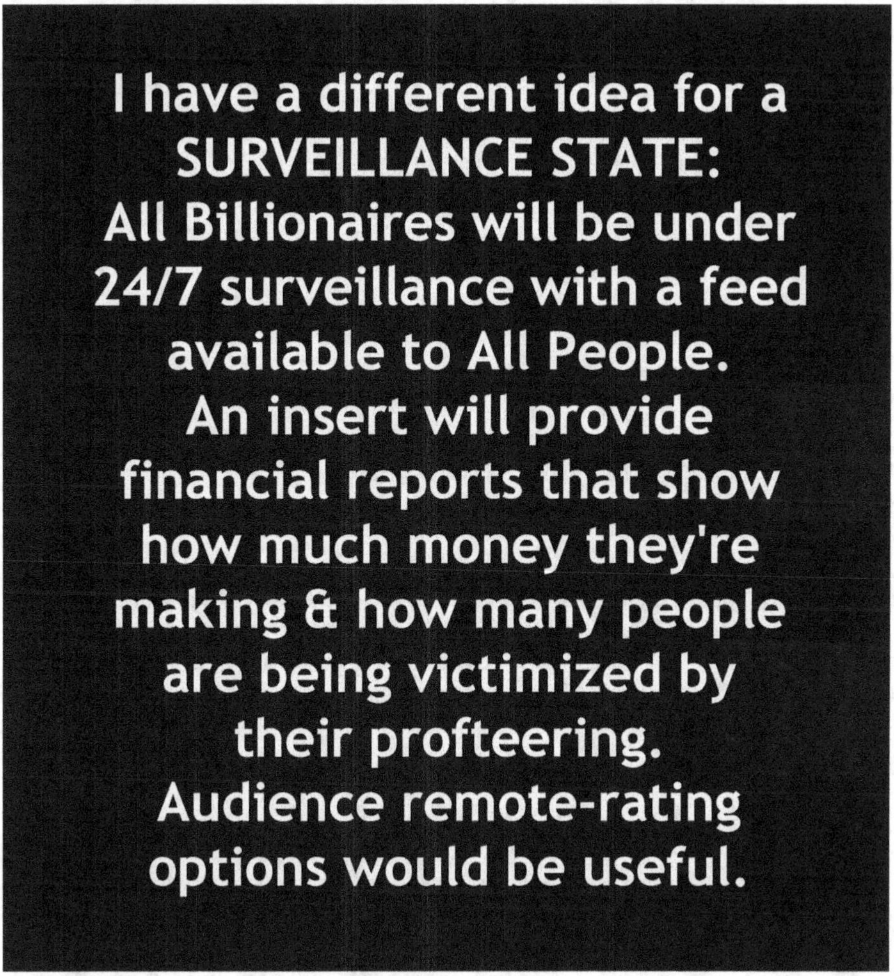

I have a different idea for a
SURVEILLANCE STATE:
All Billionaires will be under
24/7 surveillance with a feed
available to All People.
An insert will provide
financial reports that show
how much money they're
making & how many people
are being victimized by
their profteering.
Audience remote-rating
options would be useful.

Today marks the 5 month anniversary of when I 1st posted on social media about what I've been calling the PANDEMIC PANIC.

March 16, 2020
4 hrs

People are going to get angry with me, as usual, for even daring to suggest the following: What if this PANDEMIC PANIC were just an experiment in mass mind control? It's certainly working. People's behaviors are being even more transparently determined by beliefs based entirely on mediated non-experience than usual. Whether the health danger exists or not the danger of uncritical reception of 'information' from the DOCTOR GODS (who, in my experience are highly fallible) that leads to things happening for 'our own good' that might just not really be for our own good after all is an equally serious danger.

and 2 others　　32 Comments

Like　Comment　Share

****

August 16, 2020, 2:16PM (Amir-ul Kafirs to group):

HERETICS: Twilight Zone

A reminder for you: TODAY IS THE LAST DAY I'LL BE USING ANYTHING POSTED TO THE GROUP IN THE BOOK. As of tomorrow, I won't be logging any of it anymore. As such, if you have anything you want to add to end the book with, today's the day to do it. Here's a relevant Twilight Zone image that BP sent me as a txt msg:

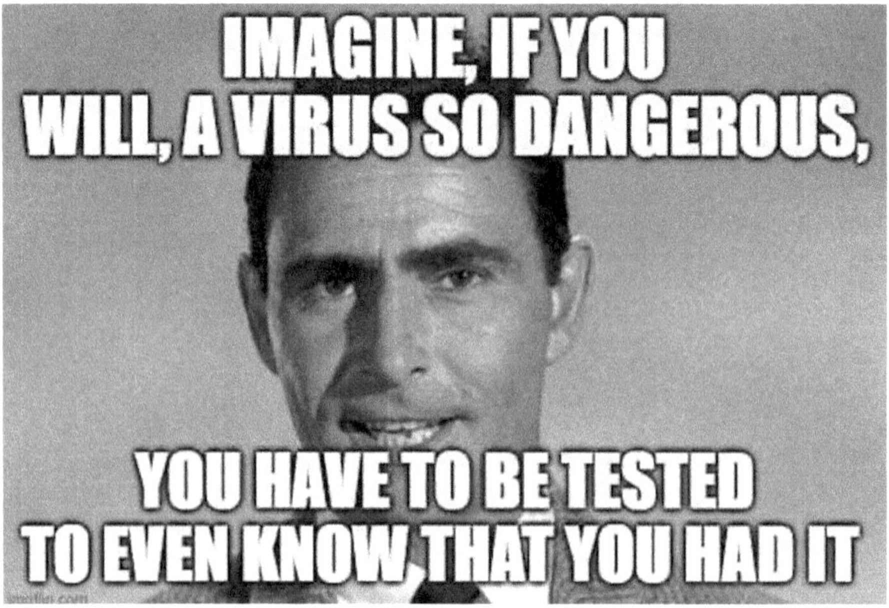

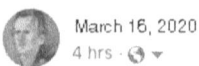

****

August 16, 2020, 22:23PM (Amir-ul Kafirs to group):

HERETICS: John Cage, "Indeterminancy", Vaccinations

I've been revisiting my huge collection of John Cage recordings in roughly chronological order & I got to "Indeterminancy". In case you're not familiar with it, in the recording I have it's Cage reading 90 stories he wrote, taking 1 minute to read each one so that some are read slow & some are read fast, etc. David Tudor plays simultaneously. Tudor's playing is supposed to be such that he's the equivalent of natural sounds coexisiting & occassionally over-riding Cage's speaking. ANYWAY, when I got to story 85 I was surprised that it was partially an *anti-vaccination* one! Here it is:

85 *

I was on an English boat going from Siracusa in Sicily
to Tunis in North Africa. I had taken the
cheapest passage and it was a voyage of two
nights and one day. We were no sooner out
of the harbor than I found that in my class no
food was served. I sent a note to the
captain saying I'd like to change to another
class. He sent a note back saying I could
not change and, further, asking whether I had
been vaccinated. I wrote back that I had
not been vaccinated and that I didn't intend
to be. He wrote back that unless I was
vaccinated I would not be permitted to
disembark at Tunis. We had meanwhile
gotten into a terrific storm. The waves were
higher than the boat. It was impossible
to walk on the deck. The correspondence
between the captain and myself continued in
deadlock. In my last note to him,
I stated my firm intention to get off his boat
at the earliest opportunity and without being
vaccinated. He then wrote back that I
had been vaccinated, and to prove it he
sent along a certificate with his signature.

****

August 16, 2020, 2:52PM (Amir-ul Kafirs to group):

HERETICS: Eugène Ionesco's "Rhinoceros"

I'm sure that at least some of you are familiar with the work of Eugène Ionesco. His play, "Rhinoceros" seems particularly relevant to our contemporary situation. Here's a summary & analysis of Act One (part one) taken offline. I emboldened & enlarged the beginning of one sentence for its particular aptness.

Summary Act One (part one)

Summary

Rhinoceros opens in a provincial town square after church on Sunday. In a grocery and a café, the mundane squabbles of bourgeois life fill the air. Jean, an upright, no-nonsense, cultured young man, chastises his slovenly, aimless friend, Berenger, for his lateness in meeting him, although Jean has only just arrived as well. Berenger thirsts for an alcoholic drink, and Jean upbraids Berenger's hungover appearance, giving him a comb and a tie. Berenger justifies his drinking as a necessary escape from the boredom of life, especially his dreary work. Jean stresses the need for will-power; he alludes to himself as the "superior man...who fulfills his duty."

The sound of a distant trumpeting interrupts the men's conversation. The sound intensifies until all characters on-stage—including a Waitress, the Grocer, the Grocer's Wife, and a Logician—see a rhinoceros off-stage and exclaim their shock. While the rhino rages nearby and the townspeople continue expressing amazement, Berenger remains unaffected.

Berenger orders alcoholic drinks for himself and Jean. Jean presses him to see what he thinks of the rhinoceros, but Berenger cares little about the disturbance. The waitress brings the drinks, and Jean again chastises his friend for drinking at noon. Berenger lies and says he ordered water and the waitress made a mistake. At another table, the Logician explains to an Old Gentleman what a syllogism is (a three-part logical statement with a main proposition, a secondary one, and a conclusion). Jean accuses Berenger of day-dreaming for lack of interest, and Berenger proclaims, "Life is a dream." Berenger tiredly comes up with a number of meager explanations for the rhino's appearance. Jean angrily refutes these and reproaches Berenger for mocking him. Berenger denies this, but lets Jean bully him; he soon accepts Jean's opinions of the rhino and agrees to abstain from liquor.

Daisy, the pretty typist from Berenger's office, passes by the men. Berenger likes her, and in his nervousness spills his drink on Jean. Berenger explains in greater depth why he drinks: when sober, he doesn't recognize himself, but when drunk, he can escape and then identify himself. While Jean lectures Berenger about strength and will-power, the Logician gives a long-winded and eventually incorrect example of a syllogism to the Old Gentleman that concerns cats and paws. Jean refutes Berenger's further descriptions of his alienated misery, labeling them contradictory.

Analysis

Ionesco explodes a number of profound ideas on to the stage, most of which are situated in the existentialist philosophy of Soren Kierkegaard, Jean-Paul Sartre, and others. The concepts of free will and responsibility are introduced and defined here. Jean is a paragon of will, of having the power to shape oneself according to one's desires. Berenger is his opposite, an alcoholic slacker who cannot even be roused by the unusual appearance of a rhinoceros. Berenger evades responsibility and himself, as is most saliently demonstrated in his attitudes toward alcohol: he lies about ordering liquor and he drinks to escape himself. Yet responsibility is not such a clear-cut issue; while Berenger arrives late to meet Jean, so does Jean. The latter, however, finds a way to justify it.

Ionesco said he wrote the play as a response to the widespread conversion of supposedly free-thinking humans to fascist ideals before and during World War II. Jean's reference to himself as the "superior man" borrows from Friedrich Nietzsche's vision of a "super-man" who is beyond conventional human morality. This super-man, Nietzsche believed, would lead the world. (The concept of a man above morality was critiqued in Fyodor Dostoevsky's*Crime and Punishment.*) Adolf Hitler exploited (and abused) Nietzsche's ideas heavily in convincing Germans that the Aryans were a master race whose destiny was to control the world. Ionesco's contribution to understanding how millions were swayed is focused in his dissection of a collective consciousness (later referred to in the play as "collective psychosis"). Ionesco posits the existence of a universal mentality that compromises the individual mind. These minds, as Berenger's does in this scene, evade responsibility and willful choice. They allow external ideas to enter without an internal check; as Jean says of Berenger, "There are certain things which enter the minds of even people without one." For Berenger, alcohol is his means for mental escapism, and the false sense of identity that alcohol confers upon him suggests why the ensuing rhinoceros-metamorphoses (and, by symbolic extension, conversions to fascism) are so seductive. Escaping oneself, or belonging to another group, Berenger implies, somehow allows the individual to feel as if he is more himself, a better, stronger, potential self. Still, the benefits of collective consciousness are given their due here; the newly unified community comes together to discuss the rhino.

- https://www.sparknotes.com/drama/rhinoceros/section1/

I made a movie called "Robopaths" that uses footage from the film version of "Rhinoceros":

382. "Robopaths"
- research probably started around late 2007, edit finished May 20, 2012
- a pastiche assembled by tENTATIVELY, a cONVENIENCE inspired by the Lewis Yablonsky term
- A/V sources used (roughly in the order in which I decided to add them to the project):
"Mother Night" movie by Keith Gordon based on the book by Kurt Vonnegut, 1996
"Colour of War VI: Adolf Hitler" movie from TWI/Granada Television - 2004
"Obedience" taken from A/V Geeks' "Science!" compilation
"Uncle Bernie's Farm" from The Mothers of Invention's "Absolutely Free" record composed by Frank Zappa
"Mother People" from The Mothers of Invention's "We're Only in it for the Money" record composed by Frank Zappa
"Mechanical Man" from "Lie" record - composed by Charlie Manson, performed by Manson + The Family
"Modern Times" movie by Charlie Chaplin, 1936
"Architecture of Doom" movie by Peter Cohen, 1989
"Joe" movie by John G. Avildsen, 1970
"Why does Herr R Run Amok?" movie by Michael Fengler & Rainer Werner Fassbinder, 1977
"Human Leech" from the "on the loose" record by Coyle and Sharp, 1964
"You Too can be a Puppet" from "Flahooley" musical, lyrics by E. Y, Harburg, music by Sammy Fain, 1951
"Seven Beauties" movie by Lina Wertmuller, 1975
"Anaconda Targets" movie by Dominic Angerame, 2004
"Punishment Park" movie by Peter Watkins, 1971
"Sweet Movie" movie by Duan Makavejev, 1974
"Otmar Bauer zeigt:" ("Otmar Bauer presents:") movie, 1969
"For the Love of... Part I" (2007-8) & "Threnody" (1992 rev. 2008) - electroacoustic compositions by Mark Steven Brooks from "Dam(n)age" CD
"Judgment at Nuremberg" movie by Stanley Kramer, 1961
"Rapture" installation by Shirin Neshat, 1999
"The South Bank Show (with Shirin Neshat)" tv show by Susan Shaw, 2001
"Hell's Ground" movie by Omar Ali Khan, 2007
"The Crooked E" movie by Penelope Spheeris, 2003
"Holy Smoke" movie by Jane Campion, 1999
"The Cult of the Suicide Bomber" movie starring Robert Baer, 2005
"Obsession: Radical Islam's War Against The West" movie by Wayne Kopping, 2006
"Rock Slyde" movie by Chris Dowling, 2010
"Rat Race" movie by Jerry Zucker, 2001
"Superstar: The Karen Carpenter Story" movie by Todd Haynes, 1987
"Terror's Advocate" movie by Barbet Schroeder, 2007
"Life and Debt" movie by Stephanie Black, 2001
"Entartete Musik - music suppressed by the third reich" movie from Beata Romanowski

for Decca Records, 1993
"Amen." movie by Costa-Gavras, 2002
"The Stranger" movie by Orson Welles, 1946
"The Boys from Brazil" movie by Franklin J. Schaffner, 1978
"Manufacturing Consent - Noam Chomsky and the Media" movie by Mark Achbar & Peter Wintonick, 1992
"Shoah" movie by Claude Lanzmann, 1985
"Conspiracy" movie by Frank Pierson, 2001
"Nazi War Criminal goes on Trial" newsreel, 1961
"EYE-TRACKING" movie by tENTATIVELY, a cONVENIENCE, 1988
"The Hunt for Adolf Eichmann" movie from Dan Setton & Ron Frank, 1994
"The House on Garibaldi Street" movie by Peter Collinson,1979
"The Man Who Captured Eichmann" movie by William A. Graham, 1996
"Work Will Make You Free Trade" movie by tENTATIVELY, a cONVENIENCE, 2000
"The Killing Fields" movie by Roland Joffé, 1984
"A" movie by Mori Tatsuya, 1998
"Rhinoceros" movie based on the play by Eugene Ionescu, 1974
"Beginning Responsibility - Lunchroom Manners" movie by Coronet Instructional Films, 1960
"Soapy the Germ Fighter" movie by Avis Films
"Shy Guy" movie by Coronet Instructional Films, 1947
"Kansas vs Darwin" movie by Jeff Tamblyn, 2007
"Flock of Dodos" movie by Randy Olson, 2007
"Man in the Glass Booth" movie by Arthur Hiller, 1975
"The Wonderful, Horrible Life of Leni Riefenstahl" movie by Ray Mller, 1993
"This Film Is Not Yet Rated" - Kirby Dick, 2006
"Come and See" - Elem Klimov, 1985
"The Kaiser's Lackey" movie by Wolfgang Staudte, 1951
"Interpreting The Kaiser's Lackey" - movie by Michael Aronson, 2007 Assistant Professor of History and German & Scandinavian Studies University of Massachusetts Amherst: Andrew Donson]
"The 5000 Fingers of Dr. T" movie by Dr. Seuss & Roy Rowland, 1952
"Monty Python's Flying Circus: Episode 1: Whither Canada" tv program by Monty Python's Flying Circus, 1969
"The Pentagon Wars" movie by Richard Benjamin, 1998
"Backwards Masking in Rocks" movie by tENTATIVELY, a cONVENIENCE, 2008
"Women in Love" movie by Ken Russell, 1969
- text sources used:
Robopaths - People As Machines - Lewis Yablonsky, 1972
Joey: A "Mechanical Boy" (Scientific American Offprint: Scientific American, March 1959) - Bruno Bettelheim
Eichmann in Jerusalem - A Report on the Banality of Evil - Hannah Arendt, 1963
http://en.wikipedia.org/wiki/Reinhard_Heydrich
"The Other Possibility" (*Die andre Mglichkeit*) , Let's Face It (originally in Ein Mann

Gibt Auskunft) - Erich Kastner, 1930
Four Arguments for the Elimination of Television - Jerry Mander, 1978
"How corporations became 'persons' - The amazing true story of a legal fiction that undermines American democracy." - Tom Stites, May 1, 2003 - http://www.uuworld.org/ideas/articles/157829.shtml
Little Superman (Der Untertan) - Heinrich Mann, 1914
- editing notes here
- 1:48:20
- on my onesownthoughts YouTube channel here: https://youtu.be/-PR7C8nFKtA
- on the Internet Archive here: https://archive.org/details/Robopaths

I think this is one of the best movies I've ever made. Below is a still from it that incorporates "Rhinoceros" footage.

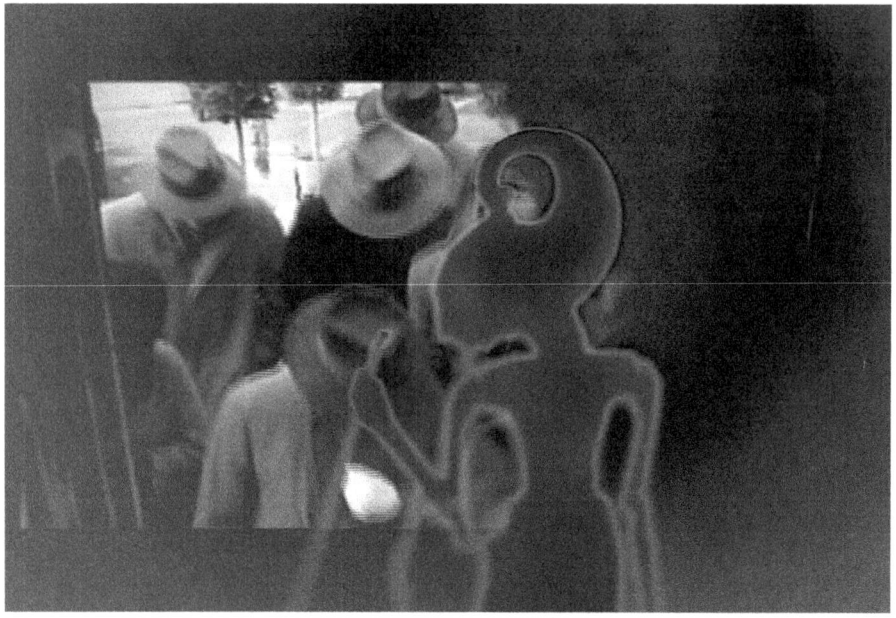

I include this still because it shows a scene I was describing to a friend yesterday because of its relevance to our current masked society. In the play, people are implied to be turning into rhinos (fascists) or to be being replaced by rhinos. The protagonist, who's upset by this, is exiting a street-car & everyone he sees has become 'faceless' because all of their hat-brims are positioned so that their faces aren't seen. The puppet silhouette is the narrator for this scene in my use of it in "Robopaths".

****

August 16, 2020, 4:42PM (Amir-ul Kafirs to group):

HERETICS: March emails

OKAY!

I finished the 2nd chapter today. It's a condensation of the March emails. It's blessedly short, only 39 pages. I think it's actually exciting reading. The main things I still have to edit are the April, May, June, July, & August emails now. Given that they constitute several thousand pages I'm not sure how long I can continue working on this without snapping. If anyone's interested in Chapter 2 let me know & I'll send a PDF of it. Then you'll be able to see how many changes I've had to make to hide people's identities, avoid redundancy (incompletely), correct errors, & reformat, etc. It's quite a task.

****

August 16, 2020, 5:07PM (Amir-ul Kafirs to BP):

Re: A sample of how I'm dealing with your emails

On Aug 16, 2020, at 4:52 PM, BP wrote:

Looks good! Though I am surprised you are using anything I wrote at all. I didn't expect it, but all cool.

Well, if you'd rather I not do so just say so. Otherwise, I like keeping a little of you in the mix because you have your own voice & it adds variety. There're only 6 of us so it helps give the writing some freshness when it switches from voice-to-voice. Everybody's reasonably different from each other.

If timing was different I may have tried to write a proper piece. I have so much swimming inside me. But it ain't gonna happen!

****

August 16, 2020, 5:09PM (Dick to group):

I have been putting up my stickers

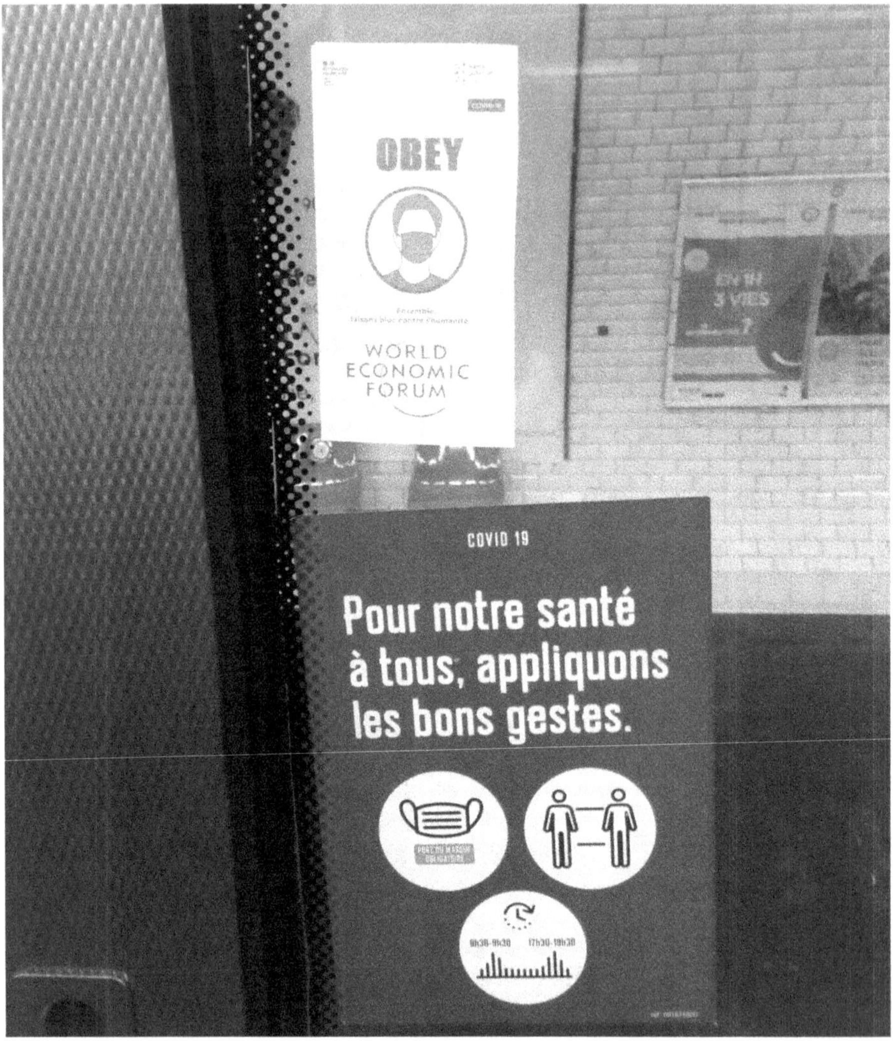

****

August 16, 2020, 5:32PM (Amir-ul Kafirs to group):

I have been putting up my stickers

What an amazing coincidence! You weren't in PGH recently were you? I found a similar image inside a Port-a-Pot in a public park today over a pretty digusting toilet:

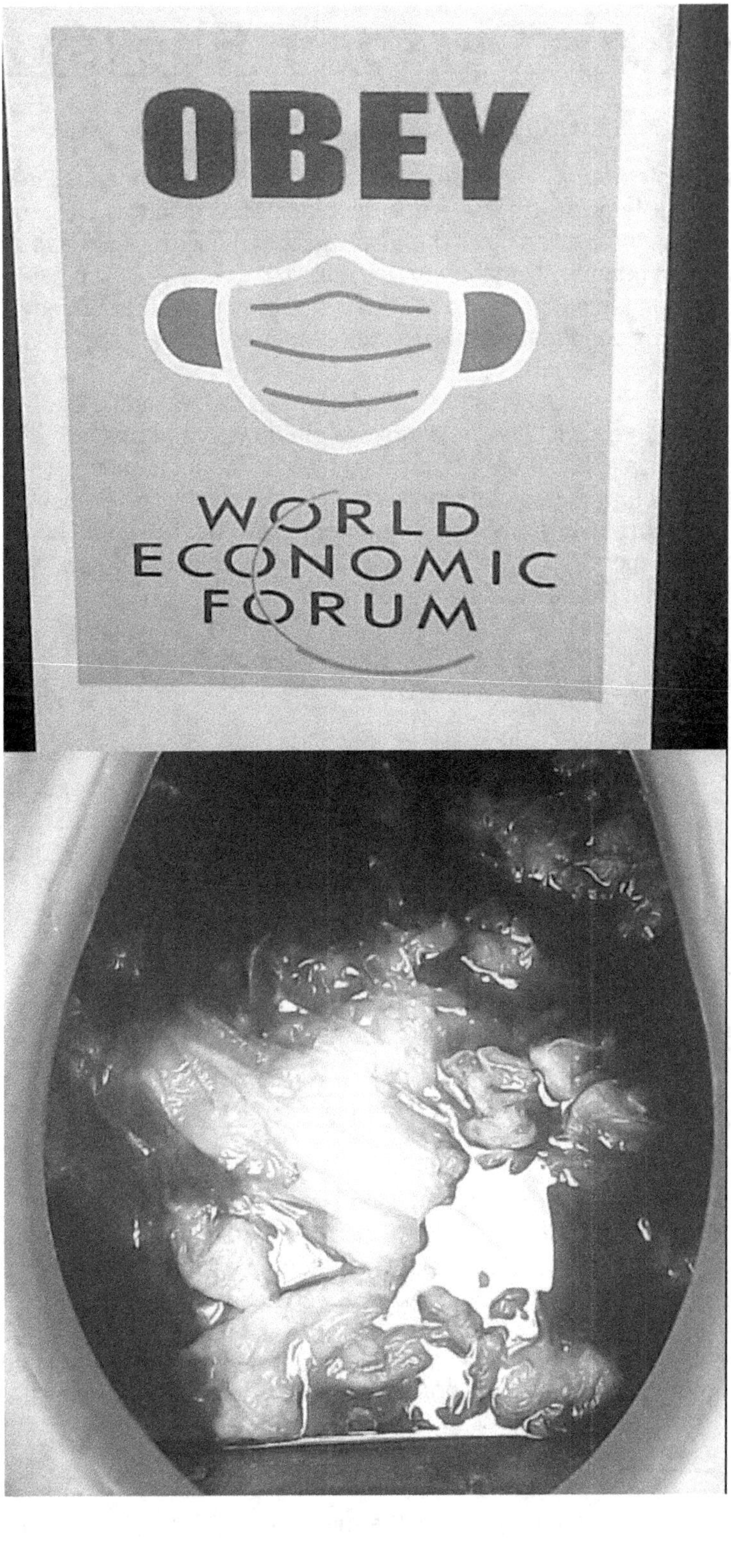

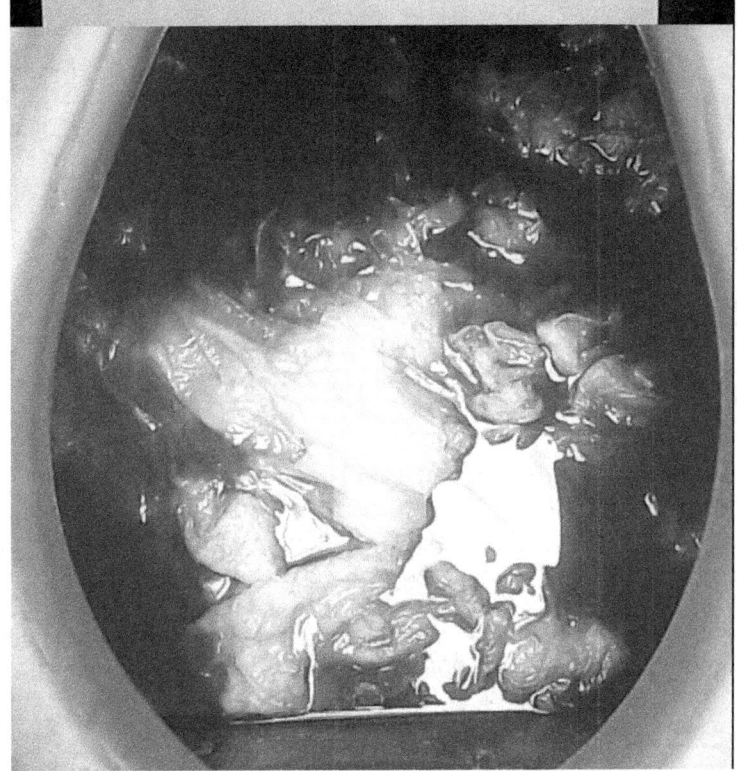
OBEY
WORLD
ECONOMIC
FORUM

Editor's Personal Backstory

- Amir-ul Kafirs

I was born September 4, 1953. My mother told me, many decades later, that it cost $25 for her to give birth to me in a hospital. According to a December 9, 2019 "Business Insider" article: "The average cost these days to have a baby in the US, without complications during delivery, is $10,808 — which can increase to $30,000 when factoring in care provided before and after pregnancy." (https://www.businessinsider.com/how-much-does-it-cost-to-have-a-baby-2018-4)

According to an online US Inflation Calculator, $25 in 1953 is the equivalent to $241.68 in 2020, a cumulative inflation rate of 866.7%. (https://www.usinflationcalculator.com) That's spectacular enough on its own but it doesn't account for the hospital birthing cost being roughly **44 times as much as the inflation increase.** An obvious argument justifying this would be to say that health care has increased by leaps and bounds in the last 66 years. The question is: Has it increased 44 times as much?

According to the abstract of a Spring, 2008, paper entitled ""Maternal Death in the United States: A Problem Solved or a Problem Ignored?" by Ina May Gaskin, CPM, MA":

"The United States has a higher ratio of maternal deaths than at least 40 other countries, even though it spends more money per capita for maternity care than any other. The lack of a comprehensive, confidential system of ascertainment of maternal death designed to record and analyze every maternal death continues to subject U.S. women to unnecessary risk of preventable mortality. Maternal deaths must be reviewed to make motherhood safer. The United Kingdom's Confidential Enquiry into Maternal and Child Health is considered the "gold standard" of national professional self-evaluation." - https://www.ncbi.nlm.nih.gov/pmc/articles/PMC2409165/

According to a January 9, 2020 article entitled "The 'staggering' out-of-pocket cost of giving birth in America":

"The average out-of-pocket cost for giving birth in the United States increased from $3,069 in 2008 to $4,569 in 2015, largely due to the rise of high-deductible health plans, according to a study published Monday in Health Affairs." - https://www.advisory.com/daily-briefing/2020/01/09/childbirth

According to the same inflation calculator used before, inflation would account for birth charges being $201.59 in 2008, a cumulative inflation rate of 706.4%. That leaves $2,867.41 unaccounted for. I suggest that GREED is a major factor and that this GREED moves counter to the general good health.

And hence I begin my questioning of the medical industry in the United States, the nation where, I suggest, DOCTOR GODS are excessively worshipped and used as a pretext for pulling the biggest coup in my lifetime.

Sometimes I wonder if I was born a hermaphrodite. My cock is somewhat smaller than average & has a very neat scar from the tip straight down to my asshole. Is it a surgical scar? Dr. John Money, a pioneering gender assignment doctor whose work I have my doubts about, was in the Baltimore area, where I was born, in 1953. It's remotely possible that I was born ambiguously gendered, "intersex" as it were, & surgically gender-assigned to be male. As far as I know, the appendix is located in the same place for both men & women. And, yet, when I had my appendix out, at age 48, I was told by the surgeon that it was a good thing that they didn't just stick a suction tube in me to suck it out but chose to cut me open instead because my appendix was not in the normal place. Why? This suspicion about my birth is highly tenuous. I contacted the hospital where I was born to ask if they had any records of an operation on me as a baby but they didn't. I wouldn't really expect them to admit to this anyway because such operations have long since been criticized as unethical & legally open to suit. I asked both my parents too & they were as worthless as always. My mom had a reaction like "Doesn't it work?" & provided no useful information otherwise except to deny an operation. My father just told me no. If a doctor had told my mom that it was for my own good to perform a lobotomy on me she might've just gone along with it, doctor knows best, my dad just wouldn't have cared.

When I was 6, in 1959 or 1960, my parents were told by representatives of the MEDICAL INDUSTRY that I needed a tonsilectomy. I was anaesthetized with ether and my tonsils were removed. I still remember the experience of the ether being as if I were receding backwards into a tunnel away from the light that was my consciousness.

The abstract for a paper entitled "The rise and decline of tonsillectomy in twentieth-century America." states:

"This article explores the rise and decline of tonsillectomy/adenoidectomy (T&A) in twentieth-century America. Between 1915 and the 1960s, T&A was the most frequently performed surgical procedure in the United States. Its rise was dependent on novel medical concepts, paradigms, and institutions that were in the process of reshaping the structure and practice of medicine. The driving force was the focal theory of infection, which assumed that circumscribed and confined infections could lead to systemic disease in any part of the body. The tonsils in particular were singled out as "portals of infection," and therefore their removal became a legitimate therapy. Nevertheless, what kinds of evidence could prove that tonsils were portals of infection? How could the effectiveness of tonsillectomy be determined? An inherent difficulty was the absence of any consensus on the criteria that would be employed to judge its efficacy. Yet tonsillectomy persisted despite ambiguous supportive evidence. Although criticisms of the procedure were common by the 1930s, its decline did not begin until well after 1945 and involved debates over the nature of evidence, the significance of clinical experience in the validation of a particular therapy, and the role of competing medical specialties." - https://www.ncbi.nlm.nih.gov/pubmed/17426070

Was the tonsillectomy necessary? I have my doubts. It seems to me that the sensation of 'having a frog in my throat', as the expression goes, has been with me most of my life and that this sensation may be a side-effect of the operation. It's my opinion that such surgery is more in the interest of medical experimentation than it is of health.

ANYWAY, it's not my intention to have so many relevant quotes meant to reinforce my position(s), it's more my intention to just tell stories from my life that reveal why I'm skeptical and heretical and philosophical in the ways that I am today. *SO*, moving on:

I don't know how old I was when my next major encounter with the medical industry was, maybe 9 or 10. The pediatrician or general practitioner that I went to told my mom that I was anemic and told her I should get iron shots. I suppose my being anemic meant that I was too tired but I don't remember that being the case. My mom bribed me by saying that everytime I cooperated with getting the shots, of which there might've been a series of 6, one per week, that I would get a comic book. That was fine with me. I don't remember being particularly scared of the shots or finding them that unpleasant or experiencing any adverse effects from them. I've been an exceptionally energetic person my whole life so sometimes I wonder whether these shots somehow contributed to that.

When I was 10 my mom went into a hospital for a month. I was told by *her* mom something like that she had gone in there for a rest & that we wouldn't be able to visit her. I don't recall realizing at the time that that probably meant that she was in a mental hospital. The story went that my mom had had her father go into a coma from a construction accident when she was 2. He died, presumably by having the life-support systems withdrawn, when she was 5. This had traumatized her & it had always been very important to her that the family that she would cofound would be a solid unit with a present & stable father. Unfortunately for her, my father could've cared less, & completely neglected the family, rarely even seeing us, always too busy with 'work' which I believe consisted in large part of his going to bars to wine & dine prospective clients — presumably exploring a sex life away from my mom in the process. My parents got separated when I was 9 & divorced when I was 10. It seems to me that this further traumatized my mom & precipitated her entry into a mental hospital.

The grandmother came by the house to feed us, I don't remember her having a very intrusive presence otherwise. Given that she was working a typical 9 to 5 job I imagine she came over before work & after work. Otherwise, I was alone with my 13 year old sister. I don't remember having any problems with not having my mom around. I don't really recall needing my mom much, it might've even been a relief not having her around because she was very OCD & intolerant of behavior outside of her stringently senseless behavioral models. An example of this, from a few years later, was when she announced a rule that we had to use the butter knife to cut a piece of butter off of the butter dish. We were then to move the butter to the side of our plate. It was then allowed that we pick up the butter again with our own knife to put it on the bread or whatever else we wanted it on. My usual reaction was to consider this ridiculous & to not comply. Non-compliance was to result in a 5¢ fine. That might not seem like much but it might've been the equivalent of a week's allowance for me, if I even had an allowance at all. Whatever money the family may've had was for my mom 1st & foremost, I was budgeted at about the level of dog food or some other lowly priority.

I was very self-disciplined & it was around this time that I started on a self-created program of scholarliness. I would give myself a task, say of finishing one portion of my homework, & then reward myself a break after the task was completed of an alotted time such as 5, 10, or 15 minutes. If this discipline grew out of the absence of an authority figure it was a positive aspect of being without parents. Such discipline is still a part of my life today & it has consistently served my purposes well. Alas, it's also set me apart, amongst other things, from almost everyone I know.

From the time of my mom's release from the hospital she was more or less continually 'sick'. I soon decided that this was both self-inflicted & that it was, as I later came to realize, a form of Munchausen Syndrome, an almost constant manipulation of other people by expecting them to feel sorry for her & to, therefore, cater to her slightest whims. This persisted for the next 56 years until she died. Naturally, this was very stressful & resulted in quite a few actual physical disorders. How much of her ailments could be claimed as at least partially originating in her *desire to be sick* is open to question & not likely to be agreed on by differing philosophies. She had colitis, kidney stones, & multiple cancers. I remember at one point her blood pressure dropped to almost zero when she was asleep & my stepdad rushed her to the ER to save her life. I have to wonder whether that was medication-related.

My mom was adamantly anti-drug but took an enormous amount of medications for most of her life. When I pointed out to her that she was on drugs every day & that she was dependent on them she emphatically denied this & didn't even understand what I was talking about. When I explained she informed me that those were her medicines & that they *weren't drugs.* After her death, I was given a list of all the drugs she was on at the time. It was something like 35 to 45 different pills a day. I hope I can find that list to display here. **[I didn't]**

The way I remember it, & I'm willing to admit that my memory is biased here, my mom went to a doctor, a clinic, or a hospital almost every week for those last 56 years. In almost every conversation that I had with her she talked about her bad health. She also told me, with great frequency, that colitis was heriditary & that I would get it & be sick with it for my whole life. I saw this as both a form of sympathetic magic, repeatedly saying something to try to make it true, & Munchausen Syndrome by Proxy, trying to make me sick both so that she could receive further pity for having a sick son AND to force a bond between us based on sickness. I don't have collitis. The older she got, the more her conversations centered around her sickness, never acknowledged as having a psychological basis, &, for perhaps the last 2 decades of her life, her impending death.

Given that she was OCD, I tried various strategies for trying to break her out of repetitive behaviors. I tried talking with her seriously, I tried joking, nothing worked. If I made a joke she just plowed right ahead on her fixed track of disease & death. At one point when she told me she was going to die I said something like: 'Yep, we all die, I'm going to die too.' That. of course, wasn't the response she wanted. I was expected to get very upset about her 'imminent' death & to cry & beg her not to die & to tell her how much I loved her & needed her. But any inclination I had to be actually sympathetic was long since worn away by the obvious manipulativeness of it all & an awareness of how harmful her behavior was to everyone around her. By the time she did eventually die, both her husbands & her daughter had preceded her. I was the only direct survivor — I think my cynicism helped me survive the constant drama.

The Junior High School that I attended had a small woods across the street from it. Sometime between ages 12 and 14 all students there were administered a vaccine because we were told that the birds that had migrated to the woods carried a disease that we had to be protected against. That seemed rather bizarre to me at the time but I didn't care that much one way or the other. That might've been around 1967. I remember the metal cylinder holding the vaccine was about 5 inches in diameter and maybe 10 inches long. The person giving the injections changed out the needle for every new person. One of my neighbors fainted when he was given the injection. I recall his fellow students finding that funny since it seemed to indicate that he was 'weaker' than the rest of us even though he was a somewhat hefty guy. I don't remember experiencing any adverse effects.

At the time, this vaccination seemed strangely unnecessary to me. I remember thinking: *Why would I be afraid of the birds?* These days, in these times of the PANDEMIC PANIC, I've been reading about previous dire predictions about Ebola, Swine Flu, the Avian Flu, and SARS and about how none of those doomsayings have come true and I'm reminded of a movie I witnessed a few years ago called "Fatal Contact: Bird Flu in America" (2006, director: Richard Pearce). It's an 'End of the World" disaster movie, meaning end-of-human-life movie, in which, obviously, the Avian Flu is the cause of death. I enjoy disaster movies, I like to see how the official responses are depicted, what the WHO does, what happens in an earthquake, in a big fire, whatever. The thing is, this is an action movie, things are exaggerated, albeit with an intent of 'realism'. It seems to me most realistic that humanity might be wiped out not by a virus but by catastrophic environmental change or military action.

I also recently acquired a copy of Mike Davis's book entitled "The Monster at our Door — The Global Threat of Avian Flu" (2005). I haven't read that yet but I did previously read Richard Preston's "The Hot Zone" about Ebola. The stories are thrilling and I reckon that many people are entranced by the morbidity.

Nonetheless, let's keep in mind that *these are **stories***, no matter how based in fact they are the final worst result hasn't come. Davis's book has an inside blurb that begins:

"FROM THE "MASTER OF DISASTER" (*THE NATION*) THE TERRIFYING STORY OF A LOOMING WORLD PANDEMIC THAT COULD KILL 100 MILLION PEOPLE."

Note the "THAT COULD KILL": that's a prediction, there've been plenty of predictions going around, I think they're contagious: 'Oh no! Watch out! He's got CONTAGIOUS PREDICTION DISEASE!!' Maybe the prophets should be quarantined. Let's put the fear-mongers under house-arrest and take away their means of communication from them. It's in the public health's best interest to not let them spread panic. People who reference exponential growth that's unchecked act like it's already happened. It seems to me that a reality check is called for in which people are reminded that predictions aren't found to be true or false until *after they've come true or not*. So far, the predictions that I've heard of locally *haven't come true* despite the so-called 'brilliance' of the doctors making them. For example, a friend who works as a respiratory therapist at a major local hospital said that his 'brilliant' head doctor predicted that by April 14, 2020, the hospital would be *full of **only COVID-19 patients***. Nope, didn't happen. Is the doctor still 'brilliant'? I speculate that he never was.

As one skeptic about the PANDEMIC PANIC expressed it:

"When previous so-called epidemics—for example, West Nile, SARS, Zika, and Swine Flu—turned out to be complete unproven duds—does this history matter?

"OF COURSE NOT. IT HAS TO BE THE VIRUS. WHAT ELSE COULD IT BE?"

- "People dying equals Coronavirus? An engineered virus?" - by Jon Rappoport - March 30, 2020

OR, as a person that I'll call *The Lord of the Flies* emailed me on March 21, 2020:

"you can't downplay this virus any more than you could downplay the Spanish Flu.

50 to 100 million died of the Spanish Flu (2.5% mortality rate)"

to which I replied:

"The difference between this and the Spanish Flu is that we look at the Spanish Flu in hindsight, it's too soon to do that with COVID-19."

I think my reponse is reasonable. The point is that to compare the Spanish Flu, something that happened 100 years ago, to COVID-19, something that we're still in the midst of, is an unworkable comparison for the simple reason that we don't have closure yet, we don't have sufficient data. One telling of the Spanish Flu story says this:

"The 1918 influenza pandemic was the most severe pandemic in recent history. It was caused by an H1N1 virus with genes of avian origin. Although there is not universal consensus regarding where the virus originated, it spread worldwide during 1918-1919. In the United States, it was first identified in military personnel in spring 1918. It is estimated that about 500 million people or one-third of the world's population became infected with this virus. The number of deaths was estimated to be at least 50 million worldwide with about 675,000 occurring in the United States.

"Mortality was high in people younger than 5 years old, 20-40 years old, and 65 years and older. The high mortality in healthy people, including those in the 20-40 year age group, was a unique feature of this pandemic. While the 1918 H1N1 virus has been synthesized and evaluated, the properties that made it so devastating are not well understood. With no vaccine to protect against influenza infection and no antibiotics to treat secondary bacterial infections that can be associated with influenza infections, control efforts worldwide were limited to non-pharmaceutical interventions such as isolation, quarantine, good personal hygiene, use of disinfectants, and limitations of public gatherings, which were applied unevenly."

- https://www.cdc.gov/flu/pandemic-resources/1918-pandemic-h1n1.html

History.com tells a similar story:

"The Spanish flu pandemic of 1918, the deadliest in history, infected an estimated 500 million people worldwide—about one-third of the planet's population—and killed an estimated 20 million to 50 million victims, including some 675,000 Americans. The 1918 flu was first observed in Europe, the United States and parts of Asia before swiftly spreading around the world. At the time, there were no effective drugs or vaccines to treat this killer flu strain. Citizens were ordered to wear masks, schools, theaters and businesses were shuttered and bodies piled up in makeshift morgues before the virus ended its deadly global march."

- https://www.history.com/topics/world-war-i/1918-flu-pandemic

Note that the Center for Disease Control says that the Spanish Flu killed "at least 50 million worldwide" while History.com states that it "killed an estimated 20 million to 50 million". A possible 30 million disagreement is pretty substantial, eh? Then there's *The Lord of the Flies*'s "50 to 100 million died of the Spanish Flu". Exaggerating a bit there, feller?

NOW, if 'downplaying' something means to diminish its massiveness then there's a big difference between the, let's say, 50,000,000 deaths of the Spanish Flu and the 263,288 confirmed COVID-19 deaths reported as of May 7, 2020 by "Our

World in Data" (https://ourworldindata.org/coronavirus). The latter has a disclaimer that says: "Limited testing and challenges in the attribution of the cause of death means that the number of confirmed deaths may not be an accurate count of the true number of deaths from COVID-19." Therefore, the number could be *more or less* by a significant amount. Still, we wouldn't "downplay" Spanish Flu deaths from 50,000,000 to 263,288 and it seems equally reasonable to me to not UP-PLAY Covid-19 deaths to a 'probable' 50,000,000 by predicting further exponential spreading. I don't know of ANYTHING that has unlimited growth, capitalism certainly doesn't, so it seems natural to me that even with the mathematically tricky 'exponential growth' (it's not as simple as 2 yields 4 yields 8, etc) it's natural for COVID-19's virile destructiveness to peak and fall. In order for COVID-19's death rate to reach that of the Spanish Flu it will have to increase by 200 times. That's an enormous amount.

"Our World in Data" further disclaims that:

"the actual total death toll from COVID-19 is likely to be higher than the number of confirmed deaths – this is due to limited testing and problems in the attribution of the cause of death; the difference between reported confirmed deaths and total deaths varies by country

"how COVID-19 deaths are recorded may differ between countries (e.g. some countries may only count hospital deaths, whilst others have started to include deaths in homes)"

That seems fair enough but there are critics who say that the number of COVID-19 deaths is *overestimated*. I've addressed to that in more detail elsewhere in this book. In the meantime consider this chart that I made a screenshot of from the CDC website on April 24, 2020:

Table 1. Deaths involving coronavirus disease 2019 (COVID-19), pneumonia, and influenza reported to NCHS by week ending date, United States. Week ending 2/1/2020 to 4/18/2020.*

Data as of April 24, 2020

Week ending date in which the death occurred	COVID-19 Deaths (U07.1)[1]	Deaths from All Causes	Percent of Expected Deaths[2]	Pneumonia Deaths (J12.0–J18.9)[3]	Deaths with Pneumonia and COVID-19 (J12.0–J18.9 and U07.1)[3]	Influenza Deaths (J09–J11)[4]	Deaths with Pneumonia, Influenza, or COVID-19 (U07.1 or J09–J18.9)[5]
Total Deaths	**24,555**	654,798	96	54,962	11,070	5,571	73,358

Note that the deaths directly attributed to COVID-19 are 24,555 and that the deaths directly attributed to pneumonia are 54,962. Pneumonia is with us all the time, I've had it twice and it is very deadly, but I've never seen the degree of fear-mongering around it that COVID-19 is generating.

But I keep digressing from my personal history.

When I was 17 to 19 I hitch-hiked around North America. My 1st trip across the US was in the fall of 1972 for a month. I decided to travel without anything other than the clothes I was wearing. I didn't take a sleeping bag or a canteen, I probably had a few dollars, maybe something like $10. I weighed 95 pounds. I slept once in a field, just in the clothes I was wearing, that was extremely uncomfortable. I walked into the Grand Canyon from the south edge carrying only a half of a paper cup of hot tea — going contrary to all the dire warnings to not enter the canyon without adequate water. I don't remember exactly how long the walk took but I think it was probably 9 hours to walk to where I spent the night by the Colorado River and then another 11 hours to climb out. I had endurance. I had the philosophy that by exposing myself to my environment I was being 'immunized' by it in mild ways. It might've been the next year that I began supporting myself as a research volunteer. For one of the studies, I think it might've been a *walking pneumonia* one, all of the volunteers had to get our antibody titers tested. There may've been 20 of us. The average titer was between 4 & 8, mine was 26. Only one person had one higher than mine. His was 52, he was a Vietnam vet. This seemed to bear out my opinion that my lifestyle of moderate exposure had strengthened my immune system.

I later learned that my own theory is essentially the same as what's known as the "Hygiene Hypothesis". Consider this abstract from a paper entitled "**The 'hygiene hypothesis' for autoimmune and allergic diseases: an update**" by H Okada, C Kuhn, H Feillet, and J-F Bach :

"According to the 'hygiene hypothesis', the decreasing incidence of infections in western countries and more recently in developing countries is at the origin of the increasing incidence of both autoimmune and allergic diseases. The hygiene hypothesis is based upon epidemiological data, particularly migration studies, showing that subjects migrating from a low-incidence to a high-incidence country acquire the immune disorders with a high incidence at the first generation. However, these data and others showing a correlation between high disease incidence and high socio-economic level do not prove a causal link between infections and immune disorders. Proof of principle of the hygiene hypothesis is brought by animal models and to a lesser degree by intervention trials in humans. Underlying mechanisms are multiple and complex. They include decreased consumption of homeostatic factors and immunoregulation, involving various regulatory T cell subsets and Toll-like receptor stimulation. These mechanisms could originate, to some extent, from changes in microbiota caused by changes in lifestyle, particularly in inflammatory bowel diseases. Taken together, these data open new therapeutic perspectives in the prevention of autoimmune and allergic diseases." - https://www.ncbi.nlm.nih.gov/pmc/articles/PMC2841828/

& from the Introduction to the same paper:

"Changes of lifestyle in industrialized countries have led to a decrease of the infectious burden and are associated with the rise of allergic and autoimmune diseases, according to the 'hygiene hypothesis'. The hypothesis was first proposed by Strachan, who observed an inverse correlation between hay fever and the number of older siblings when following more than 17 000 British children born in 1958. The original contribution of our group to the field was to propose for the first time that it was possible to extend the hypothesis from the field of allergy, where it was formulated, to that of autoimmune diseases such as type 1 diabetes (T1D) or multiple sclerosis (MS). The leading idea is that some infectious agents – notably those that co-evolved with us – are able to protect against a large spectrum of immune-related disorders. This review summarizes in a critical fashion recent epidemiological and immunological data as well as clinical studies that corroborate the hygiene hypothesis.

"The strongest evidence for a causal relationship between the decline of infections and the increase in immunological disorders originates from animal models and a number of promising clinical studies, suggesting the beneficial effect of infectious agents or their composites on immunological diseases." - https://www.ncbi.nlm.nih.gov/pmc/articles/PMC2841828/

In 1976, when I was 22 and/or 23, I was what I called a "professional asshole", a simulated patient for rectal/genital exams. I was paid reasonably well to let young nurses finger my testicles and stick their fingers up my asshole. It seems like it was around the same time that I noticed blood in my sperm so I went to a young doctor and asked what it meant. He told me I had "hematospermia" — as far as I could tell that was just Latin for "blood in my sperm". If you came to me and told me that you were coughing blood and that you were wondering what my diagnosis was would you be impressed if I said that you had "hemoptysis"? I was unimpressed by being told in Latin what I already knew in English. I don't think my cynicism about doctors had started yet, though.

Around the same time I went to a dentist to have my 'Wisdom Teeth' pulled. That wasn't very 'wise' of me because I don't remember experiencing any trouble with them. I've since come to think that maybe Wisdom Teeth are replacements for other teeth that might get worn out. I probably got this done because my mom suggested it. I should've known better. I could certainly use those 'extra' teeth now at age 66. One of the interesting things about this experience is that the dentist wouldn't give me pain killers. I had long hair at the time and I got the impression that the dentist thought I was one of those, you know, '*hippie druggies*'. Instead, he told me to put tea bags on the gaping holes in my mouth to dull the pain. I don't remember that working very well. Ironically, I didn't actually *want* pain killers but I remember the dentist making a point that *he wasn't going to give them to me*, apparently under the impression that I was craving them.

From 1976 to 1977 i subscribed to a periodical called *Madness Network News*. Its purpose was to provide a support network for people vulnerable to institutionalization for 'mental illness'. I wasn't in that category but I felt it was a cause I could learn from & support. Here's the cover of the 1st issue I received:

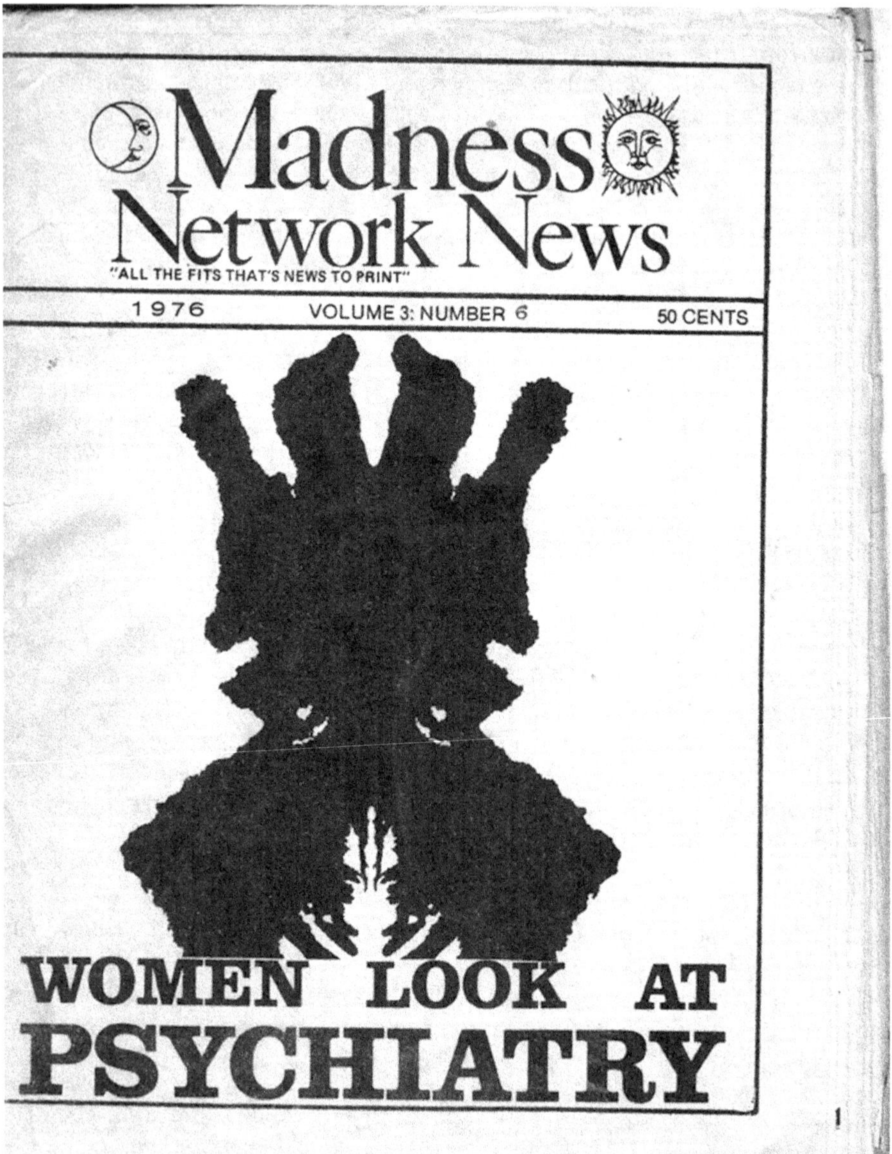

One the regular features of *Madness Network News* that I found most potentially valuable was a column called "Dr. Caligari" which described & warned against psychiatric drugs in use. The one that seemed most terrifying was PROLIXIN DECANOATE (aka fluphenazine or Prolixin-C). Read the article below & I imagine you'll find it as nightmarish as I did.

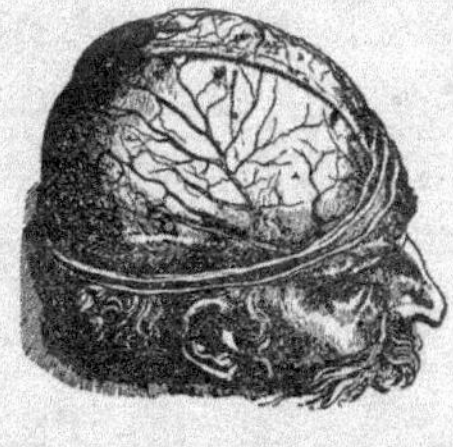

DR. CALIGARI

PROLIXIN, BIG BROTHER IN INJECTABLE FORM

"Dangers of Fluphenazine"
Dear Sir:

A new drug is being widely used in the treatment of mental illness. It is long acting and used by injection - its name is fluphenazine (Prolixin-C). Is this the thalidomide of the 70's? I would like to have the opinion of other doctors. Whilst it is still new, maybe we are lulled into a false sense of security, but are we justified in using a drug, which may take up to six weeks to eradicate from the tissues, without being sure of its safety? Its side effects alone are legion. A study of 13 papers gives the following: Common side effects reported are - lethargy, drowsiness, dizziness, muscular incoordination, parasthesia (skin numbness-C), hypotension, blurring of vision, confusion, nausea, vomiting and aches and pains. Parkinsonism is extremely common. Incidence in reports varies from 100% to 24 percent with many reports about 50 percent.

Other reported side-effects include psychotic relapse and glaucoma." (1)

"The simple fact that a number of prisoners are walking the yard in this institution like somnambulists, robots and vegetables as a result of this drug (Prolixin), should be reason enough to make people apprehensive as to the effect it is having." (2)
(quote from a petition addressed to the California Senate Committe on penal institutions by La Raza Unida, a Chicano orgaization of prisoners at California Mens Colony).

SAVES TIME

SAVES MONEY

EVEN, SAVES PEOPLE

(Prolixin ad blurb)

Prolixin (fluphenazine) is an 'anti-psychotic' consciousness constrictor with enormous implications and ramifications. When Prolixin was first developed, it was merely one more Thorazine-type drug marketed in tablet/pill form and as fluphenazine hydrochloride, a short acting injectable form with effects lasting a few days, Injectable forms of Thorazine type downers are the main form of corercive, forced drugging.

It is easy to 'mouth' pills, that is hide pills under the tongue, in the cheeks or back of throat, etc., and then spit them out later. As mentioned before a large number of people 'given' such psychiatric drugs do not like the drug's effect on body and mind and would NEVER take such drugs voluntarily. Thus, numerous techniques of avoiding such drugs have been invented by psychiatric inmates.

With liquid, or concentrate form, given as tasteless, colorless, odorless syrups in cups, or hidden in drinks or foods, it is obviously harder to avoid the drugs. However, with two to four psychiatric 'technicians' holding an unwilling psychiatric inmate and a nurse, technician or doctor "armed" with a syringe full of such drugs, avoiding forced durgging becomes almost an impossiblity. Far more frequently then those on the 'outside' would ever believe, psychiatric drugs are forcibly injected into people in the name of 'treatment', "cure" and control. This is psychiatric RAPE, and any forced treatment equals TORTURE!

It is one thing to get an injection of a mind/muscle crusher drug like Haldol, Thorazine, Stelazine, etc., with the injections' effect lasting 8-12 hours and then slowly disappearing over a day or two.* It is quite another situation when the injection contains long acting versions of these drugs immersed in oils with the drugs' effects lasting anywhere from 2-8 weeks. Prolixin Enanthate, and now the newer Prolixin Decanoate, are long acting injectable forms of Thorazine whose effects last longer than 4 weeks from one injection.

Thus, 25mg (one injection or one cc, cubic centimeter of Prolixin Decanoate), a comparitively small dose of orally taken pills, in this long acting injectable form is capable of causing muscle rigidity and zombieism for 4-6 weeks. Think of it, 4-6 weeks of mind and muscle control with only one injection lasting at most two minutes from beginning to end (longer if there is a struggle first, which there often is).

Once the injection is given the person getting this mental/muscle glue has absolutely no way of doing anything about this drug and its effects. There is no way of controlling the strength of the drug once the shot is given. Thus, after one shot of Prolixin, the next month of your life will, in effect, be controlled by other people/ the psychiatric system, i.e., psychiatrists, nurses, technicians, social workers, conservators, etc.) by means of a drug which has been deposited in your ass and which slowly seeps into your blood stream day...after day...after day...

Too often pills sit untouched

in a medicine cabinet. It's frustrating to realize that almost 50% of patients discharged from the hospital on oral medication do not take even the first dose.[1] Schizophrenic patients who "drop out" often decompensate and become unreachable.

For your unreliable pilltakers

and those who have neither the insight nor motivation for self-medication, there is more reliable therapy. Prolixin Decanoate (Fluphenazine Decanoate Injection). Because it is given by injection you know the patient is medicated. Because it is long-acting (up to 4 weeks or more of therapeutic effect from a single maintenance injection), there is a better chance the patient can be maintained as an outpatient (75% fewer readmissions in one study using long-acting injectable fluphenazines).[2]

SQUIBB Prolixin Decanoate®
Fluphenazine Decanoate Injection
helps keep the
schizophrenic patient in touch

No wonder to prison prisoners and psychiatric prisoners, Prolixin is seen as psychiatry's most deadly and damaging psychic poison, and both hated and feared. Who gives the psychiatric system the right to force injections of such drugs into people? Drugs that can cause permanent brain damage, drugs that cause suicidal drug induced depressions and despair, drugs that cause mind and muscle misery, drugs that chemically violate both

"After one month of this hell I was released to my sister, I immediately threw all the pills they gave me down the toilet. Three days later (after a shot of Prolixin-C) my whole body went rigid. I kept drooling at the mouth and my legs would not support me. The pain in my head was intense...We found out this poison they had given me, Prolixin, had to be taken with the antidote, Cogentin. The 8 weeks it took to completely eliminate this drug from my system was the horror of my life. I had a continuous sickening feeling throughout my body. Each minute of this feeling was an hour. The headaches were constant and I had no concentration, only intense irritation at anyone. I had no resistance to sheer terror. When I was living through this, I thought how merciful death would be." (3)

E.R. Squibb, the drug company that manufactures Prolixin, a big money winner, is reaping rich profits from a drug that is a horror in action for many. Prolixin ads continually emphasize how much money can be saved (cost-effectiveness, the 11th commandment of the bureaurocracy) with prolixin injections as compared to pills taken every day, psychotherapy, or other forms of 'helping'.

PROLIXIN DECANOATE
(FLUPHENAZINE DECANOATE INJECTION)

Puts control of the schizophrenic in your hands with injections 1 to 3 weeks apart or longer with an average duration of effect of about 2 weeks

Now we live in the age of legal psych[illegible] 'addiction', called 'maintenance therapy'. Prolixin clinics and Prolixin 'maintenence' is hailed by shrinks as 'the answer' to all those problems of drug refusal, the answer to social control. Prolixin is 'the answer', the simple chemical 'answer' to all the complexities of life that lead to 'freak outs' and 'freak ins'. Ultimately this simplistic way of answering complicated life situations reveals itself for what it is, drug controlled therapeutic tyranny, drug dictators in white coats and injectable forms, polypharmacracy...Hitler would have loved Prolixin!

With injections of Prolixin, 4-6 days after the injection, the highest concentration of the drug in the blood occurs. Then the blood concentration of the drug very slowly goes down over the 2-6 weeks. That is why severe muscle reactions and suicidal drug created 'depressions' are most likely to occur 4-6 days after the injection.

BLOOD CONCENTRATION OF PROLIXIN

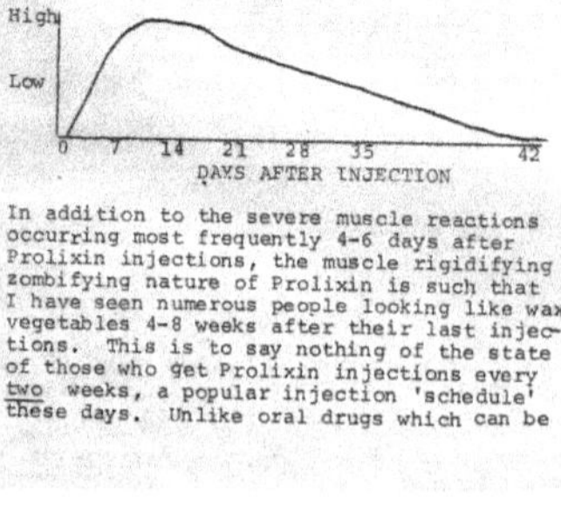

In addition to the severe muscle reactions occurring most frequently 4-6 days after Prolixin injections, the muscle rigidifying - zombifying nature of Prolixin is such that I have seen numerous people looking like waxed vegetables 4-8 weeks after their last injections. This is to say nothing of the state of those who get Prolixin injections every two weeks, a popular injection 'schedule' these days. Unlike oral drugs which can be

Controlled Drug Delivery
in schizophrenia with
PROLIXIN DECANOATE

stopped If a person has a severe muscle reaction or allergic reaction; Prolixin once injected lasts for at least a month and thus large doses of 'anti-parkinsonian' drugs must be given for Prolixin muscle reactions; inevitably they provide only a partial relief to say nothing of the dangers and drug induced 'bummers' created by the anti-parkinsonians'.

Muscle rigidity and cramps is, however, not the only damaging effect of Prolixin. Besides all the other, non-muscular side-effects, i.e., dry mouth, blurred vision, impotence, sedation, etc., Prolixin is also capable of causing severe drug created 'depressions' or drug induced states of despair and hopelessness. Again, it is often between the 4th and 6th day after the injections that such suicidal hopelessness and drug despair start to reach their height; and it is impossible to determine how many such Prolixin suicides there have now been. Disguised Drug Deaths!

"A week after admission, he received his fortnightly injection (of Prolixin-C). Twenty-four hours later, he became withdrawn, refused food, and took to his bed in mid-afternood. He appeared sad and miserable, and was unwilling to discuss his state of mind. He remained in this depressed state two days. When he returned to normal, he said that he felt the same way when he attempted suicide. A similar depressive reaction recurred when the injection was repeated a fortnight later. A check on the previous three months showed that he had an injection of fluphenazine enanthate four days before his suicidal attempt." (4)

"Case 11 - Man aged 41. Inpatient in a mental hospital f[illegible]... He was started on [illegible]d, we demar[illegible] enathate, 25 mg every month, which was changed to fluphenazine decanoate three months later. Six days after the first injection of fluphenazine decanoate, he cancelled a promising interview for a job and committed suicide by drowning on the 13th day after the injection." (5)

Today Prolixin injections are being ever more widely used. This drug 'solves' the problem of getting psychiatric and prison inmates to take their pills. Its easy to give, saves time and insures complete control. More and more community mental health centers - community control centers are starting Prolixin 'clinics'. Prolixin IS the 1984 mind/muscle control tool, here today! GONE TOMORROW!, I hope.

Caligari

Dr. Caligari - Footnotes

* This is not to imply that Haldol, Thorazine, Stelazine - etc., are not horrible drugs.

(1) D. West, "Dangers of Fluphenazine", letter to the Ed., Brit. J. Psych. 1970.

(2) La Raza Unida Statement.

(3) NAPA statement.

(4) R. deAlaraon et al, "Severe Depressive Mood Changes Following Slow-Release Intramuscular Fluphenazine Injection", Brit. Med. J. Sept., 1969, p. 565.

(5) Ibid. p. 565.

21

Around this same time, I was earning a pittance as a research volunteer at a hospital in East Baltimore. 20 years later, I wrote the following (herein somewhat abridged & otherwise edited) article describing the experience. Since I was being used as a guinea pig for drugs to be considered for administration to mental patients & since I was generally against such drugs I put particular emphasis on discouraging the drugs that I thought might be most harmful to people in a psychically fragile condition. Note also, that the information gotten from most of the 'volunteers' would have been faked &/or otherwise worthless.

Stimulants/Depressants

- an account of being a mad scientist w/in the context of Research Volunteering in Baltimore in 1976 (EV)

- written November 16th to 18th, 1996 (EV)

- tENTATIVELY, a cONVENIENCE

Stimulants/Depressants

In 1976, I was a research volunteer for 3 studies involving stimulants & depressants at what was then known as City Hospital. I think it's called Francis Scott Key Medical Center now & it may've partially been taken over by the Johns Hopkins real estate moguls.

Given that I'm writing this 20 yrs later there are bound to be inaccuracies. W/ this in mind, I warn the reader that a few things that are written w/o qualifiers about the uncertainty of my memory have the qualifiers eliminated for the avoidance of tedium rather than because they're "unnecessary" (there, now, wasn't that a tediously qualifying sentence?).

In each study, I was given 3 capsules. These cd either be stimulants, depressants, or placebos. I was never told wch. In the 1st one we were expected to hang around for a certain amt of time (perhaps 2 hrs) & to then fill out a form asking questions about how we felt. Then we were free to go unless we were feeling the effects "too much" - then we were expected to stay until we came down. Unfortunately, we only got pd for the 2 hrs - so, of course, no-one stuck around no matter how much under the influence they were. After all, all of the volunteers were probably there because they liked taking drugs & thought it wd be just fine to be pd to do it. I assume that the reason why we didn't get pd for the extra time was not only because the researchers were being cheap but also because they figured the subjects wd try to con them whenever they wanted more money. This wd've probably been the case.

It was common practice for the guinea pigs to fill out the forms before they'd felt any effects so that they cd sneak out & not have to hang around the hospital. So much for the accuracy of the results. I, on the other hand, wasn't there just to get a buzz - I was there to put my data into the pharmacological-industrial complex.

I've been interested in "Methodical Madness" for a long time - too long to summarize it in 25 words or less to any satisfactory degree. Basically, I find the concepts used to describe mentally alienated people to be inadequate. What is schizophrenia? What is psychopathia? Is paranoia always so paranoid? Etc, etc.. I've studied the creations of many "outsider artists" - having gone to both Bern & Lausanne in Switzerland just to look at the "L'Art Brut" museum collections there.

In '76, I subscribed to a magazine called "Madness Network News" - a mostly anti-psychiatric publication generally aimed at ex-mental-institution-inmates (wch, fortunately, I'm not). MNN featured a regular column by "Dr. Caligari" wch warned about the effects of drugs used in mental hospitals. A particularly frightening one was called Prolixin Decanoate (a.k.a. Fluphenazine). According to Caligari's October 26th, '76 article:

"Prolixin Enanthate, and now the newer Prolixin Decanoate, are long acting injectable forms of Thorazine whose effects last longer than 4 weeks from one injection.

"Thus, 25mg (one injection or one cc, cubic centimeter of Prolixin Decanoate), a comparitively small dose of orally taken pills, in this long acting injectable form is capable of causing muscle rigidity and zombieism for 4-6 weeks. Think of it, 4-6 weeks of mind and muscle control with only one injection lasting at most two minutes from beginning to end (longer if there is a struggle first, which there often is)."

Imagine being a sensitive person already highly frustrated by restraints & lack of love being subjected to such a chemical strait-jacket! A high percentage of suicides were reputed to occur after regaining muscle control enough to do so when coming off Prolixin. Is it any wonder? Variations on such drugs are still being tested by such places as PharmaKinetics in Baltimore (&, presumably, elsewhere).

My partial purpose in participating in studies whose purpose I suspected to be the development of drugs to be forced on people unsuccessful at fitting into "normal" society enough to prevent their institutionalization was to throw a conceptual monkey wrench sympathetic to the so-called "insane" into the works.

The 2nd study was one in wch I was given the usual 3 pills & then, after an hr's wait for the drugs to come on, put in a rm the size of a closet for 2 hrs. In the rm was a chair, a table surface attached to the walls on 3 sides in front of the chair, a pad of lined paper, a microphone, & a newspaper to distract myself w/. There might've also been a mirror that was see-thru glass on the other side - so that the researchers cd observe the subject's behavior.

I was supposed to talk & simultaneously write down what I was saying as constantly as I cd during those 2 hrs. Given that this was a time in my life when I was most intensively experimenting w/ language, my output must've seemed very bizarre indeed. E.g.: I used abbreviations of my own creation - such as TAWAS (Talking And Writing Approximately Simultaneously) to describe what I was expected to do for the study. I frequently quoted songs by such groups as The Mothers of Invention, The Fugs, Cab Calloway, The Velvet Underground, Captain Beefheart and the Magic Band, etc.. - usually w/o attributing them as quotes. I used puns in various languages. Imagine how "schizophrenic" I wd've seemed w/o my providing any explanations. As I TAWASed on June 23rd, '76: "..the situation described by (henceforth abbreviated - the word by, i.e. - via an x - oh, the irony of long explanations, or, whatever, of short abbreviations)".

Think of this more recent text as well as the older ones. I've used various fairly common abbreviations that are probably still unknown to many readers or unacceptable to lingual "conservatives" (what I like to think of as UNCONSCIOUS ANTI-PHILOLOGISTS):

the use of #s as homonym substitutes for words or just as short versions of their written out form: "2" for "to", "too", or "two", "b" for "be" or "bee", etc..

the use of symbols instead of words: "#" instead of "number".

the use of "wch" for "which", "cd" for "could", "wd" for "would", "amt" for "amount", "w/" for "with", "w/o" for "without", "ft" for foot, "thru" for "through", "hr" for "hour", "wk" for "week", "yr" for "year", "rm" for "room"; or, slightly stranger, "'ve" for "have", etc..

the use of "x" for "by" (as in the measurement abbreviation: e.g.: 2x4 board).

the use of latin abbreviations such as: "e.g." for "for example", "i.e." for "that is", "viz." for "namely", "ca." for approximately (especially as applied to dates), "cf." for "compare", "etc" for "and so on", etc.., etc..

I was very deliberately developing texts at the time that systematically eliminated much "normal" language in favor of a more "original" one of my own. To a person unaccustomed to playing w/ language, using abbreviations, etc, I wd've seemed like someone who was a very bad speller. Instead, I was far more particular about the meanings embedded in the eccentric etymologies than the average english professor is ever likely to be.

After all, I'd read Joyce's "Finnegans Wake" & was becoming familiar w/ sound poetry & visual poetry & concrete poetry, etc.. (perhaps not all of this by then - but my interests were similar. I'm reminded of the stories of people put in mental institutions because the "health care" officials were too ignorant to realize that the inmate's native language was something other than english & thought, therefore, that they were speaking "nonsense".

On the subject of such horrors, I have one friend whose aunt was given a lobotomy because the English-speaking doctors got permission from her predominantly Polish-speaking mother to do so. The mother agreed, misunderstanding what a lobotomy was.. The point of all this is that I felt that a sortof "diplomat" between the people that these drugs were aimed at & the doctors who administer them was needed.

For this 2nd study I had to come in every Monday thru Friday for 3 hrs. The pay was ridiculously miniscule considering that it took up a substantial amt of time in what wd've been the average working hrs for most people. One interesting sidenote is that one of the other subjects wrote a note inviting the other volunteers to a party & hid the note in the microphone cover so that the researchers cdn't find it & take it away. I found it but it was too late for me to go to the party. The mike was connected to a tape recorder in a rm on the other side of the (semi-hypothetical mirror). As such, comparisons between what I said & what I wrote cd be made.

After this study was over, I asked for copies of what I'd written. I figured that I'd have some use for them some day. The researchers were cooperative enough to give copies of some of them to me. I wonder wch ones they left out? Of course, when I was on speed, I'd TAWAS more & when I was on downs I'd TAWAS less. These papers were dated & had my name on them & had an estimate of the word count. This estimate was simply an average of 10 words per line multiplied by the line count. Too bad my average word count per line was something more like 13 to 15. So much for accuracy - but, I suppose the generalization was adequate.

Only 24 days are represented from what was probably about a 40 day study. Of these, the word count (using their estimates) goes between the extremes of 40 to 2,530! The following transcripts are from these 2 extremes:

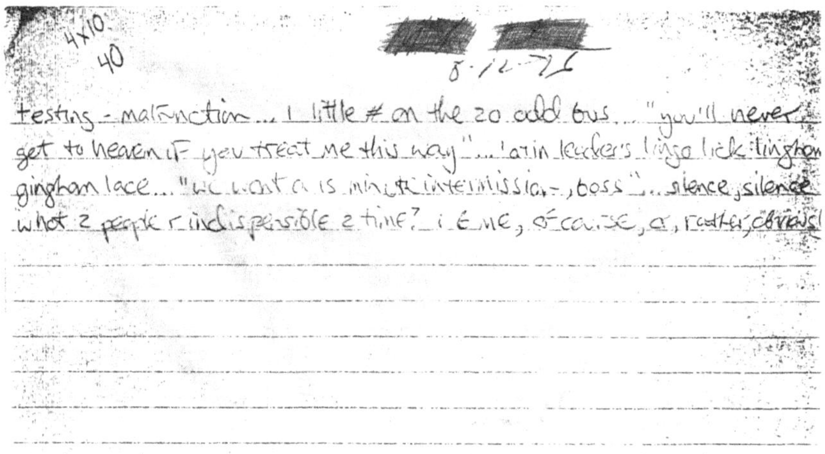
4x10
40
[redacted]
8-12-76
testing - malfunction... 1 little # on the 20 odd bus... "you'll never
get to heaven if you treat me this way"... latin leader's lingo lick lingham
gingham lace... "we want a 15 minute intermission, boss"... silence, silence
what 2 people r indispensible 2 time? i & me, of course, or, rather, obvious!

August 12th, 1976:

testing - malfunction... 1 little # on the 20 odd bus... "you'll never
get to heaven if you treat me this way"... latin leaders lingo lick lingham
gingham lace... "we want a 15 minute intermission, boss"...silence, silence
what 2 people r indispensible 2 time? i & me, of course, or rather, obviously

These transcripts are copies of the same amt of words per line in the original so that if anyone cares to compare the handwritten original w/ this typed version the comparison will be easier. I probably somewhat routinely tested the mike - sometimes using the pun substitution of "testes" for "testing" - what wd a humorless doctor make of that? I had to take the bus back & forth to the hospital (not always so easy on the return trip - completely blotto & stepping onto a bus full of loud schoolkids). The above sections in quotes are from Cab Calloway. "latin leaders" etc.. - a little liposuction from the pro-philologists' CAMP. How loaded even these 52 words can be..

T 2530 6-29 [redacted]

white light white light goin messin up my mind white light don't u know it's
gonna make me go blind white heat white heat tickles me down 2 my toes
white light hey now goodness knows have mercy...another contrived beginning
or rather planned beginning - today's dose is very strong - i can barely write
INTESNSITAT - i may b producing, primarily, exclamations, today - Whew!
i could feel this coming on after 20 minutes - at most, probably - I'm so
hyper now that the distance between my output & my emotions? is immense
2 the extent that the involvement seems merely superficial - i'll b using
cursive writing again today - 4 speed's sake - & the formal continuity
will b a rapid one distinguished X a non-planned frenetic-ness - a lack
or rather an absence of planned focal points etc. O'K! this is incredible
... few fade-away dots today - when i stop writing/talking it'll be easily
attributable 2 my refraining from using totally illegible writing - but, perhaps
i won't refrain - since i haven't been told that legibility is a prime requirement - i've only assumed - Whew! - this is so fast - it b exciting
but the residue will probably b minimal as will be the punctuation
increasingly so? white light goin messin up my mind - this'll overtake
le scribbles - 2 the non-perception - i was irritated X [illegible]'s
labeling the schizophrenic labels merely scribbles - although i haven't
read the section yet so i can't say that my impression of his reaction
is well founded - the schizophrenic scribble is comprehensibly explainable
X the inequality - inability of the hand 2 cope with the rapidity of the
mind - the schizophrenic usually - thinks incredibly rapidly - i.e.
is extremely conscious - sensitive - the scribbles are an alternative
expressive method - compensating 4 said awareness rapidity - an
acronym or rather abbreviation that i've created 2 express this
represent this state of mind is Thoughts Too Quick - Expressions
Archaic - i.e. TTQ-EA - that's very appropriate at this moment
TTQ-EA - CWMCRT - i've tried 2 develop a language

& June 29th, 1

page 1:

white light white light goin messin up my mind white light don't u know it's
gonna make me go blind white heat white heat tickles me down 2 my toes
white light hey now goodness knows have mercy...another contrived beginning
or rather planned beginning - today's dose is very strong - i can barely write
INTENSITAT - i may b producing, primarily, exclamations, today - Whew!
i could feel this coming on after 20 minutes - at most, probably - I'm so
hyper now that the distance between my output & my emotions? is immense

2 the extent that the involvement seems merely superficial - i'll b using cursive writing again today - 4 speed's sake - & the formal continuity will b a rapid one distinguished x a non-planned freneticness - a lack or rather an abcense of planned focal points etc. DING! this is incredible ...few fade-away dots today - when i stop writing/talking it'll be easily attributable 2 my refraining from using totally illegible writing - but, perhaps i won't refrain - since i haven't been told that legibility is a prime requirement - i've only assumed - Whew! - this is so fast - it's exciting but the residue will probably b minimal as will be the punctuation increasingly so? white light goin messin up my mind - this'll eventually be scribbles - 2 the nonperceptive - i was irritated x prinzhorn's labelling the schizophrenic labels merely scribbles - although i haven't read the section yet so i can't say that my impression of his reaction is well founded - the schizophrenic scribble is comprehensibly explainable x the inequality - inability of the hand to cope with the rapidity - ie. is extremely conscious - sensitive - the scribbles are an alternative expressive method - compensating 4 said awareness rapidity - an acronymn or rather abbreviation that i've created 2 express this represent this state of mind is Thoughts Too Quick - Expressions Archaic - ie. TTQ-EA - that's very appropriate at this moment TTQ-EA - CWMCRT - i've tried 2 develope a language

[There were 8 more pages for this one but I've eliminated them for the purposes of this book]

Oi Veh! Where was I? So much for transcribing the muddy waters from streams-of-consciousnesses past! I tried to keep spelling mistakes intact - after all, I was whipping thru this expereince much too quickly to take time out to spell any more carefully. Have you ever tried to handwrite what you're saying simultaneously w/ saying it while you're being watched by researchers who're going to try to evaluate how "insane" the drugs they've given you have "made you"? I recommend it highly (sortof)..

Question marks in brackets: "[?]" when they're spaced far apart from the rest of the text are meant to indicate that I'm not sure I transcribed the last word correctly. When they're normally spaced in relation to the rest of the text it means that I cdn't figure out what the word there was at all.

This ramble began w/ lyrics from The Velvet Underground's song "White Light/White Heat" & goes on to mentioning Stockhausen's "Intensitat" ("Intensity"). Other references are to Hans Prinzhorn's book entitled "Artistry of the Mentally Ill" from 1926 & reputed to be the 1st book to study the value of such art w/o passing judgement on the mental condition of the artists. Finally, I refer to José Argüelles' book "The Transformative Vision" wch I was quite interested in at the time.

As is probably obvious, I was under instructions to not scribble or draw - nonetheless, scribbling was the closest I cd get to accurately transcribing the energy flow of the more intensive speeding. I've since published a tape by Franz Kamin entitled "Scribble Music Sampler". Franz also has a book called "Scribble Death". For me, he's one of the insufficiently discovered "greats" of composer poets. Much of Franz's concerns seem to parallel mine. It's only been in the process of rereading/writing this stimulants residue in order to make it more legible that this aspect of my connection w/ Kamin has become clear in a certain way..

I doubt that I'll ever publish the entire set of stimulants/depressants texts. Just the nuisance of trying to read my handwriting so that I can retype it is enough of a discouragement. I may, however, someday try to edit out the more inspired passages & still retain the drug-ride feel. I sure as FUCK ain't doin' it tonight tho'!

The 3rd study involved taking the pills & drinking alcohol! Vodka & Tonic. Then I had to sit in a room with another guy & a newspaper for 2 hrs. This room was definitely monitored thru one-way glass. The purpose of the study was to find out how the drugs & booze effected socializing. My partner was picked on the basis of maximum compatibility w/ me. Pickin's must've been slim because this guy & I had a very hard time thinking of anything to say to each other.

He played mellotron in a band. Mellotron, for those of you who don't remember it, was a keyboard instrument mainly used for simulating string sections for schmaltzy rock & pop bands. I mainly associated it w/ The Moody Blues (who I still think are wretched) & King Crimson's 1st couple of records (wch I like even though they're pretty melodramatic). We were put together because we were both "musicians" (or some such). I doubt that I ever even bothered to describe my experiments w/ prose & graphic scores, etc..

He was also a “vanner” - competition to bikers. He was part of a group in wch everbody had a van. They threw parties at public places & bikers wd come & they'd fight. That was about the most interesting thing I ever found to talk with him about - good for about 10 minutes.. After that, we both sat uncomfortably for the next hr or 2. It was worse than being in the closet!

All in all, I definitely did not favor the depressants & gave a great deal of input warning doctors against their administration to people who feel a desperate need for more psychic space & more ability to feel un-supressed/depressed..

****

Sometime between 1977 & 1979 a young scientist friend of mine had gotten a job painting an apartment. The apt was in a vvveeerrrryyyy expensive building in the Mount Vernon section of Baltimore. This building was owned by a famous surgeon. My friend wanted help with the painting & asked me. He told me that the pay was extremely low, way below what an actual professional painter would've gotten, & that the surgeon had estimated how long it should take us to do the job & that the estimate was also ridiculously low. My scientist friend informed the surgeon that the estimate was too low but the surgeon was adamant & we needed money so we took the job anyway. I had only done one painting job before, I don't know if my friend had ever done one. We did the job, it took longer than the estimate, we got paid only for the amount of hours the surgeon was willing to pay, his estimate, for the low amount he was willing to part with. We were disgusted but we weren't professional painters either so we took the money & that was that.

Very shortly thereafter, the surgeon was in the news. He had performed a spine operation, his speciality. He'd estimated that the operation would take something like 7 hours to perform, instead it took something like SEVENTEEN hours. Instead of this being interpreted as a sign of his poor estimating he was somehow lauded as a hero for persevering. My friend & I had a good laugh over that as we speculated whether he just stuck to charging for 7 hours, etc. The patient died 2 weeks later. Did the surgeon refund the money? Go to prison for murder? For manslaughter? Was the operation even necessary? This may've been when my cynicism about doctors started in earnest.

In what was probably the early '80s, friends of mine who had a video company were hired by a dentist to make a movie about his dentistry. As I understood it, his purpose was to make it so that people would be less afraid of dentists & would, therefore, take better care of their health. In order to demonstrate this, he focused on a patient whose teeth were in very bad shape because he'd neglected them. The patient was clearly nervous about being there. The dentist convinced him that he needed to have all of his teeth pulled & told him he would be completely anaesthetized. If I remember correctly, he was partially anaesthetized instead — with the dentist explaining to the camera, but not the unsuspecting patient, that full anaesthesia was too dangerous. The video shows the man's teeth being pulled out one-by-one while blood gushes out profusely & the patient screams in agony & terror. The video I saw may not have been the video that was ultimately made for the dentist, I don't know. At any rate, anyone afraid of the dentist would've been absolutely convinced that dentists are sadistic insensitive maniacs after watching this one.

A humorous aside is that in 1989 I was at a party where I was flirting with a woman. Spontaneously, I bit her. As it turned out, she had a *thing* for biting & that was just the right thing to do to result in our hooking-up. When we were talking about this later, I learned that *her dentist had been the one that the above-mentioned video was of!!*

Sometime around 1982, a punk rock musician friend of mine went to a doctor because his testicles hurt. The doctor squeezed his scrotum, my friend screamed. According to my friend's telling of it, the doctor then told him that *that shouldn't have hurt*, that he was a 'pussy', & that he 'smoked too much pot'. In short, the doctor told him that he was just imagining things & that he didn't need any medical help. Not long thereafter, my friend's scrotum turned black & he rushed to the Emergency Room in agony & fear. When the doctor there saw his scrotum he asked him why he'd waited so long to seek help & told him that immediate surgery was required. My friend lost one testicle as a result because a blood vessel leading to it had gotten knotted causing the blood supply to be cut off. Is the doctor who originally 'advised' him atypical? I tend to think that the answer is NO, that there're many doctors whose prejudices against their patients lead to poor diagnosis & negligent treatment. Add greed & megalomania to that & things become even more problematic.

And what about sadism? Doctors are routinely depicted as people who choose a difficult profession because they're deeply caring about their fellow humans. But how many of them actually choose to be doctors because they can get filthy rich off of experimenting on people with very little accountability? How many are downright sadists?

I have a friend whose grandfather was (still is?) a doctor. His daughter, my friend's mom, when she was a child, said she didn't want to go to school that day because she felt sick. Her father, the doctor, apparently thinking that she was malingering, 'taught her a lesson' by taking her to the hospital where he worked & unnecessarily removing her appendix. Was/is he a sadist?! I unequivocally say: YES.

I have another friend who reports that they were raped by their doctor as a child. I've known entirely too many people who were raped as children. Most or all of them were somewhat permanently traumatized by the experience. It's my opinion that adults in positions of power & authority are more likely to perpetrate this crime. Simply being a patriarch might often be enough. One friend was raped by a CIA agent, another by a fireman, another by her banker grandfather. In the Marquis de Sade's 120 Days of Sodom in which kidnapped children are kidnapped, tortured, raped, & murdered, the four main perpetrators are: The Duc de Blangis, The Bishop, The Président de Curval, & Durcet, a banker. Not surprisingly, this association of people in power with abusiveness was as prevalent in 1785 as it is now. Of course, de Sade's take on that is ambiguous insofar as he was an aristocrat & insofar as these characters may be described as his 'heros' (or 'anti-heros').

As of June 19, 2020, there are 294 doctors listed on an online US Department of Justice, Drug Enforcement Agency "Cases Against Doctors" website (https://apps2.deadiversion.usdoj.gov/CasesAgainstDoctors/spring/main?execution=e1s1). Here're a few examples:

AGRAWAL, Pankaj, MD	Sicklerville	NJ	06-27-2008	03-25-2009	Pled Guilty

Distribution of Oxycodone and Money Laundering	Agrawal was sentenced to 63 months incarceration, followed by three years supervised release.	Surrendered 07-28-2008	According to court documents, Pankaj Agrawal, MD, age 62, of Sicklerville, NJ, pled guilty in U.S. District Court, District of New Jersey, to one count Distribution Oxycodone and one count Money Laundering. Between January 2005 and June 2008, Agrawal knowingly and intentionally distributed and dispensed to several individuals Oxycodone, specifically Percocet tablets.

ARMASHI, Hussam, MD	Spring Hill	FL	02-22-2005		Warrant

Sexual Battery on Person Incapacitated	Outstanding Warrant - No Adjudication	Surrendered 09-08-2006	According to court documents, Hussam Armashi was charged with with intentionally administering a narcotic, anesthetic, or intoxicating substance to a female patient who was under his care that resulted in the patient's mental or physical incapacitation, and then attempting to engage the patient in sexual activity without her consent and causing her injury. There continues to be an active, outstanding arrest warrant for Armashi in Hernando County, FL. Anyone who has information pertaining to Armashi's whereabouts is encouraged to contact the nearest Drug Enforcement Administration office or the Hernando County Police Department.

BASS, Harriston, MD	Las Vegas	NV	12-20-2006	03-05-2008	Conviction

Murder in the Second Degree; Sale of Schedule II Controlled Substances; and Unlawful Possession with Intent to Sell Schedule II Controlled Substances	Bass was sentenced to ten years to life incarceration, with a credit of 57 days time served.	Revoked 05-19-2009	According to court documents, Harriston Bass, MD, age 54, of Las Vegas, NV, was found guilty in the District Court of Clark County, Nevada, of one count murder in the second degree; 49 counts of sale of a Controlled Substance; and six counts of possession of a Controlled Substance for purpose of sale. Bass prescribed Controlled Substances to young adults and juveniles without a medical indication at their homes and hotels/casinos in Las Vegas. Several young adults overdosed and/or died as a result of Bass' prescribing and dispensing patterns.

FELDMAN, Edward N, MD	Pinellas Park	FL	01-06-2015	02-24-2016	Jury Conviction

Conspiracy to Distribute and Dispense Oxycodone, Methadone, Alprazolam, Diazepam; Distributing and Dispensing of Oxycodone, Methadone, Alprazolam, Diazepam Resulting in Death; Conspiracy to Commit Money Laundering; Illegal Monetary Transactions	Feldman was sentenced to 25 years incarceration, followed by three years supervised release. During the period of supervised release, Feldman is prohibited from engaging in any occupation relating to healthcare, including the prescribing and dispensing of Controlled Substances. Feldman was also ordered to forfeit both properties used for his medical practices in Tampa and Pinellas Park, multiple luxury vehicles, as well as cash and other valuables totaling over $600,000 in partial satisfaction of a Preliminary Order of Forfeiture totaling $6,787,104. Feldman has appealed.	Jury Conviction 12-06-2016	According to court documents, beginning from an unknown date no later than October, 2009 and continuing through December, 2014, Feldman operated with his wife, Kim Xuan Feldman, a medical practice under the name Feldman Orthopedic and Wellness Center located in Tampa, FL and subsequently Pinellas Park, FL. During this period, Feldman and his wife conspired to distribute and dispense and did distribute and dispense Oxycodone and Methadone, Schedule II Controlled Substances, and Alprazolam and Diazepam, Schedule IV Controlled Substances, outside the scope of professional practice and without a legitimate medical purpose. Feldman and his wife also launder the proceeds from their illegal distribution and dispensing through the purchase of property and deposits in various investment accounts.

Since these are DEA cases they mostly revolve around illegal sales of controlled substances. Many of the cases involve oxycodone &/or hydrocodone. Cases also involve murder, manslaughter, & various acts of sexual abuse. The Sackler family, the people who own Purdue Pharma have had 26,000 lawsuits against them for manufacturing, misrepresenting, & selling OxyContin which has resulted in more than 400,000 deaths in the last 2 decades. After pledging $3,000,000,000.00 to address this problem they declared that a judge must block further suits against them or they would withdraw the pledge. Poor babies.

One could claim that the above list of successfully prosecuted doctors indicates due vigilence & that the number of doctors who're actual criminals is very small. I disagree. It's my opinion that drug-pushing is part & parcel of what doctoring in the US, at least, is all about.

From 1990 to 1991, my girlfriend was someone who was an AIDS activist, she was bisexual & felt a special affinity for queer struggles. As such, she chose for her dentist a woman who was intending to surgically transition to a man. One day this dentist told her something like that she had to have all her teeth pulled. She came home to me very upset. I suggested that she get a 2nd opinion. She did, the 2nd dentist told her that her teeth were fine, that she didn't need to have them all pulled. She didn't go back to the 1st dentist anymore. It's my opinion that the sex-transitioning dentist needed money for her operation & was willing to subject her patients to the most extreme & expensive 'treatments' in order to quickly raise this money.

After this girlfriend & I broke up, one of the people she dated was a med student. My ex- told me a story which I, unfortunately, only remember very vaguely. It went something like this: the med student had deliberately poisoned a friend of his as a child, possibly killing him, & was never suspected or caught for it. As I recall, this was 'the reason why he wanted to become a doctor'. In retrospect I don't know whether that meant that he was hoping to continue committing such crimes & thought that being a doctor would help enable this OR whether that meant that he wanted to help people in atonement. This med student was a bit jealous of me because I had made a sexual movie with the girlfriend when we'd been together. One day I was at his apartment when he told me he liked to get high with a clear chemical that he had a small vial of. I forget what name he gave me for it. He asked me if I'd like to try it. Mindful that this was similar to how he'd poisoned his childhood friend, I demured.

There's a 4 volume set of books by Philippe Aziz entitled Doctors of Death. The 4 volumes are themed: (1) Karl Brandt the Third Reich's Man in White; (2) Joseph Mengele the Evil Doctor; (3) When Man Became a Guinea Pig for Death; (4) In the Beginning Was the Master Race. The subject of the books are obvious: nazi doctor experimentation on humans. Bayer, well-known for its invention of aspirin, was also active in nazi medical crimes:

"As part of the IG Farben conglomerate, which strongly supported the Third Reich, the Bayer company was complicit in the crimes of the Third Reich. In its most criminal activities, the company took advantage of the absence of legal and ethical constraints on medical experimentation to test its drugs on unwilling human subjects. These included paying a retainer to SS physician Helmuth Vetter to test Rutenol and other sulfonamide drugs on deliberately infected patients at the Dachau, Auschwitz, and Gusen concentration camps. Vetter was later convicted by an American military tribunal at the Mauthausen Trial in 1947, and was executed at Landsberg Prison in February 1949. In Buchenwald, physicians infected prisoners with typhus in order to test the efficacy of anti-typhus drugs, resulting in high mortality among test prisoners.

"Bayer was particularly active in Auschwitz. A senior Bayer official oversaw the chemical factory in Auschwitz III (Monowitz). Most of the experiments were conducted in Birkenau in Block 20, the women's camp hospital. There, Vetter and Auschwitz physicians Eduard Wirths and Friedrich Entress tested Bayer pharmaceuticals on prisoners who suffered from and often had been deliberately infected with tuberculosis, diphtheria, and other diseases." - https://encyclopedia.ushmm.org/content/en/article/bayer

It appears that crimes committed in the name of 'health' aren't looked down on by the law very much because Bayer is still alive & well today.

& let's not forget the Nurses of Death:

"CARING CORRUPTED - The Killing Nurses of The Third Reich"

https://youtu.be/Rz8ge4aw8Ws

"Cizik School of Nursing has created a REMI Platinum Award-winning documentary film that tells the grim cautionary tale of nurses who participated in the Holocaust and abandoned their professional ethics during the Nazi era. The 56-minute film, Caring Corrupted: the Killing Nurses of the Third Reich, casts a harsh light on nurses who used their professional skills to murder the handicapped, mentally ill and infirm at the behest of the Third Reich and directly participated in genocide."

In 1995, I was in Canada & I decided to go to a doctor to consult about several small complaints. I was even poorer than usual at the time & I only had $75 Canadian to my name, roughly $54.74 US at the time. Accustomed to the outrageous high prices of US medical practices when I went to the Canadian doctor I explained that I only had $75 & asked him how much he could do for me for that little. He laughed & said something like 'You must be from the US, that's 3 times what it'll cost you to get everything done you're asking for.'

I moved to Pittsburgh in 1996. In that year I applied for something like 100 jobs of all sorts, including at a Rite Aid & as a Security Guard. I was desperate. I didn't get hired for any of them. I had plenty of skills but it didn't take long to realize that nepotism & croneyism were the name of the game in Pittsburgh. In the meantime, I qualified for some sort of state health insurance that I don't even remember asking for. I made something like $3,000 that year — the exact amount of my rent. It was a leeeaaaaannnnn year.

I resorted to selling my body for medical research. I'd done that before, it wasn't so bad. I was rejected from one of the studies because they said I'd tested positive for hepatitis. This alarmed me so I went to a hospital to get further tested. It was unclear whether the initial test was a false positive & what type of hepatitis I might have. All I wanted was a blood test & the state health insurance was to pay for it. What I didn't know was that the hospital was in a bad financial situation & they were trying to milk as much money out of patients as they could. This was to become a familiar story.

At the hospital they wanted to perform other tests on me before giving me the blood test. I didn't ask for them or want them. One day I had to go in for a physical. I was handed a paper to sign before I could get the physical. I read it & it was asking for me to *authorize surgery*. I told them I didn't need surgery, that I was just trying to find out if I had hepatitis & that I was just there for a physical. The nurse very aggressively told me that if I didn't sign the paper I wouldn't be allowed to have anything done there at all. I refused, left, & never went back. I did eventually learn that I didn't have hepatitis. The hospital went bankrupt soon thereafter.

Back at the medical research place I learned that there was going to be a very well-paying study. However, when I inquired about it with one of the nurses she seemed very nervous. She told me that I'd have to agree to something like not having sex during the time of the study, which was to be spaced out over months, & that I had to agree to not have sex for 6 months *after the study*. That seemed rather extreme. It eventually came out that when the drug to be tested had been tested on monkeys that their babies had been born without brains. Thanks you to the nurse for warning me off about this one. I was *desperate* but I wasn't *that desperate*.

In 1997, I was in Hungary when the crown on my front tooth broke off & I swallowed it. I went to a dentist who replaced the crown for the equivalent of $50 US. As far as I could tell, he did as good a job as anyone I might've gone to in the US for **much cheaper**. I've since been told that Hungarian dentists are world-reknowned.

In the late 1990s or early 2000s I developed an abscess under one of my teeth. The pain got to be so intense that I would scream involuntarily. Finally, after work one weekend I was in so much pain that I went to the Emergency Room. I'd wanted to hold out until the dental school was open on Monday but I couldn't stand the pain anymore. At the ER I was told that I had to get my blood pressure & temperature taken. I said that I didn't want that done, that I was just there to get a pain-killer. They insisted that they wouldn't see me if I didn't get it done. I asked how much that would cost & explained that I was very poor & that I would try to pay the bill but that I didn't want to get anything done to me that I didn't need. They told me that they didn't know how much it would cost. Out of desperation I eventually relented.

After a bit of a wait, I was sent to an examination room. After another wait an intern came in. I explained the problem & he said he'd give me an injection of a local anaesthetic. He explained that *he'd never done this before so he hoped he'd get it right.* When I asked him how long the anaesthetic would last he said something like 3 days. It might've lasted for as little as 15 minutes, at any rate, it wasn't long. He gave me a prescription for a pain killer & suggested that I NOT fill it at the hospital because it would be VERY EXPENSIVE there so he suggested an outside pharmacy. I told him that I was very poor & that I was worried about how much all this was going to cost. He told me that he *wasn't worried about whether he'd get paid.* That was all well & good but the hospital was definitely concerned with that.

Anyway, that was it, temperature & blood pressure taken, an intern giving an injection & a prescription. Soon thereafter, I got the bill. It was something like $1,500. That was probably over a month's pay for me for what amounted to about 15 minutes worth of work by hospital staff. The temp & pressure taking was a fixed fee of $160. I don't remember what the itemization for the rest of it was. I was outraged & refused to pay, I complained, they reduced the bill by something like $200. That wasn't enough, I still refused to pay. When I tried to get a mortgage to buy a house in 2006 I was told I was ineligible for the mortgage because I had an outstanding hospital bill. I paid it. To me, that bill was robbery.

Ater this visit to the ER I still had the abscess so I went to the dental school. Dental schools have the reputation of being affordable for poor people with the risk run being that the student who does the work may botch it. That risk is real but the cost isn't cheap. I was told that the only thing to be done about the abscess was to have my tooth pulled. It seemed to me that the abscess could be drained some other way but I was told that that wasn't possible. Eventually I was sent in to see someone to pull the tooth & he did so, I heard the tooth crack in the process. After, I asked for the tooth, explaining that it'd been in my body for all these years & that I felt sentimental about it. He told me that it was now toxic waste & that he wasn't allowed to give it to me. He also explained that it was shattered, that the problem with it had been that it had a major crack, he continued to try to talk me out of it but eventually he gave me the tooth. It wasn't shattered, the only small crack in it might've just been from his pulling it.

In the summer of 2002, I started getting sick. Usually I just figure that staying in bed, getting plenty of rest, drinking more water than usual will make me better so I tried that at 1st. I just kept getting worse, I was coughing intensely. This went on for about 3 weeks. I don't go to doctors very often, especially since they're expensive & I've been poor my whole life, so I just stayed home & continued to go to work. I kept a diary, below are some abridged extracts:

Subject: thru the valley of the shadow of death
Date: Sun, 01 Sep 2002 11:09:45 -0400
From: anonymous <anon@fyi.net>

Dramatic, huh?

friday, august 9:
@ a party I notice a big mosquito bite in the crook of my arm,
it doesn't itch, I subconsciously attach importance to it.
perhaps that night I dream that I've been injected
w/ a fever & I feel the fever taking over my body.

saturday, august 10:
I work @ the museum & know I'm getting sick,
I go to my friend's place to start editing my movie
about being sexually obssessed.
his computer isn't working right & all of the work I do is lost,
my sickness starts to intensify, I redo the work
in a much simpler way & then go home.
I try to sleep @ ____'s but am too sick & only sleep maybe 2 hrs.
my dreams are mechanical - I imagine like a replicating virus.

tuesday, august 13:
I take off work, the fever's gone down slightly
& I think I'm getting better but the coughing's way more extreme.
very violent coughing, still can't sleep more than
a couple of hrs per night, dreaming something like
that every time I cough (or something) a sortof box
comes out of the "side" (my side?)
- I have to do something but don't know the
appropriate response? - still very mechanical.
I assume these dreams are telling me exactly what I need to know
about my health & how to deal with it
but I don't understand them.

thursday, august 15:
I've been assuming that I have a virus but it's strange
because usually with a virus/flu I have fever, coughing,
& RUNNY NOSE - & all at the same time.
this time there's no runny nose & the condition
seems to be moving in stages.
if it were a flu it would've been over by now.
still extreme coughing, still can't eat,
still can't sleep much, still slightly feverish.

monday, august 19:
I can barely talk anymore & am laying on a piece of foam
on the floor, I'm against going to drs & especially against
going to the emergency room where I know
they'll try to rob me of as much money as possible
& that the visit will result in constant harrassment by bill collectors.
I tell ____, barely able to breath at this point:
"wait.....until.....tomorrow....." - squeezing each word out
barely audibly - 1 word per breath.

She replies that I'll be dead by tomorrow.
She's right, I probably wd've died that night.
The neighbor drives me & ____ to the ER
where I'm admitted pretty quickly.

tuesday, august 20:
after CAT scans & x-rays & blood-draws & what-not,
it's decided that I have both pneumonia & appendicitis
& that I shd have my appendix removed.
basically, the choice seems to be: do this or die
- I don't want an appendectomy but I'm too weak
to be able to work thru this in any satisfactory way.
the drs open me up & then can't find my appendix
- maybe it was hiding: the little bugger!
they find it & remove it.
post-op, I'm on an IV for the 1st time of my life,
I have a "pain button" - a button I can push
to give myself morphine injections
- they're surprised I don't use it very much
- it doesn't seem to effect the pain at all anyway.
the IV rehydrates me & gives me anti-biotics,
I don't want anti-biotics but my body's been doing
a bad job of fighting the pneumonia (a losing battle)
so I go along w/ it.
it's too painful to move so I'm trying to piss
in a plastic container for that purpose but I fail,
a smiling young nurse uses a device to learn that my bladder is,
indeed, full & I get a catheter for the 1st time
& the piss rushes out for what seems like a very long time
(10 minutes or more?), the catheter doesn't bother me.

wednesday, august 21:
even w/ morphine I still can't sleep for the most part.
constant hospital routine, taking blood in the middle
of the night & such things, the money person calls the room
at something like 9:30AM, I can barely talk - only during gasps,
she says she'll visit me the next day, ____ visits me every day,
I have to concentrate to breathe, the drs are encouraging me
to use this simple breathing device to strengthen my lungs,
I'm expected to suck in hard enough to reach something like 2000,
I can barely make the counter move to 250,
it's very hard to breath.

thursday, august 22:
my bowels beneath the incision area have been non-functional
since the operation, the drs explain that they've
"gone into shock", I think the drs are nervous waiting for
the organs to start working again, they keep asking whether I've farted,

it's the 1st time anyone's ever WANTED me to fart,
at 4:30AM I feel gas start to move in these bowels
- it's as if a switch has been turned on
& an exploratory gas has been sent out to test the way,
25 minutes later I fart.
still hard to breath, incision still makes bending
at the waist almost impossible for me to do.

saturday, august 24:
day 15. I'm asking about when I can leave,
they're thinking of running another CAT scan on me
because they think there's something strange about my bowels,
I'm half-jokingly waiting to be told that
I don't have a human interior,
they decide against the CAT scan & I'm told I'll
probably be able to leave the next day, I'm off the IV,
my arms & hands are bruised from so many needles.

saturday, august 31:
I go to work again, I'm still sick
but much better, getting to work wasn't hard.
It's been 3 wks - the longest I've ever been sick by far.
At times I've felt like the woman in the original
"Carnival of Souls" - somewhat like I've died
& am in some sort of limbo,
my emotions have been mixed, if there had been noone to care
about me I wd've let myself die
- I wdn't've gone to the ER.
For the 1st few days after the operation I referred to my self as "dead",
I wasn't just being dramatic - it was really how I felt:
as if I'd really died & whatever was left wasn't really me,
I seem to be over that, my body's still reacting:
rashes are covering my legs & arms,
my scrotum's been bright red, my orgasms
have felt weirdly strangled
- at least I still get erections.

Sometime no earlier than 2005, I bit into a sandwich that had a toothpick in it & cracked the crown I'd gotten in Hungary. Since this only bothered my vanity I didn't do anything about it. Eventually, my vanity won out & I decided to go to the dental school to get a new crown put on. Once there, I was assigned a very young student who had little experience. I then became her guinea pig. I was told that before I could get a crown I'd have to get various other things done. These were all things the student needed experience with, none of them were what I had come there for. I explained that I had very little money & that I was only there for one thing. What I wanted or was there for was of no importance to the dentists. I was coldly informed that we'd do things *their way* or not at all. Unsure of what this would entail I went along with it at 1st in the hope that only one unnecessary procedure would precede my getting what I wanted. By the time of the 3rd unnecessary procedure there was no end in sight. By then I'd spent $450 with another $350 or more to be expected. I informed the instructor that it would've been cheaper for me to fly to Hungary to get it done than it was to go their route. The instructor was highly offended & escalated her already rude conduct.

Finally, the day arrived when I was to see the dentist who specialized in crowns. While I waited for the student & the dentist I saw a disheveled looking man come in. The receptionist talked to him barely hiding her contempt. It occurred to me that he might be the dentist. He was. When I went in to be examined by him he handled me as if he were looking at the teeth of a horse or a slave for sale. It was obvious that I was barely considered worthy of any politeness. While he was roughly pulling my lips back he said something like: 'Your enamel Is almost gone! What kind of chemicals are you putting in your mouth?!' The question, as I understood it, was to imply that an obvious low-life such as myself was probably huffing glue or gasoline or some such. I said something like: 'None. Maybe my drinking soda is a problem.' He snorted at that as if I was obviously lying. I wasn't.

After he'd released my mouth I rapidly left the room with the student following me. Out in the foyer, near the stairwell & in sight of a receptionist I said 'I am NEVER coming back here again. That man is INSANE & I don't think I'm the only one around here who thinks that!! He should NOT be allowed to touch patients.' I said this loudly enough so that the receptionist could hear. I wanted my anger to be apparent. The student, who was actually pretty nice, said 'Unfortunately, I have to study with him.' It was obvious that she understood how ill-treated I'd been. I said 'Look, you're a nice person & I wish you the best of luck but I *will not tolerate being so rudely treated!!'* Then I left, I've never been back to the dental school itself since. I did go back to an adjunct of it where a friend of mine who'd graduated from the school was employed. While I was sitting there being worked on I saw the abusive dentist go past looking very nervously at me. I like to think that the incident with me & the student's having to report about it damaged his career.

Living in continual poverty, despite working for a living, led to my finding out about clinics. Many of these had sliding scales, were otherwise cheap, or could be free if one pleaded penury. I engaged with 3 of them. At one of them the hours were very limited, maybe from 1:30PM to 4:30PM. I went there, it was cold out & raining, but the doctor hadn't arrived by 1:30 so the prospective patients were waiting in line out in the rain. That couldn't have helped their health much. Finally, the doctor arrived, an hour later, at 2:30 & I eventually got to see him in the company of 2 oncology med students. I told him that I was worried about my kidneys because they'd been hurting me lately & because my urine was particularly foul-smelling. He punched the skin over where my kidneys were, asked if that hurt & when I told him that it didn't he told me that my kidneys were fine. The doctor, however, was obviously far from fine. He told me that he'd recently had back surgery, he seemed very depressed. He also told me that he was a doctor at a university where he prescribed drugs for the students. I got the impression that that was pretty much it, a student would come in & say that they were depressed &/or stressed & he'd prescribe some pills. I wasn't impressed.

The doctor then informed me that I should go to the psychiatrist in the cliniic & get drugs prescribed for me because I'd been moving my hands too much while we were talking. Apparently, he took this to be a symptom of psychomotor agitation or some such. I didn't bother to explain that I'm a drummer & that when I'm bored & have nothing better to do I often practice on my legs. Instead, I explained to him that there's nothing wrong with my mind & that I didn't require any psychiatric prescriptions. It was obvious to me that he was there at the clinic to get a tax write-off, that he had close to no medical knowledge, & that what he had to offer was the chance to become addicted to drugs that would enable him to get kickbacks from the pharmaceutical companies. This man was more of a menace to patients than anything else — but poor people are expected to grovelingly accept whatever crap is handed us & be 'grateful' for it — but, as I like to say, ***Before you decide against biting the hand that feeds you ask why it has so much food in the 1st place.***

A partial take-away from the above is that one should not *automatically accept the diagnosis of a doctor.* Doctors have a mindset that defines everything in terms of disorders & diseases. This is a form of morbidity. Think of something like "restless legs syndrome": how easy it would be to misdiagnose this!

"**Restless legs syndrome** (**RLS**) is generally a long-term disorder that causes a strong urge to move one's legs. There is often an unpleasant feeling in the legs that improves somewhat by moving them. This is often described as aching, tingling, or crawling in nature. Occasionally, arms may also be affected. The feelings generally happen when at rest and therefore can make it hard to sleep. Due to the disturbance in sleep, people with RLS may have daytime sleepiness, low energy, irritability, and a depressed mood. Additionally, many have limb twitching during sleep.

"Risk factors for RLS include low iron levels, kidney failure, Parkinson's disease, diabetes mellitus, rheumatoid arthritis, and pregnancy. A number of medications may also trigger the disorder including antidepressants, antipsychotics, antihistamines, and calcium channel blockers." - https://en.wikipedia.org/wiki/Restless_legs_syndrome

I sometimes move my legs quickly while I'm sitting or laying down. Is this a "syndrome", in other words does it have to be diagnosed in terms of bad health? In my opinion, NO! Perhaps my body just isn't ready for repose, maybe it feels a need to go walking or is otherwise just manifesting a state of energeticness.

And what about SAD?, Seasonal Affective Disorder? Is it symptomatic or a "disorder" if we feel depressed when there's very little sun & it's cold? Or is that just a natural part of an instinct for hibernation that we defy with electricity, heat, & the rat race? HPD?, Histrionic Personality Disorder? That's a perfect one for natural-born performers. Instead of being praised for their performative abilities, they're chastised for their attention-grabbing.

But in the era of the PANDEMIC PANIC it's "asymptomatic" that takes the prize for stupidest & most pernicious demonizing of the positive: instead of being "healthy", by most accounts a good thing, the healthy person becomes "asymptomatic", a human time-bomb of potential contagion. The purpose is pure capitalism: pronounce any & every quality that a person might have, say a highly functional immune system, 'impossible' according to 'expert' opinion & further stipulate *that the only positive qualities a person might have* ***have to be purchased from a qualified rich person.*** Forget your immune system, all it's doing is making you a threat to others. PAY 'YOUR' DOCTOR ENORMOUS SUMS TO MAKE IT SO YOU'RE NOT ANYTHING OTHER THAN A WALKING PLAGUE, an abomination in the eyes of the DOCTOR GODS.

It was around 2007 or 2008 that I tried a different clinic, the closest one I could find to where I live, still perhaps 2 or 3 miles away. I was worried that as a man in my 50s I might have prostate cancer & I wanted to be checked for it. I was informed over the phone that the clinic was only or primarily for women but when I explained that I didn't have a car, that I'd be using a bike, & that I was worried about cancer they said that it was ok for me to come in. I eventually saw a woman doctor who brought another doctor in with her before sticking her finger up my ass. She explained that this was for protection against sexual harrassment or some such. I didn't care, I just wanted to be checked for prostate cancer. I wasn't sure whether she was protecting herself against me or whether she was protecting herself against a sexual misconduct lawsuit or whatever. She explained that my prostate felt fine, that if I had cancer it would feel hard. She also explained that the prostate cancer medications could be more harmful than the cancer itself, saying that one could live a long life with prostate cancer but that the treatment would have side-effects like impotence & incontinence. This was when I decided that **this was a good doctor to go to**.

In 2008, I got pneumonia for the 2nd time. The clinic doctor that I liked prescribed an antibiotic for it. I asked for the weaker antibiotic because I wanted to learn what the minimum I could get by on was. She told me I could get a prescription for the stronger antibiotic if the weaker one didn't work. Alas, the weaker one wasn't enough & I got sicker. Pneumonia is very debilitating. I didn't have a car so I went to the clinic on my bike, riding in the cold rain. I got there near opening time, there was no-one in the waiting room. I paid $15 & was ushered into an examination room where I was told that a doctor would see me in 10 minutes. I was very weak. The door to the room was left open, there was nothing happening in the central hallway that it was off of. This was a small clinic so if there were any patients there they would have had to walk past my exam room. At some point, there was an announcement over the intercom in the room telling me that a doctor would be right with me. Eventually someone closed the exam room door, once again telling me that a doctor would be with me soon. I was fading fast. After an hour & a half of waiting, I was so exhausted that I lay on the examination table so that I could rest better. As far as I could tell, there was still nothing happening outside the room in the rest of the clinic.

After one hour & 40 minutes a doctor came in & said: "Hello, I'm Doctor _________, How are you?" I said: "I'd be better if you hadn't left me waiting for an hour & forty minutes." She was shocked! How dare a lower class person criticize a doctor's behavior?! She said: "Are you sick?" I said: "Yes, I have pneumonia." She explained to me that she had been making a special exception by seeing me because she wasn't my regular doctor & that this wasn't my regular doctor's day. I wasn't aware that I had a "regular doctor". In other words, I'd just seen whomever was available in the past & it had turned out to be the same woman who I liked 2 times. This new doctor then informed me that since I had "attacked" her, as she literally put it, she would not attend to me. Then she left the room. So much for the Hippocratic Oath. This precious little megalomaniac would keep me waiting as long as she liked, she wouldn't have cared if I dropped dead in the meantime. I had to demand my $15 back, which I certainly needed, & then I left to once again ride my bike home in the cold rain with pneumonia.

By the time I got home, I was too weak to go to any of the other clinics, which were much further away. I enlisted a friend to drive me to one where I was well-treated, I got the antibiotics, took them, & recovered. After that I started taking vitamins for a year or more until I couldn't afford them anymore. I haven't had pneumonia since. In the meantime, I sent a detailed complaint letter to the medical instituiton that the offending doctor worked for (note the differences between my memory as recounted above and my description in the letter):

March 8, 2008

Open Letter to ________ _____ Health _________, _____

I've been a patient at _____ ____ ___________ Health several times in the past year & a half. In general I've found the staff friendly & competent. I like them. As such, I was extremely offended by what I consider to've been abusive behavior by _____ ____'s Doctor ___________ on Friday, March 7th, 2008. This letter explains:

Four weeks ago I twisted my knee. As that was healing my immune system was down & I got pneumonia. This made me very sick. I went to the _____ ____ & Doctor _______ prescribed Doxycycline anti-biotics for me. I chose the cheap kind because I don't have much money, the doctor told me that they're good but also warned that there was a slight chance they might not be good enough. I took them for 2 weeks, got better, but after they ran out I started getting sick again. I made an appointment for 10:15AM, Friday, March 7th, to get a prescription for a stronger anti-biotic.

When I arrived at 10:10, there was no-one else in the waiting room & I was shown to an examination room within 10 or 15 minutes where I was told that Doctor ___________ would be right with me. I waited until 11:00 & then opened the door because I thought they might've forgotten me. A nurse saw me & reassured me that I hadn't been forgotten. I went back in the room & about 10 minutes later, a voice over the intercom told me the doctor would be right there. Another 20 minutes or so elapsed, I wasn't feeling very good so I lay down on the examination table.

Ten minutes or so later the doctor came in & said: "I'm Dr __________, how are you?" to which I replied: "I'd be better if you hadn't left me waiting here for an hour & a half." After which, she refused to treat me on the grounds that I had "attacked" her. I told her that I wasn't attacking her but that I thought that I deserved an apology. I said: "Why don't you just apologize & then let's move on." This, apparently, was expecting too much. She said "Do you need medical care?" I said "Yes, I have pneumonia." Her reply, "You've just met me, you've attacked me, I'm not going to give you medical care." I said: "Let me get this straight: Because I think you should apologize for being an hour & a half late for our appointment, you are refusing to give me medical care?" At which point she left.

Now doctors are almost always late. Few are an hour & a half late. Some, like Doctor _______, have the courtesy to apologize - at which point I accept the apology & we get down to business. One of the apparent reasons why doctors are always late is because they seem to value their own time & not that of the patient.

I then went home & proceeded to call other clinics to arrange an appointment to get the stronger anti-biotics. I also had to arrange for someone to drive me there. A couple of hours later, after a great deal of stress, it was taken care of.

In my opinion, Doctor __________ saw herself as the "good charitable doctor" & saw me as some sort of lesser poor person. As such, I was expected to be slavish in response to her even being willing to help me. When I actually DARED to criticize her for being late - something that would be entirely reasonable in most contexts (including this one) - she refused me service because she apparently thought I needed to be 'put in my place'.

Pneumonia can be fatal. I've been sick for 4 weeks. That's an extraordinarily long time for me. This immature doctor could not have cared less. Apparently all that mattered was that she should NEVER be criticized by a patient such as myself - regardless of whether the criticism was deserved.

Do you think that Doctor ___________ is a good doctor for a clinic? I don't. Her decision to deny me health care was an act of malignant neglect & reckless endangerment - all because a sick person was irritated by her lack of consideration. ___________'s refusal of treatment was point-blank criminal.

It seems to me that the purpose of a Community Health clinic is to conscientiously provide healthcare for people regardless of their ability to pay. Many doctors realize that health care prices are artificially inflated purely for the sake of profit by people who do not have health care as their main interest.

In the more modern version of the Hippocratic Oath, doctors vow: "*To practice and prescribe to the best of my ability for the good of my patients, and to try to avoid harming them.*" Doctor ___________ has clearly forgotten this oath.

Doctor ___________, at a very minimum, should send me a written apology. More appropriately, ___________ should no longer work there & her name should be removed from the entranceway to the building.

Sincerely,

________ __ _______

I received the following token reply in which, of course, no action was mentioned to be taken to chastise the doctor.

[redacted] HEALTH [redacted]

$ 00.41

[redacted]

1S213$1032

[redacted] HEALTH [redacted]

March 12, 2008

[redacted]

Dear Mr. [redacted]

Thank you for notifying us of your complaint. We strive to provide you with the best possible service, and when you feel that it fails to meet your expectations, it's important for us to know.

We're sorry that you received service that prompted you to contact us with a complaint, and we regret any inconvenience or frustration that your experience has caused you. We understand that all physicians may not react to the same situation the same and for that we apologize. As you know many things can hold our physicians up from being on time to scheduled appointments. However, we are confident that our physicians make every effort to be there as scheduled for their patients. We try to ensure that our staff conducts itself in a manner that reflects the high regard that we have for our patients, we hope that this will not happen again.

Your care that you receive is important to us, and we hope that you'll continue to give us opportunities to serve you.

Thank you again for bringing these matters to our attention.

Sincerely,

[redacted]

Associate Administrator

Cc: [redacted]

Dissatisfied, I also informed the doctor I liked that this had happened. I never went back to that clinic & my preferred doctor wasn't working there anymore but was, instead, only at a big hospital.

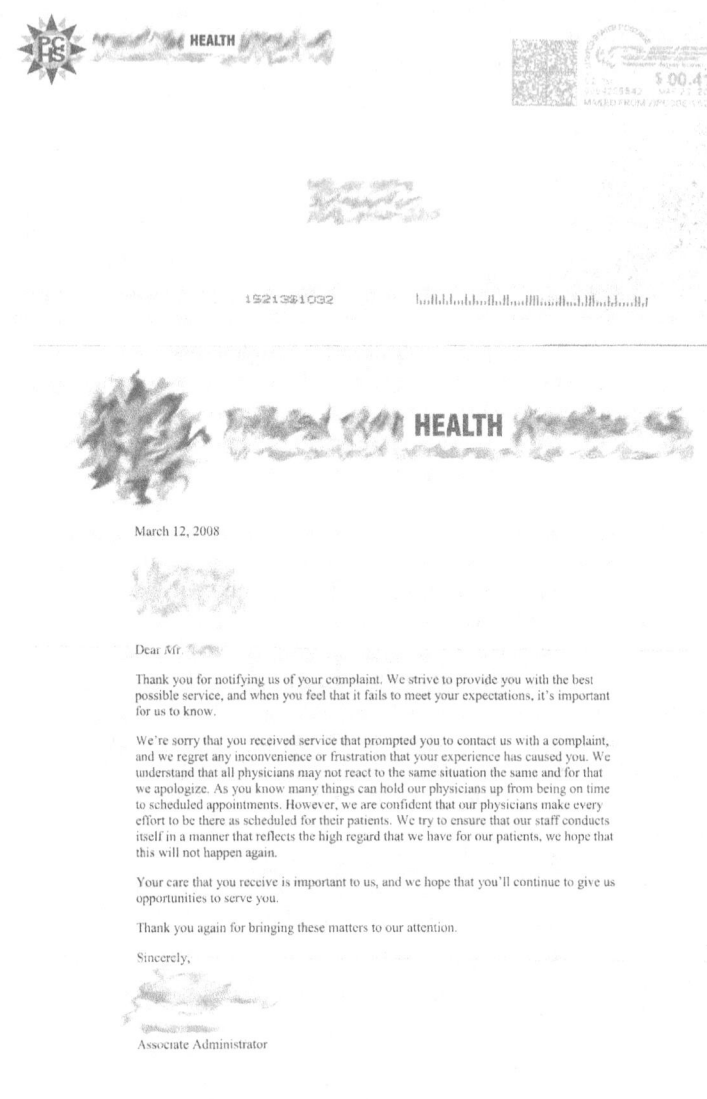

In 2010, I had become lovers with someone who wanted me to get tested for STDs. I went to the free STD clinic, a place that I dislike because everyone waiting there is usually so unhappy. I had been there a few times before, always testing negative for anything except herpes, which I knew I had. This time was different, instead of being shown into a room with one nurse, I went into a room with a young woman I was introduced to as a doctor & a rough looking man who seemed more likely to be a hired thug than some sort of medical assistant. The 'doctor' looked terrified to even be in the same room with me. She was literally backed into the corner the furthest away from where I was & was standing in a ballet position. When I was asked whether I used condoms & told them no she became even more visibly scared. What exactly was she afraid of? That I'd kill the man & rape her in her eyesocket? Her fear seemed that extreme. What they were doing there & why I was seeing them instead of one of the usual personnel was unclear to me. The man poked me with a needle, for no apparent purpose, & I had to wonder whether he was giving me a tiny injection of something. I was thinking of the infamous U.S. Public Health Service (USPHS) Syphilis Study at Tuskegee (1932-72) in which 399 African-American sharecroppers in Macon Country, Alabama were *untreated* for syphilis when they thought they were being treated. Were these 2 there to experiment on 'unsafe' 'low-lifes' such as they apparently perceived me to be? As usual, everything I was tested for came back negative.

In December of 2012, I was having tooth pain again. A wealthy friend of mine recommended her dentist. I went to him, he gave my teeth a cursory 15 minute examination, told me I needed a root canal & said a friend of his would "do it cheaply, only $1,300." Well, when you're a dentist, $1,300 might seem cheap but, for me, that was way beyond anything I could afford. I told him I'd get a 2nd opinion. That visit cost me $75. Another friend of mine suggested a dentist in a more working class neighborhood. That was a good suggestion. The new dentist asked me if I wanted to keep my teeth, I said YES. She said I might need a root canal eventually but that I'd be ok with a filling for now. She drilled a hole between 2 very tightly together teeth, filled it & sent me on my way for $60. Hhmm.. $1,375 vs $60. Alas, the filling fell out fairly quickly so I went back. The dentist said she didn't charge for replacing a filling that'd fallen out that she put in so she drilled some more, put in a new one, & I was on my way again at no expense. 8 years later, those teeth are in bad shape but at least I still have them & I haven't gotten a root canel.

In the beginning of 2013 I was informed by my supervisor at one of my 8 jobs that I could no longer have multiple jobs within the mega-institution I was working for & that I couldn't work more than 25 hours a week. Given that I was dependent on breaking those conditions to even barely survive, this was bad news for me. I asked him why? He said he didn't know, that's just what he was told. As soon as I had access to a computer I did a little research. It didn't take long to discover what the problem was.

The problem was the Affordable Health Care Act — lauded by many as a breakthrough in Socialized Health Care & lambasted by many for the same reason. I never really understood it as anything particularly beneficial to me. Nonetheless, I decided to give it a chance & I got health insurance for the 1st time since something like 30 years before. THEN the nightmare began.

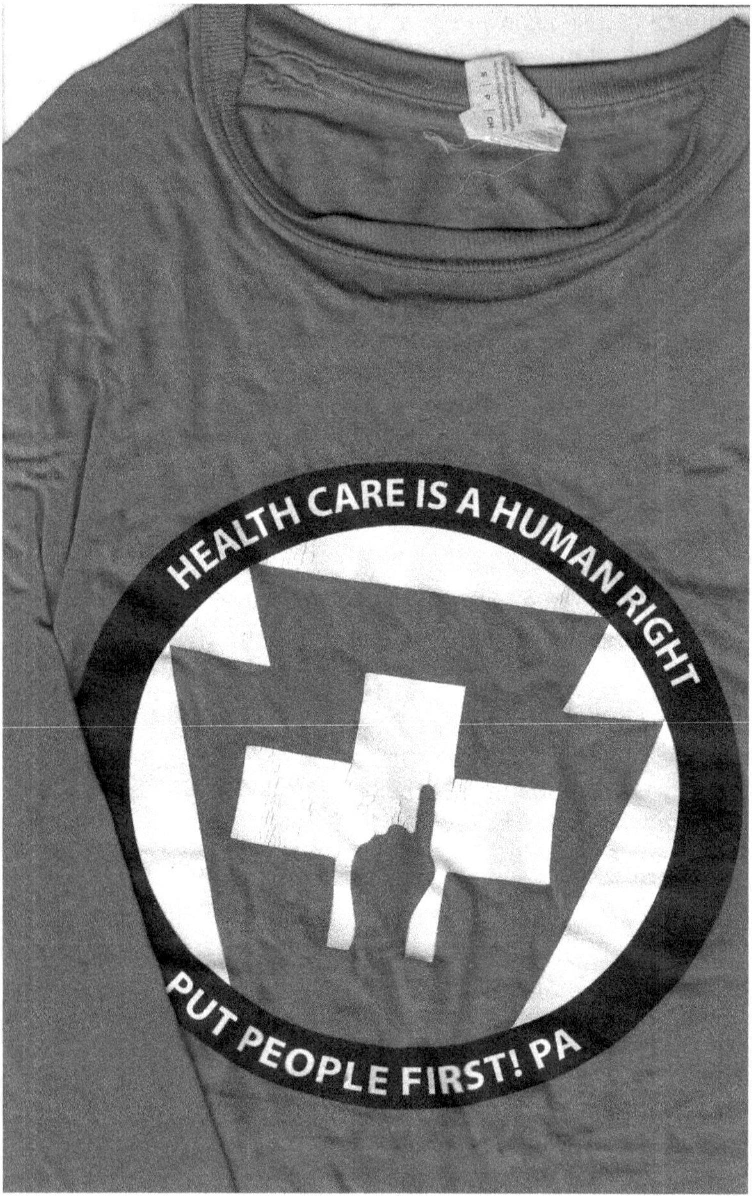

Here's a movie I made of my talking on the phone to one of the employees whose job it was to help me with this:

419. "**HealthCare NightMare**"
- shot at the Who Unit? December, 2014E.V.
- A glimpse into the dysfunctionality of HeathCare.gov & into the failure of the "Affordable Health Care Act" to be much more than yet-another scam to rob American citizens

- 13:25
- on my onesownthoughts YouTube channel here: http://youtu.be/tjB3QBz4LAc

On July 27, 2016 a group of health care activists called "Put People First! PA" drove to Harrisburg, the state capitol, to attend & testify before a regulatory hearing at which it was to be decided whether the health insurance companies should have their demands for dramatic rate increases met. I attended to deliver a short speech about my experiences with the AHCA. Here it is below:

Statement for Public Hearing on Health Care Premiums

for the Wednesday, July 27, 2016 Hearing in Harrisburg, PA

First off, I want to say that health insurance *does not equal* health care. All it equals is paying middlemen to officiate *the possibility* of health care. But that *possibility* may be so reduced by ridiculously high deductibles that it boils down to paying the middlemen *to be middlemen* & very little else.

I had Blue Cross / Blue Shield health insurance until about 1984. The premium was around $40 monthly. I discontinued it because I was poor & in good health. 30 years later, when I was forced by law to get health insurance again, a comparable policy cost around $400 a month.

What happened in those intervening 30 years? According to the Bureau of Labor Statistics, $40 in 1984 had the equivalent buying power of $91 in 2014. Obviously, the incredible escalation of insurance premiums cannot be accounted for by inflation alone.

I suggest that GREED is the main explanation for this dramatic increase. The result of the ACA has been that people are forced to pay for something that seems to be completely unregulated otherwise. This enables the health insurance companies to make their prices outrageous.

In 2014, I chose a health insurance plan that cost me around $50 a month but was supplemented by the government tax credit for something like an additional $310.

By 2015, my health insurance went up by another $50 monthly I had to pay. When it came time for my much-needed tax refund, about 85% of it was being taken away to pay for health insurance because the government said that they were overpaying their part. As such, my premium for 2014 worked out to be about $100 instead of the $50 monthly I'd agreed to paying.

As a result of not getting my tax refund because of health insurance, I was struggling to pay my other bills. How could I possibly cut back any further? Eating only one meal a day was about all that was left to me.

SO, for the entire summer of 2015 I only ate one meal a day. I also *didn't use the insurance ONCE the entire year*. I didn't visit a doctor, I didn't buy any medicines, I didn't go to the hospital. I **hoped** that my insurance premium would go down.

NOPE, it went up again! By another $50 monthly! Making matters worse, I was informed that the government would no longer pay for this particular insurance. Therefore, my premium, if I kept that insurance, would be over $450 a month that I personally would have to pay! That would be more than all my other monthly bills **combined** (excluding food) *for something I hadn't even used that year!!*

I cancelled the insurance & got a policy with a $16 monthly premium & a deductible of over $6,000 - in other words, something I'll pay for but will never use. Continuing to make matters worse, when it came time to get my 2015 tax refund, the government took about 80% of what I was expecting - to pay for health insurance - making my personal premium for something I never used $150!

PLEASE, regulate the health insurance providers. ***THEY ARE OUT OF CONTROL!!!!!*** - And/or give us the ability to OPT OUT of the ACA.

It's my understanding that the insurance companies were granted enormous rate increases despite anything that the public had to say on the matter. That made the regulatory hearing par for the course as far as my knowledge of such things goes. One of the main problems I have had with the AHCA is that it made not having health insurance ***illegal***. It was, & still is, my opinion that this move increased the surveillance state significantly AND that it was setting the stage for future police actions done in the name of 'health', for our own good. My prediction was even more accurate than I expected.

In June of 2013, I installed a huge, vvveeeerrrrryyyyy heavy exhibit at a museum I worked for. This involved me pulling & pushing giant stones, weighing as much as a ton, using a pallet jack. Sure, I had help.. but I was doing the lion's share of the work & by the time the job was over I was having trouble walking because I'd put so much pressure on my feet. I went to the doctor I liked, now at the hospital. She told me I had plantar fasciitis, she said she had it too from being on her feet all day. I reminded her of who I was & told her I knew she was the doctor for me when she talked about treatment being worse than the condition treated. We particularly bonded over her saying "Less is more." She suggested that I exercise the bottoms of my feet by rolling a tennis ball underneath them. This was exactly the type of drug-free non-costly therapy I was looking for. She asked me when she'd see me again & I told her something like "hopefully never" given that I was trying to stay in good health. She asked me to hug her before I left. Alas, when I did want to see her again, 6 years later, she'd moved on to a different state.

In 2014 I was working on my house & my backyard extensively. In the process of weed-whacking the jungle, I got poison ivy for the 1st time in my life. For me, it was as if the plants were fighting back with chemical warfare. I applied cream to my hands but I seemed to have poison ivy on my eyelid too & I was afraid to rub cream on that. I went to a medical place & explained the problem, my poison ivy wasn't that bad but I was afraid for my eyesight & afraid of getting the oil on a valuable object at one of my museum jobs. I was told that I could get a steroid injection & then be prescribed steroids in pill form. I'd never had steroids before & didn't have any opinion about them.

When it was time to give me the injection I was told that it was best to get it in the hip, in this case, my right hip. When I asked why I was told that "it's not as painful this way." I got the injection & went home & started taking the pills in the recommended dosage, it might've been twice a day. I'd been warned that the steroids might make me sleepy. Instead, I was very wide awake all night, I felt great. Within a few days, however, I started getting severe pains radiating out from where the injection had been given. It wasn't long before any pressure on my hip & leg joints, such as by standing, was excrutiatingly painful. I started crawling around my house, standing was too painful — even then I was often in so much pain that I screamed uncontrollably.

At the same time, a friend came to visit that I hadn't seen in decades. I warned him over the phone of my situation & once he got here he drove me to the ER. Once there, I was put in a wheelchair & taken to an examination room where a doctor told me he didn't know what was wrong with me but thought I should take some drugs for it. I explained to him that I thought that the steroids were the problem & that I didn't want any more drugs. He told me that was "impossible". I was given many X-Rays & when the doctor looked at them he said he still didn't know what was going on but speculated that I have Reactive Arthritis but that he didn't know what I was reacting to. That made sense to me & I told him that I was reacting to the steroids. Once again, he told me that that was impossible. Then he asked me if I still needed the wheelchair. I found that astounding since nothing whatsoever had been done to alleviate my need to not walk. I made it back to my friend's car in the wheelchair & we left.

I immediately STOPPED taking the steroids. By the next day my pain was down to about 50% of what it had been. It was still extremely painful to walk but I wasn't screaming anymore. By the day after that the pain had halved again. It was now bearable. By the next day I could walk enough to go on another political trip to Harrisburg. My opinion that the steroids were triggering the reactive arthritis was vindicated for me. I'll never get a steroid injection again & I doubt that I'll ever take the pills again either. The bill for the trip to the ER was astronomical, of course, but the insurance that I had that 1st year was good enough to make my part affordable (barely).

In 2018, I was working a job at a museum. I was feeling fine & I went to lunch. One of the specials of the day was a dish with chunks of beef. I got it & started to eat it. Within seconds I started having a reaction to it that was causing me to feel like my throat was blocked & I started gagging convulsively. I'd had this experience once before in a restaurant with a beef stew or some such that also had chunks of beef. This gagging & difficulty with breathing went on for a while & I was very uncomfortable. It wasn't long before I started vomiting. I saw a security guard & told him I was having trouble breathing. After about 20 minutes of this an ambulance crew came. I didn't really want to go with them but the last time this had happened to me it hadn't gone on for so long. Because of this I consented to go with them to a hospital Emergency Room.

I was vomiting into a trash pail the whole time although after 10 minutes or so of that very little was actually coming up anymore. I got to an examination room where I speculated that perhaps I was having an allergic reaction. The doctor informed me that I would be breaking out in hives if that were so. She told me she didn't know what was happening. I learned later from one of my security guard friends that the guard that I'd spoken to said that I was on drugs. Given that I don't even take aspirin or smoke pot & rarely drink the guard had no reason to speculate to this effect except for whatever prejudices he had. The doctor told me that I might have Esophageal Spasms but that the cause of those is unknown. I didn't know what to make of it all but the reflex gagging went on for 45 minutes until it just stopped suddenly while the doctor was there. The doctor left soon thereafter & I was just left to sit by myself in the examination room. Since the gagging had stopped, I wanted to leave but didn't even know where I was in relation to the exit. I left the room & started wandering the hallways looking for the way out. Staff seemed surprised to see me walking about but I was eventually shown the exit. I called a coworker who considerately came & picked me up & took me to my car. When I got home I looked up Esophageal Spasms but it didn't seem quite right. I tried to eat beef cubes one other time & immediately started having a bad reaction so I just threw the food away. I haven't eaten beef cubes since & I haven't had the problem since.

In the summer of 2019, I was abusing sugar more than I ever had before. I wasn't handling the heat well, I was even poorer than usual & cola & ice cream were a cheap solution to my need for stimulation & cooling. I've always had muscle cramps, Charlie Horses, as they're known, but only very rarely, maybe a few times a year. They had been excrutiatingly painful until when I was around 50 & I discovered that all I had to do was bend back the big toe of the leg with the cramp & it immediately went away. This summer, I started having frequent cramps every day. My legs also felt like there were almost constant electrical explosions in them, little spasms in multiple places. I could barely move my legs without getting a cramp so I was resorting to the big toe pulling cure all day long. Any cut on my leg took forever to heal. My feet were extremely dry, as if I'd been walking in hot sand. I could barely stay awake for more than 2 or 3 hours at a time. I had to urinate so regularly that even when I went to sleep it was no relief because I'd have to get up to piss & I'd get a painful cramp. As such, I rarely slept for more than an hour or 2 at the most. Predictably, combined with all this I was extremely depressed — I was so poor I couldn't even reliably pay bills & have enough food to eat, let alone do anything like go to a movie or buy something for myself. I essentially had almost no friends & the few that were willing to do anything with me were people I was lucky to see once a month *at best.* Times were very grim. Sugar was one of the only pleasures in my life. Nonetheless, I knew I was ruining my health.

Since I'd suspected for some time that I was probably Diabetic Type 2 I decided to make an appointment to see a doctor. I had just turned 66 & had gone out with 2 friends in succession the night before the appointment. With the 1st friend I'd drunk 2 beers & I have a taste for strong beer. With the 2nd friend I was drinking wine & we went for a walk. The 2nd friend is an alcoholic so our walk was basically a beeline to her favorite bar. I told her that I didn't want another drink but she insisted & since I rarely have a chance to hang out with her I acquiesced & drank one more beer before I went home. The next morning when I woke up my legs were numb, it was horrible, it was worse than ever.

I walked to the doctor's office as a part of my intention to get more exercise. When I got there, I explained that I had Medicare, parts A & B, but that I didn't know what it covered. I told the receptionist that if it didn't cover this doctor's visit that I wouldn't go, that I'd turn around & leave because I was completely broke & couldn't afford it if my Medicare didn't cover it. She said that she was pretty sure that it covered it. I should've turned around & left. There was one other receptionist I had to see & I went through the same routine with her. She, also, was pretty sure my Medicare would cover it.

A doctor's assistant of some sort saw me next in the examination room & put me through the intial process of getting weighed & getting my blood-pressure taken, etc. The doctor appeared & the assistant left. The doctor asked questions & I explained what I was there for & described what my diabetes symptoms were. She agreed that I probably was diabetic. I told her that I didn't want medication & that I wanted to solve the problem with diet & exercise. She told me that that was "IMPOSSIBLE". I had told her that I don't use condoms so she insisted that I get all STD blood-tests. I explained that I'm a serial monogamist, that I'd been tested before my last girlfriend, & that I knew that I only have herpes. She continued to pressure me to get STD bloodtests, I replied that as long as it was paid for by my Medicare that I would do it. She said she thought it would be. When I explained my aversion to drugs & made further philosophical explanations such that I'm a naturist she rolled her eyes in mockery of my opinions. This didn't endear her to me OR work as peer pressure. She was most definitely NOT my peer or anywhere close.

She spent the entire time trying to browbeat me into shooting insulin, which I was told I had to do IMMEDIATELY, & to get other tests. Her whole approach was to try to make me be terrified of my apparent imminent death. I explained to her that I'm not particularly afraid of dying but that I'm worried about having the quality of my life lowered. Having to inject insulin every day would definitely do that. She impressed me as basically just a drug pusher who was trying to extract money from me, I didn't think she really had my health in mind. Eventually she told me that I could get my blood drawn in another office downstairs. After she left & her assistant returned the latter informed me I actually couldn't get my blood drawn today but that I could make an appoinment to get it done.

At the 2nd receptionist's desk I went through more rigamarole & was directed to the blood-drawing office in the same building. I think it was at this point that I may've gotten wrong directions. I found the blood-drawing office, signed in, & waited for someone to see me. When I was called in they asked me if I had an appointment, I said I didn't but that I'd been told I could make one there. The phlebotomist told me that I couldn't. When I asked her how to make an appointment she said she didn't know but that there was a brochure in the lobby that would tell me how to do it. I looked in the lobby, found the brochure & found that it had NO appointment-making info. Everyone except for the doctor's assistant had been wrong.

I got home & found the relevant info online & made an appointment for the following Monday. I got my blood drawn then & started getting phone calls from the doctor &/or her assistant by the next day. The assistant seemed *astounded* that I'd gotten those blood tests for the STDs when I didn't HAVE any STDs. She must've wondered why on Earth I would do such a thing when I was just there to ask about diabetes. Yeah. I was informed that I did have Diabetes Type II & that I had to immediately start injecting insulin. I reiterated to the doctor that I didn't want to & explained that I'd try diet & exercise 1st & that if there wasn't any significant improvement in a month that I'd reconsider the insulin.

In the next day or so I made an appointment with a dietician at the same medical center. She gave me some useful advice about what to eat. She also gave me a blood sugar testing kit & explained what I must do with it. I started my regimen of good eating, cutting out sugar altogether, & daily walking for exercise. I monitored my blood sugar. Below are my 1st & last readings:

Wednesday [FASTING], September 11, 2019, 1:30PM: **229 (9.5%)**; 9PM: **136 (< 6.5)**; Thursday, October 10, 2019, 7:35AM: **96**

Within FIVE DAYS I got rid of my symptoms. Within TWO WEEKS I got my blood sugar down to an acceptable level. This was what the doctor had told me was "impossible". When I communicated this to the medical center I was told that I must've been "pre-diabetic", a fine bit of back-pedaling to someone who was told they were close to death before. In the meantime, when I tried to get more sticks for pricking myself when I was checking my blood-sugar I was told that there was a problem with my Medicare paying for it & that the doctor was tring to work it out. The pharmacist told me that I DID have needles there (for injecting insulin) & that there were also pills that were a substitute for injectable insulin. I explained that I hadn't asked for OR wanted either of them. Nonetheless, every time I went back I was reminded that they were there waiting for me to pick them up.

Roughly 6 months later I decided to cancel my Medicare part B assistance because I was having to pay for it and it was reducing my Social Security to something like $450 to $500 a month. As soon as I did this I was informed that, in fact, Medicare *had not* covered my visit & that I would possibly be billed for something like $1,300. Much or most of that was for the STD blood tests that I never wanted in the 1st place. I haven't been billed for it yet, perhaps the doctor had a crisis of conscience. Whatever the case, I will NEVER go back there, certainly NOT to that doctor & I've repeatedly informed representatives of the medical center who've called to harass me that this is the case. I did make a movie about my diabetes & my treatment of it that you can find here:

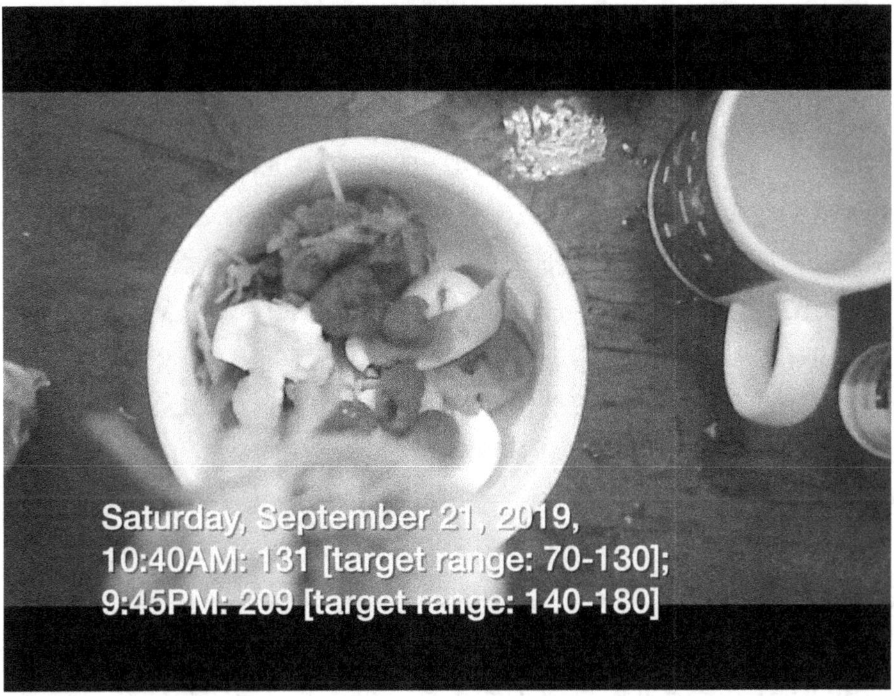

606. "**Diabetes Type 2**"
- 1:22:42
- custom HD 1920 X 1440
- on my onesownthoughts YouTube channel here: https://youtu.be/2GLu66dgpKI

SO, *YES*, I've developed a 'bad attitude' toward doctors over the decades but this last one was the one that convinced me completely that to many doctors patients are just ignorant scum whose primary purpose in life is to be used as walking ATMs.

- Amir-ul Kafirs; finished August 1, 2020

Afterword

"Tell the American people the truth about the virus, even when it's hard."

Okay, since the Donald put me in charge I'll tell you.

Humans die. It's sad for the loved ones. But there is this thing called death that gets the best of us. If you can't handle that, please isolate, give up your position in life to someone that is less afraid. There will be thousands...millions waiting in line for your job. At this point in time we have data on the virus. World-wide. One can parse the data and manipulate it in any way one chooses. I tend to see that the people who die are elderly and/or have diabetes and hypertension issues. Do you fall into those categories? If so, ask friends and family to look out for you. Hunker down. Do you have a loved one that falls into those categories? We almost all do. We should look out for them. But if they don't want to, let them enjoy their twilight years. It seems young people are resistant to this covid thing. Let us hand the world to them then. It's been drilled into my aged skull that we are robbing the children of their future due to our selfish ways. Then lets give it up. Let us give it to them NOW. We must sacrifice so that they may live a full life. Godspeed. Bless you.

Yours, Secretary of Love, **BP**

When I was a child I often wondered how anyone could have ever been a Nazi. All the adults around me had experienced WWII so the question was timely. The Nazis were the bad guys that the adults had fought against. I still have the "Service Man" star that my grandmother hung in the window when my grandfather, a merchant marine, was off on a ship somewhere delivering supplies. Anyway, I could never understand how people could start rounding up jews, the crippled, gypsies, political dissidents, and homosexuals etc and push them into gas ovens. How? It's seemed impossible! People aren't that different afterall and no one I knew would do such a thing. But recent events have been instructive. Now I believe I understand: No one ever says "I am a fascist" instead they say "I am a good citizen". That's how it works. Then after awhile they start to look around at the people who they think aren't "good citizens", that is people who don't follow the party line, and then things take a turn for the worse. "Why don't they do what's right??!!" becomes the question... then these "troublesome" people become the enemy, too. I can't hide the fact that's what I feel is happening now in a sort of proto-form. The only thing missing is some event that makes adherence to the party line obligatory... The Nazi's had the burning of the Reichstag.
Well, I'm waiting to see what the so-called 1% come up with. - **Dick Turner**

I'm going to comment on the book COVID-19 The Great Reset by klaus schwab and thierry malleret. I have not read it as I dont have so much time at the moment. I came across it from one of my (new since CV19) FukBook friends, Kim Hill. Here is the text she posted.
This book, by the founder of the World Economic Forum (the institution that partnered with the WHO to declare a pandemic of international concern in March, and is behind the call to impose lockdowns on the majority of the world's population) states openly that the virus itself is of little concern, and that lockdown measures will continue indefinitely to push through automation and digital technologies that benefit corporations at the expense of the poor and the third world.
The billionaires are not hiding that they benefit from the pandemic response while millions are being starved, deprived of their livelihoods, and kept apart from their families and communities.
The CDC and UN have stated openly that many more people have died or become ill, and will continue to do so, as a result of lockdown measures that have been affected by the virus itself.
Non-cooperation and saying I Do Not Consent are not going to stop this. The whole system that allows this violence to continue needs to be burned to the ground. The media, education, political, legal, banking, trade, medical and industrial systems all need to go.
An excerpt:
"In one form or another, social- and physical-distancing measures are likely to persist after the pandemic itself subsides, justifying the decision in many companies from different industries to accelerate automation.
After a while, the enduring concerns about technological unemployment will recede as societies emphasize the

need to restructure the workplace in a way that minimizes close human contact.

Indeed, automation technologies are particularly well suited to a world in which human beings can't get too close to each other or are willing to reduce their interactions. Our lingering and possibly lasting fear of being infected with a virus (COVID-19 or another) will thus speed the relentless march of automation, particularly in the fields most susceptible to automation.

In 2016, two academics from Oxford University came to the conclusion that up to 86% of jobs in restaurants, 75% of jobs in retail and 59% of jobs in entertainment could be automatized by 2035.

These three industries are among those the hardest hit by the pandemic and in which automating for reasons of hygiene and cleanliness will be a necessity that in turn will further accelerate the transition towards more tech and more digital.

There is an additional phenomenon set to support the expansion of automation: when "economic distancing" might follow social distancing. As countries turn inward and global companies shorten their super-efficient but highly fragile supply chains, automation and robots that enable more local production, while keeping costs down, will be in great demand.

The process of automation was set in motion many years ago, but the critical issue once again relates to the accelerating pace of change and transition: the pandemic will fast-forward the adoption of automation in the workplace and the introduction of more robots in our personal and professional lives.

From the onset of the lockdowns, it became apparent that robots and AI were a "natural" alternative when human labour was not available. Furthermore, they were used

whenever possible to reduce the health risks to human employees. At a time when physical distancing became an obligation, robots were deployed in places as different as warehouses, supermarkets and hospitals in a broad range of activities, from shelf scanning (an area in which AI has made tremendous forays) to cleaning and of course robotic delivery – a soon-to-be important component of healthcare supply chains that will in turn lead to the "contactless" delivery of groceries and other essentials.
As for many other technologies that were on the distant horizon in terms of adoption (like telemedicine), businesses, consumers and public authorities are now rushing to turbocharge the speed of adoption."
This is from the Conclusion to the book, page 247.
"There is no denying that the COVID-19 virus has more often than not been a personal catastrophe for the millions affected by it, and for their families and communities. However, at a global level, if viewed in terms of the percentage of the global population affected, the corona crisis is (so far) one of the least deadly pandemics the world has experienced over the last 2000 years. In all likelihood, unless the pandemic evolves in an unforeseen way, the consequences of COVID-19 in terms of health and mortality will be mild compared to previous pandemics. At the end of June 2020, COVID-19 has killed less than 0.006% of the world population. To put this low figure into context, the Spanish flu killed 2.7% of the world's population and HIV/AIDS 0.6%"
She also posted a link where you can download a digital version
http://93.174.95.29/main/818DC49A2DE2256A0E019CDF93AF984C

- **Phil Bradley**

The Marx Brothers famously quipped, "Who ya gonna believe, me or your own eyes?" In Louisiana, our daily COVID-19 briefings have taken on the same spirit. Our hospitals were never overrun, the lockdown did not stop the spread, and "two more weeks" of restrictions has become six months. At some point, we must hold our leaders accountable with their own facts.

The data from Louisiana Department of Health clearly shows that the mask mandates and bar closures are not responsible for the fall in cases. COVID-19 cases peaked on July 13, the same day these additional restrictions went into effect. In fact, cases fell 26% in the next two-weeks before they would have had any impact in the case counts; however, the Governor was quick to claim credit. This follows a pattern of "confirmation bias" whereby any decrease in cases is attributed to enhanced restrictions while failures are blamed on the people's lack of compliance. The truth is that any policy enacted at the peak of an epidemic will be followed by decreasing case counts. The Governor could have mandated we all wear tin foil hats on July 13th, and the cases would have still decreased. False interpretations of the data have unnecessarily prolonged interventions that have no justification in observed results.

The current decrease in COVID-19 in Louisiana is more accurately attributed to the development of herd immunity in the population. That the hardest hit areas, particularly New Orleans, largely escaped the second wave of summer infections supports this explanation. Around the world in New York, Sweden, and England, the same phenomenon has been observed. After an expansive outbreak, the virus subsides. This outcome is also consistent with thousands of years of human experience in epidemiology.

The government should provide accurate, objective information from which citizens can assess their own risk, not doomsday predictions and half-truths to control behavior through fear. Turning neighbors against each other for the sake of enforcement is just as egregious. These actions undermine faith in government and infringe on the freedoms that define us as a people. The observed data does not support the current mandatory restrictions, and they should be eliminated in favor of voluntary recommendations. Individuals and businesses should decide the safest and most practical way to conduct themselves. COVID-19 has a CDC-estimated .65% mortality rate, and the median age of a COVID-related death in Louisiana is 76. These facts should be used to focus policies on protecting the most vulnerable, not close bars and kindergartens.

The Aztecs sacrificed thousands of people every year to make sure the sun would rise each morning. Let us not make the same mistakes.

Richard Nelson
State Representative
R- Mandeville

What's my Take-Away from this?!

- Amir-ul Kafirs

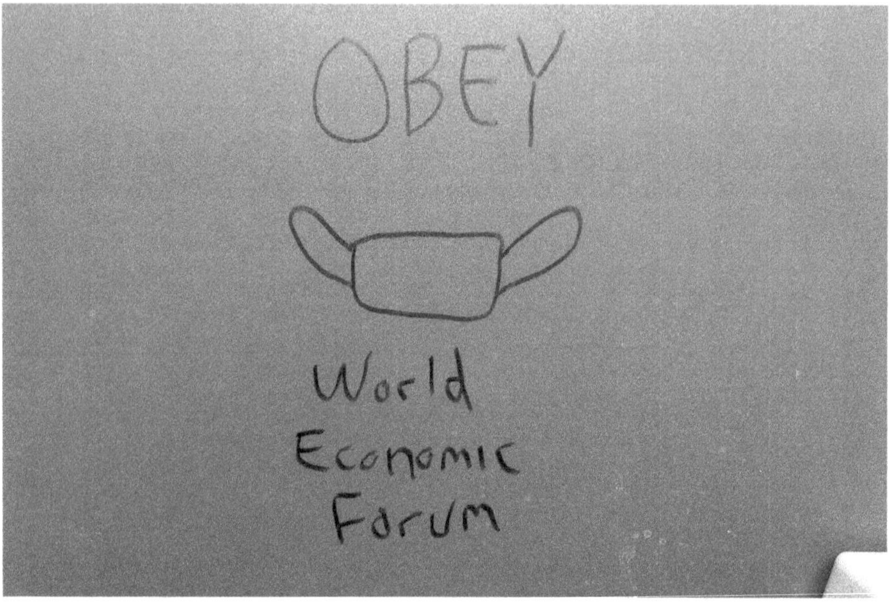

As of today, August 30, 2020, this rough draft of the Unconscious Suffocation book is now roughly 1,200 pages long & given that NO-ONE I KNOW reads more than a few books a year (including professors) & that very few people I've EVER KNOWN have read anything over 500 pages long *at most*, the likelihood of anyone reading all of this is almost nil. As such, having this book be so long will probably be considered totally foolish. Who knows? Maybe someday it'll be compared to Juan Antonio Llorente's A Critical History of the Inquisition of Spain & might be of some use to scholars (if there are any left by then).

Alas, in order to even edit it to this length I've had to go through something like 4,000 pages of material — not to mention the many videos that aren't measurable in page length. I may edit it further, I may not — my patience with the subject is long since exhausted. & that's part of the problem: there *is no closure in sight* & that, in itself, is exhausting.

My initial observation that this PANDEMIC PANIC is an experiment in Mind Control has been more than born out & the Mind Control could even be said to be of *unprecedented magnitude*.

It's my opinion, & I think it's based in reasonably substantial research, that the greediest & most domineering economic forces have been steadily working toward creating the mess that we're currently in the midst of for a very long time & that the WEF (World Economic Forum) is the main gathering of these forces. Their "The Great Reset" is a plan for reorganizing the world along lines in which the majority of the human population are simply to be controlled without any say in the process at all. The arrogance of such planning is mind-bogglingly megalomaniacal & represents a belief among a very small elite that they are 'qualified' to determine how the rest of us live.

There are people who will dismiss such an idea as "Conspiracy Theory". These people are thoughtless & ill-informed, essentially brainwashed. If any such detractors would like to give me a copy of their own book on the subject I'd be willing to read it. That marks a difference between these (not really) hypothetical beings & myself. I'll read a variety of opinions & consider them, they won't.

Why? Because most people are so intellectually lazy that in today's era of texts that're identified in terms of how long they take to read, anything over 15 minutes is too much for them to be bothered with. A decade ago, I was stunned when I was visiting a publisher & a scholar who was present remarked with wonder in his voice that a mutual friend *actually read books from cover-to-cover*. That truly astounded me! Did he mean that *he didn't?!* How on earth could he be a scholar?! I've read something like 5,000 books from cover-to-cover.

Another factor in the mix is that lazy pseudo-intellectuals don't read anything that isn't spoon-fed them by the 'news'-feed that goes along with their accepted subculture, their peer-group. When they have a possible encounter with something outside that prearranged diet they consult with Fact Chokers to see if it's ok to read the off-diet item. If it challenges the dominant narrative in any way, the censors will say it's been 'debunked' or some such nonsense & the potential reader or viewer will immediately reject the new material as invalid. This is a particularly convenient process for people who are only pretending to have a mind because then they don't have to *even try to understand an alternate viewpoint* & they're even given talking points to 'justify' their lack of open-mindedness.

In this day & age, such people ask for 'the science' to justify opinions questioning the PANDEMIC PANIC. But are they scientists? Not usually. Do they ever read science articles in ordinary circumstances? Not usually. 'Science' has long since become the new religion & having its representatives go through the rituals, reciting what might be called the equivalent of a mass in Latin is enough to give 'authority' to any propaganda, no matter how insidious. The worshipper, the 'science' sheep, wouldn't have understood Latin & don't understand the detailed specialized medical lingo anyway but the mere recitation of it is somehow 'proof' that it represents 'reality'.

I find it glaringly obvious that the PANDEMIC PANIC is a preplanned manipulation of the economy to detroy as much human independence from an oligarchy as possible. I find it highly improbable that the virus, if that's what it is, is anything other than a pretext for creating this situation.

What can be better for Mind Control than an *invisible threat?!* — one where one needn't even know anyone who's been sick or know of anyone who's died — what's 'important' is that there're constant reminders *everywhere* that this 'plague' is real, regardless of whether that's true or not.

Making matters worse, is the obviously highly politicized dividing of people into two camps: the 'good caring people' & the 'selfish psychopaths'. Such a division is specious in the extreme but it's worked wonders for turning what were formerly fairly reasonable nice people into *incredibly pompous & condescending self-righteous & self-congratulatory Thought Police*. These people viciously attack any questioning of the MONOLITHIC NARRATIVE by people such as myself as if we're completely hideous *subhumans*. I deliberately use the term "subhuman" because it's one the Nazis used & I find these new neoilliberals to be neo-nazis with a new disquise. Many of these people were formerly friends of mine, some even have reputations as 'non-conformists' & 'creative' people. I think they can kiss those delusions goodbye. Most of them have been so easily flicked into submission to a ridiculous narrative that calling it a post-hypnotic suggestion is almost too flattering.

What's happened, in my admittedly not particularly humble opinion, is that an ability to assess reality has been so undermined by an addiction to uncritically accepted streams coming from primary tools, their 'smart' phones & their computers, that they've completely lost track of any ability to see what's actually around them in their non-computer environment. This has been commented on in many ways in this book.

I seriously doubt that very many people have gone to the trouble that the 6 people who contributed to this book have gone through to try to get an understanding of what's happening around us. Entirely too many people have been happy to just have time off from work with that lovely stimulus check as the bribe for being brainless. If you really want to be such a zombie then so-be-it but don't expect the HERETICS to willingly join you.

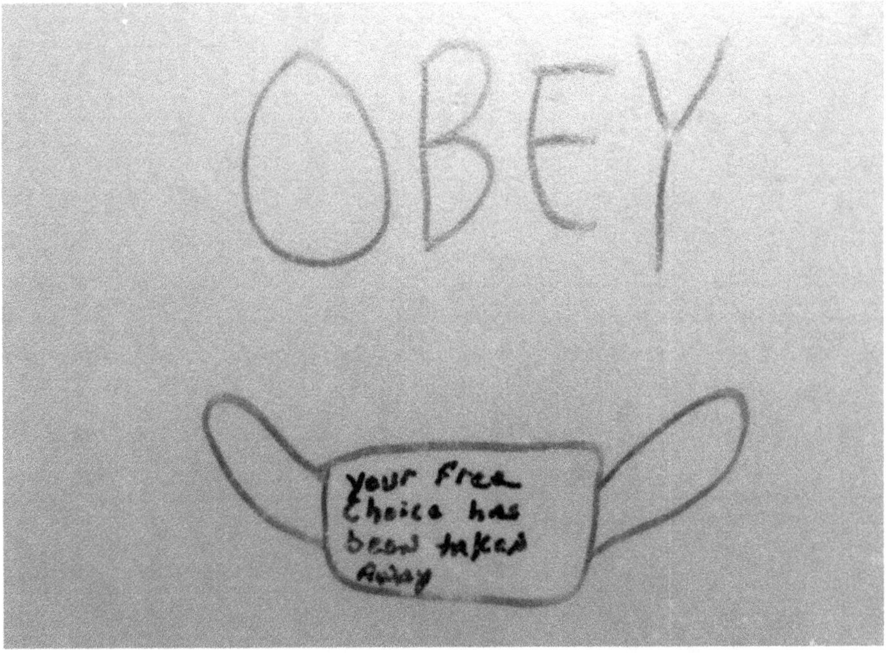

www.ingramcontent.com/pod-product-compliance
Lightning Source LLC
Chambersburg PA
CBHW071211290426
44108CB00013B/1159
9780578743592